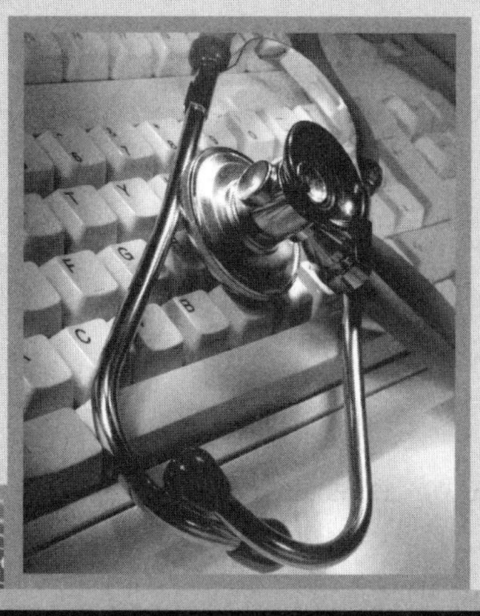

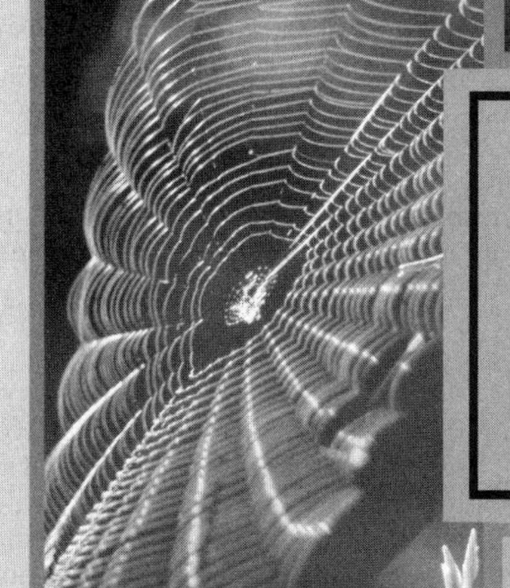

Textbook of

Functional Medicine

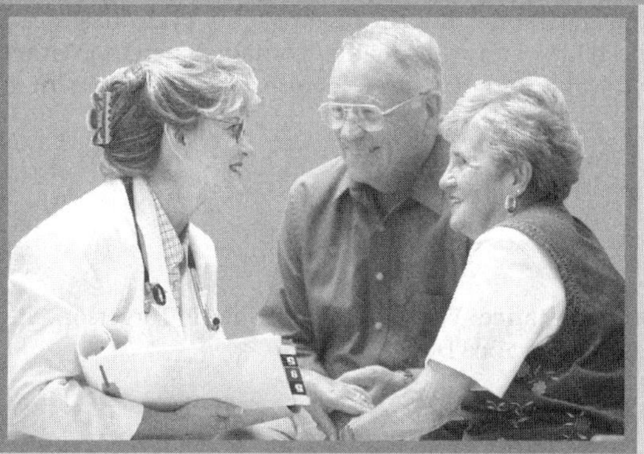

David S. Jones, MD
Editor in Chief

Institute for Functional Medicine
Gig Harbor, WA

David S. Jones, MD, Editor in Chief
Sheila Quinn, Managing Editor

4411 Pt. Fosdick Dr NW, Ste 305
P. O. Box 1697
Gig Harbor, WA 98335
800-228-0622
www.functionalmedicine.org

Disclaimer
Health care is a complex and constantly evolving field. No publication can be assumed to encompass the full scope of information that an individual practitioner brings to his or her practice and, therefore, this book is not intended to be used as a clinical manual recommending specific treatments for individual patients. It is intended for use as an educational tool, to broaden the knowledge and perspective of the practitioner. It is the responsibility of the healthcare practitioner to make his or her own determination of the usefulness and applicability of any information contained herein. Neither the publisher, the editors, authors, nor reviewers assume any liability for any injury and/or damage to persons or property arising from the use of information to be found in this publication.

ISBN No. 0-9773713-0-1

Production Team
Editorial and project assistance: Virginia Kolano, Sherrie Torgerson, Stephanie Roberts
Design: D.K. Luraas, Clairvoyance Design
Graphics: Lynn Siefken
Indexing: Marilyn Anderson

Marketing Team
Laurie Hofmann
Trish Eury
Janet Matkin
Virginia Kolano

Contributing Authors, Reviewers, and Editors

Contributing Authors

B. Jayne Alexander, DO
Bruce N. Ames, PhD
Sidney MacDonald Baker, MD
Peter Bennett, ND
Jeffrey S. Bland, PhD
John Cline, BSc, MD
Daniel Cosgrove, MD
Walter J. Crinnion, ND
Gary Darland, PhD
Joel M. Evans, MD
William J. Evans, PhD
William B. Ferril, MD
Leo Galland, MD
Michael D. Gershon, MD
Patrick Hanaway, MD
Bethany Hays, MD
Robert J. Hedaya, MD
Mark C. Houston, MD
Mark A. Hyman, MD
Mary James, ND
David S. Jones, MD
Joseph J. Lamb, MD
Robert H. Lerman, MD, PhD
Edward Leyton, MD
Peter Libby, MD
DeAnn Liska, PhD
Jay Lombard, MD
Dan Lukaczer, ND
Michael D. Lumpkin, PhD
Michael Lyon, MD
Woody R. McGinnis, MD
Carolyn McMakin, MA, DC
David Musnick, MD
Joseph E. Pizzorno Jr., ND
Lara Pizzorno, MA Div, MA Lit, LMT
James O. Prochaska, PhD
Janice M. Prochaska, MSW, PhD
Sheila Quinn, BS
Robert Rountree, MD
Barb Schiltz, MS, RD
Virginia Shapiro, DC
Michael Stone, MD, MS
Nancy Sudak, MD
Thomas Sult, MD
John M. Tatum, MD
Alex Vasquez, DC, ND
David Wickes, DC
Catherine Willner, MD

Author biographical sketches are available in the Appendix.

Reviewers

Mark Bostrom, DO, ND
David Buscher, MD
Oscar Umahro Cadogan
Sharon Dennis, DO
Jeanne Drisko, MD
Ilia Elenkov, MD, PhD
Marilyn Gage, MD
David Haase, MD
Aviad Haramati, PhD
Tori Hudson, ND
Trent Nichols, MD
Adam Perlman, MD, MPH
David Perlmutter, MD
Paul Reilly, ND
David Riley, MD
Pamela Smith, MD
R. W. Watkins, MD

Editors

David S. Jones, MD, Editor in Chief
Sheila Quinn, BS, Managing Editor

The Institute for Functional Medicine appreciates the vision, dedication, and outstanding contributions of the above-named individuals, without whom this book would not have been possible.

Acknowledgements

The Institute for Functional Medicine gratefully acknowledges the generosity of the following individuals and organizations, whose donations supported the development of this book.

The Allegheny Foundation
Francis Maes, DC

The Park Foundation
Alan Velasquez

Alpha Plus AB
Anonymous
Arlington Family Practice
Center for Healthy Living & Longevity
Richard Combs, MD
Felecia Dawson, MD
Sharon Dennis, DO
Marilyn Gage, MD
Bethany Hays, MD
Ted Hull
Sandra Hyland, RPT & Glenn Hyland, MD
Soram Singh Khalsa, MD
Joseph Lamb, MD, PC
Seung J. Lee, PhD
Frank Lipman, MD
Vincent Marinkovich, MD
Thomas Morledge, MD
Coco Kelapa Newton, MPH, RD, CCN
Jean & Scott Rigden, MD
Sarah Ryterband, MD
Tamara Sachs, MD
Karyn Shanks, MD
Thomas Sult, MD
Heidi Wittels, MD

Mel Alter, LPh, CCN
Gerald Andreoli, DC
Thomas Archie, Jr, MD
Sidney Baker, MD
James Bean, MD
Michael Bernui, DO
Carol Beveridge, PhM, RNCP
Lucie Blouin, ND
Catherine Bock, ND
J. Alexander Bralley, PhD
Graham Broughton, PhD
Gaetan Brouillard, MD
Julie & Michael Bryant, DC
Donald Buehler, MD
Louis Cady, MD
Phil Cappellano
Center for Nutrition & Therapy
Stephen Chiarello, MD
Margaret Christensen, MD
Andrea Cohen, MD
COREhealth
Karen Coshow, ND
Lester Ducote, Jr, MD
Anthony Edwards, MD
Lance Farber, DC, CCN
Stuart Ferraris, DDS
Marjorie Fisher
John Flaxel, MD
Jay Foster, PhD, CCN
Bruce Gollub, MD
Nellie Grose, MD, MPH
Martha Grout, MD
David Haase, MD
Rolf Habersang, MD
Michael Hall
Laurie Hofmann
Bruce Homstead, MS
Brian Chungi Hong, MD
Dominique Hort, DC, CCN, ND
Craig Jordan, DC
Jeffrey Kauffman, MD
Christine M. Keenan, RN
Judith Knapp, BS, RD, LDN
Jacob Kornberg, MD
Paul Le Por, DO
Leonard Leo, DC, DCN, DHerb
Kam Wah Leung, MD
Sandra T.K. Leung, DC
Diana Little, MD
Alan Mackenzie, DDS
Craig Mackey, DC
Sandra Magin, OMD, LAc
Carolyn McMakin, DC
Joseph Meese, BSPh
Christina Minger, EdD, LPC
Margaret Mitchell, MD
C.B. Moore, MD
Maureen & Jerold Morantz, DC
Jane Murray, MD
Rebecca Murray, ARNP, MSN, FNP
Loretta Naylor
Thomas O'Bryan, DC
Tyler Parham, DC, DACBN
Penelope Potter, MD
Kathleen M. Power, DC
Mitchell Pozega
Andrea Cole Raub, DO
Dalinda Reese, MD
Linda Rodriguez, NC, CPT, CNC
Nancy Russell, MD, ABHM
J. Michael Ryan, MD
Naina Sachdev, MD
Kristina Sargent, DC
Sedona Center for Complementary Medicine
James Seeba, OMD, LAc
Herbert Slavin, MD
John Slizeski, DC, PC
Leonard Smith, MD
Pamela Smith, MD
Len Sperry, MD
Ann Stanger, MD
Mary Stock, RPh, CCN
Michael Stone, MD, MS
David L. Sulkosky, DDS
Paige Thibodeau
Valori Treloar, MD
Charles Tucker, DDS
Kevin T. Wand, DO
Elizabeth Wanek, MD
Alan Weiner, DO
Annemarie S. Welch, MD
Ronald Williams, DDS
Victoria M. Wood, RD
Gerald Wyker, MD
Conradine Zarndt
Gary Zimmerman, DC

Lester Adler, MD
Anne Allison, RN
Richard Bahr, MD
Thomas Barnard, MD
John Bender, ND
Deborah Bernstein, MD
Dan Beskind, MD
John Biggs, BSC, RNCP
Barbara Bradley, DC
David Brubaker
John Cline, MD
Beverly Copeland, MD
Creative Health Institute
Ruth DeBusk, PhD, RD
John Decosmo, III, DO
Jeanne Drisko, MD
Maria Engel
Andreas Fikioris
Christy Fritz
Marianne Genetti
Thomas Giammatteo, DC
Leland Green, MD
Steven Green, DDS
Curt Hamilton, CCN
Anne Hines, MD
Stephen Inkeles, MD
Dolores Kent, NC
Nat Kirkland, Jr, MD
Arlyn LaBair, MD
Robert Lee, DO
Pierrette Lefebvre, MD
Sanford Levy, MD
Bobbi Lewis, MS, RD
Rosalba Lopez, PhD
Frank Melograna, MD, PC
Memphis Star Health Services
Devin Mikles, MD
Thomas Miller, DC
Phillip Mosbaugh, MD
Jeffrey Mueller, MD
James Mumma, DC
Kathy Mumma, DC
Richard Ng, MD
Edward Noa, DC
Mark Olsen, MD
Margaret Peterson, MD
Gerald Phillips, MD
Kim Piller
Patricia Power, NUTR
Renovare Clinic, PA
Donald Riemer, MD
Michael Rothman, MD
Elizabeth Schultz, DO
Susan Solomon, MD
Leslie Stewart, DC
Nancy Sudak, MD
John Thomson, PhD, DA
Martin Towbin, MD
Ruth Leyse Wallace, PhD
Woodrow Weiss, MD
Janelle White, MD
Katherine Worden, DO, PC
Kathy Wurster, DC
Kristofer Young, DC
Allen Zak, DC

Preface

Clinicians who focus on the management of complex, chronic disease have not chosen an easy path. This book describes an approach to improving patient outcomes across a wide range of chronic health conditions through careful analysis of common underlying pathways that interact to produce disease and dysfunction or health and vitality. Outstanding content has been contributed by experts from diverse disciplines that traditionally do not integrate their knowledge within a single text. The approach to disease management and health promotion described herein represents the evolution of the functional medicine model over the past fifteen years through the voices of its leaders.

Functional medicine reflects a systems biology approach to health care: a comprehensive analysis of the manner in which all components of the human biological system interact functionally with the environment over time.[1] Over the past century, biology and medicine have focused heavily upon understanding the physiology and biochemistry of individual organs, cells, and molecules. Traditionally, researchers and clinicians have explored one component of various biological systems at a time.[2] In clinical practice, this process usually leads to the differential diagnosis. In drug discovery, it helps us understand how individual compounds interact with a specific drug target in human physiology. From these investigations has emerged an exceptional knowledge base. We are now poised to comprehend the common underlying pathways of health and disease as never before. We can acknowledge that most diseases are rarely the result of a single physiological problem localized to a single organ.[3] Rather, most chronic disease results from the complex interactions of multiple organ systems and multiple physiological and biochemical pathways with environmental influences and genetic predispositions. This knowledge demands a new clinical approach to prevention and treatment.

Two challenging questions that have stimulated the development of functional medicine have emerged over the past two decades: *How are the body's physiological systems linked together? And how is their function influenced by both environment and genetics?* The recognition that these two questions are inextricably linked to each other has become much clearer with the discovery that the human genome contains far fewer genes than expected and that much of our biological uniqueness is related to the "non-coding" region of the genome—the region that controls systems of gene expression.[4] In essence, we have learned that our complex phenotype cannot be adequately understood by exploring one gene at a time (although that exploration is a vital part of building our knowledge). *Systems of genetic expression* give rise to our biological complexity and they need to be understood from an integrated perspective.

Health care is an enterprise focused on the alleviation of human suffering caused by disease and dysfunction. Disease has its start as a functional impairment (a *dys*function) that, left untreated, becomes a diagnosable disease that later can become the cause of death. Each disease has a past, a present, and a future tied to the progressive loss of function and vitality. James Fries in his landmark article on aging, morbidity, and natural death termed this the "loss of organ reserve."[5]

This functional systems biology approach to understanding the origin of disease is now being encouraged by the National Institutes of Health under the new program, *NIH Roadmap*, as a route to accelerate medical discoveries that will improve health.[6] "In this set of NIH Roadmap initiatives, researchers will focus on the development of new technologies to accelerate discovery and facilitate comprehensive study of biological pathways and networks." It is presently driving research in immunology, neurology, cardiology, endocrinology, and radiology.

Three characteristics define the systems biology approach to medicine: emergence, robustness, and modularity.[7] *Emergence* represents the specific characteristics that are displayed in a complex system that are not demonstrated by its individual parts and cannot be predicted from an understanding of the individual parts alone. In the functional medicine model, this has been termed the "web-like interconnections" of physiological processes and biochemical pathways. *Robustness* is the ability that complex biological systems have to maintain homeostasis in the face of changing environmental conditions. In functional medicine, this is termed "homeodynamics." The greater the degrees of physiological freedom individuals have, the more robust their health. For example, very simple EKG patterns are indicative of cardiac disease, whereas the more chaotic fine structure of heart rhythm (i.e., a homeodynamic pattern) is associated with cardiovascular fitness. *Modularity* refers to a system that is comprised of functional units working together to produce an outcome that cannot be produced by any of the units working independently. An example of this concept in functional medicine is the view of the immune, endocrine, and nervous systems as parts of one super-system, the neuroendocrineimmune system. Only by looking at that system as a whole, and not at each of its units in isolation, can the practitioner fully understand the complex presentation of multiple signs and symptoms that patients so often exhibit.

Seventy-eight percent of healthcare expenditures are now for the treatment of chronic diseases, and most physicians are not adequately trained to deal with these complex problems.[8] In functional medicine, it is our conviction that developing a healthcare system that *effectively* manages (and prevents) chronic disease will depend upon our ability to apply a systems biology approach to medicine. Functional medicine incorporates many aspects of this approach, each of which plays a vital role.

Identifying and following biomarkers of function that can be used as indicators of the onset of disease, and also as markers of the success of interventions, is an extremely important activity in functional medicine. Using a patient-centered rather than a disease-centered model emphasizes the importance of eliciting the patient's story, and incorporates mindfulness and the narrative tradition.[9] Recognizing that the extent and severity of chronic conditions in middle to late life are, to a large extent, the outcome of environmental insults received at any point from conception forward allows for a focus on long-term prevention to be integrated into clinical practice.[10] Harnessing the healing power of the mind-body interaction is also important to functional medicine clinicians, as developed from scientific progress in the field of psychoneuroimmunology.[11]

In looking back at the history of medicine in the 20th century, the origin of this concept of function can be credited to a large degree to the work of Dr. Hans Selye.[12] His pioneering work related to the functional endocrinology of what he termed "stress" and its relationship to chronic diseases as diverse as peptic ulcer, hypertension, and heart disease created a new medical model for disease arising out of dysfunction, rather than from infectious organisms or inborn errors of metabolism. He put a physiological mechanism behind the concept that "it is more important to know what kind of person has the disease, than what disease the person has."[13]

Voices from all aspects of our society are merging into a unified call for a new model to address chronic health conditions. A 2005 article in *The New England Journal of Medicine* pointed out that children being born today may be the first generation in the history of the United States with a lower life expectancy than their parents.[14] This prediction comes at a time when the United States spends twice as much per capita for health as any other country, but is 17th in the world in terms of health outcomes. Another 2005 *NEJM* study reported that Medicare is in great danger from the increasing prevalence of age-related chronic diseases, which it does not have the resources to address.[15] The former chairman of Intel Corporation, Dr. Andrew Grove, recently commented in the *Journal of the American Medical Association* that innovation in medicine is slow and that a new model is needed to address the serious health concerns of the country.[16]

Functional medicine is an effective response to this call for a new model of care. It was born out of collaborations among clinicians of many different disciplines and specialties, clinical laboratory specialists, health sciences researchers, health educators, health policy professionals, and healthcare administrators to address the rising incidence and cost of chronic disease. Over the past fifteen years, functional medicine has become an experienced voice in these discussions.

This textbook is the result of our belief that a teaching tool is necessary to assist dedicated practitioners to develop competency with the functional medicine model, and to stimulate and support the emergence of new approaches to the education of future clinicians in all healthcare disciplines. It is our hope that this textbook is but the first edition of what will be an evolving chronicle of the successful development and implementation of the functional medicine model for the effective prevention and treatment of chronic diseases.

Many individuals and organizations provided financial support for the development of this book, and many clinicians, educators, and scientists contributed to the content. For their vision, their commitment to excellence, and their generosity, we dedicate this book to them.

Jeffrey S. Bland, PhD, FACN
Founder and Board Chair
The Institute for Functional Medicine

References

1. Bork P, Serrano L. Towards cellular systems in 4D. Cell. 2005;121:511-13.
2. Kirschner MW. The meaning of systems biology. Cell. 2005;121;503-04.
3. Liu ET. Systems biology, integrative biology, predictive biology. Cell. 2005;121:505-06.
4. Marks J. What it Means to be 98% Chimpanzee. The University of California Press, Los Angeles, 2001.
5. Fries J. Aging, natural death and the compression of morbidity. N Engl J Medicine. 1980;303:130-5.
6. http://nihroadmap.nih.gov/buildingblocks/
7. Aderem A. Systems biology: Its practice and challenges. Cell. 2005;121:511-13.
8. Holman H. Chronic disease—the need for a new clinical education. JAMA. 2004; 292:1057-9.
9. Connelly JE. Narrative possibilities: using mindfulness in clinical practice. Perspect Biol Med. 2005;48:84-94.
10. Fogel RW. Changes in the disparities in chronic diseases during the course of the 20th century. Perspect Biol Med. 2005;48:S150-S165.
11. Hoffman GA, Harrington A, and Fields HL. Pain and the placebo: what we have learned. Perspect Biol Med. 2005; 48:248-65.
12. Selye H. Forty years of stress research: principal remaining problems and misconceptions. Can Med Assoc J. 1976;115:53-6.
13. Osler W. Masters in medicine: nurse and patient. RI Med J. 1971;54:33-6.
14. Olshansky SJ, Passaro DJ, Hershow RC, Hayflick L, et al. A potential decline in life expectancy in the United States in the 21st century. N Engl J Med. 2005;352:1138-45.
15. Anderson GF. Medicare and chronic conditions. N Eng J Med. 2005;353:30508.
16. Grove A. Efficiency in the health care industries. JAMA. 2005;294:490-1.

Contents

Section I Introduction

Section II Principles of Functional Medicine

Section III The Building Blocks

Section IV Fundamental Physiological Processes

Section V Fundamental Clinical Imbalances

Section VI A Practical Clinical Approach

Section VII Putting It All Together

Appendix

Index

Section I
Introduction

Chapter 1
The Vision and Mission of The Institute for Functional Medicine

David S. Jones, MD and Sheila Quinn

The Institute for Functional Medicine is a nonprofit, tax-exempt 501(c)3 educational organization that educates physicians and other healthcare practitioners in improving the management of complex, chronic disease through the use of functional medicine. IFM is accredited by the Accreditation Council for Continuing Medical Education (ACCME) to provide continuing medical education for physicians. In addition to live CME courses, IFM publishes books, course syllabus and audio recordings from live courses, and hosts an online Member Forum. Detailed information about the Institute and its educational activities can be found at www.functionalmedicine.org.

IFM's long-term goals are perfectly described in a statement by Peter F. Drucker: "The product (*of the nonprofit organization*) is neither a pair of shoes nor an effective regulation. Its product is a changed human being. The nonprofit institutions are human-change agents."[1]

Vision Statement

The vision of the Institute for Functional Medicine is to improve the health of individuals worldwide by continuous improvement in healthcare practices.

Mission Statement

The mission of the Institute is to improve patient outcomes through prevention, early assessment, and comprehensive management of complex, chronic disease. We achieve this mission by:

1. Developing the functional medicine knowledge base as a bridge between research (both emerging and established) and clinical practice;
2. Teaching physicians and other healthcare providers the basic science and clinical applications of functional medicine;
3. Communicating with policy makers, practitioners, educators, researchers, and the public to disseminate the functional medicine knowledge base more widely.

Purpose Statement

The Institute provides continuing medical education for physicians and other healthcare professionals, publishes books and other educational materials, and offers clinicians a Forum for the shared exploration of emerging research and clinical applications to improve patient care and outcomes.

Statement of Need

The U.S. healthcare system fails to address the needs of many of our citizens. Many physicians have lost their passion for patient care;[2] patients are disenchanted sufficiently with the focus of their health care to seek alternatives to conventional care in steadily increasing numbers;[3,4] the numbers of uninsured grow as employers reduce their premium share or opt out of providing employee health insurance because of costs;[5,6] and the U.S. ranks 37th in quality of health outcomes[7] despite spending $1.6 trillion per year on health care.[8]

Research suggests that the sense of futility experienced by many healthcare providers stems from a loss of meaning and empowerment in the therapeutic relationship, created (in part) as our chaotic healthcare system has shifted focus from quality issues to cost issues.[9,10,11,12,13] A paradigm shift is required to re-enchant the practice of medicine for both the healthcare provider and the patient (the consumer of health care).[14] It has been suggested that the holism inherent in the therapeutic relationship, plus an expansion of medical thinking beyond the diagnosis and the prescription pad, will re-involve the healthcare provider in the dual function of critical thinking and mindful involvement with the whole life of the patient.[15,16,17]

The Institute for Functional Medicine is committed to helping practitioners and patients achieve this important goal. Since IFM's first incorporation in 1996, it has been dedicated to reducing the fragmentation of health care with a rigorous, science-based continuing educational program whose primary focus is on improving patient outcomes through more effective prevention, early assessment, and comprehensive management of complex, chronic disease. As our mission statement indicates, IFM intends to be just such a change agent as Drucker described, helping to better the health of people worldwide by changing the way health care is practiced.

This textbook represents an important step in achieving IFM's mission—putting into the hands of healthcare providers around the world a consistent, documented view of the philosophy, concepts, underlying science, and clinical applications of functional medicine so that, together, we can work toward the continued development of this extremely important approach to patient care.

References

1. Peter F. Drucker, Managing the Nonprofit Organization (New York: HarperCollins, 1990), p. xiv.
2. Hurd NE. Physician, heal thyself. Minnesota Medicine. July 2002:85. [Accessed at http://www.mnmed.org/publications/MNMed2002/July/Hurd.html]
3. Eisenberg DM, Davis RB, Ettner SL, et al. Trends in alternative medicine use in the United States, 1990-1997: results of a follow-up national survey. JAMA. 1998;280(18):1569-75.
4. Centers for Disease Control and Prevention, US Dept of Health and Human Services. Advance Data from Vital and Health Statistics. Complementary and Alternative Medicine Use Among Adults: United States, 2002. Number 343, May 27, 2004.
5. Cooper PF, Vistnes J. Workers' decisions to take-up offered health insurance coverage: assessing the importance of out-of-pocket premium costs. Med Care. 2003;41(7 Suppl);III35-III43.
6. Ku L. The number of Americans without health insurance rose in 2001 and continued to rise in 2002. Int J Health Serv. 2003;33(2):359-67.
7. O'Connor, K. We can corral health costs by keying on prevention. Seattle Times, June 7, 2002.
8. Levit K, Smith C, Cowan C, et al. Health spending rebound continues in 2002. Health Aff. 2004;23(1):147-59.
9. Kenagy JW, et al. Toward a value-based health care system. Am J Med. 2001;110:158-63.
10. Chassin MR, Galvin RW. The urgent need to improve health care quality: Institute of Medicine national roundtable on health care quality. JAMA. 1998;280:1000-05.
11. Branch WT. Is the therapeutic nature of the patient-physician relationship being undermined? Arch Intern Med. 2000;160:2257-60.
12. Remen, RN. Recapturing the soul of medicine. West J Med. 2001;174:4-5.
13. Marton, KI. Commentary: The secret to satisfaction: empowerment for all. West J Med. 2001;173:18-19.
14. Institute for the Future. Health and Health Care 2010: The Forecast, the Challenge (2nd Edition). http://www.iftf.org/features/library.html. Chapter 18: Expanded Perspective on Health: Beyond the Curative Model, pg 337.
15. Dacher ES. Reinventing primary care. Altern Ther Health Med. 1995;1(5):29-34.
16. Chiong W. Diagnosing and defining disease. JAMA. 2001;285:89-90.
17. Johns MM. The time has come to reform graduate medical education. JAMA. 2001;286:1075-76.

Chapter 2
What is Functional Medicine?

- ▸ ***Introduction to Functional Medicine***
- ▸ ***History of Functional Medicine***

Introduction to Functional Medicine

David S. Jones, MD, Jeffrey S. Bland, PhD, Sheila Quinn

A 2003 article in the *British Medical Journal*[1] generated the following editorial comment: "It is almost a daily occurrence for primary care doctors to encounter patients whose symptoms are probably not due to discernible organic cause." Many of these symptoms appear to be related to chronic inflammatory complaints of unknown origin. Because no specific disease can unequivocally be attached to these complaints, the following question arises: What physiological processes/mechanisms result in the expression of these signs and symptoms? Could their underlying "organic cause" be related to altered function in the absence of observed pathology?

A major challenge for medicine in the 21st century will be to move toward a thorough understanding of physiological mechanisms that underlie disease rather than simply labeling later-stage effects with the names of diseases. "What should we say to patients with symptoms unexplained by disease?" asks the article associated with the editorial comment quoted above. The authors suggest that, for most patients, using the term "functional," as in "functional illness," would be more socially acceptable than "medically unexplained symptoms."

Historically, the term "functional" has been used pejoratively in medicine. It has implied either a disability associated with geriatric medicine or a psychiatric problem. Now, the term "functional" is being used to describe a manifestation of changes in basic physiological processes that produce symptoms of increasing duration, intensity, and frequency. These symptoms often represent the first signs of a later-stage, pathophysiologically definable disease. So, the term becomes applicable not only to diseases of unknown origin, but to early alterations in function that clearly move a patient toward chronic disease over the course of a lifetime.

A new model of medicine is emerging to describe these altered physiological processes that presage the onset of histopathologically defined disease. This model takes the term "functional" beyond psychosomatic illness to define a state of chronic dysfunction associated with altered physiological processes that create a physiological alarm state.

What is Functional Medicine?

Functional medicine is a dynamic approach to assessing, preventing, and treating complex chronic disease. Functional medicine helps clinicians identify and ameliorate dysfunctions in the physiology and biochemistry of the human body as a primary method of improving patient health. Functional medicine acknowledges that chronic disease is almost always preceded by a lengthy period of declining function in one or more of the body's systems. Returning patients to health requires reversing (or substantially improving) the specific dysfunctions that have contributed to the disease state. Those dysfunctions are, for each of us, the result of lifelong interactions among our environment, our lifestyle, and our genetic predispositions. Each patient, therefore, represents a unique, complex, and interwoven set of influences on intrinsic functionality that have set the stage for the development of disease or the maintenance of health.

The Functional Medicine Domain

One way to conceptualize where functional medicine falls in the continuum of health and health care is to examine the functional medicine "tree."

In its approach to a patient care model for complex, chronic disease, functional medicine encompasses the whole domain represented by the graphic shown in Figure 2.1, but concentrates on the section below Organ System Diagnosis, which differentiates it from the conventional medical model. Assessment and treatment *first* address the patient's core clinical imbalances, fundamental physiological processes, environmental inputs, and genetic predispositions, rather than heading straight for the diagnosis. (These elements are explored in detail and thoroughly documented in separate sections of this book. Here in the *Introduction*, we provide an overview of the content and concepts.) Diagnosis is not excluded from the functional medicine model, but the emphasis is on understanding and improving the functional core of the human being as the starting point for intervention. Functional medicine practitioners reason that scientific evidence strongly indicates that impaired physiological processes, if not corrected, lead to significant clinical imbalances in essential body systems. If left in a dysfunctional state, those clinical imbalances often progress to more significant signs and symptoms that may be the precursors or actual indicators of a disease state that can be diagnosed. Improving balance and functionality in these basic processes creates momentum toward health.

Conventional medicine normally acts either when a diagnosis can be made, or when signs and symptoms are severe enough (or the patient is persistent enough) to demand a clinical intervention. Functional medicine practitioners certainly do intervene when a diagnosis has already been made, but they also evaluate functionality at a much earlier stage, often averting (or deferring for a substantial period of time) the disease outcome or its secondary effects. And, in all cases, functional medicine clinicians focus on restoring balance to the dysfunctional systems by strengthening the fundamental physiological processes that underlie them, and by adjusting the environmental inputs that nurture or impair them. This approach leads to therapies that focus on restoring health and function, rather than simply controlling signs and symptoms.

Functional medicine could be characterized, therefore, as "upstream medicine" or "back to basics"—back to the patient's life story, back to the processes wherein disease originates, and definitely back to the desire of healthcare practitioners to make people well, not just manage symptoms.

Principles

These basic principles characterize the functional medicine paradigm:

- An understanding of the *biochemical individuality* of each human being, based on the concepts of genetic and environmental uniqueness;
- Awareness of the evidence that supports a *patient-centered* rather than a disease-centered approach to treatment;
- The search for a *dynamic balance* among the internal and external factors in a patient's body, mind, and spirit;
- Familiarity with the *web-like interconnections* of internal physiological factors;
- Identification of *health as a positive vitality*—not merely the absence of disease—emphasizing those factors that encourage the enhancement of a vigorous physiology; and
- *Promotion of organ reserve* as the means to enhance the health span, not just the life span, of each patient.

Each of these principles is discussed in depth in the *Principles* section, and the evidence supporting their inclusion is presented there.

Environmental Inputs

Environmental inputs (at the base of the medicine tree graphic) include the basic building blocks of life, as well as the primary influences on them. When we talk about influencing "gene expression," we are interested in the interaction between "environment" in the broadest sense and any genetic predispositions with which a person may have been born. Many environmental factors that affect genetic expression are (or appear to be) a matter of choice (such as diet and exercise), but others are very difficult for the individual patient to alter or escape (air and water quality, toxic exposures), and still others may be the result of unavoidable accidents (trauma, exposure to harmful microorganisms in the food supply through travel). Some factors that may appear modifiable are heavily influenced by the patient's economic status—if you are poor, for example, it may be impossible to choose more healthful food, decrease stress in the workplace and at home, or take the time to exercise and rest properly.

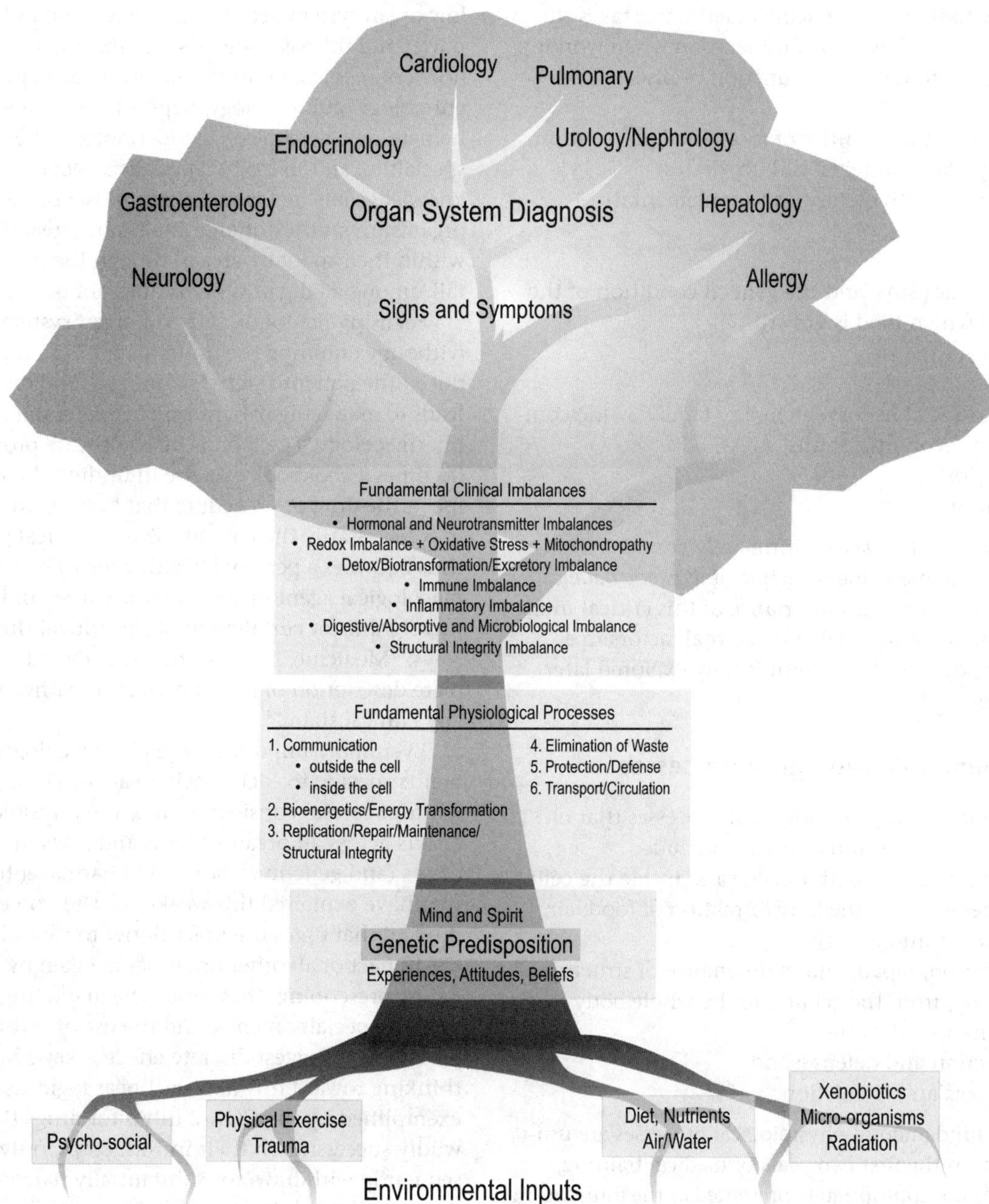

Figure 2.1 **The continuum of health and health care**

Whatever the nature of these "inputs," their influence on the human organism is indisputable, and they are often powerful agents in the search for health. Ignoring them in favor of the "quick fix" of writing a prescription means the cause of the underlying dysfunction may be obscured, but is usually not eliminated. The functional medicine practitioner takes the elements listed below into consideration when working with a patient to reverse dysfunction or disease and restore health:

- Diet (type and quantity of food, food preparation, calories, fats, proteins, carbohydrates)
- Nutrients (both dietary and supplemental)
- Air
- Water
- Microorganisms (and the general condition of the soil in which food is grown)
- Physical exercise
- Trauma
- Psycho-social factors (including family, work, community, economic status, stress)
- Xenobiotics
- Radiation

Environmental inputs are intimately connected with the functional medicine principle of *dynamic balance* mentioned above. The importance of this critical interweaving between internal and external factors in a patient's body, mind and spirit is fully explored later in the book.

Fundamental Physiological Processes

The fundamental physiological processes that ultimately determine health or disease include:

- communication, both outside and inside the cell;
- bioenergetics, or the transformation of food, air, and water into energy;
- replication, repair, and maintenance of structural integrity, from the cellular to the whole body level;
- elimination of waste;
- protection and defense; and
- transport and circulation.

These fundamental physiological processes are usually taught in the first two years of medical training, where they are appropriately presented as the foundation of modern, scientific medical care. However, subsequent training in the clinical sciences often fails to fully integrate this rich understanding of the underlying functional mechanisms of disease with therapeutics and prevention. In the second two years, conventional clinical training heavily emphasizes teaching/learning based on organ system diagnosis.[2] This approach—aggregating the patient's signs and symptoms into groupings that follow organ system declensions—has given us both the power and the weakness of specialization (e.g., the breakdown of medicine into cardiology, neurology, gastroenterology, pulmonology, nephrology, dermatology, hematology, hepatology, endocrinology, the surgical specialties, and so forth). Specialists become exceedingly knowledgeable in a well-defined subset of the human organism, but they often evaluate and treat diseases within their specialty area as though the inevitable cross-talk among all organ systems does not occur.

Focusing predominantly on organ system diagnosis without examining the underlying physiology that produced the patient's signs, symptoms, and disease often leads to managing patient care by matching diagnosis to pharmacology. The job of the healthcare provider then becomes a cookbook exercise in finding the right "recipe"—the drug or procedure that best fits the diagnosis (not necessarily the patient). Every medical problem thus becomes a personal health issue in search of a pharmacological agent or surgical procedure[3] and that leads to a significant curtailment of the critical thinking pathways: "Medicine, it seems, has little regard for a complete description of how a myriad of pathways result in any clinical state."[4]

Even more important, the pharmacologic treatments specific to each specialty are often implemented without careful consideration of the physiological effects across all organ systems and physiological processes (and genetic variations).[5] Pharmaceutical companies have exploited this weakness. Did you ever see a drug ad that urges the practitioner to carefully consider the impact of all other drugs being taken by the patient before prescribing a new one? The marketing of drugs to specific specialty niches, and the use of sound bite sales pitches that suggest discrete effects, skews healthcare thinking toward this narrow, linear logic, as notably exemplified by the COX-2 inhibitor drugs that were so wildly successful on their introduction, only to be subsequently withdrawn or substantially narrowed in use due to collateral damage.[6,7]

Pharmacological and medical hardware interests also strongly influence the research that is done and the information that reaches physicians about new drugs and procedures.[8,9,10] Our national research establishment—both private and governmental—is heavily focused on drug development and medical devices technology, rather than multifactorial, individualized, lifestyle-focused interventions. Physicians (and now patients as well) are subjected to the disproportionate impact the drug industry's ad campaigns have on information about treatment approaches for disease—everything is centered on taking a drug,[11] rather than helping patients change behavior. By controlling research topics,[12] selecting what data will be published,[13,14] and dominating continuing medical education programs,[15,16,17] the pharmaceutical industry often replaces complex thinking with more simplistic approaches relying on pharmaceuticals.[18] Even our less commercial research models (at NIH, for example) all too often concentrate on "single disease—single agent—single outcome" methodologies. Examination of lifestyle and the attendant physiological and health consequences seldom receive needed research support because the medical-industrial complex that surrounds conventional training and practice is driven by these powerful commercial interests. (Lifestyle approaches are also more difficult to study prospectively, but the work certainly can be done with the will and the resources.)

Fortunately, a stronger voice from within the ranks of medical educators and practitioners is emerging on behalf of re-evaluating the influence of commercial interests on our healthcare system—from education to research to clinical practice.[19,20] Many mainstream publications are including articles by leading medical thinkers that patient-centered health care requires a broader focus than simply labeling the problem (diagnosis) and selecting the right drug.[21]

The functional medicine approach to assessment, both before and after diagnosis, charts a course using different navigational assumptions. Every health condition instigates a quest for information centered on understanding when and how the specific biological system(s) under examination spun out of control to begin manifesting dysfunction and/or disease. Analyzing all the elements (information from the patient's story, signs, symptoms, and laboratory assessment) through a matrix focused on functionality requires critical thinking that is quite different than matching diagnosis with drug and hardware interventions. A deeper understanding of biochemistry and physiology is required of a functional medicine practitioner. The foundational principles of how the human organism functions—and how its systems communicate and interact—are essential to the process of linking ideas about multifactorial causation with the perceptible effects we call disease or dysfunction.

To assist clinicians in this process, functional medicine has adapted and organized a set of *core clinical imbalances* that function as the intellectual bridge between the rich basic science literature delineating physiological mechanisms of disease (first two years of medical training) and the clinical studies, clinical experience, and clinical diagnoses of the second two years of medical training. The core clinical imbalances serve to marry the mechanisms of disease with the manifestations and diagnoses of disease. (Re-examine the medicine tree graphic to appreciate how the core clinical imbalances fit within the total framework of health care.)

Core Clinical Imbalances

The practice of functional medicine is characterized by an examination of the core clinical imbalances that underlie the expression of disease. Those imbalances arise as *environmental inputs* such as diet, nutrients (including air and water), exercise, toxins, and trauma *are processed* (see above list of the fundamental processes involved) through a unique set of *genetic predispositions*, attitudes, and beliefs. The *core clinical imbalances* that arise from malfunctions within this complex system include:

- *Hormonal and neurotransmitter imbalances*
- *Oxidation-reduction imbalances and mitochondropathy*
- *Detoxification and biotransformational imbalances*
- *Immune and inflammatory imbalances*
- *Digestive, absorptive, and microbiological imbalances*
- *Structural imbalances* from cellular membrane function to the musculoskeletal system

Imbalances such as these are the precursors to the signs and symptoms by which we detect and label (diagnose) organ system disease. These imbalances arise from dysfunction or defect within the fundamental physiological processes that cut across all organ systems, and they alert the healthcare provider to pay attention to the full expression of disease and dysfunction. Each of these imbalances is explored in considerable detail later in the book, and the underlying evidence supporting this approach to patient care is thoroughly discussed.

The most important precept to remember about functional medicine is that restoring balance—in the patient's environmental inputs and in the body's fundamental physiological processes—can be both a precursor and a concomitant activity to evaluating and treating chronic illness, and to improving health. It involves much more than treating symptoms.

Short Description of Functional Medicine

Functional medicine is dedicated to prevention, early assessment, and improved management of complex, chronic disease by intervening at multiple levels to correct core clinical imbalances and thereby restore each patient's functionality and health to the greatest extent possible.

History of Functional Medicine

David S. Jones, MD and Jeffrey S. Bland, PhD

If contrast is the essence of vision, then clearly delineating the differences between present day conventional medicine and functional medicine will help improve our understanding of the road being pioneered by functional medicine.

In his commentary in 2003, *The Medicine We Are Evolving*,[22] Sidney MacDonald Baker, MD, postulates that current conventional medicine rests on two primary principles:

1. The fundamental subject of medical concern is disease;
2. The inquiry as to health rests first on the naming of the patient's disease.

He points out that treatment is then prescribed for the disease without rigorous consideration of the patient's unique individual needs, which may include the need to be rid of something toxic, allergenic or infectious, or the need to add something vital that is missing, or both.

Dr. Baker describes the difference between the acute-illness legacy of conventional medicine and today's functional medicine model that is focused on prevention and treatment of chronic, complex illnesses (the dominant medical problems experienced in our modern, industrialized, hygienic society):

> How do we think differently? The emerging school of thought [*functional medicine*] does not deny the usefulness to the patient and physician of diagnostic groups that allow us the comfort of knowing "what you've got." We are careful to keep in mind that a diagnosis is an idea we form about groups of people and properly belongs to the group, not an individual. Making a diagnosis in the realm of chronic illness—such as the many conditions of chronic inflammation whose proud names end in "-itis," and autism, schizophrenia, depression, anxiety, cardiovascular disease, and a host of otherwise eponymous, classical, and respectable diseases—is for us not the end of a diagnostic road, but the first step, to be followed by the ... [*consideration of unique individual needs*]. These questions are not applied to "curing the disease" but to healing the person.
>
> This approach is based on the recognition that individuality ... [*has*] a spiritual as well as a biological foundation in the sense that each of us is a unique creature. Hence our patients are denied dignity when given a group identity (diagnosis) and a group treatment (the "treatment of choice" for that diagnosis).[23]

Functional medicine evolved from a medical paradigm that, instead of emphasizing the primacy of diagnosis and pathology, focuses on the antecedent events that precede the onset of diagnosis (*cf.* the notion of "upstream medicine," discussed above under *The Functional Medicine Domain*). Leo Galland, MD, elaborated this principle first in the early 1990s in his unpublished, but widely disseminated paper, *Patient-Centered Diagnosis: A Guide to the Rational Treatment of Patients as Individuals*,[24] later expanded and published in 1997 as *The Four Pillars of Healing*.[25] Patient-centered diagnosis depends on knowledge of the mediators, triggers, and antecedents of the patient's specific disease (discussed in detail in Chapter 8). According to Dr. Galland, arriving at an accurate, detailed, structured assessment of the patient requires a collaborative context within which the patient's story includes:

> aspects of the patient that had previously been ignored. We were interested in the effects of the common components of life: a patient's thoughts and beliefs, home or work environment, exposure to potential toxins, and allergens, food and drink, stressful life events, social interactions, patterns of physical activity.

The evaluation investigates past history, including family history and clues regarding genetic and social inheritance, the environmental/emotional conditions affecting the patient's health, and those factors that continue to mediate the dysfunction and/or disease. The patient's narrative always includes clues that will eventually inform the physician about the underlying mechanisms of dysfunction, without "segregation of biological and psychosocial dimensions."[26] This model derives from the integration of research in molecular biology and behavioral psychology about the influences that lead to the clinical manifestation of disease. One approach of this kind has been labeled the "biopsychosocial model," and it helps clinicians understand "how suffering, disease, and illness are affected by multiple levels of organization, from the societal to the molecular."[27]

Starting in the early 1980s, Jeffrey Bland, PhD, first developed the fully elaborated model of functional medicine that now includes both the *six principles* and the *fundamental clinical imbalances* that underlie the dysfunctional devolution of health into disease. Writing in the preface of his 2004 seminar series syllabus,[28] Dr. Bland states:

> It amazes me that this accumulated body of information ... now comprises more than 2000 pages and 5000 referenced articles demonstrating the importance of diet, nutritional intervention, lifestyle and environment on both the prevention and management of virtually every chronic disease ... . We are involved in what Thomas Kuhn termed a "paradigm shift" in our understanding of the origin and treatment of age-related chronic diseases. The discovery of the code of the human genome and the recognition that our function is determined by much more than just our genome is a revolution in thinking. Our health and disease patterns after infancy are not "hardwired" deterministically by our genes, but rather a consequence of the interaction of genetic uniqueness with environmental factors. Our experiences wash over our genes to give rise over time to how we look, act, feel and our disease pattern. This is truly a change in thinking about the origin of disease that requires a similarly bold change in how we treat disease.

This model emerges from the groundwork of six great innovators who carved out from the domain of molecular medicine the foundational concepts underpinning functional medicine. The six pioneers of this new medical paradigm are Archibald Garrod (1902), Linus Pauling (1949), Roger Williams (1956), Abram Hoffer (1957), Hans Selye (1979), and Bruce Ames (2002). Let us pause and reflect on the contributions of these six pioneers who have improved our understanding of the human organism and the factors that contribute either to ongoing health or to the progression toward chronic, degenerative diseases.

Archibald Garrod, MD

Dr. Garrod was first to discover the diseases of genetic metabolism in the early 20th century. (He investigated the genetic metabolism diseases of infancy.) Although those diseases originated in the genes, he said, the ultimate expression of the diseases depended on the exposure of those genes to factors in the environment. He discovered alkaptonuria, which led to the understanding of phenylketonuria and the role of the phenylalanine-restricted diet in its management. In 1902, Dr. Garrod wrote, "It might be claimed that what used to be spoken of as a diathesis of a disease is nothing else but chemical individuality. It is nearly true to say that the factors which confer upon us our predisposition and immunities from disease are inherent in our very chemical structure, and even in the molecular groupings which went to the making of the chromosomes from which we sprang."[29]

Linus Pauling, PhD

Dr. Pauling made extraordinary contributions to the way we view the origin of disease. His article in *Science* magazine in 1949 on the origin of sickle cell anemia taught us that single gene mutations could contribute to disorders that cut across organ systems and produce multiple symptoms. In this article he introduced the term "molecular medicine."[30] Dr. Pauling explained that in sickle cell anemia, a single point gene mutation on the heavy chain of the globin molecule of hemoglobin could contribute to a conformational change in the way the hemoglobin molecule was structured in three dimensions. That conformational change affected the way oxygen bound to the heme portion of the hemoglobin molecule and changed the relationship between the molecule and its oxygen absorption/desorption. The change in shape of that molecule changed the shape of the red cell, because hemoglobin made up about three-quarters of the volume of a red cell. The red cell then became sickle-shaped, and this sickle would "cut" its way through the vasculature, creating the pain and disability of sickle cell crisis.[31]

Dr. Pauling predicted in 1949 that the molecular origin of disease would have extraordinary implications. As we learned more about the origin of these diseases, he believed, we would find ways to modify the expression and function of these genes to prevent the expression of disease. In 1997, 48 years after Dr. Pauling proposed this model of the potential power of molecular medicine, a paper in *The New England Journal of Medicine* validated his thesis. That article explained that administering hydroxy urea intravenously to patients who carried the genetic trait of sickle cell anemia could prevent the hemoglobinopathies associated with this genetic disorder.[32] Hydroxy urea upregulated the expression of fetal hemoglobin in these patients and "diluted" the amount of sickle cell hemoglobin, resulting in a reduction of sickle cell crisis.

Roger Williams, PhD

Dr. Roger Williams, a professor of biochemistry at University of Texas at Austin and past President of the American Chemical Society, discovered members of the B-complex vitamin family, including pantothenic acid. Dr. Williams's book, *Biochemical Individuality*, published in 1956, proposed a role of various nutrients in preventing what he called "genetotrophic diseases."[33] Genetotrophic diseases are those for which genetic uniqueness creates demands for specific nutrients beyond the average to facilitate optimal function and prevent premature disease. Dr. Williams theorized that when those specific needs are not met in a given individual, disease results.

Dr. Williams believed the major chronic degenerative diseases of aging—heart disease, stroke, cancer, diabetes, and arthritis—were related to genetotrophic imperfections. In his model, the unique genes of each individual require different levels of nutrition and a specific lifestyle for optimal health. The consequences of not meeting the specific needs of the individual are expressed, over several decades, as degenerative disease "of unknown origin." In the category of what he called genetotrophic diseases, Dr. Williams even included diseases of mental illness, childhood diseases, behavior disorders, and alcoholism. He believed they all were related to the mismatch of genes and environment. At a genetic level, the individual needed a different level of nutrients to promote proper phenotypic expression. If that need was not met, the resulting undernutrition would manifest as chronic disease in midlife. This very powerful concept revolutionized our thinking about the origin of age-related diseases.[34]

In defending his concept of biochemical individuality, Dr. Roger Williams said, "Nutrition is for real people. Statistical humans are of little interest. People are unique. We must treat real people with respect to their biochemical uniqueness."

Abram Hoffer, MD, PhD

As a psychiatrist who also held a doctorate in organic chemistry, Dr. Hoffer in the 1950s provided a unique perspective on mental illness. He discovered in the urine of schizophrenics unique chemicals that represented the oxidative byproducts of adrenaline.[35] He found that these substances produced central nervous system toxicity. As a result of these discoveries, Dr. Hoffer proposed that certain forms of mental illness resulted not from bad early childhood experiences, but as a consequence of altered brain chemistry.[36] He found that increased doses of the common B vitamins, niacin and pyridoxine, could treat these conditions in some schizophrenic patients.[37] Dr. Hoffer, with the synthesis of a new idea that incorporated biochemical genetic individuality, nutritional modulation of gene expression, and functional physiology, provided the bridge that allowed psychiatry to enter the field of biologically based, functional therapy.

Hans Selye, MD, PhD

As the father of the physiological definition of the word "stress," Dr. Selye introduced to both medical professionals and healthcare consumers the role of the mind in the function of the body.[38] Dr. Selye's tremendous insight gave birth to the rapidly evolving field of psychoneuroimmunology, which is redefining the way health practitioners view the impact of lifestyle and behavior on health. The combination of the physiology of stress and the understanding of the influence of perceived stress on genetic expression served as a powerful driver for the evolution of functional medicine.

Although Dr. Selye was never awarded a Nobel Prize for his contributions, many historians of 20th century medicine believe his insights on the role of behavior and environment in health represent one of the most important factors shaping the new medicine.

Bruce Ames, PhD

Dr. Bruce Ames, Professor of Biochemistry and Molecular Biology, and Director of the National Institute of Environmental Health Science Center, University of California, Berkeley, published his landmark paper in 2001.[39] His team's research provides the bench science to substantiate Williams's postulates on genetotrophic diseases. Ames shows in his encyclopedic review paper that "as many as one-third of mutations in a gene result in the corresponding enzyme having an increased Michaelis constant, or *K*m (decreased binding affinity), for a coenzyme, resulting in a lower rate of reaction." Some people carry polymorphisms[i] that are more critical in determining the outcome of their health history. He goes on to argue that studies have shown that administration of higher than dietary reference intake (DRI) levels of cofactors (specific vitamins and minerals) to these polymorphic genes restores activity to near-normal and even normal levels. He concludes, "Nutritional interventions to improve health are likely to be a major benefit of the genomics era."

The functional medicine model rests on the stout shoulders of these worthy researchers and clinicians. They pioneered the concepts that postulated that many agents modify gene expression in such a way as to create different phenotypes. They provided the breakthrough science that demonstrates that significant influences in this process include diet, exercise, stress, environmental, and lifestyle factors.

Molecules of functional importance transmit messages and receptors receive them. The transmitters are the molecules we call the mediators. The receivers are the membrane receptor binding and soluble receptor sites that translate the messages into altered gene expression and altered function. It is possible to manipulate both the messages and their reception on the basis of things we do every day, by the way we think, act, eat, and feel, by where we live, the nature of our relationships and our spiritual belief systems. All these factors influence the mediating molecules and can lead to an expanding health paradigm. An informational rubric encompasses communicating and receiving the right messages to be in synchrony with our genes to give rise to healthy function.

These six individuals pioneered the new medicine for the 21st century by establishing the scientific basis for recognizing that our genes generally do not determine our disease. The awareness that our environments are powerful agents influencing the genetic expression of both health and disease represents a major shift in medical thinking.[40] The utility of this model within the medical paradigm is no longer in question. It is just a question of how long it will take for this model to be fully integrated within the standard practice of medicine.

[i] A polymorphic gene is an alternate form of a *wild* gene present in >1% of the population. The most common polymorphic genes are single nucleotide polymorphisms (SNPs) that result in translational proteins and enzymes with decreased functionality. We all share at least 99.9% of the nucleotide code of our species' genome. The SNPs are what make us unique within our species. The translation of our genome message that includes our SNPs results in our individual phenotype. [Burghes, et al. Science. 2001;293: 2213–14.]

References

1. Stone J, Wojcik W, Durrance D, et al. What should we say to patients with symptoms unexplained by disease? The "number needed to offend." BMJ. 2003;3:89-90.
2. Magid CS. Developing tolerance for ambiguity. JAMA. 2001;285(1):88.
3. Ely JW, Osheroff JA, Gorman PN, et al. A taxonomy of generic clinical questions: classification study. BMJ. 2000; 321:429-32.
4. Rees J. Complex disease and the new clinical sciences. Science. 2002; 296:698-701.
5. Radford T. Top scientist warns of "sickness" in US health system. BMJ. 2003;326:416.
6. Vioxx: lessons for Health Canada and the FDA. CMAJ. 2005;172(11):5.
7. Juni P, Nartey L, Reichenbach S, et al. Risk of cardiovascular events and rofecoxib: cumulative meta-analysis. The Lancet. 2004;364:2021-29.
8. DeAngelis C. Conflict of interest and the public trust. JAMA. 2000;284(17):2237-38.
9. Prosser H, Almond S, Walley T. Influences on GPs' decision to prescribe new drugs—the importance of who says what. Fam Pract. 2003:20(1):61-68.
10. Als-Nielsen B, Chen W, Gluud C, Kjaergard LL. Association of funding and conclusions in randomized drug trials: A reflection of treatment effects or adverse events? JAMA. 2003;290(7):921-28.
11. Goodman B. Do drug company promotions influence physician behavior? West J Med. 2001;174:232-33.
12. DeAngelis CD, Fontanarosa PB, Flanagin A. Reporting financial conflicts of interest and relationships between investigators and research sponsors. JAMA. 2001;286(1):89-91.
13. Melander H, Ahlqvist-Rastad J, Meijer G, Beermann B. Evidence b(i)ased medicine—selective reporting from studies sponsored by pharmaceutical industry: review of studies in new drug applications. BMJ. 2003;326:1171-75.
14. Lexchin J, Bero LA, Djulbegovic B, Clark O. Pharmaceutical industry sponsorship and research outcome and quality: systematic review. BMJ. 2003;326:1167-76.
15. Relman AS. Separating continuing medical education from pharmaceutical marketing. JAMA. 2001;285(15):2009-12.
16. Relman AS. Your doctor's drug problem. New York Times, November 18, 2003. Opinion. Accessed at [http://www.nytimes.com/2003/11/18/opinion/18RELM.html?pagewanted=print&position=], 11/19/03.
17. Drug-company influence on medical education in USA. (editorial) The Lancet. 2000;356:781.
18. Connor S. Glaxo chief: Our drugs do not work on most patients. Common Dreams News Center, December 8, 2003. Accessed at [www.commondreams.org/cgi-bip/print_cgi?file=headlines02/1208-02.htm], 12/17/03.
19. DeAngelis CD, Fontanarosa PB, Flanagin A. Reporting financial conflicts of interest and relationships between investigators and research sponsors. JAMA. 2001;286(1):89-91.
20. Relman AS. Separating continuing medical education from pharmaceutical marketing. JAMA. 2001;285(15):2009-12.
21. Radford T. Top scientist warns of "sickness" in US health system. BMJ. 2003;326:416.
22. Baker, SM. The medicine we are evolving. Integr Med. 2003;(1)1:14-15.

23. Ibid.
24. Galland L. Patient-centered diagnosis: A guide to the rational treatment of patients as individuals. 1991. Unpublished.
25. The Four Pillars of Healing: How the New Integrated Medicine—The Best of Conventional and Alternative Approaches—Can Cure You. New York: Random House, 1997.
26. Galland L. Patient-centered diagnosis: A guide to the rational treatment of patients as individuals. 1991. Unpublished.
27. Borrell-Carrio F, Suchman AL, Epstein RM. The biopsychosocial model 25 years later: principles, practice, and scientific inquiry. Ann Fam Med. 2004;2:576-82.
28. Bland J. Nutrigenomic modulation of inflammatory disorders: Arthralgia, coronary heart disease, PMS, and menopause-associated inflammation: 2004 Seminar Series. Gig Harbor, WA: IFM, 2004. www.functionalmedicine.org
29. Garrod, A. The incidence of alkaptonuria: a study in chemical individuality. Lancet. 1902;2:1616-20.
30. Pauling L, Itano H, Singer SJ, Wells I. Sickle cell anemia, a molecular disease. Science. 1949;110: 543-48.
31. Itano H, Pauling L. A rapid diagnostic test for sickle cell anemia. Blood. 1949;4:66-68.
32. Lubin B. Sickle cell disease and the endothelium. N Engl J Med. Nov. 1997;337(22):1623-25.
33. Williams R. Biochemical Individuality. New York: John Wiley and Sons, 1956.
34. Williams R, Deason G. Individuality in vitamin C needs. Proc Nat Acad Sci USA. 1967;67:1638-41.
35. Hoffer A. Epinephrine derivatives as potential schizophrenic factors. J Clin Exp Psychopathol Q Rev Psychiatry Neurol. 1957;18(1):27-60.
36. Hoffer A. Chronic schizophrenic patients treated ten years or more. Journal of Orthomolecular Medicine. 1994;9(1):7-34.
37. Hoffer A. Effect of niacin and nicotinamide on leukocytes and some urinary constituents. CMAJ. 1956;74:448-51.
38. Selye H. Stress and the reduction of distress. J S Carolina Med Assoc. 1979:562-66.
39. Ames BN, Elson-Schwab I, Silver EA. High-dose vitamin therapy stimulates variant enzymes with decreased coenzyme binding affinity (increased Km): relevance to genetic disease and polymorphisms. Am J Clin Nutr. 2002;75:616-58.
40. Bland J. Genetic Nutritioneering. Lincolnwood, IL: Keats, a division of NTC/Contemporary Publishing Group, Inc., 1999.

Chapter 3
Why Functional Medicine?

- ***Importance of Improving Management of Complex, Chronic Disease***
- ***Our Aging Population and the Centrality of Diet, Lifestyle, and Environment***
- ***Functional Medicine Incorporates Genomics***

Importance of Improving Management of Complex, Chronic Disease

David S. Jones, MD and Sheila Quinn

The Larger Context

Despite the fact that non-genetic factors that are *modifiable*—including diet, overweight, inactivity, and environmental exposures such as smoking—account for 70–90% of mortality in the U.S.,[1] physician education, training, and reimbursement are most often focused on treating disease using drugs and surgery rather than comprehensive patient-centered treatments focused on the individual. For example, as reported in a study published in the *British Medical Journal*,[2] clinical questions in primary care can be categorized into a limited number of generic types and frequency. The four most common question types were:

1. What is the drug of choice for condition x?
2. What is the cause of symptom x?
3. What test is indicated in situation x?
4. What is the dose of drug x?

This shortsighted approach to health care should give us all cause for serious concern, because it is perpetuating a system that is far too costly and increasingly ineffective for the prevention and management of chronic diseases whose root causes are to be found in a much more complex perspective on patients' lives.

A Critical Problem

The gap between emerging research in basic sciences and integration of new knowledge into clinical practice is often astonishingly large—particularly in the area of complex, chronic illness.[3] This is one of the reasons that today's healthcare providers are not adequately trained to manage the increasing burden of complex, chronic disease.

The 20th century took on—and, to a great extent mastered—the challenges of providing health care for acute conditions (injury and life-threatening illness). Knowledge and technology grew apace, and so did costs; measures no one thought possible 100 years ago have become readily available. Organ transplants, re-attachment of severed limbs, life-support systems, new drugs, infection control procedures, laparoscopic explorations and surgeries—the list is extensive. But at the same time that our healthcare system was becoming dependent on advances in acute care, other influences were superseding acute conditions as the greatest threats to American health: increasingly stressful and sedentary lifestyles,[4,5,6] industrial pollution[7] of air, water, and earth[8] leading to devitalized (and sometimes dangerous[9,10,11]) food, overconsumption (rising rates of obesity) but undernutrition,[12] and fragmented family and community ties (social isolation[13,14,15]). These influences have helped to create an overwhelming burden of chronic disease that we do not yet train our healthcare providers to treat or prevent effectively.[16] Among other contributing factors:

- Disease prevention has too often been conceptualized as immunization and early diagnosis, an approach that is far too limited. Effective prevention of chronic disease today requires understanding individual genetic vulnerabilities (20–30% of chronic disease risk) and the effect of lifestyle upon those individual variations (70–80% of the risk).

- Physicians highly trained primarily in conventional diagnosis and treatment (drugs, surgery, radiation) are not well qualified to apply prevention-focused interventions such as nutrition, diet, and exercise to help patients minimize their risk of suffering from one or more of the major chronic diseases in America (heart disease, diabetes, autoimmune disease, mental illness, and cancer).[17]
- In addition to prevention strategies, many complex, chronic diseases are very responsive to dietary and various lifestyle interventions.[18] But clinicians without these skills are literally at the mercy of the pharmaceutical industry. "Doctors are taught about drugs by agents of the pharmaceutical industry, which works hard to persuade them to select the newest and most expensive medications—even in the absence of scientific evidence that they are any better than older, less costly ones."[19] Or, we would add, even in the presence of evidence that many non-drug interventions are therapeutically effective and significantly less expensive.[20,21]

Increasing Economic Burden

The American healthcare system is predicated on a huge myth—that the more a society spends on health care, the better the health of its population will be. We justify having—*by far*—the costliest healthcare system in the world by deluding ourselves that we therefore also have the best health in the world. However, our romance with ever newer and more expensive drugs, technology, and surgeries has not achieved what we have been led to expect. Consider just a few of the many significant statistics available on this subject:

National health expenditures:

- increased 69% between 1990 and 2000, to a per capita cost of $4,637, which is 68.5% higher than our closest competitor (Germany) and more than 2½ times as much as the UK;[22,23]
- increased at a rate 4–5 times that of inflation in most years of that decade (a time of relatively low inflation in other industries);[24]
- were disproportionately affected by the cost of prescription drugs, which were responsible for 21% of the cost increases in Year 2000, while representing only 9% of total spending;[25] and
- are expected to rise to $3.1 trillion over the next 10 years (from a level of $1.4 trillion in 2001).[26]

What does the American public get for this exorbitant price tag?

- A nation with 43.6 million uninsured in 2002[27] (while every other westernized nation provides basic coverage to all its citizens).
- An excessively high serious medical error rate (highest among U.S., Canada, the UK, Australia, and New Zealand), including (in 1994) 160,000 deaths from adverse drug reactions (ADRs).[28]
- An unacceptable portion (45%) of Americans failing to receive "indicated care"[29] including, notably, preventive care.
- A healthcare system that is thought by many to be "in imminent danger of collapse."[30]

Add to this volatile mix, the projection that one-third of the people born in the year 2000 will eventually have diabetes[31]—perhaps the most costly of the chronic diseases when all its comorbidities and secondary complications are considered[32]—and we believe that no further evidence is necessary to justify a sea change in our approach to health care. There will be many ideas about the best changes to consider, but this textbook is being written, in part, to ensure that all those who are interested in the assessment, prevention, and treatment of chronic disease know what functional medicine has to offer.

There are, of course, other powerful societal drivers for the problems described above. Among them are the demand for fast and easy, high-fat, high-sugar foods; the demand for expensive testing (such as CAT scans or MRIs) and expensive drugs; the increasingly sedentary nature of most jobs (tied to a desk) and personal lifestyles (centered around television and other passive entertainment experiences). It is important that all sectors share the responsibility for empowering healthful choices—the individual and his/her family, the workplace, the residential and civic communities, the marketplace, and the healthcare system. This book addresses needs that exist within the healthcare system, but does not in any way discount the vital influence of other elements of society. We do, however, call upon clinicians to let their voices and their work be stronger and more insistent in the call for prevention and health, rather than concentrating their formidable knowledge, intelligence, and skills on after-the-fact interventions.

Functional Medicine and the Chronic Care Model

In the inaugural issue of the *Annals of Family Medicine,*[33] the lead editorial focused on the need for a new paradigm for the primary care disciplines. The present intellectual framework[i] taught in our medical education system fails to address the web-like interactions of multiple comorbidities for chronically ill patients. The power of organ-system medicine and the scientific research based on this model have brought us to the doorstep of the 21st century where, despite huge advances in disease detection, pharmacology, and surgical interventions, we are ill-equipped for the century's greatest challenge—an aging population with ever-increasing rates of (largely preventable, often reversible) chronic disease. The dominance of the existing heuristic (rule of thumb and experience) and reductionist model has fragmented medical care into specialty and sub-specialty care, which drives costs upward[34] and conflicts with the need for a comprehensive, integrated approach to chronically ill patients with multiple comorbidities.

In Grumbach's insightful editorial, *Chronic Illness, Comorbidities, and the Need for Medical Generalism,*[35] he opens: "It is said that when students enter medical school, they care about the whole person, and by the time they graduate, all they care about is the hole in the person. Current medical education inculcates many of the dominant values of modern medicine, reductionism, specialization, mechanistic models of disease and faith in a definitive cure." He suggests that the dominant paradigm now being taught is most applicable in the context of acute illness (e.g., trauma and infection). However, the dominant illnesses of the 21st century are and will be the chronic diseases (e.g., diabetes, heart disease, arthritis, and dementia, among others). In this context, the reductionist model fails to address (what he believes is) the most germane issue: "Cure is rarely possible, but improved functional status with amelioration of symptoms of pain and dysfunction and longer life (health span) through a thorough understanding of secondary prevention is possible." He goes on to describe the paradigm shift in the intellectual matrix needed for integrated care for the chronically ill:

> These studies demonstrate the futility of reductionistically carving up patients on the basis of individual conditions and sending them to the diabetes program on Monday, the cardiac program on Tuesday, the arthritis program on Wednesday, and the depression program on Thursday. What is needed is a model of care that addresses the whole person and integrates care for the person's entire constellation of comorbidities. This generalist approach does not deny the value of specialty care, which can offer expertise and unique services to the care of patients with chronic illness. But the generalist approach affirms a central role for the primary care clinician as the coordinator and integrator of specialty care and other referral services, working in partnership with the patient and other health care personnel to optimize overall physical functioning, mental health, and well-being.[36]

IFM has been an innovator in this field for more than two decades. Functional medicine is not a unique and separate body of knowledge, but it does represent a different way of applying the scientific and clinical information that emerges from the research literature and from the clinical practices of many disciplines. Functional medicine emphasizes a definable and teachable *process* of integrating multiple knowledge bases within a pragmatic intellectual matrix that focuses on functionality at several levels as the key to health. Functional medicine uses the patient's story as an essential tool for integrating diagnosis, signs and symptoms, and evidence of clinical imbalances into a comprehensive approach to improve both the patient's environmental inputs and his or her physiological function. It is a clinician's discipline, and it directly addresses the need to transform the practice of primary care.

Functional medicine can substantially improve the existing Chronic Care Model,[37] which comprises six basic elements to foster productive interactions between patients and providers:

1. Patient self-management support;
2. Delivery system design (team-based delivery of care);
3. Decision support (consistent with scientific evidence and patient preferences);
4. Clinical information system (organizes individual patients and patient populations to receive appropriate levels of care);
5. Organizational support; and
6. Community support.

[i] The intellectual framework and filter taught and then used by primary care practitioners will, from here on, be called the intellectual matrix.

The strength of the Chronic Care Model is the acknowledgment that optimal care relies on healthcare team building involving the top levels of the organization as well as the caregivers, and integrating support for patient self-management. However, what is missing and central to success in this effort is an intellectual matrix that can filter research and clinical evidence to achieve a coherent focus applicable to the *unique* set of signs and symptoms presented by the *individual* patient. No such matrix now exists outside of the functional medicine model. The Chronic Care Model is still grounded in the heuristic, organ-system based, reductionist thinking that is inadequate to the task.[38] As presently configured, that model will run into the same wall: chronic illness and multiple comorbidities are difficult to handle because the *fundamental, underlying clinical imbalances* have not been clearly delineated as the starting point for understanding chronic, complex illness. Even the coordination of resources as described in the Chronic Care Model will inevitably fall significantly short of the goal if the focus of this integrated collaboration is not properly identified. Functional medicine helps to identify the proper focus from a multidisciplinary, patient-centered model that all caregivers can learn and apply.

The Chronic Care Model appears to assume that the best we can do for a patient with chronic disease and comorbidities is to minimize the progression of the disease through the consistent and complete application of existing standards of care. There's no implicit or explicit anticipation of actually restoring health, and no recognition that unless we can restore health (to varying degrees in different patients), the huge impact of chronic disease on the healthcare system and the economy will be virtually unchecked. One might summarize the problem in this manner:

- if assessment and treatment are not fully integrated with prevention,
- if therapeutic interventions are not expanded to include a primary emphasis on diet, exercise, and lifestyle,
- and if health and disease are not perceived as existing on a continuum, along which the patient's placement can move towards health (even in the presence of significant chronic disease and comorbidities),
- then the emphasis is always going to be on palliative care, and the costs are always going to be excessive.

Functional medicine directly addresses the restoration of health, looking for common factors among various symptoms, diagnoses, and comorbidities that can be affected by intervening to improve function at the cellular level and the organ level. The functional medicine matrix takes into direct consideration the patient's lifestyle and diet, genetic predispositions, and core clinical imbalances, seeking a multifactorial and individualized approach that will reach beneath symptoms to restore function and generate momentum toward health. Too often the patient care process is seen as complete when a diagnosis is achieved and a drug is prescribed. In functional medicine, the diagnosis is the beginning of the journey, and the patient's past and continuing story is the central driver.

Our Aging Population and the Centrality of Diet, Lifestyle, and Environment

David S. Jones, MD and Sheila Quinn

Healthy Aging Matters

Researchers have estimated "the cost to our society resulting solely from the triad of coronary heart disease, diabetes, and obesity alone is nearly half a trillion dollars!"[39] Since most of the chronic disease burden occurs in the last decades of life, the importance of healthy aging can, therefore, hardly be overstated. However, it isn't an aging population, per se, that increases the economic burden on the healthcare system. It's an older population that has either more disease, or more years of life with disease, or both. Booth et al.[40] point out that "the advances made against modern chronic diseases over the past 30 years have come to a halt." Today in North America and most of the westernized world, people are living longer and, for many, those additional years are filled with the cost and effort of managing multiple chronic diseases. We have no idea whether or not there is an upper limit to life expectancy—all past predictions about such limits have been exceeded, in a steady, linear climb of about 2.5 years per decade for the past 150 years.[41] So, we may as well assume that the upper boundary will continue to advance, which means we will be providing expensive, intensive healthcare services to a growing number of older citizens who will be living with more heart disease, more diabetes, and more arthritis, cancer, and other complex chronic diseases for 30–40 years, rather than 10–20.

At least, that's what current projections indicate. There are many who believe, however, that a different goal is within our reach: "In the ideal case, the healthy citizens of a modern society will survive to an advanced age with their vigor and functional independence maintained, and morbidity and disability will be compressed into a relatively short period before death occurs ... ."[42] There is research to support this hypothesis: "Not only do persons with better health habits survive longer, but in such persons, disability is postponed and compressed into fewer years at the end of life."[43] And, even more to the point, successful aging is often the result of factors under at least some personal control: "our weight, our exercise, our education ... our abuse of cigarettes and alcohol ... our relationship with our spouse, and our coping styles can [all] be modified. A successful old age ... may lie not so much in our stars and genes as in ourselves."[44]

To be sure, there is much about the process of aging that we cannot yet understand or control. Aging is certainly associated with increasing incidence of disease and disability on a population-wide basis. However, research is making it increasingly clear that there are many behaviors (diet, exercise, stress reduction)[45,46,47,48] and treatments (antioxidants, essential fatty acids, minerals, certain amino acids, the B vitamins, and much more)[49,50,51] that can counteract the functional decline that leaves us vulnerable to disease and disability as we age.[52] Functional medicine helps to bring this knowledge into clinical practice, both for prevention and for treatment.

Centrality of Diet and Exercise in Prevention and Treatment

A healthcare system that is primarily dependent on the prescription pad for therapeutic success will inevitably be far more costly in the long run[53] than one that brings lifestyle and environment to the fore. Diet, exercise, stress reduction, and active lifestyles are the most effective—and least costly—tools for lifelong disease prevention; there are numerous studies that validate this assertion, providing data on everything from pancreatic cancer[54] to sarcopenia[55] to very costly diseases such as heart disease and diabetes.[56,57] (We do not mean to discount the huge impact of broad societal influences such as a strong economy, an educated and well-compensated workforce, and supportive communities, but discussion of those issues is beyond the scope of this book.) Research is emerging in a continuous and expanding stream to demonstrate the therapeutic effectiveness of lifestyle interventions for the treatment of many chronic diseases.

Using type 2 diabetes as an example can help us understand more clearly what's at stake. Consider the following facts:

- The incidence of diabetes is rising rapidly—it's a red flag bearing the message that something important has gone awry.[58]
- "100% of the increase in prevalence of type 2 diabetes and obesity in the U.S. during the latter half of the 20th century must be attributed to a changing environment interacting with genes, since 0% of the human genome has changed during this time period."[59]
- Diabetes is being diagnosed in ever younger patients—so we will be paying for their care for many, many more years if we don't act now.[60,61]
- It is a very costly disease. In 2002, the total cost of diabetes was $132 billion/year—$92 billion in direct medical costs and $40 billion in disability, work loss, and premature mortality.[62] This is a 35% increase over the 1997 total.[63] In just five years, we added $34 billion/year to the healthcare budget from diabetes alone. (If this doesn't scare us, what will?)
- Diabetes has many genetic links and new information is emerging all the time about how those can be identified.[64,65,66] Clinicians will increasingly be paying attention to genes at risk through ethnicity and family history, thus bringing genomics (environment acting on genes) into play.[67]
- Diabetes increases the risk of many other chronic diseases, including various neurological conditions,[68,69] heart disease,[70,71] kidney disease,[72,73] stroke,[74] and cancer.[75,76] Today's growth in the incidence of diabetes will lead directly to increases in many other diseases as the diabetic population ages.
- For most type 2 diabetics, the disease can be prevented, delayed, or reversed.[77,78]

It's hard to read this condensed set of facts about diabetes and not wonder, "What's gone wrong?" This is a (mostly) preventable disease, about which a great deal is known; it causes great human suffering if not prevented;

it costs us tens of billions of dollars each year; and it's now hitting our children. What is standing in the way of turning this around? It's certainly not a lack of information—even a quick search of the literature turns up hundreds of relevant research articles in every field from endocrinology to epidemiology to psychology.

At the risk of offering an oversimplified explanation, one reason seems intuitively obvious: We do not have a healthcare system, or healthcare practitioners, with the skills, time, and will to do what needs to be done. We have a healthcare system that forces practitioners to focus on seeing the most patients in a day, for the smallest investment of professional time and effort, with quick access to drugs (and highly vulnerable to pharmaceutical industry pressure and patient demands). This scenario cannot help but obscure the real answers to the problem.

Functional medicine offers a way to change this scenario. Practitioners can begin approaching patient care from a different perspective, with a broader set of tools, and with an empowered patient as ally and partner. Helping the doctor—and the patient—to fully understand the critical factors that affect functionality, aging, disease, and health over a lifetime will help create a more cost-effective healthcare system, and lead to longer health spans for our citizens.

Functional Medicine Incorporates Genomics

Jeffrey S. Bland, PhD

Genomics—The Genetics-Environment Interface

April 25, 2003 represented the 50th anniversary of the publication describing the structure of DNA, in the journal *Nature*, by Watson and Crick.[79] That classic paper contained the prophetic comment, "It has not escaped our attention that the specific pairing (of the DNA bases) we have postulated immediately suggests a possible coping mechanism for the genetic material." This paper, and companion papers that appeared in the same issue of *Nature* by Wilkins, Strokes, and Wilson, and Franklin and Gosling, created a paradigm shift in medicine that has taken 50 years to be integrated into its curriculum. **The concept that disease mechanisms originate at the molecular biological level and are related to intricacies of interaction between the environment and genes and their expression heralded a new age in medicine.** The seeds that were planted then are only now coming into bloom.

Rabinowitz and Poljak commented in 2003 that we are seeing the emergence of a new primary-care model built on the molecular medicine discoveries of the last 50 years.[80] This primary-care model integrates the concept of host/environment interaction in framing a better understanding of the origin of disease and its potential treatment, individualized to the patient. Until very recently, we have tended to believe that diseases are "hard-wired" into our genes as a consequence of genetic uniqueness. This belief has caused us to forget or overlook the important variable of environment and its role in modulating the expression of genes. As these authors point out:

> These (molecular genetic) developments, however, raise the concern that both physicians and patients could fall into a trap of biological determinism, believing that one's genetic and metabolic makeup far outweighs the role of environmental factors in disease. Such thinking fails to acknowledge that most health outcomes are the result of interactions between host factors and environmental factors.[81]

Although the human genome contains only between 30,000 and 35,000 genes, millions of variations of these genes, called single nucleotide polymorphisms (SNPs), exist within the gene pool. These polymorphisms occur as variations in which the least common allele is present in at least 1% or more of the population. Researchers have found that when these SNPs are present in a gene it means a person has two different genes coding for the same function. Only recently have we understood that many of these SNPs lead to differences in the phenotype of an individual, and that how these differences may be expressed depends upon environmental factors.

One major environmental factor that modifies gene expression is the individual's nutritional status. Both macro- and micronutrients can influence the expression of genes, the translation of the genetic message into active protein, and that protein's ultimate influence in controlling metabolic function.[82,83,84,85,86]

The effective integration of these concepts into the educational model so that patient assessment and treatment can be personalized to the patient's own genetic uniqueness represents a great challenge for modern medicine. It has been postulated that medical nutrition education is very near a "tipping point" that will herald rapid changes in the existing system vis-à-vis these exciting concepts.[87] Functional medicine has been addressing these issues and training clinicians to understand and use the concepts for many years.

(According to Gladwell, the tipping point is the moment when an idea, trend, or social behavior crosses a threshold, "tips," and spreads like wildfire.[88] Broad examples from medicine include the discovery of the polio vaccine, the identification of insulin as a treatment for type 1 diabetes, the 1964 Surgeon General's Report on the health effects of cigarette smoking, and the McGovern Committee and the 1979 Surgeon General's Report on Health Promotion and Disease Prevention. Another tipping point may be the changes stemming from the Human Genome Project that are leading to a new definition of medical nutrition education.)

As evidence that we are near the tipping point in medical education, Tel Aviv University recently incorporated into its medical curriculum a course titled "Introduction to Pharmacogenomics: Towards Personalized Medicine."[89] As investigators learn how different individuals metabolize substances based on their genetic uniqueness, we learn more about the important roles specific nutrients play in modifying the expression of metabolic patterns in the individual. Diet, lifestyle, and environment have significant influence on the way an individual can metabolize specific substances based upon his or her genetic uniqueness. We are seeing the first applications of genomic medicine in the area of pharmacogenomics. Pharmacogenomics is defined as the unique metabolism of various substances based on an individual's genetic uniqueness. A great deal of research is being done to study individual variations in reactions to drugs and that body of research will contribute enormously to our understanding of personalized medicine.

Nutrigenomics

Linus Pauling was a pioneer in alerting physicians to the importance of nutrients in modulating physiological processes at the biomolecular level and ultimately giving rise to the phenotype of health or disease. The interface between genomics and nutrition is now defined as the field of "nutrigenomics." As Kozma observed:

> Information from the Human Genome Project will dramatically change health care for the dietetic and nutrition discipline. Approaches to risk assessment including obtaining family history, diagnosis, prevention, early intervention, and management of nutritional issues will evolve through the application of nutritional genomics. Dietetic and nutrition specialists will increasingly require knowledge of genomics, gene-environment interactions, the expanding role of pharmacogenomics in drug and food therapies, and genetic applications to clinical practice.[90]

The development of nutrigenomic concepts will assist clinicians in understanding the varied responses of different patients to specific nutritional therapies. An example is the wide inter-individual variation in blood lipid and lipoprotein responses to dietary change.[91] A diet that is low in fat and high in unrefined complex carbohydrate may in one individual be effective in lowering total blood lipids. In another individual with a different genotype, however, the same diet may actually increase specific members of the lipid and lipoprotein families. Similarly, some individuals, when placed on a higher-protein, low-carbohydrate diet, may have reductions in their blood lipid profiles, while others may have elevations of blood lipids on the same diet.

Fogg-Johnson and Kaput provide a good restatement for us to consider:

> Effects of the Human Genome Project are surfacing in anticipated and unanticipated areas. One of the key discoveries from the project is the existence of individual differences in gene sequences that result in differential response to environmental factors, such as diet. Those genetic differences, single nucleotide polymorphisms (SNPs, pronounced snips), are the key genetic enabler of the emerging scientific discipline called nutrigenomics or nutritional genomics. ... The science of nutrigenomics is the study of how naturally occurring chemicals in foods alter molecular expression of genetic information in each individual.[92]

Since approximately 1990, nutrition research has undergone a gradual shift in focus from epidemiology and physiology to molecular biology and genetics. This shift has resulted in a growing realization that we cannot understand the effects of nutrition on health and disease without determining how nutrients act at the molecular level. Müller and Kersten note: "There has been a growing recognition that both macronutrients and micronutrients can be potent dietary signals that influence the metabolic programming of cells and have an important role in the control of homeostasis."[93]

In every respect, the transition occurring within medical nutrition is epic in its impact and scope. Nutrition-focused practitioners are at a pivotal point in the history of their practice. Kauwell's observations are particularly pertinent: "Armed with the findings of the Human Genome Project and related research, dietetics practitioners will have the potential to implement more efficient and effective nutrition intervention strategies aimed at preventing and delaying the progression of common chronic diseases."[94]

Genomics and Proteomics: Importance for the Future of Nutrition Intervention

A central feature of this paradigm shift in medical nutrition is the recognition that not all genes within the human genome are expressed in every cell simultaneously. Instead, the expression is selective to the cell type and cell environment. The study of the synchronous activation of families of genes to yield various proteins that ultimately regulate metabolic function is called "proteomics."

A large body of information exists about the number of genes, chromosomal localization, gene structure, and gene function. Scientists are only now beginning to understand the orchestrated way the proteins expressed from these genes control metabolism.[95] For example, researchers have found that in some cells only 50% (approximately) of the genes transcribed to form the specific messenger RNA (mRNA) are translated into active proteins. The action point in the control of cellular physiology is therefore the combination of genetic transcription (expression), active protein formation, and control of metabolism that has been termed the "phenome."

The phenotype of the cell is a complex process or system of interacting events related to genetic expression, protein synthesis, protein activation, and metabolic regulation. By evaluating genetic expression through the production of specific mRNAs, the synthesis of specific proteins from those mRNAs, and ultimately the effect of those proteins on metabolic function, we can establish biomarkers of health and disease. From this understanding, we can evaluate the role of specific nutrients on this process in the individual patient. Although this may at first seem to be a daunting task, new screening technologies and powerful systems of bioinformation analysis are emerging to hasten the day when such interventions are a real option in clinical care.

Toward a Systems Biology Approach

As we write in 2005, the systems biology approach[ii] for analyzing individual effects of nutrients on function is not yet available, but a number of clearly identified relationships that connect specific SNPs, nutrient sensitivity, and disease risk are now understood. Petricoin and Liotta predicted in 2003 that clinical applications of proteomics, which involve the use of molecular genetic technologies at the bedside, will result in patient-tailored therapies.[96]

Work at the Institute for Systems Biology in Seattle, Washington, has demonstrated the success of an integrated system for understanding cellular physiology based on the interaction of genomic expression, proteomics influences, and their role in controlling metabolism.[97] Although this work is in its early stages, the "proof of concept" that a systems biology approach can be used for evaluating the impact of genetic expression, proteomic activity, and their roles in controlling metabolism, supports an optimistic perspective for the future of personalized and functional medicine.

Upstream vs. Downstream Medicine

In the last few decades, much medical research has focused primarily on discovering specific molecules that inhibit enzyme function "downstream" in a complex physiological process. The search for molecules with the selective ability to inhibit specific enzyme-mediated steps, such as angiotensin-converting enzyme inhibitors (ACE inhibitors), selective serotonin reuptake inhibitors (SSRIs), H2 blockers, and selective cyclooxygenase-2 inhibitors (COX-2 inhibitors), has succeeded in fueling the growth of the multi-billion dollar pharmaceutical industry (not without serious consequences for some patients with some of these drugs).

Genomic and proteomic research has begun to demonstrate, however, that rather than blocking specific enzymes downstream in a complex biological system associated with a specific disease, it can be even more effective to develop new approaches that would selectively regulate the expression of various alarm molecules upstream in the metabolic process that are associated with the disease. The emphasis of such research is to identify tissue-selective "upstream" modulators of

[ii] Systems biology seeks to explain complex biological systems, such as the cell, through the integration of many different types of information.

genomic and proteomic expression. The objective is to identify ways to normalize the functional changes associated with early disease risk without adversely affecting other tissues engaged in similar metabolic processes.

The Rise of Personalized Medicine

This revolutionary shift in thinking suggests that substances consumed in the diets of various cultures for thousands of years may have profound influence on gene expression and proteomic outcome. It may also help explain the epidemiological observations that certain diets are associated with reduced disease risk. As Willett pointed out, the integration of extensive epidemiological research with the discoveries being made in nutrigenomics will give rise to a new personalized medicine using diet, lifestyle, and environment as principal tools in both prevention and treatment of specific chronic diseases.[98] Burke wrote, "Evidence is now emerging of the complex interactions between genes and the environment in the causation of many diseases, and the study of the interactions represents the next important step in genomic research. Efforts to understand the molecular mechanisms that underlie complex diseases will build on insights and strategies developed in the study of single-gene diseases."[99]

From these concepts, new clinical tools and programs are emerging to help apply medical nutrition in ways that will make it more effective in improving patient outcomes, and that approach is a key component of the functional medicine model, and thus an urgently needed element in modern clinical care.

References

1. "For most diseases contributing importantly to mortality in Western populations, epidemiologists have long known that nongenetic factors have high attributable risks, often at least 80 or 90%, even when the specific etiologic factors are not clear." Willett WC. Balancing life-style and genomics research for disease prevention. Science. 2002; 296:695-97.
2. Ely JW, Osheroff JA, Gorman PN, et al. A taxonomy of generic clinical questions: classification study. BMJ. 2000;321:429-32.
3. " ... the gap between the clinician and the basic scientist has increased, not diminished, in the last quarter century." Rees J. Complex disease and the new clinical sciences. Science. 2002:296:698-701.
4. Manson JE, Skerrett PJ, Greenland P, VanItallie TB. The escalating pandemics of obesity and sedentary lifestyle. A call to action for clinicians. Arch Intern Med. 2004;164(3):249-58.
5. Kaplan JR, Manuck SB. Ovarian dysfunction, stress, and disease: a primate continuum. ILAR J. 2004;45(2):89-115.
6. Ishizaki M, Morikawa Y, Nakagawa H, et al. The influence of work characteristics on body mass index and waist to hip ratio in Japanese employees. Ind Health. 2004;41(1):41-49.
7. Pohanka M, Fitzgerald D. Urban sprawl and you: how sprawl adversely affects worker health. AAOHN J. 2004;52(6):242-46.
8. Valent F, Little D, Bertollini R, et al. Burden of disease attributable to selected environmental factors and injury among children and adolescents in Europe. Lancet. 2004;363(9426):2032-39.
9. Weisburger JH. Hazards of fast food. Environ Health Perspect. 2004;112(6);336.
10. Hightower J. Methyl mercury reference dose: response to Schoen. Environ Health Perspect. 2004;112(6);337-38.
11. Silbergeld EK. Arsenic in food. Environ Health Perspect. 2004;112(6):338-39.
12. Fletcher RF, Fairfield KM. Vitamins for chronic disease prevention in adults. JAMA. 2002;287(23):3127-29.
13. Albus C, Jordan J, Herrmann-Lingen C. Screening for psychosocial risk factors in patients with coronary heart disease—recommendations for clinical practice. Eur J Cardiovasc Prev Rehabil. 2004;11(1):75-79.
14. O'Keefe JH, Poston WS, Haddock CK, et al. Psychosocial stress and cardiovascular disease: how to heal a broken heart. Compr Ther. 2004;30(1):37-43.
15. Linfante AH, Allan R, Smith SC, Mosca L. Psychosocial factors predict coronary heart disease, but what predicts psychosocial risk in women. J Am Med Womens Assoc. 2003;58(4):248-53.
16. Yach D, Hawkes C, Gould CL, Hofman KJ. The global burden of chronic diseases: overcoming impediments to prevention and control. JAMA. 2004;291(21):2616-22.
17. "Recent evidence has shown that suboptimal levels of vitamins, even well above those causing deficiency syndromes, are risk factors for chronic diseases such as cardiovascular disease, cancer, and osteoporosis. A large proportion of the general population is apparently at increased risk for this reason ... . Physicians often do not ask about vitamin use. Patients may not volunteer information about their vitamin use, fearing that the physician would disapprove of unconventional use of vitamins." Fairfield KM, Fletcher RH. Vitamins for chronic disease prevention in adults. JAMA. 2002;287:3116-26.
18. Herman WH, Hoerger TJ, Brandle M, et al. The cost-effectiveness of lifestyle modification or metformin in preventing type 2 diabetes in adults with impaired glucose tolerance. Ann Intern Med. 2005;142:323-32.
19. Relman AS. Your doctor's drug problem. The New York Times, November 18, 2003.
20. Brody S, Preut R, Schommer K, Schurmeyer TH. A randomized controlled trial of high dose ascorbic acid for reduction of blood pressure, cortisol, and subjective responses to psychological stress. Psychopharmacology (Berl). 2002;159(3):319-24.
21. Renaud S, Lanzmann-Petithory D. Dietary fats and coronary heart disease pathogenesis. Curr Atheroscler Rep. 2002;4:419-24.
22. California HealthCare Foundation and Wilson, KB. Health Care Costs 101. October 2002.
23. Davis K, Cooper BS. American Health Care: Why So Costly? Invited Testimony before the Senate Appropriations Committee, Subcommittee on Labor, Health and Human Services, Education and Related Agencies; Hearing on Health Care Access and Affordability: Cost Containment Strategies. June 11, 2003.
24. California HealthCare Foundation and Wilson, KB. Health Care Costs 101. October 2002.
25. Ibid.

26. Centers for Medicare and Medicaid Services (CMS). Report published in online Health Affairs Journal. [http://www.healthaffairs.org/WebExclusives/Heffler_Web_Excl_020703.htm] Accessed February 10, 2003.
27. The Commonwealth Fund. Top 20 Health Policy Stories/Issues of 2003. [http://www.cmwf.org/programs/topten_2ndpg.asp] Accessed December 23, 2003.
28. Lazarou J, Pomeranz BH, Corey PN. Incidence of adverse drug reactions in hospitalized patients: A meta-analysis of prospective studies. JAMA. 1998;279(15):1200-05.
29. McGlynn EA, Asch SM, Adams J, et al. The quality of health care delivered to adults in the United States. N Engl J Med. 2003;348(26):2635-45.
30. Bloom, F. (President, American Association for the Advancement of Science) BBC News, February 14, 2003. [http://news.bbc.co.uk/1/hi/in_depth/sci_tech/2003/Denver_2003/2760101.stm] Accessed 8/1/2003.
31. Centers for Disease Control, June 15, 2003.
32. Simpson SH, Corabian P, Jacobs P, Johnson, JA. The cost of major comorbidity in people with diabetes mellitus. CMAJ. 2003;168(13):1661-67.
33. Stange KC, et al. Ann Fam Med. 2003;1(1):2-4. The *Annals* is published through a collaborative effort by 6 family medicine organizations to address the need for the development of an integrated body of knowledge and a generalist paradigm.
34. Davis K, Cooper BS. American Health Care: Why So Costly? Invited Testimony before the Senate Appropriations Committee, Subcommittee on Labor, Health and Human Services, Education and Related Agencies; Hearing on Health Care Access and Affordability: Cost Containment Strategies. June 11, 2003.
35. Grumback K. Chronic illness, comorbidities, and the need for medical generalism. Ann Fam Med. 2003;1(1):4-7.
36. Ibid.
37. Bodenheimer T, Wagner EH, Grumbach K. Improving primary care for patients with chronic illness. JAMA. 2002;288:1775-79.
38. Starfield B, Lemke KW, Bernhardt T, et al. Comorbidity: implications for the importance of primary care in 'case' management. Ann Fam Med. 2003;1(1):8-14.
39. Booth FW, Gordon SE, Carlson CJ, Hamilton MT. Waging war on modern chronic diseases: primary prevention through exercise biology. J Appl Physiol. 2000; 88:774-87.
40. Ibid.
41. Oeppen J, Vaupel JW. Broken limits to life expectancy. Science, 2002;296:1029-31.
42. Campion EW. Aging better. N Engl J Med. 1998; 338(15):1064-66.
43. Vita AJ, Terry RB, Hubert HB, Fries J. Aging, health risks, and cumulative disability. N Engl J Med. 1998;338:1035-41.
44. Vaillant GE, Mukamal K. Successful aging. Am J Psychiatry. 2001;158(6):839-47.
45. Campbell AJ, Robertson MC, Gardner MM, et al. Randomised controlled trial of a general practice programme of home based exercise to prevent falls in elderly women. BMJ. 1997;315:1065-69.
46. Stewart KJ. Exercise training and the cardiovascular consequences of type 2 diabetes and hypertension. JAMA. 2002;288(13):1622-31.
47. Engelhart MJ, Geerlings MI, Ruitenberg A, et al. Dietary intake of antioxidants and risk of Alzheimer disease. JAMA. 2002; 287(24):3223-29.
48. Armstrong AM, Chestnutt JE, Gormley MJ, Young IS. The effect of dietary treatment on lipid peroxidation and antioxidant status in newly diagnosed noninsulin dependent diabetes. Free Rad Biol Med. 1996;21(5):719-26.
49. Roberts K, Dunn K, Jean SK, Lardinois CK. Syndrome X: Medical nutrition therapy. Nutr Rev. 2000; 58(5):154-60.
50. Oakley GP. Eat right and take a multivitamin (Edit). N Engl J Med. 1998;338(15):1060-61.
51. Ames BN. Micronutrients prevent cancer and delay aging. Toxicol Lett. 1998;102-103:5-18.
52. McMurdo MET. A healthy old age: realistic or futile goal? BMJ. 2000;321:1149-51.
53. Gross DJ, Schoeldelmeyer SW, Raetzman SO. Trends in manufacturer prices of brand name prescription drugs used by older Americans—first quarter 2004 update. AARP Issue Brief, June 2004.
54. Gapstur SM, Gann P. Is pancreatic cancer a preventable disease? JAMA. 2001;286(8):967-68.
55. Roubenoff R, Castaneda C. Sarcopenia—understanding the dynamics of aging muscle. JAMA. 2001;286(10):1230-31.
56. Hu FB, Manson JE, Stampfer MJ, et al. Diet, lifestyle, and the risk of type 2 diabetes mellitus in women. N Engl J Med. 2001;345(11):790-97.
57. Diabetes Prevention Program Research Group. Reduction in the incidence of type 2 diabetes with lifestyle intervention or metformin. N Engl J Med. 2002;346(6):393-403.
58. Narayan KMV, Boyle JP, Thompson TJ, et al. Lifetime risk for diabetes mellitus in the United States. JAMA. 2003; 290(4):1884-90.
59. Booth FW, Gordon SE, Carlson CJ, Hamilton MT. Waging war on modern chronic diseases: primary prevention through exercise biology. J Appl Physiol. 2000; 88:774-87.
60. Dabelea D, Hanson RL, Bennett PH, et al. Increasing prevalence of Type II diabetes in American Indian children. Diabetologia. 1998;41:904-10.
61. Fagot-Campagna A. Emergence of type 2 diabetes mellitus in children: epidemiological evidence. J Pediatr Endo Metab. 2000;13:1395-1402.
62. National Diabetes Information Clearinghouse (NDIC). [http://diabetes.niddk.nih.gov/dm/pubs/statistics/index.htm] Accessed 12/30/2003.
63. National Diabetes Information Clearinghouse (NDIC). [http://www.niddk.nih.gov/health/diabetes/pubs/dmstats/dmstats.htm] Accessed 7/8/2002.
64. Sale MM, Freedman BI, Langefeld CD, et al. A genome-wide scan for type 2 diabetes in African-American families reveals evidence for a locus on chromosome 6q. Diabetes. 2004;53(3):830-37.
65. Zouari Bouassida K, Chouchane L, Jellouli K, et al. Polymorphism of stress protein HSP70-2 gene in Tunisians: susceptibility implications in type 2 diabetes and obesity. Diabetes Metab. 2004;30(2):175-80.
66. Rich SS, Bowden DW, Haffner SM, et al. Identification of quantitative trait loci for glucose homeostasis: the insulin resistance atherosclerosis study (IRAS) family study. Diabetes. 2004;53(7):1866-75.
67. Kaufman FR. Type 2 diabetes mellitus in children and youth: a new epidemic. J Pediatr Endocrinol Metab. 2002;25(Suppl2):737-44.
68. Ott A, et al., Diabetes mellitus and the risk of dementia—The Rotterdam Study. Neurology. 1999;53:1937-42.
69. Klein JP, Waxman SG. The brain in diabetes: molecular changes in neurons and their implications for end-organ damage. Lancet. 2003;2:548-54.
70. Greenland P, Knoll MD, Stamler J, et al. Major risk factors as antecedents of fatal and nonfatal coronary heart disease events. JAMA. 2003;290:891-97.
71. Khot UN, Khot MB, Bajzer CT, et al. Prevalence of conventional risk factors in patients with coronary heart disease. JAMA. 2003;290:898-904.
72. Rychlik I, Sulkova S. Diabetes mellitus and chronic renal insufficiency. Vnitr Lek. 2003;49(5):395-402. [Article in Czech]
73. Mohanram A, Toto RD. Outcome studies in diabetic nephropathy. Semin Nephrol. 2003;23(3):255-71.

74. Espinola-Klein C, Rupprecht HJ, Blankenberg S, et al. Influence of impaired fasting glucose on the incidence and prognosis of atherosclerosis in various vascular regions. Z Kardiol. 2004;93(Suppl4):IV48-55. [Article in German]
75. Moschos SJ, Mantzoros CS. The role of the IGF system in cancer: from basic to clinical studies and clinical applications. Oncology. 2002;63(4):317-32.
76. Hu FB, Manson JE, Liu S, et al. Prospective study of adult onset diabetes mellitus (type 2) and risk of colorectal cancer in women. J Natl Cancer Inst. 1999;91:542-47.
77. Centers for Disease Control: Diabetes Public Health Resource. CDC Statements on Diabetes Issues. [http://www.cdc.gov/diabetes/news/docs/lifetime.htm] Accessed 12/31/2003.
78. Hu FB, Manson JE, Stampfer MJ, et al. Diet, lifestyle, and the risk of type 2 diabetes mellitus in women. N Engl J Med. 2001;345(11):790-97.
79. Double helix 50th anniversary collection. Nature. 2003;422(6934):787-929.
80. Rabinowitz PM, Poljak A. Host-environment medicine. A primary care model for the age of genomics. J Gen Intern Med. 2003;18:222-27.
81. Ibid.
82. Darnton-Hill I, Margetts B, Deckelbaum R. Public health nutrition and genetics: implications for nutrition policy and promotion. Proc Nutr Soc. 2004;63(1):173-85.
83. Bauer M, Hamm A, Pankratz MJ. Linking nutrition to genomics. Biol Chem. 2004;385(7):593-96.
84. Desiere F. Towards a systems biology understanding of human health: interplay between genotype, environment and nutrition. Biotechnol Annu Rev. 2004;10:51-84.
85. Ruden DM, De Luca M, Garfinkel, MD, et al. Drosophila nutrigenomics can provide clues to human gene-nutrient interactions. Annu Rev Nutr. 2005;25:499-522.
86. Pool-Zobel BL, Selvaraju V, Sauer J, et al. Butyrate may enhance toxicological defence in primary, adenoma and tumor human colon cells by favourably modulating expression of glutathione S-transferases genes, an approach in nutrigenomics. Carcinogenesis. 2005:Mar 3;[Epub ahead of print].
87. Kushner RF. Will there be a tipping point in medical nutrition education? Am J Clin Nutr. 2003;77:288-91.
88. Gladwell M. The Tipping Point: How Little Things Can Make a Big Difference. Boston; Little, Brown: 2000.
89. Gurwitz D, Weizman A, Rehavi M. Education: teaching pharmacogenomics to prepare future physicians and researchers for personalized medicine. Trends Pharmacol Sci. 2003;24(3):122-25.
90. Kozma C. The interface between genomics and nutrition. Top Clin Nutr. 2003;18(2):73-80.
91. Masson LF, McNeill G, Avenell A. Genetic variation and the lipid response to dietary intervention: a systematic review. Am J Clin Nutr. 2003;77:1098-111.
92. Fogg-Johnson N, Kaput J. Nutrigenomics: an emerging scientific discipline. Food Technol. 2003;57(4):60-67.
93. Muller M, Kersten S. Nutrigenomics: goals and strategies. Nat Rev Genet. 2003;4:315-22.
94. Kauwell GP. A genomic approach to dietetic practice. Are you ready? Top Clin Nutr. 2003;18(2)81-91.
95. Daniel H. Genomics and proteomics: importance for the future of nutrition research. British J Nutr. 2002;87(suppl 2):S305-S11.
96. Petricoin EF, Liotta LA. Clinical applications of proteomics. J Nutr. 2003;133:2476S-484S.
97. Ideker T, Thorsson V, Ranish JA, et al. Integrated genomic and proteomic analyses of a systematically perturbed metabolic network. Science. 2001;294:929-34.
98. Willett WC. Balancing life-style and genomics research for disease prevention. Science. 2002;296(5568):695-98.
99. Burke W. Genomics as a probe for disease biology. N Engl J Med. 2003;349:969-74.

Section I

Introduction

Chapter 4
Training Clinicians in New Approaches to Care

Sheila Quinn and David S. Jones, MD

Functional Medicine: A Model of Integrated Care to Address Systemic Health Issues

Functional Medicine Can Be Taught

Functional medicine synthesizes and applies scientific evidence from the biomedical research literature in fields such as biochemistry, physiology, immunology, and nutrition. Unlike alternative medical disciplines (such as acupuncture or chiropractic or naturopathic medicine), it does not require that conventional providers master different language/tools of health care, nor does it require that alternative providers give up the tenets of their respective disciplines. It can be taught to, and used by, all healthcare providers with a background in the basic medical and clinical sciences, regardless of the particular profession a practitioner belongs to (within the limits of specific training and licensure, of course). This makes functional medicine uniquely suited to multidisciplinary, integrated clinical settings, as well as to use by individual practitioners.

This textbook is organized around the information and approach that IFM uses to teach clinicians, and exemplifies the kind of clinical thinking and patient management that characterize many functional medicine practitioners:

- A thorough understanding of the core context and concepts of functional medicine (*Principles Section*) helps to distinguish the functional medicine approach.
- Teaching functional medicine often requires refreshing and expanding the clinician's knowledge of biochemistry and physiology (*Fundamental Physiological Processes Section*).
- A strong appreciation for the importance of environmental inputs (*Building Blocks Section*) is vital to an understanding of functional medicine, for we are equally concerned with whether the raw materials of health (or disease), including genetic predispositions, are present in the patient's life.
- An emphasis is placed on learning to assess and improve underlying functional imbalances in six core areas that comprise the "engines" that drive the patient toward health or disease (*Fundamental Clinical Imbalances Section*).
- The more didactic information presented in the first five sections is brought into context for the provider in *A Practical Clinical Approach.* Here the functional medicine matrix—a tool for simplifying the complex science into a manageable clinical approach—is the underlying structure. This section demonstrates how to obtain, sort, and qualify the different kinds of patient information so as to generate a strong indicator to the clinician of the most useful way to "pull on the web" of interconnecting issues presented by the patient.
- Finally, the last section, *Putting it All Together,* helps clinicians understand some of the most important patient care issues that are commonly experienced in functional medicine.

Thus, functional medicine can be taught to any clinician who has an open mind and an eagerness to twist the kaleidoscope and look at patient care from new angles. It is a matter of acquiring, analyzing, classifying, and prioritizing information in different ways, and then applying therapeutic (or preventive) measures that are aimed at correcting the imbalances that underlie organ-system disease. If the clinician doesn't address the underlying imbalances—and understand how they arise and how they can be ameliorated—it is much less likely that restoration of health will be the ultimate outcome. Functional medicine approaches patient care with the confidence that restoring and maintaining health are achievable goals.

Functional Medicine is Discipline-Neutral

Functional medicine is discipline-neutral—the field is accessible to any health practitioner who has a fairly standard western medical science background. There are significant advantages to this "neutrality," particularly as the nation's healthcare system becomes more and more open and adaptive to integrated care concepts:

- Patients with chronic disease often use multiple care-givers from a variety of fields. It is extremely valuable to the patient (and to the efficient delivery of care) when those practitioners have a common "language" for discussing patient health. Functional medicine creates a unifying mind-set and information architecture about health and disease, regardless of widely varied clinician training and skills.
- Although the science underlying functional medicine is complex, the application of therapeutic and prevention-oriented approaches is often relatively straightforward; patients can understand it and so can practitioners from many different backgrounds. Functional medicine creates a more level playing field between and among patients and providers.
- We have had a very hierarchical healthcare system for many years in the United States; as a result, turf battles between professions are common and patients often get caught in the crossfire. With the cross-disciplinary nature of functional medicine, those problems can be minimized or eliminated.

Functional medicine is firmly grounded in scientific principles and data but adopts a flexible, eclectic perspective on medicine. The use of dietary interventions, clinical nutrition, exercise therapy, mind-body-spirit issues, botanical medicines, physical medicine, and even energy medicine (e.g., acupuncture) can all be integrated into functional medicine teaching and practice when the science warrants it. The use of drugs and/or surgery does not disappear, but lifestyle interventions assume a certain primacy (where appropriate)—both because of their lower cost and because of their long-term role in restoration of health and prevention of disease (or complications of disease).

Conventional providers and alternative providers alike are able to integrate functional medicine thinking into their existing knowledge base because underneath the superstructures created by the many professions, an abiding interest in "functionality"—how things work and what to do when they don't—is a shared terrain. Some learners may not have a strong science background, and may thus need to intensify their knowledge of biochemistry and physiology, but some with a strong science education may have to learn clinical nutrition and to appreciate the contributions of (for example) botanicals and chiropractic.

In these diverse ways, functional medicine helps create a bridge between conventional and alternative practitioners and approaches—a place where there is mutuality of ideas and interests, and where the patient's needs can come first. This common meeting ground will enhance the delivery of integrated care and contribute to the development of respectful and productive professional relationships among healthcare providers.

Focused Training is Needed to Change the Existing Model of Care

The postgraduate healthcare education industry encompasses many different methods of delivering information to clinicians: textbooks, journal articles, and professional conferences are among the most common. The sizable investment made in these activities year after year ought to create a significant obligation to demonstrate that they substantially improve the care that patients receive. Unfortunately, emerging research is demonstrating quite convincingly that the changes created by conventional continuing medical education or CME (journal articles and conferences) are much less significant than most practitioners realize. Consider just a few selected quotations:

- "lecture results in only the lowest level of behavioral change."[1]
- "the best predictor of knowledge of blood pressure treatment [for example] is a physician's year of graduation from medical school."[2]
- "Unfortunately, most of the clinical questions generated at the point of care go unanswered."[3]
- "traditional medical care delivery methods are failing to adapt by responding too slowly to rapidly changing new medical evidence."[4]
- "[M]any of the implications from research, although black and white to the researcher, are not immediately compelling to the practitioner … ."[5]

- "Uneven uptake of research findings—and thus inappropriate care—occurs across different health care settings, countries and specialties ... ."[6]
- "Didactic sessions do not appear to be effective in changing physician performance."[7]

And, very significantly:

- "In addition to being disconnected temporally and spatially from the actual delivery of care, CME has too often failed to deliver the most important and useful information to clinicians: patient-oriented evidence on common or important problems that has the potential to change practice."[8]

This disconnection from "evidence that matters" is of great concern to IFM and to functional medicine leaders and practitioners. We spend a lot of time and effort—unsupported by the deep pockets of the pharmaceutical industry or the organizational backing of medical schools, societies, or hospitals—developing courses and symposia that deliver information. We work diligently to ensure the clinical relevance of that information and to focus on the problems that cost the healthcare system the most in dollars and cost patients the most long-term distress—complex, chronic disease. But if this is not the most effective way to deliver "patient-oriented evidence that matters" (POEMs) then we want to change it.

Meeting that challenge head-on has brought us to this book. While information alone may not change clinician behavior very significantly, high quality information is an absolutely essential ingredient in the mix—necessary, but not sufficient. Developing a comprehensive textbook—where the evidence base is clearly demonstrated and the clinical connections to that evidence are made clear—seems an important step. Delivering this comprehensive information base so that clinicians can learn at their own pace, in their own homes and offices, and in response to clinical questions that arise at the point of care, may enable us to increase our effectiveness and—a prime consideration—perhaps redirect the focus of our onsite courses to more interactive, clinically specific education.

We hope that the book's users will take on a personal "commitment to change." There is evidence to show that "physicians who expressed a commitment to change were significantly more likely to change"[9] their actual behavior. We offer help with understanding how to change in Chapter 36—it may be structured as "helping patients to change unhealthy behaviors," but it is just as useful in making any kind of personal change, in one's life or one's practice.

We think of you—the current and future functional medicine practitioners—as our partners in developing the information base and improving the effectiveness of the training. Please stay in communication with us about what really does—and does not—make a difference in the way you actually practice and how your patients have fared.

Mentoring and Follow-Up Are Needed in Addition to CME

If it can be established, as we believe and have expounded on at some length in Part I of this Introduction, that certain changes are urgently needed in our current healthcare system, particularly for complex chronic disease, then the question immediately arises, "If information alone is insufficient, how can such change be achieved?" There are several important pathways to address:

1. **Change the way physicians and other practitioners are taught.** As noted above, we do know that how a physician is taught is often an extremely powerful predictor of how he/she will practice. A lot of CME effort is devoted to trying to change and update what was learned in medical school. New practitioners should be emerging from their training already prepared to practice effective, integrated care in multidisciplinary settings. The *Textbook of Functional Medicine* can contribute by providing a broader view of the underlying mechanisms of health (and disease prevention), by linking the basic sciences and the research literature with effective clinical approaches, and by strengthening the priority that is placed upon understanding the key influences on gene expression.
2. **Find ways to make continuing medical education more effective.** While the research on effectiveness of CME is not voluminous, it does present a rather alarming assessment of CME effectiveness in changing physician behavior (see above). The picture goes something like this: didactic presentations may improve knowledge but are unlikely to change behavior;[10] single interventions on a particular subject are much less likely to change behavior than multiple, varied interventions (rare);[11] complex changes are more difficult than simple ones;[12] information that is not relevant to questions that

arise at the point of care is unlikely to change behavior;[13] even CME that changes physician behaviors with some efficacy may not change patient outcomes;[14] practitioners may find change difficult if the system within which they practice is not proactive and responsive;[15] and yet physicians still like CME.[16] They attend it with great regularity and frequency, rely on it for their continued learning, and are often quite willing to make a commitment—in the moment of learning—to change.[17]

How can this massive, nationwide (costly) effort to bring good continuing education to the fore, and to use information as an effective change agent, be enhanced? There are certainly many more questions than answers on this vital topic, but two findings that have emerged with some consistency are these: mentoring is an important element and follow-up is critical. Practitioners need continuing contact with skilled and respected colleagues who can give feedback on new information and ideas, and whose collaboration can be sought about key clinical questions that directly affect patients.[18]

IFM provides you—the reader of this book—and other interested practitioners considerable support for the effective integration of functional medicine into practice through its vibrant, interactive online community (www.functionalmedicine.org). On the fully searchable IFM Member Forum (information about membership is available at http://www.functionalmedicine.org/membercommunity/becomemember.asp), you can participate in a variety of ways:

- **Engage with the experts** who post as Forum Hosts on "Topic of the Week." Cases are presented, emerging evidence is discussed, and stimulating questions are posed. Some discussions involve dozens of respondents and are highly interactive. Forum Hosts are a valuable resource for all functional medicine practitioners, even experienced ones.
- **Post a question or issue of your own.** Is a particular patient troubling you, or are there conditions or approaches you want clinical guidance on? Any member can initiate a post (although you may want to search the Forum first to see whether the topic has been explored before). You are likely to receive very thoughtful and generous responses from your colleagues. Over time, you will get to know these professionals, and you can begin independent dialogues by emailing directly to those whose expertise is most helpful to you.
- **Review the regular "Article of the Week"** postings by the Forum Consultant, who will also chime in on Forum Host or member postings by offering links to key research or relevant articles.
- **Speak up about functional medicine.** Share your education and clinical experiences with colleagues and patients. If you are an experienced functional medicine practitioner, offer to mentor a colleague who is new to the field. Recommend this book to your local hospital library, or buy an extra copy and donate it to the school where you received your professional training. In other words, expand the functional medicine community through your own efforts. The opinion of a respected colleague can be very influential.

References

1. Stancic N, Mullen PD, Prokhorov AV, et al. Continuing medical education: what delivery format do physicians prefer? J Cont Ed Health Prof. 2003;23:162-67.
2. Sackett DL, Richardson WS, Rosenberg W, Haynes RB, eds. Evidence-based medicine: how to practice and teach EBM. 1st Ed. New York: Churchill-Livingstone, 1997.
3. Ebell MH, Shaughnessy A. Information mastery: integrating continuing medical education with the information needs of clinicians. J Cont Ed Health Prof. 2003;23:S53-S62.
4. Prather SE, Jones DN. Physician leadership: Influence on practice-based learning and improvement. J Cont Ed Health Prof. 2003;23:S63-S72.
5. Lomas J. Teaching old (and not so old) tricks: effective ways to implement research findings. In Dunn EV, Norton PG, Stewart M, Tudiver F. Disseminating Research/Changing Practice. Thousand Oaks, CA: Sage; 1994.
6. Foy R, Eccles M, Grimshaw J. Why does primary care need more implementation research? Fam Pract. 2001;18(4):353-55.
7. Davis D, O'Brien MAT, Freemantle N, et al. Impact of formal continuing medical education: do conferences, workshops, rounds, and other traditional continuing education activities change physician behavior or health care outcomes? JAMA. 1999;282(9):867-74.
8. Ebell MH, Shaughnessy A. Information mastery: integrating continuing medical education with the information needs of clinicians. J Cont Ed Health Prof. 2003;23:S53-S62.
9. Wakefield J, Herbert CP, Maclure M, et al. Commitment to change statements can predict actual change in practice. J Cont Ed Health Prof. 2003;23:81-93.
10. Stancic N, Mullen PD, Prokhorov AV, et al. Continuing medical education: what delivery format do physicians prefer? J Contin Educ Health Prof. 2003;23(3):162-67.
11. Robertson MK, Umble KE, Cervero RM. Impact studies in continuing education for health professions: update. J Contin Educ Health Prof. 2003;23(3):146-56.
12. Grol R, Grimshaw J. From best evidence to best practice: effective implementation of change in patients' care. Lancet. 2003;362:1225-30.

13. Cervero RM. Place matters in physician practice and learning. J Contin Educ Health Prof. 2003;23(Suppl 1):S10-S18.
14. Markert RJ, O'Neill SC, Bhatia SC. Using a quasi-experimental research design to assess knowledge in continuing medical education programs. J Contin Educ Health Prof. 2003;23(3):157-61.
15. Grol R, Grimshaw J. From best evidence to best practice: effective implementation of change in patients' care. Lancet. 2003;362:1225-30.
16. Stancic N, Mullen PD, Prokhorov AV, et al. Continuing medical education: what delivery format do physicians prefer? J Contin Educ Health Prof. 2003;23(3):162-67.
17. Wakefield J, Herbert CP, Maclure M, Dormuth C, et al. Commitment to change statements can predict actual change in practice. J Contin Educ Health Prof 2003;23(2):81-93.
18. Grol R, Grimshaw J. From best evidence to best practice: effective implementation of change in patients' care. Lancet. 2003;362:1225-30.

Chapter 5
Changing the Evidence Model

- *Functional Medicine and the Emerging Research Base*
- *Clinical Decision Making—A Functional Medicine Perspective*

Functional Medicine and the Emerging Research Base

David S. Jones, MD

Understanding the Limitations of the Randomized Controlled Trial (RCT)

The scientific method disciplines the creative process of human inquiry. In the applied biological sciences (e.g., clinical medicine) prior to World War II, evaluation of emerging therapeutics was mainly the purview of recognized leaders in the medical profession, based primarily on their clinical impressions, without the touchstone of any systematic controls.[1] To temper the quality of evidence and render a "truer" judgment with less personal bias, elite postwar researchers developed the randomized controlled trial (RCT) protocol. The major characteristics of this method include blinded assessment (of subjects, investigators, or both) in the presence of a placebo control, random assignment to comparable groups, and inferential statistics as a surrogate for establishing causation.[2]

This methodology (RCT) found its most ardent advocates in the sphere of pharmacological therapeutic interventions, specifically drug studies (using, most often, single agents). With development of powerful pharmaceuticals, the imperative for a scientifically rigorous methodology for asking systematic questions about efficacy, benefits, risks, and causation has proved ever more important (*cf.* the thalidomide tragedy of the late 1950s and the early 1960s[3] and the unpredicted results of the more recent HERS RCT research vis-à-vis female hormone replacement therapy[4]). In the ensuing 60 years, the advocates for the RCT model have worked assiduously to understand RCT study designs, including identification of pitfalls and types of bias.[5,6,7,8,9]

The proponents of the RCT as the gold standard for unbiased research results have moved forward in the applied medical fields, both in primary and specialty care. They have developed systems for grading recommendations based on a "research quality scale" that ranks methodologies in descending order of accepted best evidence:[10,11]

- Systematic reviews and meta-analyses of RCTs
- RCTs
- Non-randomized intervention studies
- Non-experimental studies
- Expert opinion

The very influential schema called *evidence-based medicine* (EBM) has emerged using these hierarchical assumptions as foundational suppositions:

> A new paradigm for medical practice is emerging. Evidence-based medicine de-emphasizes intuition, unsystematic clinical experience, and pathophysiologic rationale as sufficient grounds for clinical decision making and stresses the examination of evidence from clinical research. Evidence-based medicine requires new skills of the physician including efficient literature searching and the application of formal rules of evidence evaluating the clinical literature.[12]

Evidence-based practice requires the integration, patient by patient, of the physician's clinical expertise and judgment with the best available relevant external evidence. Sackett in 1996 described EBM in this way: "Evidence based medicine is the conscientious, explicit, and judicious use of current best evidence in making decisions about the care of individual patients. The practice of evidence based medicine means integrating individual clinical expertise with the best available external clinical evidence from systematic research. ... Good doctors use both individual clinical expertise and the best available external evidence and neither alone is enough."[13] The process of evidence-based medicine is summarized below.[14,15]

- Select specific clinical questions from the patient's problem(s).
- Search the literature or databases for relevant clinical information.
- Appraise the evidence for validity and usefulness to the patient and practice.
- Implement useful findings in everyday practice.

As discussed in several of the aforementioned papers, the combining of these elements can be viewed as a Venn diagram (Figure 5.1), where the best outcomes occur when all three elements are represented.

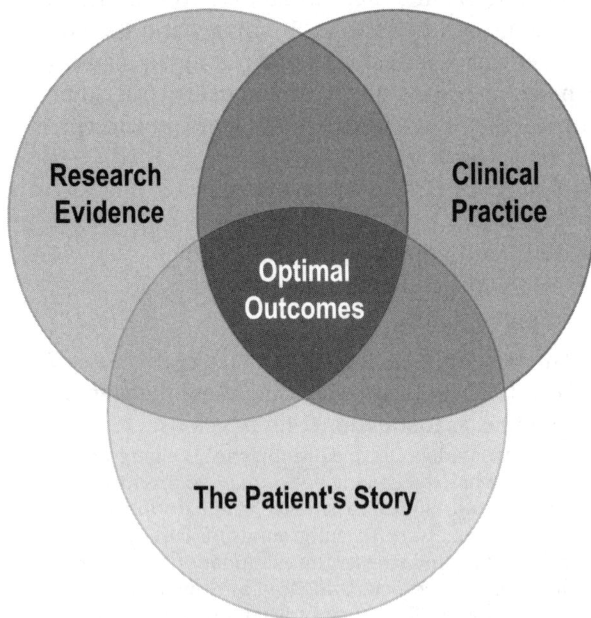

Figure 5.1 **Optimal outcomes: Applying evidence-based medicine to the real world**

Arguments in favor of evidence-based medicine include the following:[16,17]

- Increasingly available new evidence can and should lead to major changes in patient care.
- Practicing physicians often fail to obtain available relevant evidence.
- Medical knowledge and clinical performance deteriorate over time without the leavening of newer evidence influencing clinical decisions.
- Traditional continuing medical education (CME) is inefficient and generally does not improve clinical performance without a disciplined methodology of inclusion of new evidence into clinical practice.
- The discipline of evidence-based medicine can keep the physician up-to-date.

The clinical application of basic research has been slowed by two major issues. The *first problem* that has impeded the successful application of EBM to the daily specifics of patient care is the complex nature of the translation of research studies to the individual patient's unique clinical problem(s)—what Larry Weed called knowledge coupling.[18,19,20] John Hampton, Professor of Cardiology, University Hospital, Nottingham, England, in a review titled "Evidence-based Medicine, Opinion-based Medicine, and Real-world Medicine," reasons: "Clinical trials will tell us what treatments are effective, but not necessarily which patients should receive them ... . Treatment must always be tailored to the individual patient."[21] Added to this methodologic conundrum are the real-world exigencies of daily clinical practice that make it virtually impossible to collate and filter all relevant evidence prior to direct application to the unique needs of the patient. Imagine a clinic where, after each therapeutic encounter—thorough history taking accompanied by a complete physical exam—a problem list is developed that is then carefully subjected to a medical literature search and analysis. The practice of clinical medicine will not tolerate the inertia of such a process.[22] These practicalities of real-time clinical practice have slowed the integration of new research into the clinical care of patients who are often in desperate need of interventions based on emerging evidence.

To assist the practicing physician's effective inclusion of new evidence into daily practice, both government-sponsored and commercially affiliated organizations have moved EBM forward with a collation of filtered studies called *Problem Oriented Evidence that Matters* (POEMs).[23] It is now possible to search these specific databases, or self-developed relevant databases that review groups of studies that directly link research findings with specific clinical problems. The development of robust and thorough databases of POEMs is an ongoing commitment of institutions throughout the industrialized world.[24,25]

A *second major issue* has proved to be a Gordian knot that has not yet been unraveled. If medical care were as simple as identifying the clinical problem followed by the prescription of an appropriate single pharmacologic agent, then the EBM system, as presently configured and applied, would work if appropriate POEMs were available for each medical problem. However, the dream and heritage from half a century of medicalization of the daily health problems of our patients have *not* proved remedial to the widely accepted notion of "better living through chemistry."[26] (Most POEMs and most studies in the Cochrane Collection are research trials of pharmacologic therapeutic interventions.) In fact, acute medical problems are the only medical problems that appear to predictably respond as envisioned by the conventional medical paradigm. However, greater than 70% of health problems presenting to clinicians today are chronic, complex medical issues[27] for which the underlying assumptions of the RCT and medical education based on this assumption simply fail to provide satisfactory answers.

Halsted Holman, MD, of Stanford Medical School, editorialized in JAMA in 2004: "Chronic disease is now the principal cause of disability and use of health services and consumes 78% of health expenditures."[28] Within this population with chronic, complex illness, non-genetic factors that are *modifiable* by lifestyle changes—including diet, overweight, inactivity and environmental exposures such as smoking—account for 70–90% of mortality in the U.S.[29] Add to this the projection from the Centers for Disease Control (CDC) that one-third of the people born in the year 2000 will eventually have diabetes,[30] which is probably the most costly of the chronic diseases when all of its comorbidities and secondary complications are considered.[31] With similar disturbing statistics in hand, Holman goes on to point out that, "Chronic disease requires a practice of medicine quite different from that used for acute disease ... Unfortunately, few if any schools are preparing their students adequately for the roles they and their patients need to play."

Despite these sobering facts, physician education, training, and reimbursement, as well as research designs for clinical studies that physicians will depend upon for clinical decision making, continue to be focused on treating chronic disease using drugs and surgery rather than comprehensive patient-centered treatments focused on the individual. It becomes easier to see that the *second major issue* impeding the application of emerging research is the absence of an adequate filtering system (evidence design) and application architecture (or information matrix) for the focus of 21st century medical needs: complex, chronic illness. Funding of research continues to be primarily focused on pharmacologic answers to these complex, chronic problems, leaving the discerning clinician without the EBM tools and information for addressing their patients' complex needs.

In a cogent paper in *The Lancet* (van Weel and Knottnerus, 1999),[32] the difficulties of using evidence in the context of the individual patient with complex, chronic illness are discussed and specific obstacles are identified:

- EBM tends to concentrate on research methodology and reduce clinical practice to the technical implementation of research findings.
- Comorbid conditions are the usual justified reason for the exclusion of patients from RCTs, so the very patients most in need of usable evidence (e.g., those with complex, chronic conditions) are often not in the cohorts of patients being studied, leaving the findings from the research trials very limited in their applicability.
- In general practice, treatment usually consists of various elementary interventions. Combinations of evidence-based interventions do not sum to a plan that is evidence-based. Interactions between single interventions may increase or decrease their efficacy (even under ideal trial conditions) when cobbled together into a comprehensive plan.
- Clinical research does not focus on the overall outcome of composite interventions because of the complexity of such studies and the absence of well-developed tools for studying such approaches.
- Drug interventions have been studied more extensively than non-pharmacological interventions, in part due to the technical and methodological difficulties in the design of RCTs for non-drug interventions.
- This situation is a particular problem in general practice, where the use of educational, dietary, and lifestyle interventions is attractive because of their resonance with the principle of "maximum effect using minimum resources."

- The structure of RCT methodology assumes the consequences of individual variability in response to treatment will "wash out" if the subject pool is large enough and the statistical analyses sophisticated enough. While this may be true for populations, it seriously limits the applicability of the research in primary care, which is delivered one patient at a time.

According to van Weel and Knottnerus, the driving force behind EBM should be a coherent system of fundamental research of pathophysiology *and* humanities, combined with careful clinical observations, on which systematic (RCT-based) evidence of effectiveness is superimposed. Existing clinical practice should be supported or, if erroneous, corrected on the basis of this coherent system.

They go on to propose that "two complementary approaches are needed to strengthen the evidence base of non-pharmacological interventions and complex multifaceted strategies. First, the generic characteristics of complex interventions must be acknowledged as essential for its evaluation. Second, a methodology to allow the assessment of complex effects should be further developed."[33] They share the concern that EBM has de-evolved into primarily a discussion of "research methodology and [has] reduce[d] clinical practice to the technical implementation of research findings."

Dr. David Mant in his seminal paper, "Can Randomized Trials Inform Clinical Decisions about Individual Patients?" takes a slightly different tack in exploring the irony that the RCT combines strength of concept for the population being studied with weakness of specific application to the individual patient:[34]

> The paradox of the clinical trial is that it is the best way to assess whether an intervention works, but is arguably the worst way to assess who will benefit from it. ... However, the nub of the argument for me is that randomized controlled trials are primarily about medical interventions and not patients. In clinical trials, patients are randomized to allow a comparison of intervention efficacy unbiased by the individuality of the patient. This methodological approach provides society with powerful protection against witch-doctoring, and helps us eliminate the inefficiencies in the provision of medical care described by Cochrane. But the methodological minimization of information on effectiveness in relation to the individual patient leaves an evidence gap for clinicians.

Dr. Alan Feinstein, from the Department of Medicine, Yale University, in his article, "Problems in the 'Evidence' of 'Evidence-based Medicine,'" echoes similar reservations.[35] Larry Culpepper and Thomas Gilbert, in their *Lancet* commentary, "Evidence and Ethics," focus this same reservation in the primary-care arena of patient care.[36] In summation, the reductionist simplicity of the double-blind, placebo-controlled trial frequently does not work for the significant questions now facing 21st century primary care practitioners in the one-on-one decision making characteristic of clinical medicine. The statistical and mathematical sophistication needed for multi-variable analysis of the clinical context of patients with complex, chronic illness, in the inter-face between the patient's unique environmental context, and the patient's unique genomic card-catalogue of possibilities, simply does not now exist. We are in the transitional stage of realizing that our tools of evidence are inadequate to the challenge posed by emerging evidence from our scientific community that demonstrates that the world works through complex mechanisms operating simultaneously. These complex questions cannot be reduced to the relatively simple single-agent, single-condition research for which the RCT methodology is so well suited.[37,38,39]

We cannot continue to ignore where the truly significant questions reside, regardless of the difficulty and elusiveness of the answers needed to address the problems inherent in chronic, complex diseases. The RCT tool was developed during a specific period in our medical history and worked well to adjudicate between the traditionalists who claimed that clinical experience trumped bench science and the scientists who perceived the value in systematic inquiry. Major strides in treatment have occurred in the intervening 50 to 60 years as a result of the shift in opinion toward the use of RCT methodology. But we are now at another nodal decision point, unique to our cultural and medical evolution. We need a more sophisticated tool to shed light on the nature of the web-like interweaving of mechanisms at work in the chronic, complex illnesses under scrutiny.[40,41]

Complex Conditions, Complex Models

The emerging research on underlying mechanisms of dysfunctional processes that lead to diagnosable disease has outpaced the ability of existing clinical research methods to keep up with useful evaluation of the information. The complexity of the developing "explanatory models" has been serially addressed in the *Annals of Fam-*

ily Medicine, a peer-reviewed medical journal "dedicated to advancing knowledge essential to understanding and improving health and primary care," including the development of methodology and theory for addressing this conundrum.[42] In the article, "The Biopsychosocial Model 25 Years Later: Principles, Practice, and Scientific Inquiry,"[43] the authors critique the limitations of the conventional biomedical model and the research methodologies that evolve from this model, and preview the evolving model of "complexity and causality" and the nested model of "structural causality":

> Few morbid conditions could be interpreted as being of the nature "one microbe, one illness"; rather, there are usually multiple interacting causes and contributing factors. Thus, obesity leads to both diabetes and arthritis; both obesity and arthritis limit exercise capacity, adversely affecting blood pressure and cholesterol levels; and all of the above, except perhaps arthritis, contribute to both stroke and coronary artery disease. Some effects (depression after a heart attack or stroke) can then become causal (greater likelihood of a second similar event). ... These observations set the stage for models of circular causality that describe how a series of feedback loops sustain a specific pattern of behavior over time.[44,45,46] Complexity science is an attempt to understand these complex recursive and emergent properties of systems[47,48] and to find interrelated proximal causes that might be changed with the right set of interventions.[49]

David Deutsch, in *The Fabric of Reality*, describes the need for a next step in using the science of underlying mechanisms of disease in the clinical setting of medicine:

> The science of medicine is perhaps the most frequently cited case of increasing specialization seeming to follow inevitably from increasing knowledge, as new cures and better treatments for more diseases are discovered. But as medical and biochemical research comes up with deeper explanations of disease processes (and healthy processes) in the body, understanding is also on the increase. More general concepts are replacing more specific ones as common, underlying molecular mechanisms are found for dissimilar diseases in different parts of the body. Once a disease can be understood as fitting into a general framework, the role of the specialist diminishes. ... Physicians ... can look up such facts as are known. But [more importantly] they may be able to apply a general theory to work out the required treatment, and expect it to be effective even if it has never been used before.[50]

The real question facing every discerning, informed clinician in a patient-oriented clinic[51] is how to bring relevant, graded, emerging scientific evidence to the complex list of problems made unique by the patient's gene map of susceptibilities/potentialities that, in turn, communicates constantly with the ever-changing environment within which the patient lives. No RCT can possibly inform, *in a specific way*, the appropriate clinical roadmap for assessment and planning for therapeutic interventions in this complex environment.[52]

Dr. Richard Horton, editor-in-chief of *The Lancet*, addressed this issue in an editorial titled, "The Precautionary Principle":

> We must act on facts, and on the most accurate interpretation of them, using the best scientific information. That does not mean we must sit back until we have 100% evidence about everything. Where the state of the health of the people is at stake, the risks can be so high and the cost of corrective action so great, that prevention is better than cure. We must analyze the possible benefits and cost of action and inaction. Where there are significant risks of damage to the public health, we should be prepared to take action to diminish those risks even when the scientific knowledge is not conclusive, if the balance of likely costs and benefits justifies it.[53]

One such intermediate tool that addresses this second major problem in applying emerging scientific evidence to clinical problems has been developed. This algorithm for critically assessing interventions in the context of complex, chronic illness has the mnemonic "STEPed Care":

Safety (an analysis of adverse effects that patients and providers care about),
Tolerability (pooled drop-out rates from large clinical trials),
Effectiveness (how well the intervention[s] work and in what patient population[s]), and
Price (costs of intervention, but also cost-effectiveness of therapy).[54]

Clinicians who are armed with this tool can arrange the emerging evidence about underlying mechanisms of disease in the clinical context of their patients' problems and can apply this matrix of STEPed Care, bringing the best of new evidence to the unique needs of their patients.

To do more is to place patients in danger, teetering on the insubstantial edge of research, but to do less is unconscionable. For example, starting in the 1970s emerging research suggested that public health measures to insure folate nutriture for women in the childbearing years, especially prior to conception, could markedly affect the incidence of spina bifida as well as other congenital neural tube anomalies in newborns.[55,56,57,58,59]

However, it was not until March 1996 that the U.S. Food and Drug Administration (FDA) authorized addition of folic acid to enriched grain products. By 2001, a report in *JAMA* substantiated a 19% reduction in the birth prevalence of neural tube defects following the FDA's decision.[60] This delay of over two decades was and is unjustified. Discerning practitioners were applying the principles inherent in the STEPed Care process 15 years before the mandated action of the FDA, bringing to their patients of childbearing age and to their newborns the critical benefits of emerging research about folic acid at a much earlier actionable point.

Drs. Mark Hyman, Joseph Pizzorno, and Andrew Weil wrestled with this dilemma in the reconfiguration of the medical research perspective at this branching point in our evolution of medical technologies. In their 2004 commentary in *Alternative Therapies*, they propose a middle ground approach for best addressing the real problems both clinicians and patients face at this time:[61]

> Medical science is imprecise and the tools of analysis and research are imperfect despite our best intentions. No statistical model or research methodology can accurately predict the outcome in all humans who vary greatly in habits and genes. Medicine has in recent years been humbled in its hunger to help by its mistakes including hormone replacement therapy,[62] which in the end hurt rather than helped the heart, the "lipids only hypothesis" of cardiovascular disease that ignores the important role of inflammation,[63] and the belated,[64] sober end to our love affair with COX-2 inhibitors.
>
> Uncertainty is common in medicine. In the face of uncertainty, we must take a broader view, step back from the canvas of individual studies and meta-analyses and view the landscape of medicine and scientific inquiry as a whole, while understanding the limitations and value of different tools of research. We require all the tools in order to create sense and be sensible in a shifting sea of data points. The goal of seeking an informed balanced overview is to help us create understanding from knowledge, to sort through the facts and place them in the context of biologic principles, against the backdrop of all we know. Then we ask ourselves if the new data fit into the landscape or appear like a polar bear in a desert. We must also recognize that the questions we ask, how we ask them, and why, all inform the answers we receive.
>
> The responsibility of the scientist is to filter the research, place it in context, provide hope where appropriate and caution where necessary, but most importantly to be an informed, measured guide to a public seeking to gain health and ameliorate suffering.

We are also at a branch point in the evolution of clinical medicine where the "dissonance that exists between public and profession is intensifying."[65] Horton describes his answer to this dilemma as follows: "Application, synthesis, and reflection—these are my personal wishes for a renaissance in clinical medicine. It is not concerned with hierarchies of evidence; it is not dependent on up-to-date literature alone as the arbiter of clinical decision making; it does not proselytize a bottom-line approach to the reading of new research. Rather, it is about preferring interpretations to conclusions, external validity to internal validity, context to the highly controlled—and artificial—experimental environment."[66] Our patients are clamoring for this "renaissance" and the "largely skeptical and indifferent response to them has isolated physicians within an unattractive provincial and narrow island of medicine, a medicine that has become intellectually self-admiring of its scientistic purity and, as a consequence, self-deluding and self-defeating."[67]

We are again facing a paradigm shift,[68] ironically birthed by the original attempt to construct an evidence-based medical system. Thomas Kuhn[69] has described scientific paradigms as ways of looking at the world that define both the problems that can legitimately be addressed and the range of admissible evidence that may bear on their solution.

> When defects in an existing paradigm accumulate to the extent that the paradigm is no longer tenable, the paradigm is challenged and replaced by a new way of looking at the world. Medical practice is changing, and the change, which involves using the medical literature more effectively in guiding medical practice, is profound enough that it can appropriately be called a paradigm shift.[70]

The practice of EBM needs to return to its original mission of integrating evidence to inform clinical experience and to expand the understanding of basic mechanisms of health and disease.[71,72] This will help to reverse the decade-long plunge into the narrow focus on "the discussion of research methodology, reducing clinical practice to the technical implementation of research findings."[73,74] Alternate study designs and statistical methodologies are now being evaluated for analyzing complex data sets.[75]

A middle ground has been defined, creating a broader appreciation for the clarity that RCTs can bring without the obsequious and inappropriate hegemony that has characterized the debate over the last decade.[76] As concluded by Larry Dossey in his "Notes on the Journey": "One of the greatest impediments to progress in science is to assume that our fundamental concepts are basically complete. They have never been."[77]

We still have miles to go in our journey to understand the appropriate scientific methods that can reliably discipline the creative process of human curiosity about efficacy, benefits, risks, and causation of human suffering and its remediation. The new paradigm will recursively inform and redirect the EBM paradigm shift developed during the 1990s. IFM and functional medicine are already adapted to this changing model, making use of both existing and emerging research, and educating clinicians to bring the best of both worlds to their patients. It is our hope that this textbook will provide convincing evidence of the value of that mission.

Clinical Decision Making—A Functional Medicine Perspective

Joseph E. Pizzorno, Jr., ND

Introduction

As 21st century health care moves from a disease-based approach to a more patient-centric system that can address biochemical individuality to improve health and function (see Chapter 8), clinical decision making becomes more complex. Accentuating the problem is the lack of a clear standard for this more complex functional medicine approach. While there is relatively broad agreement in Western medicine for what constitutes competent assessment of disease and identification of related treatment approaches, the complex functional medicine model posits multiple and individualized diagnostic and therapeutic approaches, most or many of which have reasonable underlying science and principles, but which have not been rigorously tested in a research or clinical setting. (For a discussion of the limitations of the current RCT model in testing multifactorial and individualized approaches, see the preceding discussion in this chapter.) This has led to non-rigorous thinking and sometimes to uncritical acceptance of both poorly documented diagnostic procedures and ineffective therapies, resulting in less than optimal clinical care.

In this discussion, we will address the challenges of clinical decision making in a functional medicine practice, looking at various models of human decision making and identifying strategies to improve their application in the healthcare setting.

Challenges for the Functional Medicine Clinician

The personalization of care achievable through the functional medicine approach is the only real solution to the crisis of chronic disease facing us today. (This subject has been explored deeply in Chapters 1 through 4.) However, to practice this form of medicine is difficult, complex, and requires higher standards of decision making by clinicians. The functional medicine approach to diagnosis demands not only that we determine what disease the patient is suffering from, which can be challenging, but also what the patient's underlying physiological dysfunctions are, and the underlying cause(s), which is a complex process.

Sumatriptan or Magnesium?

Consider the clinician who wants to practice the best medicine and therefore reads not only standard medical journals but also the nutrition research. The clinician decides to compare sumatriptan to magnesium for a patient suffering migraine headache. Looking at a meta-analysis of various triptans in the treatment of migraine patients, the clinician would conclude that 100 mg of sumatriptan is likely effective in 59% of patients.[78] (Efficacy is defined as relief of headache pain within two hours.) Being a responsible clinician, he/she would also consider adverse drug reactions and would see that the placebo-subtracted proportion for patients with at least one adverse drug reaction (ADR) is 13%; for at least one central nervous system symptom, 6% (3.0–9.0%); and for at least one chest symptom, 1.9% (1.0–2.7%). The clinician might compare these data with other triptans, and choose rizatriptan instead, since it shows somewhat better efficacy and consistency, and similar tolerability.

In contrast, looking at the research for magnesium, the clinician would find a response of 41.6% from oral magnesium. This reduction in attack frequency in the magnesium group compared to 15.8% in the placebo group might be compelling, but the incidence of ADRs of diarrhea (18.6%) and gastric irritation (4.7%) would likely preclude use.[79] Not surprisingly, the conventional practitioner would very likely make an EBM decision and choose rizatriptan over magnesium.

However, digging deeper would show a dramatic difference in response to magnesium based on serum ionized magnesium levels (IMg^{2+}). Eighty-nine percent of those responding to intravenous magnesium showed low pretreatment serum magnesium levels, while only 37.5% of non-responders had a low IMg^{2+} level.[80] Digging even deeper, the clinician would notice that magnesium is twice as effective if the patient also suffers a prodromal aura.[81]

Conventional diagnosis of migraine is pretty straightforward, although atypical presentations are probably more common than previously recognized.[82] The causes, however, are myriad. A research team at SaluGenecists, Inc. performed a comprehensive review of the research literature (over 10,000 research articles studied; 1,000 cited) and identified at least 27 different physiological dysfunctions that can lead to the clinical presentation of migraine headache. Patients get to migraine via complex, individual pathways. Further, there are research reports to be studied concerning approximately 40 different "natural medicine" approaches to migraine (nutritional, herbal, and lifestyle therapies). And 20 environmental toxins may need to be evaluated in order to normalize physiological dysfunctions. The clinical decision-making process has now become far more complex than simply diagnosing migraine and prescribing a triptan! This two orders of magnitude increase in complexity dramatically increases the need for rigorous decision making.

Considering a human's approximately 4,000 enzyme systems, 1,000 chemical mediators (these two numbers are my estimates, I could not find an actual count), 2,000,000 possible single nucleotide polymorphisms (SNPs), approximately 250 nutrients known to be important in human health, and several thousand endogenous and exogenous xenobiotics, the true size of the challenge becomes readily apparent.

Clinical Decision Making

How Good Are We at Critical Thinking?

How do we expand upon the current disease-based diagnosis and treatment model to achieve a clinically effective understanding of the biochemical, physiological, and environmental uniqueness of our patients? What diagnostic challenges does this expanded model create for clinicians? One of the most important services a clinician provides his or her patients is decision making. Disease diagnosis, physiological function assessment, determining optimal treatment, limiting adverse drug reactions—all involve critical thinking skills.

How do clinicians make diagnostic and therapeutic decisions? What influences clinical decision making? What data contribute to accurate decisions? What induces errors into a clinician's decisions? How can we improve the accuracy and reliability of clinical thinking? What happens when the complexity becomes too great? While we seldom think about the *process* of decision making, our ability to do it efficiently and accurately impacts our every interaction with patients. Unfortunately, research has shown that clinical critical thinking skills need more attention in order to avoid systematic logic errors and misinterpretation of the actual predictive value of various types of patient information.

Improving the reliability of the information clinicians use to make decisions is obviously critical. To that end, evidence-based medicine has become a recurrent theme in the medical research and academic literature. A recent survey showed that virtually all (122 of 126) LCME-accredited (Liaison Committee on Medical Education) medical schools included EBM as a required course of at least 20 hours.[83] However, formal courses devoted specifically to critical thinking are rare. Utilizing the AAMC (American Association of Medical Schools) curriculum search tools found only six institutions with courses that included one of the terms "decision" or "critical" or "analytic," and the hour allocations were low. Obviously, critical thinking is informally taught in many courses and clinical rotations. Nonetheless, it seems to receive limited formal attention. A survey of 417 U.S. internal-medicine residency programs found formal clinical decision-making training (critical appraisal, searching for evidence, posing a question, and applying it in decision-making) in only 99 of 269 (37%) institutions that responded.[84]

A Cochrane review of the research evaluating the effect of teaching critical thinking skills to healthcare professionals already caring for patients found a remarkable 25% improvement in clinical accuracy.[85] However, the Cochrane review also said there were too few properly designed and conducted studies to be confident in the size of the improvement or its actual clinical significance. Nonetheless, the well-documented evidence of frequent clinician error and its role in the incidence of suboptimal care and adverse clinical outcomes is compelling. One widely reported epidemiological study that reviewed published reports found that 4 to 18% of consecutive outpatient visits result in adverse effects, with one study asserting that up to 69% of the adverse events were preventable with better decision making.[86]

It appears undeniable that patients receive a lower quality of care than would be expected considering the high level of practitioner training and the huge body of research now available. The need for accurate decision making is even more critical when clinicians adopt the principles and practices of functional medicine.

What Can We Learn From Artificial Intelligence (A.I.) Research?

One way to improve critical thinking skills is to better understand how humans make decisions. As computers became available with enough power to mimic human thinking processes, researchers had to rigorously dissect how humans make decisions. While most of the early research centered on the creation of chess programs that could match human masters, of particular relevance here is the effort to duplicate the thinking processes of healthcare professionals.

Interest in this area increased dramatically with the publication of Mycin (1980), an "expert system" that came out of research at Stanford University in the late 1970s. What caught the imagination of the A.I. and healthcare communities was that, for blood-borne infections, Mycin outperformed not only medical students and residents, but also infectious-disease fellows and medical-school faculty (see Table 5.1). How did it do this? By having logicians and programmers work with a group of infectious disease experts to exhaustively determine all the "rules" they used to determine which bacterial species caused a blood-borne infection and the optimal intervention for its eradication. Converting their knowledge into software logic required that the clinicians exhaustively think through how they make decisions. This level of rigor resulted in better decision making, not only because the model was able to incorporate the best thinking of many experts, but also because it applied those rules consistently with every patient.

According to Enrico Coiera (Foundation Chair in Medical Informatics, Faculty of Medicine, University of New South Wales, Australia), "If physiology literally means 'the logic of life,' and pathology is 'the logic of disease,' then health informatics is the 'logic of healthcare.'"[87]

Table 5.1 **Mycin vs. Students and Clinicians (1980)**

Health care expert	Score
Perfect score	80
Medical student	24
Resident	36
Actual hospital outcome	46
Infectious disease fellow	48
Medical school faculty	34–50
MYCIN	52

There are now over 70 A.I. tools in use in conventional medicine to improve diagnosis (actually outperforming clinicians in some areas), avoid drug interactions, interpret x-rays and laboratory tests, teach medical students, and perform other tasks (see Judith Federhofer's excellent review at www.computer.privateweb.at/judith). We can continue to learn much about the mechanics of medical decision making and areas of potential error by formally coding our decision-making processes into computer programs. These programs consistently reproduce our thinking processes so that they can be subjected to evaluation. By identifying where our decisions lead to correct or incorrect outcomes, we can refine our thinking and improve our use of evidence and patient data.

Artificial Intelligence—Many Ways of Thinking

Studying the types and diversity of artificial intelligence systems (called expert systems when they are used to duplicate experts in a field of study) that have been developed to mimic human thinking is very informative. In general, five types have been used in medicine (there are actually many more types of A.I., but these are the most common in health care):

- Rules-based systems
- Case based reasoning (CBR)
- Neural networks
- Fuzzy logic
- Bayesian networks

This discussion may appear daunting, but we will draw from it some straightforward guidance. Busy clinicians can't be expected to calculate all the probabilities before making recommendations for each patient, but their critical thinking skills can be improved by understanding better how decisions are made.

Rules-based Systems

Rules-based systems are fairly straightforward. They look like flow charts with "If ... then" statements. Many clinical guidelines are based on this model. Figure 5.2 shows a diagram modified from a flow chart developed by Herb Joiner-Bey, ND for Nancy Sudak, MD's article on a functional medicine approach to migraine headache, published in volume 2.6 of *Integrative Medicine: A Clinician's Journal*. Each branch point is simply an "If ... then" logic statement. This matches human reasoning well in simple cases, especially when pathognomonic decision points are available (like Koplik's spots in measles).

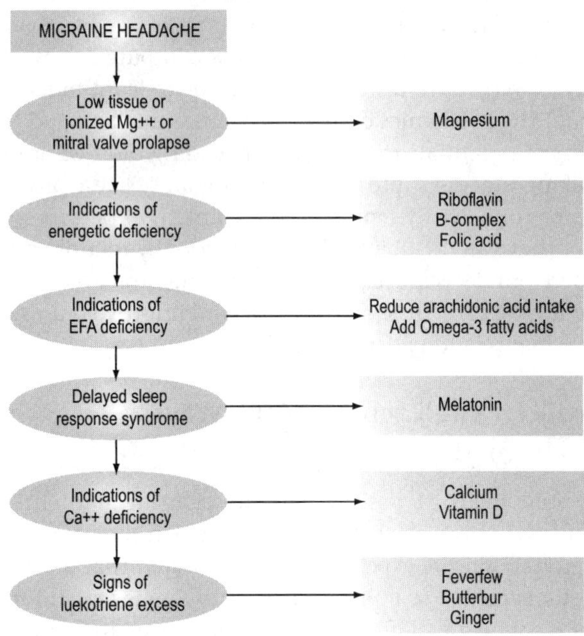

Figure 5.2 **Migraine flow chart**

Case-based Reasoning

Case-based reasoning (CBR) starts by accumulating and evaluating a large number of "solved" cases to determine the characteristics of the successfully treated patients. It then tries to match new patients with patients in the database. This method duplicates human pattern matching pretty well, i.e., once you've seen a patient with classic migraine, others are easy to recognize.

Neural Networks

Neural networks make no effort at understanding how humans think nor do they develop algorithms. Rather, they look at human decision making as a "black box." By using a large number of examples of desired behaviors, they attempt to match input (signs and symptoms) to outputs (diagnoses or therapies). The computer software is set up to be similar to the parallel processing architecture of the brain. This process may match human thinking at a very early age, but does not help us much when trying to understand adult reasoning processes.

Fuzzy Logic

The concept of fuzzy logic puts me in awe of human creativity. The idea here is to look at particular information and attempt to determine the level of uncertainty. It could be described simply as a rules system with probabilities or uncertainties added.

Bayes Inference

An expert system used frequently in medical diagnostic systems is Bayesian inference, based on the probability theory of the Rev. Thomas Bayes, an 18th century mathematician. This heuristic reasoning system makes inferences based on the rigorous mathematics of the predictive value of information. His formula for determining the predictive value of information can be simply stated as:

$$P(D|F) = P(F|D)*P(D) / P(F)$$

where:

D =	Decision (e.g., disease)
F =	Finding (e.g., symptom)
P(D) =	The *a priori* probability of the decision (e.g., the incidence of a disease in the general population)
P(F) =	The *a priori* probability of the finding (e.g., the incidence of a symptom in the general population)
P(D|F) =	Probability of the decision given the finding
P(F|D) =	Probability of the finding, given the presence of the decision

The Bayes formula can be restated in terms of sensitivity and specificity:

$$P(D|F) = P(D)*TP / (P(D)*TP + (1-P(D))*FP)$$

Or

$$P(D|F) = P(D)*TP/P(F)$$

That looks pretty complicated, but the main take-away is that the probability of the decision's accuracy is inversely proportional to the *a priori* probability of the finding. In other words, the more prevalent a piece of information (a finding or symptom) is in the population, the less predictive it is in a specific patient. Intuitively, this makes sense.

As you may recall from your study of statistics long ago, the issues of sensitivity and specificity are extremely important. They are frequently used in laboratory medicine where they provide us guidance on the usefulness of specific tests. For example, a lab test may be very sensitive, i.e., is abnormal very frequently when the disease is present. However, if it has a high false positive (low specificity, where FP = 1-specificity), meaning the result is frequently abnormal even when the disease is *not* present, it is not very useful.

The value of this kind of an inference-based expert system is that it mimics human thinking well (human brains are remarkably effective inference engines). If the mathematically rigorous Bayes thinking is used, decisions can be more accurate, and long chains of logic can be used (see Figure 5.3). This is the method used by casinos to calculate odds and by the Mars Lander to pick a site and land on it safely. Equally important, this system can be used to map human biochemistry, and we can learn a lot from it about the strengths and weaknesses of human thinking processes.

The Role of Uncertainty in Medical Error

A strong case can be made that underappreciation of uncertainty is a major cause of error in medicine.[88] McNeil has argued that the major hidden barriers to better health care result from a lack of discussion about the impact of uncertainty in medicine.[89] She enumerates three sources of uncertainty that cloud decision making:

1. uncertainty as a result of lack of convincing evidence,
2. uncertainty about the applicability of research evidence to clinical care, and
3. uncertainty about interpretation of data.

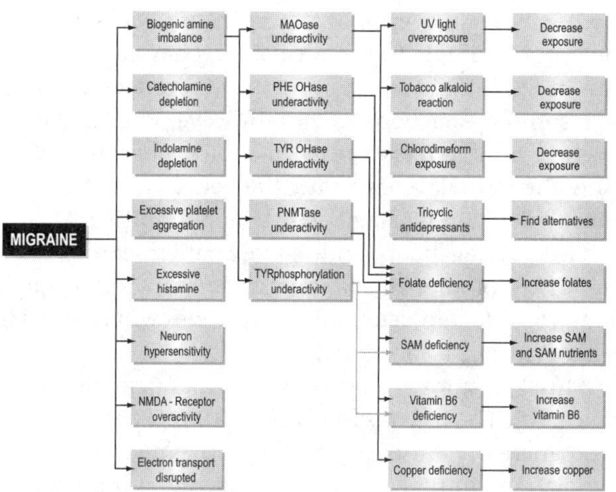

Figure 5.3 **Bayesian inference network**

Note: Each arrow indicates a Bayesian inference.

Others have asserted that the failure to learn how to make decisions under uncertainty is the leading cause of excessive diagnostic testing and inappropriate treatments.[90] Obviously, reliable evidence is critical for effective decision making. *However, too often evidence is confused with decision making.* The quality of evidence is now evaluated (several EBM scales exist, typically ranking evidence from 1 for meta-analysis to 5 for anecdotal evidence), which may be helpful, but clinical decision making is not only about the ranking of evidence; it is also about making choices in the face of uncertainty. The failure to train doctors about clinical uncertainty has been called "the greatest deficiency of medical education throughout the twentieth century."[91]

Lessons from the Reverend Bayes

Rigorously dealing with uncertainly is exactly the problem addressed by the Bayes probability formulas. Consciously utilizing the false positive to balance the true positive in order to accurately portray the true level of uncertainty significantly improves the reliability of decision making. It does this by removing our overestimation of the certainty of decisions, pointing to the need for more information to improve accuracy. Through the use of the true positive (sensitivity) and false positive (1-specificity), the mathematically correct strength of an inference can be determined—that is, the clinician can better understand the true predictive value of evidence.

The Bayes formula may look daunting, but its use can be surprisingly easy. In fact, there are available on the Internet simple Bayes calculators (I have one that runs in Excel that I am happy to share; contact me at: drpizzorno@salugenecists.com). However, the clinician does not need to make the calculation every time. After using the formula a few times, the needed modifications to decision making become more intuitive.

Let's look again at that migraine patient. It appears that 41.6% of migraine patients respond to oral magnesium. How do you determine which ones will respond? What evidence is most predictive?

Muscle cramps are a common sign of magnesium deficiency. The true positive (TP) is 48%. If the patient is experiencing muscle cramps with the migraine, the clinician might then assume that magnesium is very likely to work. However, muscle cramps are common in the general population (27.5%[92]) so the false positive (FP) is actually quite high, 25%. Therefore, the predictive value using the Bayes formula is that we've only increased the true confidence in magnesium being useful for the patient from 41.6% to 62%. This is still not very good, considering the potential for side effects.

Consider, instead, mitral valve prolapse as an indication of magnesium deficiency. Its TP is only 14%, which on the surface seems less compelling than muscle cramps. However, its prevalence in the population is low (4%[93]) so its FP is also low, only 3%. Therefore its predictive value is significantly higher—using the Bayes calculation, our confidence is now 80%—much more compelling! In addition, the incidence of an adverse reaction is now much less because we are now unlikely to be giving magnesium to a patient who does not need it.

This comparison is useful because we can see clearly that one piece of evidence appears on the surface to be more useful since it has high sensitivity, but it is actually much less useful than lower sensitivity evidence that has a much lower false positive.

The simple rule: If the prevalence in the general population of a piece of evidence (a symptom or other finding) is high, even though it may be highly associated, its predictive value is actually weak. Therefore, before the clinician can confidently make a recommendation, the **right kind of evidence**, i.e., that with a high ratio of TP to FP, needs to be gathered (e.g., discovering whether the patient suffers a prodromal aura, measuring magnesium levels, and so forth).

The Bayesian calculations required for accurate inferential information highlight a vulnerability in the human thinking process that is relevant to functional medicine: using only the true positive and ignoring the false positive when making complex decisions in an area of high uncertainty skews the decision-making. Stated differently, failing to consider the population prevalence of the evidence and the intervention leads to false confidence on the part of the clinician.

Summary

Uncertainty is a fact of life in healthcare. It arises from many sources: incomplete or inaccurate patient data; evidence that is not as good as we would like; and making inaccurate inferences from the evidence and data. Lack of awareness about this uncertainty principle leads to excessive confidence in our conclusions. Erroneously believing we have made a good decision results in stopping the evidence-gathering process prematurely. The clinical impact, then, is greater frequency of ineffective therapies and increased risk of ADRs.

What can clinicians do? There are three relatively straightforward steps that all healthcare practitioners can take:

1. Improve the quality of the evidence we use (the evidence to be considered ranges from more accurate eliciting of patient data to better understanding of underlying physiology and biochemistry, the influence of environment on gene expression, and the effectiveness of assessment tools and therapeutic strategies).
2. Understand the true predictive value of evidence by considering not only the true positive but also the critical false positive, i.e., become more aware of the population prevalence of the evidence and data we use and learn how to calculate their effect upon certainty.
3. Continue evidence gathering (especially evidence with a high true positive to false positive ratio) until the level of certainty supports a reasonable level of confidence in the efficacy and safety of the intervention.

Removing overassessment of accuracy from clinical decision making helps us prioritize where additional information has to be gathered so that we can provide the best possible care for our patients.

References

1. Marks HM. The progress of experiment: science and therapeutic reform in the United States, 1900-1990. Cambridge: Cambridge University Press, 1995.
2. Kaptchuk TJ. Intentional ignorance: a history of blind assessment in medicine. Bull Hist Med. 1998;72(3):389-433.
3. http://www.thalidomide.ca/en/index.html
4. Rossouw JE, Anderson GL, Prentice RI, et al. Risks and benefits of estrogen plus progestin in healthy post-menopausal women: principal results From the Women's Health Initiative randomized controlled trial. JAMA. 2002;288(3):321-33.
5. Sackett DL. Bias in analytic research. J Chronic Dis. 1979;32:51-63.
6. Slinger R, Moher D. How to assess new treatments. West J Med. 2001;174(3):182-6.
7. Jadad AR. The randomized controlled trial gets a middle-aged checkup. JAMA. 1998;279:319-20.
8. Dossey L. How should alternative therapies be evaluated? An examination of fundamentals. Altern Ther Health Med. 1995;1(2):6-10, 79-85.
9. Kiene H. A critique of the double-blind clinical trial. Part 1. Altern Ther Health Med. 1996;2(1):74-80.
10. Harbour R, Miller J. A new system for grading recommendations in evidence based guidelines. BMJ. 2001;323:334-36.
11. Guyatt GH, Sinclair J, Cook, DJ, Glasziou P. Users' guides to the medical literature: XVI. How to use a treatment recommendation. JAMA. 1999;281(19):1836-43.
12. Evidence-based medicine. A new approach to teaching the practice of medicine. Evidence-Based Medicine Working Group. JAMA. 1992;268(17):2420-25.
13. Sackett, DL. Evidence based medicine: what it is and what it isn't. BMJ. 1996;312:71-72.
14. Geyman JP. Evidence-based medicine in primary care: an overview. J Am Board Fam Pract. 1998;11:46-56.
15. Rosenberg W, Donald A. Evidence based medicine: an approach to clinical problem-solving. BMJ. 1995;310:1122-26.
16. Sackett DL. Evidence-based medicine: how to practice and teach EBM. New York: Churchill Livington, 1997:2-16.
17. Davidoff F, et. al. Evidence based medicine. BMJ. 1995; 310:1085-86.
18. Weed LL, Zimny NJ. The problem-oriented system, problem-knowledge coupling, and clinical decision making. Phys Ther. 1989;69(7):565-8.
19. Weed LL. Medical Records, Medical Education, and Patient Care. The Problem-Oriented Record as a Basic Tool. Chicago: Year Book Medical Publisher, Inc.: 1970.
20. Weel CV, Knottnerus JA. Evidence-based interventions and comprehensive treatment. Lancet. 1999;353:916-18.
21. Hampton JR. Evidence-based medicine, opinion-based medicine, and real-world medicine. Perspect Biol Med. 2002;45(4):549-68.
22. Grahame-Smith D. Evidence based medicine: Socratic dissent. BMJ. 1995;310:1126-27.
23. Definition of POEMs published in tips from other journals. Am Fam Physician. 2005;71(1):153.
24. http://www.InfoPOEMs.com
25. www.ahrq.gov/clinic/epcix.htm
26. A DuPont advertising slogan. 1939. http://heritage.dupont.com/touchpoints/tp_1939/depth.shtml
27. http://www.cdc.gov/pcd/issues/2004/apr/04_0006.htm
28. Holman H. Chronic disease—the need for a new clinical education. JAMA. 2004;292(9):1057-59.
29. "For most diseases contributing importantly to mortality in Western populations, epidemiologists have long known that non-genetic factors have high attributable risks, often at least 80 or 90%, even when the specific etiologic factors are not clear." Willett, WC. Balancing life-style and genomics research for disease prevention. Science. 2002,296:695-97.
30. Centers for Disease Control, June 15, 2003.
31. Simpson SH, Corabian P, Jacobs P, Johnson JA. The cost of major comorbidity in people with diabetes mellitus. CMAJ. 2003, 168(13):1661-67.
32. Weel CV, Knottnerus JA. Evidence-based interventions and comprehensive treatment. Lancet. 1999;353:916-18.
33. Ibid.
34. Mant D. Can randomized trials inform clinical decisions about individual patients? Lancet. 1999;353:743-46.
35. Feinstein AR, Horwitz RI. Problems in the "evidence" of "evidence-based medicine." Am J Med. 1997;103:529-35.
36. Culpepper L, Gilbert TT. Evidence and ethics. Lancet. 1999;353:829-31.
37. Ibid.
38. Hyman M, Pizzorno J, Weil A. A rational approach to antioxidant therapy and vitamin E. Altern Ther Health Med. 2005;11(1):14-17.
39. Kossman M, Bullrich S. Systematic chaos: self-organizing systems and the process of change. In: Masterpasqua F, Perna PA, eds. The Psychological Meaning of Chaos: Translating Theory into Practice. Washington, DC: American Psychological Association; 1997.
40. Cerutti A, Sinorini MG. Non-linear algorithms for processing biological signals. Comput Methods Programs Biomed. 1996; 51:51-73.
41. Smart A, Martin P, Parker M. Tailored medicine: whom will it fit? Bioethics. 2004; 18:322-42.
42. Borrell-Carrio F, Suchman AL, Epstein RM. The Biopsychosocial Model 25 years later: principles, practice, and scientific inquiry. Ann Fam Med. 2(6):576-82.
43. Borrell-Carrio F, et al. The biopsychosocial model 25 years later: Principles, practice, and scientific inquiry. Ann Fam Med. 2004; 2(6):576-82.
44. Mackie JL. Causes and conditions. Amer Philosoph Q. 1965;2:245-64.
45. Mackie JL. The Cement of the Universe. A Study of Causation. Oxford UK: Oxford University Press; 1974.
46. Bateson G. Steps to an Ecology of Mind: A Revolutionary Approach to Man's Understanding of Himself. New York, NY: Ballantine Books; 1972.
47. Fraser SW, Greenhalgh T. Coping with complexity: educating for capability. BMJ. 2001;323:799-803.
48. Miller WL, Crabtree BF, McDaniel R, Stange KC. Understanding change in primary care practice using complexity theory. J Fam Pract. 1998; 46:369-76.
49. Borrell-Carrio F, et al. The biopsychosocial model 25 years later: Principles, practice, and scientific inquiry. Ann Fam Med. 2004; 2(6):576-82.
50. David Deutsch. The Fabric of Reality. New York, NY: Penguin Press; 1997:16.
51. Little P, et al. Preferences of patients for patient centred approach to consultation in primary care: observational study. BMJ. 2001;322:1-7.
52. Mant D. Can randomized trials inform clinical decisions about individual patients? Lancet. 1999;353:743-46.
53. Horton R. Commentary: The *new* new public health of risk and radical engagement. Lancet. 1998;352(9124):251-52.
54. Abby SL, et al. Homocysteine and cardiovascular disease. J Am Board Fam Pract. 1998;11(5):391-98.

55. Speidel BD. Folic acid deficiency and congenital malformation. Dev Med Child Neurol. 1973;15(1):81-83.
56. Biale Y, Lewenthal H, Ben-Adereth N. Letter: Congenital malformations and decreased blood level of folic acid induced by antiepileptic drugs. Acta Obstet Gynecol Scand. 1976;55(2):187.
57. Laurence KM. Prevention of neural tube defects by improvement in maternal diet and preconceptional folic acid supplementation. Prog Clin Biol Res. 1985;163B:383-88.
58. Milunsky A, Jick H, Jick SS, et al. Multivitamin/folic acid supplementation in early pregnancy reduces the prevalence of neural tube defects. JAMA. 1989;262(20):2847-52.
59. From the Centers for Disease Control. Use of folic acid for prevention of spina bifida and other neural tube defects—1983-1991. JAMA. 1991;266(9):1190-91.
60. Honein MA, et al. Impact of folic acid fortification of the US food supply on the occurrence of neural tube defects. JAMA. 2001;285(23):2981-86.
61. Hyman M, Pizzorno J, Weil A. A rational approach to antioxidant therapy and vitamin E. Altern Ther Health Med. 2005;11(1):14-17.
62. Rossouw JE, Anderson GL, Prentice RI, et al. Risks and benefits of estrogen plus progestin in healthy post-menopausal women: principal results From the Women's Health Initiative randomized controlled trial. JAMA. 2002;288(3):321-33.
63. Ridker PM. High-sensitivity C-reactive protein, inflammation, and cardiovascular risk: from concept to clinical practice to clinical benefit. Am Heart J. 2004;148:S19-S26.
64. Mukherjee D, Nissen SE, Topol EJ. Risk of cardiovascular events associated with selective COX-2 inhibitors. JAMA. 2001;286(8):954-59.
65. Horton R. Interpretive medicine: a manifesto. Md Med J. 1997;Suppl:5-8.
66. Ibid.
67. Ibid.
68. Evidence-based medicine. A new approach to teaching the practice of medicine. Evidence-Based Medicine Working Group. JAMA. 1992;268(17):2420-25.
69. Kuhn TS. The structure of Scientific Revolutions. Chicago, Ill: University of Chicago Press; 1970.
70. Evidence-based medicine. A new approach to teaching the practice of medicine. Evidence-Based Medicine Working Group. JAMA. 1992;268(17):2420-25.
71. Ibid.
72. Sackett, DL. Evidence based medicine: what it is and what it isn't. BMJ. 1996;312:71-72.
73. Weel CV, Knottnerus JA. Evidence-based interventions and comprehensive treatment. Lancet. 1999;353:916-18.
74. Greenhalgh T, et. al. Learning in Practice. BMJ. 2003;326:142-45.
75. Bland, J. Alternative therapies—a moving target. Altern Ther Health Med. 2005;11(2):2-4.
76. Jonas WB. Researching alternative medicine. Nat Med. 1997;3(8):824-27.
77. Dossey L. A journal and a journey. Altern Ther Health Med. 1995;1(2):6-9.
78. Ferrari MD, Goadsby PJ, Roon KI, Lipton RB. Triptans (serotonin, 5-HT1B/1D agonists) in migraine: detailed results and methods of a meta-analysis of 53 trials. Cephalalgia. 2002;22(8):633-58.
79. Peikert A, Wilimzig C, Kohne-Volland R. Prophylaxis of migraine with oral magnesium: results from a prospective, multi-center, placebo-controlled and double-blind randomized study. Cephalalgia. 1996;16:257-63.
80. Mauskop A, Altura BT, Cracco RQ, Altura BM. Intravenous magnesium sulfate rapidly alleviates headaches of various types. Headache. 1996;36:154-60.
81. Bigal ME, Bordini CA, Tepper SJ, Speciali JG. Intravenous magnesium sulphate in the acute treatment of migraine without aura and migraine with aura. A randomized, double-blind, placebo-controlled study. Cephalgia. 2002;22:345-53.
82. Rains JC, Penzien DB, Lipchik GL, Ramadan NM. Diagnosis of migraine: empirical analysis of a large clinical sample of atypical migraine (IHS 1.7) patients and proposed revision of the IHS criteria. Cephalalgia. 2001;21(5):584-595.
83. Barzansky B, Etzel SI. Educational programs in US medical schools, 2002–2003. JAMA.2003;290:1190-96.
84. Green ML. Evidence-based medicine training in internal medicine residency programs a national survey. J Gen Intern Med. 2000;15:124-33.
85. Parkes J, Hyde C, Deeks J, Milne R. Teaching critical appraisal skills in health care settings. Cochrane Database Syst Rev. 2001;(3):CD001270.
86. Wiengart SN, Wilson RM, Gibberd RW, Harrison B. Epidemiology and medical error. BMJ. 2000;320:774-7.
87. Coiera E. Guide to Health Informatics. Arnold Publications, London, 2003.
88. Editorial. Lifting the fog of uncertainty from the practice of medicine. BMJ. 2004;329:1419-20.
89. McNeil BJ. Hidden barriers to improvement in the quality of care. N Engl J Med. 2001;345: 1612-20.
90. Haynes B. Bridging the gap between the Cochrane Collaboration and clinical practice. Plenary presentation. 12th Cochrane Colloquium, Ottawa, 3 October 2004.
91. Ludmerer KM. Time to heal. New York: Oxford University Press, 1999.
92. Naylor JR, Young JB. A general population survey of rest cramps. Age Ageing. 1994;23(5):418-20.
93. Freed LA, Levy D, Levine RA, et al. Prevalence and clinical outcome of mitral-valve prolapse. N Engl J Med. 1999;341:1-7.

Section II

Principles of Functional Medicine

Chapter 6
Functional Medicine is Science-Based

DeAnn Liska, PhD

Introduction

Lewis Thomas, the eminent physician essayist, called medicine "the youngest science" in his 1983 book of the same title. He observed at that time that such discoveries as antibiotics and the structure of DNA had made medicine more of a science, in which it could conduct experiments that test hypotheses about disease-causing agents and their curative interventions.[1] He clearly identified the 20th century promise of the "science of medicine"—suggesting that we would not only have absolute answers to what causes disease and dysfunction, but we would also be able to "cure" disease. Indeed, the 20th century did see an influx of new technologies, new pharmaceuticals, and a deeper understanding of the biochemical underpinnings of disease. Furthermore, the promise of the "cure" has been enhanced by such findings as the frank vitamin deficiency diseases that are cured by nutrient repletion and the bacterial-based infectious diseases that can be eradicated by antibiotic treatment.[2]

Western medicine, in particular, is driven by technological advances and built upon the notion that everything that is relevant can be tested, proved (or disproved), and, with those results, a direct solution can be found. However, this new "science of medicine" has not been able, so far, to stem the rising pandemic of chronic disease. Likewise, scientific literature is accumulating more and more evidence that the promise of directly curing conditions such as rheumatoid arthritis, type 2 diabetes, cancers, and Alzheimer's with a simple approach is not realistic. Moreover, the influx of new scientific information over the past several decades has continued to increase, while the ability of the average clinician to review that information and understand its relevance to a real-life patient is limited by time constraints and the sheer volume of material. The multifactorial nature of chronic conditions, along with the emerging understanding of just how biochemically unique we all are, has collided with our model of basing clinical decisions primarily, if not solely, on a narrow definition of science.

In Chapter 5 of this book, a very detailed and carefully documented analysis of the history and limitations of the current scientific research model was presented. Here, as we open our discussion of the principles of functional medicine, we will look at how one of the basic principles—that functional medicine is science based—plays out against that background.

Functional medicine embraces the challenge of incorporating the newest scientific literature into its model of clinical care; advances in our understanding of fundamental physiological and biochemical processes can only enhance the clinician's ability to treat patients with complex chronic disease. Science is a critical tool for improving our understanding of the underlying clinical imbalances that lead to disease, and also a lens through which we can examine, describe, and adapt to the biochemical individuality of each patient. It is by understanding these imbalances that clinicians can help patients change the course of a disease. Therefore, a functional medicine practitioner must stay abreast of the current literature and be willing to challenge beliefs and current dogma.

Functional medicine does not identify a single gold-standard method for considering something relevant or useful. Functional medicine practitioners incorporate many different sources of scientific information into the medical decision-making process: basic science, clinical experience, and the principles explored in this section are all important elements in the model. Using this approach requires a paradigm shift from the focus of the late 20th century—that there is a single valid model for useful evidence—to the broader view that all the relevant science and information should be reviewed and understood. Overall, that's the mission of this text—to help all of us make that leap to a new approach, wherein science and evidence in many forms are valuable to an innovative and clinically-relevant model of care.

Science and Evidence-based Medicine (EBM)

The emergence of the scientific method as central to medicine has changed the face of health care. Clinical trials have become the primary method of establishing medical benefit. The randomized, placebo-controlled, double-blind clinical trial (DB/PC RCT) has come to dominate the field. Without data from an RCT showing a statistically significant effect, an intervention is considered unproved, which many take to mean "not beneficial." This has led to the attempt to find the "best" medicine from the "perfect" data: an evidence-based approach to medicine.

Certainly, the testing of many approaches that were in common practice has made a strong and highly beneficial impact on medical practice. For example, estrogen replacement therapy (ERT) was considered a standard practice for decades. Maintaining estrogen levels in women over 50 at levels similar to those for younger women was thought to be beneficial, and early observational studies suggested that the benefit extended to the cardiovascular system. However, more recent investigations of ERT, utilizing the RCT, did not support the findings from those early observational studies, indicating instead that some women on ERT may be at increased risk for thrombotic events and stroke, especially within the first two years of beginning ERT.[3,4] The trials that showed increased risk of ERT generally included post-menopausal women who were not exhibiting symptoms of the menopause transition, such as hot flushes, whereas the benefit of exogenous hormones was observed in studies with younger women. As noted by Rosano et al.,[5] "several biological reasons may have contributed to the divergent findings from observational studies and RCTs." Older women may have fewer estrogen receptors, or a different pattern of expression of these receptors, and also may be more susceptible to inflammation and thrombotic events, factors that could alter their response to exogenous hormones, when compared to younger women.[6,7,8]

Testing a single, defined intervention is, however, different than managing a patient with one or more chronic, complex, multifactorial conditions. A comprehensive approach to preventing and treating such conditions has not been amenable to study through the RCT model. Moreover, most often, a statistically significant, "successful" therapy is effective in barely more than 50% of patients.[9,10,11,12] Even if the therapy is highly successful in a trial, studies indicate that patients in randomized controlled trials are often not typical of those seen in clinical practice.[13,14] (Indeed, with data indicating that adverse drug reactions from properly prescribed drugs rate as the fourth most common cause of death in hospitalized patients, consumers, government agencies, and practitioners are often left to question whether medicine does more harm than good.[15])

In 2002, David Brown asserted in a *Washington Post* article that "Evidence-based medicine is likely to transform the entire field."[16] The actual definition of EBM varies, but the Centre for Evidence-Based Medicine at the University of Toronto defines it as "the integration of best research evidence with clinical expertise and patient values."[17] Much of the literature about EBM, however, has centered on how best to score the evidence, creating a hierarchy in which some evidence has great value and other evidence has much less value. Although the definition of EBM includes the words "clinical expertise" and "patient values," the evidence base used is primarily, if not exclusively, drawn from RCT data. This focus on finding the "best" data often disregards the needs of the individual patient. For example, in a 1997 discussion on evidence-based disease management published in *JAMA*,[18] the relevant skills for employing EBM were described as "precisely defining a patient problem, proficiently searching and critically appraising relevant information from the literature, and then deciding whether, and how, to use this information in practice." Not only does this description focus on "precisely defining a patient problem," which is often difficult to do for multifactorial, complex conditions, but the implication that the "evidence" comes primarily (or only) from the literature directly "relevant" to that problem. The web-like nature of physiological processes seems a misfit in this type of evidence model.

While the goal of EBM is laudable (to improve clinical practice by using interventions that have stood the test of thorough investigation), the actual practice is not clear. In a study on why general practitioners do not implement so-called "best evidence" from research studies, Freeman and Sweeney[19] found the doctor-patient relationship to be particularly relevant. "Evidence is not implemented in a simple linear way, as some definitions of evidence based practice imply, but in an evolving process whereby reciprocal contributions from the doctor and the patient over time influence how evidence ultimately is used."

The following excerpts from a 1997 editorial in the *British Medical Journal* clarify some of the issues that are still with us today:[20]

> We face the problem that criteria for internal and external validity (that is, clinical applicability) may conflict. Clinical studies are usually performed on a homogeneous study population and exclude clinically complex cases for the sake of internal validity. Such selection may not, however, match the type of patients for whom the studied intervention will be considered … . Studies on the effectiveness of clinical care may also not easily attain internal validity. An example is the evaluation of the many interventions that cannot be blinded, such as many non-pharmacological procedures … . Thus, in seeking internally valid evidence that is externally valid for clinical practice, we need "medicine based" studies that include, not ignore, clinical reality and its inherent difficulties … . In reviewing clinical evidence we must be reluctant to adopt too detailed criteria for good and bad science and to freeze criteria for validity. Study methods themselves need to evolve.

Science and the Patient-centered Approach

Studying the body's function from a scientific perspective is a demanding process; bringing in the patient's perspective makes it even more complex. To bring these issues into clearer focus, we will examine a real-life case that is a matter of public record.

A Case of Chronic Fatigue Syndrome

In an essay titled "A Sudden Illness," Laura Hillebrand, author of the best-selling book *Seabiscuit: An American Legend*, describes her continuing battle with chronic fatigue syndrome, which began in 1987 before the syndrome was accepted by mainstream medicine.[21] One of her symptoms was a chronic strep infection. After a year in which she had seen several internists and a psychiatrist, and had several courses of antibiotics, she found an internist who again changed her antibiotics and, eventually, her strep appeared to improve. Her other symptoms, including debilitating, unremitting fatigue, did not. In her own words:

> I kept returning to see this doctor, hoping she could find some way to make me feel better. She couldn't, and I could see that it was wearing on her. In September, I was so weak that on a ride over to her office I had to drop my head to my knees to avoid passing out. When the nurse entered, I was lying down, holding my head, the room swimming around me. She took my blood pressure: 70/50. The doctor came in. She wouldn't look at me. "I don't know why you keep coming here," she said, her lips tight.
>
> I told her that I felt faint and asked about my blood pressure. She said that it was normal and left, saying nothing else. She then went to see my mother, who was in the waiting room. "When is she going to realize that her problems are all in her head?" the doctor said.
>
> I returned home, lay down, and tried to figure out what to do. My psychiatrist had found me to be mentally healthy, but my physicians had concluded that if my symptoms and the results of a few conventional tests didn't fit a disease they knew of, my problem had to be psychological. Rather than admit that they didn't know what I had, they made a diagnosis they weren't qualified to make.
>
> Without my physician's support, it was almost impossible to find support from others. People told me I was lazy and selfish. Someone lamented how unfortunate Borden was to have a girlfriend who demanded coddling. Some of Borden's friends suggested that he was foolish and weak to stand by me. "The best thing my parents ever did for my deadbeat brother," a former professor of his told him, "was to throw him out." I was ashamed and angry and indescribably lonely.

Hillebrand's condition had begun suddenly, with symptoms assumed to be from food poisoning. These were soon followed by swollen lymph nodes and a persistent strep infection. At the time, chronic fatigue was not recognized as a diagnosable condition by mainstream medicine. There was no "evidence base" to explain her condition, but there was science.

Patients having symptom complexes consistent with what we now call chronic fatigue syndrome have been described in the medical literature for centuries and have, at various times, been categorized with names such as post-viral fatigue and chronic Epstein-Barr virus (EBV) syndrome.[22] In fact, a few years before Hillebrand first experienced symptoms, Behan et al.[23] published an analysis of 50 cases of post-viral fatigue and concluded: "A metabolic disorder, caused by persistent virus infection and associated with defective immunoregulation, is suggested as the pathogenetic mechanism." The year in which her symptoms began, Buchwald, Komaroff and colleagues published a report in which they found abnormalities in immune cells of chronic fatigue patients.[24] In March of 1988, the first working definition of chronic fatigue syndrome was published in the *Annals of Internal Medicine*.[25] While Hillebrand was experiencing debilitating symptoms, being treated only with antibiotics for her chronic strep, and feeling very much alone, the literature available at the time actually showed that she was, in fact, not alone.

When faced with a patient such as Hillebrand (one of the "walking wounded," so familiar to clinicians everywhere), where the research base does not yet offer clear answers, it is important to remember that science is still there to help. Exploring the underlying physiological pathways that appear to be involved would be a functional medicine approach. The therapeutic plan could then be designed to support the healthy, balanced function of those pathways, while also removing any known or postulated triggers (e.g., strep infection) that are acting upon those pathways to exacerbate symptoms. A patient may not be "cured," but can have improved function. A clinician may not know the answers, but can have a place to start. In this particular case, the association with immune function was deducible from the symptom pattern experienced by Hillebrand, as well as from the available literature. The science was there in terms of indicating that a possible connection between these symptoms and immune dysfunction could exist. Unfortunately, to this date, an indisputable evidence base describing the underlying immune imbalances in chronic fatigue syndrome is still not available. Waiting for that level of evidence before treating the patient would leave many a patient still hearing their clinician say, "I don't know why you keep coming here."

Data are accumulating to show how complex these chronic conditions are. Not only do syndromes such as chronic fatigue and fibromyalgia have significant overlap in symptoms and biochemistry, but gene expression profiles indicate that differential expression patterns can be identified; these conditions may well represent sub-groups of specific metabolic imbalances.[26,27,28] In fact, in 1996, the Royal College of Physicians, Psychiatrists, and General Practitioners provided this summary of the evidence:[29]

> Chronic Fatigue Syndrome (CFS) is not a single diagnostic entity. It is a symptom complex which can be reached by many different routes. The conceptual model of CFS needs to be changed from one determined by a single cause/agent to one in which dysfunction is the end stage of a multifactorial process. Although it is important to recognize the role of factors that precipitate the condition, greater understanding is required of factors that predispose individuals to develop the illness, and those that perpetuate disability.

Simply stated, not every CFS patient will be the same and the focus on underlying pathways is now being seen as the way to medically manage CFS. In the functional medicine approach, the focus on those sciences that elucidate underlying pathways and clusters of symptoms is absolutely critical to prevention and treatment of complex chronic disease. These "functionalities" in physiology and biochemistry help us to identify varying patterns within a given diagnostic category and undertake a search for common underlying factors in patients with a number of different debilitating symptoms, conditions, or diseases.

Applying Science in Clinical Practice

Many evidence-based evaluations target whether a single intervention works. This is a different question than evaluating whether a patient improves in a clinical practice. Therefore, although published research is helpful as a guide, it is often not directly reflective of what a clinician faces when working with an individual patient. Moreover, the development of research methodologies has focused heavily on single-agent interventions, such as pharmaceuticals. Many of the integrative approaches that take into account the entirety of a patient's experience (e.g., diet, lifestyle, environmental exposure) are not amenable to being studied using these methodologies. As stated in a discussion in *The Lancet*:[30]

> Drug interventions have been studied more extensively than non-pharmacological interventions, because of requirements for drug registration and the technical and methodological difficulties in the design of RCTs for non-drug interventions. This situation is a particular problem for general practice. According to the principle of "maximum effect, minimum resources," patients' education, diets, and lifestyles are, in theory, particularly attractive. Generally, such interventions cannot be assessed under adequately masked conditions, so "contamination" of trial groups will threaten internal validity. So, it is not surprising that a literature search fails to find convincing evidence of effectiveness of avoidance of house-

> dust mite allergens. However, absence of proof of effect is different from proof of lack of effect. Even if there is insufficient clinical research available to support its case, exposure to allergen has a key role in the pathophysiology of airways inflammation. Consequently, the concept of asthma makes avoidance of allergens a logical measure even in the absence of direct support from a RCT.

Advances in our understanding of how the body functions at the most basic level are integral to functional medicine. Science-based functional medicine, then, is the incorporation of science within the context of the patient's experiences and biochemical individuality. It is not a prescription that can be tested in a simple RCT; it is not a clinical algorithm directing that each patient with condition X is treated with a clearly-defined therapy. Functional medicine urges the practitioner to become adept at the art of reviewing the best and most recent scientific research, both basic and clinical sciences, as part of the process of developing a personalized approach for a patient-centered practice of medicine. As stated by Aaron and Buchwald:[31]

> Finally, describing an illness as "unexplained" should not be taken to mean "unexplainable" or "imaginary." Researchers and providers involved with patients who have unexplained clinical conditions would do well to remember Osler's statement that the study of medicine "begins with the patient, continues with the patient and ends ... with the patient."

Summary

Functional medicine looks at the emerging science, and digs deep into the way these findings influence our ideas about how the body functions at the physiological and biochemical level. Functional medicine uses the core clinical imbalances as the matrix upon which to organize the science, and includes basic science, clinical trials, case reports, and clinical experience (anecdotal data) to understand a patient's situation. In functional medicine, clinical trials are one piece of the puzzle, not the only source of evidence.

Functional medicine requires an active interaction with the scientific literature. It requires a clinician to keep up with new findings in human physiology and biochemistry; it requires a clinician to integrate the current findings into the model of how problems begin and where the imbalances may lie; it requires a thought process that cannot be directly correlated to an evidence-scoring system. It requires science to continue deepening our understanding about the complexities of life and the various effects of our actions. Functional medicine relies on science and incorporates it deeply into patient-centered care in an analytical and integrative model.

References

1. Thomas L. The Youngest Science. New York:Viking Press. 1983.
2. Liska DJ, Bland JS, Medcalf D. Evaluating the benefits of functional foods. In: Yalpani M, ed. New Technologies for Healthy Foods & Nutraceuticals. Shrewsbury, MA: ATL Press. 1997:287-300.
3. Staren ED, Omer S. Hormone replacement therapy in postmenopausal women. Am J Surg. 2004;188(2):136-49.
4. Samsioe G. HRT and cardiovascular disease. Ann NY Acad Sci. 2003;997:358-72.
5. Rosano GM, Vitale C, Lello S. Postmenopausal hormone therapy: lessons from observational and randomized studies. Endocrine. 2004;24(3):251-54.
6. Ibid.
7. Harman SM, Brinton EA, Clarkson T, et al. Is the WHI relevant to HRT started in the perimenopause? Endocrine. 2004;24(3):195-202.
8. Wagner JD, Kaplan JR, Burkman RT. Reproductive hormones and cardiovascular disease mechanism of action and clinical implications. Obstet Gynecol Clin North Am. 2002;29(3):475-93.
9. Connor S. Glaxo chief: Our drugs do not work on most patients. Interview with Allen Roses, worldwide vice-president of genetics at GlaxoSmithKline (GSK), December 10, 2003. Accessed at http://www.ghchealth.com/glaso-chief-our-drugs-do-not-work-on-most-patients.html on August 14, 2005.
10. Goldstein DB, Tate SK, Sisodiya SM. Pharmacogenetics goes genomic. Nat Rev Genet. 2003;4(12):937-47.
11. Nicol MJ. The variation of response to pharmacotherapy: pharmacogenetics—a new perspective to 'the right drug for the right person'. Medsurg Nurs. 2003;12(4):242-49.
12. Kirsch I. The emperor's new drugs: An analysis of antidepressant medication data submitted to the U.S. Food and Drug Administration. Prevention & Treatment. 2002;5:1-11.
13. Geyman JP. Evidence-based medicine in primary care: an overview. J Am Board Fam Pract. 1998;11:46-56.
14. Zarin DA, Young JL, West JC. Challenges to evidence-based medicine: A comparison of patients and treatments in randomized controlled trials with patients and treatments in a practice research network. Soc Psychiatry Psychiatr Epidemiol. 2005;40:27-35.
15. Lazarou J, Pomeranz BH, Corey PN. Incidence of adverse drug reactions in hospitalized patients: a meta-analysis of prospective studies. JAMA. 1998;279:1200-05.
16. Brown D. First, Do the Trials. Then, Do No Harm. http://www.washingtonpost.com/ac2/wp-dyn/A38313-2002Aug2?language=printer Accessed 8/15/02.
17. What is EBM? http://www.cebm.utoronto.ca/intro/whatis.htm Accessed January 8, 2005.
18. Ellrodt G, Cook DJ, Lee J, et al. Evidence-based disease management. JAMA. 1997;278:1687-92.
19. Freeman AC, Sweeney K. Why general practitioners do not implement evidence: qualitative study. BMJ. 2001;323:1-5.
20. Knottnerus A, Dinant GJ. Medicine based evidence, a prerequisite for evidence based medicine. BMJ. 1997;315:1109-10.
21. Hillebrand, L. A Sudden Illness. From: The New Yorker. July 7, 2003.

22. Clauw DJ, Chrousos GP. Chronic pain and fatigue syndromes: overlapping clinical and neuroendocrine features and potential pathogenic mechanisms. Neuroimmunomodulation. 1997;4:134-53.
23. Behan PO, Behan WM, Bell EJ. The postviral fatigue syndrome—an analysis of the findings in 50 cases. J Infect. 1985;10:211-22.
24. Caligiuri M, Murray C, Buchwald D, et al. Phenotypic and functional deficiency of natural killer cells in patients with chronic fatigue syndrome. J Immunol. 1987;139:3306-13.
25. Holmes GP, Kaplan JE, Gantz NM, et al. Chronic fatigue syndrome: a working case definition. Ann Intern Med. 1988;108:387-89.
26. Aaron LA, Buchwald D. A review of the evidence for overlap among unexplained clinical conditions. Ann Intern Med. 2001;134:868-81.
27. Powell R, Ren J, Lewith G, et al. Identification of novel expressed sequences, up-regulated in the leucocytes of chronic fatigue syndrome patients. Clin Exp Allergy. 2003;33:1450-56.
28. Vernon SD, Unger ER, Dimulescu IM, et al. Utility of the blood for gene expression profiling and biomarker discovery in chronic fatigue syndrome. Dis Markers. 2002;18:193-99.
29. Wessely S. Chronic fatigue syndrome. Summary of a report of a joint committee of the Royal Colleges of Physicians, Psychiatrists and General Practitioners. J R Coll Physicians Lond. 1996;30:497-504.
30. van Weel C, Knottnerus JA. Evidence-based interventions and comprehensive treatment. Lancet. 1999;353:916-18.
31. Aaron LA, Buchwald D. A review of the evidence for overlap among unexplained clinical conditions. Ann Intern Med. 2001;134:868-81.

Chapter 7
Biochemical Individuality and Genetic Uniqueness

- ***Functional Medicine and Biochemical Individuality: A Paradigm Shift in Medicine***
- ***Development of the Knowledge Base in Biochemical Individuality***

Functional Medicine and Biochemical Individuality: A Paradigm Shift in Medicine

Mark Hyman, MD, Sidney MacDonald Baker, MD, David S. Jones, MD

Discovery consists of seeing what everybody has seen and thinking what nobody has thought.
—Albert Szent Gyorgyi,
1937 Nobel Laureate in Physiology and Medicine: the scientist who isolated vitamin C

Introduction[i]

In the *Structure of Scientific Revolutions*,[1] Thomas Kuhn analyzed the process of changing scientific paradigms. He described how in each discipline of science, new advances and theories are slow to be adopted but, once accepted, they assume the position of "normal science." They become foundational to collective beliefs and theories in a new iteration of scientific leaders. Overturning "normal science" often requires decades of accumulated evidence to succeed against the old theories that wane as their ability to explain new data is eroded. Medicine is replete with examples of "normal science" becoming obsolete in retrospect. With change, the newer theories that have been ignored—not because of lack of merit but because of their poor fit with the established paradigm—clearly present a more robust model of explanation.[2]

There are many examples of resistance to change in the history of medicine. A few medical vignettes can serve to illustrate the unnecessary delays common to incorporating new discoveries into practice:

- When Edward Jenner developed the therapeutic technique of vaccinating against smallpox in 1797, the Royal Society of London scolded him for risking his reputation on something "so much at variance with established knowledge, and withal so incredible."
- When the Hungarian physician, Ignaz Semmelweis, discovered that physicians' unwashed hands caused fatal infections among new mothers at the University of Vienna in the 1850s, he lost his academic position, dying disgraced.
- When the American writer and physician, Oliver Wendall Holmes, published an article on the prevention, through hand washing, of "childbed fever," his observations brought him bitter abuse.
- Alexander Fleming discovered penicillin in 1929. But there was a delay of 12 years before he, W.H. Florey, and E.B. Chain first used it therapeutically.[3] Together, with their scientific teams, they changed the concept of *anti*-biotics.
- Kilmer McCully, the prodigy pathologist from Harvard, first proposed the role of folate deficiency and the resultant homocysteinemia connection to cardiovascular disease in the late 1960s.[4] His hypothesis caused his banishment from the pathology department at Harvard Medical School and Massachusetts General Hospital because of the clear conflict his theory represented to the then-dominant

[i] This part of Chapter 7 was adapted by David Jones, MD, from two articles: Hyman M. Paradigm shift: The end of "normal science" in medicine; Understanding function in nutrition, health, and disease. Alt Ther. 2004;10(5):10-93. Baker SM. The medicine we are evolving. Integrative Med. Dec 2002/Jan 2003;1(1):14-15. Many thanks to Doctors Hyman and Baker, and to both journals, for permission to adapt these publications.

cholesterol model of atherosclerosis. Fortunately, he endured, working in relative obscurity at a small Veterans Administration hospital in Rhode Island, eventually vindicated by research from Europe. His model, in the current context of cardiovascular disease as primarily an expression of inflammation, has added to our understanding of metabolic and immunological connections to the development of atheromatous plaque, as well as other diseases associated with aging.

Medicine is also replete with discarded therapies that were well accepted at the time, such as the removal of the colon or all the teeth to treat chronic disease, or, more recently, low-fat diets for weight loss and the prevention of cardiovascular disease,[5] and/or conventional hormone therapy for prevention of heart disease in postmenopausal women.[6,7] We are again at the edge of a major transitional period.

Chronic Disease and the Failure of the Current Medical Paradigm

One of the most compelling, current problems in medicine is the failure of the conventional model of medical diagnosis and treatment to successfully address the burden of *chronic disease* that affects 125 million Americans in our society. Our current approach does not attempt, in a systematic manner, to effectively diagnose and treat the underlying causes of chronic disease, found in the complex interaction of genes, lifestyle, and environment. As a nation, we spend $1.6 trillion on health care each year. This represents 15% of our gross national product (GNP) or approximately $5,000 per person per year, or more than double the percent of GNP spent by any other nation on health care. Despite this, we are 12th out of 13 industrialized nations in 16 major indicators of the health status of a population, such as life expectancy and infant mortality.[8,9] In fact we are 27th in life expectancy; Cuba is 28th.

Yet that may not be the most problematic issue. Recent data point to the dangers of the medical care that evolves from our current paradigm. Our own healthcare system can do great harm. Our system of disease management has been estimated to be anywhere from the 1st to the 3rd *leading cause of death* in our hospitalized patient population,[10] resulting from hospital infections,[11,12] atypical drug reactions,[13] bedsores,[14] medical errors,[15] negligence,[16] unnecessary procedures, and surgery.[17] The cost attributed to the harm caused by the chaos in our medical system has been estimated at over $200 billion.

There are other significant problems endemic to our medical system and conventional medical paradigm:

1. The randomized controlled trial (RCT) is fundamentally ill-suited to the assessment of lifestyle and nutritional interventions, individualized therapies, and long-latency deficiency diseases.[18] (This topic is addressed, from a variety of perspectives, in both Chapter 5 and Chapter 6.)
2. The lack of publication of negative medical trials[19] promotes a positive bias in the medical literature, suggesting an unrealistic proportion of successes and supporting the primacy of pharmacological interventions.
3. Direct-to-consumer pharmaceutical marketing,[20,21] and heavy marketing of off-label uses of medications to physicians, including conventional hormone replacement therapy,[22] create misinformation and encourage inappropriate prescribing practices by healthcare providers.[23,24]
4. The many financial conflicts of interest[25,26] inherent in the practice of funding research by private industry skews the emphasis on what should be studied, and leads to suppression of conclusions that don't suit the funding source.[27,28,29,30] One of the well-known examples of the latter was the research-based comparison between generic thyroxine and Synthroid. The pharmaceutical company prevented the publication of the study that they had funded because the outcome was not favorable to the trade name drug.[31,32] With the exception of the National Institutes of Health and some private foundations, most of the research agenda is set by the pharmaceutical industry.
5. The funding, control and orchestration of most postgraduate education for physicians by the pharmaceutical industry[33,34] leads to a clear bias for the primacy of pharmacologic interventions.[35,36,37]

In addition, recent research suggests that more of the same care is not necessarily better. In areas where there are more physicians, there is a higher cost of care. There is also less patient satisfaction and worse outcomes than comparable areas with a lower cost of care.[38,39] Studies of compliance with agreed-upon standards for care and prevention show that, in spite of higher costs of medical care within the U.S., these standards are not met. There is a frequent lack of implementation of clinical science to clinical practice. For example, only 40% of patients receive aspirin after myocardial infarction.[40] A recent study of adults in 12 metropolitan areas found that only 54.9% of patients received the recommended preventive, acute, or chronic care, using 439 indicators in 30 acute and chronic conditions. The authors conclude, *"The deficits we have identified in adherence to recommended processes for basic care pose serious threats to the health of the American public. Strategies to reduce these deficits in care are warranted."*[41]

Many professionals within conventional medicine feel that the most important single reason for the deficits in our healthcare system is that we are locked into an old paradigm in medicine, "normal medicine."[42,43] The model we use to diagnose and treat disease is based on "normal" science; the single-invader, single-disease, and single-drug model of medicine. While practitioners of the healing arts are schooled in the basic sciences of anatomy, physiology, biochemistry, cell biology, genetics, epidemiology, pathology, and pharmacology—each of which encompasses its own science—no body of knowledge exists within the dominant medical culture that can be construed as "medical science."[44]

The Fallacy of Misplaced Concreteness

Lara Pizzorno, MA Div, MA Lit, LMT

Alfred North Whitehead's "fallacy of misplaced concreteness" is essentially a more logically rigorous statement of the common saying that "we err when we mistake the map for the territory." When humans interact with the world, we interpret the full experience via abstraction; we generalize from the specific observation (the "concrete") to create an idea. This is essential and logically acceptable, so long as we do not equate, and therefore significantly diminish, the actual experience with our working conception of it.

Unfortunately, we often do confound the concrete experience with the abstract idea, assuming our abstractions equal the totality of the reality. The tunnel vision which results prevents us from seeing more of what is actually before us. Science is not free of this error, with the result that new insights are typically met with hostility, and their application and benefits suppressed an average of 50 years before joining the ranks of what is considered the "standard of care."

As Whitehead cautions, "It is impossible to overemphasize the point that the key to the process of induction [the *sine qua non* of scientific reasoning], as used either in science or our ordinary life, is to be found in the right understanding of the immediate occasion of knowledge in its full concreteness ... . We find ourselves amid insoluble difficulties when we substitute for this concrete occasion a mere abstract ... . "*

Avoiding the fallacy of misplaced concreteness is not a task to be underrated by even the most scientifically adept. Such assumptions "appear so obvious that people do not know what they are assuming because no other way of putting things has ever occurred to them."

Whitehead reminds us that "Almost all really new ideas have a certain aspect of foolishness when they are first produced," possibly due to the fact that we form our systems of thought "by the rough and ready method of suppressing what appear to be irrelevant details. But when we attempt to justify this suppression of irrelevance, we find that, though there are entities left corresponding to the entities we talk about, yet these entities are of a high degree of abstraction." Whitehead identified this problem as the primary obstacle to the advancement of science; it occurs when we allow our paradigm to limit our powers of observation.

In medical terms, the fallacy of misplaced concreteness appears in the form of the abstract entities called "diseases," which are simply a constellation of symptoms that often appear together, not an actual entity. While grouping symptoms in this manner is convenient, if the abstraction controls the interaction we have with the patient, we hamper our ability to see the individual who exhibits any symptom or grouping of symptoms (disease) in his or her unique way. In addition, by narrowing our focus to an abstract entity we call "migraine" or "irritable bowel syndrome" or "diabetes," we limit our inspection of the individual's dysfunctions to a predefined set of details, thus potentially missing what may be crucial for that person.

Scientific studies that regress to the mean exemplify this fallacy. The data based on the "representative sample," having lost all the specificity that defines a real human being, are then used to provide recommendations most applicable to an equally "representative" individual, in other words, to no one at all. Such findings tell us everything we need to know about someone who doesn't exist.

Functional medicine offers us both an awareness of how the fallacy of misplaced concreteness operates to limit the effectiveness of medicine, and a way to cut through it. Only the integration of (necessarily) abstract science with concrete individual specificity—the patient-centered, individualized approach that is the hallmark of functional medicine—will enable us to provide a much more accurate and effective assessment.

*All quotations from Whitehead AN. *Process and Reality.*

We have yet to embrace the new paradigm that, for the first time, allows us to personalize medicine. We have the opportunity to focus on optimizing function and enhancing health by understanding the complex high-order functioning of the human being. The new paradigm allows us to remediate disease, not by symptom suppression, but by assessing and treating the cause of dysfunction and illness. Van Ommen, in "The Human Genome Project and the Future of Diagnostics, Treatment and Prevention," published in *The Lancet* in 1999, foretells this paradigm transition in medicine:

> The combination of large-scale gene-expression analysis with pharmacological and nutritional studies will ultimately allow the stratification of individuals by their genetically determined abilities for drug and nutrient metabolism. Tailor-made treatments and lifestyle regimens will improve the effectiveness of therapies and reduce side effects. This will apply equally to monogenic disease and more complex gene-environment interaction disorders, like cardiovascular disease, cancer, hypertension, arthritis, migraine, epilepsy, Parkinson's disease, and Alzheimer's disease.[45]

How Do We Change Paradigms?

In order to move today's model toward the future, we need to think differently. This functional school of thought does not deny the usefulness to the patient and physician of diagnostic groups that allow us to identify in some codified way "what the patient has." We are careful to keep in mind, however, that a diagnosis is an idea we form about groups of people and properly belongs to the group, not to an individual. Making a diagnosis in the realm of chronic illness—such as the many conditions of chronic inflammation whose names end in "itis," as well as autism, schizophrenia, depression, anxiety, cardiovascular disease, and a host of other recognized diseases—is for us not the end of a diagnostic road, *but only the first step*. The fundamental subject of medical concern is the human individual. The logic of inquiry rests on two questions of need:

- Does this person have an unmet individual need?
- Does this person need to be rid of something toxic, allergic, or infectious?

These principles are antithetical to the implicit emphasis of the current conventional medical paradigm, which could be described as follows:

- The fundamental subject of medical concern is disease.
- The inquiry as to health rests first on the naming of the patient's disease.
- Treatment is prescribed for the disease.

In the past, the legacy and momentum of our focus on acute illness have permitted us to remain disease-focused long after chronic illness replaced acute illness as the dominant problem in our modern, industrialized, hygienic society.[46] The medicine we are developing begins to address the following linguistic, statistical, and logical errors of the present paradigm of conventional medicine:

1. The concept that diseases are entities and can cause symptoms is entirely without scientific support. It is a linguistic error that forges a false map in the imagination of professionals and lay people.[47]
2. The idea that each patient's diagnostic and treatment options can be based on determinations of averages is a misuse of statistics when it serves as a diagnostic and therapeutic guide for each unique individual.
3. The maxim that assumptions to explain an event should not be multiplied beyond necessity (Occam's razor) is the logical partner of the one-disease, one-treatment approach of mainstream medicine, particularly in the framework of chronic illness.
4. Medicine is the only field claiming a scientific basis in which general systems theory[48]—i.e., that everything is interconnected—has not become the acknowledged basis for inquiry. Linear causality remains the accepted basis for medical etiology.

Despite the crumbling of the healthcare system around us,[49,50] we have held onto this system of differential diagnosis, biochemical homogeneity, and pharmaceutical therapy as the answer to most chronic lifestyle and long-latency nutritional deficiency diseases. However, there is an alternative model for organizing and perceiving the problems in modern terms. There are a number of organizing principles and themes that underlie nearly all disease (see Chapter 2). This new medical paradigm emerges from the basic and clinical sciences literature. The exploration of the needed shift from our current model to the origins of illness and the maintenance of health, as well as the identification of appropriate investigations, interventions, and therapies for chronic complex illnesses, both require a new intellectual architecture. The explication of a functional methodology is the central mission for this textbook.

A New Paradigm: Understanding and Enhancing Function

> The science of medicine is perhaps the most frequently cited case of increasing specialization seeming to follow inevitably from increasing knowledge, as new cures and better treatments for many diseases are discovered. But as medical biochemical research comes up with deeper explanations of disease processes (and healthy processes) in the body, understanding is also on the increase. More general concepts are replacing more specific ones as common, underlying molecular mechanisms are found for dissimilar diseases in different parts of the body. Once a disease can be understood as fitting into a general framework, the role of the specialist diminishes. Physicians ... may be able to apply a general theory to work out the required treatment, and expect it to be effective even if it has never been used before.[51]

There is much in medicine and science that we cannot perceive with our current way of seeing. A new framework and new organizational concepts are needed in a science with very few true "theories."[52] Linus Pauling remarked years ago that "although medicine is largely based on the sciences, it has not yet become a science."[53] We need a unifying theory of health and disease. We are only now on the verge of forming a clear picture of what that might look like.

A theory can be defined as "a set of facts, propositions, or principles analyzed in their relation to one another and used, especially in science, to explain phenomena."[54] Scientific theory, unlike hypothesis, is most often the result of years of investigation. Medicine has come of age and we are at the transitional edge of development of an entirely different gestalt and theory of health and disease. The science of medicine today is maturing and the old concept of the single agent (bacterium) causing a single disease (infection) treated with a single molecule (antibiotic) is being replaced by our understanding of complex, higher-order functions. We are finally able to peer into the underlying mechanisms of disease and aging, illuminated by the light of genomics, proteomics, metabolomics, and nutrigenomics.

Medicine is nearly ready to discard the old descriptive, phenomenological approach that emerged from the exigencies of medical practice in the early 20th century, where infectious disease was primary and the Pasteur model of outside invaders ruled. The organization of medicine into sub-specialties is an artifact of descriptive medicine that bears little relevance to biological principles. The current classification of diseases (ICD-9) is now less useful in understanding mechanisms and guiding innovative therapies in health and illness. Finally, we can move toward understanding and treating disease with a dynamic, functional model based on an intricate understanding of the nature of the interaction of the genome with the environment, especially in the field of nutrigenomics.[55]

The story of the role of nutrients in health and disease is a useful model to help us shift from a medical model based on pathology to one based on deviations from optimal function, with an understanding of the process of de-volution of health into chronic, complex illnesses. A fundamental change in perspective has occurred with the development of genomics, proteomics, metabolomics, and the evolution of nutrigenomics.[56] Nutrigenomics is the use of nutrients of varying and sometimes high doses to influence gene expression, with the goal of not simply treating disease, but also of optimizing function.[57] The development of the "-omics" and the applications of nutrigenomics are poised to change medicine forever from a pathology-based science to a function-based science.[58]

Example of the New Paradigm: Nutrients Beyond Deficiency Diseases

The old paradigm of diagnosis and classification of diseases into organ system pathologies (corresponding fairly closely to medical specialties) becomes less meaningful in the light of our understanding of the basic mechanisms of dysfunction in the human body. One disease may have multiple causes, and one initiating factor may cause multiple diseases. Atherosclerotic cardiovascular disease (CVD) and celiac disease provide clear examples of this concept.

We recognize cardiovascular disease by its pathology: atherosclerotic plaques. However, the development of plaques can be triggered by multiple factors. These include insulin resistance,[59] folate deficiency and hyperhomocysteinemia,[60] occult infections,[61] heavy metal toxicity,[62,63] inherited dyslipidemias, stress, and other factors that increase inflammation.[64]

The diagnosis and treatment of each of these antecedent conditions varies, and the success of medical therapy rests on making the proper assessment of the etiologic factors involved (and they are often multiple).[65] Prescribing the classic low-fat diet, usually high in refined carbohydrates, along with a beta-blocker and a statin for CVD can—counter to expectation—actually exacerbate the underlying problem in the patient with insulin resistance, or may miss entirely the key underlying mechanism (e.g., occult infection) in a different patient. Both are precursor conditions that can lead to the endpoint of CV dysfunction. Let's illustrate this point with some patient stories.

A 56-year-old patient with severe CVD, after interventions including two angioplasties and a CABG (coronary artery bypass graft), suffered a stroke. The evaluations and treatments he experienced prior to his stroke were considered "standard of care" for his diagnosis. However, with further evaluation after his stroke, through the lens of functional assessment, he was found to have a marked elevation of homocysteine (22 mmoles/liter with normal 6–8 mmoles/liter). He was tested genetically and found to have a specific genetic uniqueness, homozygous 677C to T polymorphism of MTFHR (methylenetetrahydrofolate reductase). This SNP (single nucleotide polymorphism) produces a variant enzyme that requires extraordinarily high doses of folate to facilitate coenzyme binding and MTHFR enzyme activity. His treatment plan focused on his genetic, proteomic, and metabolomic uniqueness. With appropriate nutrient intervention, his serum homocysteine equilibrated into the normal range and he has no further demonstrable progression of his atherosclerosis.[66]

Another patient report exemplifies both the functional medicine methodology as well as the problems inherent in our current disease classification system. At 57, the patient described himself in general good health, eagerly planning a climb of Mt. Kilimanjaro. However, it was noted in his comprehensive workup that he took 15 different medications: prescriptions for colitis, asthma, alopecia areata, and hypertension. He was being treated in a standard manner by an internist, a gastroenterologist, a pulmonologist, and a dermatologist, all of whom made the correct "diagnosis" and provided the appropriate medications for each diagnosis. However, by filtering the patient's signs and symptoms through the lens of underlying pathways, it was apparent that all of the patient's "diseases" had an inflammatory component that manifested across organ systems (and speciality domains). None of his physicians had searched for the underlying mechanism, nor apparently considered this assessment (an across-systems inflammatory process) relevant. Their treatments were based solely on diagnoses relevant to their specialties. An evaluation program ensued, looking for underlying mechanisms of dysfunction that could explain his disorders. With appropriate investigation, it was found that most of his diagnoses could be explained by something he was eating—gluten-containing foods—that caused the "many-headed hydra" of his inflammatory disorders.[67,68] Tests confirmed the diagnosis of celiac disease, that had been missed for over 40 years. Within six months, he was off most of his medications, lost 25 pounds, and stabilized his blood pressure. He had no more symptoms of asthma, his bowel movements normalized, and his hair grew back. A 2002 review of celiac disease in *The New England Journal of Medicine*[69] catalogued the myriad diseases that can be caused by immune-mediated gluten sensitivity, including anemia, osteoporosis, autoimmune diseases, thyroid dysfunction, schizophrenia, and psoriasis. Each of the patient's conditions could have been triggered by multiple factors; but, for him, eating gluten-containing foods was the cause of his symptoms. His genetic susceptibilities required that he not eat a particular food protein in order to maintain health and prevent triggering his symptoms.

The Diverse Roles of Nutrients

How we think about essential nutrients in general has been shaped by the vitamin deficiency diseases through which they were historically discovered. Vitamins are still defined by single deficiency diseases, such as pellagra, beriberi, scurvy, and rickets. That thinking is the basis for the current dietary reference intakes (DRIs), which recommend the minimum amount to prevent deficiency diseases, not the variable amounts needed by a polymorphic population for optimal health—sometimes hundreds of times the DRIs. Most physicians and consumers do not realize that DRIs are based simply on the minimum amount of a nutrient necessary to prevent an index deficiency disease. Applied clinical medicine has failed to recognize that nutrients are multifunctional substances with many roles. For example, in recent reviews,[70,71] vitamin D has not only been implicated in prevention of rickets, but may have a role in treating or preventing heart disease, multiple sclerosis, polycystic ovary syndrome, depression, epilepsy, type 1 diabetes, and cancer. Folate not only prevents megaloblastic anemia, but also prevents neural tube defects, and is a key factor in preventing many cases of cardiovascular disease, dementia, depression, and colon and breast cancer.[72] Magnesium plays a role in over 300 enzyme reactions.

Conventional thinking has been biased against the therapeutic use of vitamins in disease and has avoided the question of whether vitamins have a role in optimizing health.[73] Study of nutrients over the long term has been complicated by the fact that the desired outcomes being tracked involve primarily the absence of problems rather than a defined dysfunction or remediation. This is in direct opposition to pharmaceutical agents, which are meant to alter pathology. Nutrients restore normal function; they do so by optimizing normal biological functions, mostly through their actions as coenzymes in biochemical reactions.

We have approximately 30,000 genes. The most common type of variation in the human genome is the SNP, where a single base differs between individuals (being A instead of G, for example). SNPs occur about once every 1000 base pairs in the genome, making up the bulk of the 3 million variations found in the genome. The frequency of a particular polymorphism tends to remain stable in the population. (Genome information from http://www.wellcome.ac.uk/en/genome/thegenome/hg04b001.html.) These SNPs create unique biochemical needs within the population. One-third or more of them affect coenzyme-binding sites for vitamins or nutrients, and therefore have a role in disease and dysfunction.[74] Bruce Ames, in his landmark review of genetic variant enzymes and vitamin therapy, stated: "Our analysis of metabolic disease that affects cofactor binding, particularly as a result of polymorphic mutations, may present a novel rationale for high-dose vitamin therapy, perhaps hundreds of times the normal dietary reference intakes (DRI) in some cases."[75]

Our current nutritional recommendations do not accommodate the broad and varied roles of nutrients in human biology. Also absent is the consistent clinical question: "What does this individual need that she or he has failed to get?" For example, the person may need to add vitamins, minerals, essential amino acids and essential fatty acids, accessory and conditionally essential nutrients.[76] In many cases, a single nutrient may catalyze hundreds of biochemical reactions; suboptimal levels may lead to cellular and molecular dysfunction that is not recognized as a "deficiency" disease.[77] The notion that higher doses may be needed for the optimal functioning of the total organism is not widely taught, despite new evidence that suboptimal nutrient status may contribute to "long-latency" deficiency diseases that are epidemic, such as cardiovascular disease, cancer, osteoporosis, neurodegenerative disease, and immune dysfunction.[78]

Nutritional science has been seen as a secondary factor in health, something best left to the dietitian.[79] Historically, nutrition was taught at the state agricultural schools in the department of home economics. The "real" science was, of course, being pursued by the scientists at the universities, in the departments of chemistry, physics, and biology. Until recently, physicians educated within this biased system of learning have abdicated their responsibility to study the science and practice of nutrition. Clear nutritional guidelines and consensus have been hard to achieve despite emerging evidence of importance. We need to cultivate different tools of assessment and research that allow us to better answer questions about nutrition and nutraceutical therapies.[80]

Long-latency Disease: A Further Example of the New Medicine

Dr. Robert Heaney is a Professor of Medicine at Creighton University in Omaha, Nebraska. He won the 2003 E.V. McCollum Award of the American Society for Clinical Nutrition in recognition of his contributions to nutritional science and medicine, particularly in the field of osteoporosis and calcium physiology. In his E.V. McCollum Award lecture, he stated that the fundamental flaw in the establishment of recommended nutrient intakes is the presumption that if a nutrient intake is sufficient to prevent the index deficiency disease, then it is adequate for the optimal functioning of the total organism. He suggested that this narrow viewpoint overlooks two important facts. First, there are long-term consequences of lesser degrees of deficiency that may operate through similar mechanisms as the index disease; and second, there may be very different mechanisms involved in the development of long-latency deficiency diseases.

In his lecture, he also tackled the difficult question of the adequacy of the standard research tools in this area of multi-factorial causality (see also Chapters 5 and 6, plus this chapter's discussion, *How Do We Change Paradigms?*). He suggested the increased use of observational research to better infer causality in nutrition. The appropriate methodology for ferreting out the causal agents for the absence of a problem—research for benefit rather than harm—runs straight into the controversy surrounding the belief that double-blind RCTs are the gold-standard methodology for *all* scientific studies. He proposed that we can safely use the usual principles for causal inference from observational data in the nutritional context:[81]

> ... biological plausibility, correct temporal sequence, dose-response relations, experiments of nature found in inborn errors of metabolism and demonstration of causal connection in animal models. These principles are all well understood in a general way, and what ... may have been lacking up till now was the conviction within the field of nutrition that long-latency deficiency diseases exist, that they are nutritional problems, and that the use of such inferential and investigative stratagems may be both appropriate and necessary.

In the paper he adapted from his E.V. McCollum Award Lecture ("Long-latency Deficiency Disease: Insights from Calcium and Vitamin D"),[82] he lays the groundwork for a new conceptualization of the role of nutrients in health and disease. In effect, he turns nutritional science on its head by saying "prove to me that we *don't* need higher levels of nutrients for health."

> Because the current recommendations are based on the prevention of the index disease only, they can no longer be said to be biologically defensible. The pre-agricultural human diet, insofar as it can be reconstructed, may well be a better starting point for policy. ... Such a diet would have had at least some of the following features: high protein intake, low glycemic index, high calcium intake, high folic acid intake, an alkaline ash residue and high vitamin D input. It is in this nutritional context that human physiology is adapted. The burden of proof should fall on those who say that these more natural conditions are not needed and that lower intakes are safe.

He laments that nutritional science has been largely ignored by practicing physicians. His perspective finds support in Dr. Jim Kaput's more recent paper, "Nutritional Genomics: The Next Frontier in the Post Genomic Era."[83]

Dr. Heaney used the examples of calcium, vitamin D, and folate to illuminate the multi-functional nature of nutrients in complex, higher-order functioning in biology. Vitamin D has been classically associated with the prevention of rickets and osteoporosis. Current recommended levels for vitamin D intake are benchmarked to the prevention of rickets, the presumption being that if patients do not have rickets or osteomalacia, then their vitamin D intake is adequate. Evidence indicates otherwise; increasing vitamin D levels in the blood to the upper levels of the reference range improves calcium absorption efficacy by two-thirds, reducing osteoporotic fracture risk by one-third. Additionally, vitamin D has other roles. It has been shown that serum 25(OH) vitamin D concentrations are inversely associated with prostate and squamous cell cancers. The underlying mechanism for this effect appears to be as follows: people with low sun exposure or increased skin pigmentation are less able to make calcitriol (biologically active 1,25-dihydroxyvitamin D) within tissues in an amount adequate to control cell proliferation and reduce oncogenesis. Heaney hypothesizes that protective serum levels of 25(OH) vitamin D, for prevention of oncogenesis, may be much greater than current reference values.

In that same paper, he describes the multiple conditions that may arise from a single nutrient deficiency, the multifunctional nature of nutrients, and the need for higher intakes for optimal health: "*Inadequate intake of specific nutrients may produce more than one disease, may produce them by more than one mechanism, and may require several years for the consequent morbidity and mortality to be sufficiently evident to be clinically recognizable as 'disease.'*" He also suggests that the intakes of nutrients required to prevent the non-index diseases are often higher than required to prevent the index disease; for example, preventing osteoporosis requires four times the vitamin D needed to prevent rickets; similarly, preventing neural tube defects requires four times the intake of folate needed to prevent anemia.

Nutrigenomics: An Organizing Principle of the New Paradigm

Imagine a drug that could cure within days or weeks a fatal disease using a very small dose, without toxicity, and with a 100% success rate. Such a drug does not exist and probably will never exist; but this is the power and potential of nutrients. They function within the genetic and evolutionary necessities of the cell to enhance and facilitate optimal biological functioning. They are vital to our very survival. Their effectiveness in curing deficiency diseases is dramatic, but their role in the prevention and management of long-latency chronic diseases is more frequently relevant to most daily clinical practice.

Many patients worry about the dangers of medications; their compliance with pharmaceuticals is disturbingly low, as 20% of prescriptions go unfilled and 85% are never refilled.[84] The decision to see a doctor should not be measured by concern for risk and danger, but by the opportunity and anticipation of enhanced health and well being. Herein lies the potential of nutrigenomics and the new medical paradigm that allows us to understand the integrative function of complex organisms, and the essential and primary role of nutrition in maintaining that function. This new paradigm shifts us from disease treatment and disease prevention to health promotion.[85]

The study of nutrigenomics[86] spearheads a radical transformation in medicine akin to the change in physics that occurred when the deficiencies of Newtonian physics were illuminated by discoveries in quantum mechanical physics and Albert Einstein's theory of relativity. We have entered an era where genetic predisposition replaces Mendelian genetic determinism, where biochemical individuality replaces biochemical homogeneity, and where the importance of the biological terrain or internal milieu exceeds that of the external invader. However, acceptance of the change, seeing what is right in front of us, is difficult. As R.D. Laing states in *The Voice of Experience,*[87] "Our way of looking is not easily disturbed by what it sees, let alone by what it cannot see."

Kaput summarizes the concepts of nutrigenomics, a foundational component of the new functional paradigm of medicine, in a way that should give us pause and cause us to examine our outdated beliefs:

> The interface between the nutritional environment and cellular/genetic processes is being referred to as "nutrigenomics." Nutrigenomics seeks to provide a molecular genetic understanding for how common dietary chemicals (i.e., nutrition) affect health by altering the expression and/or structure of an individual's genetic makeup. The fundamental concepts of the field are that the progression from a healthy phenotype to a chronic disease phenotype must occur by changes in gene expression or by differences in activities of proteins and enzymes, and that dietary chemicals directly or indirectly regulate the expression of genomic information. We present a conceptual basis and specific examples for this new branch of genomic research that focuses on the tenets of nutritional genomics: 1) common dietary chemicals act on the human genome, either directly or indirectly, to alter gene expression or structure; 2) under certain circumstances and in some individuals, diet can be a serious risk factor for a number of diseases; 3) some diet-regulated genes (and their normal, common variants) are likely to play a role in the onset, incidence, progression, and/or severity of chronic diseases; 4) the degree to which diet influences the balance between healthy and disease states may depend on an individual's genetic makeup; and 5) dietary intervention based on knowledge of nutritional requirement, nutritional status, and genotype (i.e., "individualized nutrition") can be used to prevent, mitigate, or cure chronic disease.[88]

Nutrigenomics is a fulcrum point for placing a lever of change in our current medical paradigm. Kaput describes the robustness of this paradigm ("the next frontier in the post genomic era") as having the potential to radically change our approach to health and disease. In fact, for the first time in medicine, we have the opportunity to not only treat disease but to create a context for health. The adoption of new organizing principles and concepts that form the basis of the new medical paradigm can help us successfully navigate health and illness in the 21st century.

Development of the Knowledge Base in Biochemical Individuality

DeAnn Liska, PhD

Introduction

Our ideas of health and disease have changed dramatically in the past several decades. Once, we talked of illness as something we *caught* and could *control*; now, we talk about being susceptible to the forces around us because of our genes. Once, we understood the role of genetics in disease as important only with respect to the defined "inherited diseases of metabolism," in which a dysfunctional gene that directly leads to a disease (such as maple syrup disease, or phenylalaninemia) is passed on from generation to generation. An inherited disease of metabolism is discrete: you either have it or you don't. And, if you have it, you can manage it but you can't eradicate it.

As seen in the *Cathy* cartoon below, our understanding of "genetic predisposition" has been influenced by the concept of genetic determinism. We have believed that the genes we inherit are static and, like flood waters that grab us and pull us downstream against our will, we must succumb to a more powerful force. However (and fortunately), the emerging data from investigations that focus on understanding the integration of environmental triggers with genetic constitution indicate that we can manage most of these predispositions. Once we know where and how we are susceptible, we

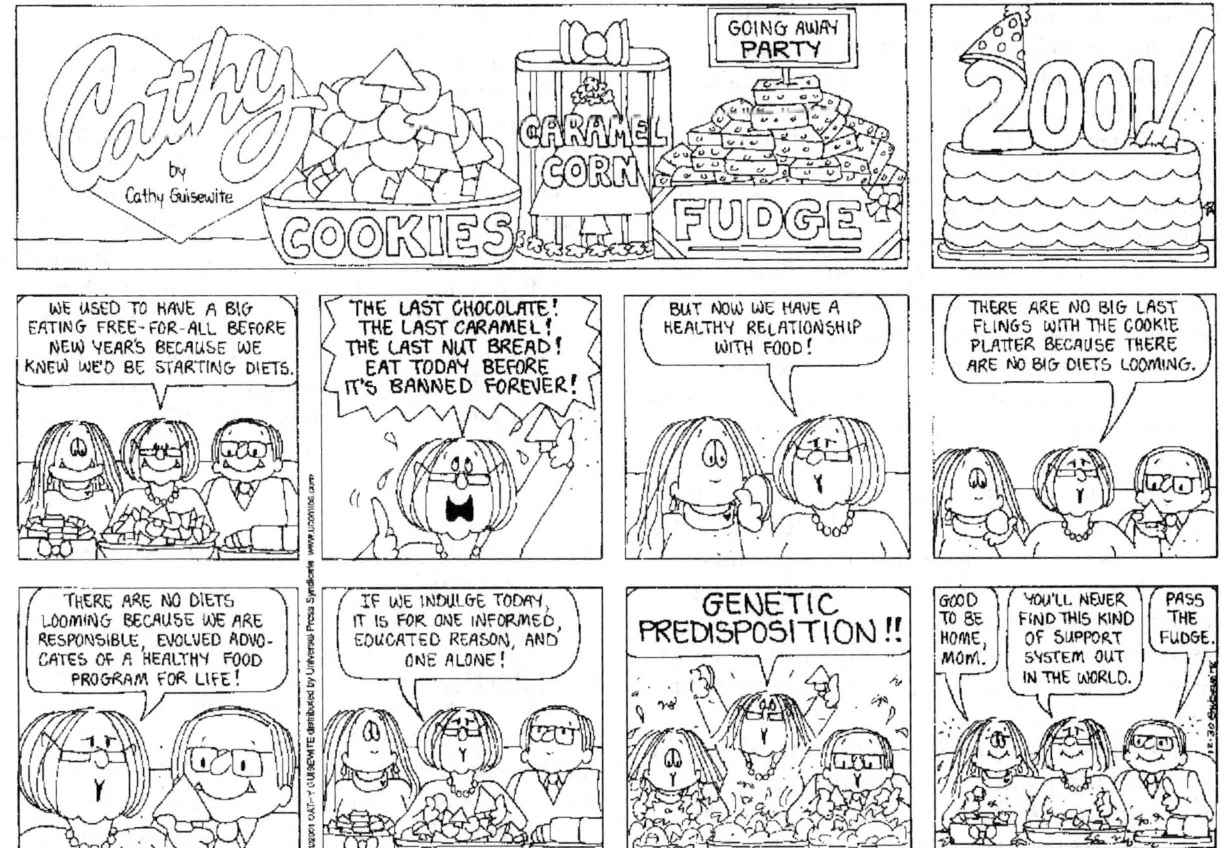

can improve the match between our environmental exposures and our own unique profiles to improve health outcome and longevity. This is the promise of 21st century medicine. And, since our genetic constitution is unique, this is the historical and scientific basis for biochemical individuality.

Biochemical Individuality in Functional Medicine

Biochemical individuality is not a new topic in functional medicine; it has been one of the underlying principles since the early 1980s. Although the unique genetic profile of an individual may be the most obvious way in which we are all "biochemically individual," in functional medicine this concept has long been defined as comprising the interaction of genetics and environment. We understand biochemical individuality to mean that each individual has a unique physiological and biochemical composition, based upon his or her individual genetic make-up, that interacts with the individual's specific environment—that continuous exposure to "inputs" (experiences, nutrients, activity, toxins, medications, etc.) that influences our genes. It is this combination of factors that accounts for the endless variety of phenotypic responses—those biochemically unique individuals we see every day in our offices and clinics. Biochemical individuality is dependent upon the DNA that is present at the moment of conception in each individual and, therefore, a discussion of biochemical individuality includes understanding how DNA is expressed and influenced.

A Brief Look at the History of Biochemical Individuality

The first work upon which the field of genetics is based came from the Augustinian monk, Gregor Mendel, who found that phenotypic traits in peas could be passed down from generation to generation. His work was published in 1866, but remained in obscurity until around 1900, when it was rediscovered and promoted by several scientists. Although the concept of genes and inheritance was taking a forefront at the time, Archibald Garrod cautioned in 1902 that the chemical behavior (metabolism) of different individuals varied in ways that were independent of genetics. Dr. Garrod discovered alkaptonuria, which led to the understanding of phenylketonuria and the role of phenylalanine-restricted diets in its management. Although he studied a classic model of inherited disease, he noted that "variations of chemical behavior ... are probably present everywhere in minor degrees" and stated "as no two individuals of a species are absolutely identical in bodily structure neither are their chemical processes carried out on exactly the same lines."[89]

The renowned biochemist, Roger Williams, PhD, was the first to use the term "biochemical individuality" in his classic book of the same name, published in 1956.[90] In this work, he described how the anatomical and physiological variations among people are related to their varied responses to the environment and to their differing nutritional needs. He pointed out that even identical twins could differ in their requirements for optimal function, based upon the fact that they developed in different environments *in utero*, a concept that is beginning to accumulate scientific support (discussed further below). In addition, he noted that, although identical twins share the same genes, their differing nutritional and developmental environments also can contribute to different expression of these genes as they grow older.

Dr. Williams came upon the idea of biochemical individuality in his work with nutrition and chronic disease. In 1950, he published an article in *The Lancet* titled "The Concept of Genetotrophic Disease," in which he proposed a role for nutrients in the prevention of chronic disease.[91] Genetotrophic diseases are those for which genetic uniqueness creates a demand for specific nutrients beyond the average intake to facilitate optimal function and prevent premature disease. Dr. Williams theorized that when those specific needs are not met in a given individual, disease results. He further proposed that the major chronic degenerative diseases of aging are genetotrophic. That is, the unique genes of each individual require different levels of nutrition and a specific lifestyle for optimal health. The consequences of not meeting the specific needs of the individual are expressed, over several decades, as degenerative disease "of unknown origin." In his model, at the genetic level, an individual has a need for a different level of nutrients to promote proper phenotypic expression. If that need is not met, the resulting "undernutrition" will manifest as chronic disease in midlife.

Although medicine did not initially embrace the concepts of genetotrophic disease and biochemical individuality, they have consistently gained more attention since the 1980s. It is now fashionable within science to talk about "individual responses." Much of this progress has come as a result of the technological advances that have allowed us to dissect DNA. Over the past two decades, individual genes have been identified and many of their functions have been described. The dogma of gene expression (Figure 7.1) was defined. The understanding of viral integration into the genes in specific cells, and the identification of mitochondrial DNA as separate but integrated in every cell have also enhanced our realization that each and every person is unique at the level of DNA.

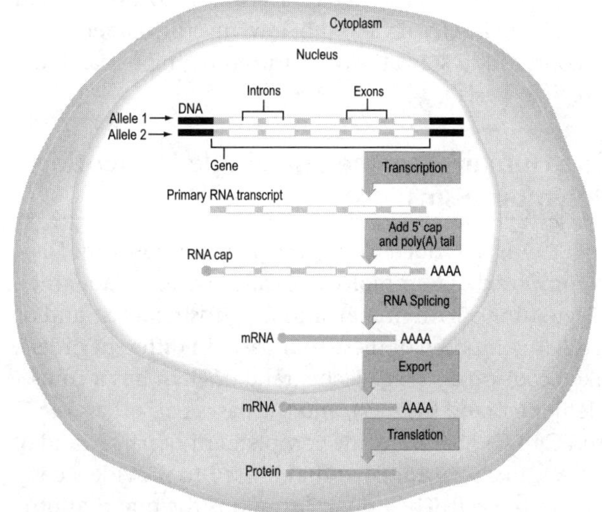

Figure 7.1 **Dogma of gene expression**

A schematic from the chromosome to gene in a cell. A gene comprises a small section of DNA on a chromosome. Each gene has two alleles (the two copies, one from each parent). A person can have two different alleles (polymorphisms), which is called a heterozygote. If the two alleles are the same, it is called a homozygote.

The Human Genome Project represented a major international commitment among scientists and provided the human genome sequence for 99% of the gene-coding DNA in April 2003, which corresponded with the 50-year celebration of Watson, Crick, and Franklin's discovery of the structure of DNA. The implications of this work, especially as they relate to medicine, are still unfolding, but they have already begun to change the way we view health and disease. As discussed in a 2003 review in the *Archives of Internal Medicine*:[92]

> The individualization of treatments has been one of the strongest therapeutic tools, while also one of the greatest challenges of the pregenomic era. Individuals with apparently identical clinical problems may respond very differently to a specific treatment, and this has generally been accepted as an insoluble problem. However, with the availability of comprehensive genetic and molecular profiles, it will probably become possible to respond to disease with individualized strategies based on genetic profiles.

The promise is to be able to fully use genetic information for individualized clinical management plans; the challenge remains to understand the multiple connections and patterns that are emerging from these data. This field is extremely active, and new findings continue to emerge each day. The areas most developed to date are briefly reviewed below, but the reader is encouraged to stay abreast of the emerging research on a regular basis.

The Human Genome and Single Nucleotide Polymorphisms

DNA is described by its base pair composition. DNA is composed of four molecules called bases: A (adenine), G (guanine), T (thymine), and C (cytosine). A strand of DNA is composed of these four bases in different orders, like beads on a string. Each strand of DNA has a complement strand (its pair), and the bases pair off as A to T, and C to G. Therefore, the complement or pair strand of DNA is like a mirror copy that is used to provide a copy within the cell. The primary strand is the one that provides the blueprint for mRNA through a process called transcription. The mRNA is then transported to the cell's nucleus, from which the protein is made in a process called protein translation (see Figure 7.2). The process of reading the DNA is called gene expression. Common definitions in the field of genetics and molecular biology are provided in Table 7.1.

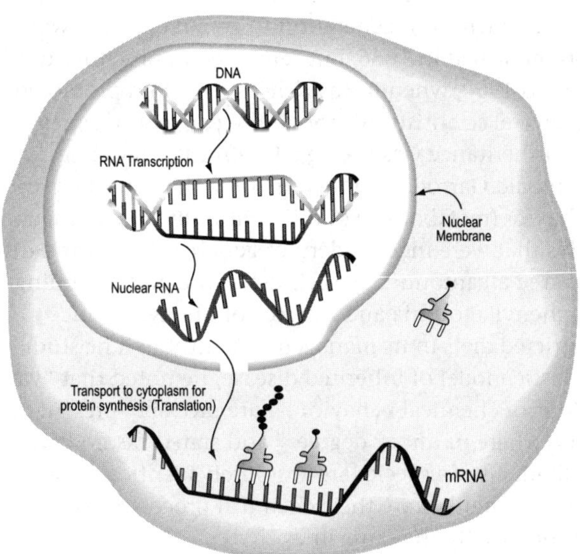

Figure 7.2 **mRNA to protein**

A schematic showing the general dogma of gene transcription and translation. A gene is transcribed into RNA, which is transported to the cytoplasm as mRNA. The mRNA carries the information of one gene, and is translated to make protein in the cell's cytoplasm.

Today, we know that the human genome is composed of approximately 3,164.7 million base pairs, which contrasts to the smallest bacterium genome of 600,000 DNA base pairs. Human DNA is arranged into 23 (physically separate) chromosomes, each of which contains between 50 million and 250 million base pairs. The human genome is estimated to encode 30,000 genes. An average gene-encoding region on human DNA is around 3,000 base pairs, but gene size can vary greatly from very small to extremely large (over 2 million base pairs). The gene density of DNA is about one gene per every 100 kilobases. The functions associated with over 50% of the discovered genes are unknown. Updates on the human genome can be obtained at the Human Genome Project Information site on the internet: http://www.ornl.gov/sci/techresources/Human_Genome/project/info.shtml.

Much of the DNA within the gene contains information that isn't transcribed, but acts to regulate the expression of the gene. This non-coding DNA is particularly important for signal transduction pathways. The amount of DNA in the human genome that directly encodes protein is only about 2% and each gene contains several areas of non-coding DNA that are involved

Table 7.1 **Definitions for Common Terminology in the Study of Genes**

Gene	The functional and physical unit of heredity passed from parent to offspring. Genes are pieces of DNA that contain the information necessary for making a cell, such as the information to make structural proteins and enzymes.
Genome	The DNA code that comprises the complete genetic composition of an organism. As an analogy, this would be the entire encyclopedia of information, or DNA, to encode one person. Each cell contains a genome, but a cell only uses the portions of the genome relevant for its specific functions.
DNA (deoxyribonucleic acid)	The chemical substance that forms the genome. DNA is composed of four specific compounds, or nucleotides: guanine (G), adenine (A), cytosine (C), and thymine (T).
mRNA (messenger RNA)	A fragment of RNA that is read from the genome (or DNA blueprint). An mRNA carries with it only the information related to one gene, so it is the molecule within the cell that transfers the information from the DNA, which contains the blueprint of all genes, for one specific gene that can then be transported to the site where the protein will be made. As an analogy, if DNA is the encyclopedia of a person's genotype, the mRNA is a photocopy of one page of that encyclopedia.
Gene expression	The process of making proteins from DNA, or reading the DNA.
Genotype	The internally encoded information of an organism (or genome).
Phenotype	The outward, physical manifestation of an organism (the interplay of environment and genotype).
Transcription	The process of making an mRNA from DNA that occurs within the nucleus of the cell. For example, during transcription, the section of DNA that contains the information for a specific gene is copied into an mRNA molecule, which is much smaller and can be transported to the site where proteins are made within the cell.
Translation	The process that occurs within the cell in which a protein is generated from mRNA. In this process, the mRNA is read by the cell's protein generation machinery to make a specific protein that can be used within the cell or transported to another site, where it will affect function.
Wild-type	The most common DNA sequence for a specific gene. This term is mainly used for comparative purposes in scientific literature to identify a standard sequence that can be compared to other sequences for identification of DNA mutations.
Mutation	A general term to describe a change in an individual's DNA sequence (genotype) from the defined wild type (the most common sequence, considered the standard for that gene). This change may or may not lead to a change in phenotype (e.g., point mutations, multiple mutations, deletions, duplications, somatic mutations).
Polymorphism	A difference in DNA sequence from the most common sequence that occurs at a consistent frequency and is maintained in the population. To be considered a polymorphism, a DNA sequence must be present in at least 1% of the population. Many polymorphisms result in proteins that are still active, but the activity differs (slower or faster) than the most common sequence.
SNPs (Single Nucleotide Polymorphisms)	A change at a singe site (single base pair) in a DNA sequence as compared to the most common sequence that occurs in at least 1% of the population. SNPs can lead to proteins that are more or less active than those from the most common sequence, and are considered to account for much of the variability seen among different individuals (i.e., biochemical individuality).

in gene regulation (see Figure 7.3). The DNA that is not contained within the genes is known to function in managing structure and conformation of the DNA, which also influence whether a gene is recognized and transcribed within a cell; however, the specific function of much of the DNA in our cells is unknown.

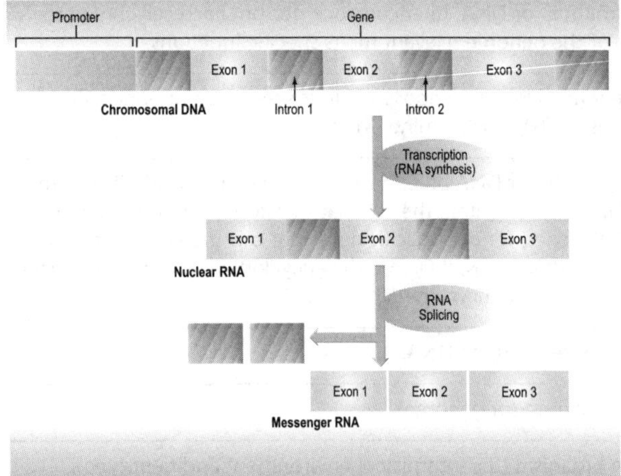

Figure 7.3 **Noncoding regions of DNA**

A schematic showing the structure of a gene. Each gene in the DNA has exons (segments that will be included in the mRNA), and introns (segments that will be selectively removed before the RNA leaves the nucleus). The role of introns in gene expression is not fully understood, but they are thought to play a role in regulation of gene expression. Some polymorphisms that affect phenotype have been shown to occur in intron sections of genes, thereby altering a protein's activity by influencing how well the gene is expressed and ultimately how much protein is actually made.

Defining the structure and sequence of the human genome has helped us understand the genetic differences that occur as mutations. A mutation is any change in DNA over the most common sequence, called the wild type. A mutation can come in many forms: a whole section of DNA may be deleted; a large section may be inserted where it doesn't belong; a small deletion or insertion can also occur. Most of these, if they are large changes, lead to observed differences in structure or function, or even death *in utero*, and they occur in less than 1% of the population. Very small changes that alter the function of an enzyme, making it more active or less able to function, but not obliterating its function completely, occur more regularly. These types of changes are generally at one base site, and so they are called single nucleotide polymorphisms; they occur in at least 1% of the population.

Because SNPs are not an embryonic lethal mutation, or an inherited single-gene mutation that leads to a severe disease or alteration of structure, they are maintained in the population and passed from generation to generation. It is estimated that around 3 million SNPs will eventually be identified; 1.8 million have already been found. SNPs can occur anywhere in the DNA, but the ones that occur on or around genes hold the most interest for researchers. Associating a SNP with a specific functional outcome holds promise for helping to personalize health care and prevention for individual patients; we may be able to intervene before a condition becomes established. [Note: Updates on SNPs can be found at the SNP Consortium Ltd. site at: http://snp.cshl.org/.]

How SNPs Alter Function

SNPs can affect the phenotype of an individual in a variety of ways. A SNP in the body of a gene may encode a protein, such as an enzyme, leading to what seems to be a minor change in structure of the protein. In many cases, this is only one amino acid change, but the change can alter the activity of the protein such that it is more active (e.g., binds its substrate more tightly) or less active. The protein may have lower stability (so that it is present but at an apparently lower concentration), or higher stability (so the protein is at an increased concentration because it is broken down less quickly). SNPs can also occur in areas of the DNA that are involved in gene regulation but may not directly alter the protein, so that the gene is transcribed more or less readily. The ultimate effect of these SNPs can be seen as "tweaks" in the metabolic pathway functions. Individuals having these SNPs may not process and excrete a toxin as quickly as the general population, or their need for a nutrient cofactor may be higher because of lowered ability to bind a specific nutrient and maintain activity.

Not all SNPs have medical significance; determining those that most influence various conditions or responses to interventions is a challenge. Moreover, most of the SNPs that are relevant will lead to only a small change, such as a decrease in an enzyme's activity, but not the on-off type of change seen with heritable disorders of metabolism. Taken together with the multifactorial nature of metabolic pathways and the myriad influences on chronic diseases, the combined effects of different SNP patterns are likely to be of greatest value in understanding susceptibility to particular diseases or conditions.

Analyzing many SNPs at once can be done using microarray technology, but understanding the myriad patterns that emerge from this analysis will take many years of work. Therefore, the integration of these new findings is being seen first in cases in which one particular change (one SNP) is found to influence a response, such as in the metabolism of a drug that occurs primarily through one specific pathway. A few areas have led the way to integrating individualized genetic information in ways that are influencing medicine today, and those are reviewed below.

Adverse Drug Reactions and Pharmacogenomics

A widely cited study published in *JAMA* in 1998[93] brought to the fore a key issue in medicine: that pharmaceutical agents are one of the most commonly identified causes of adverse events. The pharmaceutical companies develop products based on the notion that one drug will work for everyone at the same dose, the "one-size-fits-all" model. However, the meta-analysis presented in the *JAMA* article indicated that 2.2 million patients (6.7%) had adverse drug reactions (ADRs) in 1994, and 106,000 patients (0.32%) died as a result of them. Moreover, the analysis used a conservative method to reduce any contribution from errors in administration, overdose, drug abuse, therapeutic failures, and "possible ADRs" and, therefore, the findings represent only drug reactions from properly prescribed and administered drugs. The conclusion was that adverse drug reactions from properly prescribed medications represent between the fourth and sixth leading cause of death in the United States. Although this publication spurred much comment after it appeared,[94] it identified a key area of concern that had not yet been fully accepted: adverse drug reactions occur in a high number of individuals with no direct explanation.

For several years after publication of this study, a number of articles on the mechanisms of ADRs were published. Researchers began to recognize that a key factor in ADRs is biochemical individuality—specifically, variability in drug metabolism due to polymorphisms in genes for drug metabolizing enzymes.[95] At a given dose of drug, the range in variability of patient responses is 4-fold to 40-fold (i.e., 400% to 4000%).[96] The president and CEO of New Jersey-based Orchid BioSciences has been quoted as saying that "more money is spent on adverse drug response than on drug development."[97]

Not only is the issue of adverse events a major concern, but drug efficacy is also influenced by biochemical individuality and is becoming a focus of discussion in medicine. For example, in a 2003 news story, Allen Roses, the worldwide vice-president of genetics at GlaxoSmithKline, observed: "The vast majority of drugs—more than 90%—only work in 30 or 50% of the people. I wouldn't say that most drugs don't work. I would say that most drugs work in 30 to 50% of people. Drugs out there on the market work, but they don't work in everybody."[98] For example, it is known that codeine is ineffective for pain relief in about 10% of the population. In order to be efficacious, codeine must first be converted to morphine in the body, a reaction that requires the cytochrome P450 enzyme CYP2D6, and 10% of the population has a SNP in the CYP2D6 gene that results in a less active protein.[99]

The issue, then, is how to predetermine who will respond and who won't and—even more immediate—who will respond with an ADR that may be fatal. This has led to the definition of the field of pharmacogenomics or pharmacogenetics. Research in pharmacogenetics began by identifying allelic variations in genes (primarily SNPs) and has expanded to include identifying new drug targets. All definitions for pharmacogenetics revolve around how the body uses and metabolizes pharmacologic agents.

A specific example of biochemical individuality and drug response can be shown with the thiopurine S-methyltransferase (TPMT) protein, which is the enzyme that breaks down the drug 6-mercaptopurine. This drug is a chemotherapeutic agent used for acute lymphoblastic leukemia, a deadly form of cancer that afflicts approximately 2,400 children in the United States every year. Between 10 and 15% of people metabolize this drug either too quickly (resulting in lowered efficacy of a standard dose of the drug) or too slowly (resulting in accumulation of lethal levels), based upon the presence of a mutation in the TPMT gene. A genetic test now exists to determine whether this mutation is present before the drug is given to a patient.

Warfarin is a narrow-spectrum anticoagulant drug with a wide interindividual variation in dosage. The risk of serious hemorrhage during warfarin therapy ranges from 1.3 to 4.2 per 100 patient years of exposure. Therefore, it is important to find ways to quickly and effectively determine the best dosage for a patient. Warfarin is composed of two enantiomers—R-warfarin and S-warfarin—which are metabolized differently. The S-warfarin is metabolized by the 2C9 cytochrome P450 (CYP2C9), whereas the R-form is metabolized by the

CYP1A2 and CYP3A4 enzymes. The CYP2C9 gene is known to have two relatively common SNPs, one resulting in an enzyme that is only 5% as active as the wild type, and another that leads to an enzyme that is 12% as active as the wild type.

To understand the role of these polymorphisms in warfarin therapy, Aithal et al.[100] compared the SNP pattern in low-dose patients (1.5 mg per day or less) with control patients and found patients in the low-dose group were six times more likely to have a low activity SNP than the control patients. Moreover, further studies have demonstrated that using the common 5 mg per day dose initially in patients with the SNP that leads to the most compromised 2C9 activity causes an increase in the international normalized ratio and a significant risk of bleeding.[101] Patients with SNPs in 2C9 have been shown to be at greater risk for major bleeding complications in some studies, but not in all.[102,103,104] It is becoming prudent practice to genotype for CYP2C9 before beginning warfarin therapy to reduce the risk of ADRs and to decrease medical expenditures.[105,106]

These examples illustrate how findings in pharmacogenomics support the concept of biochemical individuality. The benefit to patients today is great; the potential benefit, as the knowledge base grows, is huge. In a systematic review of ADRs, Phillips et al.[107] published a list of the most common pharmaceuticals that are involved in ADRs (see Table 7.2). In this growing field, many more examples become available every year. The best resources for up-to-date information are the internet, product manufacturers, and specific laboratories that test for SNPs.

Role of Environment in Shaping Biochemical Individuality

Detoxification and Biochemical Individuality

A 2001 report suggested that between $568 billion and $793 billion is spent per year in Canada and the United States on environmentally-caused disease.[108] We are exposed to a great number of environmental compounds during the course of our lifetime (see Chapter 13 for a discussion of xenobiotics), and many of these compounds show little relationship to previously encountered compounds or metabolites. Our bodies have an extensive network of responses to manage these new and unknown substances and, because the environment is unique to each individual, these responses are at the core of what we mean by "biochemical individuality."

Table 7.2 Commonly Identified Drugs in Adverse Drug Reactions

Category	Name(s) of Drug
Beta-blockers	Atenolol, metoprolol
Angiotensin-converting enzyme inhibitor	Lisinopril
Diuretic	Furosemide, hydrochlorothiazide
Calcium channel blocker	Diltiazem, verapamil
Inotropic agent/pressor	Digoxin
NSAID	Aspirin, ibuprofen, naproxen, piroxicam
Tricyclic antidepressants	Imipramine HCl, nortriptyline HCl
Selective serotonin reuptake inhibitor	Fluoxetine
Antibiotics, antitubercular agents	Amoxicillin, erythromycin, isoniazid, rifampin
Anticoagulant	Warfarin sodium
Corticosteroid	Prednisone
Anticonvulsants	Carbamazepine, phenytoin
Antidiabetic agent	Insulin
Bronchodilators	Theophylline
Electrolytes	Potassium
Antiemetic or antihistamine	Meclizine HCl

Table was compiled from Phillips et al., JAMA. 2001;286(18):2273.

The pathways that have received the most attention to date are the phase I and phase II detoxification enzyme systems, in part because they are involved in drug metabolism and are, therefore, the focus of pharmacogenomics, but also because they are the first-line enzyme defense systems for our interaction with the environment.[109,110] Since these systems are designed to manage environmental exposure, they are also regulated by the environment. Specific detoxification pathways may be induced or inhibited depending on the presence of various dietary or exogenous compounds.[111] Gender, lifestyle habits, nutriture, and health status also influence the relative activities of various detoxification enzymes. Moreover, the detoxification enzymes show a wide variety of polymorphisms. A number of other genes are also involved with management of environmental compounds as well. (Please see Chapters 22 and 31 for more detailed discussions of the mechanisms and clinical implications of detoxification.)

Polymorphisms in enzymes encoding phase I or phase II enzymes have been associated with increased prevalence and/or risk of many conditions including asthma; cancers of the breast, prostate, lungs, esophagus, stomach, and pancreas; multiple chemical sensitivity; and cardiovascular disease.[112,113,114,115,116,117,118] Other enzymes also play important roles in our environmental exposure risks. For example, a polymorphism in the human paraoxonase (PON1) gene—which encodes a high-density lipoprotein-associated enzyme that exerts an antiatherogenic effect by protecting low-density lipoproteins (LDL) against oxidation—has been found to influence both sensitivity to specific insecticides or nerve agents, and the risk of cardiovascular disease.[119] The PON1 polymorphism has also been associated with neurological symptoms in Gulf War syndrome.[120]

Lung cancer mortality is related to smoking; however, only about 15% of the individuals who smoke will be afflicted with this cancer.[121] Tobacco smoke contains a multitude of carcinogens, but many of these carcinogens must be metabolized before they are damaging to the body. It is apparent that much variability exists in these processes.[122] For example, polymorphisms in the glutathione S-transferase (GST) gene have received much attention with respect to health risks from smoking. This enzyme is involved in detoxification of tobacco carcinogens, and studies have found that specific polymorphisms in the GST gene are related to the risk of developing coronary heart disease for smokers.[123]

Although we can cite many examples showing how the environment and specific genetic composition interact, variation in sulfur-dependent pathways is a particularly intriguing area of study. A significant number of individuals who display sensitivity to environmental compounds have impaired sulfation of endogenous compounds, particularly phenolic compounds. In addition, impairment in the sulfation detoxification pathway is associated with such conditions as Alzheimer's disease, Parkinson's disease, motor neuron disease, rheumatoid arthritis, and delayed food sensitivity.[124] Because the sulfur-dependent detoxification pathway depends upon the availability of the sulfur cofactor, and this cofactor is obtained from precursors in the diet, such as methionine, cysteine, and inorganic sulfur, this is an example of a critical interaction involving the environment, nutrition, and genetics.

Biochemical Individuality and Nutrition

Diet is known to have a major impact on chronic disease prevention and management, so it may be no surprise that the diet-gene interaction is the object of much interest from the research community. A new field of study—nutritional genomics (or nutrigenomics)—has been identified to help us understand the effect of nutrients on DNA:

> The link between diet and health is well established, but renewed interest in which dietary components are biologically active and how they exert their effects is being fuelled by the development of nutritional genomics .... Such techniques can facilitate the definition of optimal nutrition at the level of populations, particular groups, and individuals. This in turn should promote the development of food derived treatments and functionally enhanced foods to improve health.[125]

So prevalent is this understanding that it has even found its way onto the front page of consumer magazines such as *Newsweek*, which had a cover story on "Diet and Genes" in January 2005 that included discussions of the role of ingredients in broccoli (e.g., indole-3-carbinol), green tea catechins, and components of soy on gene expression.[126] Unfortunately, many of these discussions still focus on a "one-size-fits all" model for nutrition. However, the impact that the human genome project has had on the scientific knowledge underlying individualization of pharmaceutical interventions is also encompassing nutrition. Emerging data indicate we will soon be able to individualize nutrient interventions, as well as gain a much better understanding of the implications of biochemical individuality for nutrition-oriented public policy.[127,128]

Known genetic polymorphisms that affect nutrition include the hereditary hemochromatosis-linked gene (HFE), which is associated with iron overload; transferrin receptor polymorphisms that influence iron requirements; SNPs in the vitamin D receptor that are associated with bone integrity; SNPs that influence lipid metabolism and cardiovascular health, such as the apolipoproteins and LDL-receptor lipoprotein lipase; and the relationship among PPAR polymorphisms, saturated fat intake, and insulin.[129,130] Presence of specific SNPs can alter the body's metabolism in ways that can be directly observed (as with a disease like hemochromatosis or elevated lipids), or the effects can be more subtle. For example, the ability to observe what is happening at the DNA level has provided evidence that subclinical deficiencies are involved in genome instability, leading to increased DNA damage.[131] The carotenoids, vitamins C, E, and B12, folate, niacin, and zinc appear to be particularly important for genome stability.[132]

Bruce Ames, who has studied the effect of nutrients on oxidative stress and DNA integrity, has noted that as many as one-third of all mutations in a gene result in the corresponding enzyme having an increased Michaelis constant (K_m) for a coenzyme, which means the enzyme has a decreased affinity for its vitamin cofactor.[133] A decreased binding affinity results in a lower rate of reaction and, as noted by Ames, many of these effects can be ameliorated by administration of high doses of the cofactor. (Chapter 26 contains a discussion by Ames on micronutrient insufficiency.)

Perhaps the best understood example integrating findings in nutrition, genetics, and metabolism is that of folate and methylation. Folate is involved in generation of the methylation cofactor S-adenosylmethionine (SAM). A deficiency in SAM is associated with congenital abnormalities, certain cancers, cardiovascular disease, neural tube defects, and peripheral neuropathies. A deficiency in SAM results from disruption in folate metabolism. Cells are highly susceptible to folate deficiency during states of increased folate turnover since they do not accumulate excess folate. Impaired folate metabolism results from insufficient folate intake; gastrointestinal disorders that result in malabsorption; SNPs in genes encoding key pathway enzymes, especially methylenetetrahydrofolate reductase (MTHFR); increased folate catabolism; and deficiencies in vitamins B6, B12, or iron, which are also necessary in the folate-methylation pathway.[134] Of these, a SNP in the methylenetetrahydrofolate reductase (MTHFR) gene has received much research attention (see Figure 7.4).

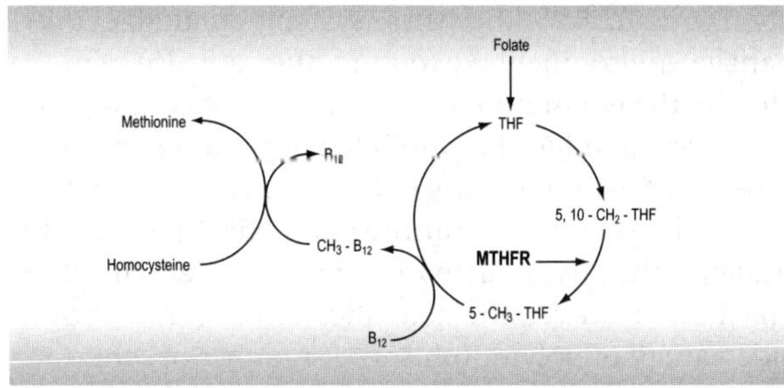

Figure 7.4 **MTHFR SNP**

Function of methylenetetrahydrofolate reductase (MTHFR). MTHFR is required for reduction of 5,10-methylenetetrahydrofolate (5,10-CH_2-THF) to 5-methyltetrahydrofolate (5-CH_3-THF) which serves as a methyl donor for the remethylation of homocysteine to methionine through methylation of cobalamin (vitamin B12) to methylcobalamin (CH3-B12). The most common SNP in this pathway is in the MTHFR, which results in a decreased activity of the MTHFR enzyme, thus influencing the balance of the homocysteine cycle.

The MTHFR polymorphism results in a thermolabile enzyme that is about 50% less active than the wild-type enzyme. Epidemiological studies have shown that this polymorphism, in the presence of low folate intake, results in elevated blood homocysteine levels and is associated with a higher risk of cardiovascular disease.[135] Silaste et al.[136] investigated the plasma homocysteine effects of a low-folate versus a high-folate diet on individuals with SNPs related to metabolism of homocysteine, including the MTHFR gene and the methionine synthase gene. The groups did not initially vary in baseline homocysteine levels. However, after the high-folate diet, although the individuals with the SNP in the MTHFR gene had a smaller increase in serum folate than those with the wild-type gene (55% compared to 85%, respectively), their blood homocysteine levels decreased more (18%) than those without the SNP (11%). A similar effect was also noted with the methionine synthase gene.

A study on the effect of diet on MTHFR polymorphisms, in which 322 men and 252 women participated, noted that about 41% of the individuals had wild-type genes at both alleles (the same gene site on each of the two chromosomes), whereas 48% had one wild-type gene and one with the SNP (heterozygotes), and 11% had SNPs on both alleles (homozygote polymorphism). The group that was homozygous for the polymorphism had higher homocysteine concentrations initially (15.8 ± 9 μmol/L) than either of the other two groups (11.3 ± 8 and 10.8 ± 9 μmol/L).[137] The study found that adherence to a Mediterranean diet was associated with reduced homocysteine in individuals with either of the alleles containing the SNP for the MTHFR, but not in those individuals who had only the wild-type genes. This study suggests that some individuals may be more responsive to specific dietary interventions than others, based upon the presence of specific DNA sequences.

Effects of Early Life on Biochemical Individuality

An intriguing area of research is the effect of early life on gene expression patterns. In a research review published in the journal *Science* in September 2004,[138] Gluckman and Hanson discuss the hypothesis that some chronic diseases in adulthood are influenced by environmental factors in the periconceptual, fetal, and infant phases of early life, a model called the "development origins of health and disease." We often think that chronic degenerative disease appears in mid-life as a consequence of something we did in mid-life, but this model suggests that very early life can influence patterns of gene expression and the risk of developing certain diseases.[139] In particular, studies in several mammalian species demonstrate that manipulation of the periconceptual, embryonic, fetal, or neonatal environment can lead to altered postnatal cardiovascular and/or metabolic function.[140,141,142] Most of these influences appear to be related to diet and include maternal undernutrition, low-protein diet, or high-fat diet. Factors such as nutrition, stress, and environmental toxins in early phases of life may combine to set in motion a trajectory leading toward dysfunction in middle age. This presents an entirely different responsibility for the healthcare system (and for all of us, as future patients); rather than just waiting until disease develops, a patient's health plan needs to begin at the time of (or even before) conception.

Epigenetic Effects

We now know that biochemical individuality is more than just a difference in gene sequence. One can easily postulate today that two fertilized eggs placed in different *in utero* environments will develop into individuals with different physiology. In a fascinating twist, studies with identical twins have also shown us that biochemical individuality can occur even when the genetics are the same and the environment is presumably the same for both individuals. This introduces the concept of epigenetic effects.

Epigenetics is the study of heritable changes in DNA function without a change in DNA sequence. Epigenetics includes mechanisms that alter activation and expression of genes, such as methylation at specific sites on DNA, histone acetylation, and modification of DNA function by RNA. Therefore, although a major focus of today's research is on identifying gene sequences and polymorphisms, it is important to heed the following caution expressed eloquently by Walter Willett,[143] from the Harvard School of Public Health:

> Genetic and environmental factors, including diet and life-style, both contribute to cardiovascular disease, cancers, and other major causes of mortality, but various lines of evidence indicate that environmental factors are most important. Overly enthusiastic expectations regarding the benefits of genetic research for disease prevention have the potential to distort research priorities and spending for health. However, integration of new genetic information into epidemiologic studies can help clarify causal relations between both life-style and genetic factors and risks of disease. Thus, a balanced approach should provide the best data to make informed choices about the most effective means to prevent disease.

Proteomics and Metabolomics

In a concept paper in the journal *Nature,* Paul Nurse,[144] from the Cell Cycle Laboratory Cancer Research at UK Lincoln's Inn Fields, London, wrote:

> Many of the properties that characterize living organisms are also exhibited by individual cells. These include communication, homeostasis, spatial and temporal organization, reproduction, and adaptation to external stimuli. Biological explanations of these complex phenomena are often based on the logical and informational processes that underpin the mechanisms involved ... . Most experimental investigations of cells, however, do not readily yield such explanations, because they usually put greater emphasis on molecular and biochemical descriptions of phenomena. To explain logical and informational processes on a cellular level, therefore, we need to devise new ways to obtain and analyze data, particularly those generated by genomic and post-genomic studies.

Clearly, today's understanding of genomics represents just the tip of the proverbial iceberg with respect to a full understanding of how the body functions and, from that, the differences among us. The genome may be the blueprint for the proteins and structures in our body, but it is the proteins that carry out functions, and the small molecules that result from protein activities that are the pillars of the signaling and communication activities throughout our bodies. Since many changes occur at once, and specific interactions or patterns can result in different outcomes, new technologies have been developed to look at multiple genes at one time. These are collectively called "microarray analysis technology" or the "gene array." These different gene expression patterns can result in a variety of different protein activity patterns. "Proteomics" is the term that has been coined to describe the study of multiple proteins at once, or protein expression/activity patterns. Proteomics is more difficult to perform from a technological standpoint, since each protein is chemically different. DNA is chemically the same; it's the pattern of bases in the DNA that changes. Gene array technology and large-scale genotyping are increasing our knowledge base every day.[145] Likewise, although proteomics is still in its infancy, technologies are also changing how medical research is being conducted.[146,147]

The greatest promise for understanding biochemical uniqueness is likely to manifest through a deeper understanding at the level of the metabolome. The scientific community is in the process of developing the technologies to quantify entire classes of metabolites; understanding the pattern of these metabolites is called "metabolomics."[148] The metabolome looks at entire biochemical pathways to understand the integrated effects of environment, toxins, nutrients, and genetics on complex metabolic regulation and tissue composition. Through the use of genomics, proteomics, and metabolomics, we can better understand, for example, the 50% concordance rate in identical twins for developing diseases such as type 1 diabetes, or the complexity of establishing breast cancer risk.[149] These technologies may even change how we look at disease. As stated by Gerling et al. in the January 2003 issue of *Archives of Internal Medicine*:[150]

> Since many different genetic defects and molecular pathways may produce clinically indistinguishable disease presentations, many disorders currently viewed as single entities may become divided into large numbers of distinct molecular diseases, with treatment increasingly targeted at the unique primary molecular defect. This will challenge currently accepted definitions of terms such as *disease*, *disorder*, and *syndrome*, as each may come to denote particular genetic components or signature molecular abnormalities, or imply an optimal mode of genetically based and/or conventional treatment. Indeed, our present difficulties in defining the gene(s) involved in many of the major diseases may be because we are studying large pools of very divergent molecular "syndromes" with the same clinical presentation. This may also explain why many treatments are only effective in certain patients.

Biochemical Individuality and the Future

Biochemical individuality is not such a new concept; it's our understanding of what it really means that is continuing to evolve. The concept of genetic predisposition is a way of indicating that we are all different, that we may have a gene that "predisposes" us to some particular condition, but the condition may not be realized unless certain other factors are also present. We are already seeing that the success of the Human Genome Project is creating a better understanding of biochemical individuality and how it can be used to improve disease prevention and management. However, fully implementing this knowledge to improve health outcomes depends on several further developments in research technology. In particular, we must develop the following technical capacities:

1. the ability to detect genetic variation that is silent or undetectable at the level of the phenotype;
2. the ability to analyze the role of epigenetics in genetic variation;
3. the ability to quantify the impact of environment on specific genetic variation patterns;
4. the ability to identify patterns of protein activities through proteomics; and
5. the ability to fully integrate changes in metabolism and entire metabolic pathways by pattern analysis.

As stated eloquently by Robert Eckhardt[151] in a review on genetics and nutritional individuality:

> The latest nutritional guidelines (Murphy 2001)[ii] incorporate recommended daily allowance for some 30 nutrients. If the metabolic pathway influencing nutritional requirements for each of these nutrients was affected independently by only two alternative alleles at a single genetic locus (almost certainly a substantial underestimate of systemic complexity), then we should expect that the number of alternative genotypes would be 3^{30} or in excess of 200 trillion; three alternative alleles would raise the level of potential diversity to 6^{30}, i.e., over a billion times higher. The advancing wave of

[ii] Murphy SP. How consideration of population variance and individuality affects our understanding of nutritional requirements in human health and disease. J Nutr. 2001;131:361S-65S.

knowledge about the human genome has confirmed the idea that each of us must be genetically unique in our nutritional needs.

Furthermore, although much of the initial focus of genomics, proteomics, and metabolomics has been on ADRs, drug metabolism, environmental interactions, and nutrient needs, research in inflammation and immune system function is also finding distinct, important differences that affect health.[152,153,154,155] Taken together, the differential effects of the genomics, environment, nutrition, and epigenetic influences indicates that we are all, clearly, biochemically individual.

References

1. Kuhn TS. The Structure of Scientific Revolutions. Chicago, Ill: University of Chicago Press; 1970.
2. Goodwin JS, Goodwin JM. The tomato effect: rejection of highly efficacious therapies. JAMA. 1984;251(18);2387-90.
3. http://www.uh.edu/engines/epi1015.htm
4. McCully K. Homocysteine, folate, vitamin B6 and cardiovascular disease. JAMA. 1998:279(5);392-93.
5. Taubes, G. The soft science of dietary fat. Science. 2001;291:2536-45.
6. Fletcher SW, Colditz GA. Failure of estrogen plus progestin therapy for prevention. JAMA. 2002;288(3):366-68.
7. Nelson HD, et al. Postmenopausal hormone replacement therapy: scientific review. JAMA. 2002;288(7):872-81.
8. Starfield B. Is US health really the best in the world? JAMA. 2000;284(4):483-85.
9. Starfield B. Deficiencies in US medical care. JAMA. 2000;284(17):2184-85.
10. Zhan C, Miller M. Excess length of stay, charges, and mortality attributable to medical injuries during hospitalization. JAMA. 2003;290:1868-74.
11. Fourth Decennial International Conference on Nosocomial and Healthcare Associated Infections. Morb Mortal Wkly Rep. 2000;49(7):138.
12. Weinstein RA. Nosocomial infection update. Special issue. Emerg Infect Dis. 1998;4(3):416-20.
13. Lazarou J, Pomeranz B, Corey P. Incidence of adverse drug reactions in hospitalized patients. JAMA. 1998;279:1200-05.
14. Barczak CA, Barnett RI, Childs EJ, Bosley LM. Fourth national pressure ulcer prevalence survey. Adv Wound Care. 1997;10:4.
15. Leape LL. Error in medicine. JAMA. 1994;272(23):1851-57.
16. Brennan TA, et al. Incidence of adverse events and negligence in hospitalized patients. N Engl J Med. 1991;324:370-76.
17. US Congressional House Subcommittee Oversight Investigation. Cost and Quality of Health Care: Unnecessary Surgery. Washington, DC: Government Printing Office. 1976.
18. Heaney R. Long-latency deficiency disease: insights from calcium and vitamin D. Am J Clin Nutr. 2003;78:912-19.
19. Fonda, D. Curbing the drug marketers. Time. July 5, 2004: p 40-42.
20. Rosenthal MB, Berndt ER, Donohue JM, et al. Promotion of prescription drugs to consumers. N Engl J Med. 2002;346(7):498-505.
21. Wolfe SM. Direct-to-consumer advertising--education or emotion promotion? N Engl J Med. 2002;346(7):524-26.
22. Fonda D. Curbing the drug marketers. Time. July 5, 2004; p 40-42.
23. Adams C, Young A. Prescription for trouble: Drugmakers pushing risky off-label uses on physicians. Nov 4, 2003, Knight Ridder, www.freep.com/news/health/drugs4_20031104.htm.
24. Mack A. Examination of the evidence for off-label use of gabapentin. J Manag Care Pharm. 2003;9(6):559-68.
25. Kassirer JP. Financial conflicts of interest in biomedical research. N Engl J Med. 1993;329:570-71.
26. Shamasunder B, Bero L. Financial ties and conflicts of interest between pharmaceutical and tobacco companies. JAMA. 2002;288(6):738-44.
27. Korn D. Conflicts of interest in biomedical research. JAMA. 2000;284(17):2234-38.
28. Choudhry NK, et al. Relationships between authors of clinical practice guidelines and the pharmaceutical industry. JAMA. 2002;287(5):612-17.
29. Nathan DG, Weatherall DJ. Academic freedom in clinical research. N Engl J Med. 2002;347:1368-71.
30. Bekelman JE, et al. Scope and impact of financial conflicts of interest in biomedical research: a systematic review. JAMA. 2003;289:454-65.
31. Dong B, Hauck W, Gambertoglio J, et al. Bioequivalence of generic and brand-name levothyroxine. JAMA. 1997;277:1205-13.
32. Rennie D. Thyroid storm. JAMA. 1997;277:1238-43.
33. Holmer A. Industry strongly supports continuing medical education. JAMA. 2001;285:2012-14.
34. Steinbrook R. Perspective: Commercial support and continuing medical education. N Engl J Med. 2005;352(6):534-35.
35. Relman A. Separating continuing medical education from pharmaceutical marketing. JAMA. 2001;285:2009-12.
36. Relman A. Your Doctor's Drug Problem. The New York Times. Nov 18, 2003.
37. Goodman B. Do drug company promotions influence physician behavior? West J Med. 2001;174:232-33.
38. Fisher ES. The implications of regional variations in medicare spending. Part 2: Health outcomes and satisfaction with care. Ann Intern Med. 2003:138(4);288-98.
39. Fisher ES. Medical care—is more always better? N Engl J Med. 2003;349(17):1665-67.
40. Lenfant C. Shattuck lecture: Clinical research to clinical practice—lost in translation? N Engl J Med. 2003;349:868-74.
41. McGlynn EA. The quality of health care delivered to adults in the United States. N Engl J Med. 2003;348:2635-45.
42. Holman H. Chronic disease—the need for a new clinical education. JAMA. 2004;292(9):1057-59.
43. Johns MME. The time has come to reform graduate medical education. JAMA. 2001;286(9):1075-76.
44. Crookshank FG. The importance of a theory of signs: critique of language in the study of medicine. Supplement II. In: Ogden CK, Richards IA. The Meaning of Meaning. New York, NY: Harcourt Brace; 1923.
45. Van Ommen GJB. The human genome project and the future of diagnostics, treatment and prevention. Lancet. 1999;354:5-10.
46. Holman H. Chronic disease—the need for a new clinical education. JAMA. 2004;292(9):1057-59.
47. Crookshank FG. The importance of a theory of signs: critique of language in the study of medicine. Supplement II. In: Ogden CK, Richards IA. The Meaning of Meaning. New York, NY: Harcourt Brace; 1923.
48. Bertalanffy L. General systems theory. New York, NY: Brazillier, 1971.
49. Radford T. Top scientist warns of "sickness" in US health system. BMJ. 2003;326:416.
50. Lundberg GD. Severed Trust: Why American Medicine Hasn't Been Fixed. New York, NY; Basic Books. 2000.
51. Deutch D. The Fabric of Reality. New York, NY: Penguin Putnam Inc.: 1997.

52. Lafaille R. Towards the foundation of a new science of health. In: Lafaille R, Fulder S, eds. Towards a New Science of Health. New York, NY: Routledge, 1993:p. 13.
53. Pauling, Linus. How to Live Longer and Feel Better. Avon Books, 1986.
54. Encarta®World English Dictionary. 1999. Microsoft Corporation. All rights reserved. Developed for Microsoft by Bloomsbury Publishing Plc.
55. Kornman KS, Martha PM, Duff GW. Genetic variations and inflammation: a practical nutrigenomics opportunity. Nutrition. 2004;20(1):44-49.
56. Chopra SS. Preparing for personalized medicine. JAMA. 2004;291(13):1640-45.
57. Kaput J, Rodriguez RL. Nutritional genomics: the next frontier in the postgenomic era. Physiol Genomics. 2004;16:166-77.
58. Kornman KS, Martha PM, Duff GW. Genetic variations and inflammation: a practical nutrigenomics opportunity. Nutrition. 2004;20(1):44-49.
59. Norhammar A. Glucose metabolism in patients with acute myocardial infarction and no previous diagnosis of diabetes mellitus: a prospective study. Lancet. 2002;359:2140-44.
60. McCully K. Homocysteine, folate, vitamin B6 and cardiovascular disease. JAMA. 1998:279(5);392-93.
61. Murat V. Chlamydia pneumoniae as an emerging risk factor in cardiovascular disease. JAMA. 2002;288:2724-31.
62. Gullar L. Mercury, fish oils and the risk of myocardial infarction. N Engl J Med. 2002;347:1747-54.
63. Yoshizawa K. Mercury and the risk of coronary heart disease. N Engl J Med. 2002;347:1755-60.
64. Ridker P. Comparison of C-reactive protein and low-density lipoprotein cholesterol levels in the prediction of first cardiovascular events. N Engl J Med. 2002;347:1557-65.
65. Kaput J. Diet-disease gene interactions. Nutrition. 2004;20:26-31.
66. Patient report from Mark Hyman, MD.
67. Hadjivassiliou M, et al. Gluten sensitivity: a many-headed hydra. BMJ. 1999;318:1710-11.
68. Fasano A. Celiac disease—How to handle a clinical chameleon. N Engl J Med. 2003;348(25):2568-70.
69. Farrell RJ, Kelly CP. Celiac sprue. N Engl J Med. 2002;346:180-88.
70. Holick M. Vitamin D: importance in the prevention of cancers, type 1 diabetes, heart disease and osteoporosis. Am J Clin Nutr. 2004;79:362-71.
71. Vasquez A, Manso G, Cannell J. The clinical importance of vitamin D (cholecalciferol): a paradigm shift with implications for all healthcare providers. Altern Ther Health Med. 2004;10(5):28-36.
72. Ames B. Cancer prevention and diet: Help from single nucleotide polymorphisms. Proc Natl Acad Sci USA. 1999;96(22):12216-18.
73. Goodwin JS, Tangum MR. Battling quackery: attitudes about micronutrient supplements in American medicine. Arch Intern Med. 1998;158(9):2187-91.
74. Ames B. Cancer prevention and diet: Help from single nucleotide polymorphisms. Proc Natl Acad Sci USA. 1999;96(22):12216-18.
75. Ames B. High dose vitamin therapy stimulates variant enzymes with decreased coenzyme binding affinity (increased Km): relevance to genetic disease and polymorphisms. Am J Clin Nutr. 2002:75:616-58.
76. Baker SM. The medicine we are evolving. Integr Med. Dec 2002/Jan 2003;1(1):14-15.
77. Fairfield K. Vitamins for chronic disease prevention in adults. JAMA. 2002;287:3116-26.
78. Ames B. A role for supplements in optimizing health: the metabolic tune-up. Arch Biochem Biophys. 2004;423:227-34.
79. Vickers A, Zollman C. ABC of complementary medicine: Unconventional approaches to nutritional medicine. BMJ. 1999;319:1419-22.
80. Heaney RP. Editorial: Vitamin D, nutritional deficiency, and the medical paradigm. J Clin Endocrinol Metab. 2003:88(11):5107-08.
81. Heaney R. Long-latency deficiency disease: insights from calcium and vitamin D. Am J Clin Nutr. 2003;78:912-19.
82. Ibid.
83. Kaput J, Rodriguez RL. Nutritional genomics: the next frontier in the post genomic era. Physiol Genomics. 2004;16:166–77.
84. Pharmaceutical Patient Compliance and Disease Management. http://www.PharmaDiseaseManagement.com.
85. Breslow L. From disease prevention to health promotion. JAMA. 1999;281:1030-33.
86. Muller M. Nutrigenomics: goals and strategies. Nat Rev Genet. 2003;4:315-22.
87. Laing RD. The Voice of Experience. New York, NY: Pantheon; 1982.
88. Kaput J, Rodriguez RL. Nutritional genomics: the next frontier in the post genomic era. Physiol Genomics. 2004;16:166–77.
89. Eckhardt RB. Genetic research and nutritional individuality. J Nutr. 2001;131:336S-39S.
90. Williams RJ. Biochemical Individuality: The basis for the genetotrophic concept. New Canaan, CT: Keats Publ. 1998.
91. Williams RJ, Beerstecher E Jr, Berry LJ. The concept of genetotrophic disease. Lancet. 1950;1(7):287-89.
92. Gerling IC, Solomon SS, Bryer-Ash M. Genomes, transcriptomes, and proteomes. Arch Intern Med. 2003;163:190-98.
93. Lazarou J, Pomeranz BH, Corey PN. Incidence of adverse drug reactions in hospitalized patients. JAMA. 1998;279:1200-5.
94. Letters to JAMA: Adverse drug reactions in hospitalized patients. JAMA. 1998;280:1741-43.
95. Phillips KA, Veenstra DL, Oren E, et al. Potential role of pharmacogenomics in reducing adverse drug reactions. JAMA. 2001;286:2270-79.
96. Cohen JS. Ways to minimize adverse drug reactions. Postgraduate Med. 1999;106:163-172.
97. Wortman M. Medicine gets personal. Tech Rev. 2001;January/February:72-78.
98. Connor S. Glaxo chief: Our drugs do not work on most patients. Accessed online December 11, 2003 at: http://news.independent.co.uk/low_res/story.jsp?story=471139&host=3&dir=505.
99. Abbott A. With your genes? Take one of these, three times a day. Nature. 2003;425(6960):760-62.
100. Aithal GP, Day CP, Kesteven PJ, Daly AK. Association of polymorphisms in the cytochrome P450 CYP2C9 with warfarin dose requirement and risk of bleeding complications. Lancet. 1998;353:717-19.
101. Palkimas MP Jr, Skinner HM, Gandhi PJ, Gardner AJ. Polymorphism induced sensitivity to warfarin: a review of the literature. J Thromb Thrombolysis. 2003;15:205-12.
102. Aithal GP, Day CP, Kesteven PJ, Daly AK. Association of polymorphisms in the cytochrome P450 CYP2C9 with warfarin dose requirement and risk of bleeding complications. Lancet. 1998;353:717-19.
103. Ogg MS, Brennan P, Meade T, Humphries SE. CYP2C9*3 allelic variant and bleeding complications. Lancet. 1999;354:1124.
104. Palkimas MP Jr, Skinner HM, Gandhi PJ, Gardner AJ. Polymorphism induced sensitivity to warfarin: a review of the literature. J Thromb Thrombolysis. 2003;15:205-12.
105. Topic E, Stefanovic M, Samardzija M. Association between the CYP2C9 polymorphism and the drug metabolism phenotype. Clin Chem Lab Med. 2004;42(1):72-78.

106. You JH, Chan FW, Wong RS, Cheng G. The potential clinical and economic outcomes of pharmacogenetics-oriented management of warfarin therapy—a decision analysis. Thromb Haemost. 2004;92(3):590-97.
107. Phillips KA, Veenstra DL, Oren E, et al. Potential role of pharmacogenomics in reducing adverse drug reactions. JAMA. 2001;286:2270-79.
108. Muir T, Zegarac M. Societal costs of exposure to toxic substances: economic and health costs of four case studies that are candidates for environmental causation. Environ Health Perspect. 2001;109 Suppl 6:885-903.
109. Ingelman-Sundberg M. Genetic susceptibility to adverse effects of drugs and environmental toxicants. The role of the CYP family of enzymes. Mutation Res. 2001;482:11-19.
110. Meyer UA, Zanger UM, Grant D, Blum M. Genetic polymorphisms of drug metabolism. Adv Drug Res. 1990;19:198-241.
111. Liska DJ. The detoxification enzyme systems. Altern Med Rev. 1998;3:187-198.
112. Tamer L, Calikoglu M, Ates NA, et al. Glutathione-S-transferase gene polymorphisms (GSTT1, GSTM1, GSTP1) as increased risk factors for asthma. Respirology. 2004;9(4):493-98.
113. Sazci A, Ergul E, Utkan NZ, et al. Catechol-O-methyltransferase Val 108/158 Met polymorphism in premenopausal breast cancer patients. Toxicology. 2004;204(2-3):197-202.
114. Nakazato H, Suzuki K, Matsui H, et al. Association of genetic polymorphisms of glutathione-S-transferase genes (GSTM1, GSTT1 and GSTP1) with familial prostate cancer risk in a Japanese population. Anticancer Res. 2003;23(3C):2897-2902.
115. Shi WX, Chen SQ. Frequencies of poor metabolizers of cytochrome P450 2C19 in esophagus cancer, stomach cancer, lung cancer, and bladder cancer in Chinese population. World J Gastroenterol. 2004;10(13):1961-63.
116. Ockenga J, Vogel A, Teich N, et al. UDP glucuronosyltransferase (UGT1A7) gene polymorphisms increase the risk of chronic pancreatitis and pancreatic cancer. Gastroenterology. 2003;124(7):1802-8.
117. McKeown-Eyssen G, Baines C, Cole DE, et al. Case-control study of genotypes in multiple chemical sensitivity: CYP2D6, NAT1, NAT2, PON1, PON2 and MTHFR. Int J Epidemiol. 2004;33(5):971-978.
118. Costa LG, Cole TB, Jarvik GP, Furlong CE. Functional genomic of the paraoxonase (PON1) polymorphisms: effects on pesticide sensitivity, cardiovascular disease, and drug metabolism. Annu Rev Med. 2003;54:371-392.
119. Ibid.
120. McKeown-Eyssen G, Baines C, Cole DE, et al. Case-control study of genotypes in multiple chemical sensitivity: CYP2D6, NAT1, NAT2, PON1, PON2 and MTHFR. Int J Epidemiol. 2004;33(5):971-78.
121. http://adam.about.com/reports/000072_3.htm
122. Miller MC III, Mohrenweiser HW, Bell DA. Genetic variability in susceptibility and response to toxicants. Toxicology Lett. 2001;120:269-80.
123. Tamer L, Ercan B, Camsari A, et al. Glutathione S-transferase gene polymorphism as a susceptibility factor in smoking-related coronary artery disease. Basic Res Cardiol. 2004;99(3):223-29.
124. McFadden SA. Phenotypic variation in xenobiotic metabolism and adverse environmental response: focus on sulfur-dependent detoxification pathways. Toxicology. 1996;111:43-65.
125. Elliott R, Ong, TJ. Science, medicine, and the future. BMJ. 2002;324:1438-42.
126. Underwood A, Adler J. Diet & Genes. Newsweek. 2005;January 17: 40-48.
127. Gibney MJ, Gibney ER. Diet, genes and disease: implications for nutrition policy. Proc Nutr Soc. 2004;63:491-500.
128. Stover PJ, Garza C. Bringing individuality to public health recommendations. J Nutr. 2002;132:2476S-80S.
129. Gibney MJ, Gibney ER. Diet, genes and disease: implications for nutrition policy. Proc Nutr Soc. 2004;63:491-500.
130. Elliott R, Ong, TJ. Science, medicine, and the future. BMJ. 2002;324:1438-42.
131. Fenech M. Micronutrients and genomic stability: a new paradigm for recommended dietary allowances (RDAs). Food Chem Toxicol. 2002;40:1113-17.
132. Fenech M. Recommended dietary allowances (RDAs) for genomic stability. Mutation Res. 2001;480-81:51-54.
133. Ames BN. A role for supplements in optimizing health: the metabolic tune-up. Arch Biochem Biophys. 2004;423(1):227-34.
134. Stover PJ, Garza C. Bringing individuality to public health recommendations. J Nutr. 2002;132:2476S-80S.
135. Gibney MJ, Gibney ER. Diet, genes and disease: implications for nutrition policy. Proc Nutr Soc. 2004;63:491-500.
136. Silaste M-L, Rantala M, Sämpi M, et al. Polymorphisms of key enzymes in homocysteine metabolism affect diet responsiveness of plasma homocysteine in healthy women. J Nutr. 2001;131:2643-47.
137. Dedoussis GV, Panagiotakos DB, Chrysohoou C, et al. Effect of interaction between adherence to a Mediterranean diet and the methylenetetrahydrofolate reductase 677C→T mutation on homocysteine concentrations in healthy adults: the ATTICA Study. Am J Clin Nutr. 2004;80:849-54.
138. Gluckman PD, Hanson MA. Living with the past: evolution, development, and patterns of disease. Science. 2004;305:1733-36.
139. Coe CL, Lubach GR. Prenatal origins of individual variation in behavior and immunity. Neurosci Biobehav Rev. 2005;29(1):39-49.
140. Rhind SM, Rae MT, Brooks AN. Environmental influences on the fetus and neonate—timing, mechanisms of action and effects on subsequent adult function. Domest Anim Endocrinol. 2003;25(1):3-11.
141. Roghair RD, Lamb FS, Miller FJ Jr, et al. Early gestation dexamethasone programs enhanced postnatal ovine coronary artery vascular reactivity. Am J Physiol Regul Integr Comp Physiol. 2005;288(1):R46-53.
142. Jones RD, Morice AH, Emery CJ. Effects of perinatal exposure to hypoxia upon the pulmonary circulation of the adult rat. Physiol Res. 2004;53:11-17.
143. Willett WC. Balancing life-style and genomics research for disease prevention. Science. 2002;296:695-98.
144. Nurse P. Understanding cells. Nature. 2003;424(6951):883.
145. Kennedy GC, Matsuzaki H, Dong S, et al. Large-scale genotyping of complex DNA. Nature Biotechnol. 2003;21(10):1233-37.
146. Liotta LA, Ferrari M, Petricoin E. Written in blood. Nature. 2003;425(6961):905.
147. Leung D, Hardouin C, Boger DL, Cravatt BF. Discovering potent and selective reversible inhibitors of enzymes in complex proteomes. Nature Biotechnol. 2003;21(6):687-91.
148. German JB, Roberts MA, Fay L, Watkins SM. Metabolomics and individual metabolic assessment: the next great challenge for nutrition. J Nutr. 2002;132:2486-87.
149. Dumitrescu RG, Cotarla I. Understanding breast cancer risk—where do we stand in 2005? J Cell Mol Med. 2005;9(1):208-21.
150. Gerling IC, Solomon SS, Bryer-Ash M. Genomes, transcriptomes, and proteomes. Arch Intern Med. 2003;163:190-98.
151. Eckhardt RB. Genetic research and nutritional individuality. J Nutr. 2001;131:336S-39S.
152. Franceschi C, Olivieri F, Marchegiani F, et al. Genes involved in immune response/inflammation, IGF1/insulin pathway and response to oxidative stress play a major role in the genetics of human longevity: the lesson of centenarians. Mech Ageing Dev. 2005;126(2):351-61.

153. Felley-Bosco E, Andre M. Proteomics and chronic inflammatory bowel disease. Pathol Res Pract. 2004;200(2):129-33.
154. Kornman KS, Martha PM, Duff GW. Genetic variations and inflammation: a practical nutrigenomics opportunity. Nutrition. 2004;20:44-49.
155. van der Pouw Kraan TC, Kasperkovitz PV, Verbeet N, Verweij CL. Genomics in the immune system. Clin Immunol. 2004;111(2):175-85.

Chapter 8
Patient-centered Care: Antecedents, Triggers, and Mediators

Leo Galland, MD

It is more important to know what person has the disease than which disease the person has.
—William Osler

The purpose of this chapter is to present an **organizational structure** for assessment of patients as unique individuals, an approach I have called person-centered diagnosis.[1] The goal of person-centered diagnosis is to enable healers to develop individualized treatment plans that are based upon an understanding of the physiological, environmental, and psychosocial contexts within which each person's illnesses or dysfunctions occur. The information you need to effectively apply this organizational structure fills the remainder of this textbook. My goal here is to describe and illustrate the structure. To create it, you must start by eliciting all of the patient's concerns. In actively listening to the patient's story, you attempt to discover the **antecedents, triggers** and **mediators** that underlie symptoms, signs, illness behaviors, and demonstrable pathology. Functional medicine is based upon treatment that is collaborative, flexible, and focused on the control or reversal of each person's individual antecedents, triggers and mediators, rather than the treatment of disease entities.

Eliciting the Patient's Story

The first step in patient-centered care is eliciting the patient's story in a comprehensive manner. It is the functional medicine practitioner's job to know not just the ailments or their diagnoses, but the physical and social environment in which sickness occurs, the dietary habits of the person who is sick (present diet and pre-illness diet), his beliefs about the illness, the impact of illness on social and psychological function, factors that aggravate or ameliorate symptoms, and factors that predispose to illness or facilitate recovery. This information is necessary for establishing a functional treatment plan.

The importance of understanding the patient's experience of his/her illness cannot be overemphasized. Extensive research on doctor-patient interactions indicates that doctors who fail to pay attention to the patient's concerns miss important clinical information. The conventional diagnostic paradigm, differential diagnosis, leads doctors to ignore or denigrate information that patients consider important, or that influences individual prognosis.[2,3,4] Not only does this ignorance impair the effectiveness of treatment,[5] it generates considerable dissatisfaction among patients.[6,7,8]

Extensive research done within the context of conventional medical care reveals what most patients know: doctors do not pay enough attention to what their patients have to say. A study done at the University of Rochester found that most patients have three reasons for visiting a physician, are interrupted within 18 seconds of starting to tell their stories, and never get the chance to finish.[9] Although doctors excuse this behavior by citing lack of time, it would have taken an average of one minute and rarely more than three minutes for a complete list of problems to be elicited.

Even when doctors know what their patients' concerns are, they typically ignore them.[10] Most patients have different ideas about their illnesses than their doctors and some form of clarification or negotiation is needed for an effective therapeutic alliance to be established.[11] A study that carefully analyzed taped transcripts of visits to a medical clinic found that patients attempted to clarify or challenge what their doctor had said in 85% of the visits. Their requests were usually ignored or interrupted.[12] Understanding the patient's perspective allows the doctor to work in a collaborative way with patients, giving information that helps the patient make healthful choices.[13] The more information the patient receives from the doctor and the more actively the patient is involved in making decisions about treatment, the higher the level of mutual satisfaction, and the better the clinical outcome.[14,15,16,17,18] A systematic review of randomized clinical trials and analytic studies of physician-patient communication confirmed a positive influence of quality communication on health outcomes.[19] Such a collaborative relationship depends upon the practitioner recognizing and acknowledging the patient's experience of the illness. Useful questions to ask include:

- How are you hoping that I can help you today?
- What do you believe is the source of your problems?
- What kind of treatment are you looking for?
- What do you most fear about your illness?
- What impact have your symptoms had on your life?

Organizing and Analyzing the Patient's Story

What modern science has taught us about the genesis of disease can be represented by three words: triggers, mediators, and antecedents. Triggers are discrete entities or events that provoke disease or its symptoms. Microbes are an example. The greatest scientific discovery of the 19th century was the microbial etiology of the major epidemic diseases. Triggers are usually insufficient in and of themselves for disease formation, however. Host response is an essential component. Identifying the biochemical mediators that underlie host responses was the most productive field of biomedical research during the second half of the 20th century. Mediators, as the word implies, do not "cause" disease. They are intermediaries that contribute to the manifestations of disease. Antecedents are factors that predispose to acute or chronic illness. For a person who is ill, they form the illness diathesis. From the perspective of prevention, they are risk factors. Knowledge of antecedents has provided a rational structure for the organization of preventive medicine and public health. Medical genomics seeks to better understand disease by identifying the phenotypic expression of disease-related genes and their products. The application of genomic science to clinical medicine requires the integration of antecedents (genes and the factors controlling their expression) with mediators (the downstream products of gene activation). Mediators, triggers, and antecedents are not only key biomedical concepts, they are also important psychosocial concepts. In person-centered diagnosis, the mediators, triggers, and antecedents for each person's illness form the focus of clinical investigation.

Antecedents and the Origins of Illness

Understanding the antecedents of illness helps the physician understand the unique characteristics of each patient as they relate to his or her current health status. Antecedents may be thought of as congenital or developmental. The most important congenital factor is gender: women and men differ markedly in susceptibility to many disorders. The most important developmental factor is age; what ails children is rarely the same as what ails the elderly. Beyond these obvious factors lies a diversity as complex as the genetic differences and separate life experiences that distinguish one person from another.

Congenital factors may be inherited or acquired *in utero*. They can most readily be evaluated from a comprehensive family history, including mother's health before and during pregnancy. Genomic analysis, which is now commercially available, can supplement the family health history as a tool for investigating unique nutritional needs or individual variability in sensitivity to environmental toxins.[20,21] The commonest single gene disorders in North America, celiac disease and hemochromatosis, may be confirmed by the presence of genetic markers, but should first be suspected from abnormalities in routine lab tests. Elevated serum ferritin concentration or transferrin saturation should prompt genetic testing for the alleles associated with hereditary hemochromatosis.[22] Increased small intestinal permeability, as measured by the inexpensive, non-invasive and under-utilized lactulose/mannitol challenge test, has a sensitivity approaching 100% for untreated celiac disease.[23] Abnormal intestinal permeability should prompt the measurement of celiac-specific immune markers in patients with chronic fatigue, autoimmune disorders, or chronic gastrointestinal complaints of any type.

Normal intestinal permeability in patients consuming gluten almost always excludes celiac disease as a consideration; however, this may not necessarily be the case for other gluten-sensitive disorders. Because celiac disease and gluten-sensitive disorders are common, have protean manifestations, and can be well controlled by nutritional interventions, intestinal permeability should be a routine component of the laboratory testing for antecedents of illness. The treatment of choice for frank hemochromatosis is phlebotomy, but mild iron overload without frank hemochromatosis is more common than the full-blown disease. These patients generally have only one of the alleles associated with the disease, but have elevated transferrin saturation and/or ferritin. They are not treated with phlebotomy, and should be treated with dietary interventions. They should not take iron or vitamin C supplements, because vitamin C reduces iron to its more toxic form.

Some familial disorders may reflect intra-uterine rather than genetic influences. Twin studies of hypertension, for example, indicate a higher concordance for blood pressure between identical twins with a common placenta than identical twins with separate placentas.[24] Presumably, the shared placenta mediates subtle nutritional influences that affect a tendency toward chronic illness in adulthood.

Post-natal developmental factors that govern the predisposition to illness include nutrition, exposure to toxins, trauma, learned patterns of behavior, and the microbial ecology of the body. Sexual abuse in childhood, for example, is associated with an increased risk of abdominal and pelvic pain syndromes among women.[25,26] Recurrent otitis media increases the risk of a child developing attention deficit disorder,[27,28] an effect that is not associated with hearing loss but may result from the effects of antibiotics on the microbial ecology of the gut.

Precipitating events are critical antecedents that closely precede the development of chronic illness. They represent a boundary in time: before this event, the person was considered healthy; since the event, the person has become a patient. Understanding the nature of the precipitating event may aid in unraveling the triggers and mediators that maintain the state of illness. The commonest precipitating events among my patients are a period of severe psychosocial distress, an acute infection (sometimes treated with antibiotics), exposure to environmental toxins at work or home, or severe nutrient depletion related to illness or crash dieting. Useful questions for uncovering precipitating events include:

- When is the last time you felt really well for more than a few days at a time?
- During the six months preceding that date, did you experience any illness or major stress, change your use of medication or dietary supplements, or make any significant life changes?

Other publications of this author present cases in which cryptogenic illness was found to be precipitated by foreign travel, antibiotic use, dietary changes,[29] smoldering infection, or the illness of a spouse.[30]

Triggers and the Provocation of Illness

A trigger is anything that initiates an acute illness or the emergence of symptoms. The distinction between a trigger and a precipitating event is relative, not absolute; the distinction helps organize the patient's story. As a general rule, triggers only provoke illness as long as the person is exposed to them (or for a short while afterward), whereas a precipitating event initiates a change in health status that persists long after the exposure ends. Common triggers include physical or psychic trauma, microbes, drugs, allergens, foods (or even the act of eating or drinking), environmental toxins, temperature change, stressful life events, adverse social interactions, and powerful memories. For some conditions, the trigger is such an essential part of our concept of the disease that the two cannot be separated; the disease is either named after the trigger (e.g., "Strep throat") or the absence of the trigger negates the diagnosis (e.g., concussion cannot occur without head trauma). For chronic ailments like asthma, arthritis, or migraine headaches, multiple interacting triggers may be present. All triggers, however, exert their effects through the activation of host-derived mediators. In closed-head trauma, for example, activation of NMDA receptors, induction of nitric oxide synthase (iNOS), and liberation of free intra-neuronal calcium determine the late effects. Intravenous magnesium at the time of trauma attenuates severity by altering the mediator response.[31,32] Sensitivity to different triggers often varies among persons with similar ailments. A prime task of the functional practitioner is to help patients identify important triggers for their ailments and develop strategies for eliminating them or diminishing their virulence.

Although the identification and elimination of triggers is not a foreign concept in conventional medicine, many physicians neglect the search. A study was conducted by telephone in which practicing physicians were asked how they would treat a new patient with abdominal pain, who had a recent diagnosis of gastritis made by a specialist in another town. Almost half were ready to put the patient on acid-lowering therapy without asking about the patient's use of aspirin, alcohol or tobacco, all of which are potential triggers for gastritis. The authors of the study concluded, "In actual practice, ignoring these aspects of the patient may well have reduced or even negated the efficacy of other therapeutic plans implemented."[33]

Mediators and the Formation of Illness

A mediator is anything that produces symptoms, damage to tissues of the body, or the types of behaviors associated with being sick. Mediators vary in form and substance. They may be biochemical (like prostanoids and cytokines), ionic (like hydrogen ions), social (like reinforcement for staying ill), psychological (like fear), or cultural (like beliefs about the nature of illness). A list of common mediators is presented in Table 8.1. Illness in any single person usually involves multiple interacting mediators. Biochemical, psychosocial, and cultural mediators interact continuously in the formation of illness.

Cognitive/emotional mediators determine how patients appraise symptoms and what actions they take in response to that appraisal.[34] They may even modulate the symptoms themselves. People in pain, for example, experience more pain when they fear that pain control will be inadequate than when they believe that ample pain management is available.[35]

Perceived self-efficacy (the belief in one's ability to cope successfully with specific problems) is a cognitive mediator that determines coping with illness. People with a high degree of health self-efficacy usually adapt better to chronic disease, maintaining higher levels of activity, requiring lower doses of pain medication, adopting healthier lifestyles, and cooperating with prescribed therapies, compared to people with low self-efficacy.[36] Self-management education is designed to enhance self-efficacy,[37] and has been shown to improve the clinical outcome for patients with several types of chronic disease, including asthma,[38] arthritis,[39,40,41] and diabetes.[42]

The biochemical mediators of disease listed in Table 8.1 are best known for their ability to promote cellular damage. Most are organized into circuits and cascades that sub-serve homeostasis and allostasis. In these networks, each mediator is multi-functional and most functions involve multiple mediators, so that redundancy is the rule, not the exception. The most striking characteristic of biochemical mediators is their lack of disease specificity. Each mediator can be implicated in many different, apparently unrelated diseases, and every disease involves multiple chemical mediators in its formation.

Table 8.1 **Common Illness Mediators**

Biochemical	Hormones Neurotransmitters Neuropeptides Cytokines Free radicals Transcription factors
Subatomic	Ions Electrons Electrical and magnetic fields
Cognitive/emotional	Fear of pain or loss Feelings or personal beliefs about illness Poor self-esteem, low perceived self-efficacy Learned helplessness Lack of relevant health information
Social/cultural	Reinforcement for staying sick Behavioral conditioning Lack of resources due to social isolation or poverty The nature of the sick role and the doctor/patient relationship

Mediator networks that regulate inflammatory and neuroendocrine stress responses have been the subject of intensive research with important clinical implications. A detailed discussion of these networks is outside the scope of this chapter, but they are addressed in Chapters 19, 23, 27, and 32; see the index for further cross-referencing. Comprehensive reviews have appeared elsewhere.[43,44,45,46] Within the framework of functional medicine, a key feature of biochemical mediators is the natural rhythm of mediator activity, which is strongly influenced by the common components of life: diet, sleep, exercise, hygiene, social interactions, solar and lunar cycles, age, and sex. Aging, illness, and chronic psychological distress upregulate activity of the inflammatory and neuroendocrine-stress response networks. Regular physical activity downregulates both.

Integrating the Patient's Story

After listening to the concerns that led each patient to seek a consultation in functional medicine, the clinician makes a series of distinctions:

1. For patients whose main concern is optimal health and prevention, ask about present and past health problems and the family health history. If these supply no indication of illness susceptibility, then turn your attention to risk factors for future illness: weight, fitness, type and level of physical activity, dietary pattern, sleep habits, use of alcohol, drugs, tobacco, firearms, environmental exposures at home and work, travel, sources of stress and pleasure, degree of involvement with others, spiritual beliefs and practices, sexual relationships, hopes and fears for the future.
2. For patients with an active health problem, always ask, "What was your health like before this problem began?" An intake questionnaire that asks about previous health problems is also helpful, because it gathers information in a different fashion concerning what the patient was like prior to the present illness. Such a tool is condition-specific, not open-ended. The two approaches complement one another.
    a. Some patients will say that they were really healthy prior to their present illness. In that case, look for a precipitating event. If you or the patient can identify one, then ask about ongoing triggers that bear some relationship to the precipitating event. For example: if the precipitating event was marital or job stress, focus on stress-related psychological triggers. If the precipitating event was an environmental exposure, focus on ongoing exposures to volatile chemicals or mold.
    b. The most challenging patients will usually indicate that their health was poor even before their present illness. In that case, take a detailed, chronological history from birth to the present that includes information about early life experience (including illness, injury and abuse), school and work performance, diet, drug and medication use, leisure activities, travel, family life, sexual experiences, habits, life stressors, and places of residence. Because gathering this data can be very time consuming, a self-administered questionnaire completed by the patient before the interview may help to prompt responses and improve memory of remote events. For many patients with complex, chronic health problems, it may be useful to take a detailed life history **before** seeking detailed information about present symptoms. Problems that emerge from such a review have to be addressed for a successful outcome of treatment. Dealing with the present concerns by themselves almost never succeeds for patients in this group.

Whatever rapport you establish with patients initially, maintaining the therapeutic relationship usually depends upon significant improvement in symptoms or in a sense of well-being within a few days to a few weeks of the initial evaluation. This is most efficiently achieved by addressing the triggers that provoke symptoms and helping the patient decrease exposure to them. When triggers cannot be identified or avoided, then symptomatic improvement must rest on control of mediator activation. A combination of the two will usually produce the most satisfactory long-term benefits.

Assessment of Triggers

A comprehensive search for triggers requires that you know the following about your patient: each drug—prescription, over-the-counter or recreational—that the patient has used and when; nutritional habits and each dietary supplement used and when; what effects the patient noted from the use of each substance; sources of stress—life events, environmental exposures, thoughts or memories, and social interactions—and when they occurred in relation to symptoms. Elicit the patient's own ideas about possible triggers by asking, "What do you think causes or aggravates your symptoms?" The patient's observations may be insightful and accurate in ascribing causality. Of course the patient's—and the clinician's—observations can also mislead, or focus on non-essential factors. Teach patients to challenge their own observations by looking for consistency and replicability, wherever possible. Suggest alternative theories for the patient to consider and explain that the search for triggers works best as a collaborative effort between patient and doctor. The patient's ability to recognize triggers is an important step in self-care.

Food and environment supply important triggers for the practice of functional medicine. Food intolerance is a very common phenomenon, reported by 33% of the population in one large study.[47] Relatively few of these reactions (4–14%) are due to true food allergies. Most food intolerance has no clear immunologic basis. Mechanisms include sensitivity to the pharmacological effect of alkaloids, amines or salicylates in food.[48,49,50,51] Histamine poisoning from scombroid fish and tyramine-induced headache are dramatic examples.[52] Although most food intolerance is short-lived, severe chronic illness can occur, and the food trigger may elude identification unless the physician starts the investigation with a high index of suspicion. Gluten intolerance, with its protean manifestations, is probably the best example. Affecting about 2% of people of European ancestry,[53] gluten intolerance is common and often unrecognized. In addition to being the essential trigger for celiac disease, gluten sensitivity may be manifest in patients with neurological disorders of unknown cause,[54] cerebellar degeneration,[55] dermatitis herpetiformis,[56] failure to thrive,[57] pervasive developmental delay,[58] inflammatory arthritis,[59,60,61,62,63] psoriasis,[64,65] Sjögren's syndrome,[66,67] and schizophrenia.[68,69] The different presentations of gluten sensitivity may derive from genetic differences among affected patients.[70]

Published studies on food intolerance and your patients' symptoms may be found through the National Library of Medicine. If the patient has a disease diagnosis, an internet search may reveal previously observed associations between specific foods and the patient's condition. Access PubMed over the internet (www.pubmed.gov) and run a search that cross-references the name of the patient's condition with "Hypersensitivity, food" and also with "Food, adverse reactions." Both of these are Medline Subject Headings (MESH). There is no MESH listing for "Food Allergy" or "Food Intolerance." Your search will be more efficient if you list the patient's condition as it appears in MESH. A negative search does not eliminate food intolerance as a trigger for the condition being searched, but the number of positive findings may surprise you.[i]

Health effects of ambient air quality are as important as those of foods. Numerous studies conducted in U.S. cities demonstrate a close correlation between fine-particle air pollution and daily mortality rates, even at levels of pollution considered safe by the World Health Organization.[71] In the industrialized world, most people spend most of their time indoors, and indoor air pollution has become a serious cause of morbidity. Studies using experimental chambers have shown that volatile organic compounds (VOCs) released from building materials, furnishings, office machines, and cleaning products can cause irritation of the respiratory system in humans and animals at levels which are one hundred times weaker than permissible exposure levels or the World Health Organization Indoor Air Guidelines.[72,73,74] Controlled experiments with people who describe themselves as sensitive to VOCs confirm that VOC exposure causes headache, fatigue, and difficulty concentrating. People who deny such sensitivity also experience symptoms, but do not experience mental impairment when exposed. Air samples of buildings with and without "sick building" complaints have established an association between VOC exposure and human sickness.[75,76,77,78]

A questionnaire can elicit important information about environmental exposures at home and at work. The open-ended question, "Has your work or home environment been a concern to you?" should be accompanied by a checklist of potential exposures.

Microbial triggers for chronic illness present a particular challenge, as exemplified by the many facets of *Helicobacter pylori* infection. Originally isolated from the gastric mucosa of patients with gastritis and peptic ulcer disease, *H. pylori* has been implicated in the pathogenesis of NSAID gastropathy,[79] gastric carcinoma,[80] lymphoma,[81] and a variety of extra-digestive disorders, including ischemic heart disease,[82] ischemic cerebrovascular disorders,[83] rosacea,[84] Sjögren's syndrome,[85] Raynaud's syndrome,[86] food allergy,[87] vitamin B12 deficiency,[88] and open-angle glaucoma.[89] For elderly patients with open-angle glaucoma and incidental *H. pylori* infection of the stomach, eradication of *H. pylori* by antibiotics was associated with improved control of glaucoma parameters at two years.[90] The mechanism by which *H. pylori* aggravates open-angle glaucoma is unknown, but may result from the ability of *H. pylori* colonization of the gastric tract to trigger the local and systemic release of platelet-activating factor, inflammatory cytokines, and vasoactive substances.

In the case of untreated *H. pylori* infection, non-invasive screening tests, including serum antibodies,

---

[i] Medical cybrarian Valerie Rankow (vgr99@optonline.net) has assisted the author with this search strategy and with numerous other, more complex searches.

stool antigens, and C-14 breath testing, are available. For other types of infection, inquiring about the previous response of a given symptom or symptom complex to antibiotics may be useful. In 1988, physicians at the University of Minnesota conducted a study in which they administered intravenous cephalosporins to patients with various types of arthritis who also manifested antibodies to *Borrelia burgdorferi*. Most of these patients were not thought to have Lyme disease. Some met diagnostic criteria for rheumatoid arthritis, some for osteoarthritis, and some for spondyloarthropathies. The response to antibiotics was quite variable and ranged from no response to dramatic and sustained improvement. The authors noted that improvement in arthritis following antibiotics was not related to the patient's clinical diagnosis or the level of anti-*Borrelia* antibody. The best predictor of a positive response to the experimental treatment was a previous history of improvement of arthritis associated with the use of antibiotics.[91]

The most comprehensive way to ask the antibiotic question is: "During the time you have had symptom X, have you taken antibiotics for any reason? Which antibiotic? Did symptom X change while you were taking the drug?" Among patients with chronic diarrhea of unknown cause, for example, some will report that their gastrointestinal symptoms improved when taking a specific antibiotic; others will report that they worsened. The first case suggests that bacteria or protozoa sensitive to the antibiotic may be causally related to the patient's gastrointestinal problems. Repeating the antibiotic prescription can establish if this response is replicable. If so, therapy can focus on treating the microbe and understanding why a single course of antibiotics was ineffective. The second case suggests that depletion of bacteria by antibiotics and concomitant increase in antibiotic-resistant organisms, including yeasts, may be contributing to diarrhea, and treatment can focus on restoration of normal intestinal flora.

Assessment of Psychosocial Mediators

Useful questions for eliciting a person's beliefs about his/her illness are:

- What do you think has caused your problem?
- What do you most fear about your problem?
- How much control do you think you have over your symptoms?

Useful questions for eliciting information about the nature and sources of social support include:

- Are there people in whom you can confide?
- How satisfied are you with your marriage/family/friends/social life?
- How much support do you receive in dealing with your health problems?
- How often do you feel loved or cared for?

Assessment of Biochemical Mediators

Understanding the biochemical alterations associated with a conventional disease diagnosis can be helpful in understanding the biochemical mediators of each person's illness. Inflammation is believed to play a critical role not only in response to infection and in the classic inflammatory diseases, but also in the pathogenesis of coronary artery disease, diabetes, cancer, depression, and the negative health effects associated with obesity and with aging.[92,93,94,95,96,97,98] The orchestration of mediator signals in the inflammation and neuroendocrine-stress networks, as they interact with one another, is critical for normal physiological functions (e.g., the architecture of sleep, the repair of injury, and the response to infection), and for the dysfunctional physiology central to the pathogenesis of most of the major chronic diseases.[99,100,101]

Most chronic disease is associated with chronic inflammation, but the patterns of immune response that underlie inflammation are not always the same. Patients with type 1 diabetes mellitus, Crohn's disease or any other disorder categorized by granuloma formation or excessive cell-mediated immune responses are likely to have an immune response to common triggers in which the Th1 component is upregulated and not subject to the normal downregulation provided by Th2 activity. Their mediator response to inflammatory stimulation produces excessive levels of gamma-interferon (g-IFN) and interleukin-12 (IL-12), key Th1-related cytokines.[102] Patients with severe depression often show a loss of negative feedback in the HPA axis. Urinary free cortisol is elevated; the diurnal pattern may be disrupted, with increased PM cortisol secretion and blunting of dexamethasone suppression. This phenomenon appears to be driven at the level of the hypothalamus, not the adrenals, because spinal fluid corticotropin releasing hormone (CRH) is elevated.[103] Several groups of researchers in the late 1990s speculated that impaired synaptic function due to a deficit of omega-3 fatty acids may contribute to the CNS dysfunction of patients with depressive illness[104,105,106,107] (although some large recent studies do not show the same patterns[108,109]). Omega-3 fatty acid levels tend to be lower in blood samples than in control populations. The key component appears to be eicosapentaenoic acid (EPA).

To utilize the vast database of available information about biochemical disease mediators, integrative clinicians should consider three strategies. First, maintain up-to-date knowledge of disease pathophysiology by reading reviews in mainstream journals on mechanisms of disease or on specific mediators. In reading these, pay special attention to the types of mediators mentioned and their functions within the networks that involve inflammation, oxidative stress, and neuroendocrine balance. Second, attend workshops and courses that emphasize integrative physiology, sponsored by institutions like IFM, the New York Academy of Sciences, the Center for Mind-Body Medicine, and the American College for Advancement in Medicine.[110] Third, employ knowledge of the commonest biochemical imbalances in chronically ill North Americans and the influence of diet, nutrition, and dietary supplements on these imbalances.

Treatment Planning

A functional medicine treatment plan should be collaborative and dynamic. Collaborative means that patient and practitioner work together to set goals and priorities. Dynamic means that the treatment plan is adjusted as needed in response to feedback. Your knowledge of the patient's beliefs about his/her illness and perceived self-efficacy are essential for collaborative treatment. An appropriate therapeutic intervention for dysfunctional beliefs is the giving of information. Patients have an intense need for explanations about the causes of their diseases.[111] They want to know how they came to be sick, so that they can attach some meaning to the illness,[112] what to expect from the illness, and what they can do to relieve symptoms or speed recovery. Information of this type can reduce anxiety (even when the diagnosis itself is frightening), increase feelings of personal control, and improve the ability to cope with pain. People change their behaviors more readily when they receive information about the importance and the nature of the changes they need to make, help with setting goals, and measuring progress. The kind of information needed is personal, not statistical. It must answer the question, "What can I do?"

The physician can help patients who are suffering from isolation by calling this isolation to the attention of family members or friends, or by attempting to connect the patient with a support group or community agency. Possibly, there is nothing that can be done to relieve the patient's isolation, but the doctor's awareness and acknowledgment of it can be important to the patient and serve to enhance the therapeutic relationship.[113]

If potential triggers have been identified, an assessment of the patient's ability to control exposure to them is important. For patients who are reluctant to make major dietary or environmental changes, explain that each avoidance is an experiment that the patient can direct with your guidance. If eliminating foods (and reintroducing those foods as a challenge) has no effect on symptoms or measurable physiologic parameters, do not encourage the patient to persist in the avoidance of those foods, whatever the results of *in vitro* allergy tests may be. The patient will have enough work to do following a healthy diet. Food intolerance is only meaningful if its effects can be demonstrated in real life.

For microbial triggers, the decision to use prescription antimicrobial drugs or natural products with antimicrobial activity may require negotiation. If the situation is not critical, it is usually worthwhile honoring the patient's preferences and intuition.

Understanding the ways in which mediators are modulated by diet enables creative nutritional therapies to be applied. Salicylic acid, the major metabolite of aspirin, suppresses activation of the nuclear transcription factor NF-κB, an anti-inflammatory effect that is independent of cyclooxygenase inhibition[114] and may be responsible for some effects of low-dose aspirin therapy.[115] Vegetables are rich sources of natural salicylates and vegetarians may have serum concentrations of salicylic acid as high as those of people ingesting 75 mg of aspirin a day.[116]

Dietary fatty acids may have profound effects on the network of inflammatory mediators, altering prostanoid synthesis, PPAR activity, and the response to cytokines like IL-1.[117,118,119] They have subtler effects on the neuroendocrine-stress response network, modulating neuronal responses to serotonergic and adrenergic transmission.[120] Therapy with omega-3 fatty acids provides an excellent example of nutritional modulation of disease activity though alteration of biochemical mediators.[121] Three principles can guide this type of therapy. The first utilizes knowledge of the pathophysiology of specific inflammatory and CNS disorders. Using this model, omega-3 therapy has been successfully applied to the treatment of patients with rheumatoid arthritis,[122] inflammatory bowel disease,[123] coronary artery disease,[124] peripheral vascular disease,[125] dysmenorrhea,[126] cystic fibrosis,[127] migraine headaches,[128] schizophrenia,[129,130] atopic eczema,[131] and multiple sclerosis.[132,133] Because the fatty acid composition of the contemporary Western diet differs significantly from Paleolithic and ancestral diets, reflecting a marked decrease in omega-3 consumption relative to total fat, the response of so many unrelated disorders to EFA supplementation may indicate that EFAs are not merely working as nutraceutical agents, but that EFA dietary status is important for disease pathogenesis.

The second method rests upon the clinical evaluation of an individual's fatty acid status using clinical parameters that are independent of disease activity. Prasad has stated that the best test for nutritional adequacy is a functional test.[134] Determine a parameter to follow and measure how administration of the nutrient(s) in question affects that parameter. This method can be applied to the use of EFA therapy in clinical practice. Stevens et al., studying boys with ADHD and a randomly selected population of schoolchildren, found a correlation between low concentrations of omega-3 EFAs, learning and behavior problems, and symptoms associated with EFA deficiency (thirst, dry skin, and dry hair).[135,136] Evaluating the presence of these symptoms in patients and observing how they change with EFA supplementation is a quick guide to EFA status that may be used clinically to evaluate the EFA contribution to mediator imbalance. This author's method for doing this has been described elsewhere.[137] Finally, it is possible to measure the levels of fatty acids in plasma and erythrocyte phospholipids, although guidelines for the level of change in fatty acid profiles needed to produce a known clinical effect have only been reported for patients with rheumatoid arthritis, in whom clinical improvement requires that eicosapentaenoic acid (EPA) account for 5% of fatty acids in plasma phospholipids.[138]

The successful application of nutritional therapies, especially dietary interventions, and other self-care practices, as part of a therapeutic plan is very helpful in enhancing self-efficacy among patients. Enhancement of self-efficacy should always be a cardinal goal of treatment in functional medicine.

Summary

Functional medicine is essentially patient centered, rather than disease centered. A structure is presented for uniting a patient-centered approach to diagnosis and treatment with the fruits of modern clinical science (which evolved primarily to serve the prevailing model of disease-centered care). The core scientific concepts of disease pathogenesis are antecedents, triggers, and mediators. Antecedents are factors, genetic or acquired, that predispose to illness; triggers are factors that provoke the symptoms and signs of illness; and mediators are factors, biochemical or psychosocial, that contribute to pathological changes and dysfunctional responses. Understanding the antecedents, triggers, and mediators that underlie illness or dysfunction in each patient permits therapy to be targeted to the needs of the individual. The conventional diagnosis assigned to the patient may be of value in identifying plausible antecedents, triggers or mediators for each patient, but is not adequate by itself for the designing of patient-centered care.

Applying the model of person-centered diagnosis to patients facilitates the recognition of disturbances that are common in people with chronic illness. Diet, nutrition, and exposure to environmental toxins play central roles in functional medicine because they may predispose to illness, provoke symptoms, and modulate the activity of biochemical mediators through a complex and diverse set of mechanisms. Explaining those mechanisms is a key objective of this textbook.

A patient's beliefs about health and illness are critically important for self-care and may influence both behavioral and physiological responses to illness. Perceived self-efficacy is an important mediator of health and healing. Enhancement of patients' self-efficacy through information, education, and the development of a collaborative relationship between patient and healer is a cardinal goal in all clinical encounters.

References

1. Galland L, "Person-Centered Diagnosis," in Power Healing. New York:Random House, 1997, pp 52-97.
2. Reiser SJ. The era of the patient. Using the experience of illness in shaping the missions of health care. JAMA. 1993;269:1012-1017.
3. Beckman HB, Frankel RM. The effect of physician behavior on the collection of data. Ann Intern Med. 1984;101:692-696.

4. Frankel R. Talking in interviews: a dispreference for patient-initiated questions in physician-patient encounters. In Studies in Ethnomethodology and Conversation Analysis. No. 1. G Psathas, ed. The International Institute for Ethnomethodology and Conversation Analysis and University Press of America. Washington D.C. 1990:231-262.
5. Roter DL, Hall JA. Physician interviewing styles and medical information obtained from patients. J Gen Intern Med. 1987;2(5):325-29.
6. Bartlett EE, Grayson M, Barker R, et al. The effects of physician communications skills on patient satisfaction; recall and adherence. J Chronic Dis. 1984;37:755-64.
7. Smith RC, Hoppe RB. The patient's story: integrating the patient- and physician-centered approaches to interviewing. Ann Intern Med. 1991;115:470-477.
8. Sanchez-Menegay C, Stalder H. Do physicians take into account patients' expectations? J Gen Intern Med. 1994;9:404-406.
9. Beckman DB, Frankel RM The effect of physician behavior on the collection of data. Ann Intern Med. 1984;101:692-696.
10. Sanchez-Menegay C, Stalder M. Do physicians take into account patients' perspectives? J Gen Intern Med. 1994;9:404-406.
11. Freidin RB, Goldin L, Cecil RR. Patient-physician concordance in problem identification in the primary care setting. Ann Intern Med. 1980;93(3):490-93.
12. Tucket D. Meetings Between Experts: An Approach to Sharing Ideas in Medical Consultations. London and New York, Tavistock Publications, 1985.
13. Hall JA, Roter DL, and Katz NR, Meta-analysis of correlates of provider behavior in medical encounters. Med Care. 1988;28:657-75.
14. Kaplan SH, Greenfield S, Ware JE Jr. Assessing the effects of physician-patient interactions on the outcomes of chronic disease. Med Care. 1989;27 Suppl 3:S110-127.
15. Ades PA, et al, Predictors of cardiac rehabilitation participation in older coronary patients. Arch Intern Med. 1992;152:1033-35.
16. Mullen PD. Efficacy of psychoeducational interventions on pain, depression and disability in people with arthritis: a meta-analysis. J Rheumatol. 1987;14 Suppl 15:33-39.
17. Wilson SR, et al. A controlled trial of self-management education for adults with asthma. Am J Med. 1993;94:564-576.
18. Lorig KR, Mazonson PD, Holman HR. Evidence suggesting that health education for self-management in patients with chronic arthritis has sustained health benefits while reducing health care costs. Arthritis Rheum. 1993;36:439-46.
19. Teutsch C. Patient-doctor communication. Med Clin North Am. 2003;87(5):1115-45.
20. Guengerich FP. Functional genomics and proteomics applied to the study of nutritional metabolism. Nutr Rev. 2001;59:259-62.
21. Pennie W, Pettit SD, Lord PG. Toxicogenomics in risk assessment: overview of an HESI collaborative research program. Environ Health Perspect. 2004;112:417-19.
22. Pietrangelo A. Hereditary hemochromatosis—a new look at an old disease. N Engl J Med. 2004;350:2383-97.
23. Vogelsgang H, Schwarzenhofer M, Oberhuber G. Changes in gastrointestinal permeability in celiac disease. Dig Dis. 1998;16:333-36.
24. Phillips DW. Twin studies in medical research. (letter) Lancet. 1993;342:52.
25. Romans S, Belaise C, Martin J, et al. Childhood abuse and later medical disorders in women. An epidemiological study. Psychother Psychosom. 2002;71(3):141-50.
26. Lampe A, Solder E, Ennemoser A, et al. Chronic pelvic pain and previous sexual abuse. Obstet Gynecol. 2000;96(6):929-33.
27. Hagerman RJ, Falkenstein AR. An association between recurrent otitis media in infancy and later hyperactivity. Clin Pediatr (Phila). 1987;26(5):253-57.
28. Adesman AR, Altshuler LA, Lipkin PH, Walco GA. Otitis media in children with learning disabilities and in children with attention deficit disorder with hyperactivity. Pediatrics. 1990;85(3):442-6.
29. Galland, L. A New Definition of Patient-Centered Medicine. In Integrative Medicine, Principles for Practice. Edited by B. Kligler and R. Lee, 2004. New York, McGraw Hill, pp 71-101.
30. Galland, L. Power Healing. New York:Random House, 1997, pp 52-114.
31. Cernak I, Savic VJ, Kotur J, et al. Characterization of plasma magnesium concentration and oxidative stress following graded traumatic brain injury in humans. J Neurotrauma. 2000;17(1):53-68.
32. Vink R, Nimmo AJ, Cernak I. An overview of new and novel pharmacotherapies for use in traumatic brain injury. Clin Exp Pharmacol Physiol. 2001;28(11):919-921.
33. Avorn J, Everitt DE and Baker MW. The neglected medical history and therapeutic choices for abdominal pain: A nationwide study of 799 physicians and nurses. Arch Intern Med. 1991;151:694-98.
34. Kleinman A, Eisenberg L, Good B. Culture, illness and care. Clinical lessons from anthropologic and cross-cultural research. Ann Intern Med. 1978;88:251-58.
35. O'Leary A. Self-efficacy and health. Behav Res Ther. 1985;23(4):437-51.
36. Holden G. The relationship of self-efficacy appraisals to subsequent health-related outcomes: a meta-analysis. Soc Work Health Care. 1991;16:53-93.
37. Bodenheimer T, Lorig K, Holman H, Grumbach K. Patient self-management of chronic disease in primary care. JAMA. 2002;288:2469-75.
38. Wilson SR, Scamagas P, German DF, et al. A controlled trial of two forms of self-management education for adults with asthma. Am J Med. 1993;94:564-76.
39. Mullen PD, LaVille EA, Biddle AK, Lorig K. Efficacy of psychoeducational interventions on pain, depression, and disability in people with arthritis: a meta-analysis. J Rheumatol. 1987;14 (suppl 15):33-39.
40. Schiaffino KM, Revenson TA, Gibofsky A. Assessing the impact of self-efficacy beliefs on adaptation to rheumatoid arthritis. Arthritis Care Res. 1991;4:150-57.
41. Lorig KR, Mazonson PD, Holman HR. Evidence suggesting that health education for self-management in patients with chronic arthritis has sustained health benefits while reducing health care costs. Arthritis Rheum. 1993;36:439-46.
42. Litzelman DK, Slemenda CW, Langefeld CD, et al. Reduction of lower extremity clinical abnormalities in patients with non-insulin dependent diabetes mellitus. A randomized, control trial. Ann Intern Med. 1993;119:36-41.
43. Habib KE, Gold PW, Chrousos GP. Neuroendocrinology of stress. Endocrinol Metab Clin North Am. 2001;30:695-728.
44. Miller DB, O'Callaghan JP. Neuroendocrine aspects of the response to stress. Metabolism. 2002;51(6 Suppl 1):5-10.
45. Petrovsky N. Towards a unified model of neuroendocrine-immune interaction. Immunol Cell Biol. 2001;79:350-57.
46. Chikanza IC, Grossman AB. Reciprocal interactions between the neuroendocrine and immune systems during inflammation. Rheum Dis Clin North Am. 2000;26:693-71.
47. Bender AE, Matthews DR. Adverse reactions to foods. Br J Nutr. 1981;46:403-7.
48. Moneret-Vautrin DA. Food antigens and additives. J Allergy Clin Immunol. 1986;78:1039-46.
49. Kniker WT, Rodriguez M. Non-IgE mediated and delayed adverse reactions to food or additives. In Handbook of Food Allergies, ed. JC Breneman, 1987, New York, Marcel Dekker, pp 125-161.
50. Perry CA, Dwyer J, Gelfand JA, et al. Health effects of salicylates in foods and drugs. Nutr Rev. 1996;54(8):225-40.

51. Lovenberg W. Some vaso- and psychoactive substances in food: amines, stimulants, depressants and hallucinogens. In Toxicants Occurring Naturally in Foods. (2nd Ed). Eds:Committee on Food Protection, Food & Nutrition Board, National Research Council. Natl. Acad. Sci. Press. Washington DC. 1973, pp 170-188.
52. Somogyi JC. Natural toxic substances in food. World Rev Nutr Diet. 1978;29:42-59.
53. Catassi C, Ratsch IM, Fabiani E, et al. Coeliac disease in the year 2000: exploring the tip of the iceberg. Lancet. 1994;343:200-3.
54. Hadjivasssiliou M, Gibson A, Davies-Jones GAB, et al. Does cryptic gluten sensitivity play a part in neurological illness? Lancet. 1996;347:369-71.
55. Hadjivasssiliou M, Grunewald RA, Chattopadhyay AK, et al. Clinical, radiological, neurophysiological, and neuropathological characteristics of gluten ataxia. Lancet. 1998;352:1582-85.
56. Collin P, Reunala T. Recognition and management of the cutaneous manifestations of celiac disease: a guide for dermatologists. Am J Clin Dermatol. 2003;4(1):13-20.
57. Wolff A, Berger R, Gaze H, et al. IgG, IgA and IgE gliadin antibody determinations as screening test for untreated coeliac disease in children, a multicentre study. Eur J Pediatr. 1989;148(6):496-502.
58. Jyonouchi H, Sun S, Itokazu N. Innate immunity associated with inflammatory responses and cytokine production against common dietary proteins in patients with autism spectrum disorder. Neuropsychobiol. 2002;46(2):76-84.
59. Ramos-Remus C, Bahlas S, Vaca-Morales O. Rheumatic features of gastrointestinal tract, hepatic, and pancreatic diseases. Curr Opin Rheumatol. 1997;9(1):56-61.
60. Falcini F, Ferrari R, Simonini G, et al. Recurrent monoarthritis in an 11-year-old boy with occult coeliac disease. Successful and stable remission after gluten-free diet. Clin Exp Rheumatol. 1999;17(4):509-11.
61. Kallikorm R, Uibo O, Uibo R. Coeliac disease in spondyloarthropathy: usefulness of serological screening. Clin Rheumatol. 2000;19(2):118-22.
62. Slot O, Locht H. Arthritis as presenting symptom in silent adult coeliac disease. Two cases and review of the literature. Scand J Rheumatol. 2000;29(4):260-63.
63. Bagnato GF, Quattrocchi E, Gulli S, et al. Unusual polyarthritis as a unique clinical manifestation of coeliac disease. Rheumatol Int. 2000;20(1):29-30.
64. Lindqvist U, Rudsander A, Bostrom A, et al. IgA antibodies to gliadin and coeliac disease in psoriatic arthritis. Rheumatology (Oxford). 2002;41(1):31-37.
65. Michaelsson G, Gerden B, Hagforsen E, et al. Psoriasis patients with antibodies to gliadin can be improved by a gluten-free diet. Br J Dermatol. 2000;142(1):44-51.
66. Teppo AM, Maury CP. Antibodies to gliadin, gluten and reticulin glycoprotein in rheumatic diseases: elevated levels in Sjögren's syndrome. Clin Exp Immunol. 1984;57(1):73-78.
67. Collin P, Korpela M, Hallstrom O, et al. Rheumatic complaints as a presenting symptom in patients with coeliac disease. Scand J Rheumatol. 1992;21(1):20-23.
68. Dohan, FC. Is celiac disease a clue to the pathogenesis of schizophrenia? Ment Hyg. 1969;53(4):525-29.
69. Vlissides DN, Venulet A, Jenner FA. A double-blind gluten-free/gluten-load controlled trial in a secure ward population. Br J Psychiatry. 1986;148:447-52.
70. Karell K, Korponay-Szabo I, Szalai Z, et al. Genetic dissection between coeliac disease and dermatitis herpetiformis in sib pairs. Ann Hum Genet. 2002;66(6):387-92.
71. Schwartz J, Dockery DW. Particulate air pollution and daily mortality in Steubenville, Ohio. Am J Epidemiol. 1992;135:12-19.
72. Schwartz J, Dockery DW. Increased mortality in Philadelphia associated with daily air pollution concentrations. Am Rev Respir Dis. 1992;145:600-4.
73. Dockery DW, Schwartz J, Spenger JD. Air pollution and daily mortality: association with particulates and acid aerosols. Environ Res. 1992;59:362-73.
74. Dockery DW, Pope A, Xu X, et al. An association between air pollution and mortality in six U.S. cities. N Engl J Med. 1993;329:1753-59.
75. Hodgson MJ, Frohlinger J, Permar E, et al. Symptoms and microenvironmental measures in non-problem buildings. J Occup Med. 1991;35:527-33.
76. Hodgson MJ. Buildings & health. Health Environ Dig. 1993;7:1-3.
77. Norback D, Torgen M, Edling C. Volatile organic compounds, respiratory dust and personal factors related to the prevalence and incidence of SBS in primary schools. Br J Ind Med. 1990;47:733-41.
78. Hodgson M. Field studies on the sick building syndrome. In Sources of indoor air contaminants: Characterizing emissions and health impacts. Tucker WG, Leaderer BP, Molhave L, Cain WS, eds. Ann N Y Acad Sci. 1992;641:21-36.
79. Chan FK, To KF, Wu JCY, et al. Eradication of Helicobacter pylori and risk of peptic ulcers in patients starting long-term treatment with non-steroidal anti-inflammatory drugs: a randomized trial. Lancet. 2002;359:9-13.
80. Uemara N, Okamoto S, Yamamoto S, et al. Helicobacter pylori and the development of gastric cancer. N Engl J Med. 2001;345:784-89.
81. Wotherspoon AC, Dogliani C, Diss TC, et al. Regression of primary low-grade B-cell lymphoma of mucosal-associated lymphoid tissue after eradication of Helicobacter pylori. Lancet. 1993;342:575-77.
82. Mendall MA, Goggin OM, Molineaux N, et al. Relation of Helicobacter pylori infection and coronary heart disease. Br Heart J. 1994;71:437-39.
83. Markus HS, Mendel MA. Helicobacter pylori: a risk factor for ischemic cerebrovascular disease and carotid atheroma. J Neurol Neurosurg Psychiatry. 1998;64:104-7.
84. Szlachcic A, Sliwowski Z, Karczewska E, et al. Helicobacter pylori and its eradication in rosacea. Physiol Pharmacol. 1999;50:777-86.
85. Aragona P, Magazzu G, Macchia G, et al. Presence of antibodies against Helicobacter pylori and its heat-shock protein 60 in the serum of patients with Sjögren's syndrome. J Rheumatol. 1999;26:1306-11.
86. Gasbarrini A, Franceschi F, Arnuzzi A, et al. Extradigestive manifestations of Helicobacter pylori gastric infection. Gut. 1999;45 (suppl):I9-I12.
87. Matysiak-Budnik T, Heyman M. Food allergy and Helicobacter pylori. J Pediatr Gastroenterol Nutr. 2002;34:5-12.
88. Kaptan K, Beyan C, Ural AU, et al. Helicobacter pylori: is it a novel causative agent in vitamin B12 deficiency? Arch Intern Med. 2000;160:1349-53.
89. Kountouras J, Mylopoiulos N, Boura P, et al. Relationship between Helicobacter pylori infection and glaucoma. Ophthalmology. 2001;108:599-604.
90. Kountouras J, Mylopoulos N, Chatzopoulos D, et al. Eradication of Helicobacter pylori may be beneficial in the management of chronic open-angle glaucoma. Arch Intern Med. 2002;162:1237-44.
91. Caperton EM, Heim-Duthoy KL, Matske GR, et al. Ceftriaxone therapy of chronic inflammatory arthritis: a double-blind placebo-controlled trial. Arch Intern Med. 1990;150:1677-82.
92. Schmidt MI, Duncan BB, Sharrett AR, et al. Markers of inflammation and prediction of diabetes mellitus in adults (Atherosclerosis Risk in Communities study): a cohort study. Lancet. 1999;353:1649-52.

93. Visser M, Bouter LM, McQuillan GM, et al. Elevated C-reactive protein levels in overweight and obese adults. JAMA. 1999;2823:2131-35.
94. Ross R. Atherosclerosis: an inflammatory disease. N Engl J Med. 1999;340:115-26.
95. Abramson JL, Vaccarino V. Relationship between activity and inflammation among apparently healthy middle-aged and older adults. Arch Int Med. 2002;162:1286-92.
96. Maes M. Major depression and activation of the inflammatory response system. In Cytokines, Stress and Depression, edited by Danzer et al. Kluwer Academic/Plenum Publishers. New York. 1999, pp 25-46.
97. Shacter E, Weitzman SA. Chronic inflammation and cancer. Oncology. 2002;16:217-26, 229.
98. Franceschi C, Ottaviani E. Stress, inflammation and natural immunity in the aging process: a new theory. Aging (Milano). 1997;9(4 Suppl):30-31.
99. Elenkov IJ, Chrousos GP. Stress hormones, proinflammatory and anti-inflammatory cytokines, and autoimmunity. Ann NY Acad Sci. 2002;966:290-303.
100. Petrovsky N. Towards a unified model of neuroendocrine-immune interaction. Immunol Cell Biol. 2001;79:350-57.
101. Jessop DS, Harbuz MS, Lightman SL. CRH in chronic inflammatory stress. Peptides. 2001;22:803-07.
102. Libby P. Inflammation: a common pathway in cardiovascular diseases. Dialogues Cardiovasc Med. 2003;8:59-73.
103. Wong ML, Kling MA, Munson PJ, et al. Pronounced and sustained central hypernoradrenergic function in major depression with melancholic features: relation to hypercortisolism and corticotropin-releasing hormone. Proc Natl Acad Sci USA. 2000;97(1):325-30.
104. Maes M, Christophe A, Delanghe J, et al. Lowered omega3 polyunsaturated fatty acids in serum phospholipids and cholesteryl esters of depressed patients. Psychiatry Res. 1999;85(3):275-91.
105. Peet M, Murphy B, Shay J, et al. Depletion of omega-3 fatty acid levels in red blood cell membranes of depressive patients. Biol Psychiatry. 1998;43(5):315-19.
106. Adams PB, Lawson S, Sanigorski, A, et al. Arachidonic acid to eicosapentaenoic acid ratio in blood correlates positively with clinical symptoms of depression. Lipids. 1996;31 Suppl:S157-61.
107. Stoll AL, Locke CA, Marangell LB, Severus WE. Omega-3 fatty acids and bipolar disorder: a review. Prostaglandins Leukot Essent Fatty Acids. 1999;60:329-37.
108. Hakkarainen R, Partonen T, Haukka J, et al. Food and nutrient intake in relation to mental wellbeing. Nutr J. 2004;3:14.
109. Jacka EN, Pasco JA, Henry MJ, et al. Dietary omega-3 fatty acids and depression in a community sample. Nutr Neurosci. 2004;7(2):101-06.
110. www.acam.org; www.functionalmedicine.org
111. Korsch BM, Gozzi EK, Francis V. Gaps in doctor-patient communication. I: Doctor-patient interaction and patient satisfaction. Pediatrics. 1968;42:855-71.
112. Williams GH, Wood PHN. Common-sense beliefs about illness: a mediating role for the doctor. Lancet. 1986;328:1435-37.
113. Eisenberg L. What makes persons "patients" and patients "well." Am J Med. 1980;69(2):277-86.
114. Gautam SC, Pindolia KR, Noth CJ, et al. Chemokine gene expression in bone marrow stromal cells: downregulation with sodium salicylate. Blood. 1995;86(7):2541-50.
115. Giggs GA, Salmon JA, Henderson B, Vane JR. Pharmacokinetics of aspirin and salicylate in relation to inhibition of arachidonate cyclooxygenase and anti-inflammatory activity. Proc Nat Acad Sci USA. 1987;84:1417-20.
116. Blacklock CJ, Lawrence JR, Wiles D, et al. Salicylic acid concentrations in the serum of subjects not taking aspirin: comparison of salicylic acid concentrations in the serum of vegetarians, non-vegetarians and patients taking low-dose aspirin. J Clin Pathol. 2001;54:553-55.
117. Calder PC, Grimble RF. Polyunsaturated fatty acids, inflammation and immunity. Eur J Clin Nutr. 2002:56 Suppl 3:S14-19.
118. Chambrier C, Bastard JP, Rieusset J, et al. Eicosapentaenoic acid induces mRNA expression of peroxisome proliferator-activated receptor gamma. Obes Res. 2002;10:518-25.
119. Diep QN, Touyz RM, Schiffrin EL. Docosahexaenoic acid, a peroxisome proliferator-activated receptor-alpha ligand, induces apoptosis in vascular smooth muscle cells by stimulation of p38 mitogen-activated protein kinase. Hypertension. 2000;36:851-55.
120. Chalon S, Vancassel S, Zimmer L, et al. Polyunsaturated fatty acids and cerebral function: focus on monoaminergic neurotransmission. Lipids. 2001;36:937-44.
121. Simopoulos AP. Omega-3 fatty acids in inflammation and autoimmune diseases. J Am Coll Nutr. 2002;21(6):495-505.
122. Belch JJF, Ansell D, Madhok R, et al. Effects of altering dietary essential fatty acids on requirements for non-steroidal anti-inflammatory drugs in patients with rheumatoid arthritis: a double blind placebo controlled study. Ann Rheum Dis. 1988;47:96-104.
123. Stenson WF, Cort D, Rodgers J, et al. Dietary supplements with fish oil in ulcerative colitis. Ann Intern Med. 1992;116:609-14.
124. Gapinski JP, VanRuiswyk V, Heudebert GR, Schectman GS. Preventing restenosis with fish oils following coronary angioplasty. Arch Int Med. 1993;153:1595-1601.
125. Nestares T, Lopez-Jurado M, Urbano G, et al. Effects of lifestyle modification and lipid intake variations on patients with peripheral vascular disease. Int J Vitam Nutr Res. 2003;73(5):389-98.
126. Harel Z, Biro FM, Kottenhahn RK, Rosenthal SL. Supplementation with omega-3 polyunsaturated fatty acids in the management of dysmenorrhea in adolescents. Am J Obstet Gynecol. 1996;174(4):1335-38.
127. Lawrence R, Sorrell T. Eicosapentaenoic acid in cystic fibrosis: evidence of a pathogenetic role for leukotriene B4. Lancet. 1993;342:465-69.
128. McCaren T, Hitzeman R, Smith R, et al. Amelioration of severe migraine by fish oil (n-3) fatty acids. Am J Clin Nutr. 1985;41:874.
129. Yao JK, Magan S, Sonel AF, et al. Effects of omega-3 fatty acid on platelet serotonin responsivity in patients with schizophrenia. Prostaglandins Leukot Essent Fatty Acids. 2004;71(3):171-76.
130. Fenton WS, Dickerson F, Boronow J, et al. A placebo-controlled trial of omega-3 fatty acid (ethyl eicosapentaenoic acid) supplementation for residual symptoms and cognitive impairment in schizophrenia. Am J Psychiatry. 2001;158(12):2071-74.
131. Mayser P, Mayer K, Mahloudjian M, et al. A double-blind, randomized, placebo-controlled trial of n-3 versus n-6 fatty acid-based lipid infusion in atopic dermatitis. J Parenter Enteral Nutr. 2002;26(3):151-58.
132. Nordvik I, Myhr KM, Nyland H, Bjerve KS. Effect of dietary advice and n-3 supplementation in newly diagnosed MS patients. Acta Neurol Scand. 2000;102(3)143-49.
133. Bates D, Cartlidge NEF, French JM, et. al. A double-blind controlled trial of n-3 polyunsaturated fatty acids in the treatment of multiple sclerosis. J Neurol Neurosurg Psychiatry. 1989;52:18-22.
134. Prasad AS. Zinc in growth and development and spectrum of human zinc deficiency. J Am Coll Nutr. 1988;7(5):377-84.
135. Stevens LJ, Zentall SS, Deck JL, et al, Essential fatty acid metabolism in boys with attention deficit hyper activity disorder. Amer J Clin Nutr. 1995;62:761–68.

136. Stevens LJ, Zentall SS, Abate ML, et al. Omega-3 fatty acids in boys with behavior, learning and health problems. Physiol Behav. 1996;59:75-90.
137. Galland L. Power Healing. New York: Random House, 1997, pp. 156-162.
138. Clelland LG, Proudman SM, Hall C, et al. A biomarker of n-3 compliance in patients taking fish oil for rheumatoid arthritis. Lipids. 2003;38:419-24.

Chapter 9
Homeostasis: A Dynamic Balance

Joseph J. Lamb, MD

Introduction

The next principle of the functional medicine paradigm is the importance of the search for *dynamic balance* among the internal and external factors in a patient's body, mind, and spirit.

Human life is dependent upon an intricate balance of minerals,[1] water,[2] organic molecules, and high-energy chemical bonds. Ever since the coalescing of the first molecules capable of replication, and the development of the first cells capable of creating an internal environment, organisms have been characterized by cellular organization, growth and metabolism, reproduction, and heredity. They have also interacted with the external environment. From these simple beginnings have come the great diversity of all plant and animal life and the majesty of human life. Despite the vast complexity inherent in the organization of a human being, the system operates within relatively narrow limits for healthy balance, as dictated by our biochemistry.

Homeostasis and Homeodynamics

Of necessity, the cells of our bodies, with their own unique intracellular environment, are also bathed in a unique external environment: the extracellular fluid. One of the first to explore the concept of balance, the 19th century French physiologist, Claude Bernard, described the extracellular fluid as the "milieu interieur" or internal environment.[3] In 1929, Walter Cannon, the noted Harvard physiologist who first advanced the "fight vs. flight" hypothesis, formally suggested "the name homeostasis for the functional organization by which an organism will retain its original condition after a transient perturbation that is not actually damaging."[4]

Homeostasis is defined in *Stedman's Medical Dictionary* as:

1. The state of equilibrium (balance between opposing pressures) in the body with respect to various functions and to the chemical compositions of the fluids and tissues.
2. The processes through which such bodily equilibrium is maintained.[5]

This balance of chemical interactions defines how well and how long our bodies function. In their classic *Textbook of Medical Physiology*, Guyton and Hall describe this automatic process:

> The very fact that we remain alive is almost beyond our own control, for hunger makes us seek food and fear makes us seek refuge. Sensations of cold make us provide warmth. Other forces cause us to seek fellowship and to reproduce. Thus, the human being is actually an automaton, and the fact that we are sensing, feeling and knowledgeable beings is part of this automatic sequence of life … .[6]

In the conventional model, this equilibrium is often viewed at its simplest solely as a balance of internal factors alone. However, our understanding of these unique forces has evolved as our understanding of human genomics, cell signaling pathways, and the mind-body connection has developed. C.H. Waddington in 1968 "introduced the term homeorrhesis to capture the idea that what living things really hold 'constant is not a single parameter, but a time extended course of change, that is to say, a trajectory.'"[7] And in a series of papers beginning in1979, J.E.Yates described a physical biology model for the description of motion and changes at all biological levels of organization which he called homeodynamics. [8]

And yet, functional medicine envisions an even more vibrant and active dynamic. Taking into account the concepts of biochemical individuality and health as a positive vitality (not the simple absence of disease), homeodynamics is the constant and vital process of balancing external and internal factors to achieve a healthy functional state.[9]

Indeed, as described in the *Textbook of Natural Medicine*,[10]

> The term "homeodynamic" describes a range of continuously occurring metabolic and physiologic activities that enable an individual to adapt to changing circumstances, stresses, and experiences. The homeodynamics of one's health are constantly at work to enable a person to function as a unique individual. Supporting health at a homeodynamic level may require one to focus attention on cellular processes or organ function at sites that seem to be far removed from the patient's area of discomfort, and at levels that may be unusual from a conventional point of view.

The recent focus on energy production and mitochondrial dysfunction, oxidative stress, neuroexcitotoxicity, and inflammation manifested by glial activation as causes of neurodegenerative diseases provides an excellent example of this model.[11]

Inherent in this sense of balance are the mechanisms by which the organism controls and maintains this homeodynamic stability and flexibility. Classically, we know of the negative and positive feedback cycles of allopathic and functional medicine. Naturopathic and functional medicines also acknowledge that there are two internal forces, a higher and a lower drive, which maintain this unique individual internal balance. These two forces together constitute the profound self-generated ability to heal, classically known in the naturopathic tradition as *vis medicatrix naturae*. The lower drive is, in many ways, the classic automatic balance described by Guyton and Hall. This inherent internal healing mechanism can be augmented greatly by the higher drive. "The higher drive is the power of the mind and emotions to intervene and affect the course of health and disease by depressing or stimulating the internal capacities."[12]

Thus, the great diversity that creates biochemical individuality is not the simple genetically-determined outcome of biochemical interactions written into our genotypes at birth. Instead, this welcome diversity is a reflection of the interaction of genetic, environmental, and mind-body factors that allow each human to have the unique breadth of experience that characterizes human life.

A pivotal study by Lichtenstein et al., exploring the causation of cancer in a pooled cohort of monozygotic and dizygotic twins from Sweden, Denmark, and Finland, found that "statistically significant effects of heritable factors were observed for prostate cancer (42%), colorectal cancer (35%), and breast cancer (27%)."[13] While they found familial (hereditary or nonhereditary) factors for many types of cancer, the rates of concordance between twins were generally below 10%. They estimated the contribution of non-shared environmental factors for different cancers to range from 58% to 82%.

This study demonstrates that environmental inputs, including diet and nutrients, air and water, exercise, toxic load from the environment, and psychosocial factors and how we interpret them, contribute significantly to our phenotypic expression. This freedom from genetic determinism is a liberating concept of functional medicine. We are thus given the wonderful opportunity to provide our patients with patient centered, biochemically individualized lifestyle and nutritional interventions to assist them in maintaining their unique homeodynamic balance.

Homeodynamic Balance: Physiological Processes

The maintenance of this unique balance of pathophysiological processes is coordinated by a variety of communication systems, both neural and hormonal. Classically, these systems involve the secretion of a chemical messenger or hormone to act either locally (both on an intracellular as well as an intercellular level) or more distantly (intercellular level).

These chemical messengers and hormones can be classified into two distinct groups by the site of action in the target cell. The first group, including polypeptide hormones as well as monoamines and prostaglandins, does not enter the cell, but instead interacts with cell membrane receptors to signal change via second-level messengers such as cyclic adenosine monophosphate, inositol triphosphate, and diacylglycerol, and also by stimulation of the nucleotide regulatory peptides (G-proteins) that bind guanosine triphosphate.[14] The second group enters the cell and interacts with a diverse collection of nuclear receptors. These receptors, for thyroid and steroid hormones, vitamin A and D derivatives, endogenous metabolites, phytonutrients, and xenobiotics, "are structurally related and collectively referred to as the nuclear receptor super family."[15] As many of the ligands for these receptors have not been identified, these undefined receptors have been labeled the orphan nuclear receptors.

The peroxisome proliferator-activated receptors (PPARs) are one subfamily of nuclear receptors and are activated by endogenous intermediate metabolites of polyunsaturated fatty acids. PPARγ, expressed primarily in adipocytes, has a crucial role in adipocyte differentiation as well as a probable role in modulating insulin sensitivity.[16] Memisglu and his colleagues have investigated the link between a PPARγ polymorphism and dietary fat intake in relation to body mass.[17] They showed that total dietary fat intake was positively associated with body mass index (BMI) among homozygous wild-type individuals but not among carriers of a variant allele. Additionally, they demonstrated that monounsaturated fat was inversely related to BMI among carriers of the variant allele. They concluded that the PPARγ genotype modulates physiological responses to dietary fat. Conversely, environment—in the form of dietary fat intake—has direct influence on our genotype, pushing the resultant phenotype toward obesity.

Vitamins have been shown to have central roles in metabolism both as substrate and important cofactors in enzymatic conversions. Two vitamins, specifically vitamins A and D, are also messengers with specific nuclear receptors. Cantorna and her colleagues have explored the effect of vitamin D in experimental autoimmune encephalomyelitis (EAE), a mouse model for multiple sclerosis (MS).[18] They showed that development of EAE was completely prevented by pretreatment with 1,25 dihydroxyvitamin D3, and that disease progression was also prevented by treatment with 1,25 dihydroxyvitamin D3. They conclude that their findings "provide strong evidence that vitamin D status may be an important factor in determining the incidence of MS and that it is a physiologically important immune system modulator."[19]

Another example of environmental influence on metabolism and disease expression is indole-3-carbinol (I3C). I3C is an endogenous metabolite of glucosinolates in the *Brassica* family of vegetables—specifically broccoli, cauliflower, cabbage, kale, and Brussels sprouts. I3C has been found to exert a chemopreventive effect on breast cancer by inducing tumor cell apoptosis[20] and by stimulation of tumor-suppression genes.[21]

Certainly, one of the most interesting recent advances is the recognition of the diverse group of phytonutrient and environmental influences that provide information through the orphan nuclear receptors. These receptors may have developed for these specific molecules because their presence in the external environment was a measure of the safety of this outer environment. When our hunter-gatherer ancestors ate a diet rich in the appropriate phytonutrients and fatty acids, these messages of bounty signaled that it was safe to grow, to reproduce, indeed to come out of the sheltering caves. When the diet shifted, orphan nuclear receptors may have recognized the changing pattern of nutrient-based information and secreted messages of alarm and inflammation that instead stimulated pathways of conservation as they sought shelter for the dark winter months.

Further research will offer functional medicine practitioners a broader understanding of the influence of environment on our genotype and new opportunities to modulate this interaction.

Summary

Each individual is much more than the simple product of genetic expression directing the construction of shared building blocks. Instead, phenotypic expression is the unique product of an ever-changing dance between genes and environment as the individual strives to create a unique, harmonious balance.

Homeodynamic physiologic processes modulate the constant interplay of environmental inputs with our genetic programming. Modifiable lifestyle choices and nutritional choices can influence the expression of wellness or disease by our biochemically unique metabolisms.

References

1. Kurokawa K. How is plasma calcium held constant? Milieu interieur of calcium. Kidney Int. 1996;49(6):1760-64.
2. Acher R. Water homeostasis in the living: molecular organization, osmoregulatory reflexes and evolution. Ann Endocrinol (Paris). 2002;63(3):197-218.
3. Guyton AC, Hall JE. Textbook of Medical Physiology. Philadelphia: W.B. Saunders Company, 2000, p.1.
4. Yates FE. From Homeostasis to Homeodynamics—Energy, Action, Stability, Senescence. 2002. http://www.biodynamic healthaging.org/Abstracts/YatesNIAsynopsis.pdf. p.1
5. Hensyl WR (Ed.). Illustrated Stedman's Medical Dictionary. Baltimore: Lippincott Williams and Wilkins, 2000.

6. Guyton AC, Hall JE. Textbook of Medical Physiology. Philadelphia: W.B. Saunders Company, 2000, p.1.
7. Waddington CH; Towards a Theoretical Biology, Vol. One. Aldine, Chicago: Prolegomena, 1968 in Yates FE. From Homeostasis to Homeodynamics—Energy, Action, Stability, Senescence. 2002. http://www.biodynamichealthaging.org/Abstracts/YatesNIA synopsis.pdf. p.1
8. Yates FE. From Homeostasis to Homeodynamics—Energy, Action, Stability, Senescence. 2002. http://www.biodynamichealthaging.org/Abstracts/YatesNIAsynopsis.pdf. p.1
9. Pizzorno JE Jr., Murray MT. Textbook of Natural Medicine. Edinburgh; Churchill Livingstone, 1999. p.10.
10. Ibid.
11. Willner C. An overview of the pathophysiology of neurodegenerative disorders. Altern Ther Health Med. 2004;10:26-34.
12. Pizzorno JE Jr., Murray MT. Textbook of Natural Medicine. Edinburgh; Churchill Livingstone, 1999. p.57.
13. Lichtenstein P, et al. Environmental and heritable factors in the causation of cancer. N Engl J Med. 2000;343:78-85.
14. Ganong WF. Review of Medical Physiology. Stamford, Connecticut; Appleton & Lange, 1997.
15. Larsen PR, et al. William's Textbook of Endocrinology. Philadelphia; Elsevier Science (USA), 2003, p. 35.
16. Larsen PR, et al. William's Textbook of Endocrinology. Philadelphia; Elsevier Science (USA), 2003, p. 36.
17. Memisoglu A, et al. Interaction between a peroxisome proliferator-activated receptor gamma gene polymorphism and dietary fat intake in relation to body mass. Hum Mol Genet. 2003;12:2923-29.
18. Cantorna MT. et al. 1,25-dihydroxyvitamin D3 reversibly blocks the progression of relapsing encephalomyelitis, a model of multiple sclerosis. Proc Natl Acad Sci USA. 1996;93:7861-64.
19. Ibid.
20. Sarkar FH, et al. Bax translocation to mitochondria is an important event in inducing apoptotic cell death by indole-3-carbinol treatment of breast cancer cells. J Nutri. 2003;133:2434S-39S.
21. Firestone GL, et al. Indole-3-carbinol and 3-3'-diindolymethane antiproliferative signaling pathways control cell-cycle gene transcription in human breast cancer cells by regulating promoter-Sp1 transcription factor interactions. J Nutri. 2003;133:2448S-55S.

Chapter 10
Web-like Interconnections: The Complex Human Organism

- ***Web-like Interconnections of Physiological Factors***
- ***Organ System Function and Underlying Mechanisms: The Interconnected Web***

Web-like Interconnections of Physiological Factors

DeAnn Liska, PhD and Dan Lukaczer, ND

Introduction

Science is a process of unraveling a phenomenon; persistence in the process, until the phenomenon is understood at deeper levels, is absolutely necessary. The body, however, isn't like a mystery novel; there isn't one villain to be found among a number of innocent bystanders caught up in the action. The body is much more complex, continually interacting with the environment and responding in minute ways. Take something as simple as the breath we take thousands of times a day. The rhythm of breath is affected by a brief noise, stopping it for a moment, or a smell, making us take a shorter quick huff or a longer, deep inhalation. All of this we may do with little conscious awareness.

Looking in a mirror, it's easy to think that the body is solid and formed, with little change in any given moment. But we are not statues. Our bodies are fully interconnected, complex, functioning organisms in which we have a constant flow of air, fluids, and energy upon a mutable matrix; nothing is ever still inside our bodies. Every twitch, every thought, every touch of the world around us on our skin elicits a response, causing a biochemical change that influences another change and then another. This is the web of our being, and in functional medicine, we use the model of a web to understand this complexity. The web model can explain the situations in which one major imbalance influences many different functions and systems, and the situations in which no major imbalance can be found, but several pathways seem to be off-center, or skewed enough to affect overall the pattern of health. The web is multidirectional—multiple factors can underlie a single condition, and multiple conditions can be influenced by a single dysfunctional process or imbalanced system.

Therefore, instead of looking for a single "root cause" of a disease and finding the "cure" from a single pill, in functional medicine we ask what is unbalanced, what has shifted the flow of biochemical information, energy, physical structure, and emotions too far to one side or the other of a healthy range, thus skewing the web. For many conditions, especially conditions associated with aging—like Alzheimer's disease, heart disease, or various arthritic conditions—finding a single root cause that will explain all the occurrences in all people is not possible. No single culprit exists and no single pill will cure these conditions in every patient. Instead, there are many influences, and there may be many imbalances, each contributing something to the outcome. Scientists and clinicians unraveling the web are likely to find a very complex set of interrelationships among myriad factors for each of these conditions.

In functional medicine, we ask about the patterns that are present and how these patterns are aiding or taking away from optimal function. Although every person is unique, with a unique set of genes interacting with the environment in a distinct, personal way, there are some major pathways we can monitor that will help us see where the imbalances are most likely to be found. Fundamentally, we look for the major points of activity on the web that, when skewed, are likely to influence many different parts of a person's biochemistry and physiology. The applications of this principle—web-like interconnections—are deeply explored throughout the chapters in Section VI: A Practical Clinical Approach. Here, we simply present the principle for your consideration.

Web-like Interconnections of Cellular Insensitivity to Insulin Signaling

Let's look at one example of a complex underlying physiological dysfunction that can manifest in a variety of ways: the dysfunction of cellular insensitivity to insulin signaling. It is an excellent model for visualizing the interconnections of complex chronic disease. Commonly referred to as the insulin resistance syndrome or metabolic syndrome, this multifaceted condition weaves its way through a web of interactions that manifest in a multitude of dysfunctions. Over 60 years ago, Dr. H.P. Himsworth used the term "insulin insensitivity" to describe his observation that diabetes was not generally associated with low insulin levels but with cellular insensitivity to insulin.[1] It took another 40 years until a consensus was reached on this radical notion. It is now clear that the vast majority of patients with type 2 diabetes have an insulin insensitivity that impairs their ability to adequately dispose of glucose; further, this defect—if discovered before frank diabetes is present—is predictive of the development of the disease.[2,3] As prescient an observation as it was, Himsworth probably did not fully understand the broader implications of his discovery. There is now a substantial and growing body of evidence that suggests insulin resistance is an underlying biochemical imbalance in not only type 2 diabetes, but cardiovascular disease (CVD), hypertension, polycystic ovary syndrome (PCOS), and even colon and some breast cancers.

How does insulin insensitivity relate to diabetes? Fundamentally, individuals who develop type 2 diabetes have a decline in the insulin secretory response. With insulin levels declining, circulating free fatty acids (FFAs)—which are normally suppressed by insulin—then rise. FFAs, in turn, stimulate hepatic glucose production. Without the normal insulin inhibitory signal, hyperglycemia occurs as the liver continues to secrete normal amounts of glucose into a greatly expanded plasma glucose pool.[4] With increasing hyperglycemia, there is a further reduction in beta cell function (possibly as a result of glucotoxicity) and a further drop in insulin.

It is estimated that the vast majority of the 16 million people diagnosed with type 2 diabetes in the U.S. carry the underlying pathophysiology of insulin resistance.[5] Many factors play into that situation: overweight, sedentary lifestyle, dietary choices, stress, and genetics are some of the most important. While muscle and adipose tissue are generally resistant to the imbalanced insulin signal, other tissues are not, and a cascading host of metabolic consequences and dysfunction ensues. Elevated insulin directly stimulates lipogenesis in arterial tissue and enhances the growth and proliferation of arterial smooth muscle cells; hyperinsulinemia decreases fibrinolysis by stimulating plasminogen activator inhibitor 1 (PAI-1),[6,7] which is associated with an increased risk for coronary thrombosis; and hyperinsulinemia leads to increased hepatic production of triglycerides (TG) and inhibition of high-density lipoproteins (HDL). Elevated TG and depressed HDL are important risk factors for coronary heart disease (CHD). These skewed pathways ultimately result in an increased incidence of CHD.[8,9,10]

Insulin resistance also plays a key role in hypertension; as much as 50% of the hypertensive population appears to be insulin resistant.[11] It has been proposed that a large segment of essential hypertension is caused by enhanced renal sodium reabsorption in the distal tubule, which is promoted by hyperinsulinemia.[12] Hyperinsulinemia may also play a role by altering internal sodium and potassium distribution in a direction that is associated with increased peripheral vascular resistance.[13] Insulin appears to work through other mechanisms as well to increase sympathetic nervous system activity and thus peripheral resistance.[14]

Furthermore, insulin resistance and hyperinsulinemia appear to have a critical relationship to androgen hormonal modulation. Research over the past 10 years has linked insulin with PCOS.[15] Studies have shown that high circulating insulin may stimulate ovarian cytochrome P450c17α and 17,20-lyase enzymes in predisposed women, resulting in elevations in serum testosterone and free unbound testosterone, which is associated with the signs and symptoms seen in PCOS. Insulin influences the androgenic state, not only by directly affecting the metabolism of ovarian androgens, but also indirectly by regulating circulating levels of sex hormone binding globulin (SHBG). Insulin has been shown to lower the production of SHBG.[16] SHBG binds to testosterone and estrogens, making them biologically unavailable and thus lowered SHBG indirectly increases the delivery of unbound and bioavailable testosterone to tissues.[17]

Insulin resistance also appears to be related to certain forms of cancer. One hypothesis has postulated a link between colorectal cancer, insulin resistance, and hyperinsulinemia.[18] While the epidemiological data are not completely consistent, the two largest prospective studies to date do support a modest correlation between colorectal cancer risk and diabetes.[19,20] Even more recently, speculation has centered on the link between hyperinsulinemia and breast cancer.[21] It has been known for some time that exposure of breast tissue to estrogens increases the risk of estrogen receptor-positive breast cancers. It is also well established that only the estrogens that are unbound to SHBG are biologically available to receptors on target cells. As mentioned, insulin inhibits the formation of SHBG. While SHBG binds to both testosterone and estrogen, it binds preferentially to testosterone, so decreased levels of SHBG result in increased levels of free unbound estrogen.[22] A more graphic representation of these and other relationships can be seen in Figure 10.1.

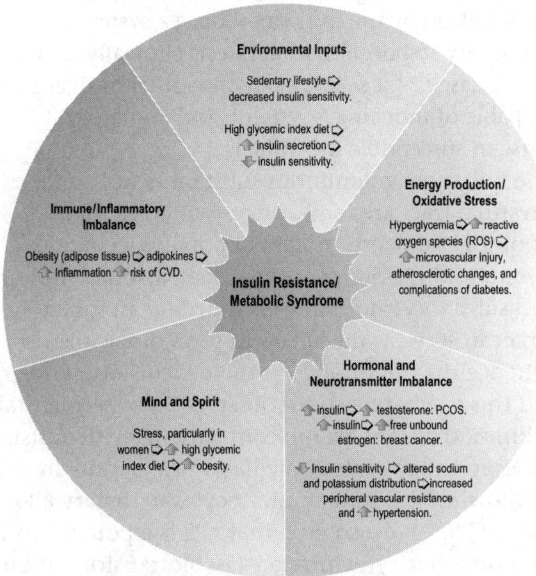

Figure 10.1 **Web-like interconnections: Insulin resistance syndrome**

Summary

As can be seen in this brief analysis, a specific dysfunction can result in myriad symptoms and can be caused by myriad factors. In this example, the imbalance is not confined to the single molecule, insulin; rather, it manifests in how the body secretes and responds to insulin. Promoting a healthy insulin response may involve many different factors. It is only by examining the web-like interconnections among these symptoms and factors that we can achieve a comprehensive assessment for the patient. As functional medicine clinicians, we examine the underlying imbalances; we ask ourselves what preceded and what triggered them; we look at upstream and downstream effects; and then we search for interventions that can affect the underlying interconnected pathways so that normal and even optimal function can be restored. Understanding how to rebalance important pathways in the body—establishing healthy and balanced web-like interconnections—is the key to reestablishing a healthy pattern of function.

Organ System Function and Underlying Mechanisms: The Interconnected Web

Alex Vasquez, DC, ND

Introduction

Understanding the scientific basis and clinical applications of functional medicine and a "whole patient" approach to health care requires that clinicians fully appreciate the interconnectedness of organ system function with biochemical and physiological processes. Simplistic models of health and disease developed decades ago may no longer be accurate or clinically useful insofar as they fail to reflect the more recently discovered complex and multifaceted interrelationships. (Figure 10.2 uses the functional medicine matrix to depict some of this complexity.) As discussed earlier in this chapter, numerous mechanisms mediate these interrelationships, including, but not limited to, those that can be described as biochemical, hormonal, neurological, immunological, piezoelectric, and physical or mechanical. Ultimately, we are forced to dissolve the artificial intellectual boundaries we have created between organ systems and expand our appreciation of individual molecules, cellular messengers, and the physiologic mechanisms that mediate intercellular communication and coordinate inter-organ function.

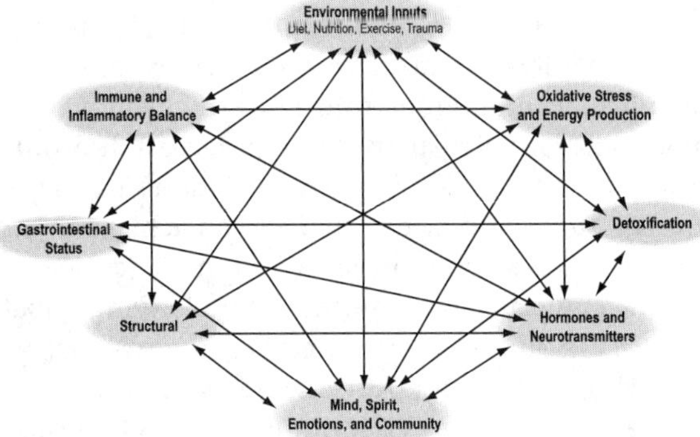

Figure 10.2 **Web-like interconnections of the functional medicine matrix**

The following discussion provides some specific examples of this profound interconnectedness that is a foundational principle of functional medicine. In this section, we will survey current research literature documenting the interconnected nature of some key organ systems and disease processes. With these examples, clinicians will better appreciate how the gastrointestinal, immune, cardiac, neurologic, and other systems interact with and depend upon each other for optimal physiologic function. Likewise, clinicians will understand more completely how essentially any dysfunction or lesion in the body can have clinically significant implications and distant adverse effects. From this perspective, individualized clinical interventions can be designed and employed to deliver better health outcomes.

Gastrointestinal Tract and Liver

While the liver and the gastrointestinal tract share an obvious anatomic connection via the portal circulation, the functional clinical implications of this connection are often not fully appreciated. Not only is the gastrointestinal tract the recipient of massive amounts of "external information" in the form of nutrients, toxicants, and allergens that weigh in at more than 1,538 pounds (700 kilograms) per year, but the gastrointestinal tract is also a reservoir for the several hundred species and subspecies of yeast, bacteria, and other microbes with the potential to modify hepatic function (e.g., detoxification) and overall health (e.g., immune response) by numerous mechanisms and with positive effects or negative consequences. (See Chapter 13 for a detailed discussion of microorganisms.)

The various organs and tissues of the gastrointestinal tract perform the complex functions of digestion, absorption, exclusion, excretion, immunologic defense, antigen sampling, and temporary storage of food residues and other substances that have been ingested. The mucosa is selectively permeable and allows the absorption of nutrients and other molecules via transcellular and paracellular routes. Compromise of mucosal integrity due to injury from antigens, infection, systemic inflammation, or toxicants such as ethanol or nonsteroidal anti-inflammatory drugs, increases absorption of potentially harmful substances that are normally excluded when mucosal integrity has not been breached. Materials that are harmless when rejected by the selectivity of the intestinal mucosa can, when inappropriately absorbed, serve as a source of inflammatory and immunogenic stimuli for the embedded macrophages in the liver (Kupffer cells) and also for the systemic immune system and the brain's embedded astrocytes and microglia. This phenomenon is clearly demonstrated by the neurological complications and focal white-matter lesions seen in the brains of patients sensitized to the dietary antigen gluten; in this scenario, it appears that dietary antigens cross a damaged mucosal lining and escape filtration by the liver to produce a systemic inflammatory response that manifests clinically as neurologic disease.[23,24] It seems likely that other antigens are also capable of inducing a systemic inflammatory response in susceptible individuals.

The two most voluminous substances in the gastrointestinal tract are food antigens and microbial metabolites and debris, notably lipopolysaccharides (LPS, endotoxin) from gram-negative bacteria. These foreign substances normally excluded by an intact mucosa can serve as mediators of physiologic disruption (hence the importance of their exclusion), and indeed this is what has been observed in experimental and clinical data. For example, in patients with autism, increases in inflammatory mediator production are seen following exposure of monocytes to dietary allergens and LPS.[25] We also note that LPS is a potent inhibitor of numerous cytochrome P450 biotransformation pathways, thus leading to impaired drug metabolism as demonstrated in recent clinical trials.[26,27] The implications of these data are profound and correlate closely with phenomena observed in clinical practice, namely that patients with irritable bowel syndrome—a condition causatively associated with both food intolerance and bacterial overgrowth of the small bowel—commonly report environmental sensitivity and medication intolerance. One plausible answer to the conundrum of the chronically unwell patient—typified by the patient with chronic fatigue or environmental illness—now becomes clear: overgrowth of the small bowel with LPS-producing bacteria leads directly to the gastrointestinal symptoms of gas and bloating, with immune system activation,[28] and also reduces hepatic clearance of metabolites, toxicants, and xenobiotics to which the patient eventually becomes sensitized (immunologically and/or non-immunologically). This explains, at least in part, the rationale for and impressive clinical efficacy associated with the implementation of clinical therapeutics that simultaneously improve intestinal microecology, improve mucosal integrity, and provide biochemical/nutritional support for the processes of detoxification.[29,30]

Gastrointestinal Tract and Immune System

Any discussion of the role of the gastrointestinal tract in relation to the immune system must include a view of the gut that is inclusive of its contents of food antigens, intraluminal microbes, and their debris and metabolic products. When the gut is simply pictured as a passive semi-sterile tube with food entering one end and feces exiting the other, then it would appear an unlikely locus of immunogenic stimulation and neurogenic inflammation that can have systemic health consequences.[31,32,33,34,35] Conversely, appreciation of the manifold quantitative and qualitative variables that can exist hidden from both the clinician's external view and the endoscopist's internal camera enables practitioners to have a more realistic perspective on the influence that gastrointestinal function, dietary antigens, and microflora can have on extra-gastrointestinal processes and overall health.[36,37]

The combination of a hypersensitive/dysregulated immune system and exposure to dietary antigens sets the stage for the clinical phenomenon commonly described as "food allergy." Diverse in frequency, duration, severity, and quality, these immune-mediated adverse reactions to foods can precipitate or exacerbate a wide range of clinical manifestations including rhinoconjunctivitis, chronic sinusitis, dermatitis, epilepsy, migraine, hypertension, joint inflammation, and mental depression.[38,39] The immunopathogenesis generally includes multiple mechanisms and is not limited to mediation via IgE antibodies and histamine. Indeed, the pathophysiology of "food allergy" is commonly seen with numerous (not singular) aberrations in physiologic function, including responses mediated by or resultant from antibodies (including IgE, IgG, and/or possibly IgA classes of antibodies), cytokine-mediated responses (e.g., TNF-α), increased intestinal permeability, occult gastrointestinal inflammation, and alterations in gastrointestinal microflora.[40] To be more complete, our conceptualization of "food allergy" must also include awareness of enterometabolic disorders (i.e., the interconnections between food, intestinal flora, and systemic health[41]) as well as contributions from neurogenic inflammation (i.e., the translation of immunogenic inflammation to a neurologic signal with systemic proinflammatory effects[42]).

Aberrations in gastrointestinal microflora can provoke a cascade of physiologic responses that may lead to widespread physiologic imbalances and result in a variety of clinical manifestations that may or may not conform to a recognized pattern or named disease even though the patient is highly symptomatic.[43] Furthermore, we can conclude from recent literature that the concept of molecular mimicry is now well established and that it provides us a model with which to apprehend the induction of immune dysfunction (especially autoimmunity) by microorganisms with immunogenic epitopes that are structurally similar to those in human tissues.[44] Thus, the link between "dysbiotic" gastrointestinal flora such as *Klebsiella pneumoniae* and systemic immune-mediated inflammatory disorders such as ankylosing spondylitis and chronic uveitis has a biological and scientific basis. Individualized assessment and treatment of such dysbiotic loci, whether in the gut, genitourinary tract, or nasopharynx, are likewise supported by current research and offer the hope of cure rather than an endless and additive cycle of anti-inflammatory and anti-rheumatic drugs. For example, evidence now shows that the systemic autoimmune disease Wegener's granulomatosis may be triggered and perpetuated by molecular mimicry with occult respiratory infections caused by *Staphylococcus aureus*, and that eradication of the infection can result in clinical improvement and reduced need for ongoing anti-rheumatic medication.[45,46,47] In addition to molecular mimicry, microbes (i.e., occult infections and environmental exposures) can also alter immune regulation by serving as a source of superantigens, which cause widespread and multifaceted immune dysfunction with resultant proinflammatory effects contributing to the exacerbation of allergy and autoimmune disease.[48]

Immune System and Cardiovascular System

The role of subclinical inflammation in the etiopathogenesis of atherosclerosis is no longer an issue of conjecture, as it has become a well-established aspect of the disease process. Even slight elevations in high-sensitivity C-reactive protein are associated with a significantly increased risk for cardiovascular morbidity and mortality in otherwise "apparently healthy" individuals.[49] With the increasing irrefutability of these data, pharmaceutical companies have scrambled to develop and sell drugs that can reduce this low-level inflammation, while physicians with a broader perspective have directed their energies toward intensifying their patient-centered search for the source(s) of inflammation in each individual patient. For example, subclinical inflammation can result from dietary indiscretion,[50] disturbed sleep,[51] and vitamin D deficiency;[52] in any of these situations, addressing the underlying causes of the inflammation with multicomponent nutritional/lifestyle interventions may deliver more effective health improvement than can the long-term use of inflammation-suppressing medications.[53,54,55]

Gastrointestinal Tract, Liver, and Neurologic Systems

The last several years have witnessed an increased appreciation for the influence that the gut and liver have on the brain, and advancements in functional assessments are now documenting analytically what was at one point known only clinically—that the status of the gut and liver have profound effects on the functioning of the brain. Evidence supporting the existence of a clinically important gut-brain interconnection has been published consistently over many decades and in major journals; see Chapters 28 (discussion by Gershon) and 31 (discussion by James) for analyses of these complex interactions. Today, among the most poignant examples are Parkinson's disease and the autistic spectrum disorders. Indeed, the strength of evidence supporting the hepato-gastrointestinal link with these "neurologic" conditions is so strong that it could be logically argued that any treatment of these conditions that does not address the hepatic and enteric aspects of these diseases is therapeutically incomplete.

Although Parkinson's disease was once considered idiopathic, we now recognize it as being a multifaceted disorder associated with defective mitochondrial function, impaired xenobiotic detoxification, and occupational and/or recreational exposure to toxicants, particularly pesticides. These associations align to create a new model for the illness based on exposure to neurotoxicants such as pesticides,[56] which are ineffectively detoxified[57] and then accumulate in the brain,[58] inducing mitochondrial dysfunction[59] and oxidative stress,[60] and leading to the death of dopaminergic neurons. Therefore, from the perspective of both prevention and treatment, the clinical approach to Parkinson's disease must include pesticide avoidance and optimization of detoxification to prevent the neuronal accumulation of neurotoxic mitochondrial poisons. The plan must also include optimization of nutritional status, antioxidant capacity, and mitochondrial function.[61]

The view that autism is a behavioral problem unfortunately continues to permeate present-day medical treatment of this condition, and many pediatricians and psychiatrists still advise only behavioral therapy and medicalization with psychoactive pharmaceuticals, particularly selective serotonin reuptake inhibitors (SSRIs).[62,63] While these interventions produce modest improvements over those seen in control groups, neither intervention remotely addresses the complex underlying physiology nor offers the possibility of cure, and SSRI use in children is highly controversial due to the association with increased incidence of suicide.[64] We now know that autism is a multifaceted disorder associated with gastrointestinal inflammation, nutritional deficiencies,[65] multiple food allergies and intolerances,[66] impairments in liver detoxification and resultant accumulation of xenobiotics, the majority of which have neurotoxic and/or immunotoxic effects.[67] Thus, autism is not a behavioral disorder *per se*; rather, it is a gastrointestinal-allergic-immunological-toxicant-nutritional-environmental disorder, and the behavioral/cognitive abnormalities are symptoms of the underlying complex and interconnected pathophysiology. See

Chapter 30 (discussion by McGinnis) for an in-depth analysis of autism and oxidative stress.

Musculoskeletal System, Neurologic System, Immune System

The adverse effects of a dysregulated immune system upon the musculoskeletal system are well known for their contributions to autoimmune diseases such as rheumatoid arthritis. In this classic scenario, the immune system is the effector, and periarticular structures, synovium, and joint surfaces are the targets of inflammatory and destructive processes that result in joint destruction and pain that affect the musculoskeletal and neurologic systems, respectively. This model holds that the direction of events flows from the immune system (autoimmunity) to the musculoskeletal system (target site) to the nervous system (perception of pain). This popular model must be updated in light of current research.

The phenomena of neurogenic inflammation and neuronal plasticity demonstrate the active, effector functions of the sensory nervous system and exemplify the extent to which the Cartesian model of the sensory nervous system (i.e., as exclusively afferent and passively receptive) is no longer valid.[68,69] Much of the musculoskeletal inflammation seen in clinical practice appears due, in large part, to inflammation that originates from and is mediated by the sensory nervous system through the release of proinflammatory mediators from sensory nerves in periarticular tissues. [70,71] Furthermore, evidence is accumulating that neurogenic inflammation can result from a heterogenous group of diverse stimuli, including allergens, environmental chemicals, and pain distant from the site of arthritis.[72,73] Likewise, evidence that intentional relaxation[74] as well as acupuncture[75] can modulate inflammatory pathophysiology indicates that psycho-emotional variables and nonbiochemical therapeutics are important clinical considerations for patients with inflammatory diseases.

Evidence also suggests that musculoskeletal therapeutics such as spinal manipulation may influence immune responsiveness. Brennan et al.[76,77] showed that chiropractic spinal manipulation resulted in an acute increase in phagocytic capacity of polymorphonuclear neutrophils, and that this result was seen only following authentic (versus sham) manipulation, and that the effect was proportional to the increase in serum levels of substance P, a multifunctional molecule that acts as a neurotransmitter as well as a proinflammatory messenger. While the clinical implications of these data are yet to be clarified, they clearly demonstrate that the immune system is sensitive to mechanical stimuli.

Beyond Biochemistry and Neurophysiology: Piezoelectricity as a Mechanism for Intersystem Connectedness

Piezoelectricity, the continuum between mechanical stress and bioelectric conduction, is a well-established aspect of organic matter, affecting all vertebrates and, therefore, humans. Notably, the nervous system in general and the spinal cord in particular demonstrate an intrinsic dipole moment that is demonstrable across species of vertebrates.[78,79] In 1977, Lipiski from Tufts University School of Medicine[80] summarized the current research of the day and speculated on the effects of spinal manipulation, yoga, and acupuncture as mediated via the body's inherent pyroelectric and piezoelectric properties. Lipinski's literature review (particularly including the work of Bassett[81]) suggests that "piezoelectricity present in many biological systems may theoretically control cell nutrition, local pH, enzyme activation and inhibition, orientation of intra- and extra-cellular macromolecules, migratory and proliferative activity of cells, contractility of permeability of cell membranes, and energy transfer." With these concepts and possibilities considered, we can construct a conceptual bridge linking mechanical stimuli such as massage, manipulation, exercise, and yoga, and (neuro)electrical stimuli such as acupuncture, meditation, prayer and intentionality, to plausible biochemical/physiological effects that translate into observed clinical benefits. This integrated model helps to explain the effects of "energetic" therapeutics such as moxibustion, acupuncture, and yoga that may be mediated by nonbiochemical physiologic mechanisms. Furthermore, this model also helps us to understand hitherto unexplainable phenomena such as the well-reported sensitivity that some people display to changes in the weather and the positioning of their bodies in relation to electromagnetic fields of the planet, electrical equipment, and power lines. Piezoelectricity may also be the physiologic conduit that transmits the effects of "distance healing," prayer, and intentionality.[82,83,84]

Summary

Human physiology is complex and treatment plans must be multifaceted to reflect this complexity. Cells, tissues, and organ systems work in concert—not in isolation—and therefore effective intervention generally requires improvement in numerous organ systems. As the artificial boundaries between organ systems dissolve, a unifying theme emerges, namely that the attainment, preservation, and re-establishment of health must be all-encompassing. Programs and paradigms related to the treatment of disease and the attainment of optimal health must reflect appreciation of environmental, physical, mental/emotional, nutritional, biochemical, hormonal, immunologic, neurologic, and gastrointestinal components of our existence that coalesce without boundaries to make the human body and our experience of life itself. Thus, new frontiers in health care will be reached not solely when new discoveries occur, but also when the integration of these discoveries into a cohesive, multifaceted, unified healthcare model prepares the way for more accurate understanding and more effective interventions. Healthcare providers of diverse backgrounds (e.g., ND, DC, MD, DO, RD, RN, LAc, and others) can and must work together to offer scientifically-based, multifactorial interventions that are adapted to the specific needs of individual patients.

References

1. Reaven GM. Insulin resistance and human disease: a short history. J Basic Clin Physiol Pharmacol. 1998;9(2-4):387-406.
2. Reaven GM. Insulin resistance in non-insulin-dependent diabetes mellitus. Does it exist and can it be measured? Am J Med. 1983;74:3-17.
3. Lillioja S, Mott D, Spraul M, et al. Insulin resistance and insulin secretory dysfunction as precursors of non-insulin-dependent diabetes mellitus. N Engl J Med 1993;329:1988-92.
4. Reaven, GM. Pathophysiology of insulin resistance in human disease Physiol Rev. 1995;75(3):473-85.
5. Centers for Disease Control and Prevention (CDC). National Diabetes Awareness Month—November 1997. Morb Mortal Wkly Rep. 1997;46:1013-1026.
6. Potter van Loon BJ, Kluft C, Radder JK, et al. The cardiovascular risk factor plasminogen activator inhibitor type I is related to insulin resistance. Metabolism. 1993;42:945-49.
7. Juhan-Vague I, Pyke SD, Alessi MC, et al. Fibrinolytic factors and the risk of myocardial infarction or sudden death in patients with angina pectoris. Circulation. 1996;94(9):2057-063.
8. Reaven GM. Are triglycerides important as a risk factor for coronary disease? Heart Dis Stroke. 1993;2:44-48.
9. Laws A, King AC, Haskell WL, et al. Relation of fasting plasma insulin concentration to high-density lipoprotein cholesterol and triglyceride concentration in men. Arterioscler Thromb. 1991;11:1636-42.
10. Assmann G, Schulte H. Relation of high-density lipoprotein cholesterol and triglycerides to incidence of atherosclerotic coronary artery disease (the PROCAM experience). Am J Cardiol. 1992;70:733-37.
11. Zavaroni I, Coruzzi P, Bonini L, et al. Association between salt sensitivity and insulin concentrations in patients with hypertension. Am J Hypertens. 1995;8:855-58.
12. Zavaroni I, Mazza S, Dall'Aglio E, et al. Prevalence of hyperinsulinaemia in patients with high blood pressure. J Intern Med. 1992;231:235-40.
13. Ibid.
14. Gans RO, Donker AJ. Insulin and blood pressure regulation. J Intern Med Suppl. 1991;735:49-64.
15. Nestler J. Insulin resistance effects on sex hormones and ovulation in the polycystic ovary syndrome. From Contemporary Endocrinology: Insulin Resistance, Edited by G. Reaven and A. Laws. Humana Press Inc., Totowa, NJ, 1999. 347-365.
16. Singh A, Hamilton-Fairley D, Koistinen R, et al. Effect of insulin-like growth factor-type 1 (IGF-I) and insulin on the secretion of sex-hormone binding globulin and IGF-I binding protein (IBP-I) by human hepatoma cells. J Endocrinol. 1990;124:R1-3.
17. Nestler JE, Powers LP, Matt DW, et al. A direct effect of hyperinsulinemia on serum sex hormone-binding globulin levels in obese women with the polycystic ovary syndrome. J Clin Endocrinol Metab. 1991;72:83-89.
18. Giovannucci E. Insulin and colon cancer. Cancer Causes Control. 1995;6:164-79.
19. Weiderpass E, Gridley G, Nyren O, et al. Diabetes mellitus and risk of large bowel cancer. J Natl Cancer Inst. 1997;89:660-661.
20. Will J, Galuska D, Vinicor F, et al. Colorectal cancer: another complication of diabetes mellitus? Am J Epidemiol. 1998;147:816-25.
21. Kaaks R. Nutrition, hormones, and breast cancer: is insulin the missing link? Cancer Causes Control. 1996;7:605-25.
22. Rosner W. The functions of corticosteroid-binding globulin and sex-hormone-binding globulin: recent advances. Endocr Rev. 1990;11:80-91.
23. Kieslich M, Errazuriz G, Posselt HG, et al. Brain white-matter lesions in celiac disease: a prospective study of 75 diet-treated patients. Pediatrics. 2001 Aug;108(2):E21.
24. Burk K, Bosch S, Muller CA, et al. Sporadic cerebellar ataxia associated with gluten sensitivity. Brain. 2001;124(Pt 5):1013-19.
25. Jyonouchi H, Sun S, Itokazu N. Innate immunity associated with inflammatory responses and cytokine production against common dietary proteins in patients with autism spectrum disorder. Neuropsychobiology. 2002;46:76-84.
26. Shedlofsky SI, Israel BC, Tosheva R, Blouin RA. Endotoxin depresses hepatic cytochrome P450-mediated drug metabolism in women. Br J Clin Pharmacol. 1997;43(6):627-32.
27. Shedlofsky SI, Israel BC, McClain CJ, et al. Endotoxin administration to humans inhibits hepatic cytochrome P450-mediated drug metabolism. J Clin Invest. 1994;94:2209-14.
28. Lin HC. Small intestinal bacterial overgrowth: a framework for understanding irritable bowel syndrome. JAMA. 2004;292(7):852-58.
29. Bland JS, Bralley JA. Nutritional upregulation of hepatic detoxification enzymes. J Appl Nutr 1992;44:2-15.
30. Bland JS, Barrager E, Reedy RG, Bland K. A Medical Food-Supplemented Detoxification Program in the Management of Chronic Health Problems. Altern Ther Health Med. 1995;1:62-71.

31. Meggs WJ. Neurogenic switching: a hypothesis for a mechanism for shifting the site of inflammation in allergy and chemical sensitivity. Environ Health Perspect. 1995;103(1):54-56.
32. Richardson JD, Vasko MR. Cellular mechanisms of neurogenic inflammation. J Pharmacol Exp Ther. 2002;302(3):839-45.
33. Kirkwood KS, Bunnett NW, Maa J, et al. Deletion of neutral endopeptidase exacerbates intestinal inflammation induced by Clostridium difficile toxin A. Am J Physiol Gastrointest Liver Physiol. 2001;281(2):G544-51.
34. Bascom R, Meggs WJ, Frampton M, et al. Neurogenic inflammation: with additional discussion of central and perceptual integration of nonneurogenic inflammation. Environ Health Perspect. 1997;Mar;105 Suppl 2:531-37.
35. Gouze-Decaris E, Philippe L, Minn A, et al. Neurophysiological basis for neurogenic-mediated articular cartilage anabolism alteration. Am J Physiol Regul Integr Comp Physiol. 2001;280(1):R115-22.
36. Inman RD. Antigens, the gastrointestinal tract, and arthritis. Rheum Dis Clin North Am. 1991;17(2):309-21.
37. Galland L. Intestinal protozoan infection is a common unsuspected cause of chronic illness. J Advancement Med. 1989;2: 539-552.
38. Vasquez A. Integrative Orthopedics: Concepts, Algorithms, and Therapeutics. The art of creating wellness while effectively managing acute and chronic musculoskeletal disorders. Updated Edition (August 2004). Houston; Natural Health Consulting Corp. WellBodyBook.com Pages 404-418.
39. Gaby AR. The role of hidden food allergy/intolerance in chronic disease. Altern Med Rev. 1998;3(2):90-100.
40. Vasquez A. Integrative Orthopedics: Concepts, Algorithms, and Therapeutics. The art of creating wellness while effectively managing acute and chronic musculoskeletal disorders. Updated Edition (August 2004). Houston; Natural Health Consulting Corp. WellBodyBook.com Pages 404-418.
41. Hunter JO. Food allergy—or enterometabolic disorder? Lancet. 1991;338(8765):495-96.
42. Meggs WJ. Neurogenic switching: a hypothesis for a mechanism for shifting the site of inflammation in allergy and chemical sensitivity. Environ Health Perspect. 1995;103(1):54-56.
43. Galland L. Intestinal protozoan infection is a common unsuspected cause of chronic illness. J Advancement Med. 1989;2: 539-552.
44. Albert LJ, Inman RD. Molecular mimicry and autoimmunity. N Engl J Med. 1999;341(27):2068-74.
45. Popa ER, Stegeman CA, Kallenberg CG, Tervaert JW. Staphylococcus aureus and Wegener's granulomatosis. Arthritis Res. 2002;4(2):77-79.
46. George J, Levy Y, Kallenberg CG, Shoenfeld Y. Infections and Wegener's granulomatosis—a cause and effect relationship? QM. 1997;90(5):367-73.
47. Van Putten JW, van Haren EH, Lammers JW. Association between Wegener's granulomatosis and Staphylococcus aureus infection? Eur Respir J. 1996;9(9):1955-57.
48. Hemalatha V, Srikanth P, Mallika M. Superantigens—Concepts, clinical disease and therapy. Indian J Med Microbiol 2004;22:204-211.
49. Koenig W, Pepys MB. C-reactive protein risk prediction: low specificity, high sensitivity. Ann Intern Med. 2002;136(7):550-52.
50. Liu S, Manson JE, Buring JE, et al. Relation between a diet with a high glycemic load and plasma concentrations of high-sensitivity C-reactive protein in middle-aged women. Am J Clin Nutr. 2002;75(3):492-98.
51. Yokoe T, Minoguchi K, Matsuo H, et al. Elevated levels of C-reactive protein and interleukin-6 in patients with obstructive sleep apnea syndrome are decreased by nasal continuous positive airway pressure. Circulation. 2003;107:1129-34.
52. Vasquez A, Manso G, Cannell J. The Clinical Importance of Vitamin D (Cholecalciferol): A Paradigm Shift with Implications for All Healthcare Providers. Alternative Therapies in Health and Medicine 2004; 10: 28-37.
53. Knoops KT, de Groot LC, Kromhout D, et al. Mediterranean diet, lifestyle factors, and 10-year mortality in elderly European men and women: the HALE project. JAMA. 2004;292(12):1433-39.
54. Topol EJ. Failing the public health—rofecoxib, Merck, and the FDA. N Engl J Med. 2004;351:1707-9.
55. Orme-Johnson DW, Herron RE. An innovative approach to reducing medical care utilization and expenditures. Am J Manag Care. 1997;3(1):135-44.
56. Ritz B, Yu F. Parkinson's disease mortality and pesticide exposure in California 1984-1994. Int J Epidemiol. 2000;29(2):323-9.
57. Menegon A, Board PG, Blackburn AC, et al. Parkinson's disease, pesticides, and glutathione transferase polymorphisms. Lancet. 1998;352(9137):1344-46.
58. Kamel F, Hoppin JA. Related Articles, Association of pesticide exposure with neurologic dysfunction and disease. Environ Health Perspect. 2004;112(9):950-58.
59. Parker WD Jr, Swerdlow RH. Mitochondrial dysfunction in idiopathic Parkinson disease. Am J Hum Genet. 1998;62(4):758-62.
60. Davey GP, Peuchen S, Clark JB. Energy thresholds in brain mitochondria. Potential involvement in neurodegeneration. J Biol Chem. 1998;273(21):12753-57.
61. Kidd PM. Parkinson's disease as multifactorial oxidative neurodegeneration: implications for integrative management. Altern Med Rev. 2000;5(6):502-29.
62. Bryson SE, Rogers SJ, Fombonne E. Autism spectrum disorders: early detection, intervention, education, and psychopharmacological management. Can J Psychiatry. 2003;48(8):506-16.
63. Couper JJ, Sampson AJ. Children with autism deserve evidence-based intervention. Med J Aust. 2003;178(9):424-25.
64. Kondro W. UK bans, Health Canada warns about antidepressants. CMAJ. 2004;171:23.
65. Wakefield AJ, Murch SH, Anthony A, et al. Ileal-lymphoid-nodular hyperplasia, non-specific colitis, and pervasive developmental disorder in children. Lancet. 1998;351(9103):637-41.
66. White JF. Intestinal pathophysiology in autism. Exp Biol Med (Maywood). 2003;228(6):639-49.
67. Edelson SB, Cantor DS. Autism: xenobiotic influences. Toxicol Ind Health. 1998;14:553-63.
68. Richardson JD, Vasko MR. Cellular mechanisms of neurogenic inflammation. J Pharmacol Exp Ther. 2002;302(3):839-45.
69. Boal RW, Gillette RG. Central neuronal plasticity, low back pain and spinal manipulative therapy. J Manipulative Physiol Ther. 2004;27(5):314-26.
70. Gouze-Decaris E, Philippe L, Minn A, et al. Neurophysiological basis for neurogenic-mediated articular cartilage anabolism alteration. Am J Physiol Regul Integr Comp Physiol. 2001;280(1):R115-22.
71. Lee JC, Salonen DC, Inman RD. Unilateral hemochromatosis arthropathy on a neurogenic basis. J Rheumatol. 1997;24(12):2476-78.
72. Bascom R, Meggs WJ, Frampton M, et al. Neurogenic inflammation: with additional discussion of central and perceptual integration of nonneurogenic inflammation. Environ Health Perspect. 1997;105 Suppl 2:531-37.
73. Meggs WJ. Neurogenic switching: a hypothesis for a mechanism for shifting the site of inflammation in allergy and chemical sensitivity. Environ Health Perspect. 1995;103(1):54-56.
74. Lutgendorf S, Logan H, Kirchner HL, et al. Effects of relaxation and stress on the capsaicin-induced local inflammatory response. Psychosom Med. 2000;62(4):524-34.

75. Joos S, Brinkhaus B, Maluche C, et al. Acupuncture and moxibustion in the treatment of active Crohn's disease: a randomized controlled study. Digestion. 2004;69(3):131-39.
76. Brennan PC, Kokjohn K, Kaltinger CJ, et al. Enhanced phagocytic cell respiratory burst induced by spinal manipulation: potential role of substance P. J Manipulative Physiol Ther. 1991;14(7):399-408.
77. Brennan PC, Triano JJ, McGregor M, et al. Enhanced neutrophil respiratory burst as a biological marker for manipulation forces: duration of the effect and association with substance P and tumor necrosis factor. J Manipulative Physiol Ther. 1992;15(2):83-89.
78. Athenstaedt H. Pyroelectric and piezoelectric properties of vertebrates. Ann NY Acad Sci. 1974;238:68-94.
79. Athenstaedt H. "Functional polarity" of the spinal cord caused by its longitudinal electric dipole moment. Am J Physiol. 1984;247(3 Pt 2):R482-87.
80. Lipinski B. Biological significance of piezoelectricity in relation to acupuncture, Hatha Yoga, osteopathic medicine and action of air ions. Med Hypotheses. 1977;3(1):9-12.
81. Bassett CA. Biologic significance of piezoelectricity. Calcif Tissue Res. 1968;1(4):252-72.
82. Byrd RC. Positive therapeutic effects of intercessory prayer in a coronary care unit population. South Med J. 1988;81(7):826-29.
83. Matthews DA, Marlowe SM, MacNutt FS. Effects of intercessory prayer on patients with rheumatoid arthritis. South Med J. 2000;93(12):1177-86.
84. Astin JA, Harkness E, Ernst E. The efficacy of "distant healing": a systematic review of randomized trials. Ann Intern Med. 2000;132(11):903-10.

Chapter 11
Health as a Positive Vitality

Nancy Sudak, MD

The Goal of Health is More than the Absence of Frank Disease

The disease model is compatible with a managed care setting, in which insurance reimbursement for services is predicated upon codified diagnoses. The problem with this practice is that it fails to acknowledge the zone of dysfunction that occurs between optimal health and diagnosable disease. Although a working understanding of disease is both critical and useful, it can be enlightening to acknowledge that a disease is not a bona fide entity, but rather a label we affix to clinical patterns of signs and symptoms. When no "disease" can be found, this model becomes less relevant, and clinicians are often at a loss to identify effective treatments beyond palliative pharmaceuticals. We lose the opportunity to transform health and move the patient back toward wellness when we adhere to this model; regenerative potential is diminished as one advances further toward chronic disease on this continuum. Clearly, waiting until disease identifies itself before developing meaningful therapeutic strategies is detrimental to our patients and costly for our healthcare system overall.

An unfortunate result of employing the disease model is that the concept of health has come to be equated with the absence of disease. Patients who return from medical evaluations relative to symptoms frequently report, "The doctor said there's nothing wrong with me." Though patients tend to be relieved when no major disease is discovered, they may also be distressed by the discrepancy between their sensation of being unwell and the physician's assertion that all findings are normal. Significant morbidity and psychological distress may ensue,[1] particularly if the physician's attitude is dismissive. Because the focus of medical education is on disease, not wellness, physicians are not specifically trained to be qualified surveyors of vitality. A comprehensive medical history should include inquiry about habits that establish health as well as behaviors that erode it. Functional medicine practitioners evaluate patients through physical findings, objective laboratory measures, and a comprehensive appraisal of an individual's environmental inputs, which typically include: dietary habits, quality of air, water and soil, toxic and infectious exposures, exercise patterns, social relationships, behavior, stress management techniques, and spiritual centering practices.

The word "health" is derived from the Old English "*hal*," meaning wholeness, being whole, hale, sound, or well.[2] In current parlance, we recognize that wholeness signifies full function of the body-mind-spirit. In this light, it is not extreme to expect to feel fully alive, vibrant, and even joyful when healthy. Since much of the population reports chronic symptoms in the absence of authenticated disease,[3] patients are led to believe that it is normal to feel unwell in the face of a clean bill of health. It is now evident that the overweight adult population in the U.S. constitutes the majority;[4] thus, it has become standard to be overweight. Obviously, the solution is not to rework our height and weight charts to accommodate an obese population, but to become conscious that what appears to be most common in our culture is not necessarily healthy. By adopting a more optimistic and functional approach to wellness, we define health as positive vitality, rather than mere absence of disease. This attitude promotes consideration of features that fortify our physiology to promote wellness, instead of concentrating on negative factors that give rise to illness.

We are aware of literally thousands of highly useful disease markers. However, ruling out disease by using laboratory measures doesn't necessarily rule in good health. Positive indicators of wellness may be found to some degree on objective testing (e.g., cellular nutrient levels, beneficial flora cultures, antioxidant levels, hormone metabolites, etc.). A diagnosis of being truly healthy will depend on favorable physical exam findings and laboratory evaluations, of course, but the patient's story of how vital and fully functional he or she feels must figure prominently in the clinician's assessment. Patients who report feeling unwell despite unrevealing evaluations tend to benefit from a functional medicine approach since broad areas of dysfunction are identifiable and treatable through supportive and restorative measures.

Importance of Functionality to Quality of Life

Illnesses and symptoms, whether acute or chronic, may generally be traced to one or more functional disturbances within the functional medicine "web." Functional status is characteristically diminished in keeping with the magnitude of symptoms. To use a simple example of immune system dysregulation, a person with an itchy patch of atopic dermatitis on one ankle is less likely to experience a decline in functionality than someone with generalized urticaria. When we are highly symptomatic, discomfort becomes a leading influence from which we cannot be readily distracted, and a greater degree of debility is anticipated. When functional capacity weakens, we can also expect quality of life to decline. Health-related quality of life is a multifaceted concept that reflects the outcome of an illness on a patient's evaluation of his or her functional status and emotional well-being. Abundant reports in the medical literature confirm the harmful impact of illness or chronic symptoms on quality of life observed in conditions such as: osteoarthritis,[5] chronic fatigue syndrome,[6] obesity,[7] insomnia,[8] childhood migraines,[9] and hip fractures.[10]

Good health—full functionality on every level—is achieved by favorable interactions between our genes and our environment. When we understand that our genes have not changed substantially from those of our Paleolithic progenitors, but that our modern environment has been radically altered since that era, we appreciate that our journey to maintain positive vitality must involve manipulating our environment advantageously to match the physiology of our genes. No two people share identical genetic activity; each individual is constantly experiencing his or her environment to produce a certain quality of life. Our daily behaviors are fundamental to the production of our internal and external environments, and represent the most powerful influences upon our physiology. These daily choices contribute directly to biochemical function and may include: diet quality and quantity, micronutrient adequacy, level of physical exercise, action of the hypothalamic-pituitary-thyroid-adrenal axis, toxic or infectious exposures, and emotional experiences of joy, fear, hostility, connectedness, etc. Negative influences include frequent application of lawn pesticides, regular ingestion of trans-fatty acids, frequently skipping meals, and excessive activation of the stress response, whereas positive influences are exemplified by purposeful avoidance of xenobiotics, adequate daily intake of pure water, essential fatty acids, antioxidants, and regular use of stress management techniques.

When we refer to an individual as being "highly functional," we are often making a judgment of someone's ability to be physically or intellectually industrious. A principal driving force behind feeling energetic, creative, and productive is vigorous cellular and biochemical function. Assessing the core clinical imbalances of a patient is predicated upon understanding the body's major molecular mediators (e.g., cytokines, immunoglobulins, antioxidants, stress hormones, neurotransmitters, fatty acids, etc.). Our health is determined by the complex interplay of these biologic modifiers as they cut across multiple organs. (See sections IV and V of this book for detailed information about these important influences.) The further we depart from daily healthy lifestyle practices, the less molecular support we provide to our metabolic functions, and if this process continues, cellular resiliency declines and we have begun to pave the road toward dysfunction and disease. We may feel less physically and emotionally lively as this path unfolds.

We can easily think of instances of how the mind affects the body. A classic example of this concept is the well-documented effect of mindfulness meditation in reducing chronic pain.[11] Another common example is the association between hostility and increased risk for myocardial infarction.[12] The effect of the body on the mind is equally observable, since physiologic variables clearly contribute to emotional and cognitive welfare. Straightforward examples of molecular mediators that modulate brain function include: blood glucose levels, neurotransmitters, essential fatty acids, and B vitamins.[13] However, less obvious biochemical mediators may have a profound impact on function. For example, if dietary intake of gluten is inappropriate for a given individual's physiology, psychiatric and emotional disturbances may be seen.[14,15] Certain people may become sluggish and unmotivated after succumbing to a carbohydrate craving. Many patients who implement a comprehensive elimination diet experience unanticipated abatement of chronic symptoms long considered part of their normal physiologic landscape. In this way, they learn that diet is an environmental input that is critically important in determining function and vigor.

Spiritual connection represents another dimension of being that affects quality of life. Though difficult to quantify in research, the role of spirituality in health care has been receiving increasing attention.[16] Geriatric patients reporting greater degrees of spirituality tended to more highly appraise their health status.[17] The American Psychiatric Association's Board of Trustees has passed a resolution stating that "it is useful for clinicians to obtain information on the religious or ideologic orientation and beliefs of their patients so that they may properly attend to them in the course of treatment." Religious commitment appears to be correlated with decreased risk for depression, substance abuse, hypertension, and other chronic health problems.[18] In a recent survey, greater than 75% of patients believed that spiritual issues should be addressed routinely in clinical care.[19] Practitioners who engage with patients' spirituality will bring more meaning to healthcare delivery and the therapeutic relationship. A practical approach to accomplishing this goal is discussed in Chapter 33.

Though conventional medicine seems to have partitioned mind and spirit from body, the functional medicine approach embraces these essential elements of wholeness as they affect one another within the matrix of core areas of function. Quality of physiologic function is generated by the performance of daily behaviors, by and large within the sphere of our control. We maximize wellness of body-mind-spirit when we consistently implement practices that strengthen our unique constitutions, and learn to reject those that seem to impair vitality and optimal function. As biochemically unique individuals, we must each determine which environmental inputs are ideal in defining our personal health.

The functional medicine model embraces the old adage "If you don't take time for your health, you'll have to take time for your illness." We understand that our daily actions collectively represent the most significant factor of control over our health. Decision-making in this regard occurs many times within a 24-hour period. When we become mindful of our immediate options to produce better health outcomes, we may ask ourselves many questions as we navigate through the day:

- Shall I eat a full breakfast or just have a doughnut during my break?
- Shall I walk to work or drive?
- Should I exercise today or sleep later?
- Which would suit my needs better—a slice of pizza on-the-run or a meal of lean protein, fresh vegetables, and whole grains that I actually sit down to eat?
- Should I watch a rerun of my favorite sit-com or go to bed earlier?
- Should I try to remain gluten-free for a few weeks to see if my headaches improve?
- Will application of lawn pesticides to kill the dandelions on my lawn affect my health and that of the planet adversely?

Once it becomes habitual to ask these questions and to mindfully implement the healthier options, making optimal choices becomes self-perpetuating. If we are paying attention, we can quickly realize how much better we feel when we show a preference for those selections better matched to our physiology.

The functional medicine paradigm illustrates the art of living well as the basis for health and well-being. Symptoms or impairment of vitality will prompt a trained practitioner to investigate for functional imbalances. Functional medicine has the potential to revolutionize healthcare delivery, not only as a result of its anticipatory and preventive nature, but because the identification and supportive treatment of underlying contributing factors is the most effective means of addressing the health of the individual. By recognizing and treating functional disturbances, physicians can guide patients toward more advantageous environmental inputs, thereby saving millions of dollars in healthcare expenditures. Functional medicine physicians routinely state that they have become re-enchanted with medical practice; once they have learned the application of nutritional biochemistry and functional physiology, they have at their disposal an extensive array of tools that are quite satisfying to implement.

References

1. Kroenke K, Arrington ME, Mangelsdorff D. The prevalence of symptoms in medical outpatients and the adequacy of therapy. Arch Int Med. 1990;150:1685-89.
2. The Century Dictionary: An Encyclopedic Lexicon on the English Language. New York: The Century Co., 1913.
3. Kroenke K, Mangelsdorff D. Common symptoms in ambulatory care: incidence, evaluation, therapy, and outcome. Am J Med. 1989;86:262-66.
4. Hedley AA, Ogden CL, Johnson CL, et al. Prevalence of overweight and obesity among US children, adolescents, and adults, 1999-2002. JAMA. 2004;291:2847-50.
5. Fontaine, K. Arthritis and health related quality of life. Johns Hopkins Arthritis. Available on-line at http://www.hopkins-arthritis.som.jhmi.edu/mngmnt/qol.html
6. Solomon L, Nisenbaum M, Reyes M, et al. Functional status of people with chronic fatigue syndrome in the Wichita, Kansas population. Health and Quality of Life Outcomes 2003;1:48.
7. Doll HA, Petersen SEK, Stewart-Brown SL. Obesity and physical and emotional well-being: associations between body mass index, chronic illness, and the physical and mental components of the SF-36 questionnaire. Obesity Res. 2000;8(2):160-70.
8. Katz DA, McHorney CA. The relationship between insomnia and health-related quality of life in patients with chronic illness. J Fam Pract. 2002;51:229-35.
9. Powers SW, Patton SR, Hommel KA, Hershey AD. Quality of life in childhood migraines: clinical impact and comparison to other chronic illnesses. Pediatrics. 2003;112:e1-e5. Available on-line at http://pediatrics.aappublications.org/cgi/reprint/112/1/e1
10. Hill SE, Williams JA, Senior JA, et al. Hip fracture outcomes: quality of life and functional status in older adults living in the community. Aust NZ J Med. 2000;30:327-32.
11. Kabat-Zinn J, Lipworth L, Burney R, Sellers W. Four-year follow-up of a meditation-based program for the self-regulation of chronic pain: treatment outcomes and compliance. Clin J Pain. 1987;2:159-73.
12. Chaput LA, Adams LS, Simon JA, et al. Hostility predicts recurrent events among postmenopausal women with coronary heart disease. Am J Epidemiol. 2002;156:1092-99.
13. Rogers PJ. A healthy body, a healthy mind: long-term impact of diet on mood and cognitive function. Proc Nutr Soc. 2001;60:135-43.
14. Correspondence, author unknown. Coeliac disease and psychiatric disorders in childhood: guilty by association. Acta Paediatr. 2001;90:1082-83.
15. Dohan FC, Martin L, Grasberger JC, et al. Antibodies to wheat gliadin in blood of psychiatric patients: possible role of emotional factors. Biol Psych. 1972;5(2):127-37.
16. Daaleman TP. Religion, spirituality, and the practice of medicine. J Am Board Fam Pract. 2004;17:370-76.
17. Daaleman TP, Perera S, Studenski S. Religion, spirituality, and health status in geriatric outpatients. Ann Fam Med. 2004;2:49-53.
18. Matthews DA, McCullough ME, Larson DB, et al. Religious commitment and health status: a review of the research and implications for family medicine. Arch Fam Med. 1998;7:118-24.
19. Plotnikoff, G. Should medicine reach out to the spirit? Understanding a patient's spiritual foundation can guide appropriate care. Postgrad Med. 2000;108(6) available on-line at http://www.postgradmed.com/issues/2000/11_00/editorial_nov.htm

Chapter 12
Healthy Aging: The Promotion of Organ Reserve

David S. Jones, MD, Jeffrey S. Bland, PhD, and Sheila Quinn

Introduction[i]

For nearly 20 years, we have used the term "organ reserve" in functional medicine as a marker for healthy aging. Our assumption has been that if we enable our patients to reduce oxidative stress and inflammation, improve the match of genes to environment, support healthy lifestyles, and improve micronutrient repletion, we will be creating greater flexibility and adaptability (degrees of freedom) in the aging human organism, enabling people to live out their years with longer periods of health and vitality and shorter periods of disease and debility prior to death. The research base, however, has yet to precisely define "organ reserve"; nor are we yet able to measure or specify the effects of all these preventive measures on the reserve capacity of our organs (hearts, lungs, livers, kidneys, brains, etc.) to respond to life's insults—illness, trauma, loss, chronic stress, and poor lifestyles. It is difficult, therefore, to describe a causal link between the concept of organ reserve and the phenomenon of healthy aging. It is, however, a useful concept—a kind of shorthand term that encompasses the physiological benefits of the functional medicine approach to health. With that caveat, let's explore some aspects of theories about aging and how we can help patients to more years of optimal health.

[i]This chapter was adapted from "Healthy aging and the origins of illness: Improving the expression of genetic potential," which was published by the authors in *Integrative Medicine: A Clinician's Journal.* Dec 2003/Jan 2004;2(6):16-25. Many thanks to the journal for permission to adapt this article.

Aging and Disease: Rectangularizing the Morbidity Curve

Suggestions from anthropological data estimate that our earliest ancestors lived on average only about 18 years, and that by the time of the Roman Empire, life expectancy was still not much over 22 years. In the interval from that point to the start of the 20th century, life expectancy at birth doubled to 45 years.[1,2] "Throughout most of the 20th century, death rates declined dramatically at every age in developed nations, and life expectancy at birth rose rapidly. For example, life expectancy at birth for U.S. females increased from 48.9 years in 1900 to 79.0 in 1995."[3]

> Ageing [sic] is a biological puzzle of long standing, particularly because it manifests itself over a wide range of biological systems, tissues and functions. ... But ageing is not a function. Ageing can be defined as an endogenous progressive deterioration in age-specific components of fitness.[4] It is not actively selected for. It is instead a secondary effect of the decline in the force of natural selection with age.[5,6] From such theory it follows that many loci, and many biochemical pathways, are expected to produce the deleterious effects of ageing, because it is a secondary side-effect of normal evolution."[7]

If it is true that the forces of natural selection lose hegemony in the years following fecundity (the aging years), but that the forces of selection have set in place the genetic mechanisms that define the biologic context of adaptive possibilities, then new models for understanding aging and constructive interventions, both in terms of public health recommendations as well as individual health care strategies, are required.

In 1980, James Fries discussed in *The New England Journal of Medicine* "a set of predictions" on aging, natural death, and the compression of morbidity.[8] In his paper, he challenged the popular notion that aging is necessarily associated with increased morbidity and disability. He also suggested that, in developed countries, with substantial improvements in public health measures, nutrition, and medical care, people would approach greater parity between "expected biological life span" and actual years of functional life. As summarized in a reflective editorial published in the same journal 18 years later: "In the ideal case, the healthy citizens of a modern society will survive to an advanced age with their vigor and functional independence maintained, and morbidity and disability will be compressed into a relatively short period before death occurs at around the age of 85 years."[9] This has become known as the *Fries hypothesis* and as the rectangularizing of the morbidity curve based on *maintenance of organ reserve*.

In 1998, again in the *NEJM*, Anthony Vita and colleagues (including James Fries) presented evidence collected from a study of 1,741 University of Pennsylvania alumni over a period of 32 years.[10] Their extensive data supported the notion that *healthful lifestyle activities* were associated with less loss of function (disability) and fewer chronic illnesses during the life span. In this study, the lifestyle factors showing the greatest correlation with differences between the upper and lower levels of risk were: 1) smoking, 2) body-mass index, and 3) patterns of exercise. An accompanying editorial summarized the findings: "In the group with the lowest level of risk, the onset of functional disability was postponed by about five years. In the group with the highest level of risk—those who had a body-mass index of 26 or higher, smoked 30 or more cigarettes per day, and got no regular vigorous exercise—there was both an earlier onset of disability and a greater level of cumulative disability, as well as more disability in the final year of life for the 10% of the cohort that had died."[11] In the Harvard Study of Adult Development, George E. Vaillant corroborated the importance of the same risk factors—smoking, obesity, and exercise—but added two emotional components, stable marriage and "mature defenses," as important differentiating factors of successful aging.[12,13]

However, subsequent analyses of the Fries hypothesis have demonstrated that the rectangularization Fries described is actually composed of two elements, mortality and morbidity, and they should be analyzed separately. Compression of *mortality* refers to an increasing concentration of *ages at death* (decreased variability of ages at death); whereas compression of *morbidity* refers to increasing concentration of illness and disability into the latter years of life.[14]

The calculations of life expectancy contain statistical Gordian knots that preoccupy many researchers in the field of aging. Behind the pure intellectual interest in aging and life expectancy lurk important public policy issues that will not be explored here.[ii] The fundamental debate is between those who believe increases in longevity will proceed more slowly in the future than they have in the past, eventually stopping entirely, and those who believe the data do not support such a conclusion. The hypothesis presented by Carnes and Olshansky,[15] postulating that animal and human data suggest that species "possess an *intrinsic mortality signature*," falls into the first category:

> Imagine a population completely protected from extrinsic causes of death, but denied access to any medical intervention that might influence (i.e., postpone the age of death) intrinsic processes—the goal for most control groups in studies involving laboratory animals. Assuming the population is representative of the species from which it came, the life expectancy for this hypothetical population is an estimate of the upper limit for the average life span of individuals within this species—an upper limit imposed by the intrinsic mortality signature.

The conundrum of *life expectancy* or *species-specific intrinsic mortality signature* rests squarely on the implicative enfolding of the natural processes of aging occurring always in real time within an incalculably complex environment that interacts with the inherent genetics and biological processes of each individual within the species. We are learning that risks of disease and age-related decline are unique to each patient, and that phenotypic expression appears to be more vulnerable to environmental pressures than to genetic influences.[16] Many in this field assert that the extension of *functional life span*[iii] and *life expectancy*[iv] as seen in the 20th century is unlikely to be duplicated in the 21st century. The large

[ii] The U.S. Social Security Administration, for example, must predict the size of future beneficiary populations. If, as some researchers believe, they are underestimating future increases in longevity, the social security system will be subject to some very significant unplanned-for financial burdens. [Roush W. Live long and prosper? *Science*. 1996;273:42-46.]

[iii] *Life span* refers to a specific individual's length of life. For example, the verified oldest-age-at-death of a member of a species establishes the *maximum* life span for that species. Therefore, maximum life span is always greater than life expectancy. The oldest fully authenticated age to which any human has ever lived is 122 years and 164 days, by Jeanne-Louise Calment. She was born in France on February 21, 1875 and died at a nursing home in Arles, southern France on August 4, 1997 (*Guinness Book of Records*).

incremental improvements in public health measures, nutrition, and medical care associated with the increases in life expectancy in the 20th century are not reproducible in the 21st century without "modifying endogenous biological processes inherent to aging." [17] Olshansky and Carnes go on to assert: "There are no life-style changes, surgical procedures, vitamins, antioxidants, hormones, or techniques of genetic engineering available today with the capacity to repeat the gains in life expectancy that were achieved during the 20th century."

However, a 2002 article by Oeppen and Vaupel[18] disputes their contentions. Using life expectancy data for the world's most long-lived populations, they show evidence of a "regular stream of continuing progress" as represented by a linear climb from 1840 to 2000. During that period, record life expectancy has broken every prediction advanced, and usually within just a few years: "Best-practice life expectancy has increased by 2.5 years per decade for a century and a half." Not to mince words, Oeppen and Vaupel conclude: "This mortality research has exposed the empirical misconceptions and specious theories that underlie the pernicious belief that the expectation of life cannot rise much further."

Wilmoth[19] concurs: "Extrapolation rides the steady course of past mortality trends, whereas popular and scientific discussions of mortality often buck those historical trends, in either an optimistic or pessimistic direction ... [E]arlier arguments about an imminent end to gains in human longevity have often been overturned, sometimes quite soon after they were put forth." In another paper published in 2000, he argued further that this contrarian view is based on data that show that "the most significant trend now affecting longevity in industrialized societies is the decline of death rates among the elderly."[20,21]

In 1999, Wilmoth and Horiuchi also demonstrated through demographic statistical methods that *rectangularization of mortality* is not a necessary and concomitant association with mortality decline.[22] Myers and Manton, in 1984, had shown that the standard deviation of deaths above age 60 in the United States increased rather than decreased between 1962 and 1979, in spite of the decline in death rates.[23] In the oldest-old populations in developed countries there has been an unexplained expansion, rather than a compression of mortality (greater variability of the *ages at death*).[24,25,26] Also, the overall rectangularity of the survival curve and the *limits of longevity* are not irrevocably linked as initially postulated by Fries in 1980. In the original theory, as the survival curve rectangularized, the limits of longevity would be substantially revealed. As shown by James Vaupel and associates,[27] as well as others,[28] as early as the 1950s and into the 1990s, there has been a general loss in the rectangularization of the survival curve as the limits of longevity have come very much into question due to the well-documented rise in improved survival at older ages.[29,30,31] For example, the number of centenarians has doubled approximately every 10 years since 1950.[32]

We enter the 21st century in need of a *general theory on population aging*,[33,34] and humbled by the awareness that "our understanding of the complex interactions of social and biological factors that determine mortality levels is still imprecise."[35] It is clear that the present sustained increase in life expectancy from birth is now due to the mortality decline at the highest ages,[36] even if as yet unexplained. We have entered a transition in population biodemographics within the developed countries where fecundity and mortality are lower and causes of death are less associated with infectious diseases and/or accidental death, and more associated with degenerative and age-related causes. Research is ongoing to delineate the subtle differences and causes of (a) life expectancy, (b) disease-free life expectancy, and (c) disability-free life expectancy.

Contemporary research has substantiated Fries' 1980 prediction that chronic illness can be postponed by changes in lifestyle, contradicting the anticipated forecast of an ever older, ever more feeble, and ever more expensive-to-care-for populace. Although his first prediction that the length of human life is fixed has proved erroneous, his second prediction that many of the "markers" of aging can be modified, has proved prescient.[37] His charge that "acute illness has ceased to be the major medical problem in the United States," and that "chronic illness now is responsible for more than 80% of all deaths and for an even higher fraction of cases of total disability" has only recently received the attention it deserved.[38]

Fries challenged the medical establishment to focus on both the elements of aging (senescence) and a strategy of postponement, rather than cure, for the chronic diseases. In order to construct therapeutic interventions

[iv] *Life expectancy* is a statistical measure of a population; it is actuarially derived and is especially sensitive to improvements in life expectancy at birth rather than later improvements in survival.

around validated elements that can enhance healthy aging and the compression of morbidity, researchers are teasing out those mechanisms that are associated with death from natural aging, as well as those consequent to chronic illness.

For most of us, death will be preceded by a decline in function, and we would all like that period of decline to be as brief as possible. Achieving that goal requires that physicians and patients alike understand what contributes to age-related decline and disease, and what mitigates against the involution of physical, psychological, and social vigor. We need a deeper understanding of the complex interaction of aging and decreased functional reserve, and the interwoven associations with illness, so that—as clinicians—we do not fail to give our patients the best possible chance for maximum health and function as they age.

Mechanisms of Aging

A number of models[v] have been proposed to account for the observable effects of aging on living organisms.[39,40,41,42,43,44,45] The model proposed by Denham Harman, MD, PhD, in 1956,[46] has developed in the intervening half century the greatest number of advocates and the most robust repository of research.[47,48] Dr. Harman proposed that the accumulated effects of oxidative damage from normal metabolism create mischief for members of all sex-dependent species after the reproductive years, although, as mentioned earlier, there may also exist extenuating factors in the oldest-old.[49,50]

A number of lines of thinking converge around Harman's *free radical theory of aging*.[51,52,53] The evolutionary biologists explain aging as a sidebar to the underlying mechanisms and processes of natural selection. As explained by Michael Rose in 1999:

> Heritable traits persist and become prevalent in a population—they are selected, in evolutionary terms—if those properties help their bearers to survive into reproductive age and produce offspring. The most useful traits result in the most offspring and hence in the greatest perpetuation of the genes controlling those properties. Meanwhile traits that diminish survival in youth become uncommon—are selected against—because their possessors often die before reproducing. ... (However) in contrast to deleterious genes that act early, those that sap vitality in later years would be expected to accumulate readily in a population, because parents with those genes will pass them to the next generation before their bad effects interfere with reproduction. (The later the genes lead to disability, the more they will spread, because the possessors will be able to reproduce longer.)[54]

These ideas have produced some very interesting research into the mitigation of the inevitable ravages of oxidative damage as the organism ages. For example, rat studies performed by Dr. Ames and his associates have shown that feeding "old rats" the normal mitochondrial metabolites *acetyl carnitine*[vi] and *lipoic acid*[vii] for a few weeks restores mitochondrial function, lowers oxidants to the level of a young rat, and increases ambulatory activity to a level usually seen only in young rats.[55,56,57]

These animal studies suggest plausible underlying mechanisms of aging as well as possible restorative interventions. Dr. Ames summarizes: "With age, increased oxidative damage to proteins and lipid membranes, particularly in mitochondria, causes a deformation of structure of key enzymes, with a consequent lessening of affinity (Km) for the enzyme substrate; an increased level of the substrate restores the velocity of the reaction, and thus restores function."[58]

Studies are now being conducted with human subjects using DNA microarray technology as an assay.[59] Young and old rat lymphocytes and young and old human leukocytes will be compared as a measure of interventional success. Ames and his associates have termed this research *searching for the metabolic tune-up*. They hope to determine the levels of micronutrients that mitigate against DNA damage. By using DNA microarray technology, the experimental interventions can be assayed for enhanced or worsened *genomic stability*. They are presently working their way through all of the established micronutrients that have shown an association between deficiency and DNA damage. However, in the end, tuning-up the metabolism will require an understanding of the cross-connections between the unique genetic constitution and the unique nutrient needs of the individual.[60] The thrust of this present

[v] Not covered here are the models based on the arrays of alleles differentiating long-lived from shorter-lived individuals within species populations, programmed aging as a specific development end point (the aging gene model), and the role of telomerase in cellular aging. (See endnotes associated with the referenced sentence.)

[vi] Carnitine is an amino acid that facilitates transport of free fatty acids across the cell membrane of the mitochondria.

[vii] Lipoic acid (a powerful antioxidant), CoQ10, tetrahydrofolate, and glutathione are part of the mitochondrial multi-enzyme complexes intricately involved with oxidative phosphorylation, cellular respiration, and Krebs cycle-derived cellular ATP/energy production within mitochondria.

research was presaged by Ames's proposal in his 1998 paper that micronutrient inadequacy is genotoxic:[61]

> Micronutrient deficiency may explain, in good part, why the quarter of the population that eats the fewest fruits and vegetables (5 portions a day is advised) has about double the cancer rate for most types of cancer when compared to the quarter with the highest intake … . Eighty percent of American children and adolescents and 68% of adults do not eat five portions a day. Common micronutrient deficiencies are likely to damage DNA by the same mechanism as radiation and many chemicals, [and] appear to be orders of magnitude more important. Remedying micronutrient deficiencies is likely to lead to a major improvement in health and an increase in longevity at low cost.

The Origins of Illness: A Mismatch between Genes and Environment

"Most of us believe we age by genetically predetermined processes that are beyond our control … and hope we have gotten the genetic luck of the draw."[62] For many years, medical professionals and the lay public alike believed that we could do little to prevent the associated illnesses of aging, as they were thought to be principally a deterministic result of our genetic inheritance.

In the past 15 years, however, as researchers have deciphered the genome locked into *Homo sapiens'* 23 pairs of chromosomes, this deterministic model of sickness has been found by most scientists in the field to be incorrect.[63] Genes do not code for specific diseases of aging.[64] Instead, they code for various strengths and weaknesses in the human constitution that give rise to resistance or susceptibility factors for age-related diseases. Some people get the "luck of the draw" and have more resistance genes to factors associated with 21st century living. For most people, however, the occurrence of illness as we age is a result of the blending of genetic susceptibility factors with environmental exposures.[65]

The multifactorial "genes for heart disease" or "genes for cancer" may never be translated into actual disease expression unless the individual plunges these less resistant genes into an environment that triggers his or her unique constitution. For example, the susceptibility within the array of "genes for heart disease" may not result in heart disease until the person eats a diet rich in saturated fat, smokes, lives a lifestyle that enhances frequent high tides of his/her stress hormones, and/or has inadequate levels of the B vitamins in his/her diet to appropriately respond to these environmental stressors.[66]

As Nada Abumrad pointed out, "Nutritional support can be tailored to the individual genotype to favor beneficial phenotypic expression or to suppress processes that lead to later pathology."[67] This recognition gives individuals much greater control over their health as they age than they would have if all sickness were simply a natural consequence of advancing age. *The pluri-potential qualities of our life depend on the vast array of information within our genome and how/what signals are—and have been—generated to induce expression from our genome.*[viii]

When Watson and Crick[68] published their benchmark research on the structure of DNA in 1953, they little suspected their discovery would initiate a revolution in medicine. They could not know it would empower *a revolution of choice* for the kind of "health probability" an individual can select, as he/she grows older.[69] Watson and Crick's discovery heralded the dawn of what has been called "genomic medicine." For clinicians it represents the age of *personalized medicine.*[70] We now know that even diseases (like cancer) that we once thought were "all in the genes" are caused by interactions between our gene matrix and environmentally derived signals transduced at the cell membrane interface and then translated through genetic processing.

From Genotype to Phenotype: The Role of Individual Susceptibility

In an article published in the *NEJM* in 2002, investigators from the Karolinska Institute in Sweden reported on 44,788 pairs of twins from their extensive health and human services registries. (One of the benefits of the socialized medical system in Sweden, Denmark, and Finland is their huge database of patients' demographics and health outcome histories.) This specific study showed that identical twins do not experience cancer at the same rate. In fact, the study reported, "Inherited genetic factors make a minor contribution to susceptibility to most types of neoplasms. This finding indicates that the environment has the principal role in causing sporadic cancer."[71]

In 1950, Roger Williams wrote a paper titled "The Concept of Genetotrophic Disease."[72] In this *Lancet*

[viii] In Matt Ridley's *(1999) GENOME: The Autobiography of a Species In 23 Chapters,* he uses the analogy of a book of life in 23 chapters to highlight the connection between what has been found in the gene mapping discoveries to this point in the genome project (30,000 to 35,000 gene sequences derived from 2.9 billion nucleotide codes in the 23 paired chromosomes).

article, Williams advanced the bold concept that a number of diseases whose origins were unknown at that time could be understood as conditions associated not with malnutrition, but with *under*nutrition based on the individual's unique genetic needs. He postulated that heart disease, cancer, diabetes, arthritis, schizophrenia, and even alcoholism could be considered to have "genetotrophic origin." Williams's concept, rooted in genetics and biochemistry, proposed that undernutrition would result in suboptimal metabolisms within susceptible individuals, which would, in turn, increase the potential for chronic illness developing over decades of living.

Medicine did not at that time embrace the genetotrophic model for the origin of disease, and the concept remained dormant for 50 years. The results of the Human Genome Project in the late 20th century and the revolution in understanding how diet and specific macro- and micronutrients influence gene expression have recently made Williams's concepts seem prescient. He appears to have predicted the transition in medicine from a largely empirical meta-science to a predictive science based on unified mechanisms of disease. We now know that the mechanisms that result in the initiation and progression of most age-related chronic illnesses have their origin, at least in part, in the genetotrophic concept.[73,74]

The recent publication of a landmark paper by Ames et al.[75] provides the bench-science substantiation needed to flesh out Williams's postulates. Ames shows in his encyclopedic review paper that "as many as one-third of mutations in a gene result in the corresponding enzyme having an increased Michaelis constant, or *K*m (decreased binding affinity), for a coenzyme, resulting in a lower rate of reaction." Some people carry polymorphisms[ix] that are more critical in determining the outcome of their health history. He goes on to argue that studies have shown that administration of higher than dietary reference intake (DRI) levels of cofactors (specific vitamins and minerals) to these polymorphic genes restores activity to near-normal and even normal levels. He concludes that "nutritional interventions to improve health are likely to be a major benefit of the genomics era."

It is also recognized now that nutritional status and specific nutrients modify drug metabolism, and the impact is unique to the genotype of the individual. Researchers have recently discovered that specific nutrients modify the expression and function of detoxification genes.[76,77,78] Cruciferous vegetables, which include broccoli, cauliflower, Brussels sprouts, and cabbage, contain nutrients called glucosinolates. These substances break down in the digestive tract to produce chemicals such as indole-3-carbinol, sulfurophane, and phenylisothiocyanate. These chemicals, in their turn, activate specific genes that help detoxify cancer-producing substances.[79] The mechanism by which specific nutrients help protect individuals with certain genotypes is just now being fully explored.

Other nutrients, such as glutathione, CoQ_{10}, vitamins C and E, the B-complex nutrients (including folic acid, B12, and B6), and the essential minerals zinc, copper, and selenium, all assist the genes in protecting against heart disease, stroke, dementias, cancer, and diabetes.[80,81,82,83,84] Genetic uniqueness may cause some individuals to require 100 times as much of a particular vitamin, mineral, or accessory nutrient as another for good health.[85] For example, "a common polymorphism exists for the gene that encodes the methylene tetrahydrofolate reductase (MTHFR) enzyme, which converts 5,10-methylene tetrahydrofolate to 5-methyltetrahydrofolate, required for conversion of homocysteine to methionine ... . Individuals with the MTHFR 677 TT genotype had a significantly higher risk of CHD, particularly in the setting of low folate status."[86] Elevated homocysteine is associated with depression, heart disease, stroke, colon and breast cancers, and dementia.[87] If susceptible individuals consume a diet that for most people would be "adequate" in these nutrients, they run the risk of developing a disease of aging such as heart disease. Kilmer McCully recently wrote: "There is an urgency to this matter. There are 500,000 people dying every year from heart disease, and millions more suffering."[88] As Willett and Stampfer pointed out in a December 2001 article in the *NEJM*, the daily consumption of a well-balanced multivitamin and mineral supplement now makes sense from a number of lines of research.[89]

We inherit more than our genes. Through custom, habit, and patterning, we also inherit nutrition and lifestyle habits. The interaction of genetic uniqueness with

[ix] A polymorphic gene is an alternate form of a *wild* gene present in >1% of the population. The most common polymorphic genes are single nucleotide polymorphisms (SNPs) that result in translational proteins and enzymes with decreased functionality. We all share at least 99.9% of the nucleotide code of our species' genome. The SNPs are what make us unique within our species. The translation of our genome message that includes our SNPs results in our individual phenotype. [Burghes, et al. Science. 2001;293:2213-14.]

lifestyle results in the illnesses many people associate with aging. A dramatic example can be seen today in the stunning increase in cases of type 2 diabetes[90,x] and the estimate that "as many as 1 in 4 apparently healthy Americans are at risk of developing 'Syndrome X,' a metabolic derangement that is a major contributor to coronary artery disease"[91] and a likely precursor to type 2 diabetes. There is clear and compelling evidence from many sources that diet and lifestyle are the culprits, since (as noted above) the human genome itself has not changed in this period of time.

Summary

People *are* living longer—that's indisputable. We know that how we live those extra years is an abiding issue. Medical education, research, and practice need to shift focus, looking at the complex issues involved in the origins of illness and healthy aging. The evidence is very strong that illness is not a predetermined consequence of aging[92,93] and that age-related decline can probably be substantially compressed (in length and in severity) by better management of the interaction between our genetic uniqueness and the overall environment to which we expose our genes throughout our lifetimes.[94] Ongoing research will help us understand the mechanisms by which the environment affects our genes, and we will be able to intervene sooner, targeting very specific risks and vulnerabilities inherent to the individual. Tailored recommendations for diet, nutritional pharmacology,[95] pharmacogenomics, lifestyle change (including "mind-body" issues), structural and physical medicine, and exercise[96,96,97] are already important in improving the expression of genetic potential, and will become more clinically useful and focused as the evidence base expands.

The doctors of the 21st century will need to understand how to assess patients' genotypes,[98,99,100] how to personalize treatment for their individual needs, configuring patient interventions to improve lifestyle and environment to minimize the risks of age-related chronic disease. We hope that this book will help the readers to do just that.

[x] Booth et al. report "a sixfold increase in prevalence of Type 2 diabetes between 1958 and 1993" and lament the fact that such ailments "usually thought only to affect individuals of middle age or older will now affect our children at a much earlier age, drastically decreasing their quality of life over a much longer period than previous generations."

References

1. Carnes BA, Olshansky SJ, Gavrilov L, et al. Human longevity: nature vs. nurture—fact or fiction. Perspect Biol Med. 1999;42(3):422-41.
2. Wilmoth JR, et al. Increase of maximum life-span in Sweden, 1861-1999. Science. 2000;289:2366-68.
3. Olshansky JS, Carnes BA, Desesquelles A. Prospects for human longevity. Science. 2001;291:1491-92.
4. Rose MR. Evolutionary Biology of Aging. Oxford Univ. Press. 1991.
5. Hamilton WD. The moulding of senescence by natural selection. J Theor Biol. 1966;12:12-45.
6. Charlesworth B. Evolution in Age-structured Populations, 2nd. Ed. Cambridge University Press. 1994.
7. Rose MR, Long AD. Ageing: The many-headed monster. Curr Biol. 2002;12(9):R311-12.
8. Fries JF. Aging, natural death and the compression of morbidity. N Engl J Med. 1980;303:130-35.
9. Campion EW. Aging better. N Engl J Med. 1998;338(15):1064-66.
10. Vita AJ, Terry RB, Hubert HB, Fries JF. Aging, health risks, and cumulative disability. N Engl J Med. 1998;338(15):1035-41.
11. Campion EW. Aging better. N Engl J Med. 1998;338(15):1064-66.
12. Vaillant GE, Aging Well. Little, Brown: Boston, 2002.
13. Vaillant GE, Mukamal K. Positive aging. Am J Psychiatry. 2001;158:839-47.
14. Wilmoth JR, Horiuchi S. Rectangularization revisited: variability of age at death within human populations. Demography. 1999;36(4):475-95.
15. Carnes BA, Olshansky SJ, Gavrilov L, et al. Human longevity: nature vs. nurture—fact or fiction. Perspect Biol Med. 1999;42(3):422-41.
16. Willett WC. Balancing life-style and genomics research for disease prevention. Science. 2002;296:695-98.
17. Olshansky JS, Carnes BA, Desesquelles A. Prospects for human longevity. Science. 2001;291:1491-92.
18. Oeppen J, Vaupel JW. Broken limits to life expectancy. Science. 2002;296:1029-31.
19. Wilmoth, JR. The future of human longevity: a demographer's perspective. Science. 1998;280:395-97.
20. Ibid.
21. Yashin AI, et al. Genes, demography, and life span: the contribution of demographic data in genetic studies on aging and longevity. Am J Hum Genet. 1999;65:1178-93.
22. Wilmoth JR, Horiuchi S. Rectangularization revisited: variability of age at death within human populations. Demography. 1999;36(4):475-95.
23. Myers, GD, Manton KG. Compression of morality: myth or reality? Gerontologist. 1984:24(4):346-53.
24. Rothenberg R, Lentzner HR, Parker RA. Population aging patterns: the expansion of mortality. Soc Sci. 1991;46(2):S66-70.
25. Wilmoth JR, et al. Increase of maximum life-span in Sweden, 1861-1999. Science. 2000;289:2366-68.
26. Rose MR, Mueller LD. Ageing and immortality. Philos Trans R Soc Lond B Biol Sci. 2000;355:1657-62.
27. Vaupel JW. The remarkable improvements in survival at older ages. Philos Trans R Soc Lond B Biol Sci. 1997;352:1799-1804.
28. Zimmer Z, et al. Changes in functional limitation and survival among older Taiwanese. 2002;56:265-76.
29. Robine JM, et al. Determining Health Expectancies. Chichester: John Wiley; 2002:75-101.
30. Oeppen J, Vaupel JW. Broken limits to life expectancy. Science. 2002;296:1029-31.
31. White KM. Longevity advances in high-income countries, 1955-96. Popul Dev Rev. 2002;28:59-76.

32. Jeune B, Vaupel JW, eds. Exceptional Longevity: from Prehistory to Present. Odense: Odense University Press; 1995:109-16.
33. Robine JM, Michel JP. Looking forward to a general theory on population aging. J Gerontol. 2004;59A(6):590-97.
34. Shock NW. Mortality and measurements of aging. In: Strehler BL, Ebert JD, Glass HB, Shock NW, eds. The biology of aging. Washington, DC: American Institute of Biological Sciences, 1960:14-29.
35. Wilmoth JR. The future of human longevity: a demographer's perspective. Science. 1998;280:395-97.
36. Vaupel JW, Carey JR, et al. Biodemographic trajectories of longevity. Science. 1998;280:855-60.
37. Fries JF. Aging, natural death and the compression of morbidity. N Engl J Med. 1980;303:130-35.
38. Holman H. Chronic disease—The need for a new clinical education. JAMA. 2004;292(9):1057-59.
39. Rose MR. Can human aging be postponed? Sci Am. December 1999:106-111.
40. Friedrich MJ. Biological secrets of exceptional old age. JAMA. 2002;288(18):2247-52.
41. Hayflick L. The future of ageing. Nature. 2000;408:267-69.
42. Guarente L, Kenyon C. Genetic pathways that regulate ageing in model organisms. Nature. 2000;408:255-62.
43. Martin GM, Oshima J. Lessons from human progeroid syndromes. Nature. 2000;408:263-66.
44. Fossel M. Telomerase and the aging cell. JAMA. 1998;279(21):1732-35.
45. Mariotti S, Sansoni P, Barbesino G, et al. Thyroid and other organ-specific autoantibodies in healthy centenarians. Lancet. 1992;339:1506-8.
46. Harman D. Aging: A theory based on free radical and radiation chemistry. J Gerontol. 1956:11:298-300.
47. Smith KC ed. Aging, Carcinogenesis, and Radiation Biology. Plenum, New York, 1976.
48. Pryor WA ed. Free Radicals in Biology (Academic, New York), Vols. 1-4. (1976-1980)
49. Beckman KB, Ames BN. The free radical theory of aging matures. Physiol Rev. 1998;78:547-81.
50. Wallace DC, Melov S. Radicals r' aging. Nat Genet. 1998;19:105-6.
51. Harman D. The aging process. Proc Natl Acad Sci U S A. 1981;78(11:)7124-28.
52. Shigenaga MK, Hagen TM, Ames BN. Oxidative damage and mitochondrial decay in aging. Proc Natl Acad Sci USA. 1994;91:10771-78.
53. Wallace DC. A mitochondrial paradigm for degenerative diseases and ageing. 2001 Ageing vulnerability: causes and interventions. Wiley, Chi Chester (Novartis Foundation Symposium 235) p 247-266.
54. Rose MR. Can human aging be postponed? Sci Am. December 1999:106-111.
55. Hagen TM, Ingersoll RT, Wehr CM, et al. Acetyl-L-carnitine fed to old rats partially restores mitochondrial function and ambulatory activity. Proc Natl Acad Sci USA. 1998;95:9562-66.
56. Hagen TM, Ingersoll RT. Liu J, et al. (R)-alpha-Lipoic acid-supplemented old rats have improved mitochondrial function, decreased oxidative damage, and increased metabolic rate. FASEB J. 1998;13:411-8.
57. Hagen TM, Wehr CM, Ames BN. Mitochondrial decay in aging: reversal through dietary supplementation of acetyl-L-carnitine and N-tert-butyl-alpha-phenylnitrone. Ann NY Acad Sci. 1998;854;214-23.
58. Ames BN. CV available from University of California Berkeley, Mailing address: CHORI, 5700 Martin Luther King Jr. Way, Oakland, CA 94609.
59. Eisen MB, Brown PO. DNA arrays for analysis of gene expression. Methods Enzymol. 1999;303:179-205.
60. Sutherland, GR. Just how long can we live? Med J Aust. 2000;173:594-96.
61. Ames BN. Micronutrients prevent cancer and delay aging. Toxicol Lett. 1998;102-103:5-18.
62. Bland JS. Genetic Nutritioneering. Keats Publishing: Lincolnwood, IL. 1999. p. 81.
63. Booth FW, Gordon SE, Carlson CJ, Hamilton MT. Waging war on modern chronic diseases: primary prevention through exercise biology. J Appl Physiol. 2000;88:774-87.
64. McMurdo M. A healthy old age: realistic or futile goal? BMJ. 2001;321:1149-51.
65. Subramanian G, Adams M, Venter JC, Broder S. Implications of the human genome for understanding human biology and medicine. JAMA. 2001;286(18):2296-307.
66. Willett, WC. Balancing life-style and genomics research for disease prevention. Science. 2002;296:695-97.
67. Abumrad N. The gene-nutrient-gene loop. Curr Opin Nutr Metab Care. 2001;4:407-10.
68. Watson J, Crick F. A structure for deoxyribose nucleic acid. Nature. 1953;171:737.
69. Willett, WC. Balancing life-style and genomics research for disease prevention. Science. 2002;296:695-97.
70. Liotta LA, Kohn EC, Petricoin EF. Clinical proteomics: personalized molecular medicine. JAMA. 2001;286(18):2211-14.
71. Lichtenstein P, Holm NV, Verkasalo PK, et al. Environmental and heritable factors in the causation of cancer—analyses of cohorts of twins from Sweden, Denmark and Finland. N Engl J Med. 2000;343(2):78-85.
72. Williams R, Beerstecher E Jr, Berry LJ. The concept of genetotrophic disease. Lancet. 1950;1(6599):287-89.
73. Bell J. The new genetics in clinical practice. BMJ. 1998;316(7131):618-20.
74. Kaprio J. Genetic epidemiology. BMJ. 2000;320:1257-59.
75. Ames BN, Elson-Schwab I, Silver EA. High-dose vitamin therapy stimulates variant enzymes with decreased coenzyme binding affinity (increased Km): relevance to genetic disease and polymorphisms. Am J Clin Nutr. 2002;75:616-58.
76. N-Acetylcysteine therapy for acetaminophen overdose. Emerg Med. 2000;8:26-32.
77. Weber A, Jager R, Klinger G, et al. Can grapefruit juice influence ethenylestradiol bioavailability? Contraception. 1996;53:41-47.
78. Pantuck EJ, et al. Stimulatory effect of brussels sprouts and cabbage on human drug metabolism. Clin Pharmacol Ther. 1979;25:88.
79. Nijhoff WA, Grubben JA, Nagengast FM, et al. Effects of consumption of brussels sprouts on intestinal and lymphocytic glutathione-S-transferases in humans. Carcinogenesis. 1995;16(61):2125-28.
80. Meydani M. Dietary antioxidants modulation of aging and immune-endothelial cell interaction. Mech Ageing Dev. 1999;111:123-32.
81. Young-in K. Methylenetetrahydrofolate reductase polymorphisms, folate, and cancer risk: a paradigm of gene-nutrient interactions in carcinogenesis. Nutr Rev. 2000;58(7):205-17.
82. Ames BN. Micronutrients prevent cancer and delay aging. Toxicol Lett. 1998;102-103:5-18.
83. Armstrong AM, Chestnutt JE, Gormleh MJ, Young JS. The effect of dietary treatment on lipid peroxidation and antioxidant status in newly diagnosed noninsulin dependent diabetes. Free Radic Biol Med. 1996;21(5):719-26.
84. Engelhart MJ, Geerlings MI, Ruitenberg A, et al. Dietary intake of antioxidants and risk of Alzheimer disease. JAMA. 2002;287(24):3223-37.

85. Ames BN. Elson-Schwab, I, Silver, EA. High-dose vitamin therapy stimulates variant enzymes with decreased coenzyme binding affinity (increased Km): relevance to genetic disease and polymorphisms. Am J Clin Nutr. 2002;75:616-58.
86. Klerk M, Verhoef P, Clarke R, et al. MTHFR 677C→ T Polymorphism and risk of coronary heat disease: a meta-analysis. JAMA. 2002;288(16):2023-32.
87. Seshadri S, Beiser A, Selhub J, et al. Plasma homocysteine as a risk factor for dementia and Alzheimer's disease. N Engl J Med. 2002;346(7):467-83.
88. McCully K, McCully M. The Heart Revolution (HarperPerennial: New York), 1999. p. 188.
89. Willett WC, Stampfer MJ. What vitamins should I be taking, doctor? N Engl J Med. 2001;345(25):1819-24.
90. Booth FW, Gordon SE, Carlson CJ, Hamilton MT. Waging war on modern chronic diseases: primary prevention through exercise biology. J Appl Physiol. 2000;88:774-87.
91. Roberts K, Dunn K, Sandra JK, Lardinois CD. Syndrome X: medical nutrition therapy. Nutr Rev. 2000;58(5):154-60.
92. Cassel CK. Use it or lose it: activity may be the best treatment for aging. JAMA. 2002;288(18):2333-35.
93. Friedrich MJ. Biological secrets of exceptional old age. JAMA. 2002;288(18):2247-52.
94. Reed DM, Foley DJ, White LR, et al. Predictors of healthy aging in men with high life expectancies. Am J Public Health. 1998;88(10):1463-68.
95. Halliwell BH. Establishing the significance and optimal intake of dietary antioxidants: the biomarker concept. Nutr Rev. 1999:57(4):104-13.
96. Friedrich MJ. Women, exercise and aging. JAMA. 2001;285(11):1429-31.
97. Tall AR. Exercise to reduce cardiovascular risk—how much is enough? N Engl J Med. 2002;347(19):1522-24.
98. Stewart KJ. Exercise training and the cardiovascular consequences of type 2 diabetes and hypertension. JAMA. 2002;288(13):1622-31.
99. Gerling IC, Solomon SS, Bryer-Ash M. Genomes, transcriptomes, and proteomes. Arch Intern Med. 2003;163:190-198.
100. Martin ER, Lai EH, Gilbert JR, et al. SNPing away at complex diseases: analysis of single-nucleotide polymorphisms around APOE in Alzheimer disease. Am J Hum Genet. 2000;67:383-94.
101. Watts G. Unmasking the secret of life. BMJ. 2002;325:736.

Section III

The Building Blocks

Chapter 13
Environmental Inputs

- *Diet and Nutrients*
- *Air and Water*
- *Physical Exercise*
- *Psychosocial Influences*
- *Trauma*
- *Xenobiotics*
- *Microorganisms*
- *Radiation*

Diet and Nutrients

Jeffrey S. Bland, PhD

Introduction

A historical review of our understanding of chronic diseases affirms that we now know these are primarily "lifestyle diseases." This gene-environment connection, in which certain genetic strengths and weaknesses are powerfully influenced by environmental choices, gives rise to the patient's health phenotype. The phenotype is a result of the interaction of the genotype with environmental factors: genomics influence proteomics,[i] which influence metabolomics, which ultimately give rise to phenomics, or how an individual looks, acts, and feels. Genes are expressed as a consequence of the environment in which they are immersed. Environment-gene interactions give rise to the expression of the diseases of the culture. No medicine or therapy can prevent the interaction between genes and environment. Unfortunately, it is not possible to attack causality in many chronic diseases without dealing with multiple environmental factors. Fortunately, we do know that the outcome, or phenotype, can be affected by modifying the environment. Yet, we are not using this information effectively to modify our approach to health care. We need this new, primary model for addressing both the prevention and management of chronic disease. That is the central theme of functional medicine.

Diet and Nutrients: The Emerging Evidence

An editorial about the relationship among environmental "inputs" such as diet, lifestyle, and longevity appeared in the *Journal of the American Medical Association*, authored by Drs. Eric Rimm and Meir Stampfer, well-respected epidemiologists at the Department of Epidemiology and Nutrition at the Harvard School of Public Health.[1] They point out that Ancel Keys, who worked at the University of Wisconsin, recently passed away. He was a pioneer in the discovery of new research methods linking nutrition and disease. He is credited for discovering that saturated fat intake is a risk factor for cardiovascular disease (CVD) and that unsaturated

[i] Proteomics applies the techniques of molecular biology, biochemistry, and genetics to analyzing the structure, function, and interactions of the proteins produced by the genes. Metabolomics provides an overview of the metabolic status and biochemical events associated with a cellular or biological system, describing their dynamic responses to genetic and environmental modulation. Phenomics attempts to integrate the information provided by these areas of study into a holistic picture of the complete organism (individual).

fat intake is associated with a lower risk of CVD. Rimm and Stampfer state:

> Nearly 50 years ago, Keys recognized the enormously divergent rates of heart disease around the world, even after adjusting for differences in age. Although coronary disease was and remains the leading cause of death in the United States and many developed and developing countries, it was almost non-existent in the traditional cultures of Crete and Japan. Rates of cancer at various sites also differ enormously—up to 100-fold—in different populations. The rapid changes in rates of many of these diseases over time and studies that show increases in chronic disease rates among migrants from traditional to Westernized cultures demonstrate that relatively swift changes in disease rates cannot be attributed solely to genetic differences between populations. Instead, they are likely due to differences in lifestyle, with dietary factors and physical activity the leading candidates ... . Although understanding of the relation of lifestyle and health outcomes will continue to be refined, information available now is sufficient to take action.

Rimm and Stampfer conclude by saying that studies on positive lifestyle practices and their mechanisms tend to be supported by the historical research record: "As a society, the United States spends billions on chronic disease treatments and interventions for risk factors. Although these are useful and important, a fraction of that investment to promote healthful lifestyles for primary prevention among individuals at all ages would yield greater benefit."[2]

Many studies from the 1990s through today emphasize the importance of diet and the environment in the prevention and management of heart disease. Pertinent studies are reported in two 2004 *JAMA* papers linking specific diets to heart disease prevention. The first is titled "Mediterranean Diet, Lifestyle Factors, and 10-year Mortality in Elderly European Men and Women."[3] This HALE Project (Healthy Ageing: a Longitudinal Study in Europe) is an interesting study. It comprises individuals enrolled in the Survey in Europe on Nutrition and the Elderly: a Concerned Action (SENECA) and the Finland, Italy, the Netherlands, and Elderly (FINE) studies. It included 1,507 apparently healthy men and 832 women, aged 70 to 90 years in 11 European countries. This cohort study was conducted between 1988 and 2000. After looking at hazard ratios of various lifestyle and diet considerations, the authors concluded that, **among individuals aged 70 to 90 years, adherence to a Mediterranean diet and healthful lifestyle was associated with a more than 50% lower rate of all-cause and cause-specific mortality.** (If we could prescribe a drug that would lower mortality of all causes by 50%, with virtually no side effects, wouldn't we all jump on that bandwagon? One has to wonder why we are not hearing a clarion call from all stakeholders for a major shift in our thinking about health care.)

A companion paper is titled "Effect of a Mediterranean-style Diet on Endothelial Dysfunction and Markers of Vascular Inflammation in the Metabolic Syndrome."[4] This study analyzes work done in the Department of Geriatrics and Metabolic Diseases in Italy. The investigators assessed the effect of a Mediterranean-style diet on endothelial function and vascular inflammatory markers in patients with metabolic syndrome. After two years, patients following the Mediterranean-style diet consumed more foods rich in monounsaturated fat, polyunsaturated fat, and fiber and had a lower ratio of omega-6 to omega-3 fatty acids. Total fruit, vegetable, and nut intake, whole grain intake, and olive oil consumption were also significantly higher in the intervention group. The levels of physical activity increased in both groups by approximately 60%, mainly by walking for a minimum of 30 minutes per day. The researchers concluded that a Mediterranean-style diet is effective in reducing the prevalence of metabolic syndrome and its associated cardiovascular risk. Reductions in high-sensitivity C-reactive protein (hs-CRP), interleukin-6 (IL-6), interleukin-7 (IL-7), and interleukin-18 (IL-18), markers for immunological functional changes, were also realized (for hs-CRP levels, p=.01 and for IL-6, p=.04). The conclusion is that implementation of an improved diet and lifestyle program results in remarkable changes in inflammatory patterns and improved insulin sensitivity. The recent "demonstration by epidemiological studies that an elevated serum IGF-I level is associated with an increased risk of developing a number of epithelial cancers,"[5] broadens the scope of concern.

Diet and the Importance of Carbohydrate Type

When we speak of the Mediterranean diet, we are not necessarily talking about a diet high in protein and low in carbohydrate. In fact, this style of diet is reasonably high in carbohydrate. However, the carbohydrate is highly unrefined, fiber-rich, and plant-phytonutrient rich, which has a different physiological effect on function than does carbohydrate in white starch or sugar. Carbohydrate is not the villain here; rather, the *type* of carbohydrate is what's important. "White" in carbohydrate (to simplify) is devoid of all the agents necessary for appropriate metabolism and physiochemical control—gastric emptying, release of glucose in a time-release fashion, and the rhythmic effect it has on the neuroendocrine-immune system through the proper release of energy molecules such as glucose and fatty acids. We should be speaking more about glycemic load and glycemic response than simply talking about percentages of protein, fat, or carbohydrate. Glucose and insulin levels can be raised postprandially by giving protein at high levels. The important feature in the construction of a diet that manages chronic disease is to balance both amount and type of macronutrients, micronutrients, and phytochemicals so that they impact the genomics of the individual with an improved health phenotype. While that balance may vary from person to person, depending on genetics and environment, there are some factors that are important for all of us; one of them is the glycemic response of the diet.[6]

Glycemic Index, Glycemic Load, Dietary Fiber Intake, and the Incidence of Type 2 Diabetes

The glycemic and insulin response after eating (more information on this can be found in Chapter 32) plays an important role in determining long-term risk of CVD. The concept that individuals carry different metabolic sensitivities to the glycemic load of the diet is supported in an article that appeared in 2004 in the *American Journal of Clinical Nutrition* ("Glycemic Index, Glycemic Load, and Dietary Fiber Intake and Incidence of Type 2 Diabetes in Younger and Middle-aged Women").[7] This is one of many papers with the same theme, documenting that a diet high in rapidly-absorbed carbohydrates and low in cereal fiber is associated with increased risk of type 2 diabetes. A diet high in fiber-rich carbohydrate from cereal fiber is associated with a lower risk of heart disease. It promotes a reduction in the relative risk of type 2 diabetes, metabolic syndrome, and insulin resistance.

Whole Grain Intake and Insulin Sensitivity

Whole grain intake is more than just carbohydrate. Grains contain a rich array of soluble and insoluble fiber, as well as hundreds of different phytochemicals. All of these influence insulin and glucose control through their effects on absorption, liver enzyme activities related to gluconeogenesis, glycogen synthesis, adipocyte physiology, centrally mediated appetite, and peripheral cells such as muscle cells. It is a much more complex story than just getting glucose from starch. We are talking about the metabolic signaling events that occur through the consumption of complex, unrefined, or minimally refined food that is high in complex carbohydrate. Quoting from a 2004 review paper that appeared in *Nutrition Reviews*:

> The apparent paradox that ad-libitum intake of high-fat foods produces weight loss might be due to severe restriction of carbohydrate depleting glycogen stores, leading to excretion of found water, the ketogenic nature of the diet being appetite suppressing, the high protein-content being highly satiating and reducing spontaneous food intake, or limited food choices leading to decreased energy intake. Long-term studies are needed to measure changes in nutritional status and body composition during the low-carbohydrate diet, and to assess fasting and postprandial cardiovascular risk factors and adverse effects.[8]

To compress morbidity, rectangularize the survival curve, and develop an effective chronic disease prevention and management program, diet must be used in an intelligent manner, and personalized to the patient's needs so as to result in an improved health phenotype.

Gluten Contamination of Commercial Oat Products

As we change environmental inputs to introduce a higher complex-carbohydrate, minimally-processed type of dietary regime, what about the relative effect that the potentially allergenic component of grains might have, including gluten and other reactive proteins? (Issues of gluten sensitivity arise throughout this book; see the index for cross-referencing.) There are certain grain-related products that are low in or devoid of gluten, such as oats. An interesting article published in *The New England Journal of Medicine* ("Gluten Contamination of Commercial Oat Products in the United States")[9] suggests, however, that certain commercially available oats are not, in fact, gluten-free. The author states that while there is quite a bit of published literature suggesting that people with celiac disease or gluten sensitivity can consume moderate amounts of uncontaminated oats, because they are low in or devoid of gluten, high variability in gluten content has been reported in batches of oats, suggesting contamination with gluten not native to oats, probably as a consequence of being processed in the same plant where wheat is processed. Gluten-sensitive individuals are urged to recognize that contamination of commercial oats in the United States with gluten grains such as wheat, barley, and rye is a legitimate concern. We should not assume that all oats are gluten-free. While they would be low in gluten relative to wheat, there may be some contamination. (This may explain why some people with gluten sensitivity have experienced a reaction to oats.)

Glycemia, Insulinemia, and Food Proteins

What about the argument that eating more protein leads to improved glucose tolerance? One paper which represents current thought is titled "Glycemia and Insulinemia in Healthy Subjects after Lactose-equivalent Meals of Milk and Other Food Proteins: The Role of Plasma Amino Acids and Incretins."[10] The authors of this paper conclude that food proteins differ in their capacity to stimulate insulin release, possibly by differentially affecting the early release of a messenger molecule called incretin. Incretin hormones and insulinotropic amino acids may stimulate higher insulin output, insulin resistance, and glycemia. This paper demonstrates that differing food proteins may have remarkably different effects on postprandial insulin and glucose levels. Those that appear to have the lowest influence on postprandial glucose are foods containing milk and soy proteins (although casein has been shown to raise postprandial insulin[11]). Food proteins that have higher postprandial glycemic responses include beef proteins and some meat and fish proteins. We need to keep in mind that the macronutrient ratio alone of carbohydrate, fat, and proteins does not really tell us what we need to know clinically about how individual foods affect particular glucose and insulin responses and, therefore, influence chronic disease risk.

Tailoring the Diet to Genetic Risk

Tailoring the diet to the patient's need can have significant positive benefits in improving the translation of the genotype into a healthy phenotype. Personalization of the diet can result in reduced inflammatory potential through normalization of neuroendocrine-immune system function (see Chapter 26 for an in-depth discussion of using diet and nutrients to reduce inflammation). The outcome of this strategy is to reduce the risk and progression of chronic disease. Here are just two examples that should alert us to the power of such an approach. Throughout the rest of this book, you will come across many more.

The 219G→T polymorphism and a diet rich in saturated fat. Certain people have specific single nucleotide polymorphisms (SNPs) and are more susceptible to the oxidative types of reactions and lipoprotein abnormalities associated with the inflammatory profile. For instance, individuals with the 219G→T polymorphism carry a much higher sensitivity to saturated fat in the diet, increasing susceptibility to inflammation and increasing the relative risk of coronary atherosclerosis, metabolic syndrome, and type 2 diabetes. Such individuals need to pay special attention to the kind of fat they ingest. They can be thought of as "yellow canaries," alerting us to the presence of higher susceptibilities in the human genome to certain types of environmental inputs.[12]

Positive role of essential fatty acids. The literature is replete with studies indicating the positive role that omega-3 balanced diets or omega-3 supplemented diets have on reestablishing proper function of the neuroendocrine-immune system and the inflammation profile. For instance, a paper in the *Journal of Nutrition* described how an α-linolenic acid-rich diet reduced inflammatory and lipid cardiovascular risk factors in hypercholesterolemic men and women.[13] DHA, as well as EPA, also has a positive role in reducing cardiovascular risk and lowering inflammatory potential in women.[14] Chronic inflammation does not result in increased risk of CVD alone, but rather relates to the whole family of chronic diseases. (A detailed discussion of essential fatty acids can be found in Chapter 27.)

Summary

At this time, we are witnessing a virtual epidemic in the increase of metabolic syndrome, type 2 diabetes, obesity, CAD, hypertension, and the epithelial cancers. The increased incidence of these conditions arises from a change in the functional metabolic state of the individual due to changing diet and lifestyle factors. One compelling perspective on these issues has been provided by Dr. Loren Cordain (and others), whose work focuses on the "growing awareness that the profound changes in the environment (eg, in diet and other lifestyle conditions) that began with the introduction of agriculture and animal husbandry ~10,000 years ago occurred too recently on an evolutionary time scale for the human genome to adjust."[15] The challenge for today's clinicians and patients is how to create a different gene expression pattern so that good health and a rectangularizing of the survival curve can be achieved in a 21st century environment. To begin with, we must apply the same level of effort to these issues that we applied in the last 100 years to acute care, with its myriad (and often miraculous) drug and surgical interventions. Nothing less will suffice.

When the wrong information is delivered to the genes in the form of a diet or lifestyle poorly matched to a person's needs, or from a toxic exposure, those genes create an environment in the body (the so-called phenotype, the phenomics of the individual) that is unwary, ill at ease, uncomfortable, and prepared to do battle. This results in chronic immunological activation or imbalance. This shift from acute threats to chronic dysfunction is the challenge of 21st century medicine. Many variables are influential—not only diet, but stress, toxins in the environment, endotoxins in the gut, chronic infection, and mechanical trauma, such as over-training in athletes. Myriad environmental factors can shift the balance in the immunological system, creating in various tissues the message of inflammation which, in turn, is related to the etiology of most chronic disease.

Air and Water

Jeffrey S. Bland, PhD

From a functional medicine perspective, physiology is in a homeodynamic state of interaction with the environment. What may appear to be "homeostasis" is, in actuality, very dynamic. An analogy is the flight of a humming bird. It can hold itself stationary, or in "stasis," at the flower to sip the nectar but, as we know from time-lapse photography, it is actually flapping its wings "dynamically" to overcome gravity. So it is with human physiology. We assume that, because blood sugar, pH, osmolarity, and cellular redox potential don't change much in the healthy individual, homeostasis is a natural set point for physiology.

At the cell biological and molecular levels, however, there is significant dynamic function going on at any one time in order to maintain what is perceived as homeostasis. Blood gases are constantly being exchanged, glucose and fats are being taken up by the cell and metabolized, hydrogen ions are moving at rapid rates across membranes, ions are being transported against gradients, and oxidation-reduction reactions are occurring at diffusion-controlled rates. All of these dynamic processes are regulated by master switches at the executive level in the control of metabolism, both locally and at the whole-person levels. This system is fueled by nutrients that support the energetics necessary to maintain homeodynamic flexibility, or "degrees of freedom."[16]

The most stable physiological system is the system with the greatest homeodynamic flexibility.[17,18] This is the state that might be defined as having the greatest potential for functional health. Redundancy is built into physiology to allow multiple processes to provide routes to the maintenance of homeostasis. The more pathways available, the greater the metabolic degrees of freedom, and the more resilient the functional physiology. As a person loses metabolic degrees of freedom, it results in the loss of "organ reserve," as defined by James Fries,[19] and increases the risk or severity of illness. An example of this is the electrocardiogram (EKG). The most complex EKG is found in the fine structure (i.e., physiological degrees of freedom) of the fit, young athlete.[20] The simplest EKG is the flat-line of a person who has lost all physiological resiliency.

The task of the functional medicine practitioner is to find ways of increasing the patient's physiological degrees of freedom which, in turn, increase functional reserve of the patient. Two environmental factors that have great impact on homeodynamic control of physiology are air and water.

Oxygen as a Limiting Nutrient

The air we breathe is composed of approximately 20% diatomic molecular oxygen. This oxygen supports aerobic metabolism. In the absence of proper oxygen delivery to the cell, metabolic degrees of freedom are significantly reduced and functional reserve is compromised. The cell, tissue, or organ that is oxygen-deprived loses its homeodynamic potential and shifts to the primitive state of anaerobic metabolism, or fermentation. In this case, the cells become more acidic and pH drops, electrolytes are disturbed, and reduction-oxidation chemistry is modified. In clinical medicine, we associate these conditions with ischemic hypoxia or, in the extreme, anoxia.[21] In these cases, oxygen becomes the limiting nutrient for function and new homeostatic levels of blood sugar, blood gases, osmolarity, and redox result that are associated with degrees of ill health or disease.[22,23]

Conditions that can result in oxygen becoming the limiting nutrient include, as examples:

- anemia
- vascular injury
- ischemic events due to vasoconstriction
- poisoning
- respiratory depression
- pulmonary dysfunction
- compromised musculoskeletal fitness

Historically, most cultures have had a traditional activity (a "therapy") designed to improve oxygen delivery to tissues, and a number of these activities have been investigated for their health effects.[24,25,26] Examples include:

- deep-breathing exercises
- yoga
- rebreathing
- dance
- physical therapy
- stress reduction (meditation)
- dietary factors to improve blood chemistry
- physical fitness training and athletic competition

At the Institutes for the Achievement of Human Potential in Philadelphia, parents of brain-injured children are taught exercises for their children that improve oxygen delivery to the brain.[27] The positive impact these therapies have on improving function in brain-injured children has been documented from hundreds of thousands of examples around the world.

Water as a Limiting Nutrient

The second most important substance in maintaining homeodynamics and functional reserve is water. The majority of the human body is composed of water. The water that makes up our body composition plays a very important role within cells in maintaining structure and function. Intercellular water binds to proteins, carbohydrates, and nucleic acids to maintain their proper function. When dehydrated, the structure of critical cellular biomolecules is adversely affected, reducing their function.[28,29] All systems are influenced by dehydration, resulting in reduced energy production, neurotoxicity, and alteration in the function of every organ. As water is lost and not replaced, the concentration of substances within cells increases, pH changes, and enzyme function is altered. Muscle cramping, sore muscles, reduced mental clarity, constipation, fatigue, and increased sensitivity to toxic substances all increase during states of dehydration. In these cases, water becomes the limiting nutrient for support of functional physiology.

The Importance of Assessing Air and Water Adequacy

In a functional medicine assessment, the adequacy of air (i.e., oxygen) and water to maintain functional organ reserve should be a first-stage priority. The use of body composition measurements using bioimpedance analysis[30] can provide information about both intra- and intercellular water status. Pulse and heart rate, along with physical assessment of oxygen saturation and tissue-specific signs of ischemia, can provide information concerning the adequacy of oxygen.

Often, clinicians assume adequacy of both oxygen and water because they are so readily available, and if the patient doesn't display overt symptoms of hypoxia or dehydration, no further evaluation is done. By concentrating on the signs and symptoms of chronic tissue deprivation of either oxygen or water, many patients who are in need of therapy in these areas will be identified. Proper intervention to improve tissue oxygen and water delivery will improve homeodynamic control and functional physiological reserve.

Health Effects of Air and Water Pollution

An extensive literature on health effects of environmental pollution is available to the interested reader. This short introduction to air and water as building blocks of health would be incomplete, however, without at least mentioning the significant impact that industrialization has had on the quality of air and water.

Water. From the fish we eat, which are now significant sources of toxins such as mercury[31] and pesticides (see, for example, the discussion on xenobiotics to be found further on in this chapter), to substances we add to water as a function of general public use[32] (chlorine, fluoride, softening agents), to bacterial or parasitic agents found as a result of contamination or overuse,[33] pure water on this planet has become a diminished resource. All of these problems have significant health implications, ranging from neurological damage[34] to respiratory problems[35] to gastrointestinal ailments.[36] Access to safe water for drinking, bathing, and normal household use is a very important part of a healthy life—one of which we are most aware when it no longer exists.

Air. "Increased levels of particulate air pollution are associated with increased respiratory and cardiovascular mortality and morbidity as well as worsening of asthma."[37] One of the most distressing aspects of air pollution is its disproportionate effect on babies and children. One study reported that "Studies on infant mortality and exposure to particles show an outstanding consistency in the magnitude of the effects, despite the different designs used"; the effect is estimated to be about a 5% increase in post-neonatal mortality for all causes and around 22% for respiratory diseases.[38] That's a heavy price to pay, and it's paid by our youngest and most vulnerable patients. That is not to imply that adults are somehow protected. A 2005 study suggested that particulate air pollutants in Scandinavia are responsible for approximately 3,500 deaths per year.[39] "The annual cost of human exposure to outdoor air pollutants from all sources is estimated to be between $40 to $50 billion … . The death toll from exposure to particulate air pollution generated by motor vehicles, burning coal, fuel oil, and wood is estimated to be responsible for as many as 100,000 fatalities annually in the United States."[40]

Summary

It can be easy to lose sight of the critical importance of adequate oxygenation and hydration of tissues as key factors in health. Air and water are taken for granted, particularly in industrialized countries and particularly by people who are mostly healthy—we breathe, we drink fluids, we give it little thought. Unfortunately, in today's world, we must pay attention to the sufficiency and quality of our air and water, and clinicians must consider whether a patient may be suffering from deprivation or contamination of these most vital building blocks to health, even when the effects may be diffuse and difficult to detect. With problems this pervasive, we cannot afford to take anything for granted.

Physical Exercise

William J. Evans, PhD

Introduction

Virtually every system in the human body is affected in some way by increasing levels of physical activity. Exercise encompasses a broad range of activities; it can be defined as increased (above resting) muscular activity and may be categorized as anaerobic (sprinting), endurance (aerobic), or resistive (weight lifting). Resistive exercise is defined as muscle contracting a few times against a heavy load or with high tension. This type of exercise is also termed progressive resistance training (PRT) when the load or intensity is progressively increased as an individual becomes stronger. PRT is distinctly different from aerobic or endurance exercise, in which muscles contract against little or no resistance. Anaerobic exercise makes use of phosphocreatine and/or glycogenolysis for energy production. This type of exercise is generally thought of as a sprinting type of exercise; however, an extremely deconditioned patient, such as an individual with chronic obstructive pulmonary disease or heart failure may perform anaerobic exercise simply by getting out of bed and walking across a room.

The adaptive response to regularly performed exercise has been repeatedly demonstrated to have remarkably beneficial effects. The list of these adaptive responses is extensive. The Centers for Disease Control and Prevention, along with the American College of Sports Medicine, has suggested that everyone should accumulate at least 30 minutes of exercise on most (preferably all) days.[41] This recommendation is based on evidence of a substantial decrease in all-cause mortality resulting from a moderate amount of increased physical activity.[42,43] The American Heart Association has stated that inactivity is a primary risk factor for cardiovascular disease.[44,45,46] Because far more Americans are inactive than those who have elevated cholesterol or who smoke, it is the predominant risk factor for heart disease in the United States. This review will focus on the acute and chronic adaptations to exercise with particular attention to substrate use and effects on risk factors for chronic disease and aging.

Aerobic Exercise

Maximal aerobic exercise capacity is termed VO_{2max}. VO_2 (volume of oxygen consumed during maximal aerobic exercise) is defined by the Fick equation:

VO_2 = Cardiac Output • Arterio - venous oxygen difference.

VO_{2max} is expressed as either:

ml O_2 consumed • kg^{-1} body weight • min^{-1} or

L O_2 consumed • min^{-1} . ml • kg^{-1} • min^{-1}

The latter formula is most often used to define an individual's aerobic capacity, as differences in body weight are controlled for.

The Fick equation demonstrates that there are two important determiners of VO_{2max}: central factors that control the delivery of oxygen to skeletal muscle and the capacity of skeletal muscle to extract and utilize oxygen for ATP during exercise. Regularly performed aerobic exercise increases VO_{2max} through the following mechanisms:

1. increased cardiac output resulting from a plasma volume expansion (approximately 15%);
2. increased stroke volume as a result of cardiac hypertrophy; and
3. improved capacity to extract and use oxygen by skeletal muscle.

This enhanced oxidative capacity of muscle is due to increased capillarization, mitochondrial density, and myoglobin content. Under most conditions, the delivery of oxygen limits maximal aerobic performance. Increasing blood hemoglobin concentration (from anemic to normal or from normal to super-normal) has been demonstrated to increase VO_{2max} and submaximal exercise performance.[47,48,49,50] Anemia due to malnutrition has been demonstrated to limit functional status and work capacity. On the other hand, aerobic exercise performance in athletes can be substantially improved by increasing hemoglobin levels above normal through the use of recombinant human erythropoietin.[51]

Maximal aerobic capacity (VO_{2max}) declines with advancing age.[52] This age-associated decrease in VO_{2max} has been shown to be approximately 1%/yr between the ages of 20 and 70 years old. This decline is likely due to a number of factors including decreased levels of physical activity, changing cardiac function (including decreased maximal cardiac output), and reduced muscle mass. Flegg and Lakatta[53] determined that skeletal muscle mass accounted for most of the variability in VO_{2max} in men and women above the age of 60 years old. A number of studies have demonstrated that the age-related decline in VO_{2max} is ameliorated by physical activity.[54,55,56,57] Bortz and Bortz[58] reviewed world records of master athletes up to age 85 for endurance events and noted that the decline in performance occurred at a rate of 0.5%/yr. They concluded that this decline of 0.5%/year may represent the effects of age (or "biological" aging) on VO_{2max} and the remainder of the decline may be the result of an increasingly sedentary lifestyle. However, Rosen et al.[59] examined predictors of this age-associated decline in VO_{2max} and concluded that VO_{2max} declines at the same rate in athletic and sedentary men and that 35% of this decline is due to sarcopenia.

Aerobic exercise has long been an important recommendation for the prevention and treatment of many of the chronic diseases typically associated with old age. These include type 2 diabetes mellitus (and impaired glucose tolerance), hypertension, heart disease, and osteoporosis. Emerging research is also demonstrating an important role for exercise in treatment and prevention of certain cancers and neurodegenerative diseases.[60,61,62,63,64,65,66]

Regularly performed aerobic exercise increases insulin action. The responses of initially sedentary young (age 20–30) and older (age 60–70) men and women to three months of aerobic conditioning (70% of maximal heart rate, 45 minutes/day, three days per week) were examined by Meredith et al.[67] They found that the absolute gains in aerobic capacity were similar between the two age groups. However, the mechanism for adaptation to regular submaximal exercise appears to be different between old and young people. Muscle biopsies taken before and after training showed a more than two-fold increase in oxidative capacity of the muscles of the older subjects, while that of the young subjects showed smaller improvements. Another study found that "Exercise training exerts antioxidative effects in the skeletal muscle in chronic heart failure, in particular, due to an augmentation in activity of radical scavenger enzymes."[68] In addition, skeletal muscle glycogen stores in the older subjects, significantly lower than those of the young men and women initially, increased significantly. The degree to which the elderly demonstrate increases in maximal cardiac output in response to endurance training is still largely unanswered. Seals and co-workers[69] found no increases after one year of endurance training while, more recently, Spina et al.[70] observed that older men increased maximal cardiac output while healthy older women demonstrated no change in response to endurance exercise training. If these gender-related differences in cardiovascular response are real, it may explain the lack of response in maximal cardiac output when older men and women are included in the same study population.[71]

Aerobic Exercise and Carbohydrate Metabolism

The two-hour plasma glucose level measured during an oral glucose tolerance test increases by an average of 5.3 mg/dL per decade, and fasting plasma glucose increases by an average of 1 mg/dL per decade.[72] The NHANES II study demonstrated a progressive increase of about 0.4 mM/decade of life in mean plasma glucose value 2h after a 75g oral glucose tolerance test (OGTT, providing a specific amount of glucose drink in a solution and measuring the changes in plasma glucose over a 2 to 3 hour period) (n = 1,678 men and 1,892 women).[73] Shimokata and co-workers[74] examined glucose tolerance in community dwelling men and women ranging in age from 17 to 92. By assessing level of obesity, pattern of body fat distribution, activity and fitness levels, they attempted to examine the independent effect of age on glucose tolerance. They found no significant differences between the young and middle-aged groups; however, the old groups had significantly higher glucose and insulin values (following a glucose challenge) than young or middle-aged groups. They concluded: "The major finding of this study is that the decline in glucose tolerance from the early-adult to the middle-age years is entirely explained by secondary influences (fatness and fitness), whereas the decline from mid-life to old age still is also influenced by chronological age. This finding is unique. It is also unexplained." However, it must be pointed out that anthropometric determination of body fatness becomes increasingly less accurate with advancing age and does not reflect the intra-abdominal and intramuscular accumulation of fat that occurs with aging.[75] The results of this study may be due more to an underestimate of true body fat levels than age, *per se*. These age-associated changes in glucose tolerance can result in type 2 diabetes and the broad array of associated abnormalities. In 1995, in a large population of elderly men and women (older than 55 years), serum glucose and fructosamine levels were seen to be higher in subjects with retinopathy compared with those without and, within the groups with retinopathy, serum glucose was significantly associated with the number of hemorrhages.[76] These relationships were independent of body composition, abdominal obesity or the presence of type 2 diabetes.

The relationship between aging, body composition, activity, and glucose tolerance was also examined in 270 female and 462 male factory workers aged 22 to 73 years, none of whom were retired.[77] Plasma glucose levels, both fasting and after a glucose load, increased with age, but the correlation between age and total integrated glucose response following a glucose load was weak: in women only 3% of the variance could be attributed to age. When activity levels and drug use were factored in, age accounted for only 1% of the variance in women and 6.25% in men.

The fact that aerobic exercise has significant effects on skeletal muscle may help explain its importance in the treatment of glucose intolerance and type 2 diabetes. Seals and co-workers[78] found that a high-intensity training program showed greater improvements in the insulin response to an oral glucose load compared to lower intensity aerobic exercise. However, their subjects began the study with normal glucose tolerance. Kirwan and co-workers[79] found that nine months of endurance training at 80% of the maximal heart rate (4 d/wk) resulted in reduced glucose-stimulated insulin levels; however, no comparison was made to a lower intensity exercise group. Hughes and co-workers[80] demonstrated that regularly performed aerobic exercise without weight loss resulted in improved glucose tolerance, rate of insulin-stimulated glucose disposal, and increased skeletal muscle GLUT 4 levels in older subjects with impaired glucose tolerance. GLUT 4 is the glucose transporter protein found in skeletal muscle. The amount and/or the activation of this transporter protein is thought to be a rate-limiting step in the transport of glucose into muscle cells. In this investigation, a moderate intensity aerobic exercise program was compared to a higher intensity program (50 vs. 75% of maximal heart rate reserve, 55 min/day, 4 day/wk, for 12 weeks). No differences were seen between the moderate and higher intensity aerobic exercise on glucose tolerance, insulin sensitivity, or muscle GLUT-4 (the glucose transporter protein in skeletal muscle) levels, indicating perhaps that a prescription of moderate aerobic exercise should be recommended for older men or women with type 2 diabetes (or at high risk for type 2 diabetes) to help to ensure compliance with the program.

Endurance training and dietary modifications are generally recommended as the primary treatment in the non-insulin-dependent diabetic. Cross-sectional analysis of dietary intake supports the hypothesis that a low-carbohydrate/high-fat diet is associated with the onset of type 2 diabetes.[81] This evidence, however, is not supported by prospective studies where dietary habits have not been related to the development of type 2 diabetes.[82,83] The effects of a high carbohydrate diet on glucose tolerance and lipoproteins have been equivocal.[84,85,86,87] Hughes et al.[88] compared the effects of a high-carbohydrate (60% CHO and 20% fat)/high-fiber (25g dietary fiber/1000 kcal) diet with and without three months of high intensity (75% max heart rate reserve, 50 min/day, 4 d/wk) endurance exercise in older, glucose-intolerant men and women. Subjects were fed all of their food on a metabolic ward during the three-month study and were not allowed to lose weight. These investigators observed no improvement in glucose tolerance or insulin-stimulated glucose uptake in either the diet or the diet plus exercise group. The exercise plus high-carbohydrate diet group demonstrated a significant and substantial increase in skeletal muscle glycogen content and, at the end of the training, the muscle glycogen stores would be considered to be saturated. Since the primary site of glucose disposal is skeletal muscle glycogen stores, the extremely high muscle glycogen content associated with exercise and a high-carbohydrate diet likely limited the rate of glucose disposal. Thus, when combined with exercise and a weight maintenance diet, a high-carbohydrate diet had a counter-regulatory effect. It is likely that the value of a high-carbohydrate/high-fiber diet lies in its effect on reducing excess body fat, which may be an important cause of the impaired glucose tolerance. Recently, Schaefer and co-workers[89] demonstrated that older subjects consuming an ad libitum high-carbohydrate diet lost weight.

There appears to be no attenuation of the response of elderly men and women to regularly performed aerobic exercise when compared to those seen in young subjects. Increased fitness levels are associated with reduced mortality and increased life expectancy. A 2005 review pointed out that these effects appear to be primarily as a result of protection against cardiovascular disease and type 2 diabetes. The authors suggest that "regular exercise induces suppression of TNF-α and thereby offers protection against TNFα-induced insulin resistance."[90] They have also been shown to prevent the occurrence of type 2 diabetes in those who are at the greatest risk for developing this disease.[91] Thus, regularly performed aerobic exercise is an important way for older people to improve their glucose tolerance.

Exercise and Weight Loss

Aerobic exercise is generally prescribed as an important adjunct to a weight loss program. Aerobic exercise combined with weight loss has been demonstrated to increase insulin action to a greater extent than weight loss through diet restriction alone. In the study by Bogardus et al.,[92] diet therapy alone improved glucose tolerance, mainly by reducing basal endogenous glucose production and improving hepatic sensitivity to insulin. Aerobic exercise training, on the other hand, increased carbohydrate storage rates and, therefore, "diet therapy plus physical training produced a more significant approach toward normal." However, aerobic exercise (as opposed to resistance training) combined with a hypocaloric diet has been demonstrated to result in a greater reduction in resting metabolic rate (RMR) than diet alone.[93] Heymsfield and co-workers[94] found aerobic exercise combined with caloric restriction did not preserve fat-free mass (FFM) and did not further accelerate weight loss when compared with diet alone. This lack of an effect of aerobic exercise may have been due to a greater decrease in RMR in the exercising group. In perhaps the most comprehensive study of its kind, Goran and Poehlman[95] examined components of energy metabolism in older men and women engaged in regular endurance training. They found that endurance training did not increase total daily energy expenditure due to a compensatory decline in physical activity during the remainder of the day. In other words, when elderly subjects participated in a regular walking program, they rested more, so that activities outside of walking decreased and thus 24-hour calorie expenditure was unchanged. However, older individuals who had been participating in endurance exercise for most of their lives have been shown to have a greater resting metabolic rate and total daily energy expenditure than did age-matched sedentary controls.[96] Ballor et al.[97] compared the effects of resistance training to that of diet restriction alone in obese women. They found that resistance exercise training results in increased strength and gains in muscle size as well as preservation of FFM during weight loss. These data are similar to the results of Pavlou et al.[98] who used both aerobic and resistance training as an adjunct to a weight loss program in obese men and demonstrated preservation of FFM.

Two important studies were carried out by Jakicic and co-workers,[99,100] examining exercise intensity and duration and their effects on weight loss. In the first study, exercise advice was provided to three groups of overweight women losing weight. All three groups were told to exercise for a total of 40 minutes each day. One group was told to perform all 40 minutes of exercise in one bout; a second group was told to perform 40 minutes of exercise in four ten-minute bouts throughout the day; and the third group was give the same advice as the second group (intermittent exercise) but was provided a motorized treadmill for their homes. They found that the duration of the exercise bout was not important. However the total number of minutes exercised per week, irrespective of the group, had the most important effect on total weight loss and maintenance of the weight loss. The second study[101] examined the effects of exercise intensity on weight loss (high vs. moderate aerobic exercise). The found that intensity had very little effect on total weight loss, but that, once again, total number of minutes exercised/week was the most important factor. These studies suggest that 150 minutes/wk may be a threshold for exercise having a significant effect on weight loss and maintenance.

Strength Training

While endurance exercise has been the more traditional means of increasing cardiovascular fitness, the American College of Sports Medicine currently recommends strength or resistance training as an important component of an overall fitness program. This is particularly important in the elderly where loss of muscle mass and weakness are prominent deficits.

Strength conditioning or progressive resistance training (PRT) is generally defined as training in which the resistance against which a muscle generates force is progressively increased over time. PRT involves few contractions against a heavy load. The metabolic and morphological adaptations resulting from resistance and endurance exercise are quite different. Muscle strength has been shown to increase in response to training between 60 and 100% of the 1 repetition maximum (1RM).[102] 1 RM is the maximum amount of weight that can be lifted with one contraction. Strength conditioning will result in an increase in muscle size and this increase in size is largely the result of increased contractile proteins. The mechanisms by which the mechanical events stimulate an increase in RNA synthesis and subsequent protein synthesis are not well understood. Lifting weight requires that a muscle shorten as it produces force. This is called a concentric contraction. Lowering the weight, on the other hand, forces the muscle to lengthen as it produces force. This is an eccentric muscle contraction. These lengthening muscle contractions have been shown to produce ultrastructural damage (microscopic tears in contractile proteins muscle cells) that may stimulate increased muscle protein turnover.[103]

Effects of Resistance Exercise and Insulin on Protein Metabolism

Hormonal and nutritional factors, particularly the availability of insulin and amino acids, have important effects in the control of muscle protein synthesis.[104,105] For example, starvation reduces the rate of protein synthesis in skeletal muscle by more than 50% compared to the rate seen in fed animals. This inhibition of protein synthesis (also seen in muscle from diabetic animals) is a result of an impairment in the initiation phase of protein synthesis.[106,107] The mechanism through which insulin regulates protein synthesis initiation involves phosphorylation of the translational regulator eukaryotic initiation factor 4E (eIF-4E)-binding protein 1 (4E-PB1).[108] Insulin-like growth factor 1 (IGF-1) results in the phosphorylation of 4E-BP1 and dissociation of the 4E-BP1 • eIF-4E complex in cells in culture (muscle cells that are grown in a medium containing appropriate nutrients and growth factors).[109] IGF-1 has also been shown to stimulate protein synthesis in rats *in vivo*[110] and in muscle in perfused hind limb preparations.[111] These studies also suggest that insulin plays a permissive role in the effect of IGF-I in stimulating muscle protein synthesis.

Studies of insulin secretion after resistance, but not endurance, exercise provide evidence for insulin's role in maintaining muscle mass. King et al.[112] and Dela et al.[113] showed that arginine-stimulated insulin secretion is decreased with endurance training. In contrast, acute resistance exercise in rats has been shown to increase insulin secretion.[114] As reviewed above, regular aerobic exercise is known to increase insulin sensitivity and glucose tolerance. In addition to its effects on insulin action, aerobic exercise training results in decreased insulin secretion.[115] Regularly performed endurance exercise in young men is associated with an insulin pulse profile in the resting fasted state characterized by less insulin secreted per burst but a similar number of bursts over a 90-minute period. These researchers suggested that training-induced elevations in target-tissue sensitivity to insulin may reduce the requirement for pulsatile insulin secretion. This coordinated response keeps glucose concentrations constant. Dela et al.[116] demonstrated that aerobic exercise training decreases both arginine- and glucose-stimulated insulin secretion, indicating, they conclude, a profound β-cell adaptation.

A single bout of concentric exercise is a recognized enhancer of insulin action, while eccentric exercise transiently impairs whole body insulin action for at least two days after the bout.[117] We have demonstrated that eccentric exercise can result in a long-term delay in the rate of glycogen synthesis.[118] The decreased insulin action and delayed glycogen synthetic rate have been shown to result from decreased rate of glucose transport rather than decreased glycogen synthase activity.[119] This transient resistance to insulin and impaired resynthesis of glycogen can result in a systemic hyperinsulinemia that may result in an increase in the rate of muscle protein synthesis. Our laboratory has demonstrated age-related differences in the insulin response to hyperglycemia following a single bout of eccentric exercise.[120] Two days following upper and lower body eccentric exercise, younger subjects demonstrated a pronounced pancreatic insulin response during a hyperglycemic clamp, while this response was blunted in healthy elderly men.

The effects of resistance exercise on insulin availability appear to be opposite those of endurance exercise and, thus, net protein accretion is stimulated with resistance exercise. Insulin has been demonstrated to have profoundly anabolic effects on skeletal muscle. In the resting state, insulin has been demonstrated to decrease the rate of muscle protein degradation. Stable isotope amino acid studies in humans[121,122] clearly demonstrate that insulin inhibits whole body protein breakdown *in vivo* and stimulates muscle protein synthesis rate in human skeletal muscle[123] and in insulin-deficient rats. However, in non-diabetic animals, this effect was not seen. Fluckey et al.[124,125] have argued that insulin is not likely to stimulate muscle protein synthesis in quiescent muscle. We have demonstrated that an insulin infusion does not increase the rate of protein synthesis in non-exercised muscle and, using a resistance exercise model, we have also demonstrated that resistance exercise did not stimulate an increase in the rate of protein synthesis. It was only with the addition of insulin that an exercise-induced increase in the rate of soleus and gastrocnemius protein synthesis was seen. This effect of insulin stimulation on the rate of protein synthesis was preserved with advancing age.

Protein Requirements and Exercise

High-intensity resistance training is clearly anabolic in both young and older individuals. Data from our laboratory demonstrate a 10 to 15% decrease in N-excretion at the initiation of training that persists for 12 weeks. That is, progressive resistance training improved N-balance; thus, older subjects performing resistance training have a lower mean protein requirement than do sedentary subjects. This effect was seen at a protein intake of 0.8g and 1.6g, indicating that the effect of resistance training on protein retention may not be related to dietary protein intake. These results are somewhat at variance with our previous research demonstrating that regularly performed aerobic exercise causes an increase in the mean protein requirement of middle-aged and young endurance athletes.[126] This difference likely results from increased oxidation of amino acids during aerobic exercise that may not be present during resistance training.

Strawford et al.[127] also demonstrated similar effects of resistance exercise training on nitrogen balance in patients with HIV-related weight loss. The investigators examined the effects of an anabolic steroid (oxandrolone, 20 mg/d and placebo) and high-intensity resistance exercise training in 24 eugonadal men with HIV-associated weight loss (mean, 9% body weight loss). Both groups showed significant nitrogen retention and increases in LBM, weight, and strength. The mean gains were significantly greater in the oxandrolone group than in the placebo group in nitrogen balance, accrual of FFM, and strength. Results were similar whether or not patients were taking protease inhibitors. These results confirm the positive effects of resistance exercise on nitrogen retention and protein requirements.

These studies, taken as a whole, demonstrate the powerful effects of resistance exercise training on protein nutriture. The anabolic effects have important implications in the treatment of many wasting diseases and conditions such as cancer, HIV infection, aging, chronic renal failure, and undernutrition seen in many very old men and women. By effectively lowering dietary protein needs, resistance exercise can limit further losses of skeletal muscle mass while simultaneously increasing muscle strength and functional capacity.

Resistance Exercise and Aging

Our laboratory examined the effects of high-intensity resistance training on the knee extensors and flexors (80% of 1RM, 3 days/week) in older men (age 60–72 years). The average increases in knee flexor and extensor strength were 227% and 107% respectively. CT scans and muscle biopsies were used to determine muscle size. Total muscle area by CT analysis increased by 11.4% while the muscle biopsies showed an increase of 33.5% in type I fiber area and 27.5% increase in type II fiber area. In addition, lower body VO_{2max} increased significantly while upper body VO_{2max} did not, indicating that increased muscle mass can increase maximal aerobic power. It appears that age-related loss in muscle mass may be an important determinant in the reduced maximal aerobic capacity seen in elderly men and women.[128] Improving muscle strength can enhance the capacity of many older men and women to perform many activities such as climbing stairs, carrying packages, and even walking.

We applied this same training program to a group of frail, institutionalized elderly men and women (mean age 90 ± 3 years, range 87-96).[129] After eight weeks of training, the 10 subjects in this study increased muscle strength by almost 180% and muscle size by 11%. More recently, a similar intervention on frail nursing home residents demonstrated not only increases in muscle strength and size, but increased gait speed, stair climbing power, and balance.[130] In addition, spontaneous activity levels increased significantly while the activity of a non-exercised control group was unchanged. In this study, the effects of a protein/calorie supplement combined with exercise were also examined. The supplement consisted of a 240-ml liquid supplying 360 kcal in the form of carbohydrate (60%), fat (23%), and soy-based protein (17%), and was designed to augment caloric intake by about 20%, and provide one-third of the RDA for vitamins and minerals. The men and women who consumed the supplement and exercised gained weight compared to the three other groups examined (exercise/control, non-exercise supplemented, and non-exercise control). The non-exercising subjects who received the supplement reduced their habitual dietary energy intake so that total energy intake was unchanged. In other words, the supplement did not add to total energy intake, but rather substituted one source of energy (the supplement) for another (their meals). More recently (in the same study population), we demonstrated that combined weight lifting and nutritional supplementation increased strength by 257 ± 62% ($p = 0.0001$) and type II fiber area by 10.1 ± 9.0% ($p = 0.033$), with a similar trend for type I fiber area (+12.8 ± 22.2%).[131] Exercise was associated with a 2.5-fold increase in neonatal myosin (a form of myosin found in growing muscle) staining ($p = 0.0009$) and an increase of 491 ± 137% ($p < 0.0001$) in IGF-1 staining. Ultrastructural damage increased by 141 ± 59% after exercise training ($p = 0.034$). Strength increases were largest in those with the greatest increases in myosin, IGF-1, damage, and caloric intake during the trial. Frail, very old elders respond robustly to resistance training with musculoskeletal remodeling, and significant increases in muscle area are possible with resistance training in combination with adequate energy intakes. It should be pointed out that this was a very old, very frail population with diagnoses of multiple chronic diseases. The increase in overall levels of physical activity have been a common observation in our studies.[132,133,134] Since muscle weakness is a primary deficit in many older individuals, increased strength may stimulate more aerobic activities like walking and cycling.

Strength training may increase balance through improvement in the strength of the muscles involved in walking. Indeed, ankle weakness has been demonstrated to be associated with increased risk of falling in nursing home patients.[135] However, balance training, which may demonstrate very little improvement in muscle strength, size, or cardiovascular changes, has also been demonstrated to decrease the risk of falls in older people.[136] Tai Chi, a form of dynamic balance training that requires no new technology or equipment, has been demonstrated to reduce the risk of falling in older people by almost 50%.[137] As a component of the National Institute on Aging FICSIT trials (Frailty and Injuries: Cooperative Studies of Intervention Techniques), individuals aged 70+ were randomized to Tai Chi (TC), individualized balance training (BT), and exercise control education (ED) groups for 15 weeks.[138] In a follow-up assessment four months post-intervention, 130 subjects responded to exit interview questions asking about perceived benefits of participation. Both TC and BT subjects reported increased confidence in balance and movement, but only TC subjects reported that their daily activities and their overall life had been affected; many of these subjects had changed their normal physical activity to incorporate ongoing TC practice. The data suggest that when mental as well as physical control is perceived to be enhanced, with a generalized sense of improvement in overall well-being, older persons' motivation to continue exercising also increases.

Province et al.[139] examined the overall effect of many different exercise interventions on reducing falls in the FICSIT trials. While separate interventions were not powered to make conclusions about their effects on the incidence of falls in an elderly population, the researchers concluded that "all training domains, taken together under the heading of 'general exercise' showed an effect on falls, this probably demonstrates the 'rising tide raises all boats' principle, in which training that targets one domain may improve performance somewhat in other domains as a consequence. If this is so, then the differences seen on fall risk due to the exact nature of the training may not be as critical compared with ... not training at all." It's important to note that in addition to regular strength and balance training, other elements play an important role in bone health and preventing falls; specifically, reducing psychotropic medication and diet supplementation with vitamin D and calcium (discussed further below) have also been shown to be effective.[140,141]

The use of a community-based exercise program for frail older people was examined in a group of predominantly sedentary women over age 70 with multiple chronic conditions.[142] The program was conducted with peer leaders to facilitate its continuation after the research demonstration phase. In addition to positive health outcomes related to functional mobility, blood pressure maintenance, and overall well-being, this intervention was successful in sustaining active participation in regular physical activity through the use of peer leaders selected by the program participants.

In addition to its effect on increasing muscle mass and function, resistance training can also have an important effect on energy balance.[143] Men and women participating in a resistance training program of the upper and lower body muscles required approximately 15% more calories to maintain body weight after 12 weeks of training when compared to their pre-training energy requirements. This increase in energy needs came about as a result of an increased resting metabolic rate, the small energy cost of the exercise, and what was presumed to be an increase in activity levels. While endurance training has been demonstrated to be an important adjunct to weight loss programs in young men and women by increasing their daily energy expenditure, its utility in treating obesity in the elderly may not be great. This is because many sedentary older men and women do not spend many calories when they perform endurance exercise, due to their low fitness levels. Thirty to 40 minutes of exercise may increase energy expenditure by only 100 to 200 kcals with very little residual effect on calorie expenditure. Aerobic exercise training will not preserve lean body mass to any great extent during weight loss. Resistance training *can* preserve or even increase muscle mass during weight loss and, therefore, may be of genuine benefit for those older men and women who must lose weight.

Bone Health

The increased calorie need resulting from strength training may be a way for the elderly to improve their overall nutritional intake when the calories chosen are nutrient-dense foods. In particular, calcium is an important nutrient to increase. Calcium intake was found to be a limiting nutrient in the diet of free-living elderly men and women in the Boston Nutritional Status Survey, which assessed free-living and institutionalized elderly men and women.[144] Careful nutritional planning is needed to reach the recommended calcium levels of 1500 mg/d for postmenopausal women with osteoporosis or using hormone replacement therapy, and 1000 mg/d for postmenopausal women taking estrogen. An increased calorie intake from calcium-containing food is one method to help achieve this goal.

In one of the very few studies to examine the interaction of dietary calcium and exercise, we studied 41 postmenopausal women consuming either high-calcium (1462 mg/d) or moderate-calcium (761 mg) diets. Half of these women participated in a year-long walking program (45 min/d, 4 d/wk, 75% of heart rate reserve). Independent effects of the exercise and dietary calcium were seen. Compared with the moderate calcium group, the women consuming a high-calcium diet displayed reduced bone loss from the femoral neck, independent of whether the women exercised.

The walking prevented a loss of trabecular bone mineral density seen in the non-exercising women after one year. Thus, it appears that calcium intake and aerobic exercise are both independently beneficial to bone mineral density at different sites.

The effects of 52 weeks of high-intensity resistance exercise training were examined in a group of 39 postmenopausal women.[145] Twenty were randomly assigned to the strength training group (2 days/week, 80% of 1RM for upper and lower body muscle groups). At the end of the year, significant differences were seen in lumbar spine and femoral bone density between the strength-trained and sedentary women. However, unlike other pharmacological and nutritional strategies for preventing bone loss and osteoporosis, resistance exercise affects more than just bone density. The women who strength trained improved their muscle mass, strength, balance and overall levels of physical activity. Thus, resistance training can be an important way to decrease the risk for an osteoporotic bone fracture in postmenopausal women.

Muscle strength training can be accomplished by virtually anyone. Many healthcare professionals have directed their patients away from strength training in the mistaken belief that it can cause undesirable elevations in blood pressure. With proper technique, the systolic pressure elevation during aerobic exercise is far greater than that seen during resistance training. Muscle strengthening exercises are rapidly becoming a critical component of cardiac rehabilitation programs, as clinicians realize the need for strength and endurance for many activities of daily living. There is no other group in our society that can benefit more from regularly performed exercise than the elderly. While both aerobic and strength conditioning are highly recommended, only strength training can stop or reverse sarcopenia. Increased muscle strength and mass in the elderly can be the first step toward increased physical activity and a realistic strategy for maintaining functional status and independence for the remaining life span.

Exercise in the Treatment of Chronic Disease

The effects of exercise in treating chronic debilitating disease are largely unexplored. For example, fatigue is the most common complaint of patients with cancer, yet the most common advice provided by oncologists is for increased rest. Just as cardiac rehabilitation has been demonstrated to provide an important mechanism for the post-myocardial infarction patient to improve fitness and reduce the risk of a second event, exercise can greatly improve fitness and reduce much of the fatigue associated with cancer and its treatment. The proven effects of resistance training to enhance nitrogen retention and increase muscle size and strength can provide positive benefits for patients with wasting diseases such as HIV infection and cachexia. Resistance exercise may prove to have powerful effects on patients with chronic renal failure who must consume low-protein diets to slow the progression of their disease. Exercise therapy for those patients forced to undergo extended periods of inactivity during dialysis could also improve functional status and decrease the fatigue associated with disuse. The potential value of a reasonable and well thought out exercise program is great and the exploration of this value should be a high priority for researchers.

Summary

Exercise exerts a powerful acute and chronic effect on virtually every system in the human body. In assessing these effects and prescribing exercise, it is important to keep in mind the very different effects of aerobic vs. resistance exercise. Both forms of exercise are recommended and should be a component of a comprehensive program of disease prevention and health promotion. Chapter 29 presents information on helping patients structure and maintain a balanced exercise program.

Psychosocial Influences

John Tatum, MD

Introduction

An examination of the building blocks of health would be incomplete without an evaluation of the pivotal role played by psychosocial influences. Even in ancient times, this view was not unknown: Hippocrates (460 BC-377 BC) is thought to have said, "It is better to know the patient who has the disease than it is to know the disease which the patient has." A substantial part of "knowing the patient" includes understanding the psychosocial influences that have shaped, and continue to influence, our patients (and ourselves). While this material is not intended to review extensively the factors and theories underlying psychological well being (there is, after all, substantial literature devoted to the field and readily accessible to the reader), we do want to emphasize the importance of the clinician's continuing attention to the subject. A further discussion of mind/body issues, including the effects of spirituality, community, and poverty on health, can be found in Chapter 33. Here, we undertake a brief review of stress, as a marker for the profound effects that psychosocial influences have on the development of each human being.

Historical Emergence of Stress as a Recognized Factor in Health

In the modern age, the first to write extensively about stress and use the term was Walter Cannon, whose work during World War I, and on into the 1930s, helped to establish the "groundwork for understanding the physiology of mind-body interactions."[146,147] Hans Selye (1907–1982), who gave full credit to Cannon's work, reintroduced the term and is considered the "father of stress," although the term was not actually used in the original short article in 1936.[148] His use of the word stress was derived from the physical sciences and engineering; through his work, the term evolved from a description of purely physical influences to encompass the biologic sphere as well.[149] His final definition of the term became: "Stress is the nonspecific response of the body to any demand made upon it."[150] In the words of one writer, "Selye's last main contribution to the stress concept was the recognition that, despite our different psychologic and cerebral reactions, both negative and positive stressors (i.e., distress and eustress) elicit virtually identical corticoid/catecholamine responses."[151] Even more specifically, "different stressors elicit different patterns of activation of the sympathetic, nervous, and adrenomedullary hormonal systems."[152] As both scientists and clinicians know, activation of those systems eventually involves the entire mind/body of the patient. The fact that thinking and psychosocial influences affect genetic expression and have long-term neurochemical consequences was demonstrated by the work of Nobel Laureate Eric Kandel, who said, "Stated simply, the regulation of gene expression by social factors makes all bodily functions, including all functions of the brain, susceptible to social influences."[153]

Selye first noticed in medical school that patients with various illnesses had many symptoms in common, such as "coated tongues, aches and pains, loss of appetite, and inflamed tonsils."[154] He later noticed a generalized syndrome in laboratory animals exposed to various noxious agents, which he described as the "general adaptation syndrome."[155] Selye distinguished distress from eustress, stating, "the fact that eustress causes much less damage than distress graphically demonstrates that it is 'how you take it' that determines, ultimately, whether you can adapt successfully to change."[156,157]

Chronic vs. Acute Stress

Since the word stress has been used in so many different ways, describing external events and internal reactions, Bruce McEwan suggested the term allostasis, as opposed to homeostasis, to describe the physiologic response of the body in the face of a challenge.[158] Robert Sapolsky, in his well-received book, *Why Zebras Don't Get Ulcers*, explains that, unlike us, the zebra has an episode of stress only when the lion is in pursuit; otherwise, he is physiologically calm.[159] Chronic stress (which most people experience) and its cumulative effects comprise what McEwan terms allostatic load. "Allostatic load does not always denote a failure of the body's efforts to cope with change or emergency. We can create it for ourselves by living in a way that makes for internal imbalance." Some examples of self-generated stress are not getting enough sleep, eating an unhealthy diet, and not getting enough exercise.[160] The importance of cumulative stress, or the allostatic load, was illustrated by the Holms and Rahe Social Readjustment Rating Scale. Points were assigned to life stressors, both positive and negative, and the higher the total number of points, the greater the likelihood of illness.[161] Further discussion of allostatic load and its effects can be found in the following section on trauma.

Health Effects of Stress

Increased stress has been associated with many health conditions that are widely discussed in the medical literature and readily accessible to the reader. Some of the most familiar (with a few interesting recent citations) include cardiovascular disease,[162,163] gastrointestinal disease,[164] and hormone dysfunctions,[165] all of which have active, ongoing explorations that continue to produce interesting data.

The etiological role of stress in disease was demonstrated in a well-designed prospective study of first-year medical students who were followed for a year. The prediction that there would be a measurable weakening of the immune system and an increase in illness at exam time was confirmed.[166] The proinflammatory cytokine IL-6 has been shown to be one mediator of stress-induced illness. The daily burden of caregivers has been recognized as particularly stressful, and the effects of that stress, including elevated IL-6 levels, have been shown to continue after the loss of the loved one.[167] Chronic stress also raises cortisol levels,[168] which have been shown to damage the brain.[169] Studies on psychosocial factors and cancer risk are inconclusive at this time.[170] Individuals under stress show less DNA repair, animals show decreases in the DNA repair enzyme methyltransferase, and examination stress increases the ability of a tumor-promoting agent to block apoptosis.[171,172]

Stress prepares the organism for an emergency, but chronic stress impairs health through a complex array of physiologic functions initiated by the release in the hypothalamus of corticotropin releasing factor (CRF). CRF triggers the release of adrenocorticotropic hormone, or ACTH, from the pituitary, which in turn causes the release of cortisol from the adrenal cortex. Cortisol helps maintain blood glucose levels but (as noted above) chronic stress or chronic administration of pharmacological cortisol preparations causes insulin resistance, hypertension, redistribution of fat in the body, decreased protein synthesis, and decreased DNA repair. Furthermore, the immune system is weakened through a decrease in the production of blood cells, antibodies, and gamma globulins, but also through an inhibition of the production of the proinflammatory interleukins IL-1, 2, and 6; tumor necrosis factor; and gamma interferon. This shift in resources from ongoing maintenance and repair of the organism to all-out defense is understandable when fleeing the lion, but harmful when chronic, as discussed eloquently by Sapolsky in *Why Zebras Don't Get Ulcers*.

Some Determinants of Individual Responses to Stress

Although chronic stress and total cumulative stress increase the chance of illness, genetic, psychological, and social factors also play important modifying roles. For example, not all rats of the same strain suffer the same degree of ill effects from the same stress. Sapolsky, professor of biology and neuroscience at Stanford University, and recipient of a McArthur Foundation "genius grant," describes a series of experiments with rats in which a second rat receives the same electric shock as the first. The second rat does not develop an ulcer if:

- there is a companion rat it can bite,
- it has a piece of wood it can gnaw on,
- it has a warning before the shock,
- it can press a lever it thinks will reduce its shock,
- the shocks are fewer than expected, and/or
- it is accompanied by a second rat it likes.[173]

Sapolsky translates these studies to humans, observing that stress-related illness is less likely to happen if:

- we have an outlet for our frustration,
- we have "a hobby" or diversion,
- we have predictive information,
- we have a real or imagined sense of control,
- we can interpret a stress favorably, and/or
- we have social connectedness.

Thus, more important than the amount of stress is one's reaction to it, and that reaction is influenced by many factors.

In his review article, "How the Mind Hurts and Heals the Body," Oakley Ray describes four classes of coping skills that improve one's ability to handle stress.[174] The first of these is knowledge. "With knowledge [or] information, comes an empowerment, a belief that the world is understandable, controllable, and friendly. Perhaps the most stressful situation is the ambiguity that comes from an awareness that one has inadequate and incomplete information."[175] If education can be seen as a measure of knowledge, and perhaps the ability to acquire knowledge, increased years of education should be associated with longevity,[176] and indeed they are. Interestingly, however, subsequent research has shown that the association with education is "explained in full by the strong association between education and income."[177] As the authors go on to point out, with a strong match to Sapolsky's list (shown above):

> Persons in lower socioeconomic strata have increased exposure to a broad range of psychosocial variables predictive of morbidity and mortality. This includes (1) a lack of social relationships and social supports; (2) personality dispositions, such as a lost sense of mastery, optimism, sense of control, and self-esteem or heightened levels of anger and hostility; and (3) chronic and acute stress in life and work, including the stress of racism, classism, and other

phenomena related to the social distribution of power and resources.

The second coping skill Ray describes is "inner resources." This refers to the "beliefs, assumptions, and predictions" one learns growing up, including whether life is seen positively or negatively.[178] Valliant and Mukamal spoke of "involuntary mental mechanisms that adaptively alter inner or outer reality in order to minimize distress."[179] Rotter introduced the important concept of locus of control,[180] and Kamen and Seligman talked of explanatory style.[181] Again, these elements map back to Sapolsky's list in a very substantive way.

Ray's third class of coping skills is social support. "In general, ... the larger the social support system is, the lower the mortality rate."[182,183] (More on this subject can be found in Chapter 33.)

The fourth class of coping skills Ray describes is spirituality (also discussed further in Chapter 33). He refers to Oxman, Freeman, and Mancheimer's 1995 study. "Those who professed no strength and comfort from religion were three times as likely to die in this six-month period as those who said they drew strength and comfort from religion. Those who did not participate in group activities were four times more likely to die than those who did."[184] Other studies have shown similar findings.[185]

There are many other psychosocial influences on health in modern life that the clinician needs to be cognizant of. Among the many that have been studied, some pertinent ones in today's highly mobile, globalized world include natural catastrophe,[186,187,188] disaster,[189] terrorism,[190,191] and immigrant status (acculturation).[192] Common experiences such as loss of a loved one, relocation, and loss of employment have been researched for decades.

Summary

This brief examination of psychosocial influences as key building blocks in patient health reveals that we cannot overemphasize the importance of taking a thorough psychosocial history as part of routine health care. Psychosocial factors influence health through the interconnected information systems of the mind, the endocrine system, the nervous system, and the immune system,[193] so the clinician cannot discount the possibility that the physical effects that brought the patient to the office may have been initiated by (triggers) and/or influenced by (mediators) psychosocial experiences. The psychosocial portion of a comprehensive traditional medical history would include birthplace and subsequent moves, parental information including parenting style, sibling information, history of abuse or neglect, academic history, sexual history, marital history, children (including miscarriages and abortions), occupational history, and history of substance abuse. Research suggests the importance of paying particular attention to stress, loss, attitude, knowledge, beliefs, social support, and spirituality, as they have a direct impact on health and outcome, as described above.

Trauma

Jayne Alexander, DO

Introduction

When a rock is dropped to the bottom of a lake it not only disrupts the column of water through which it falls, but it also alters the dynamics of the entire body of water. Similarly, trauma, typically a directed force, not only disrupts or distorts the human body along the path of impact, but also potentially alters the dynamics of the entire organism.

This discussion will consider some of the physiologic and mechanical principles involved in trauma. Clinical considerations relevant to the post-stabilization, office-based patient will be presented.

Anatomic and Physiologic Response to Trauma

Starting with embryonic development and continuing throughout life, the living human body functions in part as a spatially-oriented metabolic field engaged in the conduct of spatially-ordered metabolic processes.[194] Trauma can be viewed as a force that distorts or disrupts the body's spatial organization, or anatomy, to an extent that exceeds its ability to immediately return to its normal orientation and function.

The dominant physiologic concerns in the stabilized trauma patient are the effects of distortion mechanics, cellular breakdown secondary to frank tissue disruption, and consequent local and systemic responses. Non-incisive trauma, such as strain, spares its recipient the frank tissue disruption that occurs in incisive trauma. However, neural, vascular, and lymphatic elements that course within strained tissues are, themselves, subject to the forces of strain.[195] The resulting distortion sets the stage for mechanical compromise that can manifest as pain, swelling, and functional impairment.

Incisive and non-incisive trauma that frankly disrupts tissue integrity initiates the process of inflammation, beginning with the release of substances such as neuropeptides from peripheral nerve terminals, histamine from mast cells, prostaglandins from capillary endothelial cells, and cytokines from white blood cells.[196] Consequent increased local blood flow and increased capillary permeability contribute to fluid pooling in the extravascular space, or interstitium, and to the manifestation of edema. The presence of fibrinogen in the interstitial fluid and the infiltration of leukocytes leads to clotting, phagocytosis, and lysosomal degradation.[197]

Within three to five days of disruptive trauma, granulation tissue, which is rich in fibroblasts and small, budding blood vessels, typically begins to form. Granulation tissue fibroblasts, some of which have characteristics of smooth muscle cells, are involved in the synthesis of glycosaminoglycans and collagen, favoring the former in the early stages of healing and the latter as healing advances.[198] The neovasculature's loosely constructed interendothelial junctions allow extravasation of yet more proteins into the already protein-rich interstitium, a process that further contributes to the formation of interstitial edema.[199]

It is the critically important task of the lymphatics to remove inflammatory exudate from the interstitium.[ii,200,201] The efficiency with which that task is performed governs the length of time that the interstitium is exposed to lysosomes, proinflammatory cytokines, and other irritants. Their persistence in the interstitium can contribute to pain, via stimulation of primary afferent nociceptors, to delayed healing, and eventually to fibrosis.[202] Additionally, under conditions of venous stasis, the efficiency of lymphatic drainage inevitably affects the rate of delivery of nutriture and medication to the site of injury, as well as the rate of presentation of antigens to lymph nodes and the vigor of the subsequent immune response.[iii,203,204]

The body's response to trauma involves both the peripheral and central nervous systems. The peripheral nervous system (PNS) has two components: a somatic component, the efferent fibers of which innervate skeletal muscle, and an autonomic component which innervates most other tissues and organs.[iv] Both components carry sensory fibers, or primary afferent fibers, from somatic or visceral tissues to the central nervous system (CNS) via the dorsal horn of the spinal cord. These primary afferents are of two types—myelinated, large-caliber fibers, or A afferents, and non-myelinated, small-caliber fibers, or B afferents. The large fiber system is typically involved in discriminative touch and proprioception, and the small fiber system is involved in nociception, the detection of damaging or noxious stimuli. The small-caliber fibers, commonly referred to as primary afferent nociceptors, or PANs, are responsive to mechanical, chemical, and thermal stimulation. Low-level stimulation of PANs is perceived as crude touch or contact, whereas more intense stimulation is perceived as pain. Under conditions of repetitive stimuli, PANs are subject to sensitization—a lowering of the threshold of activation, which leads to the development of facilitation and hyperalgesia.[205]

Nociceptive information is conveyed by somatic and visceral afferents to the dorsal horn of the spinal cord, and then ascends the cord to the midbrain, primarily via the anterolateral system. The forebrain limbic system, which processes emotional content, has descending projections to the midbrain. A major area of convergence of this ascending nociceptive and descending emotional information is a cluster of norepinephrine-producing cells called the locus coeruleus (see Figure 13.1). The locus coeruleus releases norepinephrine through projections to

[ii] Among the substances found in lymph are proteins, histaminase, neutrophilic lysosomes, prostaglandin E, interleukin-1, and antigens [References 200, 201 (p. 937), and Atkinson, TP. Histamine and serotonin. In Gallin JI, et al. *Inflammation: Basic Principles and Clinical Correlates*. New York: Raven Press, 1992, p. 196.]

[iii] Of clinical significance is the understanding that osmotic and hydrostatic gradients do not account for the uptake of exudates from the interstitium by initial lymphatics. Rather, pulsatile fluid waves, consistent with arteriolar vasomotion, pass through the interstitial fluid and contribute to the opening and closing of the initial lymphatic. [Intaglietta M, Gross JF. Vasomotion, tissue fluid flow and the formation of lymph. Intl J Microcirc: Clin and Exper. 1982;1:55-65.] Once within the lymphatic vessels, the movement of lymph is supported *intrinsically* by a distension-sensitive myogenic pump, and *extrinsically* by such mechanical forces as intestinal peristalsis and thoracic respiration as well as by neural and humoral mediators. [Schmid-Schonbein GW. Microlymphatics and lymph flow. Physiol Rev. 1990;70(4):987-1028.]

[iv] The autonomic nervous system (ANS) sends fibers to all tissues except hyaline cartilage, centers of intervertebral discs, and parenchymal tissues of the CNS. [Willard, FH. Autonomic nervous system. In Ward RC, ed. *Foundations for Osteopathic Medicine*. 2nd Ed. Philadelphia: Lippincott Williams and Wilkins, 2003.]

the forebrain, the spinal cord, the hippocampus, the hypothalamus, and to cardiovascular and respiratory centers located in the brainstem.[206]

When the hypothalamus, which also receives emotional input, is stimulated by norepinephrine from the locus coeruleus, it responds by releasing both corticotropin-releasing hormone (CRH) and norepinephrine. CRH, in turn, stimulates the locus coeruleus to release more norepinephrine, thereby establishing a feed forward loop between the locus coeruleus and the hypothalamus. Additionally, CRH causes the anterior pituitary to release adrenocorticotropin (ACTH). ACTH, via systemic circulation, stimulates the release of glucocorticoids such as cortisol from the adrenal cortex, resulting in, among other things, gluconeogenesis and suppression of the release of cytokines.[207] Under normal conditions, following short-term physical or emotional stress, elevated cortisol levels will serve to downregulate this hypothalamic-pituitary-adrenal (HPA) axis. In addition to being activated by emotional stress, hormonal stimulation, and nociceptive impulses, the HPA axis is also activated by cytokines released in response to trauma, infection, histamine, and inflammation.[208] This intersystemic integration is designated as the neuroendocrine immune system.

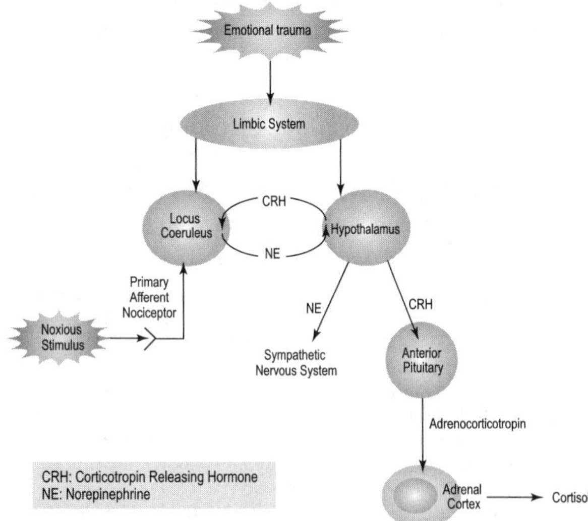

Figure 13.1 Generalized schema of effect of noxious or emotionally-charged input to the central nervous system

Release of norepinephrine from the hypothalamus increases the activity of the sympathetic nervous system (SNS). This has the effect of increasing heart rate, respiratory rate, blood pressure and cardiac output, dilating large muscular arteries and bronchioles, decreasing gastrointestinal system activity, and mediating numerous other changes that prepare the body for aggressive or defensive action.[209] Sympathetic fibers follow blood vessels to all lymphoid organs and surround T-cells, many of which have receptors for norepinephrine. Norepinephrine has the effect of increasing the rate of T-cell differentiation, enabling a short-term response to a broad array of antigens. The rate of cell division, however, is decreased, compromising the long-term effectiveness of the response.[210]

Analogous to the distorting effect that a falling rock has on the entire body of water into which it falls is the effect of trauma on the entire human organism. Various researchers and clinicians have considered the living human body as a single metabolic field,[v] a matrix field[211] or a fluid field,[212] and have considered the effects of distortion on the field as a whole. In his later years, Nobel laureate Albert Szent-Györgyi stated, "Whenever we separate two things, we lose something, something which may have been the most essential feature."[213] To the physician trained in subtle manual sensing, distortions of the whole, when present, are manually perceptible and reveal essential organizational qualities of the entire organism.

The Patient with a History of Trauma

Obtaining the History

Obtaining the history of a stabilized, office-based patient has various components. One should consider the type of trauma and the mechanical forces involved, predisposing factors or antecedents, the duration or "age" of the trauma, and the patient's overall state of health and metabolic reserve.

[v] German embryologist E. Blechschmidt describes metabolic fields as "those morphologically definable regions, at all levels of spatial resolution, which contain spatially ordered metabolic movements." This he applies to cells, tissues, organs, and the whole organism at any stage of development. [Blechschmidt, E. *The Ontogenetic Basis of Human Anatomy.* Berkeley: North Atlantic Books, 2004, p22.].

Type of trauma. Patients who are seen in the office have often experienced trauma of the momentum-inertia type, wherein a moving body or object has impacted the patient's body, exemplified by an object falling on the head; or the moving patient has impacted a stationary object, as in hitting one's head on the overhead storage compartment of an airliner. Information regarding the direction and degree of force should be obtained. Knowledge of individual vectors of force is fundamental to the diagnosis of contrecoup injuries, whiplash, and complex impact injuries. Determination of resultant vectors can guide the discerning clinician to consider areas of occult or asymptomatic trauma and potential functional compromise. Traumas that are not of the momentum-inertia type involve a variety of forces that will be addressed in subsequent sections.

Common sources of trauma that may precipitate a patient's visit to the office, and that should be solicited as part of any new patient's history, include the following:

- Birth
- Motor vehicle, pedestrian, and bicycle accidents
- Falls, sports injuries, and blows to the head
- Dental and orthodontic procedures
- Surgical procedures and wounds
- Physical, sexual, and emotional abuse including domestic violence, child and elder abuse, abusive child-rearing practices, and exposure to abuse in the role of a witness
- Loss

In obtaining a birth history, one should ascertain the duration and mechanism of labor, whether cesarean section was necessary, and whether forceps or vacuum extraction was used.[214,215] Prolonged engagement in the maternal pelvis during a long and difficult labor subjects the infant cranium to considerable compressive force, potentially resulting in cranial nerve dysfunction or plagiocephaly.[216,217,218,219] Difficulty sucking, for example, is typically the result of hypoglossal nerve irritation, a condition which can be promptly corrected by the skillful application of a decompressive manual procedure.[220] In the event of cesarean section, presurgical engagement in the birth canal requiring forceful retraction into the uterus is a scenario which, in this author's experience, has been associated with neonatal torticollis. Since, among other things, maternal HPA axis activation is associated with intrauterine growth retardation,[221] the physical and emotional health of the mother during pregnancy and her attitude toward the pregnancy should be solicited. APGAR scores and knowledge of the quality, or robustness, of the first cry are additional meaningful indicators of anatomic and physiologic health or compromise.

Auto, pedestrian and bicycle accidents, sports injuries, and falls can potentially involve open or closed head injury, fractures, sprains, and strains. Consideration of vectors of force as well as distribution of force is particularly pertinent in this form of trauma.[222,223,224] Becker states,

> "In circumstances of trauma, thousands of cells have had their inertial patterns suddenly disturbed ... into new patterns that include force factors .... Thereafter, the central nervous system must include this new data in every voluntary and involuntary use of the local areas involved and in varying degrees throughout the entire body physiology .... This is in addition to the local injuries that have been endured by the body, which are usually the only thing treated by the physician."[225]

A history of participation in ice skating, gymnastics, horseback riding, or contact sports should automatically put the physician on the lookout for the effects of trauma. Fracture need not occur for falls, blows, and other momentum-inertia type injuries to be functionally significant. Intraosseous strain typically precedes, but does not always result in, fracture. In the experience of this author, the presence of strain—interosseous, intraosseous, and that involving soft tissue—can contribute to delayed healing and to pain that persists beyond apparent healing. It therefore behooves the physician to solicit the mechanical details of even those falls and accidents that the patient appends with the assuring comment that "nothing was broken."

Many dental procedures (for example, extractions and applications of prostheses) involve the use of compressive, distractive, or torsional force, and orthodontia relies on low-grade force sustained over time to accomplish its goals. Even in the most skilled professional hands, the use of some force is inevitable. The force of extraction, for instance, may be transmitted to the mandible, maxilla, or pre-maxilla from which a tooth is removed, and with the use of excess force or torsion, the force may extend to one of the many bones with which these three articulate, potentially affecting sinus, vestibular, and cranial nerve function, and precipitating cephalgia.[226] Having a potentially similar effect is the commonly used orthodontic palate expander, which, in decompressing the maxillary arch, inevitably transmits compression to other areas of the cranium.

Surgical procedures are inherently disruptive to anatomy and physiology. A clean surgical incision in a healthy patient should undergo healing by first intention with minimal loss of tissue. Nonetheless, collagenous scars are avascular and acellular and do represent an interruption in tissue continuity. Large wounds involving extensive loss of cells undergo healing by second intention, a process that involves a more intense inflammatory reaction and more extensive wound contraction than does healing by first intention. Predictably, this process sets the stage for more extensive scarring and fibrosis.[227]

Obtaining a history of abuse and the witnessing thereof requires sensitivity and an understanding that such history may be compensatorily suppressed, unavailable to the patient's consciousness, or literally lacking in verbal narrative.[228] A tempo of interviewing should be adopted that affords patients the opportunity to assess the intent and integrity of the clinician before being called upon to reveal sensitive personal information. Once the physician is entrusted with such information, it is imperative that referral, if necessary, be made with a clearly conveyed attitude of support and respect, lest patients feel abandoned in the wake of their disclosure. Often overlooked are those who witness abuse. Witnesses are, themselves, traumatized, being caught in the psychological conflict of affiliation with either the perpetrator or the victim.[229] Of diagnosing the psychological and behavioral aftermath of abusive trauma, Herman admonishes that,

> Concepts of personality organization developed under ordinary circumstances are applied to victims, without any understanding of the corrosion of personality that occurs under conditions of prolonged terror. Thus, patients who suffer from the complex aftereffects of chronic trauma still commonly risk being misdiagnosed as having personality disorders.[230]

Loss, in the context of trauma, is unique. Unlike other forms of trauma in which the integrity of the organism is disrupted by an added force, the integrity of the organism, in loss, is disrupted by virtue of absence. In this author's experience, patients have reported pain in the midepigastric area for a number of days following loss, perhaps harkening to the "severing of heartstrings." Others having lost a spouse or intimate partner have reported a feeling of "irregularity" or concavity on the side of their body next to which the loved one slept. Clinical observations correlate. In the clinical experience of the author and her colleagues, the fluid field in patients who have experienced physical or psychological attack is often perceived as being compressed or regressed toward the physiologic midline. By contrast, in loss, there may be an actual perceived absence in an aspect of the fluid field with a compensatory shift of the midline, giving physiologic corroboration to the affectionate aphorism "my other half."

Antecedents. It is incumbent upon the physician to endeavor to determine the etiology or background related to the patient's trauma. Trauma can be preceded and precipitated by cardiovascular and cerebrovascular events, neurological phenomena such as tumor and seizure, visual impairment, and alcohol intoxication. Trauma can result from inattention secondary to fatigue, anxiety, or preoccupation. Trauma can also be a potential consequence of occupation, lifestyle, and familial or interpersonal relationships. Determining and addressing with the patient those factors which are causal or predisposing to trauma is a valuable and sometimes critical contribution of the clinician.

Long-term Consequences of Unresolved Trauma

The persistent effects of unresolved trauma manifest through a variety of mechanisms which operate locally, intersystemically, and within the patient as a whole.

Compensatory structural changes. Asymmetric falls on the buttocks, one-legged falls in holes, and forced "splits" in dance classes can dramatically shift the plane of orientation of both the body of the sacrum and the sacral base. Compensatory structural changes in the form of scoliosis can be the result.

Fibrosis. Trauma that is incisive or disruptive to tissues leads to fibrosis, the extent of which is affected in part by the efficiency of drainage of inflammatory exudate by the lymphatics in the post-traumatic period.[231] Fibrotic tissue interrupts the integrity and function of the tissues it transects, and limits the range or freedom of motion of the tissues involved. Functional impairment and discomfort, as exemplified by adhesive capsulitis and post-surgical, intra-abdominal adhesions, can ensue.

Facilitation. Spinal facilitation, a state of sensitization of the interneuronal pool, occurs as a result of prolonged or excessive stimulation of primary afferent nociceptors, as well as from direct neuronal injury or inhibitory interneuron death, and is a mechanism underlying chronic pain.[232] Maintained in a state of constant partial or subthreshold excitation, and responsive to subnormal levels of input from peripheral and autonomic PANs, facilitated levels of the spinal cord are easily stimulated. Once stimulated, signals are sent to the locus coeruleus, which invokes the locus coeruleus-norepinephrine-HPA axis and results in increased sympathetic tone and cortisol output.

Under conditions of facilitation, norepinephrine, released from the locus coeruleus in response to input from a facilitated level of the spinal cord, stimulates the hypothalamus, overpowering the normal downregulatory effect of cortisol.[233] This results in unmitigated stimulation of the hypothalamus which leads to its sustained release of norepinephrine and CRH and the consequent increase in both sympathetic tone and adrenal elaboration of cortisol.

Peripherally, the effects of facilitation may be identified by the presence of tissue texture changes, hyperalgesia, altered ease or range of motion, and anatomic asymmetry of the affected region—a constellation of findings referred to in osteopathic literature as somatic dysfunction.[234] Although a facilitated level of the cord may interact with higher centers as previously described, the facilitated reflex arc can also operate independently of higher input. Resolution of the somatic dysfunction associated with facilitation, which can be accomplished manually, allows normalization of somatic afferent input, and, barring persistent visceral input, enables normalization of HPA and autonomic function.[235]

Viscerosomatic and somatovisceral reflexes. In addition to potentially subjecting the patient to sympathetic and HPA overdrive, facilitation also predisposes the body to the establishment of viscerosomatic and somatovisceral reflexes. Facilitation of an interneuronal pool affects outflow to both visceral and somatic structures innervated by the facilitated level of the cord.[236] Thereby, facilitation that was originally established in response to persistent inflammation or mechanical irritation from an unresolved visceral trauma can, via somatic efferents, affect the skeletal muscle innervated by the same spinal level. Conversely, facilitation secondary to unresolved musculoskeletal injury can result in chronic increased autonomic stimulation of segmentally related viscera.

Allostatic load. The cumulative, long-term effect or toll taken on the body by frequent, repetitive activation of the autonomic nervous system, HPA axis, and cardiovascular, metabolic, and immune systems, or by their persistent low-grade activation to a chronically elevated baseline, is termed allostatic load.[vi,237,238] (This concept is also discussed in the preceding essay on psychosocial influences on health.) In the present discussion, it was established that somatic and visceral trauma, psychological trauma, chronic pain, inflammation, and facilitation all serve to activate the locus coeruleus-norepinephrine-HPA axis. Unresolved trauma clearly places a significant demand on the body and, over time, is a major contributor to the development of allostatic load.

The effects of allostatic load established to date are multiple. In a study involving 1,189 men and women, aged 70–79 years at outset, participants were assessed with respect to allostatic load, cognitive functioning, and physical functioning.[239] Participants with highest allostatic load scores performed most poorly with respect to cognitive and physical functioning and, on eight-year follow-up, higher baseline allostatic load scores predicted greatest loss in cognitive and physical functioning.[240] Related to an aspect of cognitive functioning is the hippocampus, which is involved in verbal and contextual memory. The hippocampus is rich in cortisol receptors, and normally participates in a feedback loop controlling release of CRH from the hypothalamus.[241,242] Persistently elevated levels of cortisol are toxic to hippocampal neurons, and lead to neuronal atrophy or death and loss of memory.[243,244]

Prolonged HPA axis activation in infancy and childhood takes its toll, inhibiting the production of growth hormone and somatomedin C.[245] This contributes to the condition of "failure to thrive," in which caloric intake does not promote weight gain. Early loss of a parent (due primarily to parental separation) and physical and sexual abuse during childhood both carry an increased risk of major depression during adulthood.[246] A history of major depression is among the strongest predictors of cardiovascular risk, depression being associated with increased resting heart rate, decreased heart rate variability, and increased plasma norepinephrine.[247] Chronic elevation of cortisol inhibits bone formation,

---

[vi] Based on the word allostasis, which is akin to the term homeodynamics. The term refers to the coordinated, broad intersystemic (particularly neuroendocrine immune) range of variability that enables the body to maintain stability in the face of protracted challenge. This is distinguished from homeostasis, which maintains discrete, physiologic parameters such as pH and electrolyte balance within a more finite operating range. (The principles of dynamic balance and homeostasis are discussed in Chapter 9.)

and women with a history of depressive illness have a greater frequency of decreased bone mineral density.[248]

Childhood abuse additionally predisposes to adult anxiety disorders, panic disorder, attempted suicide, post-traumatic stress disorder (PTSD), and likelihood of developing PTSD[vii] in response to other traumas.[249] Sensitization or hyperactivity of CRH circuits secondary to stress early in development is hypothesized to explain the psychological sequelae.[250] Females who experience PTSD from childhood sexual abuse demonstrate daily elevation of norepinephrine, epinephrine, dopamine and cortisol levels, and have a tendency toward obesity.[251] Abused females additionally have an increased rate of premenstrual syndrome, asthma, spastic colitis, and dysmenorrhea.[252] Male veterans, by comparison, who developed PTSD in combat, demonstrate an elevated norepinephrine-to-cortisol ratio, and an increased incidence of cardiovascular disease, gastrointestinal symptoms, chronic pain, and rheumatism.[253]

Chronically elevated cortisol and catecholamine levels lead to immunosuppression and decreased cellular immunity, which, in turn, leads to increased severity of the common cold and increased titers of cold-virus antibody.[254] Elevated cortisol also promotes insulin resistance.[255] This results in increased output of insulin, which has been shown to be excitatory to the sympathetic nervous system.[256] (For discussion of the inflammatory effects of increased insulin output, see Chapter 30.)

Chronic sympathetic hyperactivity elevates blood pressure and increases cardiac workload, thereby contributing to endothelial dysfunction, coronary spasm, left ventricular (LV) hypertrophy, and serious dysrhythmias. Persistently elevated blood pressure accelerates atherosclerosis, which increases the risk of myocardial infarction.[257] When coexistent with LV dysfunction, increased sympathetic tone is the most sensitive predictor of cardiac and arrhythmic mortality.[258] Increased sympathetic tone impedes development of collateral circulation following arterial occlusion.[259]

Supporting the Patient's Health

Details of treatment are not within the purview of this chapter, and clinicians of varying backgrounds will approach treatment differently. However, common goals of treatment and principles to apply in planning treatment will likely apply to most clinicians and should be addressed.

Promoting efficient exchange of all the fluids of the body is of fundamental importance. Healing is supported and adverse inflammatory and degenerative effects are averted by efficient fluid exchange. Nutrients, both endogenous and exogenous, are delivered and wastes are removed via the fluids of the body. Nutrients will not arrive at their desired destination if the destination or its access routes are in a state of stasis. Similarly, waste products and inflammatory exudates will not be removed if the routes of egress are not open and functioning.

Also fundamental to the resolution of trauma is the downregulation of afferent input. Attenuation of facilitation and elimination of the sources of nociceptive stimulation can contribute significantly to normalization by reducing input to the SNS and HPA axis. In this author's experience, this can often be accomplished by manually engaging and augmenting the corrective and generative physiologic processes that are operant in the patient's body. Ultimately, it must be acknowledged that the physician is an assistant, and the capacity for healing is inherent to the patient.

Case Studies

The following cases from the author's experience are offered in abbreviated form to illustrate potential and uncommonly considered consequences of trauma.

Case 1. Concussion and macroscopic distortion. During the winter of my freshman year in osteopathic school, one of my classmates fell on the ice, landing hard on his back and hitting the back of his head. His glasses went flying. When he retrieved them, they fit poorly, and he presumed they had been bent in the fall. In the following hours, he experienced headache, difficulty focusing, unsteadiness on his feet, and "did not feel like himself." Later that day he reported his symptoms to one of his clinical professors who, on examination, found evidence of the impact, and administered an osteopathic treatment aimed at reestablishing structural balance. Following the treatment, my classmate "felt like himself," and when he donned his glasses, they fit perfectly, indicating that it was not his glasses that had been warped, but his head. This illustrated to those of us present the capacity of the living cranium to

[vii] PTSD is characterized by hyperarousal, intrusion (vivid flashbacks and nightmares of the traumatic event), and constriction (anesthesia, detachment, passivity). [Reference 227, p35.]

deform on impact. We were left by the professor, as I will leave the reader, to consider the potential consequences of sudden distortion, or "warping," of the human cranium on such phenomena as extraocular muscle function, vestibular function, occlusion, venous sinus drainage, cranial nerve function, etc.

Case 2. Hyperthyroidism. Prior to arriving at my office, this 34-year-old mother of five was anticipating an ablative procedure for symptoms of hyperthyroidism of sudden onset two months earlier. Her history revealed that prior to, and within the same month of, her symptoms' onset she had fallen head over heels down a flight of stairs with her six-month-old daughter in her arms. On exam, her pulse was 110, speech was rapid and voice high-pitched, thyroid was palpably enlarged and she had lost 15 pounds. She complained of headache, feeling hot, "rubber legs," dyspnea, and dysarthria. Potentially relevant findings included sternoclavicular and acromioclavicular compression, upper left costovertebral compression, segmental cervical restriction and paracervical hypertonicity, occipito-temporal compression, and positional asymmetry of the temporals. Manual osteopathic treatment was administered to restore ease and function to the involved area. On follow-up four days later, the patient reported no recurrence of dyspnea, no "rubber legs," fewer headaches and improved energy; pulse was 90. Over the following weeks her condition improved and resolved.

Clinical Pearls

1. Attend to areas *where forces accumulate*, e.g., a fall on an outstretched hand may give rise to upper arm or shoulder symptoms if compressive forces are not resolved.
2. When a patient requires a boot-type cast, attempt to match its height in the other shoe. This will help to avoid low back pain and the initiation of scoliotic mechanics.
3. In managing fractures, treatment *prior* to casting aimed at decreasing or eliminating strain in interosseous, intraosseous, and soft tissues can potentially reduce the development of pain and dependent edema.
4. Solicit a history of trauma from every new patient, and consider trauma as an etiologic or contributing factor in illnesses of unknown or "idiopathic" etiology. Symptoms not typically associated with trauma may, in fact, have a traumatic etiology.

Summary

Trauma is one of many challenges presented to our patients. Its proper identification and thorough resolution can have effects that reach beyond the individual. When unresolved, trauma can dampen and defeat the human spirit. However, when resolved, trauma has the potential to impart understanding and can augment the human capacity for compassion.

Xenobiotics

John Cline, MD

Introduction

The building blocks of health include both harmful and beneficial influences upon human biology and individual genetic and biochemical uniqueness. One of the harmful environmental inputs that clinicians must pay increasing attention to is xenobiotic exposure. The word xenobiotic is defined as "a chemical substance that is foreign, and usually harmful, to living organisms."[260] Xenobiotics are also known as persistent organic pollutants (POPs), which are carbon-containing chemicals that have been introduced into the environment in ever-increasing numbers. In fact, it has been estimated that there have been over 80,000 of these chemicals introduced into the environment since World War II.[261] There is a growing body of scientific evidence documenting serious health problems that arise secondary to the exposure and accumulation of POPs in humans.[262] There are few environmental issues that have aroused more public concern than the harmful effects of POPs in the general population, especially when it concerns the health and welfare of children. Despite the volume of scientific literature published, this subject remains controversial as there are huge financial issues at stake.

History

It is interesting to note that pesticides as we know them today did not exist before World War II. Organophosphate pesticides were developed as nerve gases, and the phenoxyherbicides such as 2,4-D were designed to destroy the Japanese rice crops (with later use as a component of Agent Orange, a substance used to defoliate large areas in jungle warfare).[263] Following World

War II, these chemicals were put to use in many applications, including agricultural production, spraying of neighborhoods for mosquito eradication, and home and garden use. In the 1950s and onward, epidemiologists became concerned about the health effects of exposure to POPs. Initially, studies of wildlife communities demonstrated reproductive, developmental, endocrine, immunologic, and carcinogenic effects.[264,265,266] There were high rates of malformed genitalia, aberrant mating behavior, sterility, cancer, and immune system and thyroid dysfunction. United States epidemiologists began to notice a rise in the incidence of non-Hodgkin's lymphoma (NHL), observing that these cases were clustered in agricultural areas. This phenomenon paralleled pesticide use, causing some researchers to postulate that there was a causal link.

In 1962, Rachel Carson's book, *Silent Spring*, was truly revolutionary in bringing this issue into political and public awareness.[267] It was followed in 1996 by *Our Stolen Future*, which documented the health effects of these endocrine-disrupting chemicals.[268] In 1996, a number of governments participated in the Intergovernmental Forum on Chemical Safety and agreed upon a list of 12 POPs to be eliminated from the environment. These 12 have been dubbed "The Dirty Dozen." In 2001, the United Nations Environment Program sponsored The Binding Convention on Persistent Organic Pollutants held in Stockholm, Sweden, and there was a call for an immediate ban on 11 of the Dirty Dozen. The list of these dozen POPs and their sources are found in Table 13.1. It should be noted that DDT was still allowed to be used in developing countries to control mosquitoes in malaria prevention.

Properties of POPs

POPs are persistent because they resist photolytic, biological, and chemical degradation. They can take as long as one century to biodegrade.[269] They are carbon containing and hence organic. They are lipophilic pollutants accumulating in the fatty tissues of organisms. Furthermore, they bioaccumulate up the food chain leaving those at the top with high concentrations in their tissues. Most of the POPs are semivolatile which allows them to travel thousands of miles in the air before they settle.[270] An example of this is the Inuit of Nunavik in northern Canada. These aboriginal people consume the fat of seals, beluga and narwhal whales. These people have been found to have high body burdens of POPs.[271]

Health Effects of POPs

The available epidemiological evidence suggests that the health effects of POPs in humans are similar to those in animals in the same range of exposures. Human studies have demonstrated negative effects of POPs on neurodevelopmental, thyroid, estrogen, and immune function.[272,273,274,275] Exposures to all of the commonly used pesticides, such as phenoxyherbicides, organophosphates, carbamates, and pyrethrins, have shown positive associations with adverse health effects. Furthermore, the carcinogenic effects of certain POPs have been well demonstrated. Triazine herbicides increase breast cancer risk; carbamate and phenoxyherbicides increase lung cancer risk; use of indoor insecticides is associated with brain cancer and lymphocytic leukemia in children.[276]

In pregnant women, higher levels of polychlorinated biphenyls (PCBs) have been shown to adversely affect the brain development of their children. The affected children were initially found to have decreased visual recognition scores,[277] followed by decreased performance on short-term memory testing.[278] By age 11, these children were found to have lower average IQ scores and were delayed in reading comprehension.[279] Furthermore, there was evidence of altered gender-typical play behavior, with less masculinized play in boys and more in girls.[280] There was also decreased ability to control inappropriate responses, as is found in children with attention deficit hyperactivity disorder.[281]

There is also growing concern about the impact of flame retardants on human health. There are 175 types of flame retardants and the brominated flame retardants (BFRs) make up the majority. Tetrabromobisphenol A is the most widely used BFR. *In vitro* studies have demonstrated that it is hepatotoxic, immunotoxic, and neurotoxic. As well, it acts as an endocrine disruptor with estrogen-like properties. The primary toxic effect is as a disruptor of thyroid homeostasis.[282] Furthermore, the level of polybrominated diphenyl ethers (PBDEs, another type of flame retardant) is rising in humans, as

Table 13.1 **Environmental and Dietary Sources of Persistent Organic Pollutants (the "Dirty Dozen")**

Type	Environmental Sources	Examples of Dietary Sources
Dioxins, furans	Byproducts of petrochemical industry and chlorine bleaching in pulp and paper mills; hospital and municipal incinerators	Meat, poultry, and dairy products; sport fish (e.g., lake trout, salmon, walleye); wildlife (e.g., waterfowl and waterfowl eggs, muskrat, otter, moose, deer)
PCBs	"Fire resistant" synthetic products made before 1977, old electrical equipment, leaky containers in PCB disposal sites	Great Lakes fish (e.g., lake trout, salmon), Arctic marine mammals, breast milk
Aldrin	Pesticide used against insects in the soil to protect crops such as corn and potatoes	Dairy products, meat, fish, oils and fats, potatoes, root vegetables
Chlordane	Broad-spectrum contact insecticide used on vegetables, grains, maize, oilseed, potatoes, sugar cane, beets, fruits, nuts, cotton, and jute	Use has been severely restricted, so food does not appear to be a major pathway of exposure now; air may be a pathway because of continued use in termite control (in the United States)
DDT	Pesticide widely used during World War II to protect soldiers and civilians against diseases spread by insects	Fish, dairy products, fat of cattle, hogs, poultry and sheep, eggs, vegetables, breast milk
Dieldrin	Insecticide used to control insects in soil	Same as for aldrin
Endrin	Foliar (leaf) insecticide used on field crops such as cotton	Current dietary exposure thought to be minimal because of restricted use
Heptachlor	Nonsystemic stomach and contact insecticide used to control insects in soil	Detected in the blood of U.S. and Australian cattle in 1990; current dietary exposure thought to be minimal because of restricted use
HCB	Fungicide used for seed treatment	HCB-treated grain; current dietary exposure thought to be very low because of severely restricted use
Mirex	Stomach insecticide used to control ants, termites, and mealy bugs	Meat, fish, wild game, marine bird eggs, sea mammals
Toxaphene	Contact insecticide used primarily on cotton, cereal, grains, fruits, nuts, and vegetables and used to control ticks and mites in livestock	Dietary exposure thought to be very low because of restricted use; however, there is a local problem with some fish in Lake Superior

Legend:
PCBs = polychlorinated biphenyls
DDT = dichlorodiphenyltrichloroethane
HCB = hexachlorobenzene

Source: Contaminant profiles. In: *Health and the Environment. The Health and Environment Handbook for Health Professionals.* Ottawa: Health Canada; 1998. Cat no H46-2/98-2111. Available: www.hcsc.gc.ca/ehp/ehd/catalogue/bch_pubs/98ehd211/98ehd211.htm

recently demonstrated in a study of people living in the remote Faroe Islands. The concentration of PBDEs in human breast milk rose three fold between 1987 and 1999.[283] Breastfed Faroese children were also found to be 0.59 kg lighter and 1.5 cm shorter than non-breastfed children. The transfer through the breast milk of the contaminants methylmercury and PCBs fully explained the attenuated growth parameters.[284]

Recommendations and Summary

One of the most comprehensive reviews of the subject of xenobiotics is the document, *Systematic Review of Pesticide Human Health Effects*.[285] The conclusions are as follows:

- The scientific literature does not support the concept that some pesticides are safer than others.
- Reducing exposure is the best advice. Given the wide range of commonly used home and garden products associated with adverse health effects, the focus should be on reduction of exposure to all pesticides.

Furthermore, low-dose exposure is not necessarily safe exposure; "no evidence of harm" is not equivalent to "evidence of no harm." We are currently able to characterize the risks for only a small number of the 80,000+ POPs that have been released into our environment. There are incalculable combinations of chemicals, environmental breakdown molecules, and metabolites that need to be evaluated for safety in humans. Unfortunately, we presently have a knowledge void, and the phrase "no evidence of harmful effects" can hide the greater truth that there is simply no evidence at all.[286]

Each one of us needs to avoid exposure to POPs as much as possible and have intact and healthy detoxification systems. For the clinician, it is imperative to help patients understand this diffuse, but increasingly heavy burden our bodies are being asked to handle because it is one of the environmental inputs that has significant effects upon health. Further discussion of the clinical implications of the toxic burden, including detoxification (its processes and applications) and polymorphisms that can predispose to more significant problems, can be found in Chapter 22 and Chapter 31.

Microorganisms

Patrick Hanaway, MD

A mighty creature is the germ,
Though smaller than the pachyderm,
His strange delight he often pleases,
By giving people strange diseases.
—Ogden Nash

Introduction

Microorganisms include viruses, bacteria, fungi, protozoa, algae, and nematodes, roughly in increasing order of size. They are the oldest form of life on earth and are found virtually everywhere. Bacteria have been present on earth for more than 2.5 billion years. The combined weight of all microbial life is thought to be about 25 times more than all animal life combined.[287] Thus, humans have evolved fully in the presence of bacteria. Not only are we not alone, but we are required to live in mutual balance with this vast array of microorganisms. This relationship can be defined as symbiotic (at least one partner profits without hurting the other), commensal (partners that coexist without detriment but without obvious benefit), and pathogenic (in which there is damage to the host).

The critical interface between the human body and its internal and external environments manifests itself on many levels: the food we eat, the air we breathe, and the lifestyle we choose are all "environmental inputs" that influence our genetic material continuously. The interaction between the body (through the epidermal, respiratory, oropharyngeal, and gastrointestinal interfaces) and the myriad microbes in the environment provides benefits to both parties.

The biologic terrain where humans and microorganisms interact must remain in homeostatic balance to provide the correct milieu for the body to function optimally. In this model, bacteria and other microorganisms are not usually considered dangerous, invasive, and pathogenic. Pathogenicity among microorganisms is the exception, not the rule. Considering the huge population of bacteria and viruses in our environment and in our own bodies, it is a relatively rare occurrence that these typically symbiotic relationships become harmful. Rather, imbalanced microbial growth may be indicative of an alteration in the biologic terrain.

The symbiotic organisms living in and on us have more than 100 times the amount of genetic material that the entire human genome has.[288] The Human Genome Project tells us that at least 223 human proteins have significant homology with bacterial proteins, suggesting direct horizontal transfer from bacterial genes.[289] While the age of antibiotics has led us to focus on microbes (and bacteria in particular) as pathogens, an understanding of the co-evolution of humans and microorganisms is critical for our health and well-being.

Discussions on this point date back to ancient medical systems, but the most well-known debate on this matter was between Pasteur and Béchamp. Pasteur postulated that 'germs' were the primary cause of illness, while Béchamp argued that the 'inner terrain' was the most important factor.[290] Noted 19th century pathologist Rudolph Virchow is reported to have said, "mosquitoes seek the stagnant water, but do not cause the pool to become stagnant."[291]

Microorganisms are ubiquitous and nowhere is this more important than the critical role of the large and dynamic bacterial community present within the gastrointestinal tract. Evidence demonstrates that bacteria have co-evolved to support digestion, absorption, metabolism, and development of the immune system. Disruption of this mutual balance between the physical body and these commensal microorganisms leads to both acute and chronic disease.

Commensal Flora in the Gastrointestinal Tract

At birth, the human body is sterile. Colonization of the skin epithelia and the mucosal membranes starts immediately after birth and evolves quickly over the first days of life.[292] Many species have evolved to peacefully co-exist within the gastrointestinal tract. These species play a critical role in the dynamic education of the adaptive immune system, promoting balance and strength in the under-developed immune system.

More than a century ago, the Russian scientist Eli Metchnikov discussed the clinical importance of gastrointestinal flora. He promoted the health benefits of taking live bacterial cultures as a means of supporting the colonic microflora. Research on microbial ecology has grown rapidly since the early 1990s, particularly because of the inherent role of the gastrointestinal flora in the development of the immune system. It appears that our co-evolutionary relationship with these organisms is used as a primer for regulation of the immune system.

Colonization of gut flora begins immediately after birth and is nearly complete after the first week of life, but quantity and species vary markedly over the first six months of life.[293] More than 500 species have been noted, each with numerous strains identified by molecular probes.[294] Overall, the number of bacteria present in the gastrointestinal lumen is 10-fold greater than the number of cells in the human body,[295] with more than 100 times the human genome's DNA content.[296] Studies demonstrate that bacteria differentially colonize the neonatal and infant gastrointestinal tract based upon a number of environmental factors, including the mode of delivery (Cesarean section or vaginal delivery),[297] hygiene measures, environmental contaminants, maternal flora, age at birth, and type of feeding.[298]

Nutritional inputs from breastfeeding, bottle feeding, and introduction of solid food provide the initial substrate for growth of varying species of bacteria within the gut.[299] Other environmental factors, including more aggressive standards of hygiene, have led to a delayed development pattern and even an absence of certain groups of bacteria in the commensal flora of neonates.[300]

Hygiene Hypothesis

In 1989, Strachan[301] coined the term "hygiene hypothesis." As stated, the theory is that increased prevalence of allergy and atopic illness in industrialized countries is a result of the decrease in exposure to common infections during early life, secondary to smaller family size. A number of studies have confirmed this relationship, but there is no direct evidence for a protective role of infections. Many have attempted to extend this hypothesis, based upon epidemiologic evidence, to include the role of antibiotics, vaccines, and anti-microbial soaps, but their effects have not been proved.[302] Immunologically plausible explanations have been demonstrated.[303] Current research focuses on the role of nutrition, timing, and gut flora maturation on immunologic development.[304]

Breastfeeding has been recognized to have an important role in the nutrition of the infant. Nutritive and immunologic components of breast milk have been studied for years, but the effects of essential fatty acids and oligosaccharides as stimulants for commensal flora are now better understood. From an evolutionary perspective, the gut has been finely tuned to develop based upon the dietary presence of breast milk over the first 1–3 years of life. The immunoregulatory role of breast milk and infant nutrition has come to the fore.[305]

Colonization of Gastrointestinal Flora

There is a significant alteration in the gut flora of the neonate over the first week of life, depending upon the food source. Classically, we see the introduction of E. coli and strep species during the first few days of life, giving way to bifidobacteria, bacteroides, and clostridium. Breast-fed infants then develop a predominance of bifidobacteria, first noted by Tissier in 1905.[306] Bottle-fed infants show a more diverse pattern of colonization.[307] A number of internal and external factors influence the adherence and succession of microbes within the gastrointestinal tract, including feeding habits,[308] hygiene,[309] stress,[310] antibiotics,[311] bacteria-host communication, and gene expression.[312]

Many species have evolved to peacefully co-exist within the gastrointestinal tract. With more than 500 species identified and more than 100 trillion bacteria "in residence," the necessity of a mutually beneficial relationship is clear. While the sub-species and quantities of bacteria will vary over time, the families and species of commensal flora remain relatively constant within an individual over the course of a lifetime. The gastrointestinal microflora can, however, be modified by diet and environmental factors, and those changes can significantly affect health.

Humans and bacteria have co-evolved to offer mutual benefit. The positive health effects of these bacteria include: energy salvage from carbohydrate fermentation, synthesis of B and K vitamins, production of short-chain fatty acids (SCFAs) such as n-butyrate to act as metabolic substrate for colonocytes, lowering pH, producing anti-microbial compounds, and stimulating the immune system.[313]

Nearly 70% of the human immune system is localized in the digestive tract. The mucosal surface of the gastrointestinal tract would cover the area of a doubles tennis court (if stretched out flat), and is approximately 200x the surface area of the skin. Defense against microbes is mediated by the early reactions of innate immunity, followed by the reaction of adaptive immunity. Innate immunity includes the skin, mucosal epithelia, cytokines, and phagocytes. These non-specific defense mechanisms provide defense against common pathogens, but the innate immune response *stimulates* the adaptive immune system and influences the nature of the adaptive response.[314] The process of "oral tolerance" is an important example of this.[315] The semi-permeable gastrointestinal epithelium identifies and responds to pathogens, while minimizing the immune reaction to food antigens and commensal flora.

Through the process of co-evolution, the body has mastered a number of methods to identify microbes and develop the adaptive immune system, based upon the proper timing and presence of the bacterial stimuli. The body responds differentially to bacterial stimuli and responds to a variety of structural components on each bacterium. Recent evidence demonstrates that immunostimulatory DNA[316] may derive from the copious amounts of bacterial DNA present in the gastrointestinal tract. The epithelial mucosa is equipped with pattern recognition receptors (PRRs) that recognize bacterial DNA from commensal bacteria and modulate immune function.[317]

Thus, our immune system is dynamically educated by the presence of commensal, symbiotic, and pathogenic bacteria at the interface of the intestinal epithelium. The gut flora interacts with our innate immunity and influences the adaptive immune response in an important dialogue between our immune system and the environment. Commensal bacteria are also able to modulate expression of host genes involved in important intestinal functions, including nutrient absorption, mucosal stimulation, xenobiotic metabolism, and intestinal maturation.[318] Understanding the "cross-talk" between bacteria and the immune system helps us better understand the relative continuum between pathogenic and non-pathogenic relationships.

Altered Balance in the Human Micro-Organism Environment

Hooper and Gordon[319] have highlighted the effects of imbalance within this complex ecosystem. The increasing prevalence of allergy and atopy are associated with alterations of intestinal colonization and decreased tolerance to common food proteins and inhaled allergens. Treatment with probiotics can help to shift these symptoms back to normal.[320] The pathogenesis of inflammatory bowel disease (IBD), a condition that is becoming substantially more common, appears to involve an abnormal activation of the immune system. IBD results from an inappropriate and exaggerated mucosal immune response to normal constituents of the mucosal microflora. Host genetic background may determine the susceptibility to intestinal inflammation and normal mucosal microflora appears to maintain the inflammatory process.[321]

Overall, we see that these critical gene-environment interactions highlight immunologic dysregulation arising from the combination of varied bacterial species (commensal and pathogenic), altered adaptive immune system activation, and multiple antigenic stimuli. It appears that diet (as prebiotics and antigens) plays an important role with each of these factors.

Summary

From an evolutionary perspective, our genome has not changed over the past 50 years, but the incidence of chronic disease has become epidemic. Playing a vital role in the development of chronic diseases are the changes in our diet and various other environmental factors (see, for example, the discussion on Diet and Nutrients at the head of this chapter) that no longer provide the proper milieu for the gastrointestinal tract to properly activate the immune system. Our genetic predispositions have not prepared us to successfully manage the current lifestyle, dietary, and environmental patterns we face today. We must work to balance each of these inputs to re-align our immune systems for optimal function. As we explore the foundations of normal physiology, we must develop new therapeutic strategies to re-establish a proper relationship with our "old friends," because microorganisms are one of the key environmental inputs to health.

Radiation

Carol R. McMakin, MA, DC

Introduction

To understand the effects of environmental radiation exposure on the human system, it is important to understand that, from a biophysics perspective, the human body is an electromagnetic semiconductor matrix that allows for instantaneous communication among all cells and tissues in the system. Every physiologic process and biochemical reaction takes place in this semiconductor matrix. Every cell in the body is filled with a cytoplasmic matrix or cytoskeleton that is connected by integrins across the cell surface to every other cell surface and membrane in the body. The enzymes that create every physiologic function do not float in an intracellular soup; they are attached to the cytoplasmic matrix and perform their chemistry in a solid state context created by this intracellular structure. Water molecules line the matrix forming a system that functions as a semiconductor, sharing electrons and allowing the transmission of energy and information throughout the system.[322]

Understanding this model becomes important when considering the influences that create damage or constitute a threat to the health of the system, as well as those that may have the potential to heal.

Ionizing Radiation

The health risks of environmental x-ray exposure are well documented and easy to understand. Ionizing radioactive energy (x-rays) includes a spectrum of high-energy unseen particles that move through the cell, creating physical damage to intracellular structures. DNA seems particularly sensitive to such damage, and different organs may have different responses to exposure.[323] X-rays are useful for medical imaging because the bone and more dense body structures absorb x-rays that pass through less dense structures. The x-rays that pass through the softer tissues create the images on film that we see as diagnostic x-rays. The damaging intracellular effects of x-rays are used therapeutically in cancer treatment to destroy the DNA of malignant cells. Environmental exposure to x-rays includes the ionizing radiation produced by the sun and exposure to altitudes at which the atmospheric protection against x-ray exposure is reduced (e.g., during activities such as mountain climbing and air travel). Radon gas and natural radioactivity found in certain types of rock and brick create residential exposure risk.

Ionizing radiation is a potent carcinogen and injures living cells by damaging the DNA. X-rays create some direct damage to the DNA by splitting bonds, but most of the damage is indirectly generated by free radicals that create intracellular injury and DNA damage. Hydroxyl radicals (OH) are considered to be the most damaging of all free radicals and are created by splitting the water molecules that line the intracellular and extracellular matrix.

Immune system cells seem particularly vulnerable, as do bone marrow cells.[324] Exposure to x-rays increases the risk of breast, colon, lung and ovarian cancer, basal cell carcinoma, and leukemia. Radiation exposure reduces the level of both vitamin E and vitamin C in bone marrow.[325] The reduction may be either a direct or an indirect effect, as these vitamins are used to counteract the free radicals produced by the x-ray exposure.

Protecting the Patient

How can the clinician help patients to protect themselves from the effects of exposure to ionizing radiation? There is evidence to suggest that antioxidants and other natural substances are protective against the damaging effects of ionizing radiation.

Beta carotene: Serum concentrations of oxidized conjugated dienes (an index of lipid peroxidation) were significantly increased in children who were exposed to high levels of irradiation, as compared to children in low radiation areas, following the Chernobyl (nuclear reactor) disaster in Russia. Supplementation with natural beta carotene 40 mg per day for three months resulted in a significant decrease in serum conjugated diene levels after one and three months.[326]

Lycopene: An animal study using mice demonstrated the ability of lycopene to protect against the detrimental effects of radioactivity exposure. This protection was double that of beta carotene. This effect is likely attributable to lycopene's antioxidant properties.[327]

Lipoic acid: This study involved radiation victims in Chernobyl, Russia (the site of a nuclear reactor accident). Lipoic acid reduced free radical damage caused by radiation exposure. One group of 16 children given 400 mg of lipoic acid daily for 28 days showed significant reductions in both white blood cell free radical activity and urinary excretion of radioactive isotopes, compared to a control group of 12 children.[328]

Vitamin E: A second group of 14 children given 400 mg lipoic acid plus 200 mg vitamin E daily for 28 days showed an even greater reduction in urinary excretion as compared to both the lipoic acid and control groups.

Vitamin C improves the ability of the body to resist the toxic effects of exposure to radioactivity. Guinea pigs that were supplemented with large dosages of vitamin C (10 gram equivalent) combined with bioflavonoids were able to withstand twice the known lethal dosages of radioactivity.[329]

Cabbage, broccoli: Cabbage and broccoli were protective in reducing radiation damage and mortality from radiation exposure in animal studies. Guinea pigs exposed to whole-body x-radiation demonstrated a lower death rate and bleeding incidence when they were pre-fed on cabbage prior to receiving x-ray exposure.[330]

Ginkgo biloba: When *Ginkgo biloba* was administered to Chernobyl recovery workers, it protected them from further chromosomal damage.[331]

Melatonin is an antioxidant that protects DNA, lipids, and proteins from free-radical damage. It works by stimulating the activities of antioxidant enzymes and scavenging free radicals directly or indirectly. Among known antioxidants, melatonin is a highly effective scavenger of (OH), hydroxyl free radicals. Melatonin is distributed widely in organisms and in all cellular compartments, and it quickly passes through all biological membranes. Lymphocytes that were pre-treated with melatonin exhibited a significant and concentration-dependent decrease in the frequency of radiation-induced chromosome damage, as compared with irradiated cells that did not receive the pre-treatment.[332]

Siberian and Korean ginseng doubled the life span of rats exposed to prolonged x-rays at a total dose of 1,620 to 7,000 rads.[333]

Nonionizing Radiation

The risks of nonionizing radiation exposure are less clearly documented. The controversy arising from Robert Becker's research in the 1980s (and his books, *The Body Electric*[334] and *Cross Currents*[335]) still reverberates through the research community. Becker stated that the ever-increasing spectra of electromagnetic exposure—"electro-pollution," including FM radio waves, microwaves, and other electromagnetic fields to which humans are being exposed—create biological effects. Animal studies show chronic stress responses in animals exposed to increased levels of electromagnetic fields (EMF), demonstrated by increased body weight and alterations in neuroendocrine function. (Becker claimed that the Department of Defense interfered with research funding aimed at finding any detrimental effects from radio waves or electromagnetic fields. The military uses these EMF bands for communication and tracking.)

The commercial, legal, and financial consequences of any documented link between electromagnetic exposure and cancer are enormous. It is no wonder that researchers (such as Becker) who discover such links find themselves attacked in the public and even in the scientific press.

Robert P. Liburdy published a number of papers between 1984 and 1993 documenting the effects of electromagnetic fields on cells. In 1984 he found that radiofrequency radiation affects the immune system by altering human immunoglobulin on T and B lymphocytes. The effect takes place at power levels below the current OSHA recommended safety limit of 0.4 WKg^{-1}.[336,337]

He published several papers documenting the effects of 12 mg, 60Hz fields, such as those found in the home and workplace, on breast cancer cells. Both tamoxifen and melatonin inhibit the growth of cultured human breast cancer cells. He found that the 12 mg, 60Hz field blocked melatonin's natural oncostatic action on estrogen positive MCF-7 human breast cancer cells grown in cell culture. The next study showed the same environmental electromagnetic fields inhibit the oncostatic action of tamoxifen as well as melatonin, which implicates the estrogen receptor. The negative effect could be overridden by increasing the dose of melatonin and tamoxifen.

There is some controversy over the effects of microwave radiation (from cell phones, FM radio stations, and television transmissions) and its ability to produce specific cancers. As long as there are such huge financial and liability issues involved in the funding and publication of research on this topic, sorting out the real risks on a true scientific basis seems difficult, if not impossible, at the current time. James Oschman observes that, "the Russian standard for maximum safe microwave exposure to avoid changes in brain activity is 1000 times less than the U.S. legal maximum." Until further research is available, the reader is advised to be cautious and judicious in the selection of home and workplace locations relative to microwave and FM transmission towers, and in the use of cell phones. It has not been documented that the use of antioxidants serves the same protective function in EMF exposure as is seen in radiation exposure.

Beneficial Effects of Electromagnetic Therapies

The beneficial and therapeutic effects of electromagnetic therapies have been studied since the early 1900s. The Albert Abrams Medical Clinic in San Francisco successfully treated tuberculosis, cancer, influenza and syphilis in 1920 using frequency-specific electromagnetic therapies. Upton Sinclair expected to write an exposé on Abrams's "quackery" for *Pearson's* Magazine in 1922, but the published article was titled "House of Wonders." Sinclair was impressed by the clinical results and the hope they offered to patients. In 1934, the American Medical Association declared that electromagnetic therapies were "unscientific" and moved medicine toward the use of drugs and surgery. The study of electromagnetic therapies and the beneficial effects of electromagnetic therapeutic fields on biological systems dropped out of medical research and into the realm of biophysics.

Robert Becker's ground-breaking work (described above) on the electromagnetic nature of biological tissue and the beneficial effects of direct current (DC) fields in tissue regeneration revolutionized the treatment of non-union fractures and wound healing. The current author resurrected frequencies used in the 1920s by Abrams and others, using a battery-operated (DC) microcurrent device as a frequency generator, and began using those frequencies to treat myofascial pain and nerve pain with a technique called "frequency specific microcurrent" in 1997.[338,339] Very specific clinical responses to over 100 frequencies have been noted, including those thought to remove inflammation, remodel scar tissue, alleviate concussion, eliminate the herpes virus, and stop bleeding. Two frequencies used simultaneously produced unprecedented log scale reductions in inflammatory peptides during a 90-minute treatment in fibromyalgia patients. The changes in cytokines correlated directly with reductions in pain scores.[340]

Blinded animal research conducted at the University of Sydney by Vivienne Reeve, PhD demonstrated that the frequency to "remove inflammation" (40hz) in the "immune system" reduced lipoxygenase-mediated inflammation by 62% in four minutes in a mouse model. The reduction was time dependent and all animals responded. Three other frequency combinations tested produced no reduction in inflammation. Prescription and non-prescription anti-inflammatory medications tested with this same model reduced swelling by 45%.[341]

The research and early clinical experiences in this area are promising and suggest there is potential therapeutic benefit of electromagnetic and frequency-specific therapies.

Summary

The pervasiveness of radiation, both in the natural environment and from manmade sources, makes it a key environmental input in today's world. There are important distinctions between the effects of ionizing vs. nonionizing radiation, but overall it seems clear that less is better than more. There are foods and supplements that can help patients protect themselves from radiation damage; clinicians should become familiar with these and assist patients with known high levels of radiation exposure to take precautionary measures.

References

1. Rimm EB, Stampfer MJ. Diet, lifestyle, and longevity—the next steps? JAMA. 2004;292(12):1490-92.
2. Ibid.
3. Knoops KT, de Groot LC, Kromhout D, et al. Mediterranean Diet, lifestyle factors, and 10-year mortality in elderly European men and women. JAMA. 2004;292(12):1433-39.
4. Esposito K, Marfella R, Ciotola M, et al. Effect of a Mediterranean-style diet on endothelial dysfunction and markers of vascular inflammation in the metabolic syndrome. JAMA. 2004;292(12):1440-46.
5. Yakar S, Leroith D, Brodt P. The role of the growth hormone/insulin-like growth factor axis in tumor growth and progression: Lessons from animal models. Cytokine Growth Factor Rev. 2005;16(4-5):407-20.
6. Grossman T. Latest advances in antiaging medicine. Keio J Med. 2005;54(2):85-94.
7. Schulze MB, Liu S, Rimm EB, et al. Glycemic index, glycemic load, and dietary fiber intake and incidence of type 2 diabetes in younger and middle-aged women. Am J Clin Nutr. 2004;80:348-356.
8. McKeown NM. Whole grain intake and insulin sensitivity: evidence from observational studies. Nutr Rev. 2004;62(7):286-91.
9. Thompson T. Gluten contamination of commercial oat products in the United States. N Engl J Med. 2004;351(19):2021-22.
10. Nilsson M, Stenberg M, Frid AH, et al. Glycemia and insulinemia in healthy subjects after lactose-equivalent meals of milk and other food proteins: the role of plasma amino acids and incretins. Am J Clin Nutr. 2004;80:1246-53.
11. Westphal S, Kastner S, Taneva E, et al. Postprandial lipid and carbohydrate responses after the ingestion of a casein-enriched mixed meal. Am J Clin Nutr. 2004;80(2):284-90.
12. Moreno JA, Perez-Jimenez F, Marin C, et al. Apolipoprotein E gene promoter—219G→T polymorphism increases LDL-cholesterol concentrations and susceptibility to oxidation in response to a diet rich in saturated fat. Am J Clin Nutr. 2004;80:1404-9.
13. Zhao G, Etherton TD, Martin KR, et al. Dietary α-linolenic acid reduces inflammatory and lipid cardiovascular risk factors in hypercholesterolemic men and women. J Nutr. 2004;134:2991-97.
14. Giltay EJ, Gooren LJ, Toorians AW, et al. Docosahexaenoic acid concentrations are higher in women than in men because of estrogenic effects. Am J Clin Nutr. 2004;80:1167-74.
15. Cordain L, Eaton SB, Sebastian A, et al. Origins and evolution of the Western diet: health implications for the 21st century. Am J Clin Nutr. 2005;81:341-54.
16. Fink PW, Kelso JA, Jirsa VK, de Guzman G. Recruitment of degrees of freedom stabilizes coordination. J Exp Psychol Hum Percept Perform. 2000;26(2):671-92.
17. Reynolds D, Carlson JM, Doyle J. Design degrees of freedom and mechanisms for complexity. Phys Rev E Stat Nonlin Soft Matter Phys. 2002;66(1 Pt 2):016108.
18. Buchanan JJ, Kelso JA. To switch or not to switch: recruitment of degrees of freedom stabilizes biological coordination. J Mot Behav. 1999;31(2):126-144.
19. Fries JF. Aging, natural death and the compression of morbidity. N Engl J Med. 1980;303:130-35.
20. Biffi A, Maron BJ, Verdile L, et al. Impact of physical deconditioning on ventricular tachyarrhythmias in trained athletes. J Am Coll Cardiol. 2004;44(5):1053-58.
21. Olson EE, McKeon RJ. Characterization of cellular and neurological damage following unilateral hypoxia/ischemia. J Neurol Sci. 2004;227(1):7-19.
22. Mielke JG, Wang YT. Insulin exerts neuroprotection by counteracting the decrease in cell-surface GABA receptors following oxygen-glucose deprivation in cultured cortical neurons. J Neurochem. 2005;92(1):103-13.
23. Ziliene V, Reingardiene D, Tereseviciute N, Slavinskas R. Diagnosis of acute respiratory failure and nosocomial pneumonia. Medicina (Kaunas). 2004;40(11):1124-29.
24. Raghuraj P, Ramakrishnan AG, Nagendra HR, Telles S. Effect of two selected yogic breathing techniques of heart rate variability. Indian J Physiol Pharmacol. 1998;42(4):467-72.
25. Raub JA. Psychophysiologic effects of Hatha Yoga on musculoskeletal and cardiopulmonary function: a literature review. J Altern Complement Med. 2002;8(6):797-812.
26. Okura T, Nakata Y, Tanaka K. Effects of exercise intensity on physical fitness and risk factors for coronary heart disease. Obes Res. 2003;11(9):1131-39.
27. www.iahp.org/hurt/schedule.html
28. Rochette LM, Patterson SM. Hydration status and cardiovascular function: effects of hydration enhancement on cardiovascular function at rest and during psychological stress. Int J Psychophysiol. 2005;56(1):81-91.
29. Duning T, Kloska S. Steinstrater O, et al. Dehydration confounds the assessment of brain atrophy. Neurology. 2005;64(3):548-50.
30. Zaluska WT, Malecka T, Swatowski A, Ksiazek A. Changes of extracellular volumes measured by whole and segmental bioimpedance analysis during hemodialysis in end-stage renal disease (ESRD) patients. Ann Univ Mariae Curie Sklodowska [Med.]. 2002;57(2):337-41.
31. Webb J. Use of the ecosystem approach to population health: the case of mercury contamination in aquatic environments and riparian populations, Andean Amazon, Napo River Valley, Ecuador. Can J Public Health. 2005;96(1):44-46.
32. Rohner AL, Pang LW, Iinuma G, et al. Effects of upcountry Maui water additives on health. Hawaii Med J. 2004;63(9):264-65.
33. Yoder JS, Blackburn B, Craun GF, et al. Surveillance for waterborne-disease outbreaks associated with recreational water—United States, 2001-2002. MMWR Surveill Summ. 2004;53(8):1-22.
34. Webb J. Use of the ecosystem approach to population health: the case of mercury contamination in aquatic environments and riparian populations, Andean Amazon, Napo River Valley, Ecuador. Can J Public Health. 2005;96(1):44-46.
35. Rohner AL, Pang LW, Iinuma G, et al. Effects of upcountry Maui water additives on health. Hawaii Med J. 2004;63(9):264-65.
36. Yoder JS, Blackburn B, Craun GF, et al. Surveillance for waterborne-disease outbreaks associated with recreational water—United States, 2001-2002. MMWR Surveill Summ. 2004;53(8):1-22.

37. Frampton MW, Utell MJ, Zareba W, et al. Effects of exposure to ultrafine carbon particles in healthy subjects and subjects with asthma. Res Rep Health Eff Inst. 2004;Dec (126):1-47.
38. Lacasana M, Esplugues A, Ballester F. Exposure to ambient air pollution and prenatal and early childhood health effects. Eur J Epidemiol. 2005;20(2):183-99.
39. Forsberg B, Hansson HC, Johansson C, et al. Comparative health impact assessment of local and regional particulate air pollutants in Scandinavia. Ambio. 2005;34(1):11-19.
40. Chalupka S. Environmental health: an opportunity for health promotion and disease prevention. AAOHN J. 2005;53(1):13-28.
41. Pate, RR, M Pratt, SN Blair, et al. Physical activity and public health: a recommendation from the Centers for Disease Control and Prevention and the American College of Sports Medicine. JAMA;273:402-407,1995.
42. Blair, SN. Physical activity, physical fitness, and health. Res. Quart. Exer. Sport;64:365-376,1993.
43. Blair, SN, HW Kohl, RS Paffenbarger, DG Clark, KH Cooper, and LW Gibbons. Physical fitness and all-cause mortality. JAMA;262:2395-2401,1989.
44. Anonymous. Statement on exercise. A position statement for health professionals by the Committee on Exercise and Cardiac Rehabilitation of the Council on Clinical Cardiology, American Heart Association. Circulation;81:396-8,1990.
45. Fletcher GF, G Balady, SN Blair, et al. Statement on exercise: benefits and recommendations for physical activity programs for all Americans. A statement for health professionals by the Committee on Exercise and Cardiac Rehabilitation of the Council on Clinical Cardiology, American Heart Association. Circulation;94:857-62,1996.
46. Fletcher GF, SN Blair, J Blumenthal, et al. Statement on exercise. Benefits and recommendations for physical activity programs for all Americans. A statement for health professionals by the Committee on Exercise and Cardiac Rehabilitation of the Council on Clinical Cardiology, American Heart association. Circulation;86:340-4,1992.
47. Celsing F, J Nystrom, P Pihlstedt, B Werner, and B Ekblom. Effect of long-term anemia and retransfusion on central circulation during exercise. Journal of Applied Physiology;61:1358-62,1986.
48. Ekblom B. Factors determining maximal aerobic power. Acta Physiologica Scandinavica. Supplementum;556:15-9,1986.
49. Ekblom B, AN Goldbarg, and B Gullbring. Response to exercise after blood loss and reinfusion. Journal of Applied Physiology;33:175-80,1972.
50. Ekblom B, G Wilson, and PO Astrand. Central circulation during exercise after venesection and reinfusion of red blood cells. Journal of Applied Physiology;40:379-83,1976.
51. Berglund B, and B Ekblom. Effect of recombinant human erythropoietin treatment on blood pressure and some haematological parameters in healthy men. Journal of Internal Medicine;229:125-30,1991.
52. Buskirk ER, and JL Hodgson. Age and aerobic power: the rate of change in men and women. Federation Proc;46:1824-1829,1987.
53. Flegg JL, and EG Lakatta. Role of muscle loss in the age-associated reduction in VO2max. J. Appl. Physiol. 65:1147-1151,1988.
54. Dehn MM, and RA Bruce. Longitudinal variations in maximal oxygen intake with age and activity. Journal of Applied Physiology;33:805-7,1972.
55. Dill DB, S Robinson, and JC Ross. A longitudinal study of 16 champion runners. Journal of Sports Medicine & Physical Fitness;7:4-27,1967.
56. Pollock ML, C Foster, D Knapp, JL Rod, and DH Schmidt. Effect of age and training on aerobic capacity and body composition of master athletes. Journal of Applied Physiology;62:725-31,1987.
57. Rogers MA, JM Hagberg, WH Martin, AA Ehsani, and JO Holloszy. Decline in VO2 max with aging in master athletes and sedentary men. J Appl Physiol;68:2195-2199,1990.
58. Bortz WM 4th, Bortz WM 2nd. How fast do we age? Exercise performance over time as a biomarker. J Gerontol A Biol Sci Med Sci. 1996;51(5):M223-5.
59. Rosen M J, JD Sorkin, AP Goldberg, JM Hagberg, and I Katzel. Predictors of age-associated decline in maximal aerobic capacity: A comparison of four statistical models. J. Appl. Physiol. 84:2163-2170,1998.
60. Visovsky C, Dvorak C. Exercise and cancer recovery. Online Journal of Issues in Nursing. 2005;10(2):http://nursingworld.org/ojin/hirsh/topic3/tpc3_2.htm
61. Correa Lima MP, Gomes-da-Silva MH. Colorectal cancer: lifestyle and dietary factors. Nutr Hosp. 2005;20(4):235-41.
62. Kirshbaum M. Promoting physical exercise in breast cancer care. Nurs Stand. 2005;19(41):41-8.
63. Haydon AM, Macinnis R, English D, Giles G. The effect of physical activity and body size on survival after diagnosis with colorectal cancer. Gut. 2005;June 21;[Epub ahead of print].
64. Kiraly MA, Kiraly SJ. The effect of exercise on hippocampal integrity: review of recent research. Int J Psychiatry Med. 2005;35(1):75-89.
65. Orngreen MC, Olsen DB, Vissing J. Aerobic training in patients with myotonic dystrophy type I. Ann Neurol. 2005;57(5):754-7.
66. Perez-Avila I, Fernandez-Vietez JA, Martinez-Gongora E, et al. [Effects of a physical training program on quantitative neurological indices in mild stage type 3 spinocerebelar ataxia patients.] Rev Neurol. 2004;39(10):907-10.
67. Meredith CN, WR Frontera, EC Fisher, et al. Peripheral effects of endurance training in young and old subjects. J. Appl. Physiol. 66:2844-2849,1989.
68. Linke A, Adams V, Schulze P, et al. Antioxidative effects of exercise training in patients with chronic heart failure. Circulation. 2005;111:1763-1770.
69. Seals DR, J M Hagberg, BF Hurley, AA Ehsani, and JO Holloszy. Endurance training in older men and women: cardiovascular responses to exercise. J Appl Physiol: Respirat Environ Exercise Physiol;57:1024-1029,1984.
70. Spina RJ, T Ogawa, WM Kohrt, WH Martin III, JO Holloszy, and AA Ehsani. Differences in cardiovascular adaptation to endurance exercise training between older men and women. J Appl Physiol; 75:849-855,1993.
71. Seals DR, JM Hagberg, BF Hurley, AA Ehsani, and JO Holloszy. Endurance training in older men and women: cardiovascular responses to exercise. J Appl Physiol: Respirat Environ Exercise Physiol;57:1024-1029,1984.
72. Davidson MB. The effect of aging on carbohydrate metabolism. A review of the English literature and a practical approach to the diagnosis of Diabetes Mellitus in the elderly. Metabolism;28:688-705,1979.
73. Hadden WC, and MI Harris. Prevalence of diagnosed diabetes, undiagnosed diabetes, and impaired glucose tolerance in adults 20-74 years of age: United States, 1976-1980. In: DHHS PHS publ. no. 87-1687. Washington, D.C.: U. S. Govt. Printing Office, 1987.
74. Shimokata H, DC Muller, JL Fleg, J Sorkin, AW Ziemba, and R Andes. Age as independent determinant of glucose tolerance. Diabetes;40:44-51,1991.
75. Borkan GA, DE Hults, and F Gerzoff. Age changes in body composition revealed by computed tomography. J. Gerontol. 38:673-677,1983.
76. Stolk RP, JR Vingerling, PTVM de Jong, et al. Retinopathy, glucose and insulin in an elderly population: The Rotterdam study. Diabetes;44:11-15,1995.

77. Zavaroni I, E Dall'Aglio, F Bruschi, et al. Effect of age and environmental factors on glucose tolerance and insulin secretion in a worker population. J Am Geriatr Soc;34:271-275,1986.
78. Seals DR, J M Hagberg, BF Hurley, AA Ehsani, and JO Holloszy. Effects of endurance training on glucose tolerance and plasma lipid levels in older men and women. JAMA;252:645-649,1984.
79. Kirwan JP, WM Kohrt, DM Wojta, RE Bourey, and JO Holloszy. Endurance exercise training reduces glucose-stimulated insulin levels in 60- to 70-year-old men and women. Journal of Gerontology;48:M84-M90,1993.
80. Hughes VA, MA Fiatarone, RA Fielding, et al. Exercise increases muscle GLUT 4 levels and insulin action in subjects with impaired glucose tolerance. Am. J. Physiol. 264:E855-E862,1993.
81. Marshall JA, RF Hamman, and J Baxter. High-fat, low-carbohydrate diet and the etiology of non-insulin-dependent diabetes mellitus: the San Luis Valley Diabetes Study. Am. J. Epidemiol. 134:590-603,1991.
82. Feskens EJM, and D Kromhout. Cardiovascular risk factors and the 25-year incidence of diabetes mellitus in middle-aged men. Am. J. Epidemiol. 130:1101-1108,1989.
83. Lundgren J, C Benstsson, G Blohme, et al. Dietary habits and incidence of noninsulin-dependent diabetes mellitus in a population study of women in Gothenburg, Sweden. Am. J. Clin. Nutr. 52:708-712,1989.
84. Ebbeling CB, Leidig MM, Sinclair KB, et al. Effects of an ad libitum low-glycemic load diet on cardiovascular disease risk factors in obese young adults. Am J Clin Nutr. 2005;81:976-82.
85. Borkman M, Campbell LV, Chisholm DJ, Storlien LH Comparison of the effects on insulin sensitivity of high carbohydrate and high fat diets in normal subjects. J Clin Endocrinol Metab. 1991;72(2):432-7.
86. Garg A, Grundy SM, Koffler M. Effect of high carbohydrate intake on hyperglycemia, islet function, and plasma lipoproteins in NIDDM. Diabetes Care. 1992;15(11):1572-80.
87. Garg A, Grundy SM, Unger RH. Comparison of effects of high and low carbohydrate diets on plasma lipoproteins and insulin sensitivity in patients with mild NIDDM. Diabetes. 1992;41(10):1278-85.
88. Hughes VA, MA Fiatarone, RA Fielding, et al. Long term effects of a high carbohydrate diet and exercise on insulin action in older subjects with impaired glucose tolerance. Am. J. Clin. Nutr. 62:426-433,1995.
89. Schaefer J, AH Lichtenstein, S Lamon-Fava, et al. Body weight and low-density lipoprotein cholesterol changes after consumption of a low-fat ad libitum diet. JAMA;274:1450-1455,1995.
90. Petersen AMW, Pedersen BK. The anti-inflammatory effect of exercise. J Appl Physiol. 2005;98:1154-62.
91. Helmrich SP, DR Ragland, RW Leung, and RS Paffenbarger Jr. Physical activity and reduced occurrence of non-insulin-dependent diabetes mellitus. N. Engl. J. Med. 325:147-152,1991.
92. Bogardus C, E Ravussin, DC Robbins, et al. Effects of physical training and diet therapy on carbohydrate metabolism in patients with glucose intolerance and non-insulin-dependent diabetes mellitus. Diabetes;33:311-318,1984.
93. Phinney SD, B M LaGrange, M O'Connell, and E Danforth Jr. Effects of aerobic exercise on energy expenditure and nitrogen balance during very low calorie dieting. Metabolism;37:758-765,1988.
94. Heymsfield SB, K Casper, J Hearn, and D Guy. Rate of weight loss during underfeeding: relation to level of physical activity. Metabolism;38:215-223,1989.
95. Goran MI, and ET Poehlman. Endurance training does not enhance total energy expenditure in healthy elderly persons. Am. J. Physiol. 263:E950-E957,1992.
96. Withers RT, DA Smith, RC Tucker, M Brinkman, and DG Clark. Energy metabolism in sedentary and active 49- to 70-year-old women. J. Appl. Physiol. 84:1333-1340,1998.
97. Ballor DL, VL Katch, MD Becque, and CR Marks. Resistance weight training during caloric restriction enhances lean body weight maintenance. Am. J. Clin. Nutr. 47:19-25,1988.
98. Pavlou KN, WP Steffee, RH Lerman, and BA Burrows. Effects of dieting and exercise on lean body mass, oxygen uptake, and strength. Med. Sci. Sports. Exerc. 17:466-471,1985.
99. Jakicic JM, BH Marcus, KI Gallagher, M Napolitano, and W Lang. Effect of exercise duration and intensity on weight loss in overweight, sedentary women: a randomized trial. JAMA;290:1323-30.,2003.
100. Jakicic JM, C Winters, W Lang, and RR Wing. Effects of intermittent exercise and use of home exercise equipment on adherence, weight loss, and fitness in overweight women: a randomized trial. JAMA;282:1554-60,1999.
101. Jakicic JM, BH Marcus, I Gallagher, M Napolitano, and W Lang. Effect of exercise duration and intensity on weight loss in overweight, sedentary women: a randomized trial. JAMA;290:1323-30.,2003.
102. McDonagh MJN, and CTM Davies. Adaptive response of mammalian skeletal muscle to exercise with high loads. Eur. J. Appl. Physiol. 52:139-155,1984.
103. Evans WJ, and J G Cannon. The metabolic effects of exercise-induced muscle damage. In: Exercise and Sport Sciences Reviews, edited by J. O. Holloszy. Baltimore: Williams & Wilkins, 1991, p. 99-126.
104. Kelly J, and LS Jefferson. Control of peptide-chain initiation in rat skeletal muscle. Development of methods for preparation of native ribosomal subunits and analysis of the effect of insulin on formation of 40S initiation complexes. J. Biol. Chem. 260:6677-6683,1985.
105. Rannels DE, AE Pegg, SR Rannels, and LS Jefferson. Effect of starvation on initiation of protein synthesis in skeletal muscle and heart. Am J. Physiol. E126-E133,1978.
106. Kelly J, and LS Jefferson. Control of peptide-chain initiation in rat skeletal muscle. Development of methods for preparation of native ribosomal subunits and analysis of the effect of insulin on formation of 40S initiation complexes. J. Biol. Chem. 260:6677-6683,1985.
107. Rannels DE, AE Pegg, SR Rannels, and LS Jefferson. Effect of starvation on initiation of protein synthesis in skeletal muscle and heart. Am J. Physiol. E126-E133,1978.
108. Flynn A, and CG Proud. The role of eIF-4 in cell proliferation. Cancer Surv. 27:293-310,1996.
109. Graves LM, KE Bornfeldt, GM Argast, et al. cAMP- and rapamycin-sensitive regulation of the association of eukaryotic initiation factor 4E and the translational regulator PHAS-I in aortic smooth muscle cells. Proc. Natl. Acad. Sci. USA;92:7222-7226,1995.
110. Jacob R, X Hu, D Niederstock, et al. IGF-I stimulation of muscle protein synthesis in the awake rat: permissive role of insulin and amino acids. Am. J. Physiol. 270:E60-E66,1996.
111. Jurasinski CV, and TC Vary. Insulin-like growth factor I accelerates protein synthesis in skeletal muscle during sepsis. Am. J. Physiol. 269:E977-E981,1995.
112. King DD, MA Staten, WM Kohrt, GP Dsalsky, D Elahi, and JO Holloszy. Insulin secretory capacity in endurance-trained and untrained young men. Am. J. Physiol. 259:E155-E161,1990.
113. Dela F, KJ Mikines, BA Tronier, and H Galbo. Diminished arginine-stimulated insulin secretion in trained men. J. Appl. Physiol. 69:261-267,1990.
114. Fluckey JD, WJ Kraemer, and PA Farrell. Pancreatic islet insulin secretion is increased after resistance exercise in rats. J. Appl. Physiol. 79:1100-1105,1995.
115. Engdahl JH, JD Veldhuis, and PA Farrell. Altered pulsatile insulin secretion associated with endurance training. Journal of Applied Physiology;79:1977-85,1995.

116. Dela F, KJ Mikines, BA Tronier, and H Galbo. Diminished arginine-stimulated insulin secretion in trained men. J. Appl. Physiol. 69:261-267,1990.
117. Kirwan JP, RC Hickner, KE Yarasheski, et al. Eccentric exercise induces transient insulin resistance in healthy individuals. J. Appl. Physiol. 70:2197-2202,1992.
118. O'Reilly KP, MJ Warhol, RA Fielding, et al. Eccentric exercise-induced muscle damage impairs muscle glycogen repletion. J. Appl. Physiol. 63:252-256,1987.
119. Asp S, and EA Richter. Decreased insulin action on muscle glucose transport after eccentric contractions in rats. J. Appl. Physiol. 81:1924-1928,1996.
120. Krishnan RK, JM Hernandez, et al. Age-related differences in the pancreatic beta-cell response to hyperglycemia after eccentric exercise. Am J Physiol;275:E463-70,1998.
121. Castellino P, L Luzi, DC Simonson, M Haymond, and RA DeFronzo. Effect of insulin and plasma amino acid concentrations on leucine metabolism in man. J. Clin. Invest. 80:1784-1793,1987.
122. Tessari P, S Inchiostro, G Biolo, R Trevisan, G Fantin, MC Marescotti, E Lori, A Tiengo, and G Crepaldi. Differential effects of hyperinsulinemia and hyperaminoacidemia on leucine-carbon metabolism *in vivo*. J Clin Invest;79:1062-1069,1987.
123. Biolo G, RY Fleming, and RR Wolfe. Physiologic hyperinsulinemia stimulates protein synthesis and enhances transport of selected amino acids in human skeletal muscle. J. Clin. Invest. 95:811-819,1995.
124. Fluckey JD, LS Jefferson, TC Vary, and PA Farrell. Augmented insulin action on rates of protein synthesis following resistance exercise in rats. Am. J. Physiol. 270:E313-E319,1996.
125. Fluckey JD, WJ Kraemer, and PA Farrell. Pancreatic islet insulin secretion is increased after resistance exercise in rats. J. Appl. Physiol. 79:1100-1105,1995.
126. Meredith CN, MJ Zackin, WR Frontera, and WJ Evans. Dietary protein requirements and body protein metabolism in endurance-trained men. J. Appl. Physiol. 66:2850-2856,1989.
127. Strawford A, T Barbieri, M Van Loan, et al. Resistance exercise and supraphysiologic androgen therapy in eugonadal men with HIV-related weight loss: a randomized controlled trial [see comments]. JAMA;281:1282-90,1999.
128. Flegg JL, and EG Lakatta. Role of muscle loss in the age-associated reduction in VO2max. J. Appl. Physiol. 65:1147-1151,1988.
129. Fiatarone MA, EC Marks, ND Ryan, et al. High-intensity strength training in nonagenarians. Effects on skeletal muscle. JAMA;263:3029-3034,1990.
130. Fiatarone MA, EF O'Neill, ND Ryan, et al. Exercise training and nutritional supplementation for physical frailty in very elderly people. *The New England Journal of Medicine*;330:1769-1775,1994.
131. Singh MA, W Ding, TJ Manfredi, et al. Insulin-like growth factor I in skeletal muscle after weight-lifting exercise in frail elders. Am J Physiol;277:E135-43,1999.
132. Fiatarone MA, EF O'Neill, ND Ryan, KM Clements, GR Solares, ME Nelson, SB Roberts, JJ Kehayias, LA Lipsitz, and WJ Evans. Exercise training and nutritional supplementation for physical frailty in very elderly people. *The New England Journal of Medicine*; 330:1769-1775,1994.
133. Frontera WR, CN Meredith, KP O'Reilly, and WJ Evans. Strength training and determinants of VO2 max in older men. J. Appl. Physiol. 68:329-333,1990.
134. Nelson ME, MA Fiatarone, CM Morganti, et al. Effects of high-intensity strength training on multiple risk factors for osteoporotic fractures. JAMA;272:1909-1914,1994.
135. Whipple RH, LI Wolfson, and PM Amerman. The relationship of knee and ankle weakness to falls in nursing home residents. J. Am. Geriatr. Soc. 35:13-20,1987.
136. Wolfson L, R Whipple, J Judge, P Amerman, C Derby, and M King. Training balance and strength in the elderly to improve function. J. Am. Geriatr. Soc. 41:341-343,1993.
137. Wolf SL, HX Barnhart, NG Kutner, et al. Reducing frailty and falls in older persons: an investigation of Tai Chi and computerized balance training. Atlanta FICSIT Group. Frailty and Injuries: Cooperative Studies of Intervention Techniques [see comments]. J Am Geriatr Soc;44:489-97,1996.
138. Kutner NG, H Barnhart, SL Wolf, E McNeely, and T Xu. Self-report benefits of Tai Chi practice by older adults. J Gerontol B Psychol Sci Soc Sci;52:P242-6,1997.
139. Province MA, EC Hadley, MC Hornbrook, et al. The effects of exercise on falls in elderly patients: A preplanned meta-analysis of the FICSIT trials. JAMA;273:1341-1347,1995.
140. Kannus P, Uusi-Rasi K, Palvanen M, Paarkkari J. Non-pharmacological means to prevent fractures among older adults. Ann Med. 2005;37(4):303-10.
141. Holick MF. Vitamin D for health and in chronic kidney disease. Semin. Dial. 2005;18(4):266-75.
142. Hickey T, P A Sharpe, FM Wolf, et al. Exercise participation in a frail elderly population. J Health Care Poor Underserved;7:219-31,1996.
143. Campbell WW, MC Crim, VR Young, and WJ Evans. Increased energy requirements and body composition changes with resistance training in older adults. Am. J. Clin. Nutr. 60:167-175,1994.
144. Sahyoun N. Nutrient intake by the NSS elderly population. In: Nutrition in the Elderly: The Boston Nutritional Status Survey, edited by S. C. Hartz, R. M. Russell and I. H. Rosenberg. London: Smith-Gordon and Company, 1992, p. 31-44.
145. Nelson ME, MA Fiatarone, CM Morganti, et al. Effects of high-intensity strength training on multiple risk factors for osteoporotic fractures. JAMA;272:1909-1914,1994.
146. Jacobs GD. The physiology of mind-body interactions: the stress response and the relaxation response. J Altern Complement Med. 2001;7(Suppl 1):S83-92.
147. McEwan BS. The End of Stress as We Know It. Washington, DC: Joseph Henry Press, 2002: p. 10-11.
148. Selye H. A syndrome produced by diverse nocuous agents. Nature. 1936;138:32.
149. Szabo S. Hans Selye and the development of the stress concept. Ann N Y Acad Sci. 1998;851:19-27.
150. Ibid, p. 19.
151. Ibid, p. 21.
152. Goldstein DS, McEwen B. Allostasis, homeostasis, and the nature of stress. Stress. 2002;5(1):55-8.
153. Kandel E. A new intellectual framework for psychiatry. Am J Psychiatry. 1998;155:457-69.
154. McEwan BS. The End of Stress as We Know It. Washington, DC: Joseph Henry Press, 2002: p. 11.
155. Selye H. A syndrome produced by diverse nocuous agents. Nature. 1936;138:32.
156. Selye H. Stress without Distress. McClelland and Stewart Ltd, Toronto, 1974.
157. Selye H. Stress in Health and Disease. Butterworths, Boston, 1976.
158. McEwan BS. The End of Stress as We Know It. Washington, DC: Joseph Henry Press, 2002: p. 5.
159. Sapolsky R. Why Zebras Don't Get Ulcers. New York: WH Freeman, 1994.
160. McEwan BS. The End of Stress as We Know It. Washington, DC: Joseph Henry Press, 2002: p. 7-10.
161. Holms TH, Rahe RH. The social readjustment rating scale. J Psychosom Res. 1967;11:213-18.
162. Uchino BN, Holt-Lunstad J, Bloor LE, Campo RA. Aging and cardiovascular reactivity to stress: longitudinal evidence for changes in stress reactivity. Psychol Aging. 2005;20(1):134-43.

163. Gun Kang M, Baek Koh S, Suk Cha B, et al. Job stress and cardiovascular risk factors in male workers. Prev Med. 2005;40(5):583-88.
164. Bhatia V, Tandon RK. Stress and the gastrointestinal tract. J Gastroenterol Hepatol. 2005;20(3):332-39.
165. Berga SL, Loucks TL. The diagnosis and treatment of stress-induced anovulation. Minerva Ginecol. 2005;57(1):45-54.
166. Kiecolt-Glaser JK, Glaser R. Psychosocial moderators of immune function. Psychosom Med. 1987;49.13-34.
167. Kiecolt-Glaser JK, Kristopher JP, MacCallum RC, et al. Chronic stress and age-related increases in the proinflammatory cytokine IL-6. Proc Natl Acad Sci. 2003:15; 990-95.
168. Tull ES, Sheu YT, Butler C, Cornelious K. Relationships between perceived stress, coping behavior and cortisol secretion in women with high and low levels of internalized racism. J Natl Med Assoc. 2005;97(2):206-12.
169. Gold SM, Dziobek I, Rogers K, et al. Hypertension and HPA axis hyperactivity affect frontal lobe integrity. J Clin Endocrinol Metab. 2005; March 22, 2005 (pre-pub citation).
170. Temoshok LR. Rethinking research on psychosocial interventions in biopsychosocial oncology: an essay written in honor of the scholarly contributions of Bernard H. Fox. Psychooncology. 2004;13(7):460-67.
171. Glaser R, Thorn, BE, Tarr KL, et al. Effects of stress on methyltransferase synthesis: an important DNA repair enzyme. Health Psychol. 1985;19(5):496-500.
172. Tomei LD, Kiecolt-Glaser JK, Kennedy S, Glaser R. Psychological stress and phorbol ester inhibition of radiation-induced apoptosis in human PBLs. Psychiatry Res. 1990;33:59-71.
173. Sapolsky R. Why Zebras Don't Get Ulcers. New York: WH Freeman, 1994.
174. Ray O. How the mind hurts and heals the body. Am Psychol. 2004;59(1):29-40.
175. Ibid.
176. Kitagawa EM, Hauser M. Differential mortality in the United States: a study in socioeconomic epidemiology. Cambridge, Mass.: Harvard University Press, 1973.
177. Lantz PM, House JS, Lepkowski JM, et al. Socioeconomic factors, health behaviors, and mortality: results from a nationally representative prospective study of US adults. J Amer Med Assoc. 1997;279(21):1703-8.
178. Ray O. How the mind hurts and heals the body. Am Psychol.. 2004;59(1):29-40.
179. Vaillant GE, Mukamal K. Successful aging. Am J Psychiatry. 2001;158:839-47.
180. Rotter JB. Generalized expectancies for internal versus external control of reinforcement. Psychol Monogr. 1966;80;609.
181. Kamen L, Seligman MEP. Explanatory style and health. Curr Psych Res Rev. 1989;6:207-18.
182. Ray O. How the mind hurts and heals the body. Am Psychol. 2004;59(1): 29-40.
183. House JS, Landis KR, Umberson D. Social relationships and health. Science. 1988;241:540-45.
184. Ray O. How the mind hurts and heals the body. Am Psychol. 2004;59(1): 29-40.
185. Pargament KL, Koenig G, Tarakeshwar N, Hahn J. Religious struggle as a predictor of mortality among medically ill elderly patients: a 2-year longitudinal study. Arch Intern Med. 2001;161:1881-85.
186. Lima BR, Pai S, Toledo V, et al. Emotional distress in disaster victims. J Nerv Ment Dis. 1993;181(6):388-93.
187. Choul FH, Chou P, Lin C, et al. The relationship between quality of life and psychiatric impairment for a Taiwanese community post-earthquake. Qual Life Res. 2004;13(6):1089-97.
188. Chang CM, Connor KM, Lai TJ, et al. Predictors of posttraumatic outcomes following the 1999 Taiwan earthquake. J Nerv Ment Dis. 2005;193(1):40-46.
189. Terr LC, Bloch DA, Michel BA, et al. Children's symptoms in the wake of Challenger: A field study of distant-traumatic effects and an outline of related conditions. Am J Psychiatry. 1999;156:1536-44.
190. Schuster MA, Stein BD, Jaycox LH, et al. A national survey of stress reactions after the September 11, 2001, terrorist attacks. N Engl J Med. 2001:345(20):1507-12.
191. North CS, Nixon SJ, Shariat S, et al. Psychiatric disorders among survivors of the Oklahoma City bombing. J Amer Med Assoc. 1999;282(8):755-62.
192. Skreblin L, Sujoldzic A. Acculturation process and its effects on dietary habits, nutritional behavior and body-image in adolescents. Coll Antropol. 2003;27(2):469-77.
193. Maier SF, Watkins LR, Fleshner M. Psychoneuroimmunology. The interface between behavior, brain, and immunity. Am Psychol. 1994;49(12):1004-17.
194. Blechschmidt E, Gasser RF. Biokinetics and Biodynamics of Human Differentiation. Springfield, IL: Charles C Thomas, 1978.
195. Korr IM. The spinal cord as organizer of disease processes: some preliminary perspectives. J Am Osteopath Assoc. 1976;76:35-45.
196. Willard FH. Nociception, the neuroendocrine immune system, and osteopathic medicine. In Ward RC, ed, Foundations for Osteopathic Medicine. 2nd Ed. Philadelphia: Lippincott Williams and Wilkins, 2003.
197. Robbins S, Cotran R, Kumar V. Inflammation and Repair. In Pathologic Basis of Disease. 3rd Ed. Philadelphia: WB Saunders Company, 1984.
198. Ibid.
199. Ibid.
200. Guyton AC, Hall JE. Textbook of Medical Physiology. 9th Ed. Philadelphia: WB Saunders Company, 1996, p309.
201. Movat HZ. The Inflammatory Reaction. New York: Elsevier, 1985.
202. Witte CL, et al. Pathophysiology of chronic edema, lymphedema, and fibrosis. In Staub NC and Taylor AE, eds, Edema. New York: Raven Press, 1984.
203. Movat HZ. The Inflammatory Reaction. New York: Elsevier, 1985.
204. Measel JW. The effect of the lymphatic pump on the immune response: preliminary studies on the antibody response to pneumococcal polysaccharide. J Am Osteopath Assoc. 1982 (1);82:28-31.
205. Willard FH. Nociception, the neuroendocrine immune system, and osteopathic medicine. In Ward RC, ed, Foundations for Osteopathic Medicine. 2nd Ed. Philadelphia: Lippincott Williams and Wilkins, 2003.
206. Ibid.
207. Chrousos GP. The hypothalamic-pituitary-adrenal axis and immune-mediated inflammation. N Engl J Med. 1995;332 (20):1351-62.
208. Willard FH. Nociception, the neuroendocrine immune system, and osteopathic medicine. In Ward RC, ed, Foundations for Osteopathic Medicine. 2nd Ed. Philadelphia: Lippincott Williams and Wilkins, 2003.
209. Willard FH. Introduction. In Willard FH and Patterson MM, eds, Nociception and the Neuroendocrine-Immune Connection—1992 International Symposium. Athens OH: American Academy of Osteopathy, 1994.
210. Carreiro JE. Nociception and the neuroendocrine immune system. In An Osteopathic Approach to Children. Edinburgh: Churchill Livingston, 2003.
211. Pischinger, A. Matrix and Matrix Regulation. Brussels: Haug International, 1991.
212. Jealous JS. The fluid body. Biodynamics of Osteopathy. CD audio text, in development. 2000, 2003, 2004, 2005. www.BioDO.com. Distributed through mjlong@tampabay.rr.com.

213. Szent-Györgyi A. To see what everyone has seen, to think what no one has thought. Bio Bull. 1988;174:191-240.
214. Magoun HI. Infants and children. Osteopathy in the Cranial Field. 2nd Ed. Kirksville, MO: The Journal Printing Company, 1966.
215. Peitsch WK, Keefer CH, LaBrie RA, Mulliken JB. Incidence of cranial asymmetry in healthy newborns. Pediatrics. 2002;110(6):e72.
216. Ibid.
217. Miller RI, Clarren SK. Long-term developmental outcomes in patients with deformational plagiocephaly. Pediatrics. 2000;105 (2):e26.
218. Frymann V. Relation of disturbances of craniosacral mechanisms to symptomatology of the newborn: study of 1,250 infants. J Am Osteopath Assoc. 1966;65:1059-75.
219. Lay EM. Cranial field. In Ward RC, ed. Foundations for Osteopathic Medicine. Baltimore: Williams and Wilkins, 1997; pp 909-910.
220. Magoun HI. Entrapment neuropathy of the central nervous system. Part II. Cranial nerves I-IV, VI-VIII, XII. J Am Osteopath Assoc. 1968;67:779-87.
221. Carreiro JE. Nociception and the neuroendocrine immune system. In An Osteopathic Approach to Children. Edinburgh: Churchill Livingston, 2003, p 110.
222. Magoun HI. Whiplash injury: a greater lesion complex. J Am Osteopath Assoc. 1964;63(6):524-35.
223. Harakal JH. An osteopathically integrated approach to the whiplash complex. J Am Osteopath Assoc. 1975;74:941-55.
224. Lader E. Whiplash and related cervical trauma: its role in the development of idiopathic headache, myofascial pain, and degenerative osteoarthritis of the temporomandibular joint. The Dental Clinics of North America. July 1982.
225. Becker RE. The nature of trauma. In Life in Motion. Portland,OR: Rudra Press, 1997, pp 275-276.
226. Lay EM. The osteopathic management of temporomandibular joint dysfunction. In Gelb H, ed, Clinical Management of Head, Neck and TMJ Pain and Dysfunction. 2nd Ed. Philadelphia: WB Saunders Company, 1985.
227. Robbins S, Cotran R, Kumar V. Inflammation and Repair. In Pathologic Basis of Disease. 3rd Ed. Philadelphia: WB Saunders Company, 1984.
228. Herman JL. Trauma and Recovery. New York: Basic Books, 1997, p38.
229. Herman JL, Trauma and Recovery. New York: Basic Books, 1997, p7.
230. Herman JL, Trauma and Recovery. New York: Basic Books, 1997, p117.
231. Witte CL, Witte MH. Lymphatics in pathophysiology of edema. In Johnson, ed, Experimental Biology of the Lymphatic Circulation. Elsevier Science Publishers, 1985.
232. Willard FH. Nociception, the neuroendocrine immune system, and osteopathic medicine. In Ward RC, ed, Foundations for Osteopathic Medicine. 2nd Ed. Philadelphia: Lippincott Williams and Wilkins, 2003.
233. Carreiro JE. Nociception and the neuroendocrine immune system. In An Osteopathic Approach to Children. Edinburgh: Churchill Livingston, 2003, p 110.
234. Willard FH. Nociception, the neuroendocrine immune system, and osteopathic medicine. In Ward RC, ed, Foundations for Osteopathic Medicine. 2nd Ed. Philadelphia: Lippincott Williams and Wilkins, 2003.
235. Korr IM. The spinal cord as organizer of disease processes: (III) Hyperactivity of sympathetic innervation as a common factor in disease. J Am Osteopat Assoc. 1979;79:232-237.
236. Willard FH. Nociception, the neuroendocrine immune system, and osteopathic medicine. In Ward RC, ed, Foundations for Osteopathic Medicine. 2nd Ed. Philadelphia: Lippincott Williams and Wilkins, 2003.
237. McEwen BS. Protective and damaging effects of stress mediators. N Engl J Med. 1998;338:171-79.
238. Seeman TE , Singer BH, et al. Price of adaptation—allostatic load and its health consequences: MacArthur studies of successful aging. Arch Int Med. 1997;157(19):2259-68.
239. Ibid.
240. Seeman TE, McEwen BS, Rowe JW, et al. Allostatic load as a marker of cumulative biological risk: MacArthur studies of successful aging. Proc Natl Acad Sci U S A. 2001;98(8):4770-75.
241. McEwen BS. Protective and damaging effects of stress mediators. N Engl J Med. 1998;338:171-79.
242. Willard FH. Nociception, the neuroendocrine immune system, and osteopathic medicine. In Ward RC, ed, Foundations for Osteopathic Medicine. 2nd Ed. Philadelphia: Lippincott Williams and Wilkins, 2003.
243. Sapolsky RM, Uno H, Rebert CS, Finch CE. Hippocampal damage associated with prolonged glucocorticoid exposure in primates. J Neurosci. 1990;10(9):2897-902.
244. Willard FH. Nociception, the neuroendocrine immune system, and osteopathic medicine. In Ward RC, ed, Foundations for Osteopathic Medicine. 2nd Ed. Philadelphia: Lippincott Williams and Wilkins, 2003.
245. Carreiro JE. Nociception and the neuroendocrine immune system. In An Osteopathic Approach to Children. Edinburgh: Churchill Livingston, 2003, p 110.
246. Heim C, Newport DJ, Nemeroff CB, et al. Pituitary-adrenal and autonomic responses to stress in women after sexual and physical abuse in childhood. JAMA. 2000;284(5):592-97.
247. Curtis BM, O'Keefe JH. Autonomic tone as a cardiovascular risk factor: the dangers of chronic fight or flight. Mayo Clin Proc. 2002;77 (1):45-54.
248. McEwen BS. Protective and damaging effects of stress mediators. N Engl J Med. 1998;338:171-79.
249. Heim C, Newport DJ, Nemeroff CB, et al. Pituitary-adrenal and autonomic responses to stress in women after sexual and physical abuse in childhood. JAMA. 2000;284 (5):592-97.
250. Ibid.
251. Lemieux AM, Coe CL. Abuse-related posttraumatic stress disorder: evidence for chronic neuroendocrine activation in women. Psychosom Med. 1995;57 (2):105-15.
252. Ibid.
253. Ibid.
254. McEwen BS. Protective and damaging effects of stress mediators. N Engl J Med. 1998;338:171-79.
255. Willard FH. Nociception, the neuroendocrine immune system, and osteopathic medicine. In Ward RC, ed, Foundations for Osteopathic Medicine. 2nd Ed. Philadelphia: Lippincott Williams and Wilkins, 2003.
256. Scherrer U, Sartori C. Insulin as a vascular and sympathoexcitatory hormone. Circulation. 1997;96:4104-13.
257. McEwen BS. Protective and damaging effects of stress mediators. N Engl J Med. 1998;338:171-79.
258. Curtis BM, O'Keefe JH. Autonomic tone as a cardiovascular risk factor: the dangers of chronic fight or flight. Mayo Clin Proc. 2002;77 (1):45-54.
259. Korr IM. Hyperactivity of sympathetic innervation: a common factor in disease. The collected papers of Irvin M. Korr. Vol 2. Indianapolis IN: The American Academy of Osteopathy, 1997.
260. Webster's New World Dictionary of American English, 3rd College Edition.

261. Shea KM. Protecting our children from environmental hazards in the face of limited data—a precautionary approach is needed. J Pediatr. 2004;145:153-56.
262. Sanborn M, Cole D, Kerr K, et al. Systematic review of pesticide human health effects. Ontario College of Family Physicians. 2004:1-186. www.ocfp.on.ca.
263. Ibid.
264. Abelsohn A, Gibson BL, Sanborn MD, Weir E. Identifying and managing adverse environmental health effects: 5. Persistent organic pollutants. CMAJ. 2002;166(12).
265. Colborn T, vom Saal FS, Soto AM Developmental effects of endocrine-disrupting chemicals in wildlife and humans. Environ Health Perspect. 1993;101(5):378-84.
266. Johnson BL et al. Public health implications of persistent toxic substances in the Great Lakes and St. Lawrence basins. J Great Lakes Res. 1998;24(2):698-722.
267. Carson R. *Silent Spring*. 40th anniversary ed. New York: Houghton Mifflin; 2002.
268. Colborn T et al. *Our Stolen Future*. Toronto: Dutton; 1996.
269. Fisher BE. Most unwanted. Environ Health Perspect. 1999;107:A18-25.
270. Abelsohn A, Gibson BL, Sanborn MD, Weir E. Identifying and managing adverse environmental health effects: 5. Persistent organic pollutants. CMAJ. 2002;166(12).
271. Sandau CD, Ayotte P, Dewailly E, et al. Analysis of hydroxylated metabolites of PCBs and other chlorinated phenolic compounds in whole blood from Canadian Inuit. Environ Health Perspect. 2000;108:611-16.
272. Ribas-Fito N, Sala M, Kogevinas M, Sunyer J. Polychlorinated biphenyls (PCBs) and neurological development in children: a systematic review. J Epidemiol Community Health. 2001;55:537-46.
273. Brouwer A, Morse DC, Lans MC, et al. Interactions of persistent environmental organohalogens with the thyroid hormone system: mechanisms and possible consequences for animal and human health. Toxicol Ind Health. 1998;14:59-84.
274. Wade M. Human health and exposure to chemicals which disrupt estrogen, androgen and thyroid hormone physiology. Ottawa: Environmental and Occupational Toxicology Division, Environmental Health Directorate, Health Protection Branch, Health Canada. Available: www.hc-sc.gc.ca/ehp/ehd/bch/env_contaminants/endocrine.pdf (accessed 2002 May 13).
275. Tryphonas H. The impact of PCBs and dioxins on children's health: immunologic considerations. Can J Public Health. 1998;89(Suppl 1):S49-52.
276. Sanborn M, Cole D, Kerr K, et al. Systematic review of pesticide human health effects. Ontario College of Family Physicians. 2004:1-186. www.ocfp.on.ca.
277. Jacobson SW, Fein GG, Jacobson JL, et al. The effect of intrauterine PCB exposure on visual recognition memory. Child Dev. 1985;56(4):853-60.
278. Jacobson JL, Jacobson SW, Humphrey HE. Effects of in utero exposure to polychlorinated biphenyls and related contaminants on cognitive functioning in young children. J Pediatr. 1990;116(1):38-45.
279. Jacobson JL, Jacobson SW. Intellectual impairment in children exposed to polychlorinated biphenyls in utero. N Engl J Med. 1996;335(11):783-89.
280. Vreugdenhil HJ, Slijper FM, Mulder PG, Weisglas-Kuperus N. Effects of perinatal exposure to PCBs and dioxins on play behavior in Dutch children at school age. Environ Health Perspect. 2002;110(10):A593-8.
281. Stewart P, Fitzgerald S, Reihman J, et al. Prenatal PC exposure, the corpus callosum, and response inhibition. Environ Health Perspect. 2003;111(13):1670-77.
282. Birnbaum LS, Staskal DF. Brominated flame retardants: cause for concern? Environ Health Perspect. 2004;112:9-17.
283. Fangstrom B, Strid A, Grandjean P, et al. A retrospective study of PBDEs and PCBs in human milk from the Faroe Islands. Environ Health. 2005;4(1):12.
284. Grandjean P, Budtz-Jorgensen E, et al. Attenuated growth of breast-fed children exposed to increased concentrations of methylmercury and polychlorinated biphenyls. FASEB J. 2003;17(6):699-70.
285. Sanborn M, et al. Systematic review of pesticide human health effects. Ontario College of Family Physicians. 2004:1-186. www.ocfp.on.ca.
286. Shea KM. Protecting our children from environmental hazards in the face of limited data—a precautionary approach is needed. J Pediatr. 2004;145:153-56.
287. Xu J, Gordon JI. Honor thy symbionts. Proc Natl Acad Sci U S A. 2003;100:10452-59.
288. Macpherson AJ, Harris NL. Interactions between commensal intestinal bacteria and the immune system. Nat Rev Immunol. 2004;4(6):478-85.
289. International human genome sequencing consortium: initial sequencing and analysis of the human genome. Nature. 2001;409:860-921.
290. Manchester KL. Antoine Béchamp: père de la biologie. Oui ou non? Endeavour. 2001;25:68-73.
291. Attributed. See http://www.universal-tao.com/article/sick.html.
292. Bengmark S. Ecological control of the gastrointestinal tract: the role of probiotic flora. Gut. 1998.42:2-7.
293. Bjorksten B. Effects of intestinal microflora and the environment on the development of asthma and allergy. Springer Semin Immunopathol. 2004;25(3-4):257-70.
294. Guarner F, Magdelena JR. Gut flora in health and disease. Lancet. 2003;361:512-19.
295. Bengmark S. Ecological control of the gastrointestinal tract: the role of probiotic flora. Gut. 1998.42:2-7.
296. Macpherson AJ, Harris NL. Interactions between commensal intestinal bacteria and the immune system. Nat Rev Immunol. 2004;4(6):478-85.
297. Grolund MM, Lehtonen OP, Eerola E, Kero P. Fecal microflora in healthy infants born by different methods of delivery: permanent changes in intestinal flora after cesarean delivery. J Pediatr Gastroenterol Nutr. 1999;28:19-25.
298. Heavey PM, Rowland IR. The gut microflora of the developing infant: microbiology and metabolism. Microbial Ecol Health Dis. 1999;11:75-84.
299. Harmsen HJ, et al. Analysis of intestinal flora development in breast-fed and formula-fed infants by using molecular identification and detection methods. J Pediatr Gastroenterol Nutr. 2000;30:61-67.
300. Mackie RI, Sghir A, Gaskins HR. Developmental microbial ecology of the neonatal gastrointestinal tract. Am J Clin Nutr. 1999;69(Suppl):1035S-45S.
301. Strachan DP. Hay fever, hygiene, and household size. BMJ. 1989;299:1259-60.
302. Rook GAW, Brunet LR. Microbes, immunoregulation, and the gut. Gut. 2005;54:317-20.
303. Strachan DP. Family size, infection and atopy: the first decade of the "hygiene hypothesis." Thorax. 2000;55(Suppl):S2-S10.
304. Prescott SL. Allergy: the price we pay for cleaner living? Ann Allergy Asthma Immunol. 2003;90(Suppl 3):64-70.
305. Harmsen HJ, et al. Analysis of intestinal flora development in breast-fed and formula-fed infants by using molecular identification and detection methods. J Pediatr Gastroenterol Nutr. 2000. 30:61-67.

306. Collins MD, Gibson GR. Probiotics, prebiotics, and symbiotics: approaches for modulating the microbial ecology of the gut. Am J Clin Nutr. 1999;69(Suppl):1052S-57S.
307. Mackie RI, Sghir A, Gaskins HR. Developmental microbial ecology of the neonatal gastrointestinal tract. Am J Clin Nutr. 1999;69(Suppl):1035S-45S.
308. Harmsen HJ, Wildeboer-Veloo AC, Raangs GC, et al. Analysis of intestinal flora development in breast-fed and formula-fed infants by using molecular identification and detection methods. J Pediatr Gastroenterol Nutr. 2000;30:61-67.
309. Bjorksten B. Effects of intestinal microflora and the environment on the development of asthma and allergy. Springer Semin Immunopathol. 2004;25(3-4):257-70.
310. Bosch JA, Turkenburg M, Nazmi K, et al. Stress as a determinant of saliva-mediated adherence and coadherence of oral and nonoral microorganisms. Psychosom Med. 2003;65:604-12.
311. Teitelbaum JE, Walker WA. Nutritional impact of pre-and probiotics as protective gastrointestinal organisms. Annu Rev Nutr. 2002;22:107-38.
312. Otte JM, Cario E, Podolsky DK. Mechanisms of cross hyporesponsiveness to Toll-like receptor bacterial ligands in intestinal epithelial cells. Gastroenterology. 2004;126:1054-70.
313. Mountzouris KC, McCartney AL, Gibson GR. Intestinal microflora of human infants and current trends for its nutritional modulation. Br J Nutr. 2002;87:405-20.
314. Cellular and Molecular Immunology. Fifth Edition. Abbas & Lichtman, Ed. Saunders, Philadelphia. 2003.
315. Brandtzaeg P. Current understanding of gastrointestinal immunoregulation and its relation to food allergy. Ann N Y Acad Sci. 2002;964:13-45.
316. Van Uden J, Rax E. Immunostimulatory DNA and applications to allergic disease. J Allergy Clin Immunol. 1999;104:902-10.
317. Jijon H, Backer J, Diaz H, et al. DNA from probiotic bacteria modulated murine and human epithelial and immune function. Gastroenterol. 2004;126:1358-73.
318. Hooper LV, Wong MH, Thelin A, et al. Molecular analysis of commensal host-microbial relationships in the intestine. Science. 2001;291:881-84.
319. Hooper LV, Gordon JI. Commensal host-bacterial relationships in the gut. Science. 2001;292:1115-18.
320. Kalliomaki M, Salminen S, Poussa T, et al. Probiotics and prevention of atopic disease: 4-year follow-up of a randomised placebo-controlled trial. Lancet. 2003;361:1869-71.
321. Bouma G, Strober W. The immunologic and genetic basis of inflammatory bowel disease. Nat Rev Immunol. 2003;3:521-33.
322. Oschman JL. Energy Medicine: The Scientific Basis. Churchill Livingston, Edinburgh, 2000
323. Umegaki K, Sugisawa A, Shin SJ, et al. Different onsets of oxidative damage to DNA and lipids in bone marrow and liver in rats given total body irradiation. Free Radic Biol Med. 2001;31(9):1066-74.
324. Umegaki K, Ikegami S, Inoue K, et al. Beta-carotene prevents x-ray induction of micronuclei in human lymphocytes. Amer J Clin Nutr. 1994;59(2):401-12.
325. Umegaki K, Aoki S, Esashi T. Whole body x-ray irradiation to mice decreases ascorbic acid concentration in bone marrow: comparison between ascorbic acid and vitamin E. Free Radic Biol Med. 1995;19(4):493-97.
326. Ben-Amotz A, Yatziv S, Sela M, et al. Effect of natural beta-carotene supplementation in children exposed to radiation from the Chernobyl accident. Radiat Environ Biophys. 1998;37:187-93.
327. Kapitanov AB, Pimenov AM, Obukhova LK, Izmailov DM. Radiation-protective effectiveness of lycopene. Radiats Biol Radioecol. 1994;34(3):439-45.
328. Korkina L, et al. Antioxidant therapy in children affected by irradiation from the Chernobyl nuclear accident. Biochem Soc Trans. 1993;21:314S.
329. Clark L. Are You Radioactive? Devin-Adair Pub, 1973.
330. Kurzer MS Reduced radiation damage from ingestion of cabbage family plants. Journal of Nutrition. 1997;127(5 Suppl):1047S-49S.
331. Emerit I, Oganesian N, Sarkisian T, et al. Clastogenic factors in the plasma of Chernobyl accident recovery workers: anticlastogenic effect of Ginkgo biloba extract. Radiat Res. 1995;144:198-205.
332. Vijayalaxmi R, Reiter RJ, Meltz ML. Melatonin protects human blood lymphocytes from radiation-induced chromosome damage. Mutat Res. 1995;346(1):23-31.
333. Ben-Hur E, Fulder S. Effect of P. ginseng saponins and Eleutherococcus S. on survival of cultured mammalian cells after ionizing radiation. Am J Chin Med. 1981;9:48-56.
334. Becker RO. The Body Electric. Morrow, New York, 1985.
335. Becker RO. Cross Currents: The Promise of Electromedicine, The Perils of Electropollution. Penguin Group, Inc, New York, 1990.
336. Liburdy RP, Wyant A. Radiofrequency radiation and the immune system. Part 3. *In vitro* effects on human immunoglobulin and on murine T- and B-lymphocytes. Int J Radiat Biol Stud Phys Chem Med. 1984;46(1):67-81.
337. Oschman JL. Energy Medicine: The Scientific Basis. Churchill Livingston: Edinburgh, 2000.
338. McMakin C. Microcurrent treatment of myofascial pain in the head, neck and face. Topics in Clinical Chiropractic. 1998;5(1):29-35.
339. McMakin C. Microcurrent therapy: a novel treatment method for chronic low back myofascial pain. Journal of Bodywork and Movement Therapies. 2004;8:143-53.
340. McMakin C. Cytokine changes with microcurrent treatment of fibromyalgia associated with cervical spine trauma. Journal of Bodywork and Movement Therapies. 2005;9(3):169-76.
341. Reeve V. University of Sydney, Department of Veterinary Science, personal communication, 2003.

Chapter 14
Influence of Mind and Spirit

DeAnn Liska, PhD

Introduction

This chapter is the final entry in our Building Blocks section. We have given our attention to the effects on human health of various well-known and often well-researched biological and physical factors, and their interaction with individual genetic predispositions: diet, nutrients, air, water, exercise, trauma, xenobiotics, microorganisms, and radiation. The psychosocial realm has also been discussed, and is a source of prolific research and myriad books and articles written about common (and uncommon) clinical approaches. We now turn our attention to the impact of spirituality as one of the key building blocks of health. Here, we will briefly introduce the subject, which is just beginning to make itself felt in research and scientific writing. (Further discussion can be found in Chapter 33.)

Understanding the role of biochemical individuality (that is, genetic predisposition influenced by environment) is a cornerstone of functional medicine and has been demonstrated by such examples as the variety of differentially-regulated detoxification enzymes,[1,2,3] the relationship among body fat composition, blood pressure, and insulin resistance,[4,5,6] and the myriad influences that determine risk of conditions such as CVD.[7,8,9,10] All of these examples (and a great deal of this book) are about the physical nature of our being—the mechanisms that connect us with the physical world around us. Because these are physical, matter-based examples, we can test them. We can do genetic testing; we can devise assays to detect the result of a specific intervention. But the medicine of today involves more than just the physical, matter-based body; it also includes the spiritual experience of the patient.

Emerging Research on Spirituality and Health

As the changing research record indicates, an understanding of the role of spirituality in health and healing is attracting considerable attention of late. For example, a search of the National Library of Medicine database (PubMed) using the word "spirituality" shows that only 62 articles were published on this subject in the 20 years between 1970 and 1990, compared to 477 articles between 1990 and 2000, and more than double that number, 1226 articles, from 2000 to 2004. This increased interest was triggered by studies such as that of King and Bushwick, in which it was noted that 94% of patients admitted to hospitals believe that spiritual health is as important as physical health, and 77% believe that physicians should consider their patients' spiritual needs, but only 20% of patients reported their physicians addressing spiritual issues with them in more than just a passing fashion.[11] A 2003 study in which physicians were asked about their attitudes and preferences regarding spirituality in the medical encounter found that, of the 84.5% who indicated they should be aware of patients' spirituality, most would not ask about spiritual issues unless a patient were dying.[12] In a discussion on the role of spirituality and health, Levin makes this assertion:

> By excluding matters of spirit from clinical research and practice, physicians run the risk of leaving out a large piece of what it means to be a human being. If physicians sincerely wish to treat the whole person, they first will have to see their patients as more than just a body and a personality, or, worse, a collection of isolated organ systems.[13]

Researching the Spirituality and Health Connection: Challenges and Early Findings

Given the importance of this subject to patients and practitioners alike, it is valuable to spend a little time exploring some new findings that suggest there may be a physical, biochemical basis for spirituality. Interestingly, as with all other building blocks to health, this biochemical connection appears to be experienced differently by each of us; that is, spirituality (our experience of the divine) is another example of how we all show biochemical individuality. Moreover, the research is showing more clearly how our spirituality, life experience, and physical bodies (biochemistry) are all entwined in such a manner that ignoring one means leaving out part of the web.

First, it is beneficial to define spirituality and religion, since these terms can be interpreted differently. The Oxford dictionary defines spirituality as "of the human spirit or soul, not physical or worldly."[14] Religion, in contrast, is more limited and means "a particular system of faith and worship."[15] Therefore, spirituality is the nonphysical component of a person, whereas religion is the institutional practice, or how spirituality is codified and acted on by a group or society. These definitions help to clarify why it is often easier to observe, report on, and quantify religion than it is to assess spirituality. In fact, this is one of the primary challenges in incorporating spirituality into a science-based discussion.

There are other roadblocks as well. A primary issue is the historical conflict between "science" and "religion." Many scientists and clinicians have been taught that spirituality is unscientific, not logical, and, therefore, not relevant to a Western, science-based approach to health and disease. Certainly, history is filled with examples of how science can challenge religious beliefs, and how religion can limit scientific progress. The tone of recent research, however, is showing that the 21st century may find a way to heal the rift between science and the spiritual—or, at least, to begin examining it objectively. Even when this relationship between "science" and "religion" is difficult, a functional medicine approach of treating the patient, not just the disease, means finding ways to incorporate attention to spirituality into clinical practice in a science-based manner.

The difficulty of "measuring" spirituality challenges our current research models. Much work performed in the 1990s and early 2000s focused on spiritual practices like meditation, prayer, yoga, and quigong because those can be seen (that is, the activities can be observed, recorded, and their before-and-after effects can be assessed). For example, in a controlled trial, specific daily practice of yoga was shown to increase plasma melatonin after three months.[16] Intrinsic religiosity has also been associated with diurnal cortisol rhythm, as compared to subjects with low religiosity, who show apparent flattened cortisol patterns.[17] Davidson et al.[18] reported in 2003 that an eight-week program of mindfulness meditation before influenza vaccination led to an increase in antibody titer, as compared to non-meditating controls, which suggests an improvement in immune function with meditation.

These are but a few of many fascinating examples of the general effect spiritual practices can have on health indicators. Should we expect that each patient can benefit similarly from these practices? In functional medicine, we would say that such practices will be filtered through the patient's genetic predispositions and overall environment, so perhaps the answer is "no."

We know that stress hormone pathways and behaviors like anxiety are, at least in part, determined by certain genetic polymorphisms—that is, the polymorphic pattern of genes we inherit from our parents influences our response to stress and our susceptibility to conditions such as post-traumatic stress disorder. Continuing that train of thought, it is intriguing to speculate that at least some of these polymorphisms might also be involved in how responsive individual patients are to spiritual practices such as mindfulness meditation. Consider the finding that parallel polymorphisms in the acetylcholinesterase and paraoxonase 1 gene loci have been associated with anxiety scores.[19] Research has also documented that psychosocial stress can lead to alteration in how the acetylcholinesterase gene is spliced, which then leads to different levels of acetylcholinesterase activity in the cell.[20] Another study has reported an association between certain polymorphisms in the cytochrome P450 2D6 gene and harm avoidance; it has been postulated that this detoxification system may impact personality by influencing the generation of endogenous neurotransmitters in the brain.[21]

From these examples, it is not too far-reaching to suggest that many spiritual practices that are now being shown to influence the body's biochemistry will be experienced differently by patients with different genetic propensities. Thus, we begin to perceive the biochemical individuality of spirituality.

Possibly the most intriguing work on the interplay between biochemical individuality and spirituality has emerged from Thomas Bouchard's group at the Department of Psychology, University of Minnesota, MN. Bouchard has investigated genetics and behavior by focusing on twins reared together or apart, and has concluded that there is now strong evidence that virtually all individual psychological differences are moderately to substantially heritable.[22] In particular, he used a validated scale of intrinsic and extrinsic religiosity with 35 pairs of monozygous twins and 37 pairs of dizygotic twins reared apart and found that twin similarity could not be explained by environmental factors alone, but was only explained by a model containing genetic plus environmental factors.[23] (Note that both genetics and environment must be included for the model to be effective.)

The Temperament and Character Inventory (TCI)—a 240-question, standardized, validated, personality assessment that scores such behaviors as self-transcendence, transpersonal identification, and mysticism—has also been used to explore the interrelationship among genetics, biochemistry, and behavior. In an interesting report, Comings and colleagues obtained results suggesting an association between a polymorphism in the D4 dopamine receptor gene (DRD4) and scores on the self-transcendence scale of the TCI ($p<0.02$),[24] although this observation has not been reproduced.[25] Still, it is interesting to compare these findings with those of Newberg and colleagues, who have used neuroimaging techniques to understand the changes in brain activity during meditation. While observing cerebral blood flow during meditation in trained meditators (Buddhist monks), these researchers found an overall increase in cortical activity and suggested that this change might be related to the altered sense of space and connectedness experienced by the monks during meditation.[26] In a follow-up review of the physiology of meditation, Newberg and Iversen summarized the many studies that indicate meditation influences neurotransmitters, including increasing dopamine in the striatum, as well as increasing serum concentrations of arginine, vasopressin, GABA, melatonin and serotonin, and decreasing serum cortisol and norepinephrine.[27]

Dr. Dean Hamer, chief of gene structure at the National Cancer Institute, has published a book called "The God Gene,"[28] in which he describes studies on spirituality. He reviews a study initially targeted to better understand smoking addiction, in which he recruited 1,000 men and women and obtained TCI questionnaire scores. He reports finding a large variation among the subjects in the subscore for spirituality on the TCI. Moreover, although some have suggested that patients who are more influenced by spiritual experiences are likely to be more "temperamental" or "anxious," Hamer and colleagues found just the opposite. Subjects also provided biological samples, from which Hamer and his colleagues looked for a genetic explanation for the variation in the spiritual score on the questionnaire and keyed in on the vesicular monoamine transporter 2 gene (VMAT2). Although his work is intriguing, it has not been reproduced or thoroughly assessed by the scientific community. Furthermore, Hamer is the first to admit:

> Human behaviors, and the brain circuits that produce them, are undoubtedly the product of intricate networks involving hundreds to thousands of genes working in concert with multiple developmental and environmental events. Further advances in the field will require the development of microarray analysis that measures the activity of many different genes simultaneously. Only then will the gene hunters have a shot at achieving the promises held out by the past century of classical behavior genetics research.[29]

Spirituality as a Clinical Intervention

Integrating the spiritual into the everyday practice of medicine can be difficult. Anadarajah and Hight[30] reviewed tools for such formal assessment and integration of spirituality into medical practice and found the majority were developed for use by pastoral counselors and nurses, or as research instruments. They further commented: "Little has been written about approaches developed for use by practicing physicians in a routine medical encounter." Therefore, they designed a tool that can be incorporated into general practice: the HOPE questionnaire. A more comprehensive discussion of spiritual assessment tools can be found at http://www.gwu.edu/~cicd/toolkit/spiritual.htm (accessed Dec. 30, 2004). It is anticipated that this increased interest in the spiritual component of health will lead to many more useful tools for assessment of spirituality and, ultimately, to the ability to individualize a health plan for patients that includes the entirety of the human experience. For now, it is clear that "one size does not fit all" is true even for such practices as meditation, relaxation, and prayer; in reality, these practices will be experienced differently by each of us.

Summary

The relationship between genes, genetic expression, and spirituality is a new, intriguing area of research. Although we know that different life experiences can affect our spiritual selves, these new areas of research are showing how our unique genetic, physical selves also influence our sense of spirit and the divine (and vice versa). These studies also help us understand that patients may need different types of intervention and spiritual support; for example, some may find meditation easy to perform on their own, with a more successful result on such physical parameters as blood pressure, whereas some patients may require designated teachers or programs, not because they aren't trying hard enough, but because they aren't as "biochemically susceptible" to the effects of mediation. Clinicians will need to adapt research findings to their clinical practices—never an easy task. But surely we are all better off—patients and practitioners alike—for bringing knowledge and awareness of this important subject into both scientific inquiry and clinical practice.

References

1. Nebert DW, Russell DW. Clinical importance of the cytochromes P450. Lancet. 2002;360:1155-62.
2. Cheng P-Y, Morgan ET. Hepatic cytochrome P450 regulation in disease states. Curr Drug Metab. 2001;2:165-83.
3. Liska DJ. The detoxification enzyme systems. Altern Med Rev. 1998;3:187-98.
4. Sung KC, Ryu SH. Insulin resistance, body mass index, waist circumference are independent risk factors for high blood pressure. Clin Exp Hypertens. 2004;26:547-56.
5. Doll S, Paccaud F, Bovet P, et al. Body mass index, abdominal adiposity and blood pressure: consistency of their association across developing and developed countries. Int J Obes Relat Metab Disord. 2002;26:48-57.
6. Lukaczer D, Liska DJ. Recognizing insulin resistance syndrome. Integrative Med. 2003;2:42-48.
7. Suk HJ, Ridker PM, Cook NR, Zee RY. Relation of polymorphism within the C-reactive protein gene and plasma CRP levels. Atherosclerosis. 2005;178(1):139-45.
8. Siest G, Jeannesson E, Berrahmoune H, et al. Pharmacogenomics and drug response in cardiovascular disorders. Pharmacogenomics. 2004;5:779-802.
9. Tracy RP. Inflammation, the metabolic syndrome and cardiovascular risk. Int J Clin Pract. 2003;134 Suppl :10-17.
10. Stefanick ML, Mackey S, Sheehan M, et al. Effects of diet and exercise in men and postmenopausal women with low levels of HDL cholesterol and high levels of LDL cholesterol. N Engl J Med. 1998;339:12-20.
11. King DE, Bushwick B. Beliefs and attitudes of hospital inpatients about faith healing and prayer. J Fam Pract. 1994;39:349-52.
12. Monroe MH, Bynum D, Susi B, et al. Primary care physician preference regarding spiritual behavior in medical practice. Arch Intern Med. 2003;163:2751-56.
13. Levin J. Spiritual determinants of health and healing: an epidemiological perspective on salutogenic mechanisms. Altern Ther. 2003;9:48-57.
14. Ehrlich E, Flexner SB, Carruth G, Hawkins JM, eds. The Oxford American Dictionary. New York, NY: Avon Books. 1980:883.
15. Ibid, p. 764.
16. Harinath K, Malhotra AS, Pal K, et al. Effects of Hatha yoga and Omkar meditation on cardiorespiratory performance, psychologic profile, and melatonin secretion. J Altern Complement Med. 2004;10:261-68.
17. Dedert EA, Studts JL, Weissbecker I, et al. Religiosity may help preserve the cortisol rhythm in women with stress-related illness. Int J Psychiatry Med. 2004;34:61-77.
18. Davidson RJ, Kabat-Zinn J, Schumacher J, et al. Alterations in brain and immune function produced by mindfulness meditation. Psychosom Med. 2003;65:564-70.
19. Sklan EH, Lowenthal A, Korner M, et al. Acetylcholinesterase/paraoxonase genotype and expression predict anxiety scores in health, risk factors, exercise training, and genetics study. Proc Nat Acad Sci. 2004;101:5512-17.
20. Rossi EL. Stress-induced alternative gene splicing in mind-body medicine. Adv Mind Body Med. 2004;20:12-19.
21. Roberts RL, Luty SE, Mulder RT, et al. Association between cytochrome P450 2D6 genotype and harm avoidance. Am J Med Genet B Neuropsychiatr Genet. 2004;127:90-93.
22. Bouchard TJ Jr, McGue M. Genetic and environmental influences on human psychological differences. J Neurobiol. 2003;54:4-45.
23. Bouchard TJ Jr, McGue M, Lykken D, Tellegen A. Intrinsic and extrinsic religiousness: genetic and environmental influences and personality correlates. Twin Res. 1999;2:88-98.
24. Comings DE, Gonzalez N, Saucier G, et al. The DRD4 gene and the spiritual transcendence scale of the character temperament index. Psychiatr Genet. 2000;10:185-89.
25. Lee HJ, Lee HS, Kim YK, et al. D2 and D4 dopamine receptor gene polymorphisms and personality traits in a young Korean population. Am J Med Genet B Neuropsychiatr Genet. 2003;121:44-49.
26. Newberg A, Alavi A, Baime M, et al. The measurement of regional cerebral blood flow during the complex cognitive task of meditation: a preliminary SPECT study. Psychiatry Res. 2001;106:113-22.
27. Newberg AB, Iversen J. The neural basis of the complex mental task of meditation: neurotransmitter and neurochemical considerations. Med Hypothesis. 2003;61:282-91.
28. Hamer DH. The God Gene. New York, NY: Doubleday Press; 2004.
29. Hamer D. Rethinking behavior genetics. Science. 298;2002:71-72.
30. Anandarajah G, Hight E. Spirituality and medical practice: using the HOPE questions as a practical tool for spiritual assessment. Am Fam Physician. 2001;63:81-88.

Section IV

Fundamental Physiological Processes

Chapter 15
Communications: Intracellular and Extracellular

Gary Darland, PhD

Introduction

The Hippocratic concept of the four humors (phlegm, blood, black and yellow bile) may have been the first widely accepted concept of homeostasis. Imbalance among the four was thought to result in what today we call disease. Much more recently, homeostasis has been defined in *Dorland's Medical Dictionary* as "a tendency to stability in the normal body states (internal environment) of the organism." The definition goes on to mention that this is achieved by a system of negative feedbacks. Although implied in the latter definition, it is often overlooked that the maintenance of stability is an active process. A constant flow of information is necessary to determine the appropriate response, and energy is required to generate the response. Cells are continually monitoring both the intra- and extra-cellular environment and adjusting their biochemical processes accordingly. Unlike the implication in Dorland's definition, the responses can be either negative or positive. It's becoming increasingly apparent that many chronic diseases result from failures in these regulatory processes.

All cells, whether they are the simple prokaryotic bacteria, or the highly differentiated eukaryotic cells that comprise the human body, must be able to sense and respond to their environment. Within the eukaryotic kingdom, the biochemical mechanisms underlying these processes are nearly ubiquitous. The basics can be described rather simply, but the combinations and permutations of the interactions lead to an often bewildering complexity. It is probably not much of an exaggeration to say that at this level the "web of life" metaphor becomes reality.

There are two (at least) methods of approaching the concept of homeostasis from the standpoint of signal recognition and response. One can discuss either multiple examples briefly or go deeper into a few selected mechanisms. We have chosen the second method, and will use this space to discuss two examples of cellular communications in some detail: redox and energy sensing. We hope that these discussions will enhance the reader's understanding of similar physiological processes in other areas.

In multicelluar organisms, cellular communication occurs over varying distances. Autocrine signals are used to monitor the intracellular environment. Paracrine signals are transferred between adjacent cells. Finally, endocrine signals are produced by the endocrine glands and transmitted throughout the body. Regardless of the type of signaling, the basic molecular mechanisms are conserved. Protein receptors bind to specific molecules termed ligands and undergo a conformational change resulting in the acquisition of some biochemical activity. The acquired activity results in the transduction from the receptor to one or more effector molecules. The specifics of the process can be simple, such as opening an ion channel, but typically a cascade of reactions is involved. The term *signal transduction* is often applied to this process. In common with electronic circuitry from which the analogy is drawn, amplification, distribution, and feedback are all part of the process. Feedback is particularly important and at least one of the effector molecules can be counted upon to turn off the pathway. It is becoming increasingly apparent that one of the characteristics of many chronic diseases is defective feedback circuitry.

Signal Transduction

At the heart of signal transduction are the cellular receptors that respond to changes in the environment. Three general classes of cellular receptors exist and are described briefly below. A prerequisite for all receptors is that binding to specific ligands is necessary to affect signal transduction; in the absence of a receptor-ligand complex, the receptors are effectively shut off.

Receptor tyrosine kinases (RTKs) represent a class of receptor proteins that share four general features. They are transmembrane proteins with an extracellular binding domain that recognizes their specific ligand. For example, the insulin receptor binds specifically to insulin and this bind initiates a series of biochemical reactions that adjust the physiological state of muscle and fat cells to elevated serum glucose. Binding of the ligand to the receptor initiates a conformational change that is transmitted through the membrane to the intracellular tyrosine kinase and the regulatory domains of the receptor. (See Figure 15.1.) The tyrosine kinase domain then catalyzes the addition of a phosphate group donated by ATP to tyrosyl residues in specific substrate proteins; in many (if not most) cases, autophosphorylation occurs as well:

$$\text{Pr-TyrOH} + \text{ATP} \rightarrow \text{Pr-Tyr-OPO}_3 + \text{ADP}.$$

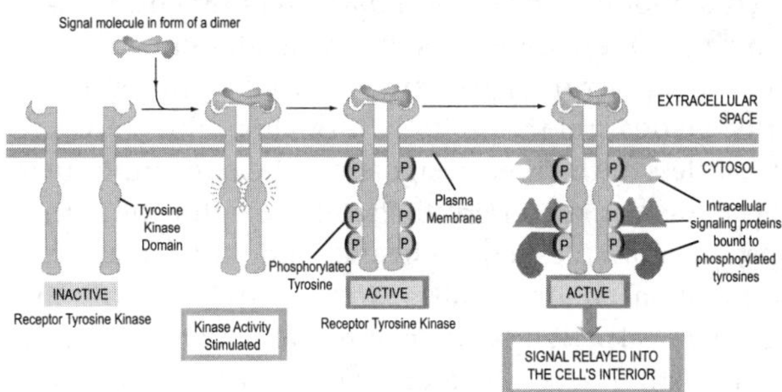

Figure 15.1 **Activation of a typical receptor tyrosine kinase**

The second class of receptors is coupled to a family of heterotrimeric ($\alpha\beta\gamma$) GTP-binding and hydrolyzing proteins (G-proteins).[1] These **G-protein coupled receptors** (GPCRs) are integral membrane proteins that also transmit extracellular signals to the cell interior. Their characteristic hallmark is the existence of seven membrane-spanning regions that enable the protein to weave its way through the cell membrane. Upon ligand binding, an interaction with G-proteins is initiated and an exchange of GDP for GTP on the α- subunit ensues. The α-ATP complex then dissociates from the trimer and initiates the signal cascade. The specific results are governed by the specific α-isoform (Figure 15.2). The effects of many of the peptide hormones, like glucagon and prolactin, are mediated through GPCRs.

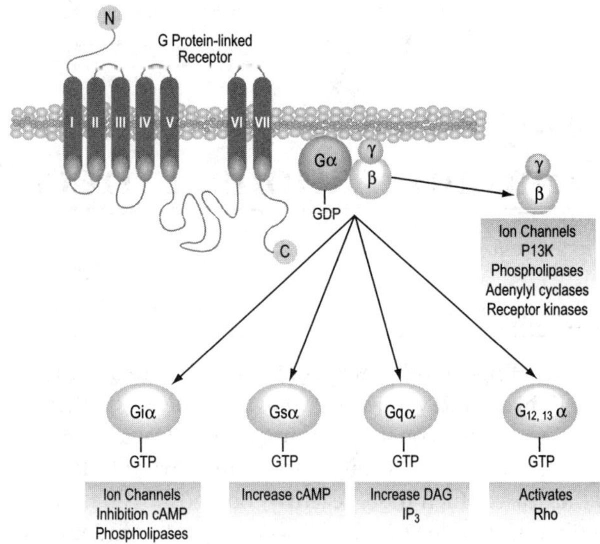

Figure 15.2 **Signal transduction through G-protein coupled receptors**

Once a "signal" is detected by the membrane receptors, it must act upon it. In order to do this, downstream biochemical pathways must be activated or inhibited. The mechanism by which this is achieved relies to a large extent on the phosphorylation/dephosphorylation of a variety of proteins. The process is often referred to colloquially as the "kinase cascade." A typical eukaryotic cell is awash in protein kinases and phosphatases. When it was discovered in the early 1960s that glycogen metabolism was to a large extent under the control of the reversible phosphorylation/dephosphorylation of glycogen phosphorylase, it was considered to be somewhat of an oddity. As more examples were discovered, the importance of kinases and phosphatases in the control of cell physiology was recognized; in 1992, the Nobel Prize in Medicine and Physiology was awarded to Edmond Fisher and Edwin Krebs. Since then, the number of protein kinases has continued to grow; it now stands at roughly 518,[2] representing over 1.7% of all known human genes, and perhaps one-third that many phosphatases.[3] It has been estimated that perhaps as many as 30% of human proteins are covalently modifiable with phosphate.[4]

The recognition that the cellular homologs of the viral oncogenes *v-src* and *v-abl* existed was followed shortly by the recognition that proteins encoded by the genes *c-src* and *c-abl*[5] were protein tyrosine kinases.[6,7,8,9] The significance of these findings soon became apparent when it was discovered[10,11] that a chromosomal translocation fused most of the *c-abl* domain with the 5′-end of *BCR* [i] (a serine/threonine kinase),[12] resulting in a more active kinase that was associated with chronic myelogenous leukemia. Targeting of the affected kinase by imatinib mesylate (*Gleevec*™) has proved to be an effective therapy[13] for this malignancy. A hint about the versatility of directing therapy toward this class of enzymes, and perhaps a hint of things to come, is a recent clinical report[14] indicating that treatment with imatinib mesylate cured a 70-year-old woman with long-standing type 2 diabetes.

Mitogens, growth factors, and a variety of other stimuli (including the inflammatory cytokines) activate the **MAPK (mitogen activated protein kinase) cascade** by binding to their respective membrane receptors (Figure 15.3). A series of kinases are activated that culminate in the activation of the "terminal" MAPKs: ERK, JNK, and p38. These then move into the nucleus and activate a transcriptional program that can lead to cell division or, at the other extreme, to programmed cell death (apoptosis). While the pathway and nomenclature can often bewilder, there is some logic inherent in the cascade. Regardless of the actual stimulus, a sequential activation of kinases occurs (see Figure 15.4) that ultimately transmits information from the cell membrane to the genome, or terminal effector proteins. Activation of all members of the cascade requires phosphorylation on multiple residues by an upstream kinase. Thus, in a typical cascade, protein kinase A (PKA) is activated by ligand binding to a GPCR. Adenyl cyclase is activated and the intracellular concentration of cAMP increases followed by the activation of PKA. MAPKKK (MAPK kinase kinase; aka MEKK) is then activated by phosphorylation catalyzed by PKA. Upon activation, it phosphorylates MAPKK, and so on.

[i] The BCR gene is the site of breakpoints used in the generation of the two alternative forms of the Philadelphia chromosome translocation found in chronic myeloid leukemia and acute lymphocytic leukemia. Online Mendelian Inheritance in Man, accessed (http://www.ncbi.nlm.nih.gov/entrez/dispomim.cgi?id=151410).

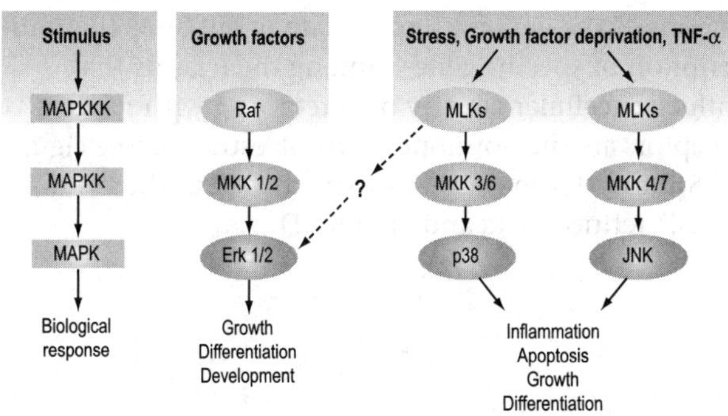

Figure 15.3 **MAPK cascade**

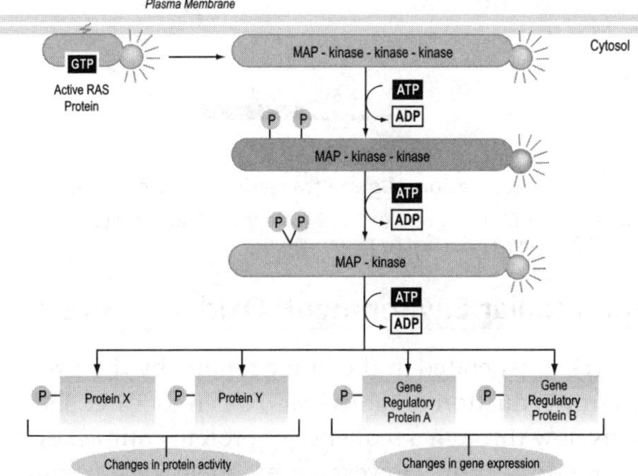

Figure 15.4 **Integration of GPCR with MAPK**

Proteins are not the only signal molecules available to the cell. Phosphatidylinositol-4,5 bisphosphate (PIP_2), a component of the cell membrane, also serves in this capacity. Phospholipases hydrolyze PIP_2, producing 1,2-diacylglycerol (DAG), which remains bound to the membrane, and inositol triphosphate (IP_3), which is soluble and released into the cytoplasm where it serves as another second messenger, analogous to cAMP. IP_3 interacts with intracellular receptors and stimulates the increase in intracellular Ca^{2+} by opening membrane calcium channels or releasing intracellular stores from the endoplasmic reticulum.

The final class of signal transducing receptors is represented by the **nuclear hormone receptor superfamily**. This group of highly conserved proteins resides in the cytoplasm and, upon binding to their (generally lipophilic) ligands, translocates into the nucleus. Upon entering the nucleus, these proteins bind to specific regions of the genome and initiate or enhance the transcription of specific genes. Among the ligands that influence cellular activity by interacting with nuclear receptors are the hormones cortisol, estradiol (see Figure 15.5), testosterone and thyroxin, as well as the "vitamins," retinoic acid and vitamin D_3.

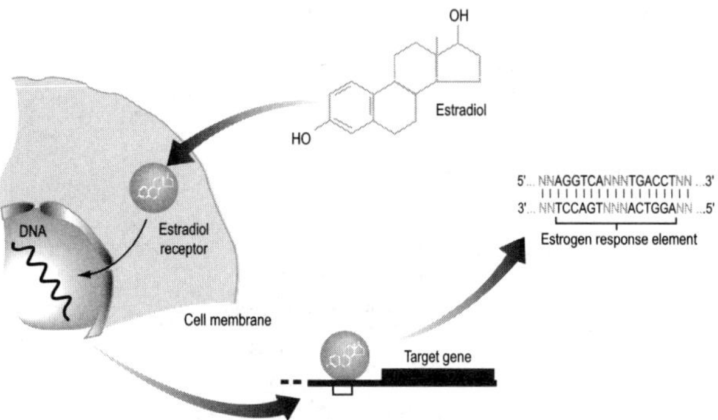

Figure 15.5 **Regulation of gene transcription by estradiol**

Source: Brown TA. Genomes, 2nd Ed., Bios Scientific Publishers Ltd: Oxford UK; 2002. Figure 12.5. Used by permission.

Intracellular Environment: Oxidative Stress

ATP is generated in the mitochondria by the two electron reduction of molecular oxygen to water. Electrons flow through a sequence of protein complexes in an orderly fashion. However, even under ideal conditions, electrons leak from mitochondria and are capable of reducing molecular oxygen to superoxide:[15,16]

$$O_2 + e^- \rightarrow O_2^-$$

It has been estimated that between 1 and 2% of molecular oxygen is consumed in this manner.[17] Under some conditions (like diabetes), mitochondrial dysfunction increases and the potential for even higher concentrations of superoxide exists.[18,19]

Superoxide in and of itself is relatively innocuous but it is a portent of more serious consequences. The enzyme superoxide dismutase catalyzes the reduction of superoxide to hydrogen peroxide:

$$2O_2^- + 2H^+ \rightarrow H_2O_2$$

Cells have a variety of mechanisms for disposing of hydrogen peroxide, including catalase and several peroxidases, the most important of which may be glutathione (GSH) peroxidase that catalyzes the reaction:

$$2GSH + H_2O_2 \rightarrow GSSG + 2H_2O$$

The reaction consumes glutathione, a sulfur containing tripeptide with a number of important cellular functions.[20] One of the more important is serving as a redox buffer to keep the cellular environment properly poised to insure proper protein folding and enzymatic activity.[21,22,23] (See Figure 15.6.) The redox state of the cell is controlled to a large (but not exclusive) extent by the GSH/GSSG couple:

$$2GSH \leftrightarrow GSSG + 2H^+ + 2e^-$$

$$E_h = E'_0 + 31.25^* [(GSSG)/(GSH)^2],$$

where $E'_0 \approx -264$ mV at 37° C and pH = 7.4.[24]

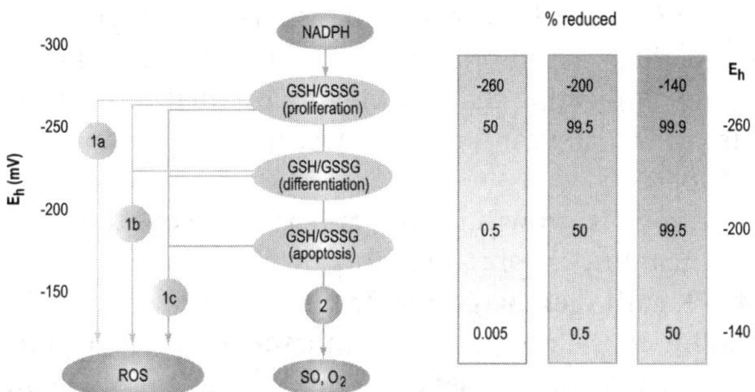

Figure 15.6 **Effect of redox state on cellular activity and protein folding**

Reprinted from Jones (2002) Meth Enz 348:93 with permission from Elsevier.

In addition to serving as a redox buffer, glutathione is consumed as a substrate in several key reactions, all depleting cellular GSH reserves: conjugation of GSH to electrophiles[25,26] and protein thiols;[27] its role in amino acid uptake [28] and drug export;[29,30] and the export of GSSG[31] as a means of maintaining E_h. If left unchecked, the cells would enter a state of oxidative stress and death would rapidly ensue (see Figure 15.1). Given the sensitivity of cells to changes in redox status, it should come as no surprise that means have evolved to keep glutathione tone in an optimum range. The reduction of GSSG is carried out by the NADPH-dependent enzyme, glutathione reductase. The primary source of NADPH is the pentose phosphate cycle and inhibition of this pathway with agents such as DHEA[32] reduces intracellular GSH.[33] The rate-limiting step in the *de novo* synthesis is the synthesis of γ-glutamyl cysteine, a reaction performed by a specific ligase. Reduction of GSH by the induction of GST with isothiocyanate[34] or by reducing the rate of GSSG reduction by depletion of NADPH[35] stimulates the synthesis of GSH. Increasing the E_h by stimulating differentiation increases the expression of glutamate:cysteine ligase[36] in an attempt to keep GSH and E_h constant. The importance of this enzyme is also illustrated by the fact that the overexpression of the enzyme in adenovirus-transformed cells protected them from the oxidative stress induced by IL-1β.[37] It is possible to increase the GSH in cells by treating with non-toxic cysteine donors like N-acetyl cysteine or L-2-oxo-thiazolidine-4-carboxylate[38] or flavonoids.[39]

Redox control of the transcription factor NF-κB is the model for redox control of gene expression.[40] In an early attempt to explain often conflicting data, Dröge and his coworkers[41] proposed that increased oxidative stress in the cytoplasm was necessary to activate translocation into the nucleus, but that reducing conditions were necessary in the cytoplasm. Despite skepticism regarding the specifics of this model,[42] data continue to appear in the literature in support of the general concept. The activity of receptors or their downstream partners can be controlled by either the redox state of the cell or by covalent modification by glutathione. Although current data often appear contradictory, it is apparent that redox signaling and glutathione have key roles to play in the regulation of transcription factors and support for the hypothesis continues to appear in the literature.[43,44,45,46,47,48,49,50]

Regulation of Metabolic Processes

All cells are confronted with the task of balancing energy production and utilization. ATP is energy currency in biological systems, so the problem becomes one of keeping the concentration of ATP at levels that are optimal for cell function. A healthy cell must maintain an ATP/ADP ratio of about 10:1.[51] In the 1960s, Atkinson rationalized and quantified this concept by introducing the term "energy charge." The enzyme adenylate kinase was a key player in the concept because, if the reaction

$$2ADP \rightarrow ATP + AMP$$

was at equilibrium, then

$$[AMP]/[ATP] = \{[ADP]/[ATP]\}^2.$$

Since the ratio of AMP/ATP varies as the square of the ADP/ATP ratio, it becomes a sensitive indicator of the health of the cell; small changes in the ADP/ATP ratio are accompanied by relatively large changes in the ratio of AMP/ATP. All of this might have remained an interesting curiosity had it not been for the discovery of a family of enzymes, AMPK/SNF1, that is universally distributed in all eukaryotes.[52,53] The mammalian AMP-activated protein kinases (AMPK) that balance anabolic and catabolic pathways are based on the ratio of AMP/ATP.

Enzyme Basics

The enzyme that was later to be named AMPK was originally isolated by Yeh and co-workers,[54] who catalyzed the 5AMP-dependent phosphorylation of acetyl CoA carboxylase (ACC), the rate-limiting step in fatty acid biosynthesis:

$$\text{acetyl-CoA} + CO_2 \rightarrow \text{malonyl-CoA}$$

Within limits, the authors were able to demonstrate the activity of AMPK increases with an increase in the ratio of AMP/ATP. The ensuing phosphorylation of ACC inhibits the enzyme, effectively shutting off fatty acid biosynthesis. As the ratio increases, kinase activity drops and ACC activity increases. When the enzyme was finally cloned and sequenced, it was discovered to be widely distributed in the eukaryotic kingdom.[55,56] The enzyme is heterotrimeric and each subunit has multiple isoforms that exhibit tissue specific distribution;[57] 12 heterotrimeric combinations are possible.

AMPK is a serine/threonine kinase that is activated by phosphorylation. Although the specifics are still somewhat sketchy, it appears that at a minimum a specific threonine residue (T^{172}) must be phosphorylated for AMPK to exhibit enzymatic activity. The identity of the specific kinase has not yet been confirmed. (The kinase is usually referred to as AMPKK but the fact that it is named does not yet mean that it has been identified.) Recently, a probable candidate has emerged, a tumor-suppressor gene, LKB1, has been shown to phosphorylate not only AMPK but thirteen other kinases with similar structure.[58] Regulation of AMPK is complex and includes not only phosphorylation but allosteric activation by AMP, which makes it a better substrate for the upstream kinase while at the same time making it a worse substrate for phosphatases. Finally, AMPKK is allosterically activated by AMP.[59]

Role of AMPK in Muscle

It is estimated that, in humans, 70% of glucose disposal occurs in skeletal muscle (the bulk of the remainder is handled largely by the liver). The glucose transporter GLUT-4 is instrumental in the uptake of glucose by muscle cells. Upon stimulation by insulin or exercise, it is recruited to the plasma membrane and facilitates glucose uptake. Emerging evidence implicates AMPK in GLUT-4 translocation in both insulin-dependent and insulin-independent pathways. During exercise, ATP is consumed and the ratio of AMP/ATP increases leading to a stimulation of AMPK. At the same time, GLUT-4 expression and activity are increased.[60] The effects are limited to the muscles affected, but systemic effects can be demonstrated by the use of 5-aminoimidazole-4-carboxamide-β-D-ribofuranoside (AICAR), an intermediate in purine biosynthesis that, upon uptake by cells, is rapidly converted into an AMP analog that stimulates AMPK. Chronic administration mimics many of the effects of exercise, increased GLUT-4 expression, membrane localization and glucose transport[61] as well as potentiating the effect of insulin. In animal models, AICAR has been shown to relieve some of the symptoms associated with metabolic syndrome,[62] an observation that makes AMPK an attractive therapeutic target.

Unlike other tissues, skeletal (and cardiac) muscle possesses a single isoform of ACC, ACC-2.[63] Like ACC-1, it becomes inactive upon phosphorylation. Since neither skeletal nor heart muscle carries out *de novo* fatty acid synthesis, the question arose as to why they should possess ACC in the first place and why should it be under such stringent control. The hypothesis was advanced[64] that its function was to generate malonyl-CoA which could then be used to regulate fatty acid oxidation. High concentrations of malonyl-CoA are known to inhibit carnitine palmitoyl transferase-1 (CPT-1) the gatekeeper of fatty acid transport into the mitochondrion. By inhibiting CPT-1, fatty acid oxidation is effectively curtailed. Under conditions where energy demand is high, such as vigorous exercise, fatty acid oxidation should not be limited by transport into the mitochondrion, where one would expect ACC-2 activity to be minimal. AMPK activation leads to phosphorylation and inactivation of ACC-2. This hypothesis has now been confirmed under several different conditions.[65,66,67,68,69] The most direct confirmation of the hypothesis was provided by Abu-Elheiga and coworkers,[70,71] who demonstrated that ACC-2 knockout mice were hyperphagic and resistant to obesity, and that fatty acid oxidation was enhanced and not inhibited by insulin.

Conditions that increase AMP, or provision of an AMP surrogate, indicate that cells are operating at a deficit under these conditions; pathways that have the potential to increase energy generation are favored. Thus, in muscle cells, glucose transport is enhanced and fatty acid oxidation increased. Both are the result of AMPK activation. As we will see below, the same principle applies to other cells of the body; while the specifics differ, the underlying principle remains the same.

The Role of AMPK in Liver

The classic targets of AMPK in the liver are ACC and HMG-CoA reductase, the first committed step on the sterol biosynthetic pathway.[72] Exposure of freshly isolated hepatocytes to AICAR results in the rapid (<10 min) inhibition of both biosynthetic enzymes.[73] In the liver, AMPK not only affects lipid biosynthesis but modulates glycogen metabolism. Infusion of AICAR into the portal vein of dogs at concentrations sufficient to stimulate AMPK stimulated glycogenolysis and hepatic glucose output even under conditions of hyperinsulinemic conditions.[74] The authors attributed the glycogenolytic effect of AMPK to some of its demonstrated effects as an inhibitor of glycogen synthase and a stimulator of glycogen phosphorylase, both of which are achieved by phosphorylation of the enzyme. It demonstrates that response of liver cells to high AMP levels can overcome the normal response of hepatocytes to insulin. The hepatic output of glucose that results from AICAR administration compares well with the stimulation of glucose uptake by muscle under the same conditions and can be rationalized as a response by the liver to reduced energy levels.

The liver is the principal organ involved in converting excess carbohydrates into fatty acids and triglycerides. This happens within minutes of exposure to elevated glucose, and is mediated in part, posttranslationally, by AMPK-activated glycolysis and lipogenesis. It has also become apparent that not only does activation of AMPK exert effects on enzyme activity through phosphorylation, but there are also marked effects on the expression of a number of glycolytic and lipogenic enzymes. Included in this list are the genes for the liver isoform of pyruvate kinase (L-PK), fatty acid synthase (FAS). It is well established that in the presence of insulin high levels of glucose stimulate the expression of genes involved in conversion of carbohydrates to lipids in the liver.[75,76] It now appears that insulin plays an indirect role in this response merely by promoting glucose metabolism; glucose metabolites are the true effector molecules. The genes regulated in this manner, such as FAS and L-PK, are characterized by a unique DNA sequence within their promoters, referred to as the carbohydrate response element (ChRE).[77,78] When activated by high concentrations of glucose metabolites, a specific transcription factor[79,80,81] binds to the promoter and transcription is initiated. Under conditions in which AMPK is activated, by AICAR[82,83] or by genetic manipulation,[84] transcription driven by ChRE is blunted.

The Role of AMPK in Adipose Tissue

Adipose tissue is the major storage site for triglycerides. Therefore, one might expect that, under conditions in which energy charge is low and AMPK is activated, lipolysis would be stimulated in order to increase systemic levels of a readily available source of energy in the form of fatty acids. Exposure of adipocytes to β-adrenergic agents stimulates hormone sensitive lipase (HSL) and the release of fatty acids from triglyceride stores. Activation of HSL is initiated by phosphorylation of the enzyme by protein kinase A (PKA).[85] Contrary to expectations, however, under conditions in which AMPK is activated,[86] the release of fatty acids from adipocytes is actually reduced. Phosphorylation of HSL by AMPK prevents phosphorylation by PKA. The explanation for this apparent paradox rests with the recognition that if fatty acid release from adipocytes exceeds the capacity of tissues such as muscle to utilize it, a futile cycle would ensue and the adipocytes would actually suffer an energy drain under conditions when demand for energy preservation is expected to be high (i.e., high AMP).

The Role of AMPK in the Hypothalamus

Thus far, we have been concerned with what might be called the local effects of AMPK activation. Since the early 2000s, an appreciation has been developing for the fact that AMPK may actually play a role in feeding behavior and, therefore, in the regulation of whole-body energy metabolism. Hints that this might be the case first appeared when it was discovered that two adipocyte-derived hormones, leptin[87] and adiponectin,[88] activated AMPK in muscle and liver, respectively.

It has been known for some time that leptin inhibits feeding behavior and that ghrelin, a peptide hormone synthesized in the stomach, stimulates feeding, and that both act, at least in part, via the same neuronal circuits. It has now been shown that both have direct effects on AMPK activity within the hypothalamus. Intraperitoneal injection of leptin inhibits, and ghrelin stimulates, AMPK activity. Furthermore, stimulation of AMPK by administering AICAR directly to the hypothalamus through an in-dwelling catheter stimulated food intake.[89] Alpha-lipoic acid (α-LA) has a history of use in diabetic neuropathy; recently it has been shown to possess anti-obesity effects that appear to be the result of the suppression of hypothalamic AMPK activity.[90] The anorexic effects of α-LA were due neither to toxicity nor leptin; the latter possibility was eliminated since the effects were observed in leptin-deficient mice (*ob/ob*). AICAR administered directly to the hypothalamus reversed the effects of α-LA. Intraperitoneal injection of α-LA to rats caused a significant decrease in the phosphorylation of both AMPK and ACC within the hypothalamus. In peripheral tissues, α-LA is known to increase glucose transport and cellular ATP levels, conditions that typically inhibit AMPK activation. While the authors did not demonstrate this effect directly, they were able to show that by manipulating the energy status within the hypothalamus they inhibited AMPK.

Studies that began in yeast and progressed to mammalian cells in order to determine how energy charge was maintained have now advanced to the state where the same basic mechanism can account, at least in part, for the control of feeding behavior and body weight in mammals.

Metabolic Syndrome: A Failure to Communicate?

As discussed in other parts of this book, there is an epidemic of metabolic syndrome and type 2 diabetes affecting nearly 50 million individuals in the United States alone.[91] The reasons for the "outbreak" are complex, but lack of exercise and poor diet top the list. The consequences are well known. However, from a physiological standpoint, the disease can be viewed as a general breakdown in cellular signaling mechanisms that evolved to maintain homeostasis. It is perhaps fair to say that the recognition that adipose tissue is a major source of signaling peptides—adiponectin, leptin, and inflammatory cytokines like IL-6 and TNF-α (as reviewed by Gimeno and Klaman[92])—has shaped a dramatic rethinking concerning the causes and therapy of the disease. It is now clear that while lowering blood glucose is necessary, it is not sufficient for managing this condition effectively.

The complexity of these signaling pathways can be gleaned from a quick glance at Figure 15.7. The diagram represents the events that are initiated when insulin binds to its receptor on the surface of an idealized cell. The end result ranges from the familiar—translocation of the glucose transporter (GLUT4) to the cell surface to facilitate glucose uptake—to activation of members of the MAPK pathway, culminating in the initiation of transcription. Along the way, interaction with RAS, a member of the GPCR kinase family, can be seen. Clearly, when a state of insulin resistance develops, it is one of the early indicators of metabolic syndrome, with the potential for a lot of chaos.

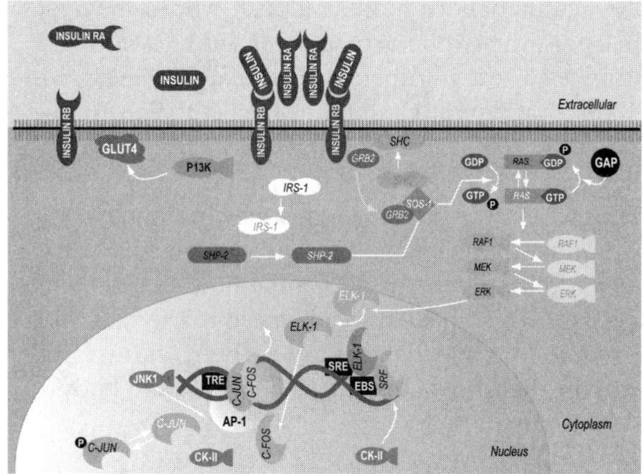

Figure 15.7 **Insulin signaling pathway**

Considerable effort is being devoted to ameliorating metabolic syndrome and type 2 diabetes by modifying insulin signaling. It should come as no surprise that many of the traditional medicines that have been used for centuries to treat diabetes have recently been demonstrated to affect these very same signaling pathways.[93] While it is not possible to discuss all the potential combinations and permutations, two targets are currently the subject of much active research and provide the potential for significant progress in treating the current epidemic. Both are subject to modification by dietary intervention, providing some confidence that pharmaceutical agents need not be the first approach.

Peroxisome Proliferator-Activated Receptors (PPARs)

PPARs are members of the nuclear hormone superfamily and, when bound to their activating ligands, they move from the cytoplasm into the nucleus, bind to specific regions of DNA (termed peroxisome proliferator response elements, or PPREs), and stimulate transcription. They differ from the steroid hormone receptors in that they tend to be promiscuous with regard to their ligands. Thus, molecules as seemingly different as arachidonic acid and pioglitazone (Actos™) are both agonists. There are three members of the family:

- PPARα is a transcription factor that activates the transcription of genes involved in fatty acid oxidation.[94]
- PPARγ is actively involved in adipogenesis, the initiation and development of adipocytes.[95,96]
- PPARδ(β) has similar ligand binding properties but its actual role in cell physiology is still largely unknown.[97]

The interest in PPARs as potential therapeutic targets derives largely from the results obtained with two classes of pharmaceutical agents. The fibrates are PPARα agonists and have proven under appropriate circumstances to be effective lipid lowering agents.[98] Insulin sensitivity has been shown to improve in response to intervention with glitazones a prototypical PPARγ agonist.[99,100] Both classes of compounds were discovered without knowing their primary targets; only later was their mode of action determined when they were found to activate the metabolism of xenobiotics.

Both classes of compound are thought to work in part by reducing circulating triglycerides. Fibrates do so by increasing the rate of disposal via stimulation of fatty acid oxidation. The PPARγ agonists are a little more subtle. By stimulating adipogenesis, they provide a site in which triglycerides may be deposited, effectively removing them from the circulation. In fact, one of the side effects of glitazones therapy is weight gain. Their paradoxical behavior (weight gain concomitant with improved insulin sensitivity) is explained by the fact that they while they induce adipogenesis, the adipocytes stay small. It is the large adipocytes that generate most of the adipocytokines that are now being recognized as major contributors to metabolic syndrome and insulin resistance.

The range of natural products known to exhibit activity as modulators of PPAR activity is impressive.[101] Activators range from the everyday (soy phytoestrogens) to the esoteric (ajulemic acid from *Cannabis sativa*). Obese Zucker rats maintained on a high-soy diet exhibited greatly improved glucose tolerance that could be associated with the ability to activate both PPARγ- and

PPARα-driven gene expression.[102] Similar results were obtained with ethanolic extracts of licorice by Mae and colleagues.[103] A wide variety of prenylflavonoids derived from licorice were found to be potent activators of PPARγ and their effects translated into decreased fasting insulin and systolic blood pressure. When one also considers that certain dietary fatty acids[104] exhibit similar effects, there can be little doubt of the potential benefit afforded by attention to diet.

Adiponectin

Adiponectin (adipocyte complement-related protein of 30 kDa, or ACRP30) is a peptide hormone that is secreted exclusively by adipocytes. Circulating levels in healthy adults range from about 2 to 17 μg/mL,[105] or nearly 0.01% of the total plasma protein. It is synthesized as 30 kDa monomer but, by virtue of a collagen-like binding domain, forms homotrimers or even higher order structures. It is induced during adipocyte differentiation and its secretion is stimulated by insulin.[106] As might be expected with such a protein, it has been shown that PPARγ agonists increase its expression and plasma concentration.[107] The authors evaluated troglitazone (Rezulin™) in middle-aged, slightly overweight (BMI 29.1 ± 0.8 kg/m^2) subjects, and found that adiponectin increased roughly two-fold. The results were duplicated in *db/db* mice, in which they were also able to demonstrate an increase in adiponectin specific mRNA. Although adiponectin is an adipocyte-specific protein, its expression and serum levels decrease with increasing obesity and/or insulin resistance.[108,109,110,111] Adiponectin improves insulin sensitivity and exhibits anti-inflammatory activity. Low levels of circulating adiponectin are thus linked *mechanistically* to insulin resistance and type 2 diabetes, rather than just being biochemical markers of an abnormal metabolic state. It's particularly interesting that, in Rhesus monkeys prone to the development of type 2 diabetes subsequent to obesity, adiponectin declines prior to the development of diabetes,[112] suggesting predictive value for this serum protein.

Adiponectin regulates glucose and lipid metabolism in muscle, liver, and adipocytes. Binding to cell surface receptors in muscle cells leads to activation of AMPK[113] and it has been shown recently in type 2 diabetics that activation of AMPK by adiponectin is impaired.[114]

In laboratory animals, a short-term intervention with a soy-protein diet increases the expression of adiponectin.[115,116] The durations of the experiments were too short (10 days) to result in significant weight loss, so it appears that soy protein is affecting adiponectin expression independently of body weight.

Summary

Evolution has resulted in the elaboration of sophisticated mechanisms to maintain cells (and whole organisms) in an optimal state. The systems are not foolproof. If balance is significantly disturbed, it can be difficult to return to a state of grace. The pathways utilized to maintain homeostasis may look bewildering (as in Figure 15.7), but in reality control is achieved by the application of relatively few mechanisms, highly elaborated to be sure, but fairly simple at their core.

One of these vital mechanisms is phosphorylation. The judicious use of kinases to modify enzymes and proteins by adding phosphate groups and thereby changing the activity, positively or negatively, is universally used by eukaryotes to control cell physiology. The second basic mechanism discussed above is the use of redox chemistry, particularly in the form of sulfhydryl groups (as for example in glutathione), to maintain the redox potential of cells in an optimal range.

If one steps back and tries to visualize the forest rather than the trees, the beauty and functional simplicity of the systems are remarkable.

References

1. Casey PJ, Gilman AG. G protein involvement in receptor-effector coupling. J Biol Chem. 1988;263(6):2577-80.
2. Manning G, Whyte DB, Martinez R, et al. The protein kinase complement of the human genome. Science. 2002;298(5600):1912-34.
3. Cohen P. The role of protein phosphorylation in human health and disease. The Sir Hans Krebs Medal Lecture. Eur J Biochem. 2001;268(19):5001-10.
4. Ibid.
5. Goff SP, Gilboa E, Witte ON, Baltimore D. Structure of the Abelson murine leukemia virus genome and the homologous cellular gene: studies with cloned viral DNA. Cell. 1980;22(3):777-85.
6. Schartl M, Barnekow A. The expression in eukaryotes of a tyrosine kinase which is reactive with pp60v-src antibodies. Differentiation. 1982;23(2):109-14.
7. Iba H, Cross FR, Garber EA, Hanafusa H. Low level of cellular protein phosphorylation by nontransforming overproduced p60c-src. Mol Cell Biol. 1985;5(5):1058-66.
8. Groffen J, Heisterkamp N, Reynolds FH Jr, Stephenson JR. Homology between phosphotyrosine acceptor site of human c-abl and viral oncogene products. Nature. 1983;304(5922):167-69.
9. Wang JY, Baltimore D. Localization of tyrosine kinase-coding region in v-abl oncogene by the expression of v-abl-encoded proteins in bacteria. J Biol Chem. 1985;260(1):64-71.

10. Heisterkamp N, Stephenson JR, Groffen J, et al. Localization of the c-ab1 oncogene adjacent to a translocation break point in chronic myelocytic leukaemia. Nature. 1983;306(5940):239-42.
11. Bernards A, Rubin CM, Westbrook CA, et al. The first intron in the human c-abl gene is at least 200 kilobases long and is a target for translocations in chronic myelogenous leukemia. Mol Cell Biol. 1987;7(9):3231-36.
12. Maru Y, Witte ON. The BCR gene encodes a novel serine/threonine kinase activity within a single exon. Cell. 1991;67(3):459-68.
13. Stone RM. Optimizing treatment of chronic myeloid leukemia: a rational approach. Oncologist. 2004;9(3):259-70.
14. Veneri D, Franchini M, Bonora E. Imatinib and regression of type 2 diabetes. N Engl J Med. 2005;352(10):1049-50.
15. Han D, Williams E, Cadenas E. Mitochondrial respiratory chain-dependent generation of superoxide anion and its release into the intermembrane space. Biochem J. 2001;353:411-16.
16. Lambert AJ, Brand MD. Superoxide production by NADH: ubiquinone oxidoreductase (complex I) depends on the pH gradient across the mitochondrial inner membrane. Biochem J. 2004;382:511-17.
17. Chance B, Sies H, Boveris A. Hydroperoxide metabolism in mammalian organs. Physiol Rev. 1979;59:527-605.
18. Kelley DE, He J, Menshikova EV, Ritov VB. Dysfunction of mitochondria in human skeletal muscle in type 2 diabetes. Diabetes. 2000;51:2944-50.
19. Lowell BB, Shulman GI. Mitochondrial dysfunction and type 2 diabetes. Science. 2005;307:384-7.
20. Meister A. Glutathione metabolism and its selective modification. J Biol Chem. 1988:263:17205-8.
21. Mosharov E, Cranford MR, Banerjee R. The quantitatively important relationship between homocysteine metabolism and glutathione synthesis by the transsulfuration pathway and its regulation by redox changes. Biochemistry. 2000;24:13005-11.
22. Miller LT, Watson WH, Kirlin WG,et al. Oxidation of the glutathione/glutathione disulfide redox state is induced by cysteine deficiency in human colon carcinoma HT29 cells. J Nutr. 2002;132:2303-6.
23. Jones DP. Redox potential of GSH/GSSG couple: assay and biological significance. Methods Enzymol. 2002;348:93-112.
24. Schafer FQ, Buettner GR. Redox environment of the cell as viewed through the redox state of the glutathione disulfide/glutathione couple. Free Radic Biol Med. 2001;30(11):1191-212.
25. Coles BF, Kadlubar FF. Detoxification of electrophilic compounds by glutathione S-transferase catalysis: determinants of individual response to chemical carcinogens and chemotherapeutic drugs? Biofactors. 2003;17(1-4):115-30.
26. Tew KD. Glutathione-associated enzymes in anticancer drug resistance. Cancer Res. 1994;54(16):4313-20.
27. Pompella A, Visvikis A, Paolicchi A, et al. The changing faces of glutathione, a cellular protagonist. Biochem Pharmacol. 2003;66(8):1499-503.
28. Cornell JS, Meister A. Glutathione and gamma-glutamyl cycle enzymes in crypt and villus tip cells of rat jejunal mucosa. Proc Natl Acad Sci U S A. 1976;73(2):420-22.
29. Borst P, Evers R, Kool M, Wijnholds J. A family of drug transporters: the multidrug resistance associated proteins. J Natl Cancer Inst. 2000;92(16):1295-302.
30. Ishikawa T. The ATP-dependent glutathione S-conjugate export pump. Trends Biochem Sci. 1992;17(11):463-68.
31. Sies H, Akerboom TP. Glutathione disulfide (GSSG) efflux from cells and tissues. Methods Enzymol. 1984;105:445-51.
32. Hollenberg PF. Mechanisms of cytochrome P450 and peroxidase-catalyzed xenobiotic metabolism. FASEB J. 1992;6(2):686-94.
33. Schafer FQ, Buettner GR. Redox environment of the cell as viewed through the redox state of the glutathione disulfide/glutathione couple. Free Radic Biol Med. 2001;30(11):1191-212.
34. Kirlin WG, Cai J, Thompson SA, et al. Glutathione redox potential in response to differentiation and enzyme inducers. Free Radic Biol Med. 1999;27(11-12):1208-18.
35. Shi MM, Kugelman A, Iwamoto T, et al. Quinone-induced oxidative stress elevates glutathione and induces gamma-glutamylcysteine synthetase activity in rat lung epithelial L2 cells. J Biol Chem. 1994;269(42):26512-17.
36. Kirlin WG, Cai J, Thompson SA, et al. Glutathione redox potential in response to differentiation and enzyme inducers. Free Radic Biol Med. 1999;27(11-12):1208-18.
37. Tran PO, Parker SM, LeRoy E, et al. Adenoviral overexpression of the glutamylcysteine ligase catalytic subunit protects pancreatic islets against oxidative stress. J Biol Chem. 2004;279(52):53988-93.
38. Schafer FQ, Buettner GR. Redox environment of the cell as viewed through the redox state of the glutathione disulfide/glutathione couple. Free Radic Biol Med. 2001;30(11):1191-212.
39. Myhrstad MC, Carlsen H, Nordstrom O, et al. Flavonoids increase the intracellular glutathione level by transactivation of the gamma-glutamylcysteine synthetase catalytical subunit promoter. Free Radic Biol Med. 2002;32(5):386-93.
40. Janssen-Heininger YM, Poynter ME, Baeuerle PA. Recent advances towards understanding redox mechanisms in the activation of nuclear factor kappa B. Free Radic Biol Med. 2000;28(9):1317-27.
41. Dröge W, Schulze-Osthoff K, Mihm S, et al. Functions of glutathione and glutathione disulfide in immunology and immunopathology. FASEB J. 1994;8(14):1131-38.
42. Bowie A, O'Neill LA. Oxidative stress and nuclear factor-kappa B activation: a reassessment of the evidence in the light of recent discoveries. Biochem Pharmacol. 2000;59(1):13-23.
43. Janssen-Heininger YM, Poynter ME, Baeuerle PA. Recent advances towards understanding redox mechanisms in the activation of nuclear factor kappa B. Free Radic Biol Med. 2000;28(9):1317-27.
44. Haddad JJ, Olver RE, Land SC. Antioxidant/pro-oxidant equilibrium regulates HIF-1a and NF-k B redox sensitivity. Evidence for inhibition by glutathione oxidation in alveolar epithelial cells. J Biol Chem. 2000;275(28):21130-39.
45. Pineda-Molina E, Klatt P, Vazquez J, et al. Glutathionylation of the p50 subunit of NF-kappa B: a mechanism for redox-induced inhibition of DNA binding. Biochemistry. 2001;40(47):14134-42.
46. Xiao GG, Wang M, Li N, et al. Use of proteomics to demonstrate a hierarchical oxidative stress response to diesel exhaust particle chemicals in a macrophage cell line. J Biol Chem. 2003;278(50):50781-90.
47. D'Alessio M, Cerella C, Amici C, et al. Glutathione depletion upregulates Bcl-2 in BSO-resistant cells. FASEB J. 2004 Oct;18(13):1609-11.
48. Barbieri SS, Cavalca V, Eligini S, et al. Apocynin prevents cyclooxygenase 2 expression in human monocytes through NADPH oxidase and glutathione redox-dependent mechanisms. Free Radic Biol Med. 2004;37(2):156-65.
49. Kabe Y, Ando K, Hirao S, et al. Redox regulation of NF-kappa B activation: distinct redox regulation between the cytoplasm and the nucleus. Antioxid Redox Signal. 2005;7(3-4):395-403.
50. Ndengele MM, Muscoli C, Wang ZQ, et al. Superoxide potentiates NF-kappa B activation and modulates endotoxin-induced cytokine production in alveolar macrophages. Shock. 2005;23(2):186-93.
51. Hardie DG, Hawley SA. AMP-activated protein kinase: the energy charge hypothesis revisited. Bioessays. 2001;23(12):1112-19.
52. Carling D. AMP-activated protein kinase: balancing the scales. Biochimie. 2005;87(1):87-91.

53. Hardie DG, Carling D, Carlson M. The AMP-activated/SNF1 protein kinase subfamily: metabolic sensors of the eukaryotic cell? Annu Rev Biochem. 1998;67:821-55.
54. Yeh LA, Lee KH, Kim KH. Regulation of rat liver acetyl-CoA carboxylase. Regulation of phosphorylation and inactivation of acetyl-CoA carboxylase by the adenylate energy charge. J Biol Chem. 1980;255(6):2308-14.
55. Carling D, Aguan K, Woods A, et al. Mammalian AMP-activated protein kinase is homologous to yeast and plant protein kinases involved in the regulation of carbon metabolism. J Biol Chem. 1994;269(15):11442-48.
56. Stapleton D, Mitchelhill KI, Gao G, et al. Mammalian AMP-activated protein kinase subfamily. J Biol Chem. 1996;271(2):611-14.
57. Rutter GA, Da Silva Xavier G, Leclerc I. Roles of 5'-AMP-activated protein kinase (AMPK) in mammalian glucose homoeostasis. Biochem J. 2003;375(Pt 1):1-16.
58. Lizcano JM, Goransson O, Toth R, et al. LKB1 is a master kinase that activates 13 kinases of the AMPK subfamily, including MARK/PAR-1. EMBO J. 2004;23(4):833-43.
59. Winder WW, Hardie DG. AMP-activated protein kinase, a metabolic master switch: possible roles in type 2 diabetes. Am J Physiol. 1999;277(1 Pt 1):E1-10.
60. Ren JM, Semenkovich CF, Gulve EA, et al. Exercise induces rapid increases in GLUT4 expression, glucose transport capacity, and insulin-stimulated glycogen storage in muscle. J Biol Chem. 1994;269(20):14396-401.
61. Jessen N, Pold R, Buhl ES, et al. Effects of AICAR and exercise on insulin-stimulated glucose uptake, signaling, and GLUT-4 content in rat muscles. J Appl Physiol. 2003;94(4):1373-79.
62. Buhl ES, Jessen N, Pold R, et al. Long-term AICAR administration reduces metabolic disturbances and lowers blood pressure in rats displaying features of the insulin resistance syndrome. Diabetes. 2002;51(7):2199-206.
63. Hardie DG, Pan DA. Regulation of fatty acid synthesis and oxidation by the AMP-activated protein kinase. Biochem Soc Trans. 2002;30(Pt 6):1064-70.
64. McGarry JD, Brown NF. The mitochondrial carnitine palmitoyltransferase system. From concept to molecular analysis. Eur J Biochem. 1997;244(1):1-14.
65. Merrill GF, Kurth EJ, Hardie DG, Winder WW. AICA riboside increases AMP-activated protein kinase, fatty acid oxidation, and glucose uptake in rat muscle. Am J Physiol. 1997;273(6 Pt 1):E1107-12.
66. Ruderman NB, Saha AK, Vavvas D, Witters LA. Malonyl-CoA, fuel sensing, and insulin resistance. Am J Physiol. 1999;276(1 Pt 1):E1-E18.
67. Winder WW, Holmes BF. Insulin stimulation of glucose uptake fails to decrease palmitate oxidation in muscle if AMPK is activated. J Appl Physiol. 2000;89(6):2430-37.
68. Ruderman NB, Saha AK, Kraegen EW. Minireview: malonyl CoA, AMP-activated protein kinase, and adiposity. Endocrinology. 2003;144(12):5166-71.
69. Roepstorff C, Halberg N, Hillig T, et al. Malonyl-CoA and carnitine in regulation of fat oxidation in human skeletal muscle during exercise. Am J Physiol Endocrinol Metab. 2005;288(1):E133-42.
70. Abu-Elheiga L, Oh W, Kordari P, Wakil SJ. Acetyl-CoA carboxylase 2 mutant mice are protected against obesity and diabetes induced by high-fat/high-carbohydrate diets. Proc Natl Acad Sci U S A. 2003;100(18):10207-12.
71. Abu-Elheiga L, Matzuk MM, Abo-Hashema KA, Wakil SJ. Continuous fatty acid oxidation and reduced fat storage in mice lacking acetyl-CoA carboxylase 2. Science. 2001;291(5513):2613-16.
72. Hardie DG, Carling D, Carlson M. The AMP-activated/SNF1 protein kinase subfamily: metabolic sensors of the eukaryotic cell? Annu Rev Biochem. 1998;67:821-55.
73. Henin N, Vincent MF, Gruber HE, Van den Berghe G. Inhibition of fatty acid and cholesterol synthesis by stimulation of AMP activated protein kinase. FASEB J. 1995;9(7):541-46.
74. Camacho RC, Pencek RR, Lacy DB, et al. Portal venous 5-aminoimidazole-4-carboxamide-1-beta-D-ribofuranoside infusion overcomes hyperinsulinemic suppression of endogenous glucose output. Diabetes. 2005;54(2):373-82.
75. Girard J, Ferre P, Foufelle F. Mechanisms by which carbohydrates regulate expression of genes for glycolytic and lipogenic enzymes. Annu Rev Nutr. 1997;17:325-52.
76. Towle HC, Kaytor EN, Shih HM. Regulation of the expression of lipogenic enzyme genes by carbohydrate. Annu Rev Nutr. 1997;17:405-33.
77. Shih HM, Towle HC. Definition of the carbohydrate response element of the rat S14 gene. Evidence for a common factor required for carbohydrate regulation of hepatic genes. J Biol Chem. 1992;267(19):13222-28.
78. Shih HM, Liu Z, Towle HC. Two CACGTG motifs with proper spacing dictate the carbohydrate regulation of hepatic gene transcription. J Biol Chem. 1995;270(37):21991-97.
79. Liu Z, Thompson KS, Towle HC. Carbohydrate regulation of the rat L-type pyruvate kinase gene requires two nuclear factors: LF A1 and a member of the c-myc family. J Biol Chem. 1993;268(17):12787-95.
80. Yamashita H, Takenoshita M, Sakurai M, et al. A glucose-responsive transcription factor that regulates carbohydrate metabolism in the liver. Proc Natl Acad Sci U S A. 2001;98(16):9116-21.
81. Koo SH, Towle HC. Glucose regulation of mouse S(14) gene expression in hepatocytes. Involvement of a novel transcription factor complex. J Biol Chem. 2000;275(7):5200-7.
82. Foretz M, Carling D, Guichard C, et al. AMP-activated protein kinase inhibits the glucose-activated expression of fatty acid synthase gene in rat hepatocytes. J Biol Chem. 1998;273(24):14767-71.
83. Leclerc I, Kahn A, Doiron B. The 5'-AMP-activated protein kinase inhibits the transcriptional stimulation by glucose in liver cells, acting through the glucose response complex. FEBS Lett. 1998;431(2):180-84.
84. Woods A, Azzout-Marniche D, Foretz M, et al. Characterization of the role of AMP-activated protein kinase in the regulation of glucose-activated gene expression using constitutively active and dominant negative forms of the kinase. Mol Cell Biol. 2000;20(18):6704-11.
85. Yeaman SJ. Hormone-sensitive lipase—new roles for an old enzyme. Biochem J. 2004;379(Pt 1):11-22.
86. Sullivan JE, Brocklehurst KJ, Marley AE, et al. Inhibition of lipolysis and lipogenesis in isolated rat adipocytes with AICAR, a cell-permeable activator of AMP-activated protein kinase. FEBS Lett. 1994;353(1):33-36.
87. Minokoshi Y, Kim YB, Peroni OD, et al. Leptin stimulates fatty-acid oxidation by activating AMP-activated protein kinase. Nature. 2002;415(6869):339-43.
88. Yamauchi T, Kamon J, Waki H, et al. The fat-derived hormone adiponectin reverses insulin resistance associated with both lipoatrophy and obesity. Nat Med. 2001;7(8):941-46.
89. Andersson U, Filipsson K, Abbott CR, et al. AMP-activated protein kinase plays a role in the control of food intake. J Biol Chem. 2004;279(13):12005-8.
90. Kim MS, Park JY, Namkoong C, et al. Anti-obesity effects of alpha-lipoic acid mediated by suppression of hypothalamic AMP-activated protein kinase. Nat Med. 2004;10(7):727-33.

91. National Center for Chronic Disease Prevention and Health Promotion web site http://www.cdc.gov/nccdphp/dnpa/obesity/trend/metabolic.htm. Accessed 16Apr2005
92. Gimeno RE, Klaman LD. Adipose tissue as an active endocrine organ: recent advances. Curr Opin Pharmacol. 2005;5(2):122-28.
93. Huang TH, Kota BP, Razmovski V, Roufogalis BD. Herbal or natural medicines as modulators of peroxisome proliferators activated receptors and related nuclear receptors for therapy of metabolic syndrome. Basic Clin Pharmacol Toxicol. 2005;96(1):3-14.
94. Chu R, Lim H, Brumfield L, et al. Protein profiling of mouse livers with peroxisome proliferators activated receptor alpha activation. Mol Cell Biol. 2004;24(14):6288-97.
95. Tzameli I, Fang H, Ollero M, et al. Regulated production of a peroxisome proliferator-activated receptor-gamma ligand during an early phase of adipocyte differentiation in 3T3-L1 adipocytes. J Biol Chem. 2004;279(34):36093-102.
96. Farmer SR. Regulation of PPAR gamma activity during adipogenesis. Int J Obes Relat Metab Disord. 2005;29 Suppl 1:S13-6.
97. Fredenrich A, Grimaldi PA. PPAR delta: an uncompletely known nuclear receptor. Diabetes Metab. 2005;31(1):23-7.
98. van Raalte DH, Li M, Pritchard PH, Wasan KM. Peroxisome proliferator-activated receptor (PPAR)-alpha: a pharmacological target with a promising future. Pharm Res. 2004;21(9):1531-38.
99. Mooradian AD, Chehade J, Thurman JE. The role of thiazolidinediones in the treatment of patients with type 2 diabetes mellitus. Treat Endocrinol. 2002;1(1):13-20.
100. Edelman SV. The role of the thiazolidinediones in the practical management of patients with type 2 diabetes and cardiovascular risk factors. Rev Cardiovasc Med. 2003;4 Suppl 6:S29-37.
101. Huang TH, Kota BP, Razmovski V, Roufogalis BD. Herbal or natural medicines as modulators of peroxisome proliferators activated receptors and related nuclear receptors for therapy of metabolic syndrome. Basic Clin Pharmacol Toxicol. 2005;96(1):3-14.
102. Mezei O, Banz WJ, Steger RW, et al. Soy isoflavones exert antidiabetic and hypolipidemic effects through the PPAR pathways in obese Zucker rats and murine RAW 264.7 cells. J Nutr. 2003; 133(5):1238-43.
103. Mae T, Kishida H, Nishiyama T, et al. A licorice ethanolic extract with peroxisome proliferator-activated receptor-gamma ligand-binding activity affects diabetes in KK-Ay mice, abdominal obesity in diet-induced obese C57BL mice and hypertension in spontaneously hypertensive rats. J Nutr. 2003;133(11):3369-77.
104. Nakamura MT, Cheon Y, Li Y, Nara TY. Mechanisms of regulation of gene expression by fatty acids. Lipids. 2004 Nov;39(11):1077-83.
105. Wong GW, Wang J, Hug C, et al. A family of Acrp30/adiponectin structural and functional paralogs. Proc Natl Acad Sci U S A. 2004;101(28):10302-7.
106. Meier U, Gressner AM. Endocrine regulation of energy metabolism: review of pathobiochemical and clinical chemical aspects of leptin, ghrelin, adiponectin, and resistin. Clin Chem. 2004;50(9):1511-25.
107. Maeda N, Takahashi M, Funahashi T, et al. PPAR gamma ligands increase expression and plasma concentrations of adiponectin, an adipose-derived protein. Diabetes. 2001;50(9):2094-99.
108. Matsubara M, Maruoka S, Katayose S. Inverse relationship between plasma adiponectin and leptin concentrations in normal-weight and obese women. Eur J Endocrinol. 2002;147(2):173-80.
109. Kern PA, Di Gregorio GB, Lu T, et al. Adiponectin expression from human adipose tissue: relation to obesity, insulin resistance, and tumor necrosis factor-alpha expression. Diabetes. 2003;52(7):1779-85.
110. Ryo M, Nakamura T, Kihara S, et al. Adiponectin as a biomarker of the metabolic syndrome. Circ J. 2004;68(11):975-81.
111. Matsuzawa Y. Adiponectin: Identification, physiology and clinical relevance in metabolic and vascular disease. Atheroscler Suppl. 2005;6(2):7-14.
112. Hotta K, Funahashi T, Bodkin NL, et al. Circulating concentrations of the adipocyte protein adiponectin are decreased in parallel with reduced insulin sensitivity during the progression to type 2 diabetes in rhesus monkeys. Diabetes. 2001;50(5):1126-33.
113. Yamauchi T, Kamon J, Minokoshi Y, et al. Adiponectin stimulates glucose utilization and fatty-acid oxidation by activating AMP-activated protein kinase. Nat Med. 2002;8(11):1288-95.
114. Chen MB, McAinch AJ, Macaulay SL, et al. Impaired activation of AMP-kinase and fatty acid oxidation by globular adiponectin in cultured human skeletal muscle from obese type 2 diabetics. J Clin Endocrinol Metab. 2005;Mar 15(preprint).
115. Nagasawa A, Fukui K, Kojima M, et al. Divergent effects of soy protein diet on the expression of adipocytokines. Biochem Biophys Res Commun. 2003;311(4):909-14.
116. Nagasawa A, Fukui K, Funahashi T, et al. Effects of soy protein diet on the expression of adipose genes and plasma adiponectin. Horm Metab Res. 2002;34(11-12):635-39.

Chapter 16
Bioenergetics and Biotransformation

Gary Darland, PhD

Introduction

Energy is the *sine qua non* of life. With the exception of green plants and some bacteria, all energy is derived by the orderly breakdown of simple organic compounds and the capture of the energy released. The major catabolic pathways for accomplishing this task are highly conserved and found in all life forms today.

All chemicals, including foods, possess intrinsic energy; if burned, heat is released and it is possible to devise an engine to transform this energy into work. In the latter half of the 19th century J. Willard Gibbs applied the first and second laws of thermodynamics and developed the concept of free energy (ΔG), a measure of the capacity of a system to perform work. Formally, the equation is

$$\Delta G = \Delta H - T\Delta S$$

It incorporates the concepts of enthalpy (H), or heat content, and entropy (S), a tendency of a closed system to approach total disorder. According to Gibbs "all systems change in such a way that free energy is minimized." By convention if $\Delta G < 0$, useful energy is produced; otherwise, energy is consumed. Any chemical reaction includes the release or consumption of energy.

In order to make useful comparisons between reactions, it is necessary to have a fixed frame of reference. Hence, the term "standard free energy change" was defined as

$$\Delta G^0 = -RT \ln K_{eq}$$

where K_{eq} is the equilibrium constant for the reaction in question, R is the gas constant (1.987 cal mol^{-1} K^{-1}), and T = 298° K (25° C). In a closed system, one that is not influenced by outside factors, chemical reactions proceed toward equilibrium.

The discussion below summarizes the primary energy-producing pathways of the cell. It is not meant to describe all of the ways in which macronutrients enter into the central metabolic pathways. It is reasonable for clinicians to ask of what relevance is the material presented below to clinical medicine. Aside from an appreciation of the beauty of the biochemistry, the answer can be as varied as medicine itself.

Perhaps consideration of the role of the micronutrient coenzyme Q (CoQ) can serve as an illustration. As described below, CoQ plays a central role in oxidative phosphorylation, the major source of ATP (energy). A deficiency of CoQ results in both a decrease in energy production and an increase in reactive oxygen species. Thus, it could be hypothesized that conditions like chronic fatigue syndrome might respond favorably to supplemental CoQ, a supposition that has been borne out in a few studies.[1,2] Furthermore, since statins inhibit the synthesis of CoQ, it is also a reasonable hypothesis that side effects of statin therapy are possible (and have, in fact, been noted).[3] Whether or not the side effects are directly related to the inhibition of CoQ—and whether the addition of CoQ to statin therapies will improve outcomes—are the subjects of ongoing research. There are some interesting studies reporting benefit for combination therapy of CoQ and statins.[4,5]

Anaerobic Catabolism of Glucose: Glycolysis

A central characteristic that distinguishes metabolic pathways from a simple chemical transformation is that the former generally involve numerous individual reactions. Since thermodynamics deals only with initial and final states, and not the path by which equilibrium is reached, the involvement of multiple reactions does not affect the amount of energy available. It does, however, permit cells to capture some of the energy for use in critical activities. The compound that serves this function is adenosine triphosphate (ATP), illustrated in Figure 16.1.

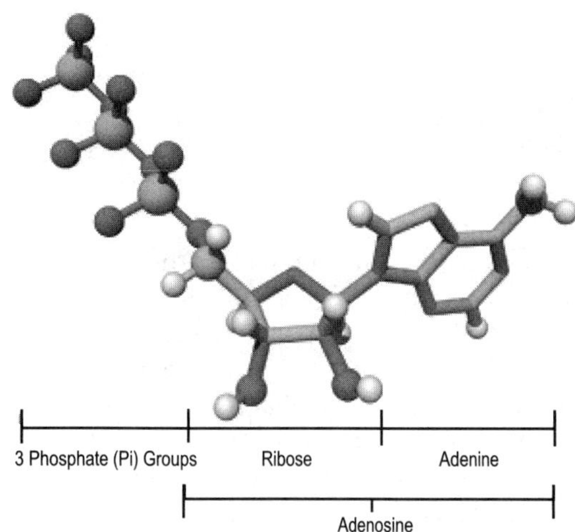

Figure 16.1 **The structure of adenosine triphosphate (ATP)**

Glycolysis, the anaerobic conversion of glucose to two molecules of lactic acid, illustrates this concept. The formula for the chemical conversion of glucose to lactic acid is:

glucose → 2 lactate + 2 H^+, $\Delta G° = -47.4$ kcal/mol,

while the same conversion performed by the glycolytic pathway results in:

glucose + 2P_i + 2ADP → 2 lactate + 2 H^+ +2 ATP, $\Delta G° = -29.7$ kcal/mol,

or a release of roughly eighteen fewer kcal/mol of glucose converted.[i] The missing energy was stored in the terminal phosphoester bond of the two ATP molecules.

ATP + H_2O → ADP + inorganic phosphate, $\Delta G° = -7.3$ kcal/mol,

or, alternatively:

ATP + H_2O → AMP+ pyrophosphate, $\Delta G° = -7.3$ kcal/mol.

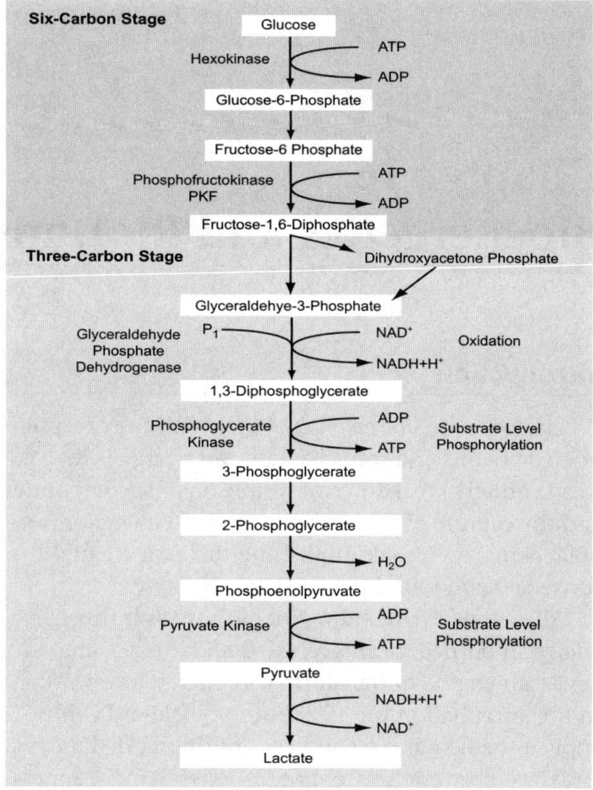

Figure 16.2 **Glycolysis or the Embden, Meyerhof and Parnas pathway**

The glycolytic pathway is ancient and has persisted virtually unchanged since shortly after the origin of life.[6] It was elucidated in the early 20th century and is often referred to as the Embden, Meyerhof and Parnas (EMP) pathway, after its discoverers. Examination of Figure 16.2 reveals two molecules of ATP are actually consumed early in the pathway in order to convert one molecule of glucose into a molecule of fructose-1,6- diphosphate:

glucose + ATP → glucose-6- P_i

fructose-6-P + ATP → fructose-1,6- di P_i.

This investment is recovered, with interest, in the two energy-producing steps in the pathway:

1,3- diphosphoglycerate + H^+ +ATP → 3- phosphoglycerate + ATP

phosphenolpyruvate + H^+ + ADP → pyruvate + ATP.

[i]Taken from H. R. Mahler and E. H. Cordes. Biological Chemistry, 2nd Edition. Harper and Row. 1971, p497.

Since there are two molecules of triose produced for each molecule of hexose, four ATP molecules are recovered after an investment of two.

The final accounting issue deals with the disposal of reducing equivalents, in the form of NADH, that are generated by the oxidation of glyceraldehyde-3- phosphate:

$$\text{glyceraldehyde-3- phosphate} + NAD^+ \rightarrow \text{1,3- diphosphoglycerate} + NADH + H^+.$$

In the absence of oxygen, this is achieved by reducing pyruvate to lactate:

$$\text{pyruvate} + NADH + H^+ \rightarrow \text{lactate} + NAD^+.$$

All of the ATP produced by glycolysis involves what biochemists refer to as "substrate level phosphorylation." The energy existing in a phosphoester bond in one molecule is preserved by transferring the phosphate group to ADP. (See Figure 16.2.)

Aerobic Oxidation of Pyruvate

The conversion of glucose to pyruvate by glycolysis generated two molecules of ATP, representing ~15 kcal/mol of energy currency for the cell. The complete oxidation of glucose to carbon dioxide and water has the potential to deliver in excess of 680 kcal/ mol of energy:

$$C_6H_{12}O_6 \text{ (glucose)} + O_2 \rightarrow 6CO_2 + 6H_2O, \quad \Delta G^0 \text{ -686 kcal/ mol}^{ii}$$

Only 2% of the available energy in glucose is captured by the cell. The aerobic oxidation of pyruvate enables the cells to generate considerably more ATP.

The Pyruvate Dehydrogenase Complex: Production of Acetyl-CoA

Under aerobic conditions, pyruvate is transported by a specific carrier protein into the mitochondria and transformed to acetyl-CoA by the multicomponent pyruvate dehydrogenase complex (PDC).

This complex enzyme consists of three distinct enzymes and is dependent upon both lipoic acid (part of the structure of coenzyme A) and thiamine pyrophosphate (TPP). The conversion begins with the oxidative decarboxylation of pyruvate by the E_1 component, a reaction requiring TPP:

$$E_1\text{-TPP} + \text{pyruvate} \rightarrow E_1\text{- TPP-acetaldehyde}.$$

[ii] Molecular Cell Biology. 4th ed. Lodish H, Berk A, Zipursky SL, et al. New York: W. H. Freeman & Co. 2000.

The product of this reaction, "active acetaldehyde," remains bound to the enzyme for subsequent reaction with the transacetylase (E_2) component:

$$E_1\text{- TPP-acetaldehyde} + E_2\text{-lipoamide(ox)} \rightarrow E_1\text{-TPP} + E_2\text{-lipoamide(red)-acetyl}$$

$$E_2\text{-lipoamide(red)-acetyl} + \text{Coenzyme A} \rightarrow \text{AcetylCoA} + E_2\text{-lipoamide (ox)},$$

which generates acetyl CoA and a reduced lipoamide moiety that remains affixed to E_2. The final step is oxidation of the lipoamide moiety by E_3, a reaction requiring both flavin adenine dinucleotide (FAD) and NAD^+:

$$E_2\text{-lipoamide (ox)} + E_3\text{-FAD} \rightarrow E_2\text{-lipoamide (ox)} + E_3\text{-FADH}_2$$

$$E_3\text{-FADH}_2 + NAD^+ \rightarrow E_3\text{-FAD} + NADH + H^+.$$

The net result of this sequence of reactions is:

$$\text{pyruvate} + \text{CoA} + NAD^+ \rightarrow \text{acetyl-CoA} + CO_2 + NADH + H^+.$$

The NADH generated can be used to reduce oxygen and generate ATP by oxidative phosphorylation (discussed below). In addition to an important role in biosynthesis reactions (such as lipid biosynthesis), acetyl CoA serves as the entry point to the Krebs cycle by which the oxidation of glucose is completed.

In addition to the enzymes described above, two other complex enzymes (whose function it is to control the flow of carbon through this central step) are also important. Pyruvate dehydrogenase kinase (PDK) and pyruvate dehydrogenase phosphatase control the activity of the PDC by catalyzing reversible phosphorylation/dephosphorylation of the E_1 subunit. When fatty acids are being rapidly oxidized, intramitochondrial levels of acetyl-CoA and/or ATP tend to be elevated. Under these conditions, PDK is activated and E_1 is phosphorylated. In the phosphorylated state E_1 is inactive and flow through PDC is blunted. Pyruvate is then used for anabolic purposes such as gluconeogenesis or amino acid biosynthesis. When the levels of ATP or ACoA decline, PDK activity decreases and PDP activity increases. The activity of pyruvate dehydrogenase is restored.[7,8] Diet and exercise are among the key modulators of the PDC.[9,10]

Krebs Cycle

The final steps in the oxidation of pyruvate to CO_2 and water are achieved by the Krebs, or tricarboxylic acid, cycle (Figure 16.3).

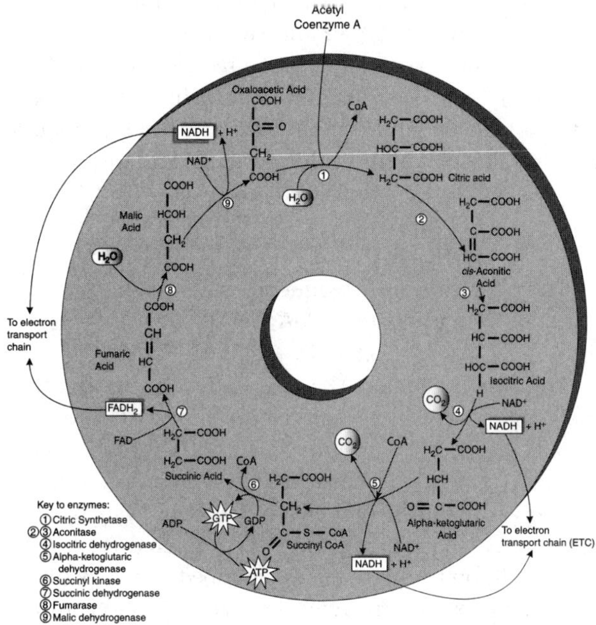

Figure 16.3 **The Krebs cycle**

It is hard to overstate the importance of the Krebs cycle cell metabolism. Not only does it play a central role in the oxidation of pyruvate, but it also serves as a source of precursors for the macromolecules that are essential to life. The eight individual reactions that comprise the cycle include three oxidative reactions that generate NADH:

isocitrate + μ-ketoglutarate + NADH + H^+

μ-ketoglutarate + NAD^+ + CoA →
succinyl- CoA + NADH + H^+

malate + NAD^+ → oxaloacetate + NADH + H^+.

The oxidation of μ-ketoglutarate is performed by an enzyme complex similar to the pyruvate dehydrogenase complex and includes the same cofactors—TPP, lipoamide and FAD.

The oxidation of succinate to fumarate is catalyzed by the flavoprotein enzyme succinate dehydrogenase:

succinate + FAD → fumarate + $FADH_2$.

The cycle includes one substrate level phosphorylation:

succinyl-CoA + GDP → succinate + GTP.

The reaction is catalyzed by the enzyme succinyl thiokinase. Energetically GTP and ATP are identical and a transphorylation reaction readily interconverts the two:

GTP+ ADP ↔ GDP + ATP.

Oxidative Phosphorylation

In addition to the complete oxidation of the carbon skeleton of pyruvate, the Krebs cycle generates eight molecules of NADH and two molecules of $FADH_2$ per molecule of glucose. The reducing equivalents must be disposed of. Mitochondria are able to achieve this and capture the energy of their oxidation as ATP by enzyme complexes located on the inner membrane of the mitochondrion that comprise the mitochondrial electron transport assembly and ATP synthase. The assembly catalyzes a series of oxidation reduction reactions, some of which are thermodynamically competent to support ATP production via ATP synthase. Proton translocation and the development of a transmembrane proton gradient provide the necessary coupling mechanism.

As in all chemical reactions, oxidation-reduction (redox) reactions involve energy. In this particular case, the amount of free energy available is expressed by the Nernst equation

$$\Delta G° = -nF\Delta E_0$$

where n represents the number of electrons and F= 23.06 kcal/volt/mol. Tables of representative values for E_0 can be found in most beginning biochemistry textbooks.

For years biochemists struggled with the mechanism by which ATP was produced in the mitochondria by the electrochemical gradient generated during the oxidation of pyruvate. The breakthrough came with the development of the chemiosmotic hypothesis by Peter Mitchell in 1961.[11] He proposed, and it has since been repeatedly confirmed, that during the oxidation of the reduced cofactors, NADH and $FADH_2$, a transmembrane proton gradient is generated. As protons move down this gradient thru complex V, F_1-F_0 ATPase, ATP is synthesized. A schematic of the process is illustrated in Figure 16.4.

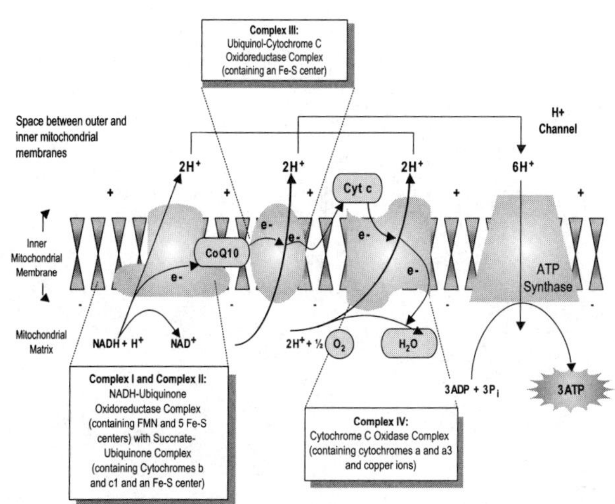

Figure 16.4 **Mitochondrial electron transport and oxidative phosphorylation**

Energy from Food

Glucose is the starting point for the central metabolic pathways described above. In order to derive energy from food, it is usually necessary to break down complex polymers of simple sugars, amino acids, or acetate. The individual components of proteins, complex carbohydrates, and fats can then enter the glycolysis (the Krebs) cycle. A wide variety of mechanisms is available to accomplish these tasks, but two are worth special consideration.

Glycogen, the principal storage form of glucose in muscle and liver, is a branched chain polysaccharide with a structure that it is similar to amylopectin, a component of starch. It consists of α–1,4 and α–1,6 glycosidic linkages between individual glucose molecules. Phosphorolysis of the α–1,4 bonds by the enzyme glycogen phosphorylase generates glucose-1-phosphate:

$$\text{glycogen}_{n+} P_i \rightarrow \text{glycogen}_{n-1} + \text{glucose-1-phosphate}.$$

The activation of glucose by ATP is not required.[iii] The interconversion of glucose-1-phosphate into glucose-6-phosphate by the enzyme phosphoglucomutase provides access to the glycolytic pathway.

Glycogen phosphorylase is a homodimeric enzyme that exists in two distinct conformational states. Under conditions where the concentration of AMP is high relative to that of ATP, the enzyme is capable of binding to glycogen and initiating the phosphorolysis of glycogen. Under normal circumstances this process is sufficient to maintain adequate glucose levels. However, under conditions of muscular exertion or stress, the activity of the enzyme can be increased. The enzyme is regulated by a reversible phosphorylation/dephosphorylation cycle. The regulation of its phosphorylation state is under the control of cAMP-dependent protein kinases and phosphatases. In the presence of epinephrine or acetylcholine, intracellular cAMP increases, thus activating glycogen phosphorylase kinase and inhibiting phosphatase. The activation leads to a rapid production of glucose-1-phosphate in the muscle, permitting accommodation of the "fight or flight" response. Uncontrolled glycogenolysis in the liver is one factor contributing to the hyperglycemic state that characterizes diabetes.[12]

Lipids and fatty acids are a major source of energy for animal cells. The oxidation of fatty acids occurs in the mitochondria. Free fatty acids are liberated from triglycerides by hydrolysis, a process catalyzed by a family of enzymes referred to as lipase. The free fatty acids are activated to their thioesters and transported into the mitochondria with the aid of carnitine palmitoyltransferase I (CPT1), carnitine-acylcarnitine translocase, and inner membrane protein CPT2.

Given the key role of carnitine in the mobilization and metabolism of fatty acids, it should come as no surprise that carnitine as its acetyl or propionyl ester has found utility in clinical situations in conditions where the efficient utilization of lipids is required.[13,14] (See Figure 16.5.)

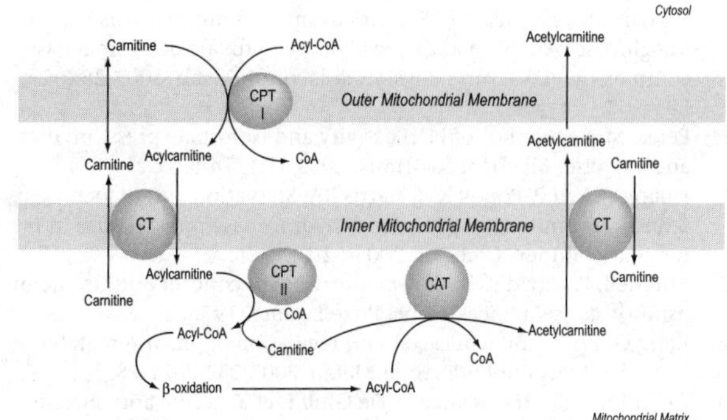

Figure 16.5 **Fatty acid oxidation**

[iii] In chemistry, one never gets something for nothing. The activation of glucose actually occurred during the synthesis of glycogen and was "stored" in the glycosidic bond.

Summary

Glycolysis and the Krebs cycle are the principal pathways by which macronutrients are converted into energy. Under anaerobic conditions, glycolysis predominates, producing lactate and ATP by substrate level phosphorylation. The process is inefficient, capturing less than 5% of the energy present in a molecule of glucose. In the presence of oxygen, however, the complete oxidation of glucose to CO_2 and water is achieved, and roughly one-third of the available energy is captured in the form of ATP. The entire process is under strict control. One of the key control points is that of the pyruvate dehydrogenase complex, the step that controls the entry of pyruvate into the Krebs cycle. Control is affected by the reversible phosphorylation/dephosphorylation of the enzyme complex.

References

1. Bentler SE, Hartz AJ, Kuhn EM. Prospective observational study of treatments for unexplained chronic fatigue. J Clin Psychiatry. 2005;66(5):625-32.
2. Werbach MR. Nutritional strategies for treating chronic fatigue syndrome. Altern Med Rev. 2000;5(2):93-108.
3. Nawarskas JJ. HMG-CoA reductase inhibitors and coenzyme Q10. Cardiol Rev. 2005;13(2):76-79.
4. Chapidze G, Kapanadze S, Dolidze N, et al. Prevention of coronary atherosclerosis by the use of combination therapy with antioxidant coenzynme Q10 and statins. Georgian Med News. 2005;(1):20-25.
5. Strey CH, Young JM, Molyneux SL, et al. Endothelium-ameliorating effects of statin therapy and coenzyme Q10 reductions in chronic heart failure. Atherosclerosis. 2005;179(1):201-6.
6. Webster KA. Evolution of the coordinate regulation of glycolytic enzyme genes by hypoxia. J Exp Biol. 2003:206:2911-22.
7. Patel MS, Korotchkina LG. Regulation of mammalian pyruvate dehydrogenase complex by phosphorylation: complexity of multiple phosphorylation sites. Exp Mol Med. 2001:33:191-97.
8. Sugden MC, Holness MJ. Recent advances in mechanisms regulating glucose oxidation at the level of the pyruvate dehydrogenase complex by PDKs. Am J Physiol Endocrinol Metab. 2003;284: E855-62.
9. Peters SJ. Regulation of PDH activity and isoform expression: diet and exercise. Biochem Soc Trans. 2003;31:1274-80.
10. Huang B, Wu P, Popov KM, Harris RA. Starvation and diabetes reduce the amount of pyruvate dehydrogenase phosphatase in rat heart and kidney. Diabetes. 2003;52:1371-76.
11. Mitchell, P. David Keilin's respiratory chain concept and its chemiosmotic consequences. Nobel Prize Lecture, 1978.
12. Jiang G, Zhang BB. Glucagon and regulation of glucose metabolism. Am J Physiol Endocrinol Metab. 2003;284:E671-78.
13. Anand I, Chandrashekhan Y, De Giuli F, et al. Acute and chronic effects of propionyl-L-carnitine on the hemodynamics, exercise capacity, and hormones in patients with congestive heart failure. Cardiovasc Drugs Ther. 1998;12:291-99.
14. Brass EP, Hiatt WR. The role of carnitine and carnitine supplementation during exercise in man and in individuals with special needs. J Am Coll Nutr. 1998;17:207-15.

Chapter 17 Digestion and Excretion

DeAnn Liska, PhD and Jeffrey S. Bland, PhD

Introduction

Every living system, whether cell, organ, whole body, or even a community of people, has to have two fundamental capacities: to bring in substances that provide energy and sustenance, and to remove waste. It is an inevitable consequence of human biology that being alive means waste is generated within the body. And, it is also a fact of life that we are exposed to innumerable substances, both beneficial and detrimental, simply by breathing, eating a meal, walking through a garden, or lying in bed. All kinds of substances are present in food, air, blankets, carpet, walls, and everything that surrounds us. Therefore, healthy function requires that the body differentiate between the good and the bad in our environment. Moreover, it is essential that the body can identify the substances necessary to maintain health and selectively take those substances into circulation, where they can nourish the cells throughout the body, while keeping out the damaging materials. To do so, the body must have protection and defense systems in place, healthy transport and circulation functions, and optimal elimination of waste.

Since this text is aimed primarily at clinicians whose professional training includes the study of normal digestive processes, we will focus our discussion here on an overview of some of the very significant ways in which normal digestive physiology is disturbed, eventually contributing to disease and bringing patients into the practitioner's office. Further perspectives on the GI tract and digestive function can be found in Chapters 24 and 28.

Over a lifetime, a person will consume over 25 tons of food, providing the body with nutrients through the digestion and absorption process. During this process, the body must maintain protection from harmful external organisms and toxins that accompany food. For example, in 1999 alone, over 1 billion pounds of pesticides were applied in the United States, and over 5.6 billion pounds were applied worldwide.[1] Pesticides are now a ubiquitous component of our environment and can be found within the home as well as in gardens and on grocery foods; even eating an organic diet cannot guarantee elimination of pesticides. Pesticide exposure is related to several types of cancers, including non-Hodgkin's lymphoma, leukemia, multiple myeloma, soft-tissue sarcoma, prostate, pancreas, lung, ovary, breast, testis, Hodgkin's disease, liver, kidney, rectum, brain and neurological system, stomach, and endometrial cancer.[2] (Further discussion of toxic exposures can be found in Chapters 13, 22, and 31.)

Conditions such as diabetes mellitus, Parkinson's disease, asthma, and hypothyroidism are also related to environmental exposures to toxic substances.[3,4,5] Toxins such as dioxin are long-lasting in the body because they are fat-soluble—they accumulate and become stored in body fat. Even pharmaceutical drugs have been found at measurable levels in rivers, drinking water, and sediments, which presumably occurs primarily from the elimination of unmetabolized drug through the urine.[6] The magnitude of these insults was discussed in a 2001 review on toxin exposure, which indicated that the expense of treating environmentally-related conditions accounts for between $57 billion and $397 billion of the healthcare economy annually in the United States and Canada.[7] Clearly, the ability to protect against these damaging substances must be part of a healthy digestion and absorption process.

Unfortunately, xenobiotics such as pesticides and pollutants aren't the only dangers that enter our system through the food we eat. Pathogens can also be present, and many individuals find that they are intolerant to certain food substances. Food allergies alone, which can be immediate (e.g., IgE-mediated) or delayed (e.g., IgG-mediated), are estimated to afflict approximately 8% of children and 2% of adults worldwide.[8] Food allergies and intolerances account for a diverse range of symptoms, from migraines and skin problems, to cardiovascular effects and gastrointestinal disorders (see Table 17.1).

Table 17.1 **Symptoms and Diseases Associated with Food Allergy and Intolerance**

System	Symptom/Disease
Cardiovascular	Edema, inflammation of the veins producing purpura, irregular heart rhythm, spontaneous bruising, urticaria, vasculitis
Gastrointestinal	Canker sores, celiac disease, chronic diarrhea, colic (babies), constipation, Crohn's disease, duodenal ulcers, gas, gastritis, indigestion, inflammatory bowel disease (IBD), irritable bowel syndrome (IBS), malabsorption, nausea, recurrent mouth ulcers, stomach ulcers, ulcerative colitis, vomiting
Genitourinary	Bed wetting, chronic bladder infections, frequent urination, nephritic syndrome
Immune	Serous otitis media
Mental/ Emotional	Attention deficit disorder, anxiety, depression, epileptic seizures, memory loss, schizophrenia
Musculoskeletal	Joint pain, myalgias, rheumatoid arthritis
Respiratory	Asthma, chronic or allergic sinusitis, constant runny nose or congested nose, nasal polyps
Skin	Eczema; itchy skin; psoriasis; red, itchy eyes; urticaria
Miscellaneous	Migraine headaches

References available in: Liska DJ, Lukaczer D. Gut restoration and chronic disease. JANA. 2002;5:20-33.

All of these examples have in common that the body must differentiate friend from foe—that is, the body must selectively identify those substances that are necessary for existence (nutrients, water, oxygen, phytonutrients, beneficial microbes) from those that are either not beneficial or, even more important, those that are detrimental. After this first step of recognition, the body must then selectively absorb and transport the necessary substances, while eliminating the detrimental materials. To do this, the body has elaborate systems for digestion and absorption, protection and defense, transport and circulation, and waste elimination.

Digestion and Absorption

From a functional medicine perspective, digestive physiology is the component of nutriture that provides the substances necessary to support bioenergetics. That is, the role of the digestive process is to prepare and separate individual nutrients from the complex food matrix that enters the body. This process begins with ingestion of the proper complement of macro- and micronutrients in the food matrix. (A more detailed description of the biochemistry of this process is provided in Chapter 16.) Individual nutrient needs can vary substantially depending upon genetics, health status and history, age, gender, environmental factors, and even location of residence. In addition, the food matrix consumed by a person is influenced by cultural background, location, access to various foods, economic and political issues, sensory and health perceptions, and habits. In much of the developed world, there is greater food diversity available year-round today than at any other period in human history. Foods can be raw, minimally processed, shelf-stable, prepackaged, prepared, nutrient-dense, or nutrient-depleted. The selection of what foods to ingest determines the quality of the diet and the ultimate influence it has on physiological function.

The proper diet is only the beginning of the process, however, since once food is ingested it must then be properly digested in order for nutrients to be absorbed. Proteins are digested to amino acids, carbohydrates to monosaccharides, and fats to free fatty acids. The digestive process is influenced by the nature of the food matrix. Minimally processed whole foods are, in general, digested more slowly than highly processed foods. This slows the release of nutrients and influences the rate at which absorption of both macro- and micronutrients occurs. A diet high in sugar and added fats will result in rapid absorption of glucose and fatty acids, creating increased demand upon the hormonal nutrient regulatory systems and enzymes such as insulin, cortisol, and insulin-like growth factor.

Clinical Implications

Clinically, these observations about digestion are important because all nutrition intervention programs need to begin with diet analysis, and the intervention prescribed must be achievable by the patient. This requires that the clinician know not only what the patient is ingesting on a routine basis, but also the context in which the person is living. A diet diary or food-frequency questionnaire should be utilized as part of the routine historical information that all health practitioners obtain on their patients. Taken with patient history, this information helps to determine amount and types of protein, fat, and carbohydrate intake and allows for the evaluation of micronutrient density (i.e., vitamins and minerals), phytonutrient intake (e.g., flavonoids, polyphenols, isoflavones, glucosinolates), accessory nutrient intake (e.g., coenzyme Q10, carnitine, taurine, lipoic acid), and fiber. This information is critically important in designing a nutrition program personalized to the patient's specific needs.

Digestion initially involves the breakdown of large molecules in food into smaller units—for example, the breakdown of protein into amino acids. Adequate stomach acid is particularly important not only for digestion, but also for protecting against pathogenic organisms and food antigens.[9,10] For example, antacid use has been shown to inhibit digestion of proteins and cause food allergy in an animal model study.[11] Stomach acid decreases with age, a condition called hypochlorhydria, which is related to the prevalence of atrophic gastritis in people over age 60. Hypochlorhydria is also associated with increased levels of *Helicobacter pylori* (*H. pylori*), an increase in proximal small intestine pH, small intestine bacterial overgrowth, and decreased secretion of intrinsic factor, which is necessary for adequate absorption of vitamin B12.[12,13,14]

The presence and secretion of adequate amounts of specific digestive enzymes is essential for healthy digestion and absorption of nutrients, and lack of any of the necessary enzymes can have local and systemic effects. Exogenous pancreatic enzymes have been shown to reduce histamine secretion and clinical symptoms associated with challenge of an allergenic food in a double-blind, placebo-controlled trial.[15] Pancreatic secretions may decrease with age, and are adversely affected by alcohol abuse, pancreatitis, cystic fibrosis, diabetes, gallstones, and inflammation.[16,17] Pancreatic dysfunction necessitates oral replacement of pancreatic enzymes, as well as bicarbonate, which acts to neutralize the chyme after it leaves the stomach. Other digestive dysfunctions include inadequate bile secretion, which has also been associated with increased mucosal infiltration of *H. pylori*.[18,19]

Water-soluble nutrients are absorbed by a different mechanism than are the fat-soluble substances. Water-soluble nutrients (carbohydrates, amino acids, and the water-soluble vitamins) are absorbed in the small intestine by transport across the brush border cells through both passive and active transport systems. Fat-soluble nutrients (the fat-soluble vitamins and fatty acids) must first undergo emulsification with bile and are then taken into the lymphatic system for later association with plasma proteins. Clearly, for adequate absorption of nutrients, a healthy small intestinal mucosa is essential. It is possible to have specific defects in either the water-soluble or the fat-soluble absorptive pathways, resulting in symptoms of specific nutrient deficiency. The GI mucosal barrier, then, is the major first line of defense against unwanted toxins, antigens, and microbes that may transition intact through the digestive process.

Protection and Defense

The GI Mucosal Barrier

The GI mucosal membrane surface is the largest interface between our internal body and the external world. It covers more than 400 square meters, which is over 200-fold greater than the surface area of the skin.[20] The GI mucosal layer has the specific charge of allowing in only health-promoting nutrients and phytonutrients, while keeping out potentially damaging molecules and pathogenic organisms; it is the protective cell layer that provides the barrier between the inside of the body and the external world, and is responsible for nutrient absorption. The GI mucosa includes the gastric epithelial layer, which covers the stomach and protects it from damaging stomach acid. This mucosa also plays an important role in protecting the stomach from ingested toxins, drugs, alcohol, and pathogens such as infectious bacteria and viruses. The mucous gel that coats the stomach is comprised of phospholipids, secreted by gastric epithelial cells, that render the surface layer resistant to damage by stomach acid.[21,22,23]

Two pathways exist for transport across the epithelium: intracellular (through cells, controlled by the cell membrane) and paracellular (between cells, controlled by the permeability of tight junctions, which are distributed around the apical membranes of enterocytes).[24] In a normal, healthy intestine, the tight junctions constitute a barrier that provides limited access for substances from the outside (lumen) to be absorbed inside the body. They force substances to go through a cell to enter into circulation (Figure 17.1). To go through a cell, most substances require specific uptake systems, such as an active transport system, which can be regulated by the body. Some substances transition through cells passively—for example, fat-soluble substances that can easily cross the cell membrane layer (see below). Since the detoxification system is very active in the intestinal mucosa, and is attached to the membrane inside the cell, the body also has a defense mechanism against this passive uptake as long as the substance goes through the cell.

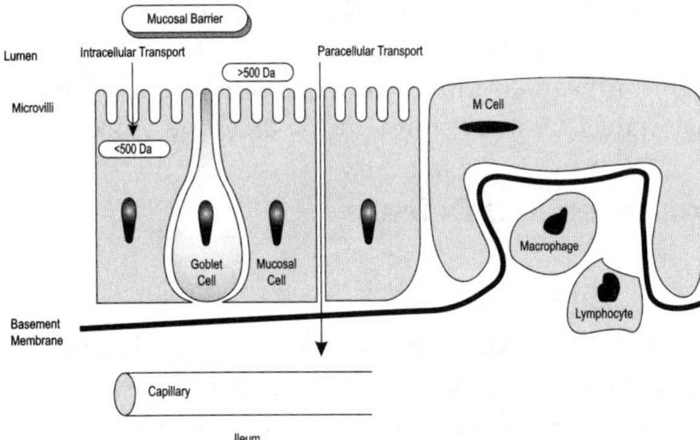

Figure 17.1 **Permeability dynamics**

Without the GI barrier, molecules of all types can pass into circulation without being detected; they can slip around the cells, thereby avoiding the body's first-line protection and defense mechanisms. In a healthy intestinal tract, the intestine's tight junctions limit the transport of large molecules (>500 Da) across the epithelium. In an unhealthy intestine, however, the tight junctions become "leaky" and these large molecules, which can include unprocessed proteins or large amino acids that have intact antigenic sites on them, can then slip into circulation. Intestinal permeability—or "leaky gut"—is the name given to the condition in which this barrier is breached and foreign antigens and other damaging substances slip around the cells and into circulation.[25,26,27,28]

Abnormal or increased intestinal permeability is commonly seen in patients presenting with intestinal inflammation, food allergies and intolerances, and celiac sprue. For example, a study of 200 children with cow's milk allergy showed a significant increase in intestinal permeability (assessed by the commonly used dual sugar permeability assay) in the children with the allergy as compared to controls.[29] Abnormal intestinal permeability has also been documented in patients after radiation or chemotherapy treatments (probably due to the killing of proliferating cells), and is induced by stress. Poor nutrient intake or absorption, or lack of enteral nutrition (e.g., parenteral nutrition) cannot support healthy regeneration of the rapidly proliferating cells in the small intestine and, therefore, can also profoundly affect the integrity of the GI barrier function.[30] Endogenous toxins, such as bacterial and fungal by-products produced by resident flora, and exogenous toxins, such as incompletely digested food, food additives, alcohol, over-the-counter drugs like NSAIDs, and foreign microbes, can also negatively influence intestinal integrity (see Table 17.2).[31,32]

In-depth discussions of GI-related processes and conditions can be found in Chapters 24 and 28.

Clinical Implications

The re-establishment of the "intelligent mucosal barrier" is achieved clinically by introducing a program that (1) *removes* potential offending antigens and toxic substances from the diet; (2) enhances digestive support with the use of exocrine pancreatic digestive aids (*replace*), where required; (3) *reinoculates* the intestinal tract with symbiotic bacteria (probiotics) and selective substrates for their metabolism such as fructooligosaccharides or arabinogalactans (prebiotics); and (4) helps to *repair* the GI mucosa by supplementing the diet with nutrients necessary for the promotion of mucosal healing, such as L-glutamine, zinc, pantothenic acid, and vitamin E. In functional medicine, we call this the 4R program (see Chapter 28).

Table 17.2 **Some Factors Associated with Intestinal Permeability**

Alcohol
Cancer radiation therapy
Corticosteroids
Excessive stress
Excessive simple sugar consumption
Fasting
Food allergies
Gastrointestinal infections
NSAIDs
Nutrient insufficiencies
Premature birth
Whole food exposure before the age of 4 months

Inhalation and the GI Tract

Most clinicians are aware of inhalant allergens and their influence on such conditions as inflammatory asthma. A functional medicine approach, however, looks for the connections among different systems: the web of interactions that may underlie a set of symptoms. As an example of this complexity, inhalant antigens have been proposed to play a role in gastroenteropathies. For example, animal studies have shown that esophageal eosinophilic inflammation occurs after intranasal allergen challenge.[33] Human studies have also suggested an interaction between the GI tract and the airways. A study in Sweden showed that adults with birch pollen allergy have increased eosinophils and cells positive for IgE in their duodenum during pollen season.[34]

Although the role of inhaled toxicant, such as carcinogens in tobacco smoke, has been accepted as a contributor to disease, emerging data suggest active and passive tobacco smoke exposure may also contribute to disease in other ways. For example, tobacco smoke has been shown to contain endotoxin, which is a very potent proinflammatory agent, and may contribute to respiratory inflammation.[35] Emerging data have also linked the fine and ultra-fine particulate matter present in air pollution to cardiovascular morbidity and mortality. Therefore, the intake of these particles during aerobic exercise should be considered, especially for patients who jog or run in urban areas and are exposed to excessive car exhaust during exercise.[36]

The Skin as a Barrier

As the external barrier, skin is under a constant barrage of insults from physical conditions, microbes, and chemicals. The skin functions much like the intestinal tract, using tight junctions as a barrier to potentially damaging environmental substances. Skin also has an extensive immune system.[37] Emerging data indicate the presence of antimicrobial peptides,[38] enabling the human epidermis to kill invading microbes. In this capacity, recognition of a pathogen by the keratinocyte triggers cytokine production that leads to elimination of the pathogen.[39]

Although an important barrier, a review of published research indicates that the study of the skin barrier may be more difficult than understanding intestinal permeability, since there is no good model system or permeability test. Studies are being published showing that supporting and enhancing the barrier function of the skin may have therapeutic potential. For example, a study was done with preterm infants in Bangladesh, who were known to have compromised skin barrier function that put them at high risk for serious infections.[40] In this study, daily massage with sunflower seed oil was compared to massage with a lanolin, petrolatum and mineral oil-based material; the infants receiving the sunflower oil massages were 41% less likely to develop nosocomial infections. In another study, the oxidation of squalene by UV exposure was reported to be significantly inhibited after one application of a skin rinse with vitamin E, as compared to the rinse without vitamin E.[41]

Immune System Surveillance and Removal Mechanisms

Immune system functionality is discussed in great depth in numerous other places in this book (see Chapters 18, 23, and 27). The brief review below highlights the vital role the immune system plays in protection and defense through the intake, processing, and excretion of external substances.

The gut-associated lymphoid tissue (GALT). Approximately 60% of the immune system, and more than 80% of the immunoglobulin-producing blasts and plasma cells, are located within the mucosa of the GI tract. This complex system is called the gut-associated lymphoid tissue (GALT).[42,43] The primary purpose of the GALT is to provide the first line of defense against foreign invaders such as food antigens and pathogenic bacteria. A major difference between the GALT and the circulatory immune system is that the GALT can produce two layers of defense to a foreign pathogen or antigen: the localized secretory IgA (sIgA) response, and the systemic IgE or IgG response. Taken together, these two responses account for the production of the majority of the body's immunoglobulins.[44]

The localized sIgA provides the first immunological response to antigens that are ingested; sIgA has been described as an "antiseptic paint" covering the intestinal tract. As the predominant immunoglobulin on the surface of the GI mucosa, sIgA can effectively prevent infection, neutralize viruses, and remove antigens before they cross the mucosal barrier and reach circulation so they can be excreted directly through the feces.[45,46] Therefore, sIgA prevents these invaders from entering the system without activating the complement or inflammatory systems.[47] Adults produce three to four grams of sIgA per day, which can also be found in saliva and colostrum.[48] A low level of total sIgA in the GI tract is associated with altered intestinal permeability and an increased uptake of food antigens, resulting in atopic symptoms.[49]

Antigens and foreign substances that escape the sIgA surveillance can enter the mucosal layer, where the GALT provides the second layer of defense. In this process, which is the classic response described in most textbooks, the interaction with the antigen-specific IgE and IgG induces a systemic immune response in which antibodies are generated, cytokines are produced, and the full immune system is engaged. Along with activation of the systemic immune system, an inflammatory response often commences at the site where the antigen has invaded. This inflammatory response closes off the area, blocking the influx of more antigens. (The activation of the inflammatory cascade is a double-edged sword because the inflammation response leads to production of reactive oxygen species, which are used to destroy invading pathogens but which can also damage healthy, intact tissue.)

The GALT is also instrumental in the development of immune tolerance to harmless antigens in the diet and commensal microbes. Oral tolerance begins in the newborn with small amounts of intact food antigens, including beta-lactoglobulin, egg, peanut, and gliadin.[50] Oral tolerance is an important process in which the body becomes able to recognize food molecules and not respond to them with a full-fledged antibody-immune response. Studies with children who have food allergies have shown compromised transforming growth factor-beta and reduced numbers of the T-helper lymphocytes that produce this cytokine (i.e., Th3 cells) in the duodenal epithelium and the lamina propria.[51,52] The oral tolerance response is also stimulated by the commensal intestinal microbes, and this relationship suggests a role of intestinal microflora in development of healthy oral tolerance response.[53,54]

The systemic immune system. The systemic immune system is composed of the circulating lymphocytes, the B cells and T cells, which circulate through the body in search of their target antigens. Initially, lymphocytes must be activated toward a specific antigen. Antigens entering the body through mucosal surfaces activate the lymphocytes that are waiting in the mucosa-associated lymphoid tissues (MALT): intranasal and inhaled antigens activate lymphocytes in palatine tonsils and adenoids; and antigens taken in through the GI tract are taken into specialized epithelial cells called M (microfold) cells (Figure 17.1), which then transport the antigen to Peyer's patches.[55] Activation via the Peyer's patches is the most common pathway for induction of the immune response. Immune responses to blood-borne antigens are usually initiated in the spleen, and responses to microorganisms in tissues are generated in local lymph nodes.

Induction of the immune system is quite complex, but current dogma indicates that two major pathways exist: cellular immunity that involves the Th1 pathway; and humoral immunity that involves the Th2 pathway. (See Figure 17.2.) The pathways are named after the T-helper cells involved in the pathway (e.g., Th1 and Th2); T-helper cells are differentiated from each other by the products they produce (that is, the specific cytokines they secrete when activated). In general, the Th1 pathway functions against invading organisms, where Th1 cells secrete interferon-γ and interleukin-2, and also involves macrophages and cytotoxic T cells that act in concert to kill the invading organisms. The Th2 pathway is induced in response to antigenic stimuli and leads to secretion of interleukins-4, -5, and -6 by T-helper cells, which support the function of the antibody-producing B-cells (see Figure 17.3).

Much literature has indicated that these two systems balance each other: when one is overexpressed, the other is inhibited. For example, glucocorticoids selectively inhibit the Th1 pathway, and shift a person toward Th2 reactions, which may lead to higher susceptibility to allergic responses.[56] Estrogens inhibit Th1 proinflammatory cytokines and stimulate Th2 cytokines, which is suggested as the reason that autoimmune diseases that involve overexpression of Th1 (e.g., rheumatoid arthritis, multiple sclerosis) frequently remit during pregnancy but exacerbate during postpartum periods.[57] Th1 and Th2 are also differentially involved in such conditions as psoriasis and atopic dermatitis, respectively.[58] Genetics is known to play a role in the robustness of Th1 or Th2 responses, as are lifestyle and nutriture.[59,60,61,62] In addition, early exposure to infectious organisms is also implicated. For example, the "hygiene hypothesis" has been proposed to account for the increasing prevalence of atopic diseases over the past decade. The hygiene hypothesis suggests that diminished exposure to childhood infections leads to a decreased Th1 response, which therefore may enhance the Th2 response in an individual.[63,64]

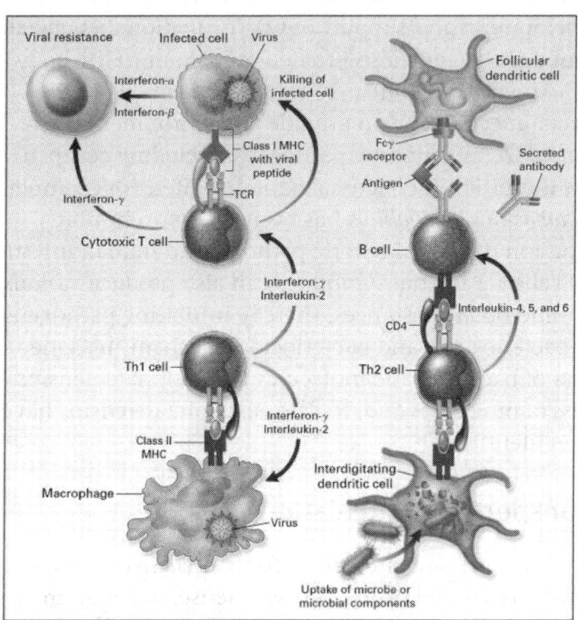

Figure 17.2 **An overview of lymphocyte responses**

From: Delves PJ, Roitt IM. The immune system—Second of Two Parts. N Engl J Med. 2000;343:108-117. Used by permission. ©2000 Massachusetts Medical Society. All rights reserved.

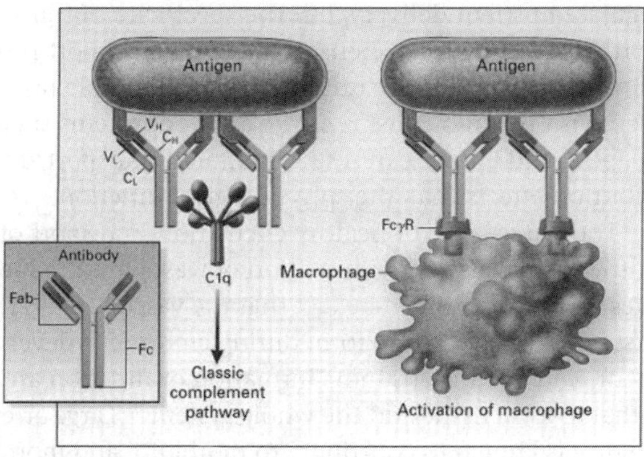

Figure 17.3 **Role of antibodies**

From: Delves PJ, Roitt IM. The immune system—Second of Two Parts. N Engl J Med. 2000;343:108-117. Used by permission. ©2000 Massachusetts Medical Society. All rights reserved.

The functioning of the immune system with respect to specific conditions will be discussed in more detail elsewhere, but important to this discussion is the understanding that many components must work together in the delicate balance of immune system function, and the immune system forms a communications link among different tissues with respect to surveillance and defense, and includes macrophage cells, T cells, and B cells. In the brain, glial cells function much as macrophages do, removing waste and providing nutrients to neurons; they are affected by several neurodegenerative conditions.[65] Because the immune system responds to foreign agents, the interplay with the environment is crucial in its regulation and activity. In addition, several of the immune system-regulated cytokines have clinical relevance (see Figure 17.2), which may show individual responses depending on a person's genetics. It is also important to note that the Th1 and Th2 responses also appear to work together to facilitate recovery from infection, and may support each other in other important ways.[66] In addition, emerging data indicate a role for a third class of T-helper cells, the Th3 cells, which downregulate Th2 responses.[67]

The Detoxification System and Defense

Drugs and toxicants have to get into the body to function and/or to produce toxic effects. By far the easiest way to evade a healthy barrier system is simply to slide through cell membranes by passive diffusion. Therefore, many drugs are designed as lipid-soluble molecules,[68] and many of the toxic substances that are found in our bodies are also lipid soluble. Small, weak acids and bases can slip into cells by riding in with water in a passive manner; however, while water-soluble (hydrophilic) molecules are taken into the water-based blood and transported to the kidneys where they can be excreted, lipid-soluble (hydrophobic) molecules cannot be directly removed via the kidneys.[69] The very nature of lipid-soluble compounds means they will be able to attach to cell membranes, which are composed of lipids, and slide through these membranes into the cell, where they can directly interact with important proteins and molecules necessary for healthy function, thus exerting damage within the cell. The primary mechanism in the body for removing lipid-soluble toxins is the detoxification system, which functions to convert lipid-soluble substances to water-soluble metabolites so they can be excreted via the urine.

After a xenobiotic is taken into the body, it first passes through the liver. Therefore, the liver is a primary site for detoxification and for the majority of detoxification enzymes, including alcohol dehydrogenase, the phase I cytochrome P450 enzymes (CYP P450), and the phase II conjugation enzymes (e.g., glucuronidases and conjugases that attach glutathione, glycine, taurine, and sulfate). (Detailed discussions of these processes can be found in Chapters 22 and 31.) The position of the liver in this sequence accounts for the statistics showing that liver injury from drugs and xenobiotics leads to 2–5% of hospitalizations from jaundice, an estimated 15–30% of the cases of fulminant liver failure, and ~40% of the acute hepatitis cases in patients older than 50.[70]

Because the detoxification enzymes show such high variability from subject to subject, the adage "one man's meat is another man's poison" is relevant to how individuals detoxify drugs, toxicants, and environmental compounds. That is, individuals relate to their environments in very individualized ways with respect to the detoxification system, and responses can vary dramatically such that one person can show intense symptoms at the same level of exposure that another person finds tolerable. Some of this variability is due to environment, lifestyle, and history, but the majority comes from genetics.[71,72] Because the detoxification system is so involved in managing environmental interactions within the body, it may be no surprise that dietary components can have significant effects on the activity of detoxification enzymes.[73,74,75]

Commensal Microflora and Defense

The beneficial symbiotic microflora that reside primarily in the large intestine have a direct impact on promoting a healthy GI tract barrier and supporting defense functions. Much research has been focused on how commensal microflora, including bifidobacteria and lactobacilli, provide beneficial effects. For example, the production of short-chain fatty acids (SCFAs) by these bacteria appears to promote growth and differentiation of intestinal mucosal cells, which results in decreased risk of colon cancer and attenuation of intestinal permeability.[76] Probiotics, which are exogenous sources of friendly bacteria, also appear to benefit patients with atopic eczema, possibly by promoting antigen degradation and healthy GI barrier function.[77] Intestinal microflora influence digestion not only through nutrient needs and the ability to digest large carbohydrates (such as fibers that escape hydrolysis in the stomach and small intestine), but also through a feedback effect on transit time. SCFAs may also protect intestinal integrity by stimulating intestinal mucosal cell turnover and intestinal mucosal blood flow.[78]

Most notably, healthy microflora is required for development and support of GALT function; beneficial symbiotic bacteria also provide protection to the body by acting as antagonists toward pathogens. They use several mechanisms to provide an environment resistant to colonization by pathogens, including competitive inhibition for bacterial adhesion sites. For example, *Lactobacillus acidophilus* has been shown to inhibit adhesion of several enteric pathogens to human intestinal cells.[79] Bacterial symbiotes can also produce various antimicrobial substances, thereby inhibiting pathogens by bacteriostatic and bacteriocidal mechanisms. One class of bacteriostatic molecules is the alpha-defensins class of molecules and, to date, six alpha-defensins have been identified.[80]

Transport and Circulation

Transport and circulation functions are not often considered a part of the body's defense, but they are instrumental in supporting the body's defense functions and providing nutrients throughout the body. Once absorbed, nutrients must be distributed to the tissues where metabolism occurs, and many nutrients have specific carrier proteins or structures that facilitate their transport. Not only does this allow the body to regulate nutrient delivery, but the specificity of transport allows a level of defense. Defects in transport proteins or specific genetic uniqueness, for example (as seen with polymorphisms of the apolipoproteins such as apo E and Lp(a)), can result in altered transport/distribution effects that alter physiological function.

The importance of healthy circulation, transport of nutrients to cells, and elimination of waste from tissue sites is shown by the mere fact that the vasculature is the first functional organ to form during embryonic development, and disruptions in its formation or function are lethal to local tissue and the whole system.[81] Large artery rigidity is known to contribute to morbidity and mortality associated with the most common chronic conditions seen today, including arterial hypertension, diabetes mellitus, and heart failure. Aortic rigidity precedes the development of arterial hypertension in individuals with borderline hypertension.[82] The microcirculation also plays an important role in defense mechanisms.

Transport of nutrients to the cells is not the end of the process. The fat-based cell membranes provide a barrier function within the body, separating the aqueous-based extracellular environment from the aqueous-based intracellular environment. Very small water-soluble molecules can slip into the cell passively in water, but the concentrations of these tend to be low. Therefore, specific transport processes are also required to get water-soluble nutrients across the fat-based cell membranes. Many of these nutrients are taken into cells through an active transport process. For example, glucose is taken into the cell from the blood via the Glut-2 or Glut-4 receptors. Dysfunctions in this uptake system can occur.

Maintenance of healthy cell membranes is essential and data have shown that the type of fat in the diet directly influences the fat in the cell membranes. Omega-3 fats have been shown to promote healthy function of membrane receptors by influencing the environment around the receptors. For example, in an animal feeding study, rats consuming omega-3 fatty acids in place of omega-6 fatty acids (in otherwise identical diets) showed lower serum triglycerides and an attenuated insulin-stimulated transport of glucose into adipocytes than the animals with the omega-6 fats.[83] Cell culture studies have shown that the amount of EPA as compared to linoleic acid influences membrane fluidity and receptor-mediated signaling through the phospholipase-C/phosphoinositol pathway.[84] A compelling series of articles has been published addressing membrane phospholipid composition and neurotransmitter function in depression and schizophrenia.[85,86] As stated in one review: "This suggests that a tight relationship exists between essential fatty acid status and normal neurotransmitter function, and that altered PUFA levels may contribute to the abnormalities in neurotransmission seen in schizophrenia."

Because cell membranes are composed primarily of fat, and many toxicants, including most drugs, are fat soluble, many of these substances can cross the cell membrane barrier without specific transport processes. Therefore, as another layer of defense, cells have an "antiporter" system for these xenobiotics, which acts to pump molecules out of the cell. This antiporter system is called P-glycoprotein, which is a product of one of the multi-drug resistant genes (MDR1 and MDR2). This system was first described in tumor cells that became resistant to chemotherapeutic agents as a result of increased expression of this transporter. The P-glycoprotein transporter is found in many tissues, such as cells in the small intestine, liver, and kidney, and at the blood-brain and blood-testes barriers.[87] P-glycoprotein functions to limit absorption of drugs and xenobiotics and to promote their excretion, but is also strongly influenced by concomitantly administered drugs.[88]

Circulation and transport of nutrients affects the functioning of the cardiovascular system, which is heavily influenced by factors such as homocysteine[89,90] that are influenced by nutrition. Many dietary factors are known to affect nitric oxide synthase, the enzyme responsible for generating nitric oxide (NO), which regulates vascular relaxation.[91] Emerging data indicate that the oxygenation state of hemoglobin also regulates NO.[92] Antioxidants in the diet can also affect oxidant stress, which can, in turn, alter endothelial function.[93]

Clinical Implications

Fat-soluble substances such as steroid hormones are transported on their own binding proteins and are vulnerable to environmental influences. For example, sex hormone-binding globulin, an important transport protein for the regulation of plasma concentration of sex steroid hormones, can be influenced by many environmental factors, including smoking, oral contraceptive use, soy isoflavone intake, stress, toxic chemical exposure, and excess alcohol intake. All of these factors can influence the relative concentration of the sex hormone-binding globulin, thereby modifying the concentration and availability of specific sex hormones, such as estrogen, testosterone, or progesterone.

In the functional medicine workup, evaluation of whether a patient may have a transport or circulatory difficulty, or a cellular resistance to the substance of concern, needs to be considered. Conditions that could modify the transport or circulation of substances include dyslipidemia, altered blood pressure or vascular reactivity, regional ischemic events, the breakdown of membrane barriers of defense, increased oxidative stress and injury, or the presence of chronic inflammation. Specific tailored therapies can be integrated into the overall treatment plan that focus on improving active transport by strengthening proper membrane barrier function and proper membrane bioenergetics so that active transport can be maintained, by supporting proper vascular endothelial function, and by enhancing cellular uptake through stimulation of membrane receptor sites and mitochondrial and nuclear signaling systems.

Elimination of Waste

Metabolism of nutrients either by the host or by enteric or opportunistic microorganisms also results in the production of metabolic by-products, or waste. These need to be properly excreted to complete the nutrient cycling process. Excretion of waste products can occur by way of solid, liquid, or gas exchange. Aerobic metabolism of glucose produces carbon dioxide and water that both need excretion. Carbon dioxide is excreted as a gas by the lungs. Water is excreted as a liquid through the kidneys, skin, and intestines, and as a vapor through the lungs and skin.

Protein metabolism results in the production of urea and sulfate, which are excreted through the kidneys. Incomplete protein metabolism results in the formation of amines such as trimethylamine, ammonia, or other middle-molecular weight nitrogenous substances that are excreted through the urine and skin. These nitrogenous compounds have strong "fishy" odors, which often characterize people with protein metabolic disorders or hepatic or GI difficulties in managing protein in the diet.

Fats are ideally metabolized and excreted as carbon dioxide, water, and phosphate (as it relates to phospholipid metabolism). Fat metabolism problems result in the excretion of fat in the stool (i.e., steatorrhea) or alterations in serum lipid levels (i.e., elevated serum cholesterol or triglycerides).

Fecal vs. Urinary Excretion

Many metabolites and dietary substances undergo further metabolic modification as they are converted to excretory products. This includes hormones, neurotransmitters, eicosanoids, vitamins, and phytochemicals, as well as xenobiotics and drugs. The principal mechanism by which these excretory products are created is through the detoxification/biotransformation pathways, although some may be secreted in kidney tubules without transformation. Most of this conversion is done in the liver, although detoxification enzymes are also present in the GI mucosa, kidneys, lung epithelial tissue, and other tissues, which can also contribute to biotransformation. Once a substance has undergone biotransformation to its conjugate, it is partitioned into either the bile for excretion in the feces, or through the kidney to be excreted in the urine. Dehydration has a serious adverse influence on detoxification and excretion due to decreased urinary output. In patients with functional impairment in excretion, copious amounts of water should be administered.

Fecal excretion also plays an important role in eliminating the remnants and cellular debris of enteric bacteria. It is estimated that there are more than two pounds of enteric bacteria in the human digestive tract. These organisms have their own natural life cycles and, when they die, their cell bodies must be excreted. Beyond that, enteric bacteria produce many metabolites that must be detoxified by the gastrointestinal biotransformation systems and excreted as secondary metabolites.

An example of the relationship between enteric bacteria and metabolites is the conversion of lignans and isoflavones by specific enteric flora into secondary metabolites such as equol. Equol is absorbed across the gastrointestinal lumen, has impact on modulating aspects of functional physiology, and is then excreted in the urine. Although the exposure to equol seems beneficial to the host, there are many other examples of enteric bacteria metabolism resulting in the formation of toxic compounds that must be biotransformed and excreted. In addition, certain enteric bacteria also possess enzymes such as beta-glucuronidase that can deconjugate detoxified substances (such as estrogen metabolites) in the colon and render them available for resorption. This places an additional burden on the detoxification and excretory systems.

Functionally, the excretory system can be improved through enhanced bowel transit time because that implies less contact time for absorption of toxic substances. This is clinically achieved by increasing the intake of insoluble fiber. Supplementing the diet with symbiotic microorganisms such as specific strains of lactobacilli and bifidobacteria can also enhance transit time. For example, the *L. acidophilus NCFM®* strain has been shown to decrease incidence of pediatric diarrhea, significantly decrease levels of toxic amines in the blood of dialysis patients with small intestine bacterial overgrowth (SIBO), and facilitate lactose digestion in lactose-intolerant individuals.[94]

Fiber can also promote transit time and healthy excretion, as well as providing other positive benefits to a patient. The fibers classed as "prebiotics" are particularly beneficial. Prebiotics are fibers that have been shown to preferentially promote commensal GI microflora, and include fructans (such as inulin and fructooligosaccharides, or FOS), arabinogalactans, and soy oligosaccharides. Some fibers have been shown to promote short-chain fatty acid production and healthy microflora in the GI, but may not be officially designated as prebiotics. For example, rice fiber has been shown to improve bile acid excretion and decrease fecal bacterial enzyme activities associated with pathogens and imbalanced flora, such as beta-glucuronidase, mucinase, and nitroreductase.[95]

It is important to emphasize the clinical benefit of introducing a dietary detoxification program that includes more whole fruits and vegetables and fiber-rich whole grains when trying to improve excretion. There are many detoxification-focused diets that increase the intake of cruciferous vegetables (broccoli, cauliflower, Brussels sprouts, and cabbage), red and orange vegetables, and whole fruits, including apples and berries. These foods contain specific phytochemicals that have been found to enhance detoxification. Fasting is not considered an optimal approach to detoxification and the improvement of excretion due to its lack of fiber content and its tendency to cause constipation. Regular exercise also helps in maintaining proper peristaltic action and promoting proper transit time.

Summary

The theme that emerges from this discussion of digestive physiology is that the delivery of fuel to the cells and the subsequent removal of waste products produced during metabolism are much more complex than just examining the presence or absence of the substance itself. Rather, in a functional medicine evaluation, one has to determine whether there are difficulties in transport of a substance once it has been absorbed, whether it is properly distributed to the appropriate tissues through circulation, and whether, once delivered, it can be taken up by cells correctly to promote proper function. Each of these processes has been found to show great genetic variability from person to person, and we now know that there are many environmental, lifestyle, and dietary variables that influence each of these steps in the maintenance of proper cellular function.

References

1. Alavanja MCR, Hoppin JA, Kamel F. Health effects on chronic pesticide exposure: cancer and neurotoxicity. Annu Rev Public Health. 2004;25:155-197.
2. Ibid.
3. Kirkhorn SR, Schenker MB. Current health effects of agricultural work: respiratory disease, cancer, reproductive effects, musculoskeletal injuries, and pesticide-related illness. J Agric Safety Health. 2002;8:199-214.
4. Sherer TB, Betarbet R, Greenmayre JT. Environment, mitochondria, and Parkinson's disease. Neuroscientist. 2002;8:192-197.
5. Muir T, Zegarac M. Societal costs of exposure to toxic substances: economic and health costs of four case studies that are candidates for environmental causation. Environ Health Perspect. 2001;109(suppl 6):885-903.
6. Zuccato E, Calamari D, Natangelo M, Fanelli R. Presence of therapeutic drugs in the environment. Lancet. 2000;355(9217):1789-1790.
7. Muir T, Zegarac M. Societal costs of exposure to toxic substances: economic and health costs of four case studies that are candidates for environmental causation. Environ Health Perspect. 2001;109(suppl 6):885-903.
8. Fogg MI, Spergel JM. Management of food allergies. Expert Opin Pharmacother. 2003;4:1025-1037.
9. Pilotto A. Aging and the gastrointestinal tract. Ital J Gastroenterol Hepatol. 1998;30:137-153.
10. Schmucker DL,Heyworth MF, Owen RL, et al. Impact of aging on gastrointestinal mucosal immunity. Dig Dis Sci. 1996; 41:1183-1193.
11. Untersmayr E, Schöll I, Swoboda I, et al. Antacid medication inhibits digestion of dietary proteins and causes food allergy: A fish allergy model in Balb/c mice. J Allergy Clin Immunol. 2003;112:616-623.
12. Baik HW, Russell RM. Vitamin B12 deficiency in the elderly. Annu Rev Nutr. 1999;19:357-377.
13. Saltzman JR, Russell RM. The aging gut: nutritional issues. Gastroenterol Clin North Am. 1998;27:309-324.
14. Kassarjian Z, Russell RM. Hypochlorhydria: a factor in nutrition. Annu Rev Nutr. 1989;9:271-285.
15. Raithel M, Weidenhiller M, Schwab D, Winterkamp S, Hahn EG. Pancreatic enzymes: a new group of antiallergic drugs? Inflamm Res. 2002;51(suppl 1):S13-S14.
16. Nakamura T, Takeuchi T, Tando Y. Pancreatic dysfunction and treatment options. Pancreas. 1998;16:329-336.
17. Kim KH, Lee HS, Kim CD, et al. Evaluation of pancreatic exocrine function using pure pancreatic juice in noninsulin-dependent diabetes mellitus. J Clin Gastroenterol. 2000;31:51-54.
18. Kawai Y, Tazuma S, Inoue M. Bile acids reflux and possible inhibition of Helicobacter pylori infection in subjects without gastric surgery. Dig Dis Sci. 2001;46:1779-1783.
19. Graham DY, Osato MS. H. pylori in the pathogenesis of duodenal ulcer: interaction between duodenal acid load, bile, and H pylori. Am J Gastroenterol. 2000;95:329-336.
20. Takahashi I, Kiyono H. Gut as the largest immunologic tissue. J Parenteral Enteral Nutr. 1999;23:S7-S12.
21. DeMeo MT, Mutlu EA, Keshavarzian A, Tobin MC. Intestinal permeation and gastrointestinal disease. J Clin Gastroenterol. 2002;34:385-396.
22. Barrios JM, Lichtenberger LM. Role of biliary phosphatidylcholine in bile acid protection and NSAID injury of the ileal mucosa in rats. Gastroenterol. 2000;118:1179-1186.
23. Wakabayashi H, Orihara T, Nakaya A, et al. Effect of *Helicobacter pylori* infection on gastric mucosal phospholipids contents and their fatty acid composition. J Gastroenterol Hepatol. 1998;13:566-571.
24. Nusrat A, Turner JR, Madara JL. Molecular physiology and pathophysiology of tight junctions IV. Regulations of tight junctions by extracellular stimuli: nutrients, cytokines, and immune cells. Am J Physiol Gastrointest Liver Physiol. 2000;279:G851-G857.
25. DeMeo MT, Mutlu EA, Keshavarzian A, Tobin MC. Intestinal permeation and gastrointestinal disease. J Clin Gastroenterol. 2002;34:385-396.
26. Nejdfors P, Ekelund M, Jeppsson B, et al. Mucosal *in vitro* permeability in the intestinal tract of the pig, the rat, and man: species- and region-related differences. Scand J Gastroenterol. 2000;35:501-507.
27. Thomson ABR, Jarocka-Cyrta E, Faria J, et al. Small bowel review—Part II. Can J Gastroenterol. 1997;11:159-165.

28. Gardner M. Gastrointestinal absorption of intact proteins. Ann Rev Nutr. 1988 ;8 :329-350.
29. Kalach N, Rocchiccioli F, de Boissieu D, et al. Intestinal permeability in children: variation with age and reliability in the diagnosis of cow's milk allergy. Acta Pediatr. 2001;90:499-504.
30. MacFie J. Enteral versus parenteral nutrition: The significance of bacterial translocation and gut-barrier function. Nutrition. 2000;16:606-611.
31. Jenkins A, Trew D, Crump B, et al. Do non-steroidal anti-inflammatory drugs increase colonic permeability? Gut. 1991;32:66-69.
32. Bjarnason I, Wise R, Peters T. The leaky gut of alcoholism: possible route of entry of toxic compounds. Lancet 1984;1:79-82.
33. Heine RG. Pathophysiology, diagnosis and treatment of food protein-induced gastrointestinal diseases. Curr Opin Allergy Clin Immunol. 2004;4:221-229.
34. Magnusson J, Lin XP, Dahlman-Höglund A, et al. Seasonal intestinal inflammation in patients with birch pollen allergy. J Allergy Clin Immunol. 2003;112:45-50.
35. Larsson L, Szponar B, Pehrson C. Tobacco smoking increases dramatically air concentrations of endotoxin. Indoor Air. 2004; 14:421-424.
36. Sharman JE, Cockcroft JR, Coombes JS. Cardiovascular implications of exposure to traffic air pollution during exercise. QJM. 2004;97:637-643.
37. Schwarz T. Skin immunity. Br J Dermatol. 2003;149(Suppl 66):2-4.
38. Gallo RL, Huttner KM. Antimicrobial peptides: an emerging concept in cutaneous biology. J Invest Dermatol. 1998;111:739-43.
39. Pivarcsi A, Kemeny L, Dobozy A. Innate immune functions of the keratinocytes. A review. Acta Microbiol Immunol Hung. 2004; 51:303-310.
40. Darmstadt GL, Saha SK, Ahmed AS, et al. Effect of topical treatment with skin barrier-enhancing emollients on nosocomial infections in preterm infants in Bangladesh: a randomized controlled trial. Lancet. 2005;365(9464):1039-45.
41. Ekanayake-Mudiyanselage S, Tavakkol A, Polefka TG, et al. Vitamin E delivery to human skin by a rinse-off product: penetration of alpha-tocopherol versus wash-out effects of skin surface lipids. Skin Pharmacol Physiol. 2005;18:20-26.
42. Takahashi I, Kiyonon H. Gut as the largest immunologic tissue. J Parenteral Enteral Nutr. 1999;23:S7-S12.
43. Brandtzaeg P. Development and basic mechanisms of human gut immunity. Nutr Rev. 1998;56:S5-S18.
44. Liska DJ, Lukaczer D. Gut restoration and chronic disease. JANA. 2002;5:20-33.
45. Lukaczer D. Secretory IgA and gastrointestinal barrier competence. Quarterly Rev Natural Med. 1996;Fall:227-229.
46. Albanese C, Smith S, Watkins S, et al. Effect of secretory IgA on transepithelial passage of bacteria across the intact ileum *in vitro*. J Am Coll Surg. 1994;179:679-688.
47. Friehorst J, Ogra PL. Mucosal immunity and viral infections. Ann Med. 2001;33:172-177.
48. Delves PJ, Roitt IM. The immune system. New Engl J Med. 2000;343:108-117.
49. Ahmed T, Fuchs GJ. Gastrointestinal allergy to food: a review. J Diarrhoeal Dis Res. 1997;15:211-223.
50. Heine RG. Pathophysiology, diagnosis and treatment of food protein-induced gastrointestinal diseases. Curr Opin Allergy Clin Immunol. 2004;4:221-229.
51. Perez-Machado MA, Ashwood P, Thomson MA, et al. Reduced transforming growth factor-beta1-producing T cells in the duodenal mucosa of children with food allergy. Eur J Immunol. 2003;33:2307-2315.
52. Chung HL, Hwang JB, Park JJ, Kim SG. Expression of transforming growth factor beta1, transforming growth factor type I and II receptors, and THF-alpha in the mucosa of the small intestine in infants with food protein-induced enterocolitis syndrome. J Allergy Clin Immunol. 2002;109:150-154.
53. Perez-Machado MA, Ashwood P, Thomson MA, et al. Reduced transforming growth factor-beta1-producing T cells in the duodenal mucosa of children with food allergy. Eur J Immunol. 2003;33:2307-2315.
54. Manickasingham SP, Edwards AD, Schulz O, Reis e Sousa C. The ability of murine dendritic cell subsets to direct T helper cell differentiation is dependent on microbial signals. Eur J Immunol. 2003;33:101-107.
55. Delves PJ, Roitt IM. The immune system. New Engl J Med. 2000;343:108-117.
56. Elenkov IJ. Glucocorticoids and the Th1/Th2 balance. Ann N Y Acad Sci. 2004;1024:138-146.
57. Salem ML. Estrogen, a double-edged sword: modulation of TH1- and TH2-mediated inflammations by differential regulation of TH1/TH2 cytokine production. Curr Drug Targets Inflamm Allergy. 2004;3(1):97-104.
58. Biedermann T, Rocken M, Carballido JM. TH1 and TH2 lymphocyte development and regulation of TH cell-mediated immune responses of the skin. J Investig Dermatol Symp Proc. 2004;9:5-14.
59. Long KZ, Nanthakumar N. Energetic and nutritional regulation of the adaptive immune response and trade-offs in ecological immunology. Am J Hum Biol. 2004;16:499-507.
60. Sudo N, Aiba Y, Oyama N, et al. Dietary nucleic acid and intestinal microbiota synergistically promote a shift in the Th1/Th2 balance toward Th1-skewed immunity. Int Arch Allergy Immunol. 2004;135:132-135. Epub 2004 Sep 2.
61. Malm C. Exercise immunology: the current state of man and mouse. Sports Med. 2004;34:555-566.
62. Nieters A, Linseisen J, Becker N. Association of polymorphisms in Th1, Th2 cytokine genes with hayfever and atopy in a subsample of EPIC-Heidelberg. Clin Exp Allergy. 2004;34:346-353.
63. Ngoc LP, Gold DR, Tzianabos AO, Weiss ST, Celedon JC. Cytokines, allergy, and asthma. Curr Opin Allergy Clin Immunol. 2005; 5(2):161-166.
64. Hussain I, Kline JN. DNA, the immune system, and atopic disease. J Investig Dermatol Symp Proc. 2004;9:23-28.
65. Kurosinski P, Gotz J. Glial cells under physiologic and pathologic conditions. Arch Neurol. 2002;59:1524-1528.
66. Bot A, Smith KA, von Herrath M. Molecular and cellular control of T1/T2 immunity at the interface between antimicrobial defense and immune pathology. DNA Cell Biol. 2004;23:341-350.
67. Akbari O, Stock P, DeKruyff RH, Umetsu DT. Role of regulatory T cells in allergy and asthma. Curr Opin Immunol. 2003;15:627-633.
68. Goodman & Gilman's: The Pharmacological Basis of Therapeutics. 9th edition. Goodman LS, Limbird LE, Milinoff PB, et al. (eds.) McGraw Hill,New York. 1996:4-6.
69. Liska D. The detoxification enzyme system. Altern Med Rev. 1998;3:187-198.
70. Sturgill MG, Lambert GH. Xenobiotic-induced hepatotoxicity: mechanisms of liver injury and methods of monitoring hepatic function. Clin Chem. 1997;43(8 Pt 2):1512-26.
71. Ingelman-Sundberg M. Genetic susceptibility to adverse effects of drugs and environmental toxicants. The role of the CYP family of enzymes. Mutation Res. 2001;482:11-19.
72. McFadden SA. Phenotypic variation in xenobiotic metabolism and adverse environmental response: focus on sulfur-dependent detoxification pathways. Toxicology. 1996;111:43-65.

73. Moskaug JO, Carlsen H, Myhrstad MC, Blomhoff R. Polyphenols and glutathione synthesis regulation. Am J Clin Nutr. 2005;81(1 Suppl):277S-283S.
74. Manach C, Donovan JL. Pharmacokinetics and metabolism of dietary flavonoids. Free Radic Res. 2004;38:771-785.
75. Harris RZ, Jang GR, Tsunoda S. Dietary effects on drug metabolism and transport. Clin Pharmacokinet 2003;42:1071-1088.
76. Scheppach W. Effects of short chain fatty acids on gut morphology and function. Gut. 1994;35(suppl 1):S35-S38.
77. Kalliomaki MA, Isolauri E. Probiotics and down-regulation of the allergic response. Immunol Allergy Clin North Am. 2004;24:739-752.
78. LeLeiko NS, Walsh MJ. The role of glutamine, short-chain fatty acids, and nucleotides in intestinal adaptation to gastrointestinal disease. Pediatr Clin North Am. 1996;43:451-469.
79. Bernet M, Brassart D, Nesser J, et al. Lactobacillus acidophilus LA 1 binds to human intestinal cell lines and inhibits cell attachment and cell invasion by enterovirulent bacteria. Gut. 1994;35:483-489.
80. Cunliffe RN. Alpha-defensins in the gastrointestinal tract. Mol Immunol. 2003;40:463-467.
81. Rossant J, Howard L. Signaling pathways in vascular development. Annu Rev Cell Dev Biol. 2002;18:541-573. Epub 2002 Apr 02.
82. Plante GE. Vascular response to stress in health and disease. Metabolism. 2002;51(6 Suppl 1):25-30.
83. Fickova M, Hubert P, Cremel G, Leray C. Dietary (n-3) and (n-6) polyunsaturated fatty acids rapidly modify fatty acid composition and insulin effects in rat adipocytes. J Nutr. 1998;128:512-519.
84. de Jonge HW, Dekkers DH, Bastiaanse EM, et al. Eicosapentaenoic acid incorporation in membrane phospholipid modulates receptor-mediated phospholipase C and membrane fluidity in rat ventricular myocytes in culture. J Mol Cell Cardiol. 1996;28:1097-1108.
85. du Bois TM, Deng C, Huang XF. Membrane phospholipid composition, alterations in neurotransmitter systems and schizophrenia. Prog Neuropsychopharmacol Biol Psychiatry. 2005;29(6):878-888.
86. Peet M, Stokes C. Omega-3 fatty acids in the treatment of psychiatric disorders. Drugs. 2005;65:1051-1059.
87. Fromm MF. Importance of P-glycoprotein at blood-tissue barriers. Trends Pharmacol Sci. 2004;25:423-429.
88. Matheny CJ, Lamb MW, Brouwer KLR, Pollack GM. Pharmacokinetic and pharmacodynamic implications of P-glycoprotein modulation. Pharmacotherapy. 2001;21:778-796.
89. Murphy MM, Vilella E, Ceruelo S, et al. The MTHFR C77T, APOE, and PON55 gene polymorphisms show relevant interactions with cardiovascular risk factors. Clin Chem. 2002;48:372-375.
90. McCully KS. Homocysteine and vascular disease. Nature Med. 1996;2:386-389.
91. Wu G, Meininger CJ. Regulation of nitric oxide synthesis by dietary factors. Annu Rev Nutr. 2002;22:61-86.
92. Gladwin MT, Crawford JH, Patel RP. The biochemistry of nitric oxide, nitrite, and hemoglobin: role in blood flow regulation. Free Radic Biol Med. 2004;15:707-717.
93. Lum H, Roebuck KA. Oxidant stress and endothelial cell dysfunction. Am J Physiol Cell Physiol. 2001;280:C719-C741.
94. Sanders ME, Klaenhammer TR. Invited Review: The scientific basis of *Lactobacillus acidophilus* NCFM® functionality as a probiotic. Dairy Sci. 2001;84:319-331.
95. Gestel G, Besancon P, Rouanet J-M. Comparative evaluation of the effects of two different forms of dietary fibre (rice bran vs. wheat bran) on colonic mucosa and faecal microflora. Ann Nutr Metab. 1994;38:249-256.

Chapter 18
The Biology of Inflammation: A Common Pathway in Cardiovascular Diseases, Part I

Peter Libby, MD

Introduction[i]

This primer on inflammation biology describes the mechanisms of innate and acquired immunity, and the key players in the inflammatory response, explicating and disentangling the connections between them—the better to argue the case that the entire spectrum of inflammatory diseases represents host defenses gone awry. A number of cardiovascular conditions, some exotic, but many common, involve an important component of inflammation, representing host defense mechanisms that can cause disease. Part I of this essay provides a general background to the biology of inflammation. The discussion will serve as a roadmap and glossary of inflammation that will facilitate placing this topic into the clinical context of cardiovascular diseases. Part II, a discussion of how these concepts influence atherosclerosis and myocardial infarction, can be found in Chapter 27.

Inflammation is Intertwined with the Vasculature

Physicians in ancient times recognized the importance of inflammation in pathophysiology. Inflammation has features easily recognizable at the macroscopic level and grossly apparent on physical examination. The Latin terminology handed down from Celsus in classical times described the cardinal features of inflammation: *rubor, tumor, calor,* and *dolor. Rubor* (redness) arises from increased local blood flow due to vasodilatation. *Calor* (heat) also likely reflects increased regional blood flow and vasodilatation. *Dolor* (pain) results from local release of inflammatory mediators that stimulate nociceptors in local nerves. *Tumor* (swelling) reflects tissue edema and often accompanies the redness and heat at sites of inflammation. Localized increases in vascular permeability, part and parcel of the inflammatory process, contribute to the local edema manifest as swelling. Aside from pain, all of these classic signs of inflammation relate to perturbations in the vasculature. Increased blood flow, vasodilatation, and increased vascular permeability characteristically accompany sites of inflammation. Considered in this context, the general pathology of inflammation falls within the province of cardiovascular pathophysiology in its most fundamental aspects.

Although known to the ancients, knowledge about the cellular basis of inflammation required advances in microscopy and tissue analysis made in the 19th century. The commercial development of aniline dyes in the textile industry stimulated the development of synthetic organic chemistry in the 1800s. The scientific "spin-off" of this commercially driven research and development included the application of newly synthesized dyes to provide contrast of stained tissues during microscopic examination. This technological advance spurred the development of cellular pathology embodied in the work of Rudolph Virchow. Armed only with stained tissue sections and keen inductive reasoning, the cellular pathologists of the 19th century worked out

[i] Adapted, with permission, from: Libby P. Inflammation: a common pathway in cardiovascular diseases. Dialogues in Cardiovascular Medicine. 2003;8(2):59-73. The original article has been divided into two parts for this book; part II can be found in Section VI: A Practical Clinical Approach, as the first piece in Chapter 27. **Acknowledgment**: Supported in part by a grant from the National Heart, Lung, and Blood Institute (HL-34636).

the involvement of leukocytes in inflammatory reactions in tissues.[1]

The 19th century also witnessed the birth of experimental pathology. The investigation of inflammatory phenomena figured prominently in the early development of this science. Elie Metchnikoff, summering in Messina, Italy, observed the engulfment by the leukocytes of marine invertebrates of foreign bodies, a process he called phagocytosis.[2] These observations and Metchnikoff's astute interpretations led to the recognition of the role of leukocytes and host defenses against foreign invaders. As the germ theory of disease developed in the latter part of the 19th century, the concept of foreign bodies extended to microbial invaders. To this day, much of the biology of inflammation consists of exchanges of messages among various classes of leukocytes and with parenchymal cells.

The molecular nature of the messages exchanged among cells during inflammatory reactions developed largely during the 20th century. During the first two-thirds of the 20th century, much work focused on the purification and elucidation of the structures of low molecular-weight mediators of inflammation. Molecules such as histamine, related to a simple amino acid, exemplified "autocoids" involved in inflammatory responses. Histamine can cause profound changes in vascular biology, including increased permeability of microvessels. Histamine also elicits the contraction of smooth muscle cells, manifest as vasoconstriction of some beds and bronchoconstriction in the airways. Small-molecule lipid mediators characterized during this period included the prostaglandins, the leukotrienes, the lipoxins, and platelet-activating factor (PAF). Some peptide mediators of inflammation of higher molecular weight, including bradykinin, also underwent purification and characterization.

In the latter third of the 20th century, the study of protein mediators of inflammation and immunity burgeoned. Advances in protein biochemistry, and eventually molecular biology, led to the identification of the cytokines, now considered major messengers in host defenses and inflammatory reactions. Originally considered products of "professional" inflammatory cells such as leukocytes, traditional concepts viewed "peripheral" cells, such as those of the vasculature or parenchymal cells of various organs, as responders to signals elaborated by leukocytes. More recently, we have come to appreciate that many cell types, notably including vascular endothelial and smooth muscle cells, can produce as well as respond to various cytokines.[3] Thus, our understanding of the complexity of the networks involved in inflammatory signaling has grown considerably as scientific knowledge has advanced.

Phagocytes: The First Line of Host Defenses

In the more than a century following Metchnikoff's definition of phagocytosis, appreciation of the importance of this process has only grown as we have filled in the cellular and molecular mechanisms. The granulocyte—or polymorphonuclear leukocyte—embodies *par excellence* the phagocyte involved in acute inflammatory reactions. In acute bacterial infections, chemotactic peptides of microbial origin such as formyl-methionyl-leucyl-phenylalanine (f-met-leu-phe) or anaphylatoxins (see below) beckoned granulocytes from the vasculature to the nidus of infection. Activated by these bacterial products and others such as endotoxin (lipopolysaccharides manufactured by certain bacteria), the polymorphonuclear leukocyte degranulates, releasing enzymes that can attack the invaders. Granulocytes also manufacture enzymes that produce molecules involved in killing microbial invaders. Various oxidases generate superoxide anion, O_2^-, an example of a bactericidal reactive oxygen species. The granulocyte also releases myeloperoxidase, an enzyme that produces hypochlorous acid (HOCl). Hypochlorous acid, more commonly known as laundry bleach, can also kill bacteria. Although bacterial products may directly initiate the recruitment of granulocytes during infection, endogenous mechanisms soon join in.

Bacterial endotoxin can stimulate the expression on the surface of vascular endothelial cells of an adhesion molecule that binds selectively to a ligand on granulocytes.[4] E-selectin, not normally expressed by resting endothelial cells, arises rapidly on endothelial cells stimulated with bacterial lipopolysaccharide or certain cytokines. E-selectin binds to sialyl Lewis X molecules on the granulocyte surface. This interaction captures the polymorphonuclear leukocyte flowing through post-capillary venules and mediates a rolling of the granulocyte on the endothelial surface.[5] Other members of the selectin family may serve similar roles in slowing the progress of the polymorphonuclear leukocyte through the microcirculation. Tarrying in venules due to selectin-mediated rolling, the leukocyte can then form firmer interactions by binding to members of another family of adhesion molecules expressed by inflamed endothelial cells: members of the immunoglobulin (IgG) superfamily.[6] These molecules, exemplified by intercellular adhesion molecule-1 (ICAM-1), arrest the rolling leukocyte, the next step in the recruitment process. Once adherent, the granulocyte receives chemoattractant signals from beyond the endothelial layer to trigger transmigration of the adherent leukocyte so that it can penetrate into the target tissue. The bacterial-derived chemoattractants, such as f-met-leu-phe, promote this directed migration. In addition, host cytokines such as interleukin-8 (IL-8), manufactured locally in response to bacterial products such as endotoxin, can unite with bacterially-derived chemoattractants to call the polymorphonuclear leukocyte into the tissue invaded by bacteria.[7,8] This schema of a local inflammatory stimulus (the bacteria) and recruitment of leukocytes by adherence transmigration, followed by activation of the effector mechanisms of the leukocyte as summarized above, applies not only to acute inflammation due to a bacterial infection, but serves as a general paradigm for localized inflammatory responses.

Of course, bacterial invasion sometimes spreads beyond the local tissue. Septicemia, or blood-borne infection, elicits a systemic or generalized host-defense reaction with profound cardiovascular consequences. Bacterial endotoxemia wreaks havoc with homeostasis of blood coagulation.[9] Endotoxin induces endothelial expression of the potent procoagulant molecule tissue factor.[10] It also augments production of inhibitors of fibrinolysis such as plasminogen activator inhibitor-1(PAI-1).[11] Such changes can give rise to disseminated intravascular coagulation, one of the dread consequences of disseminated gram-negative infection. Circulating endotoxin leads to widespread release of cytokines, such as IL-1 and tumor necrosis factor (TNF) (see below). These cytokines can induce fever, which in turn causes tachycardia. In addition, the small molecule nitric oxide (NO), produced by endothelial cells stimulated with bacterial endotoxin as well as deriving from other inflamed cells including leukocytes, can promote vasodilatation and hypotension.[12] A hyperkinetic state ensues with low resistance and high cardiac output characteristic of septic shock. This picture, all too commonly encountered clinically, represents an extreme case on a systemic or generalized scale of the acute inflammatory response to a bacterial invader.

Not all bacterial infections play out on a scale of hours to days. Chronic microbial infections represent an example of inflammatory responses that endure longer. While some of the cells and messengers in the dramatis personae of chronic inflammatory responses differ from those described above in the context of acute responses, many of the fundamental principles remain the same. Consider, for example, the classic chronic bacterial disease, tuberculosis. The pathological hallmark of infection with the tubercle bacillus is a granuloma rather than an abscess populated by polymorphonuclear leukocytes. In the granuloma, the mononuclear phagocyte, rather than the polymorphonuclear leukocyte, takes center stage. Derived from blood monocytes, the tissue macrophage becomes the key effector cell in chronic inflammatory responses. The tubercle granuloma can last for years, as opposed to the abscess populated by polymorphonuclear leukocytes in a pyogenic bacterial infection. The granuloma represents the results of the interaction of the parenchymal tissue of the infected organ with the macrophages. This pathology plays out in a similar fashion in atheroma, an example of a special case of granuloma formation considered below.

As alluded to above, recruitment of monocytes to sites of chronic infection or inflammation recapitulates on a slower scale the accumulation of granulocytes to foci of acute inflammation. In the case of the monocyte, adhesion molecules of the IgG superfamily, such as vascular cell adhesion molecule-1 (VCAM-1), interact with integrin molecules on the mononuclear cell, such as very late antigen-4 (VLA-4). Once adherent to the endothelial cell, endogenous chemoattractant molecules direct the migration of the mononuclear phagocyte into the inflamed tissue. While IL-8 favors recruitment of granulocytes, members of another chemokine family, the CXC chemokines, selectively recruit monocytes. Macrophage chemoattractant protein-1 (MCP-1) represents an example of a mononuclear phagocyte chemoattractant that helps to recruit these cells to sites of formation of granuloma for other chronic inflammatory processes.

Granulocytes, the typical effector cells of acute inflammatory responses, have eponymous granules packed with preformed mediators. When recruited to sites of acute inflammation, they degranulate, rapidly produce a reactive oxygen species through the "respiratory burst," and die, often by apoptosis.[13] At sites of chronic inflammation, the life history of the mononuclear phagocyte differs considerably. The blood monocyte, recruited to a site of chronic inflammation, differentiates into a macrophage. A variety of endogenous stimuli favor the transition of the blood monocyte into a tissue macrophage involved in chronic inflammatory responses. Molecules such as macrophage-colony stimulating factor (M-CSF) and activators of protein kinase-C promote monocyte differentiation. Equipped for prolonged combat rather than a short battle with acute invaders, the macrophage effector mechanisms typically outlast those of granulocytes.

Macrophages have a well-developed phagolysosome system that is well suited for combating chronic invaders. For example, the macrophage can engulf particulate matter such as the tubercle bacillus and transport the engulfed particle to the lysosome, an intracellular compartment filled with digestive enzymes. Often in concert with phagocytosis, the macrophage elaborates reactive oxygen species, including superoxide anion (0_2^-), NO, and hypochlorous acid.[12] The macrophage appears capable of producing these small-molecule effectors of host defenses on a more prolonged timescale than the granulocyte. The mononuclear phagocyte excels at producing higher-molecular-weight mediators as well. The macrophage, when activated, can produce large quantities of cytokines. In addition, the tissue macrophage produces abundant proteases involved in tissue remodeling, a property of particular importance in cardiovascular pathology (see below).[14,15] Pus (comprised of a mixture of live, dying, and dead granulocytes) typifies abscesses at sites of acute inflammation. In granuloma, however, rather than committing suicide, macrophages may fuse, forming giant cells whose palisade of nuclei classically characterizes the tuberculous granuloma. Prolonged persistence of the phagocytic cell predominates at sites of chronic, as opposed to acute, inflammatory responses.

The Innate Immune Response

The two general pathways of inflammation described above represent two limbs of host defense mechanisms now often described as "innate immunity." The term innate denotes instant readiness to cope with invaders, circumventing the need for an instructional period as the acquired (antigen specific) immune response requires. The types of structures on invaders that trigger the innate immune response include molecules with shared structural features, such as gram-negative endotoxin. The structures that recognize these relatively conserved structures have been called "pattern-recognition receptors." Families of pattern recognition receptors include scavenger receptors (first characterized in the context of atherosclerosis),[16] and a recently characterized family of transmembrane molecules known as toll-like receptors (TLR).[17]

Innate immunity represents a first line of defense against invaders capable of rapid deployment. Innate immunity plays out first not only within the organism, but also earlier during phylogeny. The innate immune response represents a more primitive form of host defense present in invertebrates and independent of the more selective recognition involved in adaptive immunity, a more recent development during evolution.[18] In addition to the leukocytic effector cells of acute and chronic inflammation described above, the complement system contributes importantly to innate immunity.[19,20] The alternative pathway of complement activation recognizes common patterns (for example, de-sialylated glycoconjugates on the surface of erythrocytes). Activation of complement by the alternative pathway leads to formation of the terminal membrane attack complex that can effectively punch holes in invading microbial cells. In this way, complement can kill bacterial and other invaders and, when unleashed inappropriately, host cells as well.

Cytokines: Omnipresent Organizers of the Inflammatory Response

As noted above, for most of the 20th century, attention focused on small molecules as mediators of inflammation. Over the last quarter century, we have become acquainted with large families of protein mediators of inflammation and immunity known collectively as cytokines.[21] These cytokines fall into many categories. Originally considered exclusively as products of leukocytes, many initially bore the name "interleukin." As our knowledge of the biology of cytokines has increased, so has our appreciation that many cells can elaborate these multi-functional mediators. Hence, more recently recognized families of cytokines often bear other names. Many of the cytokines categorized early on derive from mononuclear phagocytes, classifying them as monokines. Others, produced by T-lymphocytes, bore the name "lymphokine." Chemoattractant cytokines fall into families known as chemokines.[22] A related class of protein mediators known as colony-stimulating factors has overlapping characteristics with classical cytokines (e.g., interleukin-3). Therefore, discussions of cytokines often include colony-stimulating factors. The following paragraphs will introduce briefly certain of the prototypical cytokines to illustrate the properties of these important mediators. Table 18.1 shows examples of cytokines important in cardiovascular pathology and often cited in the cardiovascular literature.

Table 18.1 **Examples of Cytokines Involved in Cardiovascular Inflammation**

Cytokine	Abbreviation(s)	Important functions
Interleukin-1	IL-1	Endogenous pyrogen, T cell coactivator, proinflammatory activation of vascular cells
Tumor necrosis factor	TNF	As above, autocrine regulator of myocardiocytes
Gamma interferon	IFN-γ	Macrophage activator, inducer of histocompatibility antigens, prototype Th1 cytokine
Interleukin-10	IL-10	Often anti-inflammatory, prototype Th2 cytokine
Macrophage-colony stimulating factor	M-CSF	Macrophage activator and co-mitogen
Monocyte chemoattractant protein-1	MCP-1	Macrophage chemoattractant
CD40 Ligand	CD40L, CD154, gp39	As IL-1 but also activates caspase-1 and induces macrophage tissue factor expression
Interleukin - 18	IL-18	Gamma interferon induction

Interleukin-1: The Prototypical Monokine

As is typical, the protein now known as interleukin-1 (IL-1) represented a convergence of various activities found to reside in a small family of closely-related proteins after years of parallel work in various laboratories.[23] The molecular characterization of IL-1 arose from the identification, purification, and eventually the cDNA cloning of the active principle in mediating fever known as endogenous pyrogen. The example of IL-1 illustrates many features common to cytokines. Seldom produced by resting cells, many cell types produce this protein inducibly in response to inflammatory stimuli such as bacterial endotoxin. Initially synthesized as a 33000 dalton precursor, interleukin-1β (IL-1β), the predominant secreted form of this cytokine, requires processing to attain its full biological activity. An enzyme known as interleukin-1β-converting enzyme, or ICE, effects this conversion.[24] Interestingly, ICE represented the prototype of a new family of proteinases known as caspases, so named because they are cysteinyl proteinases that cleave at aspartyl residues (asp) in their substrates. The other isoform of IL-1, known as interleukin-1α (IL-1α), often remains associated with the cell surface and does not require proteolytic processing for biological activity.

IL-1 binds to selective transmembrane receptors. The signaling receptor for IL-1β feeds into the same intracellular pathway as the pattern recognition receptors, TLRs, alluded to above. IL-1β engagement of its signaling receptor ultimately causes activation of a transcription factor known as nuclear factor-kappa B (NFκB).[25] NFκB, when activated, binds to cognate sequences in the promotor regions of the genes encoding a wide variety of inflammatory effectors. Thus, IL-1β action unleashes a coordinate program of inflammatory mechanisms in many leukocytes and other host cells. In this way, IL-1β acts as a master regulator of the innate immune response, evoking the elaboration of many other cytokines, including augmentation of its own gene expression.[26] Like many potent biological pathways, IL-1β has an endogenous inhibitor, a structural homologue known as IL-1 receptor antagonist. This endogenous molecule competes for the signaling receptor of IL-1β, limiting its actions. Itself induced in response to inflammatory signals, the IL-1β receptor antagonist constitutes a negative feedback loop poised to prevent untrammeled amplification of this potent proinflammatory pathway

Tumor Necrosis Factor-Alpha: A Death-linked Cytokine

Tumor necrosis factor-α (TNF-α), a close cousin of IL-1β, exhibits augmented production and spectral and biological activities similar to that due to IL-1. Like IL-1β, TNF-α has several surface receptors. The active signaling receptor, however, elicits activation not only of NFκB, but also of the pathway that causes programmed cell death, or apoptosis.[27] Thus, in addition to the proinflammatory action that TNF-α has in common with IL-1β, it links to the control of cell death.

Interleukin-6: A "Messenger" Cytokine

A prominent target gene for activation by TNF-α and IL-1β, many peripheral cells, including vascular smooth muscle, can secrete copious quantities of interleukin-6 (IL-6) when stimulated by the primary proinflammatory cytokines IL-1 or TNF. IL-6 activates B cells and promotes their maturation, an important aspect of antibody production and acquired immunity. Of great interest in cardiovascular pathology, IL-6 serves as a link between the acute inflammatory response mediated by the primary proinflammatory cytokines and the systemic reaction to acute inflammation, known as the "acute-phase response."[28,29] IL-6 alters the pattern of protein synthesis by hepatocytes. After encountering IL-6, the liver shifts new protein synthesis from "housekeeping" proteins such as albumen toward production of acute-phase reactants, which serve as readily sampled systemic markers of inflammation. The acute phase reactants may also participate in inflammatory responses involved in cardiovascular pathology. For example, C-reactive protein (CRP), a classic acute-phase reactant, has garnered considerable interest recently as a prognostic or predictive indicator of cardiovascular risk.[30] In addition, CRP can activate complement and thus actively participate in innate immunity. Serum amyloid-A, another prominent acute-phase reactant, may increase hundreds of times in the plasma of patients with inflammatory states. Serum amyloid-A can bind to high density lipoprotein (HDL), impairing some of the salutary properties of this lipoprotein molecule, thus potentially increasing coronary risk prospectively.[31] Another acute-phase reactant, fibrinogen, directly participates in blood coagulation. In this manner, the acute-phase response may link to a thrombotic diathesis of considerable import in cardiovascular diseases. IL-6, as an instigator of the acute-phase response, can in this manner serve as an important link between inflammation and cardiovascular events.

Interferon Gamma: The Prototypical Lymphokine

Immune interferon, or interferon gamma (IFN-γ), contrasts with the aforementioned cytokines inasmuch as a much smaller gamut of cells produce this cytokine. Classically considered exclusively a product of activated T-lymphocytes, even after exhaustive investigations only a few cell types have proven capable of producing IFN-γ. As might be expected of a cytokine derived from a cell type prominent in adaptive immunity, IFN-γ enhances antigen presentation by augmenting the expression of major histocompatibility complex antigens important for recognition of foreign antigens.[32] However, IFN-γ also stimulates mononuclear phagocytes, among other aspects of the innate immune response. Nonetheless, the range of actions produced by IFN-γ shows considerably more selectivity than that of IL-1 or TNF, illustrating that all cytokines act promiscuously.

Macrophage Chemoattractant Protein-1: A Typical Chemoattractant Cytokine

Several families of chemokines exist. Specialists use a shorthand based on the spacing of conserved cysteine residues in the amino acid sequence of the cytokines to classify these various families. MCP-1 falls into the family of CXC cytokines, indicating that an unspecified (X) amino acid residue lies between neighboring cysteine residues.[33] Chemokines typically bind to specific membrane receptors grouped into similar families based on their ligand. The MCP-1 receptor, CXC-R2, belongs to the large family of heptahelical, or 7 membrane spanning G-protein-coupled receptors. Thus, the signaling mechanism of chemokines does not generally overlap with those of the primary proinflammatory cytokines. As the spectrum of receptors on various classes of cells varies, so does the specificity of the targets for chemoattraction of various chemokines. MCP-1, as mentioned above, binds selectively to cells of the mononuclear family. Mice lacking the receptor for MCP-1 show impaired recruitment of mononuclear phagocytes to sites of chronic inflammation.

The Lymphocytes: Major Mediators of Acquired Immunity

Thus far, our discussion of inflammatory responses has focused on innate or "ready-made" immunity. Higher organisms have added to the repertoire of host defenses a complex surveillance and effector system based on highly-variable and fine structural determinants known as acquired immunity. This name also conveys the idea that acquisition of this form of immunity requires time, rather than being prefabricated as in the case of innate immunity. The T lymphocyte orchestrates acquired immunity, which has both humoral (antibody-mediated) and cellular limbs.

Generation of the Acquired Immune Response: The Helper T Cell

A subset of T cells known as helper T cells, usually bearing the CD4 determinant, initiates most acquired immune responses by recognizing antigen via engagement of a selective cell surface receptor. The recognition of antigens by the helper T cell requires presentation on the surface of a cooperating cell, known as the antigen-presenting cell, or APC. The T cell receptor does not recognize the foreign antigen in isolation, but requires presentation in the context of a structure on the surface of the APC, the class II major histocompatibility antigen. Each individual bears his or her own mix of these highly polymorphic molecules that serve an essential role in generating the immune response. Incidentally, histocompatibility antigens bear this name because they themselves are capable of generating an immune response to organs transplanted from different members of a species, hence the term histocompatibility antigen. The engagement of the T cell's receptor for antigen causes the T cell to secrete IFN-γ, which raises the level of class II histocompatibility antigens on the surface of potential antigen-presenting cells, priming them to contribute to the generation of the acquired immune response. Engagement of the antigen receptor also causes the T cell to augment its production of a lymphokine known as IL-2, originally termed T-cell growth factor. The T cell activated by antigen also increases its expression of the cell surface that binds IL-2. Thus, the T cell that has encountered foreign antigen in the context of its own class II molecule can undergo self-perpetuated clonal expansion, producing and responding to its own growth factor, an example of an autocrine growth control loop. Expanding the population of antigen-specific T cells amplifies the response to a given foreign antigen—for example, to a virus.

The term "helper T cell" refers to the ability of the CD4 cell, when activated, to promote development of a full-blown immune response, both humoral and cellular. Stimulation of the humoral immune response involves the expression on the surface of the activated T cell of CD154, also known as CD40 ligand.[34] This surface molecule binds to a cognate receptor on the B-lymphocyte, the antigen-producing cell, causing it to mature into a plasma cell capable of secreting large quantities of antibody directed against specific antigens. The IL-2 secreted by the activated T cell serves not only in autocrine growth, but also in "paracrine growth," stimulating the proliferation of CD8 cells, also known as killer or cytotoxic T cells, the efferent limb of the cellular immune response.

Cytolytic T Cells: Effectors of the Cellular Immune Response

Stimulated by IL-2 secreted by the activated helper T cell, CD8 cells proliferate and become activated themselves. The CD8 cell recognizes foreign antigen in the context of class I MHC (major histocompatibility complex) molecules. While helper T cells recognize antigen presented on the surface of antigen-presenting cells in the context of self-class II MHC, the cytolytic T cell recognizes antigen presented in the context of class I molecules on the surface cells infected with viruses or, in the case of transplanted organs, the foreign cell itself. Recognition of the foreign antigen causes the cytolytic T cell to secrete a molecule known as perforin, which resembles the terminal membrane attack complex component of complement, and likewise can poke holes in the membrane of the cell under attack.[35] In addition, digestive enzymes, such as granzyme, arise from the activated killer T cell. The cytolytic T cell, usually bearing the CD8 antigen on its surface, also can express Fas, a TNF-like molecule, on its surface. Fas engages Fas-ligand on the cell under attack. Fas ligation, like TNF, causes activation of the cell-death cascade. The Fas pathway thus represents yet another mechanism by which the CD8-positive T cell can kill a cell that harbors a viral infection or otherwise presents foreign antigen.

B Cells: A Source of Antibody

As described above, the effector limb of cellular immunity requires contact between the cytolytic T cell and its target. Humoral responses mediated by antibody, soluble molecules, do not require such cell-cell contact. The B cell, in receipt of "help" from T cells and aided by the "messenger" cytokine IL-6, becomes a plasma cell specialized in secreting large amounts of antibody.

Antibody can serve several roles in host defenses. By binding to determinants on the surface of microbial invaders, antibody molecules can "fix" complement through the classical pathway, leading to lysis of the invading cell by mechanisms already discussed. Antibody coating the surface of bacteria also can engage the Fc-receptors on the surface of phagocytes, targeting them for engulfment and destruction. This function of antibody, known as opsonization, was likened by the Irish playwright George Bernard Shaw to putting butter on a slice of bread before eating it.[36] Antibody can also neutralize invaders such as viruses simply by binding them tightly and preventing their access to target cells.

Clinical Implications of Host Defenses Gone Awry

We have now outlined a series of host defense mechanisms ranging from primitive to highly-developed and specific, all focused on defending the organism from invading pathogens and foreign bodies. These defense mechanisms each serve important roles in health and homeostasis. Individuals with congenital or acquired deficiencies in each of these major pathways of host defenses exhibit heightened susceptibility to different types of disease. As impaired antibody responses predispose to pyogenic bacterial diseases, consider the case of the increased incidence of pneumococcal disease in splenectomized patients. Individuals with impaired cellular immunity have difficulty eliminating viruses and intracellular bacteria, as in the case of the acquired immune deficiency syndrome (AIDS). Individuals with mutations that impair their ability to make superoxide anion show susceptibility to pyogenic infections, particularly *Staphylococcus aureus*.

Unfortunately, these powerful host defense mechanisms can cause disease when expressed inappropriately or in excess. The entire spectrum of inflammatory diseases represents host defenses gone awry. The humoral and cellular immune responses, appropriately directed against foreign invaders, become pathological when turned against self, as in the case of the autoimmune diseases. Many autoimmune diseases cause vasculitis, placing them within the spectrum of cardiovascular diseases. Acute allograft rejection and the chronic vasculopathy often seen in transplanted organs represent another undesired consequence of the otherwise salubrious host-immune response. In some cases, microbial invaders may elicit an immune response that cross-reacts with an endogenous host structure. Such antigenic mimicry may account for the association of rheumatic heart disease with streptococcal infections. Recent evidence inculpates antigenic mimicry between *Chlamydia pneumoniae* and a determinant of cardiac myosin as a mechanism of autoimmune cardiomyopathy. Cholesterol emboli may activate complement, provoking an inflammatory response with often dramatic clinical consequences.

Table 18.2 lists a number of cardiovascular conditions, some exotic but many common, that involve an important component of inflammation, representing host defense mechanisms that nonetheless can cause disease. In Part II of this essay (Chapter 27), we will consider examples of some common cardiovascular diseases that specifically illustrate this principle.

Table 18.2 **Examples of Cardiovascular Diseases Involving Inflammation**

Disease	Example of Inflammatory Process in Pathogenesis
Atherosclerosis	Fibroproliferation in response to macrophage-derived mediators
Unstable angina pectoris	Inflammation characterized by elevated C-reactive protein without infarction
Atheroma disruption	Macrophage-induced collagenolysis, T cell inhibition of collagen synthesis
Vascular thrombosis	Favored by acute-phase reactants fibrinogen, plasminogen inhibitor
Myocardial infarction	Phagocyte ingestion of necrotic cells and subsequent tissue repair
Myocarditis	Leukocyte infiltration and cytokine activation of cardiocytes and endothelium
Abdominal aortic aneurysm	Prominent inflammation of the adventitia as well as intima-media
Cholesterol emboli syndrome	Complement activation
Cardiovascular complications of lupus erythematosus, scleroderma, rheumatoid arthritis, etc	Vasculitis
Rheumatic heart disease	Pancarditis
Transplantation rejection	Killer-T cell-mediated myocardiocytolysis
Allograft vasculopathy	CD4-mediated fibroproliferative response to foreign antigens
"No-reflow"	Leukocyte sludging due to activated endothelium
Restenosis post-arterial intervention	Activation of vascular cells and leukocyte recruitment provoked by injury
Infective endocarditis	Complement activation by immune complexes contribute to complications

References

1. Virchow R. Cellular Pathology. London: John Churchill; 1858.
2. Chernyak L, Tauber AI. The birth of immunology: Metchnikoff, the embryologist. Cell Immunol. 1988;117:218-233.
3. Libby P. Changing concepts of atherogenesis. J Intern Med. 2000;247:349 358.
4. Bevilacqua MP, Pober JS, Majeau GR, et al. Interleukin-1 acts on cultured human vascular endothelium to increase the adhesion of polymorphonuclear leukocytes, monocytes and related leukocyte cell lines. J Clin Invest. 1985;76:2003-2011.
5. Frenette PS, Wagner DD. Insights into selectin function from knockout mice. Thromb Haemost. 1997;78:60-64.
6. Wang J, Springer TA. Structural specializations of immunoglobulin superfamily members for adhesion to integrins and viruses. Immunol Rev. 1998;163:197-215.
7. Mukaida N, Harada A, Matsushima K. Interleukin-8 (IL-8) and monocyte chemotactic and activating factor (MCAF/MCP-1), chemokines essentially involved in inflammatory and immune reactions. Cytokine Growth Factor Rev. 1998;9:9-23.
8. Luster AD. Chemokines—chemotactic cytokines that mediate inflammation. N Engl J Med. 1998;338:436-445.
9. Libby P, Simon DI. Inflammation and thrombosis : the clot thickens. Circulation. 2001;103:1718-1720.
10. Nemerson Y, Giesen PL. Some thoughts about localization and expression of tissue factor. Blood Coagulation Fibrinol. 1998;9:S45-47.
11. Loskutoff DJ, Van Mourik JA, Erickson LA, Lawrence D. Detection of an unusually stable fibrinolytic inhibitor produced by bovine endothelial cells. Cell. Biol. 1983;80:2956-2960.
12. Nathan C, Shiloh MU. Reactive oxygen and nitrogen intermediates in the relationship between mammalian hosts and microbial pathogens. Proc Natl Acad Sci USA. 2000;97:8841-8848.
13. Fadok VA, Henson PM. Apoptosis: getting rid of the bodies. Curr Biol. 1998;8:R693-695.
14. Dollery CM, McEwan JR, Henney AM. Matrix metalloproteinases and cardiovascular disease. Circ Res. 1995;77:863-868.
15. Libby P, Geng Y-J, Aikawa M, et al. Macrophages and atherosclerotic plaque stability. Curr Opin Lipidol. 1996;7:330-335.
16. Krieger M. The other side of scavenger receptors: pattern recognition for host defense. Curr Opin Lipidol. 1997;8:275-280.
17. Medzhitov R, Janeway CA, Jr. Innate immune induction of the adaptive immune response. Cold Spring Harb Symp Quant Biol. 1999;64:429-435.
18. Kimbrell DA, Beutler B. The evolution and genetics of innate immunity. Nat Rev Genet. 2001;2:256-267.
19. Walport MJ. Complement. First of two parts. N Engl J Med. 2001;344:1058-1066.
20. Walport MJ. Complement. Second of two parts. N Engl J Med. 2001;344:1140-1144.
21. Libby P, Ross R. Cytokines and growth regulatory molecules. In: Fuster V, Ross R, Topol E, eds. Atherosclerosis and coronary artery disease. New York, NY: Lippincott-Raven; 1996:585-594.
22. Luster AD. Chemokines--chemotactic cytokines that mediate inflammation. N Engl J Med. 1998;338:436-445.
23. Dinarello C. The interleukin-1 family: 10 years of discovery. FASEB J. 1994;8:1314-1325.
24. Thornberry NA, Bull HG, Calaycay JR, et al. A novel heterodimeric cysteine protease is required for interleukin-1 beta processing in monocytes. Nature. 1992;356:768-774.
25. Collins T, Cybulsky MI. NF-kappaB: pivotal mediator or innocent bystander in atherogenesis? J Clin Invest. 2001;107:255-264.
26. Dinarello CA, Ikejima T, Warner SJC, et al. Interleukin-1 induces interleukin-1. I. Induction of circulating interleukin-1 in rabbits *in vivo* and in human mononuclear cells *in vitro*. J Immunol. 1987;139:1902-1910.
27. Strasser A, O'Connor L, Dixit VM. Apoptosis signaling. Annu Rev Biochem. 2000;69:217-245.
28. Luster AD. Chemokines—chemotactic cytokines that mediate inflammation. N Engl J Med. 1998;338:436-445.
29. Loppnow H, Libby P. Proliferating or interleukin 1-activated human vascular smooth muscle cells secrete copious interleukin 6. J Clin Invest. 1990;85:731-738.
30. Libby P, Ridker PM. Novel inflammatory markers of coronary risk: theory versus practice. Circulation. 1999;100:1148-1150.
31. Van Lenten B, Hama SY, de Beer F, et al. Anti-inflammatory HDL becomes proinflammatory during the acute phase response. Loss of protective effect of HDL against LDL oxidation in aortic wall cell cocultures. J Clin Invest. 1995;96:2758-2767.
32. Collins T, Korman AJ, Wake CT, et al. Immune interferon activates multiple class II major histocompatibility complex genes and the associated invariant chain gene in human endothelial cells and dermal fibroblasts. Proc Natl Acad Sci USA. 1984;81:4917-4921.
33. Luster AD. Chemokines—chemotactic cytokines that mediate inflammation. N Engl J Med. 1998;338:436-445.
34. Schonbeck U, Mach F, Libby P. CD154 (CD40 ligand). Int J Biochem Cell Biol. 2000;32:687-693.
35. Clark WR. Immunology. The hole truth about perforin. Nature. 1994;369:16-17.
36. Shaw G. The doctor's dilemma. Baltimore, MD: Penguin Books, Inc. 1911.

Section V

Fundamental Clinical Imbalances

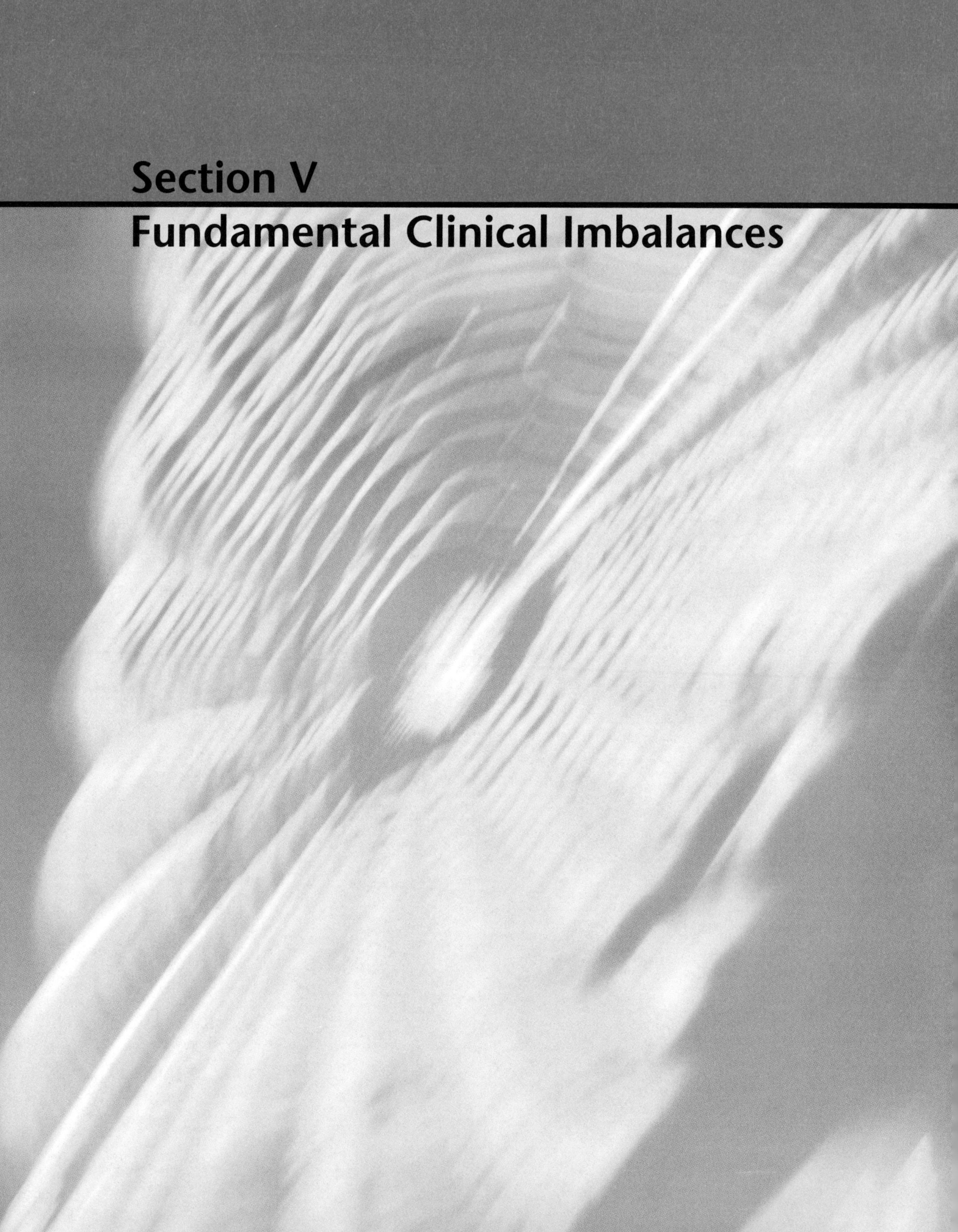

Chapter 19
Hormonal Imbalances

- *Female Hormones: The Dance of the Hormones, Part I*
- *Male Hormones*
- *The Epidemic of Insulin Insensitivity*

Female Hormones: The Dance of the Hormones, Part I

Bethany Hays, MD

Introduction

The health of the human organism is determined by its flexibility in responding to the environment, and by the balance between the breakdown and use of functional and structural chemicals and their replacement. This essential process is called metabolism. Response to the environment is determined primarily by 1) information obtained through the senses and mediated by the brain and hypothalamus (the adrenal side), and 2) information obtained from food or other environmental exposures and mediated by the immune system and the pancreas and liver (the insulin side). The research literature is replete with interesting examples of the interconnectedness of these functions.[1,2,3,4,5,6,7,8,9]

Biologic function can be broadly conceptualized into reactions of approach or avoidance:

- Negative sensory information from the environment (fear, for example) leads to an avoidance reaction that involves withdrawal, contraction, and shutting down of growth and reproduction. It is mediated by the adrenal (stress adaptive) hormones, adrenaline, and cortisol. Adrenaline is primarily activating, for fight or flight; cortisol is primarily suppressive (e.g., of the immune system, of the brain as in depression, of growth as in osteoporosis).
- Positive environmental sensory information (e.g., attraction) allows for growth and reproduction and is represented by the hormone insulin, which allows for growth and storage of energy. Insulin interacts with a number of trophic hormones (including estrogen, testosterone, DHEA, and thyroid) that balance adrenaline and cortisol in different ways. Insulin is triggered both by environmental signals (e.g., the presence of food in the GI tract) and by internal signals of glucose status.

The major hormones (adrenaline and cortisol) appear to have a critical role in maintaining life and balancing the metabolism but, by themselves, would not provide the flexibility in response to the environment that has characterized the human species. The minor hormones provide a much higher degree of flexibility. Once we have a better understanding of how these hormones "dance" with each other to balance metabolism and respond to a changing environment, we can design treatment strategies that are consistent with the body's attempt to create longevity and avoid some of the missteps previously made with regard to hormone replacement.[10]

An Evolving Model of Health Care

In medicine we have traditionally diagnosed (or named) a disease and then used that diagnosis to determine a treatment that is standardized to cover the majority of people presenting with that disease. This orientation may be partly responsible for current concerns about iatrogenic morbidity and mortality.[11,12,13,14]

The functional medicine model inverts this paradigm, placing the patient's genetic and environmental individuality as the fulcrum around which healthcare evaluation and treatment are organized. This systems biology approach allows for consideration of common mechanisms of disease across multiple systems, the importance of interactions within and between complex systems, and the role of individually variable responses. This approach supports increased personalization and precision in a patient's evaluation and care through the integration of modern genomics, proteomics, and metabolomics.

In a review article in *The New England Journal of Medicine*,[15] Wylie Burke, MD, PhD points out a number of ways in which medicine today is being transformed by the understanding of genomics and proteomics.

- Diseases are being reclassified through genomic understanding. For example, in the past, Duchenne's muscular dystrophy, Becker's muscular dystrophy, and x-linked dilated cardiomyopathy were considered distinct clinical entities, but are now being grouped as related dystrophinopathies.
- The complexity of gene-gene and gene-environment effects on disease is beginning to be appreciated at a new and deeper level. He discusses, as an example, the effect on cystic fibrosis patients of *Pseudomonas aeruginosa* interacting with the gene for mannose-binding lectin, a protein that functions in innate immune responses.
- Dr. Burke concludes: "The study of gene mutations has provided a new model of pathophysiology in which the molecular causes of disease are illuminated by genetics. Evidence is now emerging of the complex interactions between genes and between genes and the environment in the causation of many diseases, and the study of these interactions represents the next important step in genomic research."

Balance and imbalance—core concepts in functional medicine—are not precise terms. We study biochemical and physiological pathways in order to determine the mechanisms that contribute to the functionality of different organ systems. When those mechanisms do not function properly, biologic processes and pathways become dysfunctional—imbalanced. As knowledge of molecular function unfolds, it is increasingly apparent that pleiotropic effects are plentiful and, therefore, that the common pathways leading to disease have many varied routes of expression—biochemical individuality plays a very significant role.

Hormonal balance adds yet another layer of complexity to the understanding of physiologic function and malfunction. Major hormonal pathways affect basic function and survival; the minor hormones, as noted above, provide the flexibility that underlies the unique adaptivity and creativity of humans. The interactions among hormones that respond to the basic approach/avoidance decisions of the organism help bring the complex functioning of the human body into better focus.

In order to apply the concept of genomics to the diseases primarily affected by hormonal imbalances, we first need to follow these hormone molecules through their "life cycles" to describe both balance and imbalance. We will then explore how they behave and interact to affect common conditions of hormone imbalance.

The "Life Cycle" of Estrogen

Estradiol, the primary functioning estrogen, is produced primarily in the ovarian theca cell from androgenic molecules produced in the granulosa cell during the reproductive lifetime of the ovary. After menopause, estradiol is formed in small amounts in the ovary but in larger amounts in the periphery. It is produced by aromatization of testosterone by CYP 19(arom) in the ovary and other tissues,[16] or by 17 hydroxylation by EDH 17 B2 (17β-hydroxysteroid dehydrogenase type 2) of estrone in the periphery. The presence of estrogen precursors and the presence and activity of these two enzymes determine the amount of estradiol in the cell and subsequently in the circulation. Relatively small amounts (nanograms) of estrogen compared to larger amounts (micrograms) of other steroid hormones have powerful effects, so the regulation and metabolism of estrogen is potentially much more important than other adrenal or ovarian hormones. Although the main contributor to the circulating levels of estrogen prior to menopause is the ovary, after menopause a number of sites produce estrogen,[17] which can have significant local effect even if their contribution to the serum levels is small. A number of pathological tissues appear to have the ability to upregulate the production of estrogens, thereby increasing the local presence of estrogen as well.[18] The two other primary forms of estrogen are estrone and estriol. Estradiol and estrone are inter-convertible while estriol is largely a downstream metabolite and is naturally present in significant amounts only during pregnancy. The biologic potency of these estrogen forms is variable not only inherently, but also in different tissues.

Sex Hormone Binding Globulin (SHBG)

When estradiol is released into the blood stream, it binds loosely with SHBG, which is produced in the liver. The amount of SHBG is a major determinant of the amount of free estrogen and testosterone (which also binds to SHBG), and can therefore be a major determinant in the availability of these steroids and their effects on target tissues. Polymorphisms of the gene producing SHBG have been identified; they can significantly affect the amount of circulating estradiol.[19] SHBG production in the liver also responds to the amount of estrogen and testosterone circulating through the liver, with higher levels of estrogen and lower levels of testosterone increasing the production.

Estrogen Receptors

Estrogens and estrogen-like molecules function via transcription-regulating nuclear proteins called receptors. In the case of estrogen, the receptors are activated by the ligand (estrogen), forming dimers.[20] The estrogen receptor is now known to exist in at least two forms. The second estrogen receptor, designated "β," has been shown to interact in some cells with the original estrogen receptor (now designated "α") to form heterodimers. Thus, homodimers of alpha or beta receptors, heterodimers (one each of alpha and beta), and their ligands (estrogens and estrogen-like chemicals, those containing a phenolated A ring) eventually find their seat on the estrogen response elements (EREs) of the DNA, after interacting with heat shock proteins in the cytoplasm and regulatory proteins in the nucleus. It is thought that the different homodimers or the heterodimers, or perhaps cytoplasmic co-regulating proteins determine which EREs will be triggered in a given tissue.[21] Certain tissues contain higher numbers of α or β receptors. Breast, endometrium, and ovarian stroma are α-receptor-rich tissues, whereas brain, bone, intestinal mucosa endothelium, and prostate are β-receptor-rich tissues.[22] Thus, an estrogen receptor alpha homodimer found in breast or endometrium will initiate cell division, whereas an estrogen receptor beta homodimer in bone may inhibit osteoclastic cell activity.

In this way an estrogenic chemical can act as a stimulant or agonist in one tissue and as a depressant or antagonist in another. In the classic estrogen-sensitive tissues, breast and endometrium, DNA transcription of EREs codes for activities primarily related to cell division. Therefore, estrogen is a trophic or growth-producing hormone in these tissues. In other tissues such as bone, liver, endothelium, skin, and brain, alpha and beta receptor homodimers and heterodimers can have either an agonist or antagonist effect, allowing estrogen to act as either a growth stimulant or a suppressor of growth.

There are many chemical ligands to these estrogen receptors (called selective estrogen receptor modulators or SERMs) that occur in both natural and pharmaceutical forms. They may function through different interactions with the alpha- and beta-receptors forming different homo- and heterodimers. The ultimate effect in a given cell is the integration of the number and ratio of homo- and heterodimers formed, as well as the affinity of the estrogen or estrogen-like chemical for the α- or β-receptor. For instance, estrone has a higher affinity for the ER-α. This would suggest that it would be more active in breast, endometrium, and ovary, where it would have cell growth stimulating effects (less desirable in menopause and postmenopause), and less active in the ER-β containing tissues like brain, bone, and endothelium. These latter organs (brain, bone, and endothelium) are often the targets of menopausal hormone replacement and would require much higher doses of estrone to have the desired effect. This understanding provides part of a rationale for administering estradiol as a replacement hormone rather than CEE (conjugated equine estrogens), estrone, or estrone-containing combinations.

The type and number of estrogen receptors are induced by the presence of estrogen[23] and certain estrogen-like molecules such as tamoxifen,[24] and are down-regulated by progesterone via the progesterone receptor. Thus, in tissues such as the endometrium, estrogen receptors are seen in high numbers in the follicular (estrogen) phase of the menstrual cycle and are low or absent in the late luteal phase after progesterone receptors appear. In other tissues, such as breast, progesterone receptors are expressed throughout the menstrual cycle, potentially functioning to suppress estrogen receptors and suggesting that the two tissues may respond differently to progesterone stimulation. They may also respond differently in the postmenopausal state than in the premenopausal state. Clinical and epidemiological data support this hypothesis.[25,26,27,28,29,30]

For many years it was thought that estrogen only functioned through the estrogen receptor, one of a family of nuclear receptors that activate estrogen response elements on DNA. More recent research shows that the transcription of many genes is modulated by estrogen. Microarray studies showed that estrogen affects hundreds of genes in diverse cell lines and tissues. (Nearly four hundred human genes are listed in the ERGD—the Estrogen Responsive Genes Database.[31]) The gene expression profiles change in various developmental stages and disease states. In fact, a gene's responses to estrogen are dependent on many factors, including the available subtype of ER, the co-regulators, the estrogen exposure time, and the amount of estrogen. It is now known however, that estrogen has non-genomic actions on cells as well. These estrogen responses are thought to be mediated through cell membrane receptors because their rapid effects could not occur if mediated by the slower process of gene transcription.[32] Examples are the effect of estrogen on NO (nitric oxide) production, and certain functions of estrogen in the brain and pancreatic insulin cells.

Estrogen Metabolism and Phase I Detoxification

Once the estrogen molecule has engaged with the cell, it must be inactivated and excreted in order for the feedback mechanisms that control its action to function normally. In other words, for a hormone to "dance" with other hormones, it must have a flexible response pattern—i.e., be able to increase and decrease rapidly. If functioning estrogens build up in the system, the delicate ebb and flow of hormones is impaired; the resulting imbalance then affects monthly cycling, pregnancy, and lactation. Following menopause, the dance of hormones continues, but to different ends—prolonging life and supporting structural, cardiac, and neurological function. Healthy hormonal balance post menopause still requires that the levels of hormone be tightly regulated, with rapid and effective disposal of used and unnecessary estrogens.

The estrogen molecule is disposed of by the same cytochrome P450 enzyme system that is used to eliminate drugs, toxins from the environment, and biologically active or unwanted food substances. This, in combination with the very small number of estrogen molecules needed to have full estrogenization, suggests that the body views estrogen as a potentially dangerous toxin, unlike DHEA or progesterone. Emerging research is beginning to explore which estrogenic compounds and metabolites actually create the greatest risk.[33,34]

Estrogen has three major phase I detoxification fates: CYP 1A1 primarily converts estrogens to 2-OH estrogens; CYP 1B1 primarily converts estrogen to 4-OH estrogens; and enzymes of the CYP 2C family and 3A4[35] convert estrogen to 16-OH estrogens.[36,37,38,39] These three oxidized molecules have the same dangerous potential as other phase I detoxification by-products since they are reactive or "sticky" molecules. They must therefore be rapidly detoxified using a number of phase II pathways. Because of the large number of P450 SNPs (single nucleotide polymorphisms), there is great variation in the human population. The resultant diversity of intermediate metabolic end-products and the proportions among 2-, 4-, and 16-OH estrogens have been shown to have potential in predicting the risk of estrogen-related diseases such as breast, uterine, and prostate cancer.[40,41,42,43,44]

Some of these SNPs are potentially modified by the environment. The activity of CYP 1A1, for instance, can be upregulated by the glucosinolates (such as indol-3-carbinol) in Brassica vegetables.[45] This upregulation increases the precursor for a powerful anti-estrogen, 2-methoxyestrone.[46] Conversely, the activity of CYP 1B1 is responsible for the production of 4-OH estrogens, which can be rapidly converted to DNA-damaging quinones.[47] CYP 1B1 can be up- and downregulated by a number of drugs, by lifestyle factors such as avoidance of polycyclic aromatic hydrocarbons,[48] and by herbs (ginseng, an inhibitor[49]). CYP 2C and CYP 3A4 convert estrogen to 16-OH estrogen, considered to be a stronger estrogen than estradiol. The integrated effects of the biotransformation of estrogens by these P450 enzymes can be followed by assaying for 2-OH, 4-OH, and 16-OH estrogens.

Estrogen and Phase II Detoxification

Each of these phase I products must be further detoxified by phase II reactions using molecules such as methyl groups, sulfate groups, or glucuronides. The resulting phase II products are then water soluble, nonreacting, and do not have the hormonal effect of their parent molecules. As water-soluble molecules, they can be excreted in bile (primarily) or in the urine.

Sulfation: the circulating pool of estrogen. Sulfated-estrogen hormones act as another pool of estrogens; removal of the sulfate molecule by sulfotransferase (SULT) enzymes (also called EST or estrogen sulfotransferase)[50] activates estrogen. Remember that very small amounts of estrogen appear to have large effects and that estrogen is viewed by the body as a toxin. Free estradiol is kept in the ng/dl range as compared with the much higher amounts of testosterone, DHEA, and progesterone. The large pool of available SHBG-bound estrogens suggests, however, that need for estrogen can increase and decrease rapidly. Sulfation is a potentially important modulator of estrogen effect.

Methylation. Methylation capability is important in several ways relevant to women's health and is intimately tied to estrogen metabolism in the phase II detoxification of estrogens. Perhaps the most important effect of methylation in estrogen metabolism is the production of 2-methoxyestrone in the liver. 2-methoxyestrogens appear to provide protection from other more dangerous estrogen metabolites (e.g., 4- and 16-OH estrogens)[51] and are being studied as therapeutic interventions for breast cancer. Methylation adequacy can be evaluated by testing for serum homocysteine and serum or urinary methylmalonic acid. Corrective action, using appropriate doses of specific B vitamins, can be assessed by the results of these tests.

Glucuronidation. Glucuronidation of estrogens occurs through the action of UDP-glucuronosyltransferase (UGT).[52] Once the molecule is glucuronidated, it passes into the gut through the bile. In the presence of imbalanced bacteria producing excessive β-glucuronidase, the glucuronide molecule is stripped off and the estrogen reabsorbed; this process is called enterohepatic recirculation. This repeated circulation of estrogen through the liver may be a potent stimulation for production in the liver of estrogen-induced proteins such as SHBG and clotting factors. Symbiotic bacteria and adequate fiber, as well as D-glucarate, will improve glucuronidation and excretion of estrogens.[53]

The "Life Cycle" of Progesterone

Progesterone is a 21-carbon steroid and an early precursor molecule in the adrenal and ovarian steroid cascades. As such, it can be converted into estrogen, cortisol, aldosterone, and testosterone in different tissues. In physiological doses this multi-pathway metabolism seems to protect the patient from overexpression of any one end-product and contributes to the low side-effect profile of progesterone. Progesterone is produced in the adrenals in small amounts throughout life, in large amounts in the ovary following ovulation and formation of the corpus luteum, and in massive amounts by the placenta during pregnancy.

Progesterone has numerous functions, including downregulation of the estrogen receptor, inhibition of estrogen transcription activation at the DNA level, and effects on cellular adhesion, on local estrogen metabolism (such as the induction of enzymes converting E2→E1), and on sulfation.

Progesterone has been shown to stimulate cell cycle turnover in a way additive to estrogen in normal breast tissue. In a study by Soderqvist[54] of normal breast tissue (biopsy of normal volunteers without any evidence of disease or pathology) in women with hormonally proven ovulation, some women had enhanced response to progesterone and some had a paradoxical decrease in mitotic activity. The authors allude to the possibility of regional differences in response as well as mechanisms that may affect the relative risk (RR) of cancer stimulation in these women. Pike, in a review of estrogen/progestogen effects on breast cancer incidence, notes that cancer cells and pre-cancerous cells may respond differently to a particular hormonal milieu.[55] Therefore it is simplistic to say that progesterone either prevents or encourages breast cancers.

Hans Selye in the 1940s discovered that progesterone and some of its metabolites have profound anesthetic properties. These effects are thought to be primarily due to alpha 3,5,dihydroprogesterone's (allopregnanolone) actions on the GABA receptor in the brain.[56,57,58,59] These effects are so rapid (minutes) that it is unlikely they are mediated via progesterone receptor transcriptional activity. Rather, they act at a site close to or identical to that of barbiturate action. Metabolism of these brain active chemical metabolites occurs primarily in the liver. Therefore, when progesterone is administered orally, especially in high doses, significant CNS effect can be expected in some patients.

Oral routes of administration of bioidentical progesterone have a rapid intrahepatic metabolism and short serum half-life, complicating the pharmacodynamics of treating with progesterone.[60] Transdermal preparations have been shown in most studies to attain inadequate levels to create luteal phase effects and levels of hormone in the serum vary depending upon the preparation used.[61] Apparently because of selective secretion in saliva, much higher levels can be obtained in the saliva when progesterone is given transdermally rather than orally. Transdermal progesterone can deposit in the subcutaneous fat and this can be a problem for premenopausal women who need both high luteal phase levels to create the secretory changes in the endometrium and the rapid decline in hormone level leading to breakdown of the endometrial lining and menstruation. Transvaginal progesterone, on the other hand, has been shown to have a "first pass" effect in the uterus, perhaps explaining the apparent protection of the endometrial lining from overgrowth despite low serum levels of progesterone.[62]

These issues make the decision about progesterone therapy complex. Like estrogen, some of the metabolites of progesterone are more potent in certain tissues than the parent hormone. Progesterone is bound in the circulation primarily by albumin and, therefore, testosterone and estrogen levels do not determine the amount of free progesterone available to distant tissues, as they do for each other through their effect on SHBG.

Progesterone Receptors

Progesterone functions through nuclear receptors that trigger DNA transcription in a manner similar to estrogen's interaction with estrogen nuclear receptors. Like estrogen, progesterone functions differently in different tissues. In the endometrium, progesterone induces secretory activity and apoptosis, leading to breakdown of the endometrium upon withdrawal. In the breast, progesterone has been shown in *in vitro* cellular experiments to induce cell cycling followed by growth inhibition and cellular differentiation.[63,64]

The "Life Cycle" of Testosterone

Testosterone is a 19-carbon steroid formed by hydroxylation of androstenedione in the testes, the ovaries, or the adrenal glands. Testosterone is the *life-force hormone*. In both men and women it is a primary source of libido and it is associated with aggressive behavior. Although males and females start life with low levels of both estrogen and testosterone, at puberty they differentiate so that women have more estrogen and men have more testosterone. Androgens such as DHEA, androstenedione, and testosterone decline slowly over time, in both men and women.[65,66] After menopause, estrogen levels in women fall significantly, while testosterone levels continue their slow decline with age, leaving women relatively testosterone dominant after menopause. Men's testosterone levels also fall, eventually leaving them relatively more estrogen dominant and, in fact, with higher estrogen levels than women of the same age after mid-life, creating what some have suggested is a kind of androgynous de-differentiation of the sexes in old age.[67]

Testosterone is secreted in men and women in a diurnal pattern with peak output in the early morning. In women, however, testosterone is also secreted in "surges" around the time of ovulation (related to the midcycle increase in production of both estrogen and testosterone) and just before the menses (due to increased production of androstenedione from the corpus luteum[68]), correlating well with women's reported increased interest in initiating sex and fantasizing at these times. These differences should be taken into account when prescribing hormone replacement with an intention to increase libido.

Where do Postmenopausal Hormones Come From?

Using dexamethasone suppression, ACTH, and HCG stimulation to separate out the adrenal from ovarian contributions to circulating hormone levels, it is thought that most of the estrogen in plasma post menopause comes from adrenal precursors that are aromatized in extra-ovarian locations. Progesterone and 17-OH progesterone appear to have an almost exclusively adrenal origin following menopause. In fact, the ovaries and the adrenals should be considered together in most situations, as estrogen feedback may actually occur through the effect of estrogen on hypothalamic CRF-producing cells.[69] DHEA is primarily adrenal in origin, but the fact that even lower levels are seen in oophorectomized women suggests a small but significant ovarian contribution. Testosterone, DHT, and androstenedione appear to be produced in both adrenals and in the postmenopausal ovary.[70]

The Pathway from Hormonal Balance to Imbalance

As more detailed understanding of hormonal function emerges, the importance of genetic uniqueness and complex interactions between hormones and between the hormonal system and the environment becomes evident. The delicate balance among these hormones may tip into imbalance in any number of ways. However, the approach described by the functional medicine web will allow the clinician to dissect these complexities and formulate appropriate therapeutic approaches.

Immune System Modulation of Hormonal Balance

The intimate interconnections between the immune system and the endocrine system have led some to call the immune system the migratory or "portable" endocrine system.[71] It seems appropriate that the hormones intimately associated with reproduction in women would integrate with the immune system, enhancing allograft tolerance required for full fetal gestation to occur during a pregnancy. Postpartum, the complex interaction between the mother's immune system and her child's during breastfeeding protects mother and child from infection.

The effect of estrogen on the immune system is likely involved in the modulation of inflammation-based diseases such as cardiovascular disease, osteoporosis, and Alzheimer's, which increase with the drop in estrogen seen in the postmenopause period.

"During reproductive years females tend to have a more vigorous immune response: higher immunoglobulin concentrations, stronger primary and secondary responses, increased resistance to the induction of immunological tolerance and a greater ability to reject tumors and homografts."[72] Changes in resistance to infection, immune response, hormone levels and genetics may affect a variety of diseases in women. Levels of estrogen before and after menopause and levels of estriol and progesterone during pregnancy appear to affect autoimmune diseases. For instance, the augmented Th1 response during the reproductive years may explain the increased incidence but decreased severity of autoimmune diseases such as MS in women. However, hormonal changes coincident with pregnancy modulate improvement in the Th1-associated autoimmune diseases, when the Th1 and Th2 systems alternate dominance and become more "cooperative."[73] Due to the biphasic response of the immune system to estrogen, women during their reproductive years are more likely to mount a Th1 response to an infection or antigen, except during pregnancy.[74] This may explain the feeling of many women that their symptoms and signs associated with Th2 disorders began with a pregnancy. A 2004 review reported that "the Th1/Th2 balance may affect the susceptibility to or the course of infections as well as autoimmune and atopic/allergic diseases."[75]

Thus, pregnancy appears to represent a unique situation for the immune system, switching from a Th1-dominant environment to an often Th2-dominant environment. Although it has been almost universally held that pregnancy is a "high estrogen state," it is in fact a time when ovarian production of hormones is suppressed and placental production of estrogens, primarily estriol, and progesterone is high. Estriol may block the effects of estradiol on the mother's immune system, just as it blocks the negative effects of estrogen for the fetus. Progesterone has been shown to stimulate the Th2 system, which is responsible for activating B-cells and downregulating Th1. However, recent analyses of this situation have suggested that the Th1/Th2 story may be an oversimplification, and further research is needed.[76]

The Crosstalk of Other Hormones

Estrogen receptors are phosphoproteins; this means their function can be altered by changes in phosphorylation initiated by protein kinases. Substances such as growth factors activate the kinases and can therefore initiate transcription of ER-responsive genes without the presence of estrogens.[77] This "crosstalk" has been shown to take place *in vitro* between estrogen signaling pathways and dopamine, epidermal growth factor, transforming growth factor-α, insulin or IGF-1, and cyclic AMP.[78] Progesterone has been shown to upregulate this crosstalk.[79] This research suggests possibilities for the stimulation of ER-negative breast cancer cells and a mechanism for the increased incidence of breast cancer seen in the Women's Health Initiative and other studies in women on progestogens. It also suggests one possible mechanism for the increased incidence of breast cancer in women with insulin resistance and diabetes and provides some logic to the recommendation to avoid milk products (a high source of IGF-1) in cases of breast cancer.[80]

Progesterone vs. Progestins

Considerable differences exist between isomolecular *progesterone* and synthetic *progestins*. In the U.S., because most therapeutic regimens include progestins, studies in the literature must be carefully scrutinized to determine whether the *progestogen* (the term used to describe both) is (isomolecular) progesterone or a synthetic progestin.

Progesterone also plays a role in the metabolism of estrogens. Increased progesterone increases sulfatase activity, which increases free estrogen levels. Artificial progestins do not all have similar effects. Norethisterone has no effect on sulfatase activity and 19-nor-progestins such as NETA decrease sulfatase.[81] Progesterone decreases conversion of E1→E2 via 17-hydroxysteroid dehydrogenase (HSD) but does not affect aromatase activity.

Although man-made progestins clearly have a progesterone-like effect on the endometrium, are better absorbed by mouth, and have a longer half-life (with good clinical correlates such as the reversal of the incidence of estrogen-induced cancers of the endometrium virtually to the level of the placebo[82]), newer information suggests that the previous assumption that they also have the same beneficial profile in breast, blood vessels, and brain was probably a mistake. From the work of Clarkson et al.[83] in Cynomolgus monkeys, and supported by data from the PEPI trial (one of the few randomized studies in which isomolecular progesterone has been compared to progestins), medroxyprogesterone acetate (MPA) markedly attenuates the beneficial effects of estrogens on blood vessel dilating effects as well as the accumulation of collagen in diet-induced atherosclerotic plaques. They also showed that MPA increased insulin resistance. In this setting, therefore, progestins would be expected to increase the risk of coronary events and breast cancer risk seen in insulin resistance. It is not known how natural progesterone or cycling of progesterone will compare.

Progesterone has been hypothesized to be both a preventive and a priming factor in breast cancer progression. Progesterone induces apoptosis and cell differentiation, but it also promotes a switch (cross-talk) from growth driven by steroid hormones to growth driven by peptide growth factors. These two conflicting actions on the breast cell might be projected to produce two different populations. For one, progesterone would be preventive; for the other, it might induce breast cancer. It is likely that pre- and postmenopausal women represent these two populations.

It is difficult if not impossible to mimic the ovarian production of progesterone therapeutically. Because of the difficulties of formulating a well-absorbed bioidentical hormone (until the development of micronized progesterone), oral progestins were substituted for progesterone in most of the studies done on hormone replacement, including the largest RCT, the Women's Health Initiative. As stated before, a great deal of confusion exists in the literature because progestins have often been substituted in research studies for progesterone, on the assumption that they would function the same, without clarification of the substitution. So, bioidentical progesterone is often credited with producing symptoms and risks that actually are only seen with artificial progestins. Artificial progestins have numerous side effects (mood alterations, headaches, breast tenderness, and bloating[84]) not seen as often with bioidentical progesterone, and they fail to provide some of the downstream metabolites of progesterone such as the brain active steroid allopregnanolone, a known GABA receptor agonist.[85] How to formulate a clear therapeutic plan in the face of this often contradictory information is addressed in Chapter 32.

Sex Hormone Binding Globulin and Testosterone

Decreased SHBG levels are often seen in cases of hirsutism, acne vulgaris, and polycystic ovary syndrome, due to relative increases in testosterone. SHBG levels may be modestly reduced in hypothyroidism, acromegaly, Cushing's disease, obesity, and hyperprolactinemia. Growth hormone decreases SHBG. Increased SHBG is seen in hyperthyroidism, cirrhosis of the liver, estrogen dominance or low progesterone, and during pregnancy and hormone therapy. Much of the interaction between hormones is mediated by these binding globulins; therefore, therapies that affect SHBG levels should be undertaken with caution if the release or binding of free estrogen or testosterone is not an intended outcome. SHBG levels can also be used as a marker for the total amount of estrogen and testosterone traversing the liver (high levels suggest estrogen dominance and low levels suggest an increased testosterone-to-estrogen ratio). SHBG levels can also help in the estimation of the total estrogen burden when testosterone levels are normal.

"There are no agreed upon definitions of androgen deficiency in women, nor is there a clear-cut parameter, such as free testosterone level, with an accepted limit below which biochemical testosterone deficiency can be diagnosed," according to Dr. Susan Davis of Victoria, Australia.[86] According to some, the effect of testosterone in women is primarily mediated by its ability to lower SHBG, thereby increasing the levels of free estrogen. Since levels of testosterone have a positive correlation with breast cancer, [87,88] careful consideration of the benefits of the therapy is prudent before prescribing testosterone as a first line approach when women complain of decreased libido.

Low levels of testosterone should be considered in women who have undergone surgical menopause or loss of ovarian function secondary to radiation or chemotherapy, autoimmune destruction of the ovary, and in women on birth control pills, as they suppress both estrogen and testosterone from the ovary and LH from the pituitary, which reduces the stimulus for ovarian stromal production of testosterone.[89] In any event, testosterone is unlikely to have much effect on libido without "priming" by estrogen, which often solves the problem by itself.

Clearly, in some postmenopausal women on HRT the addition of testosterone has an improved effect over estrogen alone.[90] The most important role of testosterone in normal hormone function post menopause may well be its effect on relative estrogen levels. The lower levels but higher ratios of testosterone to estrogen in postmenopausal women decrease SHBG, making estrogen more available and thereby keeping the low levels of estrogens more clinically functional for longer in tissues. Glucocorticoids, growth hormone, and insulin also lower SHBG, increasing available estrogen as well as testosterone. Conversely, hormones that raise SHBG (such as thyroxine and oral estrogens) may decrease available testosterone and should be evaluated as part of the complex interrelationship of hormones before simply adding exogenous testosterone.

Testosterone is also metabolized to estrogen in peripheral tissues through the aromatase enzyme pathways in skin, bone, and brain, making estrogen available to these tissues locally without raising blood levels of estrogen. This may be particularly important in the case of bone metabolism, where testosterone may not only stimulate osteoblastic bone building but increase the estrogen inhibition of osteoclastic reabsorption.

Detoxification and Biotransformation Interactions

Sulfation of estrogens and other steroid hormones provides a second pool of circulating estrogens, making them available to tissues with sulfatase capability. Patients with inadequate dietary sulfate and those with sulfation defects may have smaller circulating levels of estrogen with higher levels of free estradiol. Supplying sulfate groups as $NaSO_4$ by oral supplementation may improve estrogen metabolism for these individuals.

Tissues with high levels of sulfatase may have elevated estrogen effects in the presence of normal blood levels of estrogen. It has been demonstrated that various progestins (promegestone, nomegestrol acetate, medrogestone, dydrogesterone, norelgestromin), tibolone and its metabolites, as well as other steroidal (e.g., sulfamates) and non-steroidal compounds, are potent sulfatase inhibitors. In other studies, it has been shown that medrogestone, nomegestrol acetate, promegestone or tibolone can stimulate the sulfotransferase activity for the local production of estrogen sulfates, leading to significant reduction in free estrogens. The integrated effect, as postulated, would lower estrogen stimulation. This has led to the concept of selective estrogen enzyme modulators (SEEMs) of the intracrine production of estrogens in breast cancer cells[91] and may explain the beneficial effect of using high-dose progestins in breast cancer.

Methylation capability is critical to catechol metabolism of dopamine, epinephrine, and norepinephrine and therefore may have effects on the incidence of depression, the interaction of estrogen and adrenaline, and the incidence of hot flashes mediated by norepinephrine in the hypothalamus. It is also clearly related to dopamine-mediated diseases such as Parkinson's.

Environmental and Nutritional Modulation of Hormonal Balance

A large body of evidence is accumulating that examines the role of xenobiotics on hormonal function through a variety of mechanisms. These substances have a phenolic A ring, similar to estradiol, that is able to interact with the ligand-binding site of the estrogen receptor.[92] To date, identified effects include alteration in the cytochrome P450 family of detoxification and biotransformation enzymes, agonist or antagonist effect to native hormones via receptor mechanisms, altered transcription of nuclear receptors through protease mediated degradation, inhibitors of histone deacetylase activity, and altered DNA methylation.[93,94,95,96] Direct, non-receptor mediated inhibition of estrogen sulfotransferases by xenobiotics has also been described.[97]

Nutritional deficiencies from inadequate intake or depletions induced by excess oxidative stress also constitute an important pathway for imbalances to develop.

For instance, zinc deficiency, which is one of the most pervasive nutrient deficiencies in industrialized societies, may have significant impact on steroid hormone function since the steroid nuclear receptors are zinc finger proteins that require zinc binding for proper function.[98] An example of induced depletion is that of B12 by xenobiotic epoxides; protection from this depletion may be provided by adequate glutathione stores.[99]

In Chapter 32, we will look at specific clinical correlates, emphasizing the web of interconnectedness in the dance of hormones and the challenges of clinical decision making based on multiple dynamically interacting variables.

Hormones and Breast Cancer

Estrogen and Breast Cancer

There has been ongoing debate between the advocates and opponents of postmenopausal hormone replacement because of the effects of estrogen and, more recently, progestogens on breast cancer incidence and cause.[100] It is difficult to determine how much of the literature is unbiased and how much is influenced by the "stakeholders." The pharmaceutical industry appears to hold the purse strings on much of medical research, both epidemiologic and basic science.[101,102]

It has been said that the fact that endometrial cancer has a dose-response relationship to estrogen, whereas the dose-response relationship between estrogen and breast cancer does not appear to be as clear, suggests that the effect of estrogen on breast cancer is not a direct causal relationship.[103] However, the presence of estrogen clearly increases the incidence of breast cancer, and there may be a time-related effect with long exposures enhancing the risk.[104,105] According to the Women's Health Initiative, the relative risk of cancer in women taking at least one form of hormone therapy (Prempro®) is 1.29, a non-statistically significant increase in the WHI, as the confidence interval (CI) included 1. However, this number is very close to a number of other studies, some of which did show statistical significance.[106,107] Furthermore, the rate of intralobular cancer has increased while the rate of intraductal cancer has remained stable from 1974 to 1998. Intralobular cancer is more associated with combination HRT, even though it has a more favorable outcome, because a majority of the tumors are estrogen sensitive.[108]

Various genes of high and low penetrance are associated with increased or decreased incidence of breast cancer.[109]

- High penetrance/low frequency: BRCA1, BRCA 2, p53, PTEN and LKB1 confer a high risk of breast cancer but do not make up the majority of cases of cancer in women since they are low frequency in the population, making up less than 10% of breast cancers.
- Low penetrance/high frequency genes, such as those coding for the CYP enzymes involved in both production and metabolism of estrogen, are less potent, increasing an individual woman's risk of cancer only slightly; however, they are probably involved in the majority of cancers.[110]
    1. 4-OH estrogens have been shown to create DNA-damaging quinones, and they may be a significant breast cancer risk factor in women bearing an upregulated polymorphism of the CYP 1B1 enzyme (research results have been mixed).[111,112,113,114] The increased risk of breast cancer caused by estrogens is likely to be mediated through the stimulation of cell cycle turnover of DNA-damaged cells. Thus, estrogen can increase 4-OH metabolite damage to DNA, but the primary contribution to breast cancer is the increase in the growth, immortalization, and failure of apoptosis of breast cancer cells.
    2. CYP 1A1 can be upregulated by environmental toxins and result in a modest increase in some women.[115]
    3. One polymorphism of 2D6 (poor metabolizers) has been associated with an increased risk of breast cancer.[116]
    4. Polymorphisms for CYP 19 (aromatase) have been shown in some cases to increase risk.[117]
- Phase II detoxification is also important genetically. The following genes for phase II conjugation have significant effect on hormone function:
    1. Glutathione transferase polymorphisms coding for major detoxification and antioxidation pathways are associated with increased breast cancer risk.[118,119,120]
    2. Polymorphisms for methylation (MTHFR and COMT) have been discussed elsewhere and are also associated with increased risk.[121,122]

3. Polymorphisms of sulfotransferase (SULT 1A1) have also been implicated in increased risk of bioactivation of both estrogen metabolites and xenobiotics.[123,124]
4. 17OH steroid dehydrogenase and upregulation of aromatase are also implicated.

- DNA repair genes such as XRCC1 399Q increase risk in African American women. Other XRCC variants are also associated with risk.[125]
- Genes associated with ER and PR receptors can affect breast cancer risk.[126,127]
- Polymorphisms for heat shock proteins (HSP70) and cytokines (TNF-α) may also confer risk.[128]

Progesterone and Breast Cancer

It was long held that because progestins protected the endometrium they must also protect the breast. Studies of cell division, however, showed a very different pattern of response in the breast as compared to the endometrium, with increased cell division during the luteal phase in breast tissue. The Women's Health Initiative (WHI) findings initially showed a statistically non-significant increase in breast cancer (RR 1.29; CI 1.0-1.59) that was not seen in the subsequent study of women on estrogens alone, where the RR was .71 (CI 0.59-1.01). This research is often used to suggest that progestins increase the risk of breast cancer and therefore should not be used postmenopausally when the uterus is not present. Interpretations of this apparent difference between progestin-treated and non-treated women do not take into account the possibility of different levels of estrogen in these two groups.

The recent publication of the WHI,[129] with its subpopulation of women who (because of prior hysterectomy) were not given progestins, suggests a considerable difference in the incidence of breast cancer between these two groups. It should be remembered, however, that estrogen levels between these two groups were not measured and were possibly different. Half of women who undergo hysterectomy have also had bilateral oophorectomy, and would therefore be expected to have lower levels of both estrogen and testosterone.[130] Estrogen levels were not measured in either arm of the WHI.[131]

Because of the conflicting information regarding the culpability of progesterone or progestins in the causation of breast cancer, it *should not* be used therapeutically in a cavalier fashion. It is likely, however, that progesterone has a protective effect in premenopausal women as the cyclic production of progesterone from the corpus luteum also induces differentiation and apoptosis, thereby maintaining the positive effects of estrogens (the maintenance of type III lobules which are less cancer prone) on the amount of at-risk tissue.[132] In postmenopausal women progesterone may have very different effects, especially when applied in high doses.[133] Pike, in a review of estrogen/progestogen effects on breast cancer incidence, notes that cancer cells and pre-cancerous cells may respond differently to a particular hormonal milieu.[134]

Insulin and Glucose Metabolism and Breast Cancer

Finally, another piece of the puzzle falls into place when we begin to consider the interrelationship of women's hormones with insulin and glucose metabolism. Women's hormones affect the ability of women to find and store energy (glucose) for pregnancy. In an environment of excess calories, particularly of low quality, this ability turns lethal. High glycemic foods increase insulin requirements, ultimately leading to insulin resistance and elevated insulin levels. Hyperinsulinemia has been shown to be a marker of increased risk of breast cancer.[135] Further supporting the interrelationship between ovarian/adrenal steroids and carbohydrate metabolism is the finding that progesterone primes the breast cell for "cross-talk" with so-called secondary hormonal factors such as the peptide growth factors.[136] Insulin, EGF, and IGF-1 may be among these growth factors.

Progestins and, to a lesser extent, progesterone induce insulin receptors, one of the protein kinase cell surface receptors that are mitogenic. While this may improve the functioning of insulin, it may also increase the mitogenic stimulation of insulin. Progestogens are also thought to increase insulin resistance, however. Progestogens also downregulate IGF-1 receptors via induction of IGF-2.[137] This may be important in the evolution of ER receptor negative tumors.[138]

Obesity in the premenopausal woman often indicates insulin resistance, which can lead to anovulation and polycystic ovary syndrome (PCOS).[139,140,141] Concomitantly, there is a higher ovarian production of estrogen, making the relative contribution of fat estrogens unimportant, but lower levels of progesterone, decreasing breast cell cross-talk with IGF and insulin. In the postmenopausal period, however, the obese woman has significantly more estrogen from fat production than the non-obese woman and, in addition, has insulin resistance, increasing the production of peptide growth factors. These findings and this model of hormone fluctuations may help explain why premenopausal obesity is associated with decreased risk of breast cancer, whereas postmenopausal obesity is linked with a higher risk of breast cancer. When progestins are added in the postmenopausal woman, an even higher risk of breast cancer is the result. However, contradicting this theory is the finding that CEE and MPA increase the risk of breast cancer only in women who are not obese.[142,143] These relationships are complex and subgroup analysis in some of the large randomized studies will have to be done before these interrelationships are clear.

Cortisol and breast cancer. The clinical supposition that women under more stress are at greater risk for cancer has been borne out by research that shows an association between abnormal adrenal function and breast cancer. Sephton et al. found that survival was diminished in women who had flattening of the diurnal rhythm of cortisol production.[144] Therefore, attention to adrenal stress is important in the outcomes of patients with breast cancer.

Table 19.1 provides a summary of breast cancer risk factors, along with an estimation of the magnitude of risk for each one, reprinted with permission from a 2005 review of the evidence.

Hormones and Heart Disease

Estrogen and NO Production

Estrogen has been shown to rapidly increase production of NO by the endothelial cell in an estrogen receptor-mediated action that is not arbitrated by the intranuclear receptor.[145] Because of its rapid effects, it has been suggested that placing an estrogen patch at the first sign of a heart attack or stroke might be a life-saving therapy for women. However, the induction in the liver of clotting factors might complicate the course of vessel occlusion unless prompt anti-coagulation was undertaken simultaneously and perhaps unless the genetics of the individual for clotting functions was known. In any event, this is not considered standard of care for women suffering symptoms of heart attack or stroke, although it holds some potential for the future. Administering estrogen to males was counterproductive in the same setting. There are other beneficial effects of estrogen on the initiation and progression of cardiovascular disease. Estrogen is known to have beneficial effects on LDL and HDL cholesterol but negative effects on triglycerides. Vascular responsiveness to estrogen appears to diminish after 10–12 years post menopause, as estrogen levels decline, and it is not clear whether it can be restored.[146] This effect of estrogen on NO and vasomotor stability has direct implication for hot flashes, sublingual estrogen having been shown to rapidly stabilize the vascular response to a hot flash,[147] and may be related to the disappearance of hot flashes after around age 60 in most women.

There is also evidence that estradiol decreases angiotensin II-induced free radical production and that it acts to upregulate manganese superoxide dismutase (SOD) and extracellular SOD in monocytes.[148]

Postmenopausal hormone replacement, especially via oral administration, has been shown by the Women's Health Initiative to have profoundly negative effects on the incidence of clotting, PE, heart attack and stroke.[149] These effects appear to be largely mediated through upregulation of the liver's production of clotting factors especially in the subset of genetically susceptible populations. Final conclusions about the cardiovascular net relative risks and benefits of estrogen in the postmenopausal woman remain to be elucidated.

The Brain and Estrogen: Depression, Anxiety, and Hot Flashes

Brain symptoms and preservation of brain function are the two most important aspects of estrogen therapy faced by the discerning practitioner. The brain symptoms that most often lead a woman to consult her practitioner and cause the practitioner to consider hormone therapy are hot flashes and depression. Hot flashes, a brain symptom caused by dysregulation of the hypothalamic temperature control mechanism, are the most troublesome symptoms of mid-life women and the ones most likely, along with the insomnia that often accompanies them, to lead women to abandon their fears of breast cancer and choose to take hormone therapy. Hot flashes are also linked to depression in postmenopausal women.[150]

Table 19.1 **Summary of Breast Cancer Risk Factors**

	Breast Cancer Risk Factors	Magnitude of Risk
Well-confirmed factors	Increasing age	++
	Geographical region (USA and western countries)	++
	Family history of breast cancer	++
	Mutations in BRCA1 and BRCA2 genes	++
	Mutations in other high-penetrance genes (p53, ATM, NBS1, LKB1)	++
	Ionizing radiation exposure (in childhood)	++
	History of benign breast disease	++
	Late age of menopause (>54)	++
	Early age menarche (<12)	++
	Nulliparity and older age at first birth	++
	High mammographic breast density	++
	Hormonal replacement therapy	+
	Oral contraceptives, recent use	+
	Obesity in postmenopausal women	+
	Tall stature	+
	Alcohol consumption (~1 drink/day)	+
Probable factors	High insulin-like growth factor I (IGF-I) levels	++
	High prolactin levels	+
	High saturated fat and well-done meat intake	+
	Polymorphisms in low-penetrance genes	+
	High socioeconomic status	+
	Factors that Decrease Breast Cancer Risk	
Well-confirmed factors	Geographical region (Asia and Africa)	--
	Early age of first full-term pregnancy	--
	Higher parity	--
	Breast feeding (longer duration)	--
	Obesity in premenopausal women	-
	Fruit and vegetables consumption	-
	Physical activity	-
	Chemopreventive agents	-
Probable factors	Non-steroidal anti-inflammatory drugs	-
	Polymorphisms in low-penetrance genes	-

++ (moderate to high increase in risk)
+ (low to moderate increase in risk)
-- (moderate to high decrease in risk)
- (low to moderate decrease in risk)

Source: Dumitrescu RG, Cotarla I. Understanding the breast cancer risk—where do we stand in 2005? J Cell Mol Med. 2005;9(1):208-221. Used by permission.

Hot Flashes

Hot flashes are associated with the dysregulation of the hypothalamic temperature regulatory system in the brain. The astute woman having hot flashes will notice that just before the hot flash begins she experiences either a sensation that it is warm or that she has had an increase in adrenaline with associated rapid heart beat, anxiety, etc. It then seems as if the temperature regulatory mechanism, which normally adjusts the body's internal temperature, has gone wild. Instead of making a minor adjustment, the temperature-rheostat seems to have only two settings: on and off. A flush is followed by sweating, increased pulse, and other disturbing symptoms such as chest tightness, anxiety, and finally coldness. These symptoms are all similar to the symptoms of overproduction of adrenaline. Although the hypothalamic temperature control mechanism appears to be *nor*adrenaline regulated, the interrelationship between these two neuropeptides and the relationship of high adrenaline or catecholamine states with women who struggle with hot flashes cannot be ignored. A third hormone also comes into play here: thyroid is known to be involved in temperature regulation. The high "adrenaline" lifestyle of the average American woman may explain why other cultures appear to suffer less with hot flashes. Estrogen and adrenaline counterbalance each other in the brain, both being brain "activators." Estrogen increases alpha adrenergic receptor density in the hypothalamus[151] and decreases it in the cortex. It decreases the seizure threshold[152] and increases serotonin availability.[153] Estrogen increases anxiety when an imbalance with the anxiolytic properties of progesterone occurs. Therefore, estrogen and catecholamines interact in the brain and estrogen levels may be one of the balancing mechanisms when catecholamine levels are tonically elevated.[154]

There is also recent evidence suggesting a direct role of hypoglycemia as the triggering event in hot flushes. Through an experimental "glucose clamp technique" study, it was demonstrated that a drop in glucose triggered a cascade mediated through norepinephrine that resulted in the compensatory hot flush. Estrogen is necessary for mRNA transcription of the glucose transport protein into the brain and loss of estrogen results in relative neuroglucopenia.[155] This raises important and practical considerations for the management of menopausal vasomotor symptoms through modulation of glucose control. It has also been suggested that the hot flash is a protective counter-regulatory mechanism in the central nervous system and that those women who do not mount a significant vasomotor response have a greater degree of cognitive impairment in the absence of estrogen.[156]

SSRIs in the treatment of hot flashes. Currently, because of the published WHI findings, many women and their doctors are resisting hormonal treatment of hot flashes. Hlakaty showed that after a few years only a subset of women continues to have difficulty with hot flashes and, significantly, these are the same women who have trouble with depression.[157] One SSRI (venlafaxine at a dosage of 75–150 mg per day[158]) reduced hot flashes 60–70%. This SSRI is both a serotonin and a norepinephrine reuptake inhibitor. Other SSRIs that have shown some effectiveness with reduction of hot flashes are paroxetine 12.5–25 mg,[159] and citalopram 20–60 mg and fluoxetine 20 mg/day.[160,161] Gabapentin 900 mg/day has also shown some effect.[162] All SSRIs and SNRIs may have sexual side effects.[163]

Adrenaline and Anxiety

Adrenaline increases anxiety, increases temperature, and can cause downregulation of the triiodothyronine receptor. When adrenaline is continuously elevated, the body tries to balance these actions by lowering estrogen and thyroid. Estrogen lowering may leave the menopausal woman with very low levels of estrogen and, through estrogen's effect on TGB, thyroid. There is evidence from the WHI and the HERS trials that women who appear to continue to struggle with hot flashes are also the women who will benefit from hormone therapy for other brain symptoms such as depression/anxiety.[164]

Depression

The World Health Organization has declared depression to be the number one illness affecting women's health overall, affecting 9–12% of women worldwide. Gender differences in the incidence of depression (twice as frequent in women[165]) and the fact that this discrepancy begins at menarche and dissipates somewhat at menopause implicates estrogen (or progesterone) in its causation. Adrenaline primarily contributes to anxiety and hot flashes; cortisol is associated with depression. Progesterone balances estrogen and has anxiolytic effects but, because of its close association with cortisol, can cause increased depression.[166]

Emotional lability, anxiety, and depression timed with the premenstrual phase of a woman's cycle are perhaps the most troublesome among the symptoms collectively known as premenstrual syndrome, or PMS. This complex of symptoms affects approximately 75% of the female population,[167] and is severe enough in up to 20% of women to require treatment.[168] In addition, "[t]hree to eight percent of women of reproductive age meet strict criteria for premenstrual dysphoric disorder (PMDD)."[169,170]

It has been recognized by many authors that these symptoms occur primarily during times of changing hormones: menarche, pregnancy and postpartum, premenstrually, and in perimenopause.[171] It makes sense that during these changes in hormone levels and balance there would be more challenges to the system's flexibility, and a less flexible system would suffer the consequences of imbalances that create symptoms. In situations where estrogen or progesterone is adapting to other hormones that are out of balance, women appear to be vulnerable to increased symptomatology. Because of the interaction of the neurotransmitters, the hypothalamic/pituitary hormones, and the nervous and immune systems, sorting out the individual woman's needs during these times of change can be daunting.

Cortisol, which is stimulated by the high adrenaline lifestyle and stress,[172] is strongly associated with many types of depression.[173,174] Since there is a predominance of the pattern of high adrenaline → high cortisol → high insulin in our culture, one can often see the pattern of high adrenaline → anxiety → high cortisol → anxious depression → depression. As the toxic upregulation of the adrenals continues, the ability to sustain adrenaline levels fails, often leading to caffeine abuse as a potent blocker of adrenaline metabolism. The dominance of cortisol leads to increasing problems with abdominal obesity, sleep disturbances, and depression. As cortisol dominance takes over and the ability to secrete adequate adrenaline declines, depression becomes the primary symptom and anxiety abates. As cortisol raises blood sugar, inducing the context for insulin resistance, weight begins to distribute throughout the body. Since this mechanism for producing insulin resistance is so ubiquitous, the apple body type, though often thought simply to be a symptom of insulin resistance, frequently is in fact a symptom of insulin resistance that is initially triggered by elevated cortisol.[175]

Estrogen becomes involved in this scenario in a number of ways. Elevated adrenaline may be balanced by depressed production of estradiol within the ovary. This is probably mediated by the effects of cortisol, which decreases estrogen effect centrally as well as peripherally. This may lead to infertility even in the presence of normal blood levels of estrogen maintained by the numerous pools to support estrogen availability. The integrated effect on the delicate balance that exists within the ovarian tissues may disturb ovulation. When estrogen is given exogenously, especially in the presence of a progestin that does not have anxiolytic effects (such as birth control pills), anxiety may be severe.[176] In a brain that is only marginally balanced, the surges of estrogen and progesterone in the luteal phase of the cycle may create the anxiety and irritability known as PMS. During this time of higher production of both estrogen and progesterone, it is likely that the imbalances between estrogen and progesterone are more pronounced. Postmenopausally, high adrenaline levels can depress an already low estrogen level below the level needed to maintain bone density and brain synaptic functions, making hormone replacement a seductive approach unless the practitioner realizes that the real pathology is the elevated adrenaline. When estrogen is added, adrenaline and cortisol may actually decrease to some extent, thus creating a balance in the over-activated brain. This can be helpful in the short term, but the ultimate goal should be to lower adrenaline and cortisol and remove excess exogenous estrogen from the picture.

Thyroid Interactions

Meanwhile, the thyroid gland reactively attempts to balance the effects of elevated adrenaline. Adrenaline is a cardiac irritant, as is thyroid.[177,178] When adrenaline is chronically elevated, the feedback mechanisms of the body attempt to counteract the negative effects on cardiac irritability by lowering T_4. This can lead to modest elevations in TSH with symptoms of hypothyroidism. Many clinicians have instigated treatment for "sub-acute or sub-clinical hypothyroidism" in this clinical context. When thyroid hormone is added in this situation, it is not unusual to see the patient "intolerant" of doses which the truly hypothyroid patient tolerates easily. The clinical approach is often to continue thyroid replacement but at a lower dose, building to larger doses slowly.

However, the complexity of the problem worsens in this clinical context. If the excess adrenaline state has not been addressed and the patient's metabolism is additionally required to accommodate the increase in thyroid hormone levels, further compromises in the dance of hormones occur. Rigidity, which is characteristic of aging, rather than the flexibility of a more youthful and adaptive system, eventuates.

Adrenaline also inhibits the function of T_3 at the receptor level. This may explain the symptomatology of the perimenopausal woman who has problems with hot flashes but in the intervals between her "surges" feels cold. A more appropriate management of hot flashes would be to address high adrenaline (avoid hypoglycemia stimuli, invoke stress reduction activities, moderate exercise, and improve sleep hygiene). To moderate temperature fluctuations, patients can wear layered clothing and instigate nasal breathing with onset of the hot flash. Moderation in the swings in estrogen can be achieved by supporting estrogen (and lowering adrenaline) through metabolic interventions (e.g., isoflavones, avoidance of xenoestrogens, improvement in biotransformation and excretion of hormones), all of which have shown some efficacy in treating hot flashes, although the evidence is very mixed.[179,180,181,182,183]

Depression, Anxiety and Hormone Therapy

Treatment of depression, which can be life threatening, is a more urgent issue and may require temporary or permanent hormone therapy. It appears that 80% of the female menopausal population will do better in the long run without prescribing estrogen. Another 20% appear to require estrogen for prevention of depression. These may be women who have undergone oophorectomy, who have autoimmune destruction of the ovary, or who have physiologic depression of estrogen production in the context of elevated adrenaline. While estrogen therapy is still the most effective treatment of hot flashes, it is not always helpful for depression and may exacerbate anxiety (as discussed above). However, when hormone levels are measured and found to be low, patients should be evaluated (and treated, if necessary) for symptoms of elevated adrenaline. If hormone levels appear to be low due to inadequate function of the ovary after menopause, replacement is in order. The goal should be physiologic replacement to the level of normal menopausal women: 15–25 ng/dL.

At this level, it may not be necessary to replace progesterone, provided that the woman is making adequate progesterone from the adrenals and does not have excessive estrogen metabolites or xenoestrogen exposure. In the absence of adequate adrenal progesterone, this imbalance should be corrected as well with bioidentical progesterone. Since progesterone is rapidly converted in the liver to allopregnanolone, a brain active GABA receptor agonist, oral administration may only be appropriate for patients with increased need for anxiolysis. Otherwise, symptoms of grogginess or even worsened depression may occur. It should be remembered that transdermal absorption is variable and vaginal and buccal absorption can be quite high, so finding the right dose and route of administration of progesterone can be difficult.[184,185]

In premenopausal women with depression, hormone therapy will more likely be aimed at balancing estrogen/progesterone levels by decreasing estrogen over-activity by improving metabolism, biotransformation, and excretion of estrogen, and by raising progesterone, thereby dampening swings in the levels of these hormones. In postpartum women, levels may need to be elevated by replacement and in perimenopausal women, also characterized by oscillating levels of these key hormones, the first intervention includes steps towards balancing metabolism.

In both pre- and postmenopausal women, it is also important to address the overactivity of the hypothalamic-pituitary axis (HPA) system, which can become unresponsive to the normal downregulation feedback of cortisol. Cortisol levels are increased when circadian rhythms are interrupted, especially sleep disturbance. Depression frequently accompanies dysfunctional sleep patterns.[186] Dexamethasone suppression testing is abnormal in this clinical context. This has been shown in animals to be lifelong and may be programmed *in utero*. It appears that a stressed mother programs her fetus to come into a stressful environment and the fetal brain develops with increased numbers of CRF (corticotropin-releasing factor) producing cells reflected in increased levels of CRF in the cerebral spinal fluid. Cortisol also fails to turn off the CRF production in the amygdala, increasing fear and anxiety responses.[187] These individuals have a lifelong struggle with overactivity of the HPA and may respond to stress-reducing techniques such as meditation, HeartMath, mindfulness-based stress reduction, yoga, energy medicine, or other therapies that teach the patient to modify the input to their HPA axis and thus lower cortisol and adrenaline. Furthermore, strategies to reduce adrenaline will also decrease both anxiety and the stimulus to cortisol production.

Hormones and Autoimmune Disease

It seems probable from the increased incidence of autoimmune disease in women that hormones (or hormonal balance) play a part in the alterations of the immune system that are involved in a number of autoimmune diseases. Estrogen appears to push the immune system in the direction of the proinflammatory Th1 pathways, except in pregnancy.

Because pregnancy is actually a high estriol/high progesterone state, estriol, functionally a weak estrogen, may actually act as a selective estrogen receptor modulator (SERM) and progesterone clearly has anti-estrogen properties. The changes in the phase II detoxification pathways associated with pregnancy have a profound effect on estrogen balance, on the ratio of 2- to 16-OH estrogen metabolites, and on individual tissues producing and metabolizing their own estrogens (such as breast, synovium, and brain). 16-OH metabolites go up in SLE and RA patients and go down in pregnancy.[188] The decrease in TNF-α during pregnancy increases apoptosis of activated immune cells (as does vitamin D). Estrogen is also thought to decrease TNF-α during pregnancy contributing, it is thought, to the improvement in MS during pregnancy. However, the full complexity of the mechanism underlying the immune response changes in pregnancy has not been worked out.

Mechanisms that initiate autoimmune disease and those that sustain it may be different. Some studies suggest that the timing of oral contraceptives is important in the later incidence of RA.[189] One model of autoimmune disease that seems to fit the available information and a functional medicine understanding of the interwoven web of functional interactions is as follows: Epitopes of triggering factors from the environment encounter the immune system and interact with the antigen-presenting system of the immune cells, especially in persons whose HLA systems are vulnerable. Estrogen and estriol appear to have a function in the presentation of antigens. Progesterone and androgens appear to be involved in apoptosis of activated immune cells; estrogen, contrarily, may be involved in sustaining the inflammatory activity of the activated T cells. The presence of adequate amounts of DHEA (suggesting the ability of the adrenals to produce appropriate amounts of cortisol) is necessary to quench the immune "fires." When adrenal stress or fatigue is present, this system fails, allowing amplification of the inflammatory pathways.

At this point, the presence of an estrogen-dominant environment further complicates the immune system's attempts to shut down the reactive furnace. Possible mediators of this process include xenoestrogens, genetic predisposing factors that increase inflammatory estrogen metabolites (such as the 16-OH or 4-OH), increased aromatase enzyme, and inflammatory cytokines such as IL-6, TNF-α, and IL-1β.[190] Il-6 inhibits ovulation by interfering with the LH pulse generator and IL-1β increases FSH and LH, further stimulating estrogen production from the ovary. Inflammatory prostaglandins induced by the proinflammatory cytokines such as PGE2 then increase aromatase, adding to the estrogen fueling of the process and creating a feed-forward inflammatory catastrophe.

RA exemplifies this cascade effect, leading to a disease of upregulated Th1. RA worsens with pathological increases in estrogen, except during pregnancy (explanation for this anomaly has been presented above). RA worsens at menopause.[191] This is also true of MS.[192] During pregnancy, estriol and progesterone may function to inhibit presentation of antigens to Th1 cells, and increase apoptosis of activated immune cells, respectively.

Systemic lupus erythematosus (SLE), a disease of upregulated Th2, is variable in its response to pregnancy, sometimes getting better but often getting much worse. In SLE, high estrogen increases Th2 activity, whereas the decrease in estrogen at menopause is usually associated with improvement in SLE symptoms.[193,194]

In some autoimmune diseases, estrogen is thought to have a biphasic effect, and there may turn out to be a bell-shaped curve with regard to the effect of estrogen on the immune system—i.e., too much or too little estrogen may be equally detrimental to the normal functioning of the immune system. In any event, it would appear that the relationship of estrogen to diseases of autoimmunity is complex and not fully worked out at this point. Statements such as the one that follows demonstrate the difficulty in interpreting information when it is not made clear whether the estrogen levels are normal prior to therapy and whether the hormone is given with the intention of achieving physiologic levels. As Salem[195] pointed out:

> The immune basis for these phenomena is poorly understood. Based on a distinctive profile of cytokine production, data accumulated thus far have revealed modulator effects for estrogen on the Th1-type and Th2-type cells, which represent two polarized forms of the effector specific immune response. Recent evidence indicates that estrogens inhibit the production of Th1 proinflammatory cytokines, such as IL-12, TNF-alpha and IFN-gamma, whereas they stimulate the production of Th2 anti-inflammatory cytokines, such as IL-10, IL-4, and TGF-beta. This can explain why estrogen suppresses and potentiates Th1- and Th2-mediated diseases, respectively. We hypothesize that exacerbation or suppression of inflammatory diseases by estrogen is

mediated by skewing Th1-type to Th2-type response. This view represents a novel mechanism for the modulator effect of estrogen on certain inflammatory diseases that can lead to beneficial or detrimental impacts depending on the type of immune response involved. Such a concept is valuable when considering the application of combination therapies that include estrogen.

Hormones and Specific Gynecological Syndromes

Endometriosis

Endometriosis occurs in up to 20% of asymptomatic women and in higher percentages of women with infertility. Historically, there have been two main theories for the initiation of endometriosis: the retrograde menstruation theory postulates that menstrual fluid carrying live endometrial cells flows retrograde out the tubes and implants on the peritoneum;[196] and the coelomic metaplasia theory suggests that transformation of totipotential cells occurs in the coelomic epithelium of the peritoneum.[197] It is possible that a combination of these is true. It has been suggested that retrograde menstruation supplies nutrients or stimulators of the endometriosis process without being the source of the endometrioid cells. This might explain why hysterectomy dramatically improves the disease for most women, although some are still found to develop endometriosis after tubal ligation or hysterectomy.

It appears that early endometriosis is regulated by different chemistry than late/established endometriosis. In early endometriosis, high levels of inflammatory cytokines, lymphocytes and macrophages are found in the peritoneal fluid, implicating inflammation or the immune system in the initiation of the disease. If the coelomic metaplasia theory is correct, a logical next question would be: what initiates the cellular transformation of the totipotential cells? Since the immune system has cells that produce the cytokines that can have an effect on DNA, and 60% of the immune system surrounds the gastrointestinal tract (which is in close approximation to the tissue affected by endometriosis), the gastrointestinal tract may also be a good place to look for an "upstream" approach to endometriosis.[198]

Recent studies have begun to dissect the mechanisms of cell transformation from totipotential cells and/or failure to remove cyclic ectopic endometrial cells in the peritoneal cavity. It has been demonstrated that IL-1 is overproduced in the peritoneal fluid and peritoneal-derived macrophages of endometriosis patients, and that this overproduction stimulates the synthesis and secretion of migration inhibitory factor (MIF) through a NFκB mechanism.[199] Upregulation of macrophage-stimulating protein (MSP) and its receptor (RON) have also been demonstrated by microarray mRNA transcription studies.[200] MSP has a dual role in preventing apoptosis and in promoting cell scatter facilitating invasion, both potentially important mechanisms in establishment and persistence of endometriosis implants. Other direct studies have also shown resistance to apoptosis in endometrial cells.[201,202]

Matrix metalloproteinase enzymes (MMPs) and their complementary tissue inhibitor metalloproteinases (TIMPs) also have altered patterns in endometriosis. The metalloproteinase system has been shown to play a key role in normal endometrial remodeling and ultimately in tissue disruption leading to menstruation.[203,204] Additionally, some xenobiotics have been shown to interfere with MMP function, possibly by interfering with the usual progesterone suppression of the MMP production.[205]

Finally, others have suggested a prominent role of oxidative stress with activated peritoneal macrophages generating increased amounts of lipid peroxides and lipid peroxide degradation products, which promote a sterile inflammatory reaction.[206]

These findings suggest a strong immune/inflammatory component of endometriosis, as well as several potential underlying mechanisms affecting the increased risk noted in women with other family members with endometriosis. Additionally, the xenobiotic effect on these underlying mechanisms may suggest a contribution to the increasing incidence of endometriosis over the past few decades. It is likely that endometriosis is the final common pathway of a variety of possible mechanisms and represents a good example of pleiotropic concept of many chronic processes, where multiple mechanisms converge to present as a common clinical disease.

If endometriosis is a benign transformation of the coelomic totipotential cells, it is logical to ask if there is a malignant form of this disease. In fact there are three cell types induced in this type of tumor of the peritoneum (including the peritoneum reflecting over the ovary). These are the three cell types of the female genital tract: the serous (tubal), endometrial (endometrium), and mucinous (cervical) cells. Benign forms of proliferation of each of these are known as endosalpingiosis, endometriosis, and pseudomyxoma peritonei, respectively. The malignant forms of these cell types are called epithelial cancers of the ovary. Understanding ovarian epithelial cancer in this way explains why we have so much trouble diagnosing ovarian cancers before they have "metastasized." In fact, they start out in multiple sites in the peritoneum and only appear to be ovarian because the largest bulk of tumor will be found in the ovary, where growth-inducing hormones such as estrogen are found. While malignant transformation of endometriosis has been seen, it is likely that the benign and malignant forms of this peritoneal disease are no more related than the benign and malignant transformation of other cell types. Further support for the connection of the gut and malignant peritoneal disease is the common finding of an association of gastrointestinal symptoms with ovarian cancer[207] and the little known association of milk (one of the most reactive foods) and ovarian cancer.[208]

As is true in a number of transformed tissues (breast cancer cells, fibroids), aromatase enzyme is found in high levels in endometriosis.[209] This would suggest that early endometriosis is transformed into late hormonally-stimulated endometriosis by the upregulation of aromatase. There is an accompanying increase in prostaglandin E2 as well, probably induced by the inflammation of the early upregulated proinflammatory cytokines.

Fibroids

Fibroids represent another abnormal cell type that seems to have the capability of upregulating estrogen in the local environment. Fibroids have a commonly seen but not reliable relationship with endometriosis.[210] The transformation of the myometrial cell by some stimulus seems to occur in families, suggesting either a genetic or common environmental initiator. Interestingly, reports are beginning to appear that also point to the ability of certain xenobiotics to upregulate estrogen receptor transcription and expression of estrogen responsive genes in myomas.[211] The reported association with endometriosis and the increased familial association of fibroids may represent a common environmental pathway or may represent an increased genetic susceptibility to xenobiotics. Once the myometrial cell is transformed, the same therapies that seem to improve diseases of estrogen sensitivity apply to the treatment for regression of fibroids.

Osteoporosis

One of the statistically significant findings of the Women's Health Initiative was the decrease in bone fractures seen in the women on hormones.[212,213] There has been a question, however, of how much estrogen is needed to produce improvement in bone strength. In a recent report by Ettinger et al.,[214] very low dose (.0014 mg) transdermal estradiol has been shown to increase bone mineral density in older women (average age 66). Ettinger points out that earlier studies showing little improvement in women with lower doses of hormone were done in surgically menopausal younger women. It would be expected that it would take a higher dose of hormone to produce normal levels of hormone in these women, as estradiol levels decline with age.

Osteoporosis is clearly an immune-associated disease. The presence of TNF-α producing T cells is essential for priming the estrogen-deficient bone environment to influence bone metabolism. In a study from the research group of Pacifici et al.,[215] it has been shown that the increased activation of TNF-α producing T cell in the ovariectomized mice is due to increased INF-gamma levels, resulting from ovariectomy-induced enhanced secretion of IL-12 and IL-18 by macrophages.[216] Therefore, the association of osteoporosis and menopause may actually be an association of changes in the immune system that are affected by changing levels of estrogen.

Summary

The research underlying the various functions of hormones, the causes and effects of dysfunction, and the influences of genetics, age, life stage, lifestyle, and environment on all the various factors is still a work in progress. Some of what has been written here may be superseded by new information by the time this book is published. However, there are some themes we can rely on for evaluating the fundamental clinical imbalances that are related to women's hormones:

- Caution is always warranted in prescribing drugs that will alter function, because the unforeseen effects, downstream, upstream, or sidestream, may be critically important.
- Each woman must be evaluated as an individual, for her particular situation may not reflect the "average" picture often described in the research.

- Effects of lifestyle and environment are powerful—stress, diet, exogenous toxins, and the possibility of nutrient insufficiencies or deficiencies (from diverse causes) should be fully evaluated.
- All hormonal effects occur *in relation* to other hormones in the body. Looking at a single hormone in isolation is usually unwise.
- The relationship of hormonal imbalance to other key aspects of the matrix—particularly immune balance and inflammation and gastrointestinal balance—must be considered. Interventions may begin at one of these other points if the preponderance of clinical evidence points that way.

Male Hormones

Daniel Cosgrove, MD

Introduction

The products of the testis have been recognized as essential to male virility and male physical characteristics since ancient times. Over 95% of circulating testosterone is made in the Leydig cells in the testis. Yet Leydig cells make up less than 10% of testicular volume. Among the seminiferous tubules are intertubular spaces with lymphatics, blood vessels, and Leydig cells. The Leydig cells receive signals and secrete testosterone. These regulatory signals include paracrine factors (e.g., cytokines, including IL-1, IL-6), corticotropin-releasing hormone (CRH), IGF-1, and various peptides and steroid hormones.

Historically, androgens have been thought to have two principal effects: *androgenic* and *anabolic* effects. *Androgenic* includes the growth, development, and maintenance of the male reproductive tract. Testosterone is required for male sexual differentiation in the fetus and in the adolescent. It is required to maintain adult male sex characteristics, and spermatogenesis. *Anabolic* effects include stimulation of somatic growth, i.e., increased muscle and bone density.

Recently, the broader and more complex role of androgens has been recognized, but is still far from fully understood. Androgens play an important role in immune function, in the development and maintenance of muscle and bone, and in erythropoiesis, i.e., bone marrow making red blood cells.[217,218,219] Testosterone can affect cardiovascular disease and emotional well-being.[220,221] Low serum testosterone levels correlate with depression and accelerated arteriosclerosis, among other disease states, but to what extent lack of testosterone plays a causative role, or is itself a manifestation of a greater imbalance, is not clear.

Synthesis

Testosterones, and all mammalian hormones, are synthesized from cholesterol through a series of enzymatic steps requiring P450 and other reactions (see Figure 19.1). Pregnenolone, 17-alpha hydroxy-pregnenolone, progesterone, DHEA, and androstenedione or androstenediol are some of the possible synthetic steps.

Although 95% of men's testosterone is made in the testis, the adrenal glands secrete DHEA and androstenedione, which are potential precursors to testosterone.[i] The most important (rate-limiting) step in "steroidogenesis" is the delivery of cholesterol into the P450 complex in the mitochondria. This is regulated by the StAR protein.[ii]

GnRH (gonadotrophin-releasing hormone) is produced in neurons in the anterior hypothalamus, adjacent to the pituitary in the brain. GnRH is secreted in pulses, which causes the pituitary to secrete luteinizing hormone (LH), also in pulses. GnRH activates LH secretion by both direct receptor protein mechanisms as well as by increasing transcription. LH pulses then stimulate testosterone production in the Leydig cell of the testis. LH affects testes in a similar manner to the GnRH effect

---

[i] The testis secretes virtually all of these precursor hormones, but their concentration in the spermatic vein is proportionately the same as their concentration inside the testis. Winters [Winters, "Androgens in Health and Disease," 2003, pg.13] has written, "One idea is these precursor steroids are secreted as unnecessary byproducts in the transformation of pregnenolone to testosterone, because none is known to have a physiological function in males" (emphasis added). This statement reflects the perception among many medical scientists that describing specific roles for these hormones, other than precursors, is speculative. There are conflicting reports and conclusions about the independent role of each of these potential precursors, especially pregnenolone and DHEA, but in recent years it has become more accepted to acknowledge that there is a complex relationship between stress and various sex steroids. Although the testicular secretion of these hormones is relatively minor, there is no doubt that DHEA circulates in the bloodstream at a concentration roughly 1000 times greater than testosterone. DHEA is often measured in mg/ml, whereas testosterone is usually measured in ng/ml. DHEA is discussed later in this chapter.

[ii] Mutations of StAR can cause an uncommon type of congenital adrenal hyperplasia, the lipoid type (LCAH). Instead of the usual virilization in most CAH, because precursors to cortisol are shifted to androgens, there is complete loss of adrenal and gonadal steroid production because the cholesterol cannot get into the mitochondria.

on the pituitary: it has immediate effects (4 hours) and delayed effects (about 72 hours) and these are thought to be a result of direct activation of cAMP, and then via upregulated genes, respectively.[222]

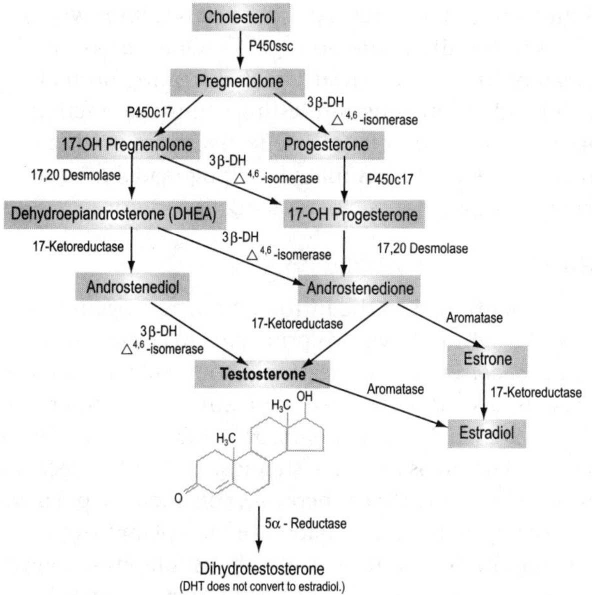

Figure 19.1 **Synthesis of the male sex hormones in Leydig cells of the testis**

Note: P450SSC, 3 -DH, and P450c17 are the same enzymes as those needed for adrenal steroid hormone synthesis. 17, 20-desmolase is the same as 17, 20-lyase of adrenal hormone synthesis. Source: Michael W. King, PhD, IU School of Medicine. From: http://web.indstate.edu/thcme/mwking/steroid-hormones.html. Used with permission.

Feedback and Modulation of Testosterone Production

Although testosterone therapy is gaining in acceptance, the concept once promoted as an anti-aging approach—that simply measuring and restoring testosterone blood levels is adequate justification for treatment—was terribly oversimplified. There are web-like complex interactions of many organs and signaling pathways with many factors affecting testosterone production, in addition to LH. Every few years, medical scientists revise their conception of the role of androgens, as understanding of their complexity improves.

A few facts to consider about testosterone production:

- Testosterone, in a sense, regulates its own production by its negative feedback inhibition of LH secretion; testosterone feedback inhibition also occurs via GnRH.[223,224,225,226] Testosterone has an effect on LH within a few hours, but also downregulates GnRH gene expression.
- Testosterone receptors and estradiol (ER-alpha) receptors are on Leydig cells and each has two specific pathways to decrease production of testosterone.[227,228,229]
- Estradiol is very important in negative feedback to decrease LH. Several studies suggest estradiol may be *required*.[230,231,232,233] Estradiol plays an important role in several functions in normal men. It is created almost entirely from aromatization of testosterone.
- T_3 directly stimulates Leydig cell hormone production in mice, partly by increasing StAR expression.[234]
- Men with prolactin (PRL) producing pituitary microadenomas have low plasma testosterone levels because pulsatile LH secretion is suppressed.[235]
- Growth hormone (GH), secreted by the pituitary, has been reported to play some role in testosterone production, but it is probably minimal. GH increases IGF-1, and there are IGF-1 receptors on Leydig cells. Testosterone levels are generally normal in men with GH deficiency[236] but men treated with GH for several months increased their plasma testosterone levels somewhat.[237]
- Corticotropin-releasing hormone (CRH), best known for its role in stimulating ACTH production from the pituitary, is secreted *by* Leydig cells and acts through high-affinity receptors on Leydig cell membranes to negatively regulate LH action by inhibiting its effect on cAMP-related androgen synthesis.[238] This could partially explain the mechanism of testosterone deficiency in stress.
- Corticosterone reduces LH-stimulated processes in rat Leydig cells[239] and may contribute to testosterone deficiency in stress.
- FSH was once thought to influence testosterone production but it appears to have a negligible effect.[240]

Effects of Androgens

Brain and Cognitive Effects

Several CNS functions are regulated by testosterone (T), including fetal sexual development and differentiation of the brain, and gonadotrophin secretion. Behavior and cognition are also modulated by T. Many of the effects of T are mediated through the androgen receptor

(AR) which is widely but selectively distributed throughout the brain.[241] Some of these effects are termed "activational" effects, and their mechanism is complex and poorly understood. Castrated rats fail to demonstrate normal sexual behavior, but the behavior is restored by T replacement.[242] Mice with age-related decreases in plasma T show a progressive impairment of spatial learning and memory related to T levels, which can be reversed with T supplementation.[243]

DHT (dihydrotestosterone) binds the AR much more tightly than T,[244] and DHT seems to also play a role in the brain.[245,246] DHT, unlike T, cannot be converted to estrogen. Estrogen, converted from T by aromatase, binds both alpha and beta estrogen receptors (ER) in the brain. Fink[247] demonstrated that both estrogen and testosterone, but not DHT, increase serotonin in parts of rat brains via specific mechanisms. Shughrue later raised the issue of the clinical importance of this relationship:

> The estrogen induction of SERT mRNA ... together with the correlation between sensitivity of ... serotonin neurons to estrogen ... provides a potential topochemical handle with which to investigate testosterone/estrogen regulation of SERT (serotonin transporter) gene expression. These findings are discussed in relation to the possible role of interactions between sex steroids and serotonin mechanisms in mood disorders, schizophrenia and Alzheimer's disease.[248]

While the animal studies and *in vitro* studies help clarify the mechanisms, many behavioral studies with humans demonstrate the effects. There have been many studies examining the relationship between androgen levels and cognitive performance, but these have produced inconsistent results.[249] In general, literature reviews and functional MRI studies suggest that men and women use different parts of the brain to process certain cognitive tasks, and these brain differences are differentiated in the fetus under the influence of hormones. In addition, the activational effects of hormones modulate the neural pathways for adults.

Cherrier and Craft[250] discuss fascinating differences in cognitive function and recruitment of various parts of the brain, relative to endogenous androgens.

> Men, on average, tend to use a Euclidean (distance) or cardinal direction (N,S,E,W) approach to spatial navigation, whereas women on average tend to use landmark references ... . [A previous study] found that when young men and women were required to learn a route on a tabletop map, men were able to learn the route in fewer trials, but women remembered more of the landmarks located along the route.[251]

Studies with exogenous androgens have inconsistent results, but general themes do appear. There is a clear pattern in those studies of humans with relatively low androgens at baseline (e.g., elderly or hypogonadal men) showing improvements in test scores of spatial ability and other beneficial, but selective, improvements in cognitive function.[252,253,254] One reason for apparent inconsistent results is that treating normal males with androgens and testing cognitive function has not been as dramatically effective at improving cognitive scores as studies that use hypogonadal men, or female-to-male transsexuals taking testosterone.

Muscle and Body-Building Effects

As mentioned in the introduction, androgens have been thought to have two principal effects: *androgenic* and *anabolic* effects. Recreational bodybuilders and athletes discovered that certain derivatives of testosterone had greater anabolic than androgenic activity, and these became known as anabolic steroids.[255,256] In the decades of the 1970s and 1980s there was considerable polarization of views about the anabolic effects of androgens. In general, the academic view was that supraphysioloigcal doses of testosterone do not further increase muscle mass or improve muscle strength, and that anabolic and androgenic activity cannot be dissociated; they are described by the same dose-response relationship, and are mediated through the androgen receptor (AR).

Recent studies have now established that, in fact, androgenic steroids, especially when "stacked" (adding multiple steroids simultaneously), definitely increase fat-free mass, muscle size, and strength,[257] and the anabolic effects persist in a linear dose-response relationship[258] over a wide range of concentrations. The androgenic effects use the AR, but involve recruitment of tissue-specific coactivators and corepressors. The mechanisms are not entirely clear since ARs in most tissues are either saturated or downregulated at physiologic testosterone concentrations.[259,260,261]

Although the potential for abuse by young athletes is considerable, the application of androgenic steroids can be helpful in various medical conditions with muscle wasting and bone loss. These include autoimmune disorders, especially in patients who have received chronic glucocorticoids,[262,263] but also HIV-infected men, patients with end-stage renal disease, ALS, and others. Many studies have demonstrated great variability in individual responses to androgens; the mechanisms are not understood.[264,265]

Bone Effects

The skeleton is a metabolically active organ, constantly undergoing remodeling under the dual control of metabolic and structural needs, and modulated by both estrogen and testosterone. Men lose bone mass with age, and hypogonadism is one cause of male osteoporosis. Low T levels are a risk factor for minimal trauma hip fracture.[266] In young men with acquired hypogonadism, T replacement increases bone density.[267] The bone-building effects of T seem to be due both to T itself, as well as to its conversion to estrogen.[268]

Cardiovascular Disease

There are reports of cardiovascular events in young male bodybuilders using high doses of anabolic-androgenic steroids (AAS).[269] Pathological data from men abusing exotic AASs should not be extrapolated to the legitimate therapeutic use of androgens, or to androgen physiology,[270] although a 2004 study reported adverse (and long-lasting) effects on apolipoproteins and lipoprotein(a) from self-administered AAS.[271]

Low endogenous testosterone is a component of the metabolic syndrome, characterized by obesity, glucose intolerance, hypertension, hypertriglyceridemia, low HDL cholesterol, a procoagulatory state, and an anti-fibrinolytic state. (Many discussions of metabolic syndrome can be found in this book; refer to the index for cross-references.) Body weight, leptin, and insulin levels decrease with testosterone treatment in hypogonadal men.[272,273,274] In general, providing exogenous T to eugonadal men lowers HDL cholesterol, but treatment of hypogonadal men does not lower HDL.[275,276]

An elevated serum level of lipoprotein(a) is an independent risk factor for heart disease. It is inherited, but not rare. Lifestyle changes such as diet and exercise have little effect upon Lp(a) serum levels. Supplementation with exogenous T in both hypogonadal and eugonadal men lowered serum Lp(a) by over 30%.[277]

Both fibrinogen and plasminogen activator inhibitor-1 (PAI-1) serum levels correlate with increased heart disease risk. Higher doses of T given to healthy men led to a sustained decrease of fibrinogen by 20% and decreased PAI-1 levels.[278] In general, these effects are most pronounced with higher doses in normal men and minimally significant in the usual replacement doses for hypogonadal men.

Perception and Androgens

Changes in testosterone in patients undergoing psychological stress. The brain itself affects GnRH, which is produced within neurons, as described above. Neurons have the obvious influence of external stimuli: vision, hearing, and perception in general. Stress results in decreased serum testosterone levels. Bernton[279] demonstrated in 1995 that Special Forces military training resulted in low testosterone. More recently, Gomez-Merino[280] reported that the immune and hormonal systems were affected by a five-day military course following three weeks of combat training. She concluded:

> The impaired secretion of dehydroepiandrosterone sulfate (DHEA-S) and prolactin, two immunomodulatory hormones, was thought to be a response to the chronic stressors. Lowered testosterone reflects a general decrease in steroid synthesis as a consequence of the physical and psychological strain.[iii]

The biochemical mechanism(s) by which "psychological strain" leads to decreased GnRH in the hypothalamus are unclear. It could be due to changes in the pulsing, or downregulated genes, as described above.

Several authors writing about sailing, especially sailing alone for long periods, describe decreased beard growth rate that returns about two days prior to arrival on shore and encountering women. Mike Golding, a well-known, world-class sailor, has written about it.

> An intriguing but little known feature of sailing singlehanded non-stop around the world is that due to the amount of time they spend alone at sea the amount of testosterone male skippers produce drops to a very low level. Aside from beard growth lack of testosterone in men can affect the pitch of the voice, temper as well a host of more complex side issues ... . "You certainly don't need to shave as much when you are out here because your beard slows down," says Golding. "And it probably changes your demeanour a little. You are less prone to getting angry. It doesn't mean you are not upset, but you don't get angry."[281]

[iii] Although most anterior pituitary hormones, including growth hormone (GH), adrenocorticotropic hormone (ACTH), luteinizing hormone (LH), and thyroid stimulating hormone (TSH), are stimulated by hypothalamic releasing factors, the secretion of prolactin (PRL) is under inhibitory hypothalamic control. Dopamine is the predominant PRL inhibitory factor and disruption of hypothalamic dopaminergic pathways or alteration of dopamine synthesis leads to hypersecretion of PRL. Increased PRL is associated with lower testosterone, but in this clinical study, PRL levels also decreased.

Testosterone and depression. Studies that have examined changes in testosterone in depressed men have yielded mixed results, but these differences may relate to variability in the populations studied (age; healthy or ill), different assays, and timing of the measures. Small studies that compare age-matched controls are subject to the considerable variability among normal males. Levitt and Joffee[282] found no difference in total and free testosterone, estradiol, and cortisol in 12 depressed males and age-related controls. Margolese[283] reviewed the literature in 2002 and found several studies reporting significant between-group differences in total testosterone levels.

Barrett-Connor[284] studied endogenous androgen levels in 856 men 50–89 years old, as well as the prevalence of depression measured with the Beck Depression Inventory (BDI). Bioavailable testosterone decreased with age, confirming two earlier studies[285,286] and BDI scores increased with age, confirming other reports of increasing prevalence of depression in older men.[287,288] However, in addition, the BDI score was significantly and inversely associated with bioavailable testosterone, independent of age, weight change, and physical activity.

Correlating *endogenous* low serum testosterone levels with depression does not necessarily mean that testosterone *supplementation* improves mood in hypogonadal men. However, Wang demonstrated that testosterone replacement does improve mood in hypogonadal men in an early small trial[289] and then confirmed it with more recent studies.[290,291]

Supraphysiological doses of testosterone treatment in eugonadal healthy men led to statistically significant increased "anger hostility scores" in a small study performed by O'Connor in England.[292] O'Connor contends that these increased scores were still well within the normal range, and that there was no increase in aggressive *behavior.*

Hypogonadism and Fertility

Testosterone has been discussed in fertility clinics for decades, but only recently has its role in anti-aging therapies become more mainstream. Fertility literature describes decreased testicular function manifested by decreased libido, decrease in ejaculate volume, infertility, and change in beard and body hair growth. Individuals with sperm counts between 10 and 20 million/ml are classified as having mild oligospermia.[293] Pregnancies in this group frequently occur, and therefore these individuals are classified as subfertile rather than infertile. Males with sperm counts below 5 million/ml have severe oligospermia. Such individuals, as well as azospermic males, require an endocrine evaluation. FSH, LH, thyroid-stimulating hormone (TSH), prolactin, testosterone, and estradiol levels are typically obtained. FSH and LH values in excess of 40 mIU/ml indicate primary testicular failure, which is refractory to treatment. Donor sperm or adoption is usually then recommended to these couples. When FSH, LH, and testosterone levels are all low, this indicates a hypothalamic-pituitary disorder, and a brain MRI is indicated.[294]

Traditionally, it has been thought that low levels of testosterone might impair sexual desire but not necessarily sexual functioning. "Administration of testosterone may increase libido but generally will not restore impaired sexual function."[295] The discrepancy here may be that the author was referring to supplementation of eugonadal men presenting with complaints of sexual dysfunction. Wang[296] reported significant increases in sexual desire, enjoyment, percent full erection, and satisfaction with erections ($p<0.001$ for all) in comparing testosterone gel supplementation to placebo in her study of 150 hypogonadal men; the effects remained from six months until the end of the treatment period. Shippen has claimed virtual resolution of erectile dysfunction in about 80% of his patients.[297] My own clinical experience with hundreds of men is that testosterone improves sexual function in hypogonadal men, but rarely is an adequate remedy alone; eugonadal men do not show the same response.

Testosterone and its Derivates

Dihydrotestosterone

There are two important androgens. Testosterone (T) is converted to dihydrotestosterone (DHT) by the enzyme 5 alpha reductase. DHT blood levels are about one tenth of T levels, but the potency of DHT in bioassays is at least twice that of T. Its activity at the local tissue level may be more important. In these respects, its function is analogous to the T_3 thyroid hormone.

DHT is *required* for prostate differentiation (fetal development) and function. Inhibitors of this enzyme are used therapeutically to diminish the development of benign prostate hypertrophy (BPH).[298] In fact, there is evidence that all men gradually develop BPH and even prostate cancer if they live long enough, and that treating with inhibitors of the 5 alpha-reductase enzyme such as finasteride (Proscar) delays the development of BPH and ameliorates some of its symptoms.[299] Saw palmetto is a popular herb available without a prescription. It has proved effective in treating symptoms of BPH.[300,301] Its primary function appears to be inhibiting the 5 alpha-reductase enzyme.

Men treated with these enzyme inhibitors do not experience muscle loss. And men with congenital absence of the enzyme have normal muscle development at puberty (although they would lack masculinization of external genitalia). It appears then that DHT is not necessary for the androgenic effect of testosterone upon muscle, so therapeutic anabolic androgens that cannot be converted to DHT are under investigation for use in patients with muscle wasting (e.g., those with HIV or ALS).

Hypogonadal men treated with testosterone cream or patches should apply the patch away from the scrotum or upper inner thigh. Apparently, 5 alpha-reductase enzyme concentrations are greater under the skin near the groin than elsewhere, and application near the scrotum leads to disproportionately higher serum levels of DHT.

DHT definitely contributes to libido and sexual arousal. Aggressive lowering of DHT, even without decreasing T, has the potential adverse effect of decreasing libido and sexual arousal.

The Role of Estrogen

Estrogen plays several crucial roles in men. Recently, the discovery of a few men lacking aromatase or estrogen receptors has led to a greater understanding of the role of estrogen. Certain theoretically predictable clinical features in these men have been described, including osteopenia, increased bone turnover, hyperinsulinemia, glucose intolerance, and abnormal lipid profiles.[302,303,304,305] Estrogen appears to increase the risk for BPH.[306]

As mentioned earlier in this chapter, estrogen has an important role in modulating brain function. Androgen and estrogen receptors are found in the brain, and aromatase locally in the brain appears to be important. In mice, aromatization of testosterone to estrogen within the developing brain activates the estrogen receptors and is necessary for normal sexual differentiation of the hypothalamic nuclei. As noted above, estrogen also appears to play a key role in negative feedback within the HPA axis by inhibiting LH secretion.

In 1998, Eugene Shippen[307] wrote a book for laymen that reflects many ideas currently held by clinicians practicing hormone therapies. He devoted an entire chapter (without references) to the role of estrogen. He suggested that aromatization of testosterone is increased with aging; with liver dysfunction, especially within the P450 system; with zinc deficiency; with excessive alcohol consumption; and with obesity. Therefore, in those patients with elevated estradiol/testosterone ratios combined with low testosterone, administering more testosterone only creates further excessive aromatization, and further increases the estradiol/testosterone ratio. Although this principle may be important in some patients, unfortunately this has led to the potentially inappropriate practice of prescribing aromatase inhibitors routinely with testosterone prescriptions.

What has been demonstrated or refuted about Shippen's claims since the publication of his book? Obesity has long been known to be associated with increased estradiol, and estrogens are synthesized in fat cells. Wang's recent study using transdermal testosterone in 163 hypogonadal men reported progressively increasing serum estradiol levels from 6 to 24 months of treatment to "the upper limit of the male reference range."[308] This was in contrast to T, DHT, LH, FSH, and SHBG serum levels, which all appeared to stabilize and become level within six months.

There has been the suggestion that zinc supplementation may decrease the risk of prostate cancer.[309] There is some evidence that zinc deficiency impairs testosterone synthesis[310] and several animal and bench studies suggest that zinc modulates testosterone,[311] but clinical studies are few, and at least one recent publication warns against the potentially toxic or pro-carcinogenic practice of "high dose" supplementation of zinc for prostate health.[312] Zinc is a normal component of seminal fluid, and severe zinc deficiency has been associated with infertility, but, otherwise, mild zinc deficiency in the Western diet is not an established cause of accelerated aromatization of testosterone to estrogen.

Acute ethanol ingestion lowers serum testosterone levels and raises LH levels, suggesting a primary effect on the testes.[313] Chronic alcoholism is associated with hepatic cirrhosis and elevated estradiol and gynecomastia.[314] Alcohol use in moderation has not been demonstrated to be a significant cause of altered estradiol/testosterone ratios. In the TromsØ study,[315] measuring hormone levels in over 1,500 patients, there was no difference between alcohol users and non-users, and no dose-response effect among users.

DHEA

The adrenal gland's production of DHEA (dehydroepiandrosterone) peaks at about age 20. Thereafter, blood concentrations of DHEA decline steadily throughout adulthood in both sexes, typically dropping to 15–20% of youthful levels in old age. This decline has led researchers to search for an association among blood levels of DHEA, signs of aging, and diseases associated with aging. Unlike testosterone, which is available only by prescription, DHEA is widely available as a supplement. The popularity of DHEA arose from a number of reports in the popular press of a study conducted by Morales et al.[316] that characterized DHEA as similar to the mythical fountain of youth. For three decades, there have been inconsistent reports about the various risks and benefits of DHEA supplementation, leaving many prudent clinicians wondering whether the hype had overshadowed good science.

Recently, there has been a tremendous outpouring of medical literature documenting many clinical benefits of DHEA, especially its anti-diabetes and anti-atherosclerosis effects,[317,318,319,320] yet clarifying its minimal or absent utility for body-building in younger men, despite ubiquitous claims on supplement-selling websites.

Although one reads repeated comments that DHEA's actions are because it converts to androgens, there is increasing evidence that DHEA has independent sites of action.[321] Moreover, DHEA has virtually no conversion to androgens in the bloodstream in men, and very little in women.

DHEA and cardiovascular disease. In 1986, Barrett-O'Connor[322] reported that *endogenous* DHEA serum levels correlated with decreasing mortality, especially age-related cardiovascular mortality. Higher endogenous levels of DHEA could have been a result of less stress or more exercise; one could not conclude that supplementing exogenous DHEA conferred benefit. Other studies failed to confirm these findings.[323]

More recently, Kawano demonstrated that DHEA supplementation (25 mg/day) in hypercholesterolemic middle-aged men (not selected for initial low serum DHEA-S) improved vascular endothelial function, measured by brachial flow index.[324] Other benefits in these same patients included improved insulin sensitivity and decreased plasminogen activator inhibitor type 1 (PAI-1) concentration. PAI-1 and decreased insulin sensitivity are well known independent risk factors for atherosclerosis. DHEA administration has reduced atherosclerotic plaque in animal studies.[325,326]

In a recent human clinical study, DHEA improved insulin sensitivity and decreased abdominal fat in both elderly men and women, leading Villareal[327] to conclude DHEA has promise as therapy for metabolic syndrome. The beneficial effect of DHEA on endothelium is apparently independent of androgen receptors. A membrane-bound, G protein-coupled receptor for DHEA has been identified in bovine vascular endothelial cells, which could be one potential mechanism.[328]

DHEA's role in mood and cognitive function. Compagnone reported in 1998 that DHEA increased dendrite growth in mice, and had other beneficial neurological functions independent of its role as a "precursor." [329] It has immediate neurotransmitter-related functions, and is not limited to its presumed traditional role as a steroid binding a cell nucleus. More recently, Suzuki and Svendson demonstrated that DHEA is involved in the maintenance and division of human neural stem cells.[330] This led to attempts at using it in clinical treatment of Alzheimer's disease, which were not successful.[331] Clinically, several studies have associated low DHEA levels with depression or decreased mood.

DHEA is not an androgen. Recently DHEA has been the subject of debate in that, unlike many androgen steroids (e.g., androstenedione), it was specifically exempted from the list of controlled substances in the Anabolic Steroid Control Act of 2004, which became law in early 2005. The legislation specifically reads:

> The term "anabolic steroid" means any drug or hormonal substance, chemically and pharmacologically related to testosterone (other than estrogens, progestins, corticosteroids, and dehydroepiandrosterone).[332]

This exemption has generated justifiable debate, due in part to the mixed reports in the medical literature about the androgenic effects of DHEA, or its ability to easily convert to more potent androgens following administration. Both DHEA and DHEA-S *can* be converted in *peripheral* tissues to androstenedione, testosterone, and dihydrotestosterone, and both are aromatized to estrogens.[333] DHEA is a chemical precursor to testosterone within cells (as is cholesterol), but several studies have confirmed that DHEA supplementation does not increase serum testosterone levels in men, but does to some extent in women.[334,335]

In general, muscle building and improved athletic performance are not an effect of DHEA. Nawata has written in *Hormone Research*, "Although DHEA and DHEA-S have few intrinsic androgenic actions, they have recently attracted widespread attention due to their beneficial anti-aging effects" (emphasis added).[336]

Virtually all testosterone is made from the testes, but DHEA found in the bloodstream is secreted by the adrenal glands. DHEA circulates at over 1,000 times the concentration of testosterone, yet DHEA does not simply convert to testosterone in the bloodstream in men, or castration would not lower testosterone. On the other hand, given even a minor conversion pathway from DHEA to testosterone, one might expect that adding DHEA exogenously might create higher androgen levels, given the high serum concentration of DHEA relative to testosterone. At least one investigator has found evidence of increased androstenedione and DHT in subjects given relatively high doses (100–250 mg) of oral DHEA.[337] Minor improvements in strength were found in elderly men supplementing with 100 mg of DHEA.[338]

The Approach to the Patient

The remainder of this discussion is drawn from knowledge gained not only from familiarity with the medical literature (as referenced previously) but also from my own experiences in developing therapeutic and prevention-oriented strategies for patients. Opinions expressed are mine.

Men with *acquired* hypogonadism (after trauma, for example) experience several well-established changes: alterations in body composition with decreased muscle mass and increased fat mass, decreased muscle strength, decreased bone mass (i.e., bone demineralization, which defines "osteoporosis" when it becomes severe), impaired red cell production, decreased libido, and erectile dysfunction. Psychological symptoms include depression, anxiety, insomnia, memory impairment, and reduced cognitive function.

Testosterone levels decrease with aging, so that 25–50% of men over 65 have levels that are more than two standard deviations below the norms for young adult men. Aging men, as a group, experience the signs and symptoms listed above for hypogonadism in young men. This epidemiological *association* does not demonstrate *causation*; one could imagine that both the lower serum levels of testosterone and these symptoms are all simply "part of the aging process." Nevertheless, as reviewed earlier in this chapter, recent studies have shown that all of the symptoms and signs listed above have been shown to improve with testosterone therapy.

Defining which older men are "androgen deficient" and merit therapy, or have decreased testosterone as a normal consequence of aging, is influenced in part by philosophy, and there is no consensus. Part of the problem is that there is no biochemical measure of androgen activity, which can vary with different target tissues. In addition, there is no single *clinical* measure of androgen effects, and different measures (libido, muscle mass, bone density) respond differently to a given dose of testosterone. Therefore, treating individual men should be based upon the identification of specific impaired androgen-dependent functions, combined with low T levels. Successful testosterone treatment in the individual patient is measured by specific clinical improvements, such as increased strength and muscle mass in a frail man with initially low T serum levels.

The decision to treat with testosterone is complicated by the fact that many psychological and/or physiological processes affect all of the signs and symptoms of hypogonadism, and could be solely the cause. For example, an obese sedentary man with poor nutrition presented with sarcopenia (i.e., decreased muscle mass), muscle weakness, increased body fat, insulin resistance, metabolic syndrome, osteopenia, and impaired cognitive function and decreased libido. An older man with these symptoms would be likely to have low serum testosterone that is partly predictable because of age alone. All of these changes have been demonstrated to improve with testosterone, yet *all* of these changes could also be a consequence of fitness and nutrition issues, and all could be improved with changes in fitness and nutrition, without using hormones (see Chapters 13, 26, and 29).

In addition to clinical manifestations of hypogonadism resulting from other causes, low serum testosterone can itself be a result of several medical conditions, including diabetes mellitus, liver disease, hemochromatosis, and obesity, especially with increased abdominal fat. Lower T levels have been associated with several medications, including ketoconazole, cimetidine, and glucocorticoids. Smoking and chronic alcohol use lower T levels.

These confounding issues may be difficult to differentiate (and multiple issues may be contributing factors). Heavy alcohol use is independently associated with bone demineralization, and it would also be expected to influence body composition, nutrition, erectile function, and mood. In addition, excessive alcohol effects testicular production of testosterone. Obviously, restoring T levels without addressing alcoholism would fail to address the fundamental cause of the imbalance.

However, in both an alcoholic and the sedentary obese man with poor nutrition, testosterone could, in combination with lifestyle changes, accelerate the improvement in all of the parameters measured.

Ideally, one would like to know what imbalances in male hormones look like clinically and how to assess them (key indicators), as well as where they come from (genetics, diet, nutrition, environmental toxins, stress, etc.). In reality, this will not be possible with the vast majority of patients, because of the enormous overlap of causes and indicators. Frequently, as the clinician begins to understand the patient as a whole person in the setting of his or her life, not simply as a series of parameters and measures to be adjusted, the most important issues may not be hormones or even nutrition, per se. In the example above, the obese sedentary man's wife died two years ago after 40 years of marriage in which she cooked and was the center of social relationships. This led to a change to a diet of fast food and processed food high in refined sugars and low in protein and phytonutrients. The subsequent depressed mood as well as social relationship changes led to decreased physical activity. His poor nutrition was compounded by new onset "stress eating," and the resulting weight gain and energy loss led to even less physical activity. The combination of these factors accelerated his osteoarthritis of the knees, which further impaired his ability to walk to the store and get adequate groceries. My point here is that hormones, like all of these parameters, can be both cause and effect. A thorough history, physical exam, and laboratory screening will help to pinpoint a more accurate and comprehensive assessment.

There may be debate about the relative importance of lifestyle interventions such as improving nutrition and fitness, decreasing stress, or improving relationships. However, it is safe to say that without addressing a number of fundamental changes, no specific targeted therapy will be adequate for this individual. On the other hand, we could agree that addressing the root cause for the patient example above means getting him into new social interaction and helping him derive meaning in his life apart from his now-deceased wife, but *solely* addressing *that* issue is unlikely to be as effective as a combined approach. Testosterone could still play a role in accelerating improvement in several of the parameters that would be followed in this individual.

Testosterone Therapy

It is illegal to prescribe androgens for sports performance or cosmetic muscle enhancement. The prudent clinician will document the diagnosis of hypogonadism, and list those symptoms and signs that support the diagnosis. Since it has been claimed that hormones cause cancer, and testosterone causes prostate cancer, careful monitoring for cancer is crucial.

Options for testosterone therapy. Testosterone is currently not available orally except as modified compounds that are hepatotoxic. Injections have been used for decades, but the inconvenience of injections, the marked swings of serum levels with peaks and troughs, and the tissue damage with potential fibrosis from repeated injections for years, make this choice inferior to topicals for most patients. Topical application is now available in a patch, and most recently as a gel (AndroGel®). One of the first patches was recommended as a scrotal patch. Any application of testosterone near the groin usually results in unwanted higher DHT levels, apparently due to an increased concentration of the 5-alpha-reductase enzyme subcutaneously near the groin. Patches are recommended for application on the upper torso, but there have been problems with tape, either in lack of adhesion or skin sensitivity. Patches are also limited for titration of the dose. The gel is increasingly the preferred delivery system, but AndroGel is expensive. Compounding pharmacies have been adding testosterone to creams for decades. I have been prescribing testosterone in creams for many years, but now that AndroGel is on the market, if the patient's insurance will reimburse for it, and he is comfortable with the diagnosis of hypogonadism for his medical and life insurance companies, the gel becomes the best choice. The inexpensive creams have the advantage of simply adding DHEA if needed. A typical prescription is testosterone 50 mg and DHEA 25 mg per gram of cream; apply one gram twice daily. Many men prefer to take a single dose, so the concentration is doubled and the cream is applied once daily, either in the morning or evening. Most men apply it in the morning.

Assessing the patient after initiating therapy. The patient should return in two weeks for a review of potential adverse effects (especially aggression) and perceived benefits, such as libido, desire to exercise, or any change in fatigue and energy. Laboratory tests can be obtained at two weeks, just to be certain the dose is not much too low or too high, but a recheck in 6–12 months will allow more accurate clinical and laboratory evaluation. At that time, clinical changes should be evident. Subjective changes in mood, well-being, libido, and erectile function should have stabilized and no longer be subject to placebo effect (as they might be immediately following the start of therapy). Body composition, weight, changes in exercise program, and muscle strength should be measured. For patients with low bone density, DEXA or CT repeat measures should wait for at least one year.

Lab measures. Virtually all published studies of testosterone use serum levels. Saliva testing for testosterone has its advocates but it has not been accepted widely.

It is important to document the last dose. If the patient takes the cream twice daily, he should withhold his morning dose and have the blood drawn in the morning, about 12 hours after the last dose. If he takes only one dose every 24 hours, be sure to consistently check a level at the same time, and be aware that comparing T levels from blood drawn 24, 12, or sometimes one hour after cream application can cause big changes in the serum level.

I recommend ordering baseline serum total and free testosterone, DHT, estradiol and DHEA-S, PSA, hemoglobin, and iron (optimally as the panel with iron and transferrin saturation) as a baseline prior to therapy. The four hormones can be remeasured 2–6 weeks later. Optimally, they should also be checked six months later (when PSA and hemoglobin should also be rechecked), and then annually thereafter. It is reasonable for the cost-sensitive patient to not remeasure all four hormones every time. Many men see their hemoglobin creep up from 15 g to nearly 20 g. At 17 g, I encourage them to give blood. The formal prescription for removing a unit is rarely necessary. Testosterone therapy is not a contraindication for most blood banks. If the patient has a strong hematopoietic response to testosterone, a unit of blood may have to be given twice annually. This may have a risk of iron deficiency but, in practice, most men have iron levels beyond what they need. Since iron is a potent oxidant, lowering the iron level through blood donation is an added benefit.

DHEA. A common mistake is ordering DHEA rather than DHEA-S, the sulfated form. DHEA-S shows more stable blood levels. Not all patients need DHEA therapy with testosterone, but some patients appear to get even lower levels of DHEA after therapy, presumably due to a feedback mechanism, and do well with both prescribed.

Estradiol measures before and after therapy can indicate how much conversion is occurring from T to estradiol, which is in part an indication of the activity of an individual patient's aromatase enzyme. Estradiol serum level of 50 pg/ml with a total testosterone of 500 ng/dl, i.e., about 10% (which is really 1% converting both measures to the same units) is fine. Prescribing anastrozole (Arimidex), which blocks this enzyme activity thus decreasing the estrogen/testosterone ratio, is very rarely necessary. Athletes using high-dose androgens for bulking up may need it, but it should not be necessary for most men with hypogonadism. Low levels of estrogen may affect neurons and bone, and may lead to loss of teeth. Rarely, there are patients with gynecomastia and/or an elevated estradiol level for whom lowering the testosterone dose may decrease its benefit. In my experience, lowering the testosterone usually works, and does not bring into the equation other potential adverse effects of another medication.

DHT is typically about 10% of T; both are often measured in ng/dL. To repeat a theme, the individual variation in conversion of T to DHT, apparently a function of 5 alpha-reductase activity, is enormous. In a few patients, DHT rises dramatically and disproportionately to T. First, insure the patient is not applying it near the groin. I recommend these patients avoid any application from waist to knees, just to be certain. Having excluded an issue of application of cream or gel, these patients, and perhaps any patient at risk of benign prostatic hypertrophy (BPH), could use saw palmetto or finasteride. Saw palmetto is available without prescription. I recommend it to nearly all men over 50 since lower DHT has been associated with decreased progression of BPH. Finasteride is sold in 1 mg doses (Propecia and others) to decrease men's hair loss from the scalp, and in 5 mg doses (Proscar and others) for BPH symptoms. Often half of the 5 mg pill works well to keep DHT levels at 10% or less of total T.

PSA should not rise as a result of testosterone therapy. Typically PSA fluctuates perhaps 0.2 ng/ml, but an increase of about that amount in six months merits a repeat test and close scrutiny. Be cautious about comparing PSA results from different labs or different techniques of measure. I measure PSA at least every six months for those patients taking any hormone therapy. For patients with PSA levels greater than 2.5, I measure free PSA (which includes total PSA in the report). Higher PSA levels suggest increase risk of prostate cancer, but *lower* free PSA levels suggest increased risk. Free PSA is usually measured with the Beckman method, whereas total PSA screening is performed with another method that may have a different total PSA value.

Testosterone measures and lab methodology. The process for measuring hormones differs among labs and often various choices are available at one lab. Testosterone levels are now available measured by "LC/MS/MS," which means liquid chromatography followed by mass spectroscopy, and then again run through mass spectroscopy. This is the gold standard. Results may be a little lower than those obtained from the traditional Centaur machine. The greatest variations come with measuring free or bioavailable T. T is nearly all bound to SHBG, and more loosely bound to albumin. Long discussions center around "bioavailable T" vs. "free T" since some T that is not totally unbound (usually with albumin) still has activity. SHBG tends to increase in men with age, but there is great variability among individuals. The lab report with "bioavailable T" often lists free T, albumin, and SHBG all as one report. Free and bioavailable are *calculated* values, and often not correct. Only a few years ago, it was discovered that SHBG has two binding sites, not one, so the calculations were wrong. In addition, genetic variations in SHBG allow for tight or loose binding of T, which result in less or more free T, but calculated values cannot take these variations into account.

The best measure of free T is with equilibrium dialysis, so that a membrane permeable to T but not to larger proteins is placed for 18 hours, and then the free T on the other side is quantified. This technique is the gold standard. The report often simply has total and free T measures listed. Beware of labs that measure free T using ammonium sulfate to precipitate out all the proteins. This methodology should be abandoned due to great fluctuations in results.

Following total testosterone only may be better than once thought. It is not subject to the tremendous variation associated with methodologies for free T. In addition, total testosterone may better reflect overall body stores.

Estradiol in men requires a sensitive, accurate measure for these low concentrations. Be sure the lab is not using the inexpensive ELISA kits for estrogen, which are not sufficiently accurate.

Philosophical Considerations

Some modern clinicians might forbid Michelangelo to paint the Sistine Chapel. The fumes from the paint and the prolonged awkward positions on the scaffolding, as well as anxiety about the work itself and arguments with patrons and assistants, would all take a toll on his health. The best physicians, however, would not forbid the work, but would help him achieve his goals with greater safety and preservation of function. Strategies might include getting a pad on the scaffolding, improving ventilation, some stretching exercises, and breathing exercises before arguments with church officials. The <u>value</u> of his work—to Michelangelo, not to others—and the overall <u>cost</u> (to him) of that work, can only be estimated after a good history and careful assessment. And only then can one make recommendations appropriate to the individual.

This little fable is meant to point out that the philosophy and belief system of the doctor influence decisions made on behalf of the patient. In terms of using hormone therapy to offset adverse effects of aging, some clinicians may believe there is a special intrinsic value in remaining natural over "artificial" and "allowing nature to take its course." Such physicians may rarely prescribe androgens. However, women and men both have diminished physical functions and greater vulnerability to injury and illness following their prime reproductive years. On average, a man loses 75% of his testosterone, and 40% of his lean muscle mass with age. Age-related frailty includes lack of balance and strength, leading to greater vulnerability and increasing risk of hip and vertebral fractures with resulting posture change (kyphosis) and lack of height. In addition, aging men as a group have less joy and more depression. An aging man with low testosterone can expect, as a result of taking testosterone, greater overall drive, including a greater desire to exercise, greater bone density, greater muscle mass and strength, improved mood, and less susceptibility to depression.

For the first time in history, life after age 60 might fairly routinely last another 30–40 years. With less frailty, thoroughly screened for cancer and heart disease, the older man now has a unique opportunity to change roles, to continue to be highly productive, and to remain physically and sexually active. Certainly, the benefits of taking testosterone must be weighed against the risks of therapy, but the risks associated with doing nothing must also be taken into consideration. Ultimately, the physician must serve the patient, helping him (with reasonable safety) to achieve his personal goals or refer him to another practitioner.

The Epidemic of Insulin Insensitivity

Dan Lukaczer, ND

Introduction

When thinking about patients from the perspective of fundamental clinical imbalances, insulin balance is a critical piece of the puzzle. In most tissues, adequate insulin secretion is necessary for proper glucose disposal and management.[339] The binding of insulin to its receptor in the cell membrane is the first step of a metabolic cascade leading to cellular glucose uptake. When insulin does not bind properly or efficiently, however, the ensuing dysfunction leads to a series of complex effects on various tissues that result in a host of metabolic abnormalities. Insulin insensitivity may be the single most important underlying metabolic dysfunction related to chronic disease. For that reason, you will find it addressed a number of times in this book, from different perspectives.

The term insulin resistance refers to a reduced sensitivity of the cell to the action of insulin. Insulin resistance or insensitivity results when normal insulin action is impaired and the cell does not "hear" the message of the insulin signaling molecule. To overcome this impairment, and to maintain glucose homeostasis, the pancreas will attempt to secrete larger and larger amounts of insulin.[340] There is great interindividual variation in the ability of insulin to mediate glucose disposal. Studies have shown that insulin sensitivity can vary up to 10-fold in non-diabetics.[341] Without this compensatory hyperinsulinemia, individuals who are insulin resistant develop glucose intolerance and diabetes. However, if the pancreas can continue to secrete large amounts of insulin, the individual then continues to maintain near-normal glucose homeostasis.

Insulin resistance and the resultant hyperinsulinemia are surprisingly common, and may be seen in as many as 25% of a normal non-diabetic population;[342] most individuals who develop insulin resistance maintain normal to near-normal glucose control. It is estimated that 60 to 70 million Americans fall into this category. However, up to 25% of these individuals will go on to develop type 2 diabetes.

Insulin Resistance and Chronic Disease

Not all individuals who are insulin resistant ultimately develop diabetes. However, those who do not are still at increased risk for a variety of other age-related diseases[343] that include coronary heart disease (CHD), stroke, polycystic ovary syndrome (PCOS), colon and breast cancer, and cognitive decline. The insulin resistance syndrome (IRS), also referred to as syndrome X or metabolic syndrome, refers to a cluster of signs and symptoms that includes: varying degrees of impaired glucose tolerance, depressed HDL cholesterol, elevated triglycerides, elevated blood pressure, and truncal adiposity. The underlying pathophysiology of the syndrome involves insulin resistance and consequent hyperinsulinemia.

As abdominal fat is increased, insulin sensitivity decreases, production of inflammatory cytokines increases, and the relative risk of heart disease, dementia, and cognitive decline all increase. Recent publications have demonstrated the relationship among lifestyle, adipocyte activity, inflammation, and chronic disease incidence.[344,345]

Diabetes

There are an estimated 16 million type 2 diabetics in the U.S. and the overwhelming majority carry the underlying pathophysiology of insulin resistance.[346] The relative severity of insulin resistance *and* impairment of pancreatic beta cell function determines the severity of hyperinsulinemia and when *or if* hyperglycemia occurs. Normally, insulin has a suppressive effect on circulating free fatty acids (FFAs). When the insulin secretory response declines, circulating FFA levels become elevated. FFAs, in turn, stimulate hepatic glucose production. Without the normal insulin inhibitory signal, hyperglycemia occurs as the liver continues to secrete normal amounts of glucose into a greatly expanded plasma glucose pool.[346] With increasing hyperglycemia there is a further reduction in beta cell function (possibly as a result of glucotoxicity) and a further fall in insulin.

Type 2 diabetes mellitus affects 90%–95% of people with diabetes and most often appears after age 40. However, it can no longer be considered an adult-onset disease, as it is now found commonly in obese teenagers.[348] The diagnosis of type 2 diabetes, impaired glucose tolerance, and impaired fasting glucose is based on both the World Health Organization[349] and the American Diabetes Association (ADA)[350] guidelines. (For an extended discussion, see Chapter 37.) According to these criteria, type 2 diabetes can be diagnosed either by an oral glucose tolerance test (2-hour post-75-gram load) with a value of 200 mg/dL or greater, or by a fasting glucose concentration of 126 mg/dL or greater. In addition, there are intermediate categories of glucose tolerance. Impaired glucose tolerance is diagnosed by a 2-hour post load oral glucose tolerance test of 140 mg/dL or greater but less than 200 mg/dL, and impaired fasting glucose is diagnosed by a fasting glucose of between 100 and 125 mg/dL. Both individuals with impaired glucose tolerance (IGT) and those with impaired fasting glucose (IFT) are at high risk of developing diabetes. From the ADA position statement:

> Recently, IFG and IGT have been officially termed "pre-diabetes." Both categories, IFG and IGT, are risk factors for future diabetes and cardiovascular disease (CVD) … . On the basis of expert opinion, screening should be considered by health care providers at 3-year intervals beginning at age 45 years, particularly in those with BMI ≥25 kg/m². Testing should be considered at a younger age or be carried out more frequently in individuals who are overweight (BMI ≥25 kg/m² [iv]) and have additional risk factors.[351]

This excellent ADA 2005 article provides an in-depth look at a very complex subject.

Coronary Heart Disease

Those individuals who maintain a compensatory hyperinsulinemia in the face of insulin insensitivity do so at great biological cost. A primary consequence is increased risk for CHD. Metabolic syndrome is associated with CHD through three mechanisms:

1. Elevated insulin directly stimulates lipogenesis in arterial tissue and enhances the growth and proliferation of arterial smooth muscle cells, contributing to arteriosclerosis.[352,353]
2. Insulin resistance and hyperinsulinemia decrease fibrinolysis by stimulating plasminogen activator inhibitor 1 (PAI-1), which is associated with an increased risk for coronary thrombosis. PAI-1 is higher in patients with CHD and is related to insulin resistance and insulin-mediated glucose disposal.[354,355]
3. Hyperinsulinemia leads to increased hepatic production of triglycerides (TG) and inhibition of high-density lipoproteins (HDL). Elevated TG and depressed HDL are important risk factors for CHD.[356,357,358]

This strong relationship between insulin, TG, and HDL apparently results from insulin's influence on the cholesteryl ester transfer protein, which promotes the movement of cholesteryl ester from HDL to very low-density lipoproteins (VLDL).[359] The higher the TG levels, the greater the losses of cholesteryl ester from HDL and the lower the plasma HDL-cholesterol concentration. Additionally, Apo A1, which is the major protein associated with HDL and independently associated with reduced risk of coronary heart disease, is catabolized in a high insulin state, further degrading HDL.

Risk of Cognitive Decline

When the balance of inflammatory mediators is shifted through altered gene expression patterns, the central set points of our physiology are being influenced—the so-called homeodynamic set points, which have to do with alterations in the neuroendocrine-immune system. This is one "super system," with parts interrelated through receptor physiology and signaling mechanisms that transfer information molecules throughout the body and modify its function. The endocrine system is changed; the immune system is changed; and the nervous system is changed, as a consequence of the shift toward inflammation. "[T]here is accumulating evidence suggesting that inflammation is the bridging link between atherosclerosis and the metabolic syndrome."[360] That is why the metabolic syndrome results in a greater risk for cognitive decline through the adverse impact of inflammatory mediators on neuronal function.[361]

[iv] May not be correct for all ethnic groups.

Hypertension and Stroke

Insulin resistance may also play a key role in hypertension. As many as 50% of the hypertensive population may be insulin resistant.[362] The sodium hypothesis of hypertension attributes increased peripheral vascular resistance to elevated *intra*cellular sodium concentrations. Based on cross-cultural comparisons, this was thought to be mainly due to increased dietary intake of sodium in salt-sensitive individuals. Intracultural studies suggest, however, that dietary salt may account for only a minor segment of increased blood pressure in the hypertensive population.[363] It has been proposed that a larger segment of essential hypertension is caused by enhanced renal sodium reabsorption in the distal tubule promoted by hyperinsulinemia.[364] Hyperinsulinemia may also play a role by altering internal sodium and potassium distribution in a direction that is associated with increased peripheral vascular resistance.[365] Insulin appears to work through other mechanisms as well to increase sympathetic nervous system activity and thus peripheral resistance.[366] This relationship between insulin and blood pressure is further supported by studies that show blood pressure drops when the insulin dose is decreased in obese hypertensive patients with type 2 diabetes.[367] Additionally, blood pressure increases when insulin treatment is initiated in diabetic patients.[368]

Polycystic Ovary Syndrome (PCOS)

Insulin resistance appears to have a critical relationship to androgen hormonal modulation. Research over the past 10 years has linked insulin resistance and hyperinsulinemia with PCOS, a disorder affecting an estimated 6% of women of reproductive age and the most common cause of female infertility in the United States.[369] Hirsutism and acne are also common consequences of this disorder. Studies have shown that high circulating insulin may stimulate ovarian cytochrome P450c17α and 17,20 lyase enzymes in predisposed women, resulting in elevations in serum testosterone and free unbound testosterone, both seen in PCOS.

Insulin influences the androgenic state directly by affecting the metabolism of ovarian androgens, and indirectly by regulating circulating levels of sex hormone binding globulin (SHBG). Insulin has been shown to lower the production of SHBG.[370] SHBG binds to testosterone and estrogens, making them biologically unavailable. Lowered SHBG therefore indirectly increases the delivery of testosterone to tissues as increased amounts of testosterone are unbound and bioavailable.[371] Studies indicate that improving insulin sensitivity and decreasing circulating insulin beneficially affects women with PCOS.[372,373]

Cancer

An area of increasing research interest is the relationship of insulin resistance to cancer. One hypothesis has postulated a link between colorectal cancer, insulin resistance, and hyperinsulinemia.[374,375] While the epidemiological data are not completely consistent, the two largest prospective studies to date do support a modest correlation between colorectal cancer risk and diabetes.[376,377] Additional support for a promoting effect of insulin on colorectal carcinogenesis has been found in animal models, thereby providing direct evidence for a possible cause-and-effect relationship between hyperinsulinemia and colorectal cancer.[378,379]

Even more recently, speculation has centered on the link between hyperinsulinemia and breast cancer.[380] It has been known for some time that exposure of breast tissue to estrogens increases the risk of breast cancer. It is well established that only the fraction of estrogens unbound to SHBG are biologically available to receptors on target cells. As mentioned earlier, insulin inhibits the formation of SHBG. While SHBG binds to both testosterone and estrogen, it binds preferentially to testosterone; therefore, decreased levels of SHBG will result preferentially in increased levels of free unbound estrogen.[381] In support of this concept, some epidemiological studies have shown that high plasma levels of unbound estrogen are associated with increased risk of breast cancer, at least among postmenopausal women.[382,383,384,385]

Summary

Insulin resistance syndrome represents one of the most important imbalances in clinical care today. It is a multifactorial health condition that has become increasingly common in industrialized societies. It affects, by conservative estimates, a quarter of the U.S. population. It initially manifests as impairments in insulin sensitivity that cause a cascade of biochemical changes resulting in increasing risk for a host of chronic degenerative diseases. Coronary heart disease, hypertension, polycystic ovary syndrome, cognitive decline, and type 2 diabetes appear to be directly related to this metabolic imbalance. Certain cancers may also be causally related. The economic costs of treating these end-stage disorders are enormous. Recognition and early treatment are, therefore, essential. Treatment of the underlying biochemical defect, loss of insulin sensitivity, and resistance to glucose disposal is of central importance. While genetic inheritance may determine propensity to the disorder, modifiable factors such as weight, exercise, smoking, diet, and nutrition play a critical role. A comprehensive strategy of lifestyle and dietary modifications along with nutrient supplementation is an important step in clinical management of this fundamental clinical imbalance.

References

1. Immumorin IG, Dong Y, Zhu H, et al. A gene-environment interaction model of stress-induced hypertension. Cardiovasc Toxicol. 2005;5(2):109-32.
2. Traustadottir T, Bosch PR, Matt KS. The HPA axis response to stress in women: effects of aging and fitness. Psychoneuroendocrinology. 2005;30(4):392-402.
3. Weber-Hamann B, Kopf D, Lederbogen F, et al. Activity of the hypothalamus-pituitary-adrenal system and oral glucose tolerance in depressed patients. Neuroendocrinology. 2005;81(3):200-4.
4. Dharia S, Parker CR Jr. Adrenal androgens and aging. Semin Reprod Med. 2004;22(4):361-68.
5. Karrow NA. Activation of the hypothalamic-pituitary-adrenal axis and autonomic nervous system during inflammation and altered programming of the neuroendocrine-immune axis during fetal and neonatal development: Lessons learned from the model inflammagen, lipopolysaccharide. Brain Behav Immun. 2005;July12:[Epub ahead of print].
6. Seibold F. Food-induced immune responses as origin of bowel disease? Digestion. 2005;71(4):251-60.
7. De Souza CT, Araujo EP, Bordin S, et al. Consumption of a fat-rich diet activates a proinflammatory response and induces insulin resistance in the hypothalamus. Endocrinology. 2005;July7:[Epub ahead of print].
8. Shernhammer ES. Rotating night shifts and risk of breast cancer in women participating in the Nurses' Health Study. J Natl Can Inst. 2001;93(20):1563-67.
9. McLean JA. Cognitive dietary restraint is associated with higher urinary cortisol excretion in healthy premenopausal women. Am J Clin Nutr 2001;73:7-12.
10. Rossouw JE, Anderson GL, Prentice RL, et al. Writing Group for the Women's Health Initiative Investigators. Risks and benefits of estrogen plus progestin in healthy postmenopausal women: principal results from the Women's Health Initiative randomized controlled trial. JAMA 2002;288:321-33.
11. Galland L. Applying Person-Centered Diagnosis to the Problem of Chronic Fatigue. 7th International Symposium on Functional Medicine, 2000. Institute for Functional Medicine, Gig Harbor, WA.
12. Schimmel EM. The hazards of hospitalization. Annals of Internal Medicine. 1964, Volume 60, pages 100-110.
13. Baker GR. The Canadian Adverse Events Study: the incidence of adverse events among hospital patients in Canada. CMAJ. 2004;170(11):1678-86.
14. Fischer G. Adverse events in primary care identified from a risk-management database. J Fam Pract. 1997;45(1).40-46.
15. Burke W. Genomics as a probe for disease biology. N Engl J Med. 2003. 349;10:969.
16. Jefcoate CR Chapter 5:Tissue Specific Synthesis and Oxidative Metabolism of Estrogens. J Natl Can Inst Monogr. 2000;27:95-112.
17. Zhu BT Functional role of estrogen metabolism in target cells: review and perspectives. Carcinogenesis. 1998;19(1):1-27.
18. Zhao Y Estrogen biosynthesis proximal to a breast tumor is stimulated by PGE2 via cyclic AMP, leading to activation of promoter II of the CYP19(aromatase) gene. Endocrinology. 1996;137:5739-41.
19. Dunning AM. Polymorphisms associated with circulating sex hormone levels in postmenopausal women. J Natl Cancer Inst. 2004;96:936-45.
20. Kim SH, Tamrazi A, Carlson KE, Katzenellenbogen JA. A proteomic microarray approach for exploring ligand-initiated nuclear hormone receptor pharmacology, receptor selectivity, and heterodimer functionality. Moll Cell Proteomics. 2005;4:267-77.
21. Monroe DG, Secreto FJ, Subramaniam M, et al. Estrogen receptor a and b heterodimers exert unique effects on estrogen- and tamoxifen-dependent gene expression in human U2OS osteosarcoma cells. Molec Endocrinol. 2005;19(6):1555-68.
22. Bland J. Nutritional Modulation of Inflammatory Disorders. Metagenics Educational Programs, Gig Harbor, WA: 2004, pg 153.
23. Verdier-Sevrain S, Yaar M, Cantatore J, et al. Estradiol induces proliferation of keratinocytes vis receptor-mediated mechanisms. FASEB J. 2004;18(11):1252-54.
24. Elkas J. Modulation of endometrial steroid receptors and growth regulatory genes by Tamoxifen. Obstet Gynecol. 2000;95:697-703.
25. Soderqvist G. Proliferation of breast epithelial cells in healthy women during the menstrual cycle. Am J Obstet Gynecol. 1997;176:123-28.
26. Cowan LD. Breast cancer incidence in women with a history of progesterone deficiency. Am J Epidemiol. 1981;114(2):209.
27. Plu-Bureau G. Percutaneous progesterone use and risk of breast cancer: results from a French cohort study of premenopausal women with benign breast disease. Can Detect Prev. 1999;23(4):290-96.
28. Mohr PE. Serum progesterone and prognosis in operable breast cancer. Br J Can. 1996;73:1552.
29. Kenemans, P. Tibolone: how does its mechanism of action translate into clinical effects? Maturitas. 2004;48(Suppl 1):13-17.
30. Chang K Influences of percutaneous administration of estradiol and progesterone on human breast epithelial cell cycle *in vivo*. Fertil Steril. 1995;63(4):783-91.
31. Tang S, Han H, Bajic VB. ERGDB: Estrogen Responsive Genes Database. Nucleic Acids Res. 2004;32(Database issue):D533-36.
32. Cordian B. Nongenomic effects of oestrogen: embryonic mouse midbrain neurones respond with a rapid release of calcium from intracellular stores. Eur J Neurosci. 1998;10(1):255.
33. Dubey RK, Tofovic SP, Jackson EK. Cardiovascular pharmacology of estradiol metabolites. J Pharmacol Exper Ther. 2004;308(2):403-9.
34. Cheng TC, Chen ST, Huang CS, et al. Breast cancer risk associated with genotype polymorphism of the catechol estrogen-metabolizing genes: a multigenic study on cancer susceptibility. Int J Cancer. 2005;113(3):345-53.
35. Modugo FA. Potential role for the estrogen-metabolizing cytochrome P450 enzymes in human breast carcinogenesis. Breast Cancer Res Treat. 2003 Dec;82(3):191-97.

36. Masson LF, Sharp L, Cotton SC, Little J. Cytochrome P-450 1A1 gene polymorphisms and risk of breast cancer: a HuGE review. Am J Epidemiol. 2005;161(10):901-15.
37. Tsuchiya Y, Nakajima M, Kyo S, et al. Human CYP1B1 is regulated by estradiol via estrogen receptor. Cancer Res. 2004;64(9):3119-25.
38. Modugno F, Knoll C, Kanbour-Shakir A, Romkes M. A potential role for the estrogen-metabolizing cytochrome P450 enzymes in human breast carcinogenesis. Breast Cancer Res Treat. 2003;82(3):191-97.
39. Knupfer H. Cyp2C and IL-6 expression in breast cancer. Breast. 2004 Feb;13(1):28-34.
40. Yager JD. Endogenous estrogens as carcinogens through metabolic activation. J Natl Can Inst Monogr. 2000;(27):67-73.
41. Meilahn EN. Do urinary oestrogen metabolites predict breast cancer? Buernsey III Cohort Follow-up. Br J Cancer. 1998;78(9):1250-55.
42. Muti P. Urinary estrogen metabolites and prostate cancer: a case-controlled study in the United States. Cancer Causes Control. 2002;13(10):947-55.
43. Sasaki M. EYP 1B1 gene polymorphisms have higher risk for endometrial cancer and positive correlations with estrogen receptor alpha and estrogen receptor beta expressions. Cancer Res. 2003;63(14):3913-18.
44. Osborne MP. Upregulation of estradiol C16a hydroxylation in human breast tissue: a potential biomarker of breast cancer risk. J Natl Can Inst. 1003;83(23):1917-20.
45. Bonnesen C, Stephensen PU, Andersen O, et al. Modulation of cytochrome P-450 and glutathione S-transferase isoform expression *in vivo* by intact and degraded indolyl glucosinolates. Nutr Cancer. 1999;33(2):178-87.
46. Seeger H. Inhibition of human breast cancer cell proliferation with estradiol metabolites is as effective as with tamoxifen. Horm Metab Res. 2004;36(5):277-80.
47. Cavalieri E. Estrogens as endogenous genotoxic agents-DNA adducts and mutations. J Natl Cancer Inst Monogr. 2000;27:75-93.
48. Keshava C. Transcriptional signatures of environmentally relevant exposures in normal human mammary epithelial cells: benzo[a]pyrene. Cancer Lett. 2005;221(92):201-11.
49. Chang TKH, Chen J, Benetton SA. *In vitro* effect of standardized ginseng extracts and individual ginsenosides on the catalytic activity of human CYP 1A1, CYP1A2, AND CYP1B1. Drug Metab Disp. 2002;30(4):378-84.
50. Parl FF. Estrogens, Estrogen Receptors and Breast Cancer. IOS Press, Washington, D.C. 2000, pg 31.
51. Thibodeau PA, Kachadourian R, Lemay R, et al. *In vitro* pro- and antioxidant properties of estrogens. J Steroid Biochem Mol Biol. 2002;81(3):227-36.
52. Pfeiffer E, Treiling CR, Hoehle SI, Metzler M. Isoflavones modulate the glucuronidation of estradiol in human liver microsomes. Carcinogenesis. 2005;July 28:[Epub ahead of print].
53. Calcium-D-Glucarate. Altern Med Rev. 2002;(4):336-39.
54. Soderqvist G. Proliferation of breast epithelial cells in healthy women during the menstrual cycle. Am J Obstet Gynecol. 1997;176:123-28.
55. Pike MC. Estrogens, progestogens, normal breast cell proliferation, and breast cancer risk. Epidem Rev. 1993;15(1):17-35.
56. Majewska MD. Steroid hormone metabolites are barbiturate-like modulators of the GABA receptor. Science. 1986;232:1004.
57. Ugale RR, Hirani K, Morelli M, Chopde CT. Role of neuroactive steroid allopregnanolone in antipsychotic-like action of olanzapine in rodents. Neuropsychopharmacology. 2004;29(9):1597-609.
58. Reddy DS. Pharmacology of endogenous neuroactive steroids. Crit Rev Neurobiol. 2003;15(3-4):197-234.
59. Weinberger DR. Anxiety at the frontier of molecular medicine. N Engl J Med. 2001;344(16):1247.
60. Grow DR. Metabolism of endogenous and exogenous reproductive hormones. Obstet Gynecol Clin North Am. 2002;29(3):425-36.
61. Lewis JG, McGill H, Patton VM, Elder PA. Caution on the use of saliva measurements to monitor absorption of progesterone from transdermal creams in postmenopausal women. Maturitas. 2002;41:1-6.
62. Leonetti HB. Topical progesterone cream has antiproliferative effect on estrogen-stimulated endometrium. Fertil Steril. 2003;79(1):221-22.
63. Hesch RD, Kenemans P. Hormonal prevention of breast cancer: proposal for a change in paradigm.Br J Obstet Gynaecol. 1999;106(10):1006-18.
64. Kumar NS. Selective down-regulation of progesterone receptor isoform B in poorly differentiated human endometrial cancer cells: implications for unopposed estrogen action. Cancer Res 1998;58(0):1860-65.
65. Dharia S. Parker CR Jr. Adrenal androgens and aging. Semin Reprod Med. 2004;22(4):361-68.
66. Guay A, Munarriz R, Jacobson J, et al. Serum androgen levels in healthy premenopausal women with and without sexual dysfunction: Part A. Serum androgen levels in women aged 20-49 years with no complaints of sexual dysfunction. Int J Impot Res. 2004;16(2):112-20.
67. Hess RA. A role for oestrogens in the male reproductive system. Nature. 1997;390(6659):509-12.
68. Davis SR. Testosterone treatment: psychological and physical effects in postmenopausal women. Menopausal Medicine. 2001;9(2):1-6.
69. Galland L. Applying person-centered diagnosis to the problem of chronic fatigue. 7th International Symposium on Functional Medicine, 2000. Institute for Functional Medicine: Gig Harbor, WA.
70. Vermeulen A. The hormonal activity of the postmenopausal ovary. J Clin Endocrinol Metab. 1976;42:247.
71. Yale Department of Ob/Gyn website. Sex hormones and the immune system. http://info.med.yale.edu/obgyn/reproimmuno/projects/hormones.html
72. Ibid.
73. Wilczynski JR. Th1/Th2 cytokines balance yin and yang of reproductive immunology. Eur J Obstet Gynecol Reprod Biol. 2005;May 11:Epub ahead of print.
74. Ostensen M, Forger F, Nelson JL. Pregnancy in patients with rheumatic disease: anti-inflammatory cytokines increase in pregnancy and decrease post partum. Ann Rheum Dis. 2005;64:839-44.
75. Elenkov IJ. Glucocorticoids and the Th1/Th2 balance. Ann NY Acad Sci. 2004;1024:138-46.
76. Ragusa A, de Carolis C, dal Lago A, et al. Progesterone supplement in pregnancy: an immunologic therapy? Lupus. 2004;13(9):639-42.
77. Bland J. Nutritional Modulation of Inflammatory Disorders. Metagenics Educational Programs, Gig Harbor, WA: 2004, pg 154.
78. Ibid.
79. Lange CA. Hypothesis: Progesterone primes breast cancer cells for crosstalk with proliferative or antiproliferative signals. Endocrinology 1999;13(6):829.
80. Plante J. Your Life In Your Hands. Thomas Dunne Books 2000, New York, NY.
81. Soderqvist G. Effects of sex steroids on proliferation in normal mammary tissue. Ann Med. 1998;30:511-524.
82. The Writing Group for the PEPI Trial. Effects of hormone replacement therapy on endometrial histology in postmenopausal women. JAMA 1996;275:370-75.

83. Register TC, Adams MR, Golden DL, Clarkson TB. Conjugated equine estrogens alone, but not in combination with medroxyprogesterone acetate, inhibit aortic connective tissue remodeling after plasma lipid lowering in female monkeys. Arterioscler Thromb Vasc Biol. 1998;18(7):1164-71.
84. Fitzpatrick L. "Where do We Go From Here ... Unopposed Estrogen?" The Female Patient Supplement, February 2004, pg.3.
85. Majewska MD. Steroid hormone metabolites are barbiturate-like modulators of the GABA receptor. Science. 1986;232:1004.
86. Ibid.
87. Dorgan JF. Relation of prediagnostic serum estrogen and androgen levels to breast cancer risk. Cancer Epidemiol Biomarkers Prev. 1996;5:533-39.
88. Zeleniuch-Jacquotte A. Relation of serum levels of testosterone and dehydroepiandrosterone sulfate to risk of breast cancer in postmenopausal women. Am J Epidemiol. 1997:145:1030-38.
89. Davis SR. Testosterone treatment: psychological and physical effects in postmenopausal women. Menopausal Medicine. 2001;9(2):1-6.
90. Davis SR. The use of testosterone after menopause. J Br Menopause Soc. 2004;10(2):65-69.
91. Pasqualini JR. The selective estrogen enzyme modulators in breast cancer: a review. Biochem Biophys Acta. 2004;1654(2):123-43.
92. Witorsch RJ. Endocrine disruptors: can biological effects and environmental risks be predicted? Regl Toxicol Pharmacol. 2002;36(1):1180.
93. Tabb, M, Blumberg, B. New modes of action for endocrine disrupting chemicals. Mol Endocrinol. 2005;July 21:[Epub ahead of print].
94. Wozniak AAL, Bulayeva NN, Watson, CS. Xenoestrogens at picomolar to nanomolar concentrations trigger membrane estrogen receptor-alpha-mediated Ca2+ fluxes and prolactin release in GH3/B6 pituitary tumor cells. Environ Health Perspec. 2005;113(4):431-39.
95. Bulayeva NN, Watson, CS. Xenoestrogen-induced ERK-1 and ERK-2 activation via multiple membrane-initiated signaling pathways. Environ Health Perspect. 2004;112(15):1481-87.
96. Moggs JG. Molecular responses to xenoestrogens: Mechanistic insights from toxicogenomics. Toxicology. 2005;Jul 1:[Epub ahead of print].
97. Fisher JS. Are all EDC effects mediated via steroid hormone receptors? Toxicology. 2004;205(1-2):33-41.
98. Prasad AS. Zinc: an overview. Nutrition. 1995;11(1 Suppl):93-99.
99. Watson WP, Munter T, Golding BT. A new role for glutathione: protections of vitamin B12 from depletion by xenobiotics. Chem Res Toxicol. 2004;17(12):1562-67.
100. Levgur M. Hormone therapy for women after breast cancer: a review. J Reprod Med. 2004 Jul;49(7):510-26.
101. Lexchin JR. Implications of pharmaceutical industry funding on clinical research. Ann Pharmacother. 2005;39(1):194-97.
102. Lemmens T. Confronting the conflict of interest crisis in medical research. Monash Bioeth Rev. 2004;23(4):19-40.
103. Thorneycroft IH. Unopposed Estrogen and Cancer "Where do We Go From Here ... Unopposed Estrogen?" The Female Patient Supplement, February 2004: pg.19.
104. Collaborative Group on Hormonal Factors in Breast Cancer. Breast cancer and hormonal contraceptives: collaborative reanalysis of individual data on 53,297 women with breast cancer and 100,239 women without breast cancer from 54 epidemiological studies. Lancet. 1996;347:1713-27.
105. Collaborative Group on Hormonal Factors in Breast Cancer. Breast cancer and hormone replacement therapy: collaborative reanalysis of data from 51 epidemiological studies of 52,705 women with breast cancer and 108,411 women without breast cancer. Lancet. 1997;350:1047-59.
106. Ewertz M, Mellemkjaer L, Poulsen AH, et al. Hormone use for menopausal symptoms and risk of breast cancer. A Danish cohort study. Br J Cancer. 2005;92(7):1293-97.
107. Lee SA, Ross RK, Pike MC. An overview of menopausal oestrogen-progestin hormone therapy and breast cancer risk. Br J Cancer. 2005;May 17:Epub ahead of print.
108. Li CI, Moe RE, Daling JR. Risk of mortality by histological type of breast cancer among women aged 50-79 years. Arch Intern Med. 2003;163:2149-53.
109. Dumitrescu RG. Understanding breast cancer risk-where do we stand in 2005? J Cell Mol Med. 2005;9(1):208-21.
110. Ibid.
111. Zimarina TC, Kristensen VN, Imianitov EN, Bershtein LM. [Polymorphisms of CYP1B1 and COMT in breast and endometrial cancer.] Mol Biol (Mosk). 2004;38(3):386-93.
112. Wen W, Cai Q, Shu XO, et al. Cytochrome P450 1B1 and catechol-O-methyltransferase genetic polymorphisms and breast cancer risk in Chinese women: results from the Shanghai Breast Cancer Study and a meta-analysis. Cancer Epidemiol Biomarkers Prev. 2005;14(2):329-35.
113. Lord SJ, Mack WJ, Van Den Berg D, et al. Polymorphisms in genes involved in estrogen and progesterone metabolism and mammographic density changes in women randomized to postmenopausal hormone therapy: results from a pilot study. Breast Cancer Res. 2005;7(3):R336-44.
114. Rajapakse N, Butterworth M, Kortenkamp A. Detection of DNA strand breaks and oxidized DNA bases at the single-cell level resulting from exposure to estradiol and hydroxylated metabolites. Environ Mol Mutagen. 2005;45(4):397-404.
115. De Jong M. Genes other than BRCA1 and BRCA2 involved in breast cancer susceptibility. J Med Genet. 2002;39:225-42.
116. Ibid.
117. Hirose K. The CYP19 gene codon 39 Trp/Arg polymorphism increases breast cancer risk in subsets of premenopausal Japanese. Cancer Epidemiol Biomarkers Prev. 2004;13(8):1407-11.
118. Ibid.
119. Albin N. Main drug-metabolizing enzymes systems in human breast tumors and peritumoral tissues. Cancer Res. 1993;53:3541-46.
120. Gudmundsdottir K. GSTM1, GSTT1, and GSTP1 genotypes in relation to breast cancer risk and frequency of mutations in the p53 gene. Cancer Epidemiol Biomarkers Prev. 2001;10:1169-73.
121. Campbell IG. Methylenetetrahydrofolate reductase polymorphism and susceptibility to breast cancer. Breast Cancer Res. 2002;4:R14.
122. Ergul E. Polymorphisms in the MTHFR gene are associated with breast cancer. Tumour Biol. 2003;24:286-90.
123. Han DF, Zhou X, Hu MB, et al. Sulfotransferase 1A1 (SULT 1A1) polymorphism and breast cancer risk in Chinese women. Toxicol Lett. 2004;150(2):167-77.
124. Coughtrie MW. Sulfations through the looking glass—recent advances in sulfotransferase research for the curious. Pharmacogenomics J. 2002;2(5):297-308.
125. Smith TR. DNA-repair genetic polymorphisms and breast cancer risk. Cancer Epidemiol Biomarkers Prev. 2003;12:1200-4.
126. Gold B. Estrogen receptor genotypes and haplotypes associated with breast cancer risk. Cancer Res. 2004;64:8891-900.
127. De Jong M. Genes other than BRCA1 and BRCA2 involved in breast cancer susceptibility. J Med Genet. 2002;39:225-42.
128. Ibid.
129. Anderson GL, Limacher M, Assaf AR, et al. Effects of conjugated equine estrogen in postmenopausal women with hysterectomy: the Women's Health Initiative randomized controlled trial. JAMA. 2004;291(14):1701-12.
130. Gross CP. Factors affecting prophylactic oophorectomy in postmenopausal women. Obstet Gynecol Survey. 2000;55(3):147-48.

131. Anderson GL, Limacher M, Assaf AR, et al. Effects of conjugated equine estrogen in postmenopausal women with hysterectomy: the Women's Health Initiative randomized controlled trial. JAMA. 2004;291(14):1701-12.
132. Russo J. Developmental, Cellular and Molecular Basis of Human Breast Cancer. Chapter 1 in: Russo J, Journal of the National Cancer Institute Monographs No. 27, 2000.
133. Anderson E. Cellular homeostasis and the breast. Maturitas. 2004;48(Suppl 1):13-17.
134. Pike MC. Estrogens, progestogens, normal breast cell proliferation, and breast cancer risk. Epidem Rev. 1993;15(1):17-35.
135. Stoll BA. Essential fatty acids, insulin resistance and breast cancer. Nutrition and Cancer. 1998;31(1):72-77.
136. Lange CA. Hypothesis: progesterone primes breast cancer cells for crosstalk with proliferative or antiproliferative signals. Mol Endocrinol. 1999;13(6):829-36.
137. Goldfine ID. Progestin regulation of insulin and insulin-like growth factor 1 receptors in cultured human breast cancer cells. Breast Cancer Res Treat. 1992;22:69-79.
138. Lange CA. Hypothesis: Progesterone primes breast cancer cells for cross-talk with proliferative or antiproliferative signals. Mol Endocrinol. 1999;13(6):829-36.
139. Ross R, Janssen I, Dawson J, et al. Exercise-induced reduction in obesity and insulin resistance in women: a randomized controlled trial. Obes Res. 2004;12(5):789-98.
140. Kahl KG, Bester M, Greggersen W, et al. Visceral fat deposition and insulin sensitivity in depressed women with and without comorbid borderline personality disorder. Psychosom Med. 2005;67(3):407-12.
141. Schroder AK, Tauchert S, Ortmann O, et al. Insulin resistance in patients with polycystic ovary syndrome. Ann Med. 2004;36(6):426-39.
142. Morimoto LM, White E, Chen Z, et al. Obesity, body size, and risk of postmenopausal breast cancer: the Women's Health Initiative (United States). Cancer Causes Control. 2002;13(8):741-51.
143. Lahmann PH, Hoffmann K, Allen N, et al. Body size and breast cancer risk: findings from the European Prospective Investigation into Cancer and Nutrition (EPIC). J Cancer. 2004;111(5):762-71.
144. Sephton SE, Sapolsky RM, Kraemer HC, Spiegel D. Diurnal cortisol rhythm as a predictor of breast cancer survival. J Natl Cancer Inst. 2000;92(12):994-1000.
145. Caulin-Glaser T. 17b estradiol regulation of human endothelial cell basal nitric oxide release, independent of cytosolic Ca2+ mobilization. Circ Res. 1997;81(5):885-92.
146. Sarrel P. "Vasomotor and Vascular Considerations." Where Do We Go From Here ... Unopposed Estrogen? The Female Patient Supplement, February 2004.
147. Sarrel PM. Ovarian hormones and the circulation. Maturitas. 1990;12(13):287-98.
148. Strechlow K, Rotter, S, Wassmann S, et al. Modulation of antioxidant enzyme expression and function by estrogen. Circ Res. 2003;93(2):170-77.
149. Rossouw JE, Anderson GL, Prentice RL, et al. and the Writing Group for the Women's Health Initiative Investigators. Risks and benefits of estrogen plus progestin in healthy postmenopausal women: principal results from the Women's Health Initiative randomized controlled trial. JAMA. 2002;288:321-33.
150. Hlatky MA. Quality-of-life and depressive symptoms in postmenopausal women after receiving hormone therapy: results from the Heart and Estrogen/Progestin Replacement Study (HERS) trial. JAMA. 2002;287(5):591-97.
151. Quesada A, Etgen AM. Functional interactions between estrogen and insulin-like growth factor-I in the regulation of a1B-adrenoceptors and female reproductive function. J Neurosci. 2002;22(6):2401-8.
152. Foldvary-Schaefer N, Harden C, Herzog A, Falcone T. Hormones and seizures. Cleve Clin J Med. 2004;71(Suppl 2):S11-18.
153. Amin Z, Canli T, Epperson CN. Effect of estrogen-serotonin interactions on mood and cognition. Behav Cogn Neurosci Rev. 2005;4(1):43-58.
154. Personal communication with Diana Schwarzbein, MD.
155. Dormire S, Reame NK. Menopausal hot flash frequency changes in response to experimental manipulation of blood glucose. Nurs Res. 2003;52(5):338-43.
156. Ratka, A. Menopausal hot flashes and development of cognitive impairment. Ann NY Acad Sci. 2005;102:11-26.
157. Hlatky MA. Quality-of-life and depressive symptoms in postmenopausal women after receiving hormone therapy: results from the Heart and Estrogen/Progestin Replacement Study (HERS) trial. JAMA. 2002;287(5):591-97.
158. Evans ML, Pritts E, Vittinghoff E, et al. Management of postmenopausal hot flushes with venlafaxine hydrochloride: a randomized, controlled trial. Obstet Gynecol. 2005;105(1):161-66.
159. Stearns V, Beebe KL, Iyengar M, Dube E. Paroxetine controlled release in the management of menopausal hot flashes: a randomized controlled trial. JAMA. 2003;289(21):2827-34.
160. Suvanto-Luukkonen E, Koivunen R, Sundstrom H, et al. Citalopram and fluoxetine in the treatment of postmenopausal symptoms: a prospective, randomized 9-month, placebo-controlled, double-blind study. Menopause. 2005;12(1):18-26.
161. Loprinzi CL, Sloan JA, Perez EA, et al. Phase III evaluation of fluoxetine for treatment of hot flashes. J Clin Oncol. 2002;20(6):1578-83.
162. Guttuso T Jr. Hot flashes refractory to HRT and SSRI therapy but responsive to gabapentin therapy. J Pain Symptom Manage. 2004;27(3):274-76.
163. Brizendine L. Managing menopause-related depression and low libido. OBG Management. 2004;6(8):29.
164. Hlatky MA. Quality-of-life and depressive symptoms in postmenopausal women after receiving hormone therapy: results from the Heart and Estrogen/Progestin Replacement Study (HERS) trial. JAMA. 2002;287(5):591-97.
165. Spinelli MG. Depression and hormone therapy. Clin Obstet Gynecol. 2004;47(2):428.
166. Costa E, Silva JA. Overview of the field. Metabolism Clinical and Experimental. 2005;54(Suppl 1):5-9.
167. MedlinePlus Medical Encyclopedia: Premenstrual Syndrome. Accessed 5/23/05 at http://www.nlm.nih.gov/medlineplus/ency/article/001505.htm
168. Halbreich U. The diagnosis of premenstrual syndromes and premenstrual dysphoric disorder—clinical procedures and research perspectives. Gynecol Endocrinol. 2004;19(6):320-34.
169. Halbreich U. Borenstein J, Pearlstein T, Kahn LS. The prevalence, impairment, impact, and burden of premenstrual dysphoric disorders (PMS/PMDD). Psychoneuroendocrinology. 2003;28(Suppl3):1-23.
170. Kaur G, Gonsalves L, Thacker HL. Premenstrual dysphoric disorder: a review for the treating practitioner. Cleve Clin J Med. 2004;71(4):303-5, 312-13, 317-18.
171. Spinelli MG. Depression and hormone therapy. Clin Obstet Gynecol. 2004;47(2):428.
172. Kalantaridou SN, Makrigiannakis A, Zoumakis E, Chrousos GP. Stress and the female reproductive system. J Reprod Immunol. 2004;62(1-2):61-68.
173. Tafet GE, Smolovich J. Psychoneuroendocrinological studies on chronic stress and depression. Ann NY Acad Sci. 2004;1032:276-78.
174. Portella MJ, Harmer CJ, Flint J, et al. Enhanced early morning salivary cortisol in neuroticism. Am J Psychiatry. 2005;162(4):807-9.

175. Lindmark S, Lonn L, Wiklund U, et al. Dysregulation of the autonomic nervous system can be a link between visceral adiposity and insulin resistance. Obes Res. 2005;13:717-28.
176. Lund TD, Rovis T, Chung WC, Handa RJ. Novel actions of estrogen receptor-beta on anxiety-related behaviors. Endocrinology. 2005;146(2):797-807.
177. Carvalho-Blanco SD, Kim BW, Zhang JX, et al. Chronic cardiac-specific thyrotoxicosis increases myocardial -adrenergic responsiveness. Mol Endocrinol. 2004;18(7):1840-49.
178. Zhong JQ, Dorian P. Epinephrine and vasopressin during cardiopulmonary resuscitation. Resuscitation. 2005;Jul 19:[Epub ahead of print].
179. Krebs EE, Ensrud KE, MacDonald R, Wilt TJ. Phytoestrogens for treatment of menopausal symptoms: a systematic review. Obstet Gynecol. 2004;104(4):824-36.
180. Neff MJ. NAMS releases position statement on the treatment of vasomotor symptoms associated with menopause. Am Fam Physician. 2004;70(2):393-94, 396, 399.
181. Crisafulli A, Marini H, Bitto A, et al. Effects of genistein on hot flushes in early postmenopausal women: a randomized, double-blind EPT- and placebo-controlled study. Menopause. 2004;11(4):400-4.
182. McKee J, Warber SL. Integrative therapies for menopause. South Med J. 2005;98(3):319-26.
183. Brooks JD, Ward WE, Lewis JE, et al. Supplementation with flaxseed alters estrogen metabolism in postmenopausal women to a great extent than does supplementation with an equal amount of soy. Am J Clin Nutr. 2004;79:318-25.
184. Sturpe D. Transdermal progesterone ineffective. J Fam Pract. 2003;52:362-63.
185. Lewis JG, McGill H, Patton VM, Elder PA. Caution on the use of saliva measurements to monitor absorption of progesterone from transdermal creams in postmenopausal women. Maturitas. 2002;41:1-6.
186. Galland L. Applying Person-Centered Diagnosis to the Problem of Chronic Fatigue. 7th International Symposium on Functional Medicine, 2000. Institute for Functional Medicine, Gig Harbor, WA.
187. Ibid.
188. Weidler C. Patients with rheumatoid arthritis and systemic lupus erythematosus have increased renal excretion of mitogenic estrogens in relation to endogenous anti-estrogens. Rheumatol. 2004;31(3):489-94.
189. Doran MF, Crowson CS, O'Fallon WM, Gabriel SE. The effect of oral contraceptives and estrogen replacement therapy on the risk of rheumatoid arthritis: a population based study. J Rheumatol. 2004;31:207-13.
190. Cutolo M, Sulli A, Capellino S, et al. Sex hormones influence on the immune system: basic and clinical aspects in autoimmunity. Lupus. 2004;13(9):635-38.
191. Jolly M. Hormone replacement therapy in rheumatoid arthritis. J Rheumatol. 2004;31(7):1462-63
192. Smith R, Studd JW. A pilot study of the effect upon multiple sclerosis of the menopause, hormone replacement therapy and the menstrual cycle. J R Soc Med. 1992;85(10):612-13.
193. Sanchez-Guerrero J, Villegas A, Mendoza-Fuentes A, et al. Disease activity during the premenopausal and postmenopausal periods in women with systemic lupus erythematosus. Am J Med. 2001;111(6):464-68.
194. Askanase AD. Estrogen therapy in systemic lupus erythematosus. Treat Endocrinol. 2004;3(1):19-26.
195. Salem ML. Estrogen, a double-edged sword: modulation of Th1- and Th2-mediated inflammations by differential regulation of Th1/Th2 cytokine production. Curr Drug Targets Inflamm Allergy. 2004;3(1):97-104.
196. Quinn M. Endometriosis: the consequence of neurologic dysfunction? Med Hypotheses. 2004;63(4):602-8.
197. Okamura H, Katabuchi H. Detailed morphology of human ovarian surface epithelium focusing on its metaplastic and neoplastic capability. Ital J Anat Embryol. 2001;106(2 Suppl 2):263-76.
198. Skoog SM, Foxx-Orenstein AE, Levy MJ, et al. Intestinal endometriosis: the great masquerader. Curr Gastroenterol Rep. 2004;6(5):405-9.
199. Cao WG, Morin M, Metz C, et al. Stimulation of macrophage migration inhibitory factor expression in endometrial stromal cells by interleukin 1,{beta} involving the nuclear transcription factor NF{kappa}B. Biol Reprod. 2005;May 1:[Epub ahead of print].
200. Matsuzaki S, Canis M, Pouly JL, et al. The macrophage stimulating protein/RON system: a potential novel target for prevention and treatment of endometriosis. Mol Hum Reprod. 2005;11(5):345-49.
201. Lebovic DI, Mueller MD, Taylor RN. Immunobiology of endometriosis. Fertil Steril. 2001;75(1):1-10.
202. Dmowski WP, Gebel H, Braun, DP. Decreased apoptosis and sensitivity to macrophage mediated cytolysis of endometrial cells in endometriosis. Hum Reprod Update. 1998;4(5):696-701.
203. Sharpe-Timms KL, Cox, KE. Paracrine regulation of matrix metalloproteinase expression in endometriosis. Ann NY Acad Sci. 2002;955:147-156; discussion 157-8, 396-406.
204. Bruner-tran KL, Rier SE, Eisenberg, E, Osteen KG. The potential role of environmental toxins in the pathophysiology of endometriosis. Gynecol Obstet Invest. 1999;48(Suppl 1):45-56.
205. Zhou HE, Nothnick WB. The relevancy of the matrix metalloproteinase system to the pathophysiology of endometriosis. Front Biosci. 2005;10:569-75.
206. Murphy AA, Santanam N, Parthasarathy S. Endometriosis: a disease of oxidative stress? Semin Reprod Endocrinol. 1998;16(4):263-73.
207. Goff BA. Frequency of symptoms of ovarian cancer in women presenting to primary care clinics. JAMA. 2004;291(22):2755-56.
208. Cramer DW. Characteristics of women with a family history of ovarian cancer. I. Galactose consumption and metabolism. Cancer. 1994;74:1309-17.
209. Wolfler MM, Nagele F, Kolbus A, et al. A predictive model for endometriosis. Hum Reprod. 2005;20(6):1702-8.
210. Hemmings R, Rivard M, Olive DL, et al. Evaluation of risk factors associated with endometriosis. Fertil Steril. 2004;81(6):1513-21.
211. Hodges LC, Hunter DS, Bergerson JS, et al. An *in vivo/in vitro* model to assess endocrine disrupting activity of xenoestrogens in uterine leiomyoma. Ann NY Acad Sci. 2001;948:100-11.
212. Cauley JA, Robbins J, Chen Z, et al. Effects of estrogen plus progestin on risk of fractures and bone mineral density: the Women's Health Initiative randomized trial. JAMA. 2003;290(13):1729-38.
213. Lindsay R. Hormones and bone health in postmenopausal women. Endocrine. 2004;24(3):223-30.
214. Ettinger B, Ensrud KE, Wallace R, et al. Effects of ultralow-dose transdermal estradiol on bone mineral density: a randomized clinical trial. Obstet Gynecol. 2004;104(3):443-51.
215. Cenci S, Toraldo G, Weitzman MN, et al. Estrogen deficiency induces bone loss by increasing T cell proliferation and lifespan through IFN-g-induced class II transactivator. Proc Natl Acad Sci U S A. 2003;100(18):10405-10.
216. Roggia C. Role of TNF-alpha producing T-cells in bone loss induced by estrogen deficiency. Minerva Med. 2004;95(2):125-32.
217. Rovensky J, Radikova Z, Imrich R, et al. Gonadal and adrenal steroid hormones in plasma and synovial fluid of patients with rheumatoid arthritis. Endocr Regul. 2004;38(4):143-49.
218. Untergasser G, Madersbacher S, Berger P. Benign prostatic hyperplasia: age-related tissue-remodeling. Exp Gerontol. 2005;40(3):121-28.

219. Hero M, Wickman S, Hanhijarvi R, et al. Pubertal upregulation of erythropoiesis in boys is determined primarily by androgen. J Pediatr. 2005;146(2):245-52.
220. Wang C, Cunningham G, Dobs A, et al. Long-term testosterone gel (AndroGel) treatment maintains beneficial effects on sexual function and mood, lean and fat mass, and bone mineral density in hypogonadal men. J Clin Endocrinol Metab. 2004;89(5):2085-98.
221. Wang C, Swerdloff RS, Iranmanesh A, et al. Transdermal testosterone gel improves sexual function, mood, muscle strength, and body composition parameters in hypogonadal men. J Clin Endocrinol Metab. 2000;85:2839-53.
222. Saez JM, Forest MG. Kinetics of human chorionic gonadotropin-induced steroidogenic response of the human testis. I. Plasma testosterone: Implications for human chorionic gonadotropin stimulation test. J Clin Endocrinol Metab. 1979;49:278-83.
223. Takahashi PY, Liu PY, Roebuck PD, et al. Graded inhibition of pulsatile luteinizing hormone secretion by a selective gonadotropin-releasing hormone (GnRH)-receptor antagonist in healthy men: evidence that age attenuates hypothalamic GnRH outflow. J Clin Endocrinol Metab. 2005;90(5):2768-74.
224. Velduis JD, Iranmanesh A, Keenan DM. Erosion of endogenous testosterone-drive negative feedback on pulsatile luteinizing hormone secretion in healthy aging men. J Clin Endocrinol Metab. 2004;89(11):5753-61.
225. Winters SJ, Clark BJ. Testosterone synthesis, transport, and metabolism. In Bagatell CJ, Bremner WJ (Eds): Androgens in Health and Disease. Humana Press: Totowa, NJ, 2003.
226. Veldhuis JD, Zwart A, Mulligan T, Iranmanesh A. Muting of androgen negative feedback unveils impoverished gonadotropin-releasing hormone/luteinizing hormone secretory reactivity in healthy older men. J Clin Endocrinol Metab. 2001;86:529-35.
227. Winters SJ, Clark BJ. Testosterone synthesis, transport, and metabolism. In Bagatell CJ, Bremner WJ (Eds): Androgens in Health and Disease. Humana Press: Totowa, NJ, 2003.
228. Pelletier G, Labrie C, Labrie F. Localization of oestrogen receptor alpha, oestrogen receptor beta and androgen receptors in the rat reproductive organs. J Endocrinol. 2000;165(2):359-70.
229. Pelletier G, El-Alfy M. Immunocytochemical localization of estrogen receptors a and b in the human reproductive organs. J Clin Endocrinol Metab. 2000;85(12):4835-40.
230. Smith EP, Boyd J, Frank G, et al. Estrogen resistance caused by a mutation in the estrogen-receptor gene in a man. N Engl J Med. 1994;331:1056-61.
231. Morishima A, Grumbach MM, Simpson ER, et al. Aromatase deficiency in male and female siblings caused by a novel mutation and the physiological role of estrogens. J Clin Endocrinol Metab. 1995;80(12):3689-98.
232. Finkelstein JS, Whitcomb RW, O'Dea LS, et al. Sex steroid control of gonadotropin secretion in the human male. I. Effect of testosterone administration in normal and gonadotropin-releasing hormone-deficient men. J Clin Endocrinol Metab. 1991;73:609-20.
233. Finkelstein JS, Whitcomb RW, O'Dea LS, et al. Sex steroid control of gonadotropin secretion in the human male. II. Effect of estradiol administration in normal and gonadotropin-releasing hormone-deficient men. J Clin Endocrinol Metab. 1991;73:621-28.
234. Manna PR, Tea-Sempre M, Huhtaniemi IT. Molecular mechanisms of thyroid hormone-stimulated steroidogenesis in mouse leydig tumor cells. Involvement of the steroidogenic acute regulatory (StAR) protein. J Biol Chem.1999; 274:5909-18.
235. Winters SJ, Troen P. Altered pulsatile secretion of luteinizing hormone in hypogonadal men with hyperprolactinemia. Clin Endocrinol (Oxf.). 1984; 21:257-63.
236. Juul A, et al. Effects of growth hormone replacement therapy on IGF-related parameters and on the pituitary-gonadal axis in GH-deficient men. Hormone Res. 1998;49:269-78.
237. Carani C, Granata AR, De Rosa M, et al. The effect of chronic treatment with GH on gonadal function in men with isolated GH deficiency. Eur J Endocrinol. 1999;140:224-30.
238. Dufau ML, Tinajero JC, Fabbri A. Corticotropin-releasing factor: an anti-reproductive hormone of the testis. FASEB J. 1993;7:299-307.
239. Sankar BR, Maran RR, Sivakumar R, et al. Chronic administration of corticosterone impairs LH signal transduction and steroidgogenesis in rat Leydig cells. J Steroid Biochem Mol Biol. 2000;72:155-62.
240. Winters SJ, Clark BJ. Testosterone Synthesis, Transport and Metabolism. In: Bagatell CJ, Bremner WJ, editors. Androgens in Health and Disease. 2004. P.16.
241. Janne OA, Palvimo JJ, Kallio P, Mehto M. Androgen receptor and mechanism of androgen action Ann Med. 1993;25:83.
242. Putnam SK, Du J, Sato S, Hull EM. Testosterone restoration of copulatory behavior correlates with medial preoptic dopamine release in castrated male rats. Horm Behav. 2001;39(3):216-24.
243. Wolf OT. Cognitive functions and sex steroids. Ann Endocrinol (Paris). 2003;64(2):158-61.
244. Grino PB, Griffin JE, Wilson JD. Testosterone at high concentrations interacts with the human androgen receptor similarly to dihydrotestosterone. Endocrinology. 1990;126:1165-72.
245. Cherrier MM, Craft S. Androgens and cognition. Chapter 15 in Bagatell CJ, Bremner WJ (Eds): Androgens in Health and Disease. Humana Press: Totowa, NJ, 2003.
246. Cherrier MM, Anawalt BD, Herbst KL, et al. Cognitive effects of short-term manipulation of serum sex steroids in healthy young men. J Clin Endocrinol Metab. 2002;87(7):3090-96.
247. Fink G, Sumner B, Rosie R, et al. Androgen actions on central serotonin neurotransmission: relevance for mood, mental state and memory. Behav Brain Res. 1999;105:53.
248. Shughrue P, Scrimo P, Lane M, et al. The distribution of estrogen receptor-beta mRNA in forebrain regions of the estrogen receptor-alpha knockout mouse. Endocrinology. 1997;138(12):5649-52.
249. Ly LP, Jimenez M, Zhuang TN, et al. A double-blind, placebo-controlled, randomized clinical trial of transdermal dihydrotestosterone gel on muscular strength, mobility, and quality of life in older men with partial androgen deficiency. J Clin Endocrinol Metab. 2001;86(9):4078-88.
250. Cherrier, Craft. Androgens and Cognition. In Androgens in Health and Disease, ed. Bagatell and Bremner, 291-304. Towata, NJ: Humana Press, 2003.
251. Cherrier, Craft. p.295.
252. Hooven CK, Chabris CF, Ellison PT, Kosslyn SM. The relationship of male testosterone to components of mental rotation. Neuropsychologia. 2004;42(6):782-90.
253. Cherrier MM, Plymate S, Mohan S, et al. Relationship between testosterone supplementation and insulin-like growth factor-I levels and cognition in healthy older men. Psychoneuroendocrinology. 2004;29(1):65-82.
254. Driscoll I, Hamilton DA, Yeo RA, et al. Virtual navigation in humans: the impact of age, sex, and hormones on place learning. Horm Behav. 2005;47(3):326-35.
255. Verroken M. Ethical aspects and the prevalence of hormone abuse in sport. J Endocrinol. 2001;170:49-54.
256. Dawson RT. Drugs in sport—the role of the physician. J Endocrinol. 2001;170:55-61.
257. Hartgens F, Kuipers H. Effects of androgenic-anabolic steroids in athletes. Sports Med. 2004;34(8):513-54.
258. Maravelias C, Dona A, Stefanidou M, Spiliopoulou C. Adverse effects of anabolic steroids in athletes: A constant threat. Toxicol Lett. 2005;158(3):167-75.

259. Antonio J, Wilson JD, George FW. Effects of castration and androgen treatment on androgen-receptor levels in rat skeletal muscles. J App Physiol. 1999;87:2016-19.
260. Dahlberg E, Snochowski M, Gustafsson JA. Regulation of the androgen and glucocorticoid receptors in rat and mouse skeletal muscle cytosol. Endocrinology. 1981;108:1431-40.
261. Rance NE, Max SR. Modulation of the cytosolic androgen receptor in striated muscle by sex steroids. Endocrinology. 1984;115:862-66.
262. Reid IR, Wattie DJ, Evans MC, Stapleton JP. Testosterone therapy in glucocorticoid-treated men. Arch Intern Med. 1996;156:1173-77.
263. Reid IR, Ibertson HK, France JT, Pybus J. Plasma testosterone concentrations in asthmatic men treated with glucocorticoids. Br Med J. 1985; 291:574-77.
264. Bhasin S, Woodhouse L, Casaburi R, et al. Testosterone dose-response relationships in healthy young men. Am J Physiol Endocrinol Metab. 2001;281:E1172-81.
265. Singh AB, Hsia S, Alaupovic P, et al. The effects of varying doses of T on insulin sensitivity, plasma lipids, apolipoproteins, and C-reactive protein in healthy young men. J Clin Endocrinol Metab. 2002;87(1):136-43.
266. Stanley HL, Schmitt BP, Poses RM, Deiss WP. Does hypogonadism contribute to the occurrence of minimal trauma hip fracture in elderly men? J Am Geriatr Soc. 1991; 39:766-771.
267. Behre HM, Kliesch S, Leifke E, et al. Long-term effect of testosterone therapy on bone mineral density in hypogonadal men. J Clin Endocrinol Metab. 1997; 82:2386-2390.
268. Schiavi RC. Androgens and sexual function in men. In: Oddens BJ, Vermeulen A, eds. Androgens and the Aging Male. Parthenon, New York, 1996. P.111-128.
269. SaderMA, Griffiths KA, McCredie RJ, et al. Androgenic anabolic steroids and arterial structure and function in male bodybuilders. J Am Coll Cardiol. 2001;37(1):224-30.
270. Wu, FCW, von Eckardstein A. Androgens and coronary artery disease. Endocr Rev. 2003;24(2):183-217.
271. Hartgens F, Rietjens G, Keizer HA, et al. Effects of androgenic-anabolic steroids on apoliproteins and lipoprotein (a). Br J Sports Med. 2004; 38(3):253-9.
272. Behre HM, Simoni M, Nieschlag E. Strong association between serum levels of leptin and testosterone in men. Clin Endocrinol. 1997; 47:237-240.
273. Sih R, Morley JE, Kaiser FE, and et al. Testosterone replacement in older hypogonadal men: a 12-month randomized controlled trial. J Clin Endocrinol Metab. 1997; 82:1661-1667.
274. Wang C, Swerdloff RS, Iranmanesh A, et al. Transdermal testosterone gel improves sexual function, mood, muscle strength and body composition parameters in hypogonadal men. Testosterone Gel Study Group. J Clin Endocrinol Metab. 2000; 85:2839-2853.
275. Rockhold RW. Cardiovascular toxicity of anabolic steroids. Ann Rev Pharmacol Toxicol. 1993; 33:397-520.
276. Wang C, Swerdloff RS, Iranmanesh A, et al. Transdermal testosterone gel improves sexual function, mood, muscle strength and body composition parameters in hypogonadal men. Testosterone Gel Study Group. J Clin Endocrinol Metab. 2000; 85:2839-2853.
277. Marcovina SM, Lippi G, Bagatella CJ, Bremner WJ. Testosterone-induced suppression of lipoprotein (a) in normal men: relation to basal lipoptrotein (a) level. Atherosclerosis. 1996; 122:89-95.
278. Anderson RA, Ludlam CA, Wu FC. Haemostatic effects of supraphysiological levels of testosterone in normal men. Thromb Haemost. 1995; 74:693-697.
279. Bernton E, Hoover D, Galloway R, Popp K. Adaptation to chronic stress in military trainees. Adrenal androgens, testosterone, glucocorticoids, IGF-1, and immune function. Ann New York Acad Sci. 1995 Dec.29; 744:217-231.
280. Gomez-Merino D, Chennaoui M, Burnat P, et al. Immune and hormonal changes following intense military training. Mil Med. 2003 Dec;168(12):1034-1038.
281. Golding, Mike. The Westass Chronicles. Accessed at: http://wetass-chronicles.com/2004/12/moist-and-odiferous-vignette-from.html
282. Levitt AJ, Joffee RT. Total and free testosterone in depressed men. Acta Physiatr Scand 1988; 77:346-348.
283. Margolese HC. The male menopause and mood: testosterone decline and depression in the aging male—is there a link? Journal of Geriatric Psychiatry and Neurology 2000; 13:93-101.
284. Barrett-Connor E, Von Muhlen DG, Kritz-Silverstien D. Bioavailable testosterone and depressed mood in older men: The Rancho Bernardo Study. Journal of Clinical Endocrinology and Metabolism. 1999; 84(2):573-577.
285. Vermeulen A. Androgens in the aging male. Clinical Endocrinol Metab. 1991; 73:221–224.
286. Davidson JM, Chen JJ, et al. Hormonal changes and sexual function in aging men. Journal of Clinical Endocrinology and Metabolism. 1983; 57:71-77.
287. Murrell SA, Himmelfarb, S, et al. Prevalence of depression and its correlates in older adults. Am J Epidemiol. 2003; 88(11):5074-5086.
288. Blazer D, et al. The association of age and depression among the elderly: an epidemiological exploration. J Gerontol. 1991; 46:M210-M215.
289. Wang C, Alexander G, Berman N, et al. Testosterone replacement therapy improves mood in hypogonadal men—a clinical research center study. Journal of Clinical Endocrinology and Metabolism. 1996; 81(10):3578-3583.
290. Wang C, Swerdloff RS, Iranmanesh A, et al. Transdermal testosterone gel improves sexual function, mood, muscle strength and body composition parameters in hypogonadal men. Testosterone Gel Study Group. J Clin Endocrinol Metab. 2000; 489:(5):1-28.
291. Wang C, Cunningham G, Dobs A, et al. Long-term testosterone gel (AndroGel) treatment maintains beneficial effects on sexual function and mood, lean and fat mass, and bone mineral density in hypogonadal men. J Clin Endocrin Metabol. 2004;89(5):2085-98.
292. O'Connor D, Archer J, Wu FC. Effects of testosterone on mood aggression and sexual behavior in young men: a double-blind placebo controlled cross-over study. Journal of Endocrinology and Metabolism. June 2004; 89(6)2836-2847.
293. WHO Laboratory Manual for the Examination of Human Semen and Sperm-Cervical Mucus Interaction, 4th Ed. Cambridge Univ Press: Cambridge, 1999. Accessed at http://www.endotext.org/male/male7/maleframe7.htm. Endotext.org is a web-based source of information on endocrine disease directed to physicians.
294. Illions EH, Valley MT, Kaunitz AM. Infertility: A clinical guide for the internist. Women's health issues, part II. Med Clin N Am. 1998;82(2):271-95.
295. Noble J (Ed). Textbook of Primary Care Medicine, 3rd ed., 2001. Mosby, Inc. p 474.
296. Wang C, Cunningham G, Dobs A, et al. Long-term testosterone gel (AndroGel) treatment maintains beneficial effects on sexual function and mood, lean and fat mass, and bone mineral density in hypogonadal men. J Clin Endocrin Metabol. 2004;89(5):2085-98.
297. Shippen, Eugene and Fryer, William. The Testosterone Syndrome: The critical factor for energy, health and sexuality—reversing the male menopause. NY: M. Evans and Company, Inc. 1998.
298. Andriole G, Bruchovsky N, Chung LW, et al. Dihydrotestosterone and the prostate: the scientific rationale for 5alpha-reductase inhibitors in the treatment of benign prostatic hyperplasia. J Urol. 2004;172(4 Pt 1):1399-1403.
299. Chiu KY, Yong CR. Effects of finasteride on prostate volume and prostate-specific antigen. J Chin Med Assoc. 2004;67(11):571-4.

300. Comhaire F, Mahmoud A. Preventing diseases of the prostate in the elderly using hormones and nutriceuticals. Aging Male. 2004;7(2):155-69.
301. Gerber GS, Fitzpatrick JM. The role of a lipido-sterolic extract of Serenoa repens in the management of lower urinary tract symptoms associated with benign prostatic hyperplasia. BJU Int. 2004;94(3):338-44.
302. Grumbach MM, Auchus RJ. Estrogen: consequences and implications of human mutations in synthesis and action. J Clin Endocrinol Metab. 1999;84:4677-94.
303. Smith EP, Boyd J, Frank G, et al. Estrogen resistance caused by a mutation in the estrogen-receptor gene in a man. N Engl J Med 1994; 331:1056-1061.
304. Morishima A, Grumbach MM, Simpson ER, et al. Aromatase deficiency in male and female siblings caused by a novel mutation and the physiological role of estrogens. J Clin Endocrinol Metab. 1995; 80(12):3689-3698.
305. Dobs AS, Schrott H, Davidson MH, et al. Effects of high-dose simvastatin on adrenal and gonadal steroidogenesis in men with hypercholesterolemia. Metabolism. 2000; 49:1234-1238.
306. Barrack ER, Berry SJ. DNS synthesis in the canine prostate: effects of androgen and estrogen treatment. Prostate. 1987; 10:45-56.
307. Shippen E, Fryer W. The Testosterone Syndrome: The critical factor for energy, health and sexuality—reversing the male menopause. NY: M. Evans and Company, Inc. 1998.
308. Wang C, Cunningham G, Dobbs A, et al. Long-term testosterone gel (AndroGel) treatment maintains beneficial effects on sexual function and mood, lean and fat mass, and bone mineral density in hypogonadal men. Journal of Endocrinology and Metabolism. May 2004; 89(5):1-28.
309. Kristal AR, Stanford JL, Cohen JH, et al. Vitamin and mineral supplement use is associated with reduced risk of prostate cancer. Cancer Epidemiol Biomarkers Prev. 1999;8:887-92.
310. Schuetz P, Peterli R, Ludwig C, Peters T. Fatigue, weakness and sexual dysfunction after bariatic surgery—not an unusual case but an unusual cause. Obes Surg. Aug. 2004; 14(7):1025-1028.
311. Kim JS, Yun CH. Inhibition of human cytochrome P450 3A4 activity by zinc (II) ion. Toxicol Lett. 2005 Apr.28; 156(3)341-350.
312. Moyad MA. Zinc for prostate disease and other conditions: a little evidence, a lot of hype, and a significant potential problem. Urol Nurs. 2004 Feb; 24(1):49-52.
313. Ren JC, Banan A, Keshavarzian A, et al. Exposure to ethanol induces oxidative damage in the pituitary gland. Alcohol. 2005;35(2):91-101.
314. Koc M, Polat P. Epidemiology and aetiological factors of male breast cancer: a ten years retrospective study in eastern Turkey. Eur J Cancer Prev. 2001;10(6):531-4.
315. Bjørnerem A, Straume B, Midtby M, et al. Endogenous sex hormones in relation to age, sex, lifestyle factors, and chronic diseases in a general population: The TromsØ Study. J Clin Endocrinol Metab. 2004;89(12):6039-47.
316. Morales AJ, Nolan JJ, Nelson JC, Yen SSC. Effects of replacement dose of dehydroepiandrosterone in men and women of advancing age. J Clin Endocrinol Metab. 1994; 78:1360-1367.
317. Villareal DT, Holloszy JO. Effect of DHEA on abdominal fat and insulin action in elderly women and men: a randomized controlled trial. JAMA. 2004 Nov 10; 292 (18):2243-8.
318. Williams MR. Dehydroepiandrosterone increases endothelial cell proliferation *in vitro* and improves endothelial function *in vivo* by mechanisms independent of androgen and estrogen receptors. J Clin Endocrinol Metab. 2004;89(9):4708-15.
319. Kawano H. Dehydroepiandrosterone supplementation improves endothelial function and insulin sensitivity in men. J Clin Endocrinol Metab. 2003;88(7):3190-5
320. Nasrallah MP. The value of dehydroepiandrosterone sulfate measurements in the assessment of adrenal function. J Clin Endocrinol Metab. 2003;88(11):5392-8.
321. Williams M, Komesaroff P. Dehydroepiandrosterone increases endothelial cell proliferation *in vitro* and improves endothelial function *in vivo* by mechanisms independent of androgen and estrogen receptors. J Clin Endocrinol Metab. 2004;89(9):4708-15.
322. Barrett-Connor E, Khaw KT, Yen SSC. A prospective study of dehydroepiandrosterone sulfate, mortality and cardiovascular disease. N Engl J Med. 1986; 315:1519-24.
323. LaCroix AZ. Dehydroepiandrosterone sulfate, incidence of myocardial infarction, and extent of atherosclerosis in men. Circulation 1992; Vol 86: 1529-1535.
324. Kawano H, et al. Dehydroepiandrosterone supplementation improves endothelial function and insulin sensitivity in men. J Clin Endocrinol Metab. 2003;88:3190-95.
325. Arad Y, Badimon JJ, Badimon L, et al. Dehydroepiandrosterone feeding prevents aortic fatty streak formation and cholesterol accumulation in cholesterol-fed rabbit. Arteriosclerosis. 1989; 9:159-166.
326. Gordon GB, Bush DE, Weisman HF. Reduction of atherosclerosis by administration of dehydroepiandrosterone. J Clin Invest. 1988;82:712-720.
327. Villareal DT, Holloszy JO. Effect of DHEA on abdominal fat and insulin action in elderly women and men: a randomized controlled trial. JAMA. 2004 Nov 10; 292 (18):2243-8.
328. Williams M, Komesaroff P. Dehydroepiandrosterone increases endothelial cell proliferation *in vitro* and improves endothelial function *in vivo* by mechanisms independent of androgen and estrogen receptors. J Clin Endocrinol Metab. 2004;89(9):4708-15.
329. Compagnone NA, Mellon SH. Dehydroepiandrosterone: a potential signaling molecule for neocortical organization during development. Proc Natl Acad Sci USA. 1998; 95(8):4678-83.
330. Suzuki M, et al. Mitotic and neurogenic effects of dehydroepiandrosterone (DHEA) on human neural stem cell cultures derived from the fetal cortex. Proc Natl Acad Sci USA. 2004; 101(9):3202-7.
331. Wolkowitz OM. DHEA treatment of Alzheimer's disease: a randomized, double-blind, placebo-controlled study. Neurology. 2003 Apr 8; 60(7):1071-6.
332. Kornblut, Anne and Wilson, Duff. How One Pill Escaped the List of Controlled Steroids. New York Times. Apr 17, 2005.
333. Longcope C, Dehydroepiandrosterone metabolism. J Endocrinol. 1996;150:S125-127.
334. Morales AJ, Nolan JJ, Nelson JC, Yen SSC. Effects of replacement dose of dehydroepiandrosterone in men and women of advancing age. J Clin Endocrinol Metab. 1994; 78:1360-1367.
335. Yen SSC, Morales AJ, Khorram O. Replacement of DHEA in aging men and women. Ann NY Acad Sci. 1995; 774:128-42.
336. Nawata H, et al. Adrenopause. Hormone Research. 2004;62(Suppl. 3):110-14.
337. Bowers L. Oral dehydroepiandrosterone supplementation can increase the testosterone/epitestosterone ratio. Clinical Chemistry. 1999;45:295-97.
338. Morales AJ. The effect of six months treatment with a 100 mg daily dose of dehydroepiandrosterone (DHEA) on circulating sex steroids, body composition and muscle strength in age-advanced men and women. Clin Endocrinol (Oxf). 1998 Oct; 49(4):421-32.
339. Adamo M, LeRoith D, Simon J, Roth J. Effect of altered nutritional states on insulin receptors. Annu Rev Nutr. 1988;8:149-166.
340. Flier J. An overview of insulin resistance In: Moller DE, ed. Insulin Resistance. Chichester, U.K. Wiley: 1993.
341. Reaven G, Brand R, Chen Y, et al. Insulin resistance and insulin secretion are determinants of oral glucose in normal individuals. Diabetes. 1993;42:1324-32.

342. Reaven, GM. Pathophysiology of insulin resistance in human disease Physiol Rev. 1995;75(3):473-85.
343. Reaven GM. Role of insulin resistance in human disease. Diabetes. 1988;37:1495-1507.
344. Avogaro A, deKreutzenberg SV. Mechanisms of endothelial dysfunction in obesity. Clin Chim Acta. 2005;Jun 24;[Epub ahead of print].
345. Villareal DT, Holloszy JO. Effect of DHEA on abdominal fat and insulin action in elderly women and men. JAMA. 2004;292(18):2243-48.
346. Trends in the prevalence and incidence of self-reported diabetes mellitus—United States, 1980-1994. Morb Mortal Wkly Rep. 1997;46:1013-26.
347. Reaven GM. Pathophysiology of insulin resistance in human disease. Physiol Rev. 1995;75(3):473-85.
348. Skidmore PM, Yarnell JW. The obesity epidemic: prospects for prevention. QJM. 2004;97(12):817-25.
349. Screening for Type 2 Diabetes. Report of a World Health Organization and International Diabetes Federation meeting. © 2003, World Health Organization Department of Noncommunicable Disease Management, Geneva.
350. American Diabetes Association. Standards of medical care in diabetes. Diabetes Care. 2005:28(Supp 1):S4-36.
351. Ibid.
352. Okopien B, Stachura-Kulach A, Kulach A, et al. The risk of atherosclerosis in patients with impaired glucose tolerance. Res Commun Mol Pathol Pharmacol. 2003:113-114:87-95.
353. Kaplan RC, Strickler HD, Rohan TE, et al. Insulin-like growth factors and coronary heart disease. Cardiol Rev. 2005:13(1):35-39.
354. Potter van Loon BJ, Kluft C, Radder JK, Blankenstein MA, Meinders AE. The cardiovascular risk factor plasminogen activator inhibitor type I is related to insulin resistance. Metabolism. 1993;42:945-49.
355. Juhan-Vague I, Pyke SD, Alessi MC, et al. Fibrinolytic factors and the risk of myocardial infarction or sudden death in patients with angina pectoris. Circulation. 1996;94(9):2057-63.
356. Reaven GM. Are triglycerides important as a risk factory for coronary disease? Heart Dis Stroke. 1993;2:44-48.
357. Laws A, King AC, Haskell WL, et al. Relation of fasting plasma insulin concentration to high-density lipoprotein cholesterol and triglyceride concentration in men. Arterioscler Thromb. 1991;11:1636-42.
358. Assmann G, Schulte H. Relation of high-density lipoprotein cholesterol and triglycerides to incidence of atherosclerotic coronary artery disease (the PROCAM experience). Am J Cardiol. 1992;70:733-37.
359. Swenson TL. The role of the cholesteryl ester transfer protein in lipoprotein metabolism. Diabetes Metab Rev. 1991;7:139-53.
360. Ziegler D. Type 2 diabetes as an inflammatory cardiovascular disorder. Curr Mol Med. 2005;5(3):309-22.
361. Yaffe K, Kanaya A, Lindquist K, et al. The metabolic syndrome, inflammation, and risk of cognitive decline. JAMA 2004;292(18):2237-42.
362. Zavaroni I, Coruzzi P, Bonini L, et al. Association between salt sensitivity and insulin concentrations in patients with hypertension. Am J Hypertens. 1995;8:855-58.
363. Luft FC. Salt and hypertension at the close of the millennium. Wien Klin Wochenschr. 1998:110(13-14):459-66.
364. Zavaroni I, Mazza S, Dall'Aglio E, et al. Prevalence of hyperinsulinaemia in patients with high blood pressure. J Intern Med. 1992;231:235-240.
365. Ibid.
366. Gans RO, Donker AJ. Insulin and blood pressure regulation. J Intern Med. 1991;229(suppl 2):49-64.
367. Tedde R, Sechi LA, Marigliano A, et al. Antihypertensive effect of insulin reduction in diabetic hypertensive patients. Am J Hypertens. 1989;2:163-70.
368. Randeree HA, Omar MA, Motala AA, Seedat MA. Effect of insulin therapy on blood pressure in NIDDM patients with secondary failure. Diabetes Care. 1992;15:1258-63.
369. Nestler J. Insulin resistance effects on sex hormones and ovulation in the polycystic ovary syndrome. From Contemporary Endocrinology: Insulin Resistance Edited by G. Reaven and A. Laws Humana Press Inc., Totowa NJ, 1999. 347-365.
370. Singh A, Hamilton-Fairley D, Koistinen R, et al. Effect of insulin-like growth factor-type 1 (IFG-I) and insulin on the secretion of sex-hormone binding globulin and IGF-I binding protein (IBP-I) by human hepatoma cells. J Endocrinol. 1990;124:R1-3.
371. Nestler JE, Powers LP, Matt DW, et al. A direct effect of hyperinsulinemia on serum sex hormone-binding globulin levels in obese women with the polycystic ovary syndrome. J Clin Endocrinol Metab. 1991;72:83-89.
372. Nestler JE, Jakubowicz DJ. Decreases in ovarian cytochrome P450c17a activity and serum free testosterone after reduction in insulin secretion in women with polycystic ovary syndrome. N Engl J Med. 1996;335:617-23.
373. Velazquez EM, Mendoza S, Hamer T, et al. Metformin therapy in polycystic ovary syndrome reduces hyperinsulinemia, insulin resistance, hyperandrogenemia, and systolic blood pressure, while facilitating normal menses and pregnancy. Metabolism. 1994;43:647-54.
374. Giovannucci E. Insulin, insulin-like growth factors and colon cancer: a review of the evidence. J Nutr. 2001;131:3109S-20S.
375. Giovannucci E. Insulin and colon cancer. Cancer Causes Control. 1995;6:164-79.
376. Weiderpass E, Gridley G, Nyren O, et al. Diabetes mellitus and risk of large bowel cancer. J Natl Cancer Inst. 1997;89:660-61.
377. Will JC, Galuska DA, Vinicor F, et al. Colorectal cancer: another complication of diabetes mellitus? Am J Epidemiol. 1998;147:816-25.
378. Tran TT, Medline A, Bruce WR. Insulin promotion of colon tumors in rats. Cancer Epidemiol Biomarkers Prev. 1996;5(12):1013-15.
379. Corpet DE, Jacquinet C, Peiffer G, Tache S. Insulin injections promote the growth of aberrant crypt foci in the colon of rats. Nutr Cancer. 1997;27:316-20.
380. Kaaks R. Nutrition, hormones, and breast cancer: is insulin the missing link? Cancer Causes Control. 1996;7:605-25.
381. Rosner W. The functions of corticosteroid-binding globulin and sex-hormone-binding globulin: recent advances. Endocr Rev. 1990;11:80-91.
382. Han C, Zhang HT, Du L, et al. Serum levels of leptin, insulin, and lipids in relation to breast cancer in China. Endocrine. 2005;26(1):19-24.
383. Frasca F, Pandini G, Vigneri R, Goldfine ID. Insulin and hybrid insulin/IGF receptors are major regulators of breast cancer cells. Breast Dis. 2003;17:73-89.
384. Bernstein L, Ross RK. Endogenous hormones and breast cancer risk. Epidemiol Rev. 1993;15:48-65.
385. Toniolo PG, Levitz M, Zeleniuch-Jacquotte A, et al. A prospective study of endogenous estrogens and breast cancer in postmenopausal women. J Natl Cancer Inst. 1995;87:190-97.

Chapter 20
Neurological Imbalances

Catherine Willner, MD

Introduction

It is important to understand some of the ways in which the nervous system is different from other organ systems in the body—and the extent to which its failure to function can be a devastating consequence both to the individual and to society. The cells and tissues of the human nervous system share many features in common with all other cellular structures in the body. In this sense, all principles of functional medicine can be applied in situations where the predominant problem faced by a clinician seems to be one that is neurological. In fact, it would be the most appropriate application of the principles of functional medicine to optimize functioning *before* a specific disease related to genomic or environmental risk can be identified. However, getting to that ideal requires understanding the nervous system in terms of the unique biochemistry, physiology, and pathology that sometimes set it apart from other systems. These issues deserve special attention.

Functional medicine approaches the nervous system as one part of a web of interconnectedness of all bodily systems and functions and assesses how to optimize processes that permit healthy functioning of the whole organism. Functional neurology considers this web as it impacts the ability of the nervous system to perform optimally in all of its functions. It is sometimes a struggle to make the leap between traditional neurology and these paradigms, but it is also a very exciting challenge. We will look briefly at certain aspects of traditional neurological assessment, explore some unique characteristics of the nervous system, and then discuss the application of this knowledge to functional neurology.

Traditional Neurological Assessment

Neurologists are taught very precisely to label in space (anatomy), function (physiology and pathology), and time (pathophysiology of acute, subacute, and chronic), and to consider genetics and the environment (though we are traditionally taught little in terms of how to impact the latter two elements). Often, those disorders that we recognize as being impacted by environmental influences are considered as irreversible or too delayed to alter when they result from certain toxic exposures or severe deficiencies. There are, of course, exceptions, such as disorders associated with B12 deficiencies, or metabolic changes that occur with acute or chronic alcohol exposure, or the cognitive and other neurological changes associated with altered thyroid status. We are taught that these can be at least partially reversed by treatment if they are recognized early, and their recognition is a core aspect in traditional neurological training. However, in many circumstances, by the time these disorders have actually resulted in diagnosable conditions involving the nervous system, the damage is quite severe. Traditional neurology is only beginning to respect the more subtle aspects of metabolic dysfunction and to apply methods to assess or prevent early failure in the system (e.g., the use of folate to prevent neural tube defects).

Assessment of the temporal sequence of pathophysiological events is often useful in diagnostic considerations. Acute events, particularly those that occur suddenly such as stroke, migraine or seizure, are different than the subacute (infection, demyelinating disorders like multiple sclerosis) or chronic progressive disorders that involve cognition and memory (dementias), movement, or other bodily functions. Those are usually considered the system disorders: Parkinsonism, cerebellar disorders, autonomic failure, peripheral neuropathies, and various combinations (multisystem diseases or atrophy). Disorders that cause progressive loss of the functions of the nervous system have been traditionally labeled *neurodegenerative*. Some of these chronically progressive disorders are listed in Table 20.1.

Table 20.1 **Traditional Neurodegenerative Disorders**

Dementias (Alzheimer's, Pick's, Lewy body disorders)
Idiopathic Parkinson's disease
Parkinson plus syndromes (dementia, the most frequent)
Cerebellar degeneration (olivopontocerebellar atrophy)
Shy-Drager syndrome (autonomic failure)
Progressive supranuclear palsy
Motor neuron disorders (e.g., ALS)
Hereditary peripheral neuropathies

Because we are living longer as a population, and because our population as a whole is aging, many people are surviving much longer with these diagnoses, although the impact on the patient's quality of life and the economic burden on society are both significant. However, it is important to take into consideration that other disorders, not specifically considered neurodegenerative, also are costly to manage. For example, the toll in terms of work attendance, activities of daily living, and pain caused by migraine alone is quite high.[1] The availability of progressively more expensive pharmaceuticals to treat this disorder has not solved the underlying problem, although it brings symptom relief to many.[2] As with almost every other traditionally labeled "neurological disease" or disorder, *prevention* of stroke, migraine, epilepsy, multiple sclerosis, peripheral neuropathy, the dementias, and the degenerative system disorders should be as important as management.

Function and Structure: The Nervous System

Probably the most important task performed by the nervous system in a general sense is communication, which permits coordination of adaptive responses both within the brain and throughout the entire organism. This permits, for example, *awareness* (perception) of both internal and external environments and *performance* in those environments. Rapid adjustment or fine tuning of both awareness and performance is a function of the unique features of that communication system. Though such processes are present in most other organ systems, the nervous system is unique because of the rapidity with which it can alter function, and also because of the greater distances from the origins of many signals. It is also unique because it permits awareness of and interaction with the environment (consciousness, memory, cognition). This system of communication requires electrical potentials as well as chemical interactions from neurotransmitters or substances more traditionally considered hormonal. And, the nervous system allows us to perceive and to react both at a conscious level and with autonomic activity, where conscious awareness is not required.

There are certain features of the nervous system that warrant consideration in this discussion:

- The nervous system has **unique energy requirements** that include fairly consistent access to oxygen and to glucose, though other carbon-based fuels can be accommodated. It is a demanding metabolic environment with high energy requirements partly because of the generalized need to maintain electrochemical gradients to allow generation of action potentials appropriately and to allow receptors to function normally. Mitochondrial function, as the source of this energy, is key to optimization of function.
- The method of communication at synapses by neurotransmitters and receptors requires continuous recycling of both the chemicals and their receptors. This requires a normally functioning genome as well as access to substrate to make the enzymes, the neurotransmitters, and the receptors.
- Maintenance of the membrane structure system is critical to normal performance of neurons and the surrounding complex cellular system of glial cells. Discussion of their complex functions is beyond our scope, but one of their major functions is to provide insulation by forming myelin, which permits electrical activity to travel appropriately to the correct destination at speeds in the range of 100 m/s.
- As a result of that need for insulation, both in the brain and at a distance, through the fiber tracts and the peripheral nervous system, the concentration of lipid is unique and high, both as cell membrane components and in the myelin, which insulates axons (the processes sent out by cells to accomplish this communication). The relatively high content of polyunsaturated fatty acid (PUFA) places the

brain at significant risk for lipid peroxidation secondary to free radical damage.

- It is also important to remember that the neurons are, for the most part, postmitotic tissues. Though potential for regeneration (especially in the periphery) and plasticity of surviving neurons is one of the strong points of the system, the limited ability of the nervous system to regenerate or replace damaged cells does have serious consequences.
- Certain regions of the brain, specifically the substantia nigra and the striatum, have very high concentrations of iron, which also increases the risk of peroxidation.
- Finally, the nervous system is relatively segregated from the rest of the body—from the bloodstream in particular by the blood-brain and blood-nerve barriers.[3] This segregation necessitates a separate source for immunological protection and defense, mostly provided in the CNS by the glial cells. When the system fails, the consequences can be devastating. (Neuroimmunology is a very complicated and fascinating subject. The gut, with its unique role of interaction with the external environment, has similar types of barriers and unique defenses and many of the same principles of functional medicine can be applied. See *The Gut Liver Axis* in Chapter 31).

A short summary of the features discussed above is presented in Table 20.2. Now, let's consider some of the consequences of these features and how functional neurology might approach the task of enhancing or protecting these functions, particularly in situations where the nervous system might be vulnerable. Our specific focus will be on the consequences of oxidative dependence—free radical damage, neurotoxicity, and apoptosis (cell death).

Table 20.2 **The Nervous System—Unique Features**

High energy requirements, mitochondrial dependence
High metabolic turnover, excitatory transmitters
Post-mitotic state
High lipid content (specialized membranes, PUFA)
Transmembrane electrochemical gradient
Region-specific mineral concentration (Fe)
Sequestration (BBB/BNB/myelin)

Neurological Vulnerability: Oxidative Dependence and Free Radical Stress

The nervous system, with its high metabolic requirements, uses about 20% of the oxygen provided from ventilation. Oxygen and oxygen species are used in the body for several different functions, including their role in the respiratory chain for energy production, as ATP is manufactured by alteration of carbon bonds to form water and carbon dioxide. Oxidation also plays a role in defense against destruction or damage caused by foreign substances and free radical attack.

Free radical formation is a necessary and essential function of these systems; however, when the system is not balanced, that function fails. There are elaborate mechanisms of protection from free radical damage for the brain and body:[4] enzymes such as SOD (superoxide dismutase—requiring Zn, Cu, Mn), glutathione peroxidase (requiring Se), and catalase (requiring Fe); dietary antioxidants (Vitamins C and E, among others); and endogenous antioxidants (coenzyme Q10, carnitine, lipoic acid).

There are risks in this setting that are both genetic and environmental. In both acute and chronic disorders, there is evidence that both energy metabolism deficits and glutamate-mediated excitatory transmitter dysfunction may be causative and integral to damage by reactive oxygen and nitrogen species.[5]

The Basics of Oxidative Stress and Neuronal Function

The respiratory chain provides the mechanisms for production of energy through the formation of high-energy phosphate bonds. (The basics of bioenergetics are discussed in Chapter 16.) The system is a complex one, involving membranes, enzymes, cofactors, substrates, and the cellular organelles called mitochondria, which are maternally inherited and contain their own DNA (mtDNA is discussed further in Chapter 21). Getting down to absolute basics, the neurons, like every other cell in the body, utilize carbon-based atoms and oxygen to produce energy for the production of enzymes, neurotransmitters, and structural components of the cell (such as complex receptors). One of the most important functions of this system is the maintenance of an electrochemical gradient or membrane potential, which is unique for cell systems that can generate an "action potential" or other electrical charge. The action potential is the basis for the rapid communication capacity of the nervous system. As mentioned above, the necessity to provide insulation or sequestration for the electrical charge is supported by the formation of myelin, which is a complicated lipid structure produced by glial cells in the central nervous system and by Schwann cells in the periphery. These supporting cells (including the glia) perform many other protective functions as well by processing or storing many of the neurotransmitters in the system when they are not acting as receptors.

Energy is required to accomplish all of these tasks. When the mitochondria fail to produce adequate energy, the result will be suboptimal function at many levels in the cells within the system in general.[6] However, in addition to the impact that might be caused by inadequate energy availability for normal functioning, there is also the risk posed by the process of extracting such energy. The work of producing energy via the mitochondria has a price that includes generating free radicals and other products that have to be handled by the system. Free radicals are dangerous to many targets, especially the mitochondrial DNA and lipid-laden membranes (which are especially available in the nervous system). If not appropriately managed, free radicals cause oxidative stress, a topic that is discussed in greater depth in Chapters 21 and 30. A list of common targets for free radical damage is presented in Table 20.3.

Table 20.3 **Free Radical Targets**

Lipid cell membranes
Cell receptor complexes
Enzymes
Structural proteins (neurofilaments)
DNA
Mitochondrial buffering*
Viruses, bacteria*

*Normal functions

The generally recognized diseases associated with mitochondrial disorders, which were traditionally referred to as mitochondrial encephalomyopathies, are now more commonly called mitochondrial cytopathies[7] to emphasize the multisystem nature of the dysfunction. The most common of these are summarized in Table 20.4. There are disorders now known to be associated with defects in each of the five complexes classically described within the mitochondria.[8] Though most of the proteins and subunits of the mitochondria are actually encoded by nuclear DNA, there are 13 critical polypeptide subunits of the electron transport complexes that are formed by mitochondrial DNA.[9] The actual mitochondrial dysfunction can be anything from a specific point mutation in mitochondrial DNA to large-scale deletions or duplications. The inheritance is variable from maternal, both dominant and recessive, to acquired or sporadic mutations. Many changes in function that occur with aging are thought to be related to the consequences of oxidative stress or various toxic insults, to which the mitochondria seem to be particularly predisposed because of their relative absence of DNA-repairing enzymes.[10]

Table 20.4 **Mitochondria-related Disorders**

Kearns-Sayre syndrome (ophthalmoplegia, retinal pigmentation, conduction block, dementia)
LHON (Leber's hereditary optic neuropathy; subacute blindness in young adults)
MELAS (mitochondrial myopathy, encephalopathy, lactic acidosis, and stroke-like episodes)
MERRF (myoclonic epilepsy, ragged red fibers)
CPEO (chronic progressive external ophthalmoplegia)
Pearson's syndrome (sideroblastic anemia, pancreatic dysfunction, death in infancy)
NARP (neuropathy, ataxia, retinitis pigmentosa syndrome)
Maternally inherited myopathy with cardiomyopathy (spares the CNS)

The heterogeneity of these disorders is related to the specific dysfunction, but the major organ systems involved are those that are most dependent on oxidative metabolism: the brain and muscle (skeletal and heart) are the most frequently affected, though other tissues like the kidney and liver are also clearly at risk. The abnormality most often discussed in the skeletal muscle is the development of mitochondrial proliferation with abnormal morphology (which, along with patchy atrophy, gives the appearance of "ragged red" fibers on trichrome staining). Interestingly, these changes are not seen frequently with nuclear DNA changes, but are quite common with disorders produced by abnormalities of the mitochondrial DNA.

Glutamate Excitotoxicity and Cell Dysfunction

Glutamate, probably the most abundant free amino acid in the central nervous system, is the main excitatory amino acid (EAA) neurotransmitter in the CNS.[11] Though the majority of glutamate is actually housed within the neuronal storage vesicles, there are high quantities in the extracellular space. The other major excitatory substance is aspartate. Analogous to the double-edged sword of mitochondrial respiratory chain free radical production, these EAA neurotransmitters are critical to the brain's plasiticity of function. However, in excess, they are toxic to neurons. There are two major receptor types for glutamate, ionotropic and metabotropic. Ionotropic receptors are grouped into two major subtypes: NMDA (N-methyl-D-aspartate) and non-NMDA receptors (the AMPA-kainate receptor). The metabotropic receptor is coupled to cyclic GMP and modulates production of intracelluar messengers, which also influence the ionotropic glutamate receptors. Under normal circumstances, when adequate energy and cell function permit the electrochemical gradient to maintain a normal membrane potential, the NMDA receptor is blocked by magnesium. Loss of the gradient results in loss of the magnesium ion blocking the NMDA receptor, which, when activated by glutamate, results in influx of calcium into the neuron. Under normal circumstances, this reaction is self limiting. In models of neurotoxicity, there is an escalating cascade of damage leading to cell death.[12]

This same scenerio of excitatory neurotoxicity is postulated in the mechanisms of ischemic and hypoxic damage as seen with stroke or hemorrhage. In this setting, rather than a clear-cut loss of energy and change in gradient potential altering the receptor for glutamate, it is suspected that there might actually be increases in the amount of glutamate because of failure of the surround to modulate the substance.[13] The consequence is overactivation of the receptor due to excess amounts of glutamate, then ultimately cell failure. Both sodium and calcium are increased intracellularly in this setting.

Exogenous glutamate receptor agonists are known to produce neurotoxicity. One of the best understood models comes from clinical insights about lathyrism,[i] characterized especially by spastic paralysis of the hind or lower limbs. Lathyrism results from an AMPA glutamate receptor agonist found in the foods known to be associated with this condition; it produces a clinical syndrome similar to or mimicking ALS, predominantly with upper motor neuron changes.

Once the receptor cell is activated, glutamate is normally recycled by active transport back into glial cells or it is to some extent sequestered in neurons.[14] Its elevation extracellularly can cause continued reactivation of both NMDA and non-NMDA receptors, thereby allowing increased levels of calcium to enter the neuron. Calcium is normally buffered by intracellular buffering proteins such as calbindin or parvalbumin. However, when the buffering capacity is exceeded, the excess calcium ions may catalyze the activity of specific destructive enzymes that are not normally activated. These include xanthine oxidase, nitric oxide synthase, and phospholipase, all of which produce free radicals, including reactive oxygen and nitrogen species.[15]

Sustained elevation of calcium in particular is thought to initiate toxic consequences, including activation of catabolic enzymes such as proteases, phospholipases, and endonucleases that damage enzymes, membranes, and DNA.[16] These can be rapidly lethal. High intracellular calcium also leads to uncoupling of the mitochondrial reactions, resulting in further production of free radicals as well as energy failure. Other activations include initiation of protein kinase and lipid kinase cascades, which include, for example, activation of calcium calmodulin kinase (CaMK) and other kinases that modify the function of ion channels, including the NMDA and AMPA/kainate receptors.[17] High intracellular calcium leads to formation of free radicals by several other mechanisms as well, including calcium-dependent activation of phospholipase A2, which liberates arachidonic acid, leading to further free radical production and lipid peroxidation.

Glutamate Excitotoxicity and Free Radical Production: The Feed-Forward Loop

During normal cell function, stimulation of the NMDA receptors leads to activation of nitric oxide synthase (NOS). The release of nitric oxide that occurs as L-arginine is oxidized to citrulline by NOS is a short-lived reaction and self limiting under normal circumstances.[18] Nitric oxide is a potent vasodilator and a free radical species itself, but is not thought to cause severe damage in normal physiology. As with other reactions, its normal role in metabolism is necessary for health. Once increased excitotoxicity leads to calcium-altered

[i]The grass pea, *Lathyrus sativus*, ... [has] a high content of β-N-oxalyl-L-alpha, β diaminopropionic acid (ODAP), the compound considered to incite the condition known as "lathyrism," an irreversible paralysis, if the seeds are consumed in excessive amounts ... . From http://www.hort.purdue.edu/newcrop/proceedings1993/V2-256.html#Grasspea.

enzyme systems and free radical generation, there is damage of all the cell components mentioned above. Superoxide (O_2^-), produced by xanthine oxidase, reacts with nitric oxide (NO), produced by NO synthase, to form peroxynitrite ($ONOO^-$), one of the most potent reactive nitrogen species; it causes nitration of intracellular proteins containing tyrosine.[19] These changes result in further damage to structural and enzyme proteins and increase the demand on the mitochondria, which further upregulate in response, but cannot adequately counter the production of their own free radicals, resulting in even more damage. Peroxynitrite is also indicted in other reactions within neurons,[20] including DNA deamination, strand breaks, mutations, and damage to the mitochondrial complexes I, II and mitochhondrial aconitase. Ultimately, cell death occurs as a result of multiple system failures.

Because of the significant toxicity posed by peroxynitrite, research is being conducted concerning the role of the nitric oxide and NOS systems in the neurodegenerative disorders and their potential for manipulation to prevent this cascade of damage.[21] There are a number of disease models where induction of NOS is suspected as a trigger in the progression of pathology. Indications have been seen in the experimental model of multiple sclerosis (EAE, experimental autoimmune encephalomyelitis) and are widely demonstrated in models of cerebral ischemia for stroke. Aminoguanidine, an inhibitor of NOS, was used in the EAE model and resulted in a dose-dependent reduction of disease expression.[22] Using the MPTP model (discussed in Chapter 21), researchers have shown that pretreatment with an inhibitor of NOS (7-nitosindazole) prevented development of parkinsonism and typical cognitive changes seen in baboons exposed to MPTP.[23] Application of NOS synthase inhibitors also provided protection in cortical neuron cell cultures against the toxic effects of beta-amyloid, which is the altered protein structure known to be associated with the plaques of Alzheimer's disease.[24,25] It is also known that exposure of rat microglial cells in culture to beta-amyloid results in the release of nitric oxide, especially in conditions of inflammatory upregulation.[26] Arginine analogs have been used to interfere with this NOS pathway; however, most of the substances studied are potent vasoconstrictors that interfere with normal function, making clinical application elusive.[27]

Similar problems have been encountered in attempts to identify pharmacological substances that block the NMDA receptors. Some of the newer anti-convulsant type medications have some degree of NMDA blocking activity. Although in theory this might be protective in many settings, including acute brain injury, ischemia, or surgical stress, when direct application of NMDA inhibitors has been attempted, significant problems with memory, learning, and overall functioning have resulted.[28]

Summary

Certain unique attributes of the nervous system, in combination with the complexities of mitochondrial function and the generation of free radical species as part of normal metabolic function, lead to the recognition of a delicate balance that must be fostered to permit healthy human functioning. These insights also offer the opportunity to apply scientific principles to the optimization of CNS systems in an effort to minimize genetic and environmental risks that can result in myriad neurological disorders, from migraine to stroke to MS to parkinsonism and dementia.

References

1. Lipton R, Stewart W, Von Korff M. Burden of migraine: societal costs and therapeutic opportunities. Neurology. 1997;48(Suppl 3):S4-S9.
2. Dodick DW, Lipsy RJ. Advances in migraine management: implications for managed care organizations. Manag Care. 2004;13(5):45-51.
3. Abbott NJ. Dynamics of CNS barriers: evolution, differentiation, and modulation. Cell Mol Neurobiol. 2005;25(1):5-23.
4. Bourre JM. [The role of nutritional factors on the structure and function of the brain: an update on dietary requirements.] Rev Neurol (Paris). 2004;160(8-9):767-92.
5. Stewart VC, Heales SJ. Nitric oxide-induced mitochondrial dysfunction: implications for neurodegeneration. Free Radic Biol Med. 2003;34(3):287-303.
6. Andrews HE, Nichols PP, Bates D, Turnbull DM. Mitochondrial dysfunction plays a key role in progressive axonal loss in multiple sclerosis. Med Hypotheses. 2005;64(4):669-77.
7. Sarnat HB, Marin-Garcia J. Pathology of mitochondrial encephalomyopathies. Can J Neurol Sci. 2005;32(2):152-66.
8. Chaturvedi S, Bala K, Thakur R, Suri V. Mitochondrial encephalomyopathies: advances in understanding. Med Sci Monit. 2005;11(7):RA238-246.
9. DiMauro S, Moraes CT. Mitochondrial encephalomyopathies. Arch Neurol 1993;50:1197-208.
10. Shigenaga MK, Hagen TM, Ames BN. Oxidative damage and mitochondrial decay in aging. Proc Natl Acad Sci. 1994;91(23):10771-78.
11. Boulland JL, Levy LM. [Glutamate, glutamine and ischaemia in the central nervous system.] Tidsskr Nor Laegeforen. 2005;125(11):1479-81.

12. Vannucci RC, Brucklacher RM, Vannucci SJ. Intracellular calcium accumulation during the evolution of hypoxic-ischemic brain damage in the immature rat. Brain Res Dev Brain Res. 2001;126(1):117-20.
13. Nicholls D, Attwell D. The release and uptake of excitatory amino acids. Trends Pharmacol Sci. 1990:11:462-68.
14. Yudkoff M, Daikhin Y, Nissim I, et al. Brain amino acid requirements and toxicity: the example of leucine. J Nutr. 2005;135(6 Suppl):1531S-38S.
15. Brown RH Jr. Superoxide dismutase and familial amyotrophic lateral sclerosis: new insights into mechanisms and treatments. Ann Neurol. 1996;39:145-46.
16. Choi DW, Calcium: Still center-stage in hypoxic-ischemic neuronal death. Trends Neurosci. 1995;18:58-60.
17. Smart TG. Regulation of excitatory and inhibitory neurotransmitter-gated ion channels by protein phosphorylation. Curr. Opin. Neurobiol. 1997;7:358-67.
18. Haynes V, Elfering S, Traaseth N, Giulivi C. Mitochondrial nitric-oxide synthase: enzyme expression, characterization, and regulation. J Bioenerg Biomembr. 2004;36(4):341-46.
19. Beckman JS. The double-edged role of nitric oxide in brain function and superoxide-mediated injury. J Dev Physiol. 1991;15(1):53-59.
20. Kocak-Toker N, Giris M, Tulubas F, et al. Peroxynitrite induced decrease in Na+, K+-ATPase activity is restored by taurine. World J Gastroenterol. 2005;11(23):3554-57.
21. Hansson E, Ronnback L. Altered neuronal-glial signaling in glutamatergic transmission as a unifying mechanism in chronic pain and mental fatigue. Neurochem Res. 2004;29(5):989-96.
22. Cross AH, et al. Aminoguanidine, an inhibitor of inducible nitric oxide synthase, ameliorates experimental autoimmune encephalomyelitis in SJL mice. J Clin Invest. 1994;93:2684-90.
23. Hantraye P, et al. Inhibition of neuronal nitric oxide synthase prevents MPTP-induced parkinsonism in baboons. Nat Med. 1996;2(9):1017-21.
24. Iadecola C. Cerebrovascular effects of amyloid-beta peptides: mechanisms and implications for Alzheimer's dementia. Cell Mol Neurobiol. 2003;23(4-5):681-89.
25. Goodwin JL, Uemura E, Cunnick JE. Microglial release of nitric oxide by the synergistic action of beta-amyloid and IFN-gamma. Bran Res. 1995;692:207-14.
26. Resink AM, Brahmbhatt HP, Cordell B, et al. Nitric oxide mediates a component of B-amyloid neurotoxicity in cortical neuronal cell cultures. Soc Neurosci Abstr. 1995;21:1010.
27. Beckman JS. The double-edged role of nitric oxide in brain function and superoxide-mediated injury. J Dev Physiol. 1991;15(1):53-59.
28. Danilczuk Z, Ossowska G, Lupina T, et al. Effect of NMDA receptor antagonists on behavioral impairment induced by chronic treatment with dexamethasone. Pharm Rep. 2005;57:47-54.

Chapter 21
Oxidation-reduction Imbalances

Catherine Willner, MD

Introduction

In Chapter 20, we learned about the importance of energy to the nervous system, and we discussed its vulnerability to injury as a result of the oxidative stress that accompanies energy production. Now, we will examine in greater depth the structure, function, and genetics of the mitochondria—the energy producers of the body—and their role in certain nervous system pathologies.

The tiny cellular organelles called mitochondria are present in almost all cells, with predominance in highly metabolically active cells such as skeletal and cardiac muscle and the nervous system. The relationship between mitochondria and the cells in which they reside is a unique interdependence and has much to teach about the important principles of energy and oxidative stress and their importance in functional medicine. In this past century, the theory that mitochondria were originally bacteria that formed a symbiotic union with early prokaryotic cells has generally come to be accepted, though there were historically many alternative hypotheses as to their origin.[1,2] Among several factors arguing for their origin as "oxygen-metabolizing" early bacteria, they share many features with unicellular organisms, including morphology, consisting of two membranes and invaginations called cristae, with shapes typical of bacteria. Weighing in as perhaps the strongest argument for bacterial origin is the fact that they contain their own genetic material. For a very detailed and fascinating review of this history, as well as the current scientific status of mitochondrial functions across species, the work by Scheffler is an excellent resource.[3]

Mitochondrial Functions

Biochemical processes that occur within mitochondria are outlined in Table 21.1. The best known of these processes is oxidative phosphorylation, accomplished by the membrane-based respiratory chain, which consists of five subunits and requires a number of transporters and complex molecules. (Chapter 16 on Bioenergetics contains Figure 16.4, which depicts this mechanism.) This complex oxidizing electron transport chain is the primary source of the high-energy phosphate substrate ATP, but it is important to remember that many other functions also take place there. The citric acid cycle, amino acid biosynthesis (and, most prominently in liver tissue, the urea cycle), and fatty acid oxidation all make substrate available for oxidation within mitochondria. Additionally, calcium regulation or buffering and a series of control mechanisms for the process of programmed cellular demise (apoptosis) are also in the domain of mitochondrial control. These are biochemical processes that, in general, regulate energy metabolism and prepare for the oxidation of carbon-based structures to provide energy for other cellular functions. In an efficiently functioning mitochondrion, the downstream products of this process are ATP, carbon dioxide, and water. The presence of mechanisms impacting the ability to induce apoptosis makes sense because energy and calcium metabolism must be closely monitored to maintain normal cellular function, especially in the cells that have high-energy demands. Mitochondrial function and the ability to support normal cellular functions, especially in highly demanding neuromuscular tissues, not only change with age but are at risk from environmental, intrinsic, and genetic injuries and insults. These functions are worthy of discussion as they relate to the unique genetics and structure of mitochondria because understanding the physiology creates the potential for modifying pathology.

Table 21.1 **Mitochondrial Operations**

Oxidative phosphorylation (respiratory chain ATP production)
Citric acid cycle
Amino acid synthesis
Fatty acid oxidation
Calcium metabolism and cytoplasmic sequestration
Apoptosis

Mitochondrial Genetics

Mitochondria contain their own DNA (mtDNA) and in humans mtDNA is responsible for forming some necessary substrates for energy production. A large number of the components necessary for this process actually are formed from messages contained in nuclear DNA, especially Complex II, which is associated with succinate dehydrogenase. Many other genes that might be required for a bacterium to function independently have been relocated to or subsumed by nuclear DNA. Mitochondria have lost the ability to translate proteins as efficiently as their independently surviving counterparts. Mitochondrial DNA in the human is double stranded and circular, consisting of 16,569 base pairs;[4] it contains approximately 37 genes in comparison to the thousands of genes present in bacterial DNA. For the most part, the functions that remain the responsibility of mtDNA are associated with oxidative phosphorylation. The mitochondrial genes encode for 13 polypeptides involved in that process, as well as ribosomal RNA and transfer RNA.

Mitochondria and mtDNA are primarily maternally inherited. (There have been exceptions reported, with clinical disorders such as myopathy originating from paternally inherited mtDNA.[5]) Clinical manifestations of mitochondrial dysfunction, discussed below, are highly variable and will be expressed in both females and males, but it is predominantly the females who pass on the mitochondrial and mtDNA mutations to their progeny. There is potential for some paternal contribution to mitochondrial (dys)function because of nuclear genetics, but mtDNA is involved in producing essential components of oxidative phosphorylation and evidence has mounted during the past century that mtDNA mutations produce many of the clinical disorders related to mitochondrial dysfunction.

The expression of these disorders is complex, not only because of the interaction of mitochondrial and nuclear genetics, but also because of how mitochondria reproduce within different cell lines and tissues. The number of mitochondria within any given cell varies on the basis of energy requirements for different tissues. In the context of athletic training or increased energy demands within a specific tissue, the number of mitochondria can increase, which requires replication of the mitochondria completely unrelated to cellular division. Additionally, there is more than one mtDNA in the typical mitochondrion, which permits variable expression of mutations during replication. The co-existence of normal mtDNA alongside mtDNA with mutations, whether spontaneous or inherited, is known as heteroplasmy. In a normal person, a completely normal mtDNA genome is present in all the mitochondria (homoplasmy). In an individual carrying mutations, there will be some normal and some mutated mtDNA within the mitochondria. These interesting features of mitochondrial genetics and their interactions with different cellular components account for variations on the expression of dysfunction in different tissues, in different family members from the same mother, and in changes that occur over time. For a more in-depth discussion of these interesting phenomena, excellent reviews are available.[6,7]

Mitochondrial Structure

The content of the phospholipid bilayer is composed of two membranes, an important factor in mitochondrial function. Like all membranes, the mitochondrial membranes function better when fluidity is optimized. The inner membrane is especially unusual because of the relatively high content of protein complexes forming the respiratory chain. Cardiolipin (diphosphatidylglycerol) is thought to be unique to this inner membrane; it is highly concentrated at these sites and appears to be involved in proper functioning of the respiratory chain, where oxidative phosphorylation occurs. As mentioned above, the respiratory chain is composed of five subunits named Complex I–V. Four of the five are predominantly produced by coordinated actions of nuclear and mtDNA-generated polypeptides. Complex II is formed uniquely from nuclear transcription products. Two of its four subunits are associated with the enzyme succinate dehydrogenase, which is one of the enzymes involved in the citric acid cycle. Therefore, there is a mechanism for the respiratory chain to monitor CoA utilization and reducing equivalents (NAD and FAD) in the organelle. These substrates, nicotinamide adenine dinucleotide and flavin adenine dinucleotide, are derived from B vitamins (niacin and riboflavin). Cytochrome c and other heme-based molecules are integral to the function of the respiratory chain and are produced within the mitochondria.

Another very important structural and functional component is the ubiquinone family, specifically coenzyme Q10. Because this sterol-like structure is formed within the body using the same acetylation pathway as cholesterol, its formation can be disrupted by statin drugs, which block an early step in the metabolic pathway of its production (HMG CoA reductase). Though there may be some element of selectivity of enzymes for substrates leading to this pathway, enabling statins to impact cholesterol synthesis more dramatically, this is incompletely documented. For more detailed analysis of these processes and other functions accomplished in and by mitochondria, a number of interesting reviews can be consulted.[8,9,10,11,12]

Mitochondropathies

Disorders of mitochondrial function cross many medical disciplines simply because of the presence of mitochondria in metabolically active tissues. Though there are clearly clinical manifestations isolated to single tissues, the disorders typically attributed to mitochondrial dysfunction involve several tissues. They are intriguing because of the complex issues related to maternal inheritance in the mtDNA, tissue heterogeneity and heteroplasmy, as well as the autosomal genomics relevant to nuclear DNA. The highly energy-dependent nature of the neuromuscular system, however, naturally leads to a prominent position for these tissues in the pathophysiology of mitochondrial disorders. Many have been named or classified by the systems involved or the symptoms associated, although, as the complex genetics of mitochondria have been elucidated, there has been an effort to associate specific disorders with specific alterations in either mitochondrial or Mendelian nuclear genetics, or both. In addition to genetic explanations for failure of energy metabolism, there are also disorders associated with mitochondrial failure caused by other factors, including those associated with use of certain antibiotics that damage mitochondria[13,14] or pathological conditions such as stroke, where mitochondrial function can be altered to the point that apoptosis is triggered despite initial cellular survival following anoxic insult. There are also genetic mutations that damage other mitochondrial functions besides ATP production, including disorders of mineral storage, calcium homeostasis, and multiple cellular processes that can lead to apoptosis.

The earliest description of mitochondrial disorders associated with alterations in mitochondrial DNA was a report in the late 1980s of a mitochondrial myopathy associated with a specific large genetic deletion.[15] Leber's hereditary optic neuropathy (LHON) within one specific family was then identified to be associated with a point mutation.[16] LHON is clinically associated with rather sudden onset of blindness from optic atrophy, most often seen in males.

The more common syndromes associated with mtDNA defects, though all quite rare, have been named historically by their symptom complexes. MELAS (mitochondrial encephalomyopathy, lactic acidosis, and stroke-like episodes) typically presents during childhood with a clinical presentation that includes episodes of vomiting, headaches with migrainous features, and vascular events similar to stroke episodes (although imaging does not typically show lesions concordant with normal "vascular" strokes). The presence of lesions typical of scarring beyond vascular territories has made an argument for these being metabolically induced areas of tissue damage.[17] Over time, there is progressive loss of function. As information about the genetics of mitochondria has been uncovered, the MELAS syndrome, like other disorders, has been found to be associated with many different mutations in mtDNA.[18]

MERRF (myoclonus, epilepsy, ragged red fibers) is characterized by those clinical features, including the myopathy associated with the pathological hallmark of ragged red muscle cells on biopsy. Ataxia and cognitive decline to the point of dementia are typical, as is damage to other energy-dependent tissues, such as hearing and peripheral nerves. A list of the more common syndromes with neurological features is presented in Table 21.2.

A very intriguing case presentation of a patient with myopathy developing in adulthood emphasizes the variability associated with mitochondrial division and replication. The pathology, associated with ragged red fibers and Complex IV deficient fibers, increased over a 12-year period of study.[19] Progenitor muscle satellite cells capable of regenerating muscle tissue showed no, or only very low levels of, mutated mtDNA, leading to an intervention that seemed to reverse the presentation by stimulating these progenitor cells.[20] In tissues that do have the ability to regenerate, albeit slowly, this represents an exciting potential for possible treatment of these frequently devastating disorders. Though beyond the scope of this discussion, the treatments directed at these disorders have been rather disappointing, including use of antioxidants and nutrients to support mitochondrial structure and function.

Table 21.2 **Mitochondropathies (the more common syndromes)**

MELAS (mitochondrial encephalomyopathy, lactic acidosis, stroke-like episodes)
MERRF (myoclonic epilepsy with ragged red fibers)
LHON (Leber's hereditary optic neuropathy)
KSS (Kearns-Sayre syndrome)
CPEO (chronic progressive external ophthalmoplegia)
PS (Pearson syndrome)
NARP (neuropathy, ataxia, retinitis pigmentosa)
MILS (maternally inherited Leigh's syndrome)
AID (aminoglycoside-induced deafness)

The autosomal inheritance related to mitochondrial dysfunction is more complex simply because of the volume of functions served by nuclear DNA products and because there can be overlap of disorders of both genomes, which further complicates the clinical picture. Leigh syndrome, a disorder of infancy and childhood involving psychomotor delay, a variety of cognitive changes, and seizures, can be inherited as a recessive, x-linked or maternal disorder. Because of the large number of mitochondria and their dependence on energy, the tissues most involved include the nervous system, cardiac and skeletal muscle. Liver, kidney, and pancreas can also be involved in many of these syndromes. Exercise intolerance, frank myopathies with muscular weakness and wasting, arrhythmias, and a variety of neurological symptoms are common in these conditions. Leukoencephalopathy (white matter lesions by MRI) is fairly typical. Evaluating for dysfunction in these tissues is the starting point in the assessment of these patients, but formal neurological evaluation is very useful to delineate the nervous system features that occur so frequently. Liver and renal function should also be assessed, as well as lactate levels, which can be elevated at rest. Not all patients will present with such laboratory changes. Limited exercise can sometimes reveal early and significant elevation of lactate levels. When suspected, cellular DNA can be analyzed, including in the white blood cells. As discussed above, because Complex II is not under the control of mtDNA, a normal or elevated level of succinate dehydrogenase can be diagnostic of a mitochondrial DNA disorder in the context where the activity of other complexes is reduced.

There are genetic disorders of other types of mitochondrial function in addition to those associated directly with energy production, such as iron transport and storage. An x-linked sideroblastic anemia related to iron export has been identified and so have defects of iron storage in certain presentations of Friedrich's ataxia. A mutation recognized to be related to a deficiency of thymidine phosphorylase, leading to accumulation of thymidine, may prove to be amenable to treatment.[21] Finally, genetic and environmental disorders associated with reduced coenzyme Q10 have been identified. They do respond to replacement therapy in the absence of other significant genetic pathologies but the clinical response has not been uniform in all disorders.[22]

These disorders of mitochondrial function can be inherited maternally or develop sporadically from spontaneous mutations and must, to some extent, exhibit heteroplasmy (with some normal "wild-type" mitochondria) to permit survival. As techniques capable of quantifying mtDNA damage, especially deletions, have become available, there has been mounting evidence that progressive mitochondrial dysfunction is associated with aging and is highly variable between different tissue types and individuals.[23] Cells with high rates of turnover tend to exhibit less mtDNA damage, while cells with slower turnover, such as muscles and the nervous system, show progressive increase in the frequency of mtDNA deletions.

Oxidative Stress

Mitochondria provide high-energy substrates at a cost. The process of oxidative phosphorylation, though an efficient pathway for the production of ATP, is also a major source of free radicals, which have the potential to damage cellular components, including any and all structures that can be oxidized. Phospholipid membranes, DNA, enzymes, and other proteins are most vulnerable to this type of damage. It is estimated that up to 4% of oxygen utilized in normal mitochondria ultimately forms free radicals such as superoxide, hydrogen peroxide, and hydroxyl radicals, which obviously puts the mitochondrial membranes, cardiolipin, and mtDNA at high risk for oxidation. Though there are elaborate buffering systems in place, both at the level of the mitochondria and within the cellular matrix, these protective processes can be overwhelmed. Free radical oxygen and nitrogen processes, generated as part of normal metabolism, can also intermix to produce peroxynitrite, a particularly volatile substance with great potential for lethal damage to cellular components.

There are other sites at risk for oxidative stress in cells that utilize oxygen, including the cytochrome P450 system, peroxisomes, and cytosolic oxidases. These subcellular components have their own systems of protection, which can also be overwhelmed. As methods for assessing oxidative damage to various structures have become more available, we have learned that such damage is present in many chronic diseases, especially in those that involve neurological tissues. Because a normal membrane potential is required for propagating action potentials and for normal receptor function in neurons, the importance of healthy membranes with adequate ATP is paramount to normal neurological function. Consider, for example, the physiology of excitotoxicity mediated by the excitatory transmitters, glutamate and aspartate, which act at the NMDA (N-methyl-D-aspartate) receptor. This receptor complex allows calcium to enter the cell, which is a normal physiological mediator of numerous cellular processes. However, when the system malfunctions, the consequence of abnormal activation of these receptors is called excitotoxicity, and it can contribute to pathology and ultimately cellular demise in many different clinical settings. An excellent review of this important topic was done by Waxman and Lynch in 2005.[24]

Neurodegenerative Disorders

The hallmark of the neurodegenerative disorders is progressive loss of specific populations of neurons. Because neurons are so energy dependent and mitochondria do have a significant role in programmed cellular demise, specifically the process of apoptosis, mitochondrial dysfunction has come to be associated with such disorders.[25] Though some of the neurodegenerative disorders are indeed associated with known genetic risks, more commonly the pathophysiology identified at autopsy (and in animal models of these disorders) involves free radicals, oxidative stress, and altered calcium metabolism—that is, environmental rather than genetic common denominators. As we now understand the mitochondropathies, both genetically and mechanistically, we see that in disorders where mitochondrial dysfunction is a primary pathological manifestation, progressive neuronal loss is often a part of the process. This awareness has made the role of mitochondria in other neurodegenerative disorders a reasonable hypothesis.

One of the manifestations of LHON, involving primarily mtDNA (maternal) inheritance of a disorder of Complex I of the respiratory chain, includes involvement of the basal ganglia and clinical manifestations of dystonia, as well as extrapyramidal features typical of Parkinsonism that is responsive to dopamine therapy.[26,27] Similar mutations involving a familial multisystem degeneration, also associated with parkinsonian features, was shown to be associated with mtDNA mutations.[28] However, when looking at larger populations of patients with Parkinson's and/or Alzheimer's disease, though there were some members of these groups that had specific mtDNA mutations, there have not been any specific mutations or sets of mutations that are consistent across the groups.[29]

Further evidence of the role of mitochondrial dysfunction in neurodegenerative disorders includes syndromes presenting in infants and children. Leigh's syndrome, which occurs typically in very young patients who are normal during very early development, shows widespread subcortical degeneration involving multiple brain structures. The pathology includes demyelination, gliosis, and vascular proliferation and is associated with either mtDNA maternal inheritance or autosomally-mediated mitochondrial dysfunction. Several different types of presentations have been identified.[30,31]

Friedreich's ataxia (FRDA) is an autosomal recessive disorder presenting typically in early adulthood with clinical features of progressive limb and gait ataxia, loss of deep tendon reflexes with axonal sensory neuropathy, and pyramidal (long tract) signs. It is the most common of the hereditary ataxias. The FRDA gene has been identified and is known to code for a specific protein, called frataxin. This protein is present in significant amounts in the cerebellum and spinal cord. In the presence of the abnormal genetic response, it is not produced in adequate amounts, leading to problems with mitochondrial function due to iron accumulation. This negatively impacts the activities of respiratory chain complexes I, II, III, and the matrix enzyme aconitase. The result is mitochondrial failure, but also increased free radical oxidation because of the presence of excess free iron (which further damages enzymes).[32] Interestingly, the widely prevalent antioxidant enzyme superoxide dismutase fails to reverse this iron-based free radical damage in cell cultures, but there has been evidence of improved cellular function in cultures using other antioxidants, such as idebenone.[33]

Other examples of genetic dysfunction associated with mitochondrial mutations that lead to progressive neurological disorders include at least some of the hereditary spastic paraplegias.[34] The autosomally recessive Wilson's disease is clinically associated with liver failure, psychiatric disease, dystonia, and rigidity similar to Parkinson's symptoms. Dysfunction in a copper transport ATP-ase, one of which localizes to mitochondria, is characteristic of this condition. There have also been Complex I enzyme defects identified in the liver mitochondria of patients with this disorder.[35]

Parkinson's Disease

A closer look at Parkinson's disease was made possible when a rather sudden clinical onset in certain patients was correlated with use of an illegal analog of a narcotic, injectable meperidine, called MPTP (1-methyl-4-phenyl 1,2,3,6-tetrahydropyridine).[36] This ultimately led to animal models of drug-induced Parkinson's disease. Numerous publications about the pathology observed in these patients revealed that MTPT is neurotoxic to dopaminergic neurons by way of a reaction through the active metabolite, called MPP^+ (1-methyl-4-phenylpyridinium), which is formed by action of monoamine oxidase in glial cells. MPP enters neurons via a dopamine reuptake pathway and is identified in mitochondria, where it interferes with the activity of Complex I, leading to compromised oxidative phosphorylation and increasing the risk of oxidative damage significantly.[37] Compromise of Complex I activity has also been identified in other cells in patients with Parkinson's disease, including platelets.[38] Genetic markers for nuclear dysfunction related to Complex I have been identified.[39] There is also evidence for mtDNA contributions in certain cases.[40] However, when a larger series of Parkinson's patients was evaluated, there was no obvious concordance in these findings for consistent mtDNA mutations.[41]

What seems to be clear is that genetic mutations in Complex I activity impact some patients with later onset Parkinson's disease. A small study using very high doses of coenzyme Q10 and vitamin E did demonstrate benefit sufficient to delay treatment with L-dopa.[42] The lead author contends that larger studies are necessary before recommending use of this approach, but the study did demonstrate a dose-related effect; the best outcome used the highest dose of coenzyme Q10, comparing 300, 600 and 1200 mg over the course of 18 months. Criticisms have been levied about these early data because patients quickly reported improvement in activities of daily living, but one could argue that this would be expected if energy metabolism were improved. The extent to which this approach is neuroprotective is presently being debated and larger trials are anticipated.[43]

Part of the controversy surrounding any delineation of neuroprotective effects of antioxidants and other molecules presumed to be involved in neurotoxicity stems from the data surrounding the large clinical trials investigating the pathophysiology elucidated by the MPTP data.[44] Inhibitors of monoamine oxidase B (MAO-B), including selegiline, rasagiline, and others, have been assessed for their ability to block conversion of MTPT to MPP^+ (an oxidative reaction), as well as for their ability to block oxidative metabolism of dopamine, because of early studies in primates in the MPTP model.[45] A number of studies directed at modifying the pathology identified with MPTP have been published, leading ultimately to the large controlled trial within the Parkinson study group. The most notable of these is the DATATOP trial looking at treatment with vitamin E in the form of α-tocopherol and l-deprenyl (selegiline).[46] This large double-blind, placebo-controlled study showed no isolated benefit of vitamin E, but did confirm prior findings of delayed onset of disability using the presumed MAO-B inhibitor selegiline. Eventually, a possible dopaminergic, and hence symptomatic, effect of this agent was suspected, which clouded the interpretation. More recently, the impact of these drugs has been thought to be neuroprotective through mechanisms that block apoptosis.[47] Rasagiline has been shown to exert a number of anti-apoptotic effects.[48] In studies looking at this drug, using a design to reduce the confounding contribution of symptomatic improvement, there are early indications that it is neuroprotective.[49]

Dopaminergic cellular demise in Parkinson's disease is associated with several well-delineated mechanisms, as discussed above. These include the presence of mitochondrial dysfunction, oxidative stress, and proinflammatory cytokines suggestive of chronic inflammation; this is a neurotoxic and probably excitotoxic effect, leading ultimately to apoptosis.[50] Abnormalities in the processing of proteins in the cell, related to the ubiquitin-proteasome system, which may explain the presence of Lewy bodies in certain patients, have also been elucidated.[51,52] Environmental factors are now discussed frequently as contributing to the pathology because of findings in twin studies.[53] What seems to make most sense is that vulnerability in the function of dopaminergic neurons, which are susceptible to toxicity from compounds that could mimic the effect of MPTP, contributes to progressive cellular degeneration and mitochondrial dysfunction. This is not a well-documented primary problem in all cases, especially in those where Complex I likely plays a significant role. Efforts at identifying appropriate neuroprotective strategies include limiting the exposure to L-dopa, optimizing antioxidant therapies, and supporting mitochondrial function with the goal of reducing cellular death by apoptosis. These are now the focus of intense debate and research. Pending further research, the relative safety of higher doses of coenzyme Q10 and the use of tolerable agents that can target the MAO-B or, more likely, the propargylamine inhibitors, are the most appropriate first course of therapy. Of course, keeping the patient away from all potential neurotoxins is also vital.

Episodic Neurological Disorders

Altered energy metabolism and mitochondrial processes also participate in several other neurological syndromes, including the episodic disorders, such as migraine. A 1995 review hypothesized a possible relationship between migraine and magnesium concentrations in the brain.[54] Other episodic disorders, including seizures, have been reviewed in terms of the possible contribution of mitochondrial dysfunction and the consequences of oxidative stress leading to progressive damage.[55] Because of the paramount importance of energy for maintaining cellular function, the electrochemical gradient, and appropriate structure of the lipid bilayer within the nervous system, a role for mitochondrial dysfunction would be logical in episodic disorders such as migraines, seizures, and stroke.

Summary

Neuromuscular tissues are predominantly post-mitotic, energy-dependent tissues. As such, they are highly dependent on normal mitochondrial function. Under normal circumstances, the process of oxidative phosphorylation generates free radicals as part of the production of ATP, and these dangerous byproducts are typically managed by a system of antioxidant protection within the mitochondrion as well as within the cell. When mitochondrial function is interrupted or dysfunctional, this free radical stress escalates. Dysfunction of energy metabolism results in dysregulation of calcium within the cell, sometimes directly by changes in the NMDA receptor via mechanisms of excitotoxicity, and sometimes by other pathways. This process, which is normally buffered by mitochondria, further contributes to cellular dysfunction, escalating to produce more oxidative damage and failure of mitochondrial function. At some point, mechanisms of apoptosis, mostly governed by mitochondria, lead to cell death. These mechanisms, in addition to others associated with cellular dysfunction (like chronic inflammation), seem to be a common denominator for many neurological disorders. In virtually all neurodegenerative conditions, there are some similarities with the changes discussed above in Parkinson's disease, including those with known genetic contributions such as Huntington's disease, and the motor neuron disorders such as ALS (amyotrophic lateral sclerosis). The contributions of these various physiological processes are being assessed with the hope that these disorders can eventually be treated effectively. The ability to alter cellular dysfunction, and hence survival, is the goal of all neuroprotective strategies, and efforts to optimize energy production without the ravages of excess oxidative stress is a laudable goal. Unfortunately, approaches for modifying these various parameters, including use of antioxidants and substrates to optimize mitochondrial function, have produced mixed results in published studies.

References

1. Margulis LS. On the origin of mitosing cells. J Theoret Biol. 1967;14:225.
2. Gray MW, Doolittle WF. Has the endosymbiont hypothesis been proven? Microbiol Rev. 1982;46:1-42.
3. Scheffler IE. Mitochondria. Wiley-Liss, New York, 1999.
4. Anderson S, Bankier AT, Barrel BG, et al. Sequence and organization of the human mitochondrial genome. Nature. 1981;290:457-65.
5. Schwartz M, Vissing J. Paternal inheritance of mitochondrial DNA. N Engl J Med. 2002;347:576-80.
6. DiMauro S, Schon EA. Mechanisms of disease: mitochondrial respiratory-chain diseases. N Engl J Med. 2003;348:2656-68.
7. Smeitink J, van den Heuvel L, DiMauro S. The genetics and pathology of oxidative phosphorylation. Nature Rev Genet. 2001;2:342-52.
8. Owczarek J, Jasinska M, Orszulak-Michalak D. Drug-induced myopathies. An overview of the possible mechanisms. Pharmacol Rep. 2005;57:23-34.
9. Saris NE, Carafoli E. A historical review of cellular calcium handling, with emphasis on mitochondria. Biochemistry (Mosc). 2005;70(2):187-94.
10. Huss JM, Kelly DP. Mitochondrial energy metabolism in heart failure: a question of balance. J Clin Invest. 2005;115:547-55.
11. Xu W, Charles IG, Moncada S. Nitric oxide: orchestrating hypoxia regulation through mitochondrial respiration and the endoplasmic reticulum stress response. Cell Res. 2005;15(1):63-65.
12. Higuchi Y. Glutathione depletion-induced chromosomal DNA fragmentation associated with apoptosis and necrosis. J Cell Mol Med. 2004;8(4):455-64.
13. Kohn S, Fradis M, Robinson E, Iancu TC. Hepatotoxicity of combined treatment with cisplatin and gentamicin in the guinea pig. Ultrastruct Pathol. 2005;29(2):129-37.
14. Yu F, Yu F, Li R, Wang R. Toxic effect of Chloromycetin on the ultrastructures of the motor neurons of the Chinese tree shrew (Tupaia belangeri). Can J Physiol Pharmacol. 2004;82(4):276-81.
15. Holt IJ, Harding AE, Morgan Hughes JA. Deletions of muscle mitochondrial DNA in patients with mitochondrial myopathies. Nature. 1988;331:717-19.
16. Wallace DC, Singh G, Lott MT, et al. Mitochondrial DNA mutation associated with Leber's hereditary optic neuropathy. Science. 1988;242:1427-31.
17. Schon EA, Hirano M, DiMauro S. Molecular genetic basis of the mitochondrial encephalopathies. In Schapira AHV, DiMauro S (eds). Mitochondrial Disorders in neurology. Boston, Butterworth-Heinemann, 2002, pp 69-113.
18. DiMauro S, Schon EA. Mechanisms of disease: mitochondrial respiratory-chain diseases. N Engl J Med. 2003;348:2656-68.
19. Weber K, Wilson JN, Taylor L, et al. A new mtDNA mutation showing accumulation with time and restriction to skeletal muscle. Am J Hum Genet. 1997;60:373-80.
20. Clark KM, Bindoff LA, Lightowlers RN, et al. Reversal of a mitochondrial DNA defect in human skeletal muscle. Nature Genet. 1997;16:222-24.
21. Nishino I, Spinazzola A, Papadimitrious A, et al. Mitochondrial neurogastrointestinal encephalomyopathy: an autosomal recessive disorder due to thymidine phosphorylase mutations. Ann Neurol. 2000;47:792-800.
22. Remes AM, Liimatta EV, Winqvist S, et al. Ubiquinone and nicotinamide treatment of patients with the 3243A-G mtDNA mutation. Neurology. 2002;59:1275-77.
23. Melov S, Shoffner JM, Kaufman A, Wallace DC. Marked increase in the number and variety of mitochondrial DNA rearrangements in aging human skeletal muscle. Nucleic Acids Res. 1995;23:4122-26.
24. Waxman EA, Lynch DR. N-methyl-D-aspartate receptor subtypes: multiple roles in excitotoxicity and neurological disease. Neuroscientist. 2005;11:37-49.
25. Manfredi G, Beal MF. The role of mitochondria in the pathogenesis of neurodegenerative diseases. Brain Pathol. 2000;10:462-72.
26. Wooten GF, Currie LJ, Bennett JP, et al. Maternal inheritance in Parkinson's disease. Ann Neurol. 1997;41:265-68.
27. Simon DK, Johns DR. Mitochondrial disorders: clinical and genetic features. Ann Rev Med. 1999;50:111-27.
28. Simon DK, Pulst SM, Sutton JP, et al. Familial multisystem degeneration with parkinsonism associated with the 11778 mitochondrial DNA mutation. Neurology. 1999;53:1787-93.
29. Brown MD, Shoffner JM, Kim YL, et al. Mitochondrial DNA sequence analysis of four Alzheimer's and Parkinson's disease patients. Am J Med Genet. 1996;61:283-89.
30. Vu TH, Hirano M, DiMauro S. Mitochondrial diseases. Neurol Clin. 2002;20:809-39.
31. Petruzzella V, DiGiacinto G, Scacco S, et al. Atypical Leigh syndrome associated with the D393N mutation in the mitochondrial ND5 subunit. Neurology. 2003;61:1017-18.
32. Cavadini P, O'Neill HA, Benada O, Isaya G. Assembly and iron-binding properties of human frataxin, the protein deficient in Friedreich ataxia. Hum Mol Genet. 2002;11:217-27.
33. Schulz JB, Dehmer T, Schols L, et al. Oxidative stress in patients with Friedreich ataxia. Neurology. 2000;55:1719-21.
34. Casari G, De Fusco M, Ciarmatori S, et al. Spastic paraplegia and OXPHOS impairment caused by mutations in paraplegin, a nuclear-encoded mitochondrial metalloprotease. Cell. 1998;93:973-83.
35. Gu M, Cooper JM, Butler P, et al. Oxidative phosphorylation defects in liver of patients with Wilson's disease. Lancet. 2000;356:469-74.
36. Davis GC, Williams AC, Markey SP, et al. Chronic Parkinsonism secondary to intravenous injection of meperidine analogues. Psychiatry Res. 1979;1:649-54.
37. Langston JW. The etiology of Parkinson's disease with emphasis on the MPTP story. Neurology. 1996;47:S153-60.
38. Parker WD Jr, Swerdlow RH. Mitochondrial dysfunction in idiopathic Parkinson disease. Am J Hum Genet. 1998;13:203-11.
39. Hattori N, Yoshino H, Tanaka M, et al. Genotype in the 24-kDa subunit gene (NDUFV2) of mitochondrial complex I and susceptibility to Parkinson disease. Genomics. 1998;49:52-58.
40. Gu M, Cooper JM, Taanman JW, Schapira AH. Mitochondrial DNA transmission of the mitochondrial defect in Parkinson's disease. Ann Neurol. 1998;44:177-86.
41. Simon DK, Mayeux R, Marder K, et al. Mitochondrial DNA mutations in complex I and tRNA genes in Parkinson's disease. Neurology. 2000;54:703-9.
42. Shults CW, Oakes D, Kieburtz K, et al, and the Parkinson Study Group. Effects of coenzyme Q10 in early Parkinson disease: evidence of slowing of the functional decline. Arch Neurol. 2002;59:1541-50.
43. Schapira AHV, Olanow CW. Neuroprotection in Parkinson's disease: mysteries, myths, and misconceptions. JAMA. 2004;291:358-64.
44. Olanow CW. Oxidation reactions in Parkinson's disease. Neurology. 1990;40(Suppl3):32-37.
45. Cohen G, Pasik P, Cohen B, et al. Pargyline and deprenyl prevent the neurotoxicity of 1-methyl-4-phenyl-1,2,3,6-tetrahdropyridine (MPTP) in monkeys. Eur J Pharmacol. 1984;106:209-10.
46. The Parkinson Study Group. Effects of tocopherol and deprenyl on the progression of disability in early Parkinson's disease. N Engl J Med. 1993;328:176-83.
47. Boulton AA. Symptomatic and neuroprotective properties of the aliphatic propargylamines. Mech Ageing Dev. 1999;111:201-9.

48. Naoi M, Maruyama W, Youdim MB, et al. Anti-apoptotic function of propargylamine inhibitors of type-B monoamine oxidase. Inflammopharmacology. 2003;11:175-81.
49. Parkinson Study Group. A controlled, randomized, delayed-start study of rasagiline in early Parkinson disease. Arch Neurol. 2004;61:561-66.
50. Jenner P, Olanow CW. Understanding cell death in Parkinson's disease. Ann Neurol. 1998;44(3 Suppl 1):S72-S84.
51. McNaught KS, Olanow CW, Halliwell B, et al. Failure of the ubiquitin-proteasome system in Parkinson's disease. Nat Rev Neurosci. 2001;2:589-94.
52. Olanow CW, Perl DP, DeMartino GN, McNaught KS. Lewy-body formation is an aggresome-related process: a hypothesis. Lancet Neurol. 2004;3:496-503.
53. Tanner CM. Is the cause of Parkinson's disease environmental or hereditary: Evidence from twin studies. Adv Neurol. 2003;126:1722-33.
54. Welch KM, Ramadan NM. Mitochondria, magnesium and migraine. J Neurol Sci. 1995;134:9-14.
55. Cock HR. The role of mitochondria and oxidative stress in neuronal damage after brief and prolonged seizures. Prog Brain Res. 2002;135:187-96.

Section V

Fundamental Clinical Imbalances

Chapter 22
Detoxification and Biotransformational Imbalances

DeAnn Liska, PhD, Michael Lyon, MD, David S. Jones, MD

The Detoxification Systems—Introduction

The concept that toxins accumulate in the body and are the cause of various health problems has long been a fundamental tenet of traditional healthcare systems around the world. For centuries, societies have valued therapies that have promoted the idea of cleansing and detoxifying. From the simple water fast used since antiquity to the sometimes elaborate detoxifying regimes of spas, including saunas, enemas, hydrotherapy treatments, and dietary modifications, detoxification as a therapeutic goal has long been pursued (see Table 22.1 for common terms used in reference to detoxification).

In the early 21st century, as society has increasingly been exposed to toxic compounds in the air, water, and food, it has become apparent that an individual's ability to detoxify substances to which he or she is exposed, both exogenously (xenobiotics) and endogenously (products of metabolism), is of critical importance to overall health. Many of the xenobiotics to which we are exposed show little relationship to previously encountered compounds or metabolites, and yet healthy bodies are often capable of managing these environmental exposures through complex systems of detoxification enzymes.

Public acknowledgement regarding the extent of environmental exposure to xenobiotics is at an all-time high. For example, the EPA estimates that in 1994 alone, over 2.2 *billion* pounds of toxic chemicals were released into the environment in the United States.[1] EPA estimates for 2002 have grown to 4.7 billion pounds.[2] Moreover, it is likely that at least 25% of the United States population suffers to some extent from heavy metal poisoning.

Table 22.1 **Common Terms Used in Reference to Detoxification**

Term	Definition
Toxicology	The science that deals with reversible and irreversible noxious or harmful effects of (chemical) substances on living organisms.
Biochemical toxicology	A field of toxicology focusing on the biochemical mechanisms that underlie dysfunction or toxicity (i.e., molecular toxicology).
Xenobiotics	Chemicals or molecules that are foreign to the biologic system, originating externally (e.g., toxic substances in the environment, phytochemicals, drugs).
Detoxification	Any process of decreasing the negative impact of xenobiotics (toxic substances and nontoxins) on bodily process. The process of detoxification involves biotransformation of endogenous and exogenous molecules into excretable metabolites. The term *detoxication* is often used to refer specifically to the intracellular biotransformation process.
Induction	Initiation of transcription of a gene leading to upregulation of a particular biochemical pathway. See also *upregulation*.
Upregulation	The increased activity (following induction) of a particular biochemical pathway resulting in an increased concentration of the product(s) of that pathway.

Discovery of the Detoxification Reactions

The hypothesis that xenobiotics consumed by animals, including man, are transformed to water-soluble substances and excreted through the urine was first put forth in the late 18th century. For more than 100 years after the initial observation, research into the identification of various metabolites continued, and many conjugation reactions were identified.

In his landmark 1947 monograph, *Detoxification Mechanisms*, Roger Williams brought together many observations and defined the field of detoxification. Williams described how these non-reactive compounds could be biotransformed in two phases: functionalization, which uses oxygen to form a reactive site, and conjugation, which adds a water-soluble group to this reactive site.[4] The original terms (functionalization and conjugation) describing these two steps eventually became known as phase I and phase II detoxification, respectively. The result is the biotransformation of a lipophilic compound into a water-soluble compound that can be discharged in urine. Therefore, detoxification is not one reaction, but rather a process that involves multiple reactions and multiple players.

"The term 'cytochrome P450' first appeared in the literature in 1962. It was a microsomal membrane-bound hemoprotein without known physiological functions at that time and was characterized by a unique 450-nm optical absorption peak of its carbon monoxide-bound form ... ."[5] (A remembrance of the early work on cytochrome P450s by one of its prominent researchers was published in 2003.[6]) A high concentration of this cytochrome P450 enzyme was soon found to be localized in the liver, and researchers discovered that it was responsible for converting lipophilic (fat-loving) toxins into biotransformed intermediates that were more water soluble (the phase I process).

Later research revealed that these biotransformed intermediates undergo further biotransformation in the liver by a second series of enzymes called conjugases (the phase II process). A good review of the history of these discoveries was written by Smith and Williams in 1970.[7] The conjugases are enzymes that attach molecules such as glucuronic acid, sulfate, glutathione, glycine, taurine, or methyl groups to the biotransformed intermediates. As this research continued into the 1980s and 1990s, investigators discovered a surprising number of phase I cytochrome P450s and phase II conjugases. For example, we are now aware that endogenously-produced hormones and other signaling molecules are not only detoxified by these enzymes, allowing for elimination, but also are metabolized into other signaling molecules, allowing for more variation in the activities of these important substances.

Scientists and clinicians still face a considerable challenge in understanding detoxification. The question of how the body can handle such a range of compounds it has never seen before has led to much work aimed at exploring the protein structure and regulation of various enzymes involved in detoxification.[8,9] We now know that a battery of enzymes, each with broad specificity, is available for managing the work of detoxification: there are "at least 57 human P450s (termed isoforms) which are all encoded by separate genes ... and most cytochrome P450 genes are subject to genetic polymorphism."[10] And, "Nearly fifteen P450s are involved in the metabolism of drugs and other xenobiotics chemicals ... ."[11] The whole field is very complex and rapidly evolving.

A Broader Definition of Detoxification

The complex systems of the detoxification enzymes generally function adequately to minimize potential damage from xenobiotics. However, dysfunction may occur when these systems are overloaded or imbalanced. Some studies have suggested an association between the ability of the body to adequately transform toxic xenobiotics and metabolites, and the etiology of various puzzling disease entities, such as chronic fatigue syndrome, fibromyalgia, and multiple chemical sensitivities.[12] Research has also begun to validate the hypothesis that chronic neurologic symptoms, such as those seen in Parkinson's disease, may result from impairment of detoxification ability.[13,14,15] A link between compromised detoxification ability and certain types of cancer has been reported, although the research is still evolving.[16,17,18] Xenobiotics implicated in cancer causation include polyaromatic hydrocarbons (often abbreviated as PAH) and asbestos. It has been suggested that many cases of cancer are due to compromised ability to adequately detoxify xenobiotics, a condition that may result from a genetic tendency toward lower detoxification activity, insufficient nutrient support for detoxification, and/or excessive intake of xenobiotics or environmental carcinogens.[19,20] These accumulated data suggest that an individual's ability to remove toxins from the body may play a role in the etiology or exacerbation of a range of chronic conditions and diseases.[21] We still say "may" for all these putative interconnections, because we really do not know for certain. Research is emerging all the time that casts doubt on earlier findings and opens new avenues for future investigations.[i] Linking detoxification to a specific disease in a research study is nearly impossible with today's tools, since the detoxification enzyme system is so complex and individualized, and is involved in supporting so many functions in the body. As in countless other areas of medicine, however, clinicians must still make decisions for their patients in the light of the best information available.

New functional assessment tools are now available to significantly enhance our understanding of biochemical differences between individuals. These tools allow clinicians to quantitatively analyze the body's ability to adequately detoxify the compounds to which it is exposed. Moreover, as our understanding of the underlying biochemical mechanisms involved in the regulation and nutritional support of the detoxification systems continues to deepen, the connections to disease are becoming clearer, and clinicians are gaining a better understanding of how to develop a therapeutic detoxification program.

Biotransformation

The conversion (biotransformation[22]) of toxic substances into non-toxic metabolites (and their subsequent excretion) takes place primarily at two major sites, although many systems are ultimately involved. The majority of detoxification occurs in the liver and secondarily in the intestinal mucosal wall. Some also occurs in other tissues, but to a lesser extent. As mentioned previously, the phase I and phase II processes biochemically transform toxic substances into progressively more water-soluble, and therefore excretable, substances through a series of chemical reactions (Figure 22.1).

Bioinactivation vs. Bioactivation

Biotransformation leads to changes in a molecule, increasing its water solubility and, in most cases, hastening its excretion. Many biotransformation reactions may also be considered bioinactivation or detoxification reactions. Bioinactivation generally means a decrease in the intensity of the toxic effect of a molecule because its presence is more transient and the toxic nature of the molecule is often reduced.

However, biotransformation reactions may also result in products that are more toxic than the parent compound. Such reactions are referred to as bioactivation reactions. Bioactivation reactions are more likely to occur in phase I of the biotransformation system. Let's look at an example of how this happens:

- The introduction of a polar moiety, which accompanies phase I reactions, is intended to prepare the molecule for conjugation reactions (phase II). However, this intermediate state is often more reactive than the original molecule, and it may interact with components of biological systems (e.g., proteins or DNA). For example, the organophosphate pesticide parathion is transformed into paraoxon by a phase I oxidation reaction. The resulting molecule is several times more potent a neurotoxin than its parent molecule.
- In a subsequent reaction, paraoxon can be hydrolyzed, as a result of which, the toxic effect on its target enzyme acetylcholinesterase is lost.
- Thus, the first biotransformation reaction, the oxidation to paraoxon, results in bioactivation, while the second reaction, the hydrolysis, results in bioinactivation.

Exposure

All organisms are exposed constantly and unavoidably to exogenous xenobiotics, as well as to the byproducts of metabolism, which can also be toxic. Fat solubility (lipophilicity) enables these substances to be absorbed and it also makes elimination of many xenobiotics a major challenge. Elimination of xenobiotics is most often determined by their conversion (biotransformation) to water-soluble chemicals by enzymes in the liver and other tissues that facilitate their elimination.

[i] Most of the research available on these topics is epidemiological, animal research, or bench science, so our knowledge of real effects in real people is still very limited. Animal research has been emphasized because animal models of drug research are accepted as evidence of human effects. However, a 2004 review article by MacDonald in *Toxicological Sciences* (v. 82:3-8) is replete with examples of highly significant differences between animal and human metabolism of drugs, particularly for "false positives": "Positive findings in long-term rodent studies do not necessarily predict human hazard." Guengerich observed in a 2003 review (*Molecular Interventions*, v. 3(4):194-204) that "The relevance of P450 modulation to cancer risk has not been easy to establish in humans ... ." He reports that early research linking lung and prostate cancers, for example, to P450 alterations has not been reproducible.

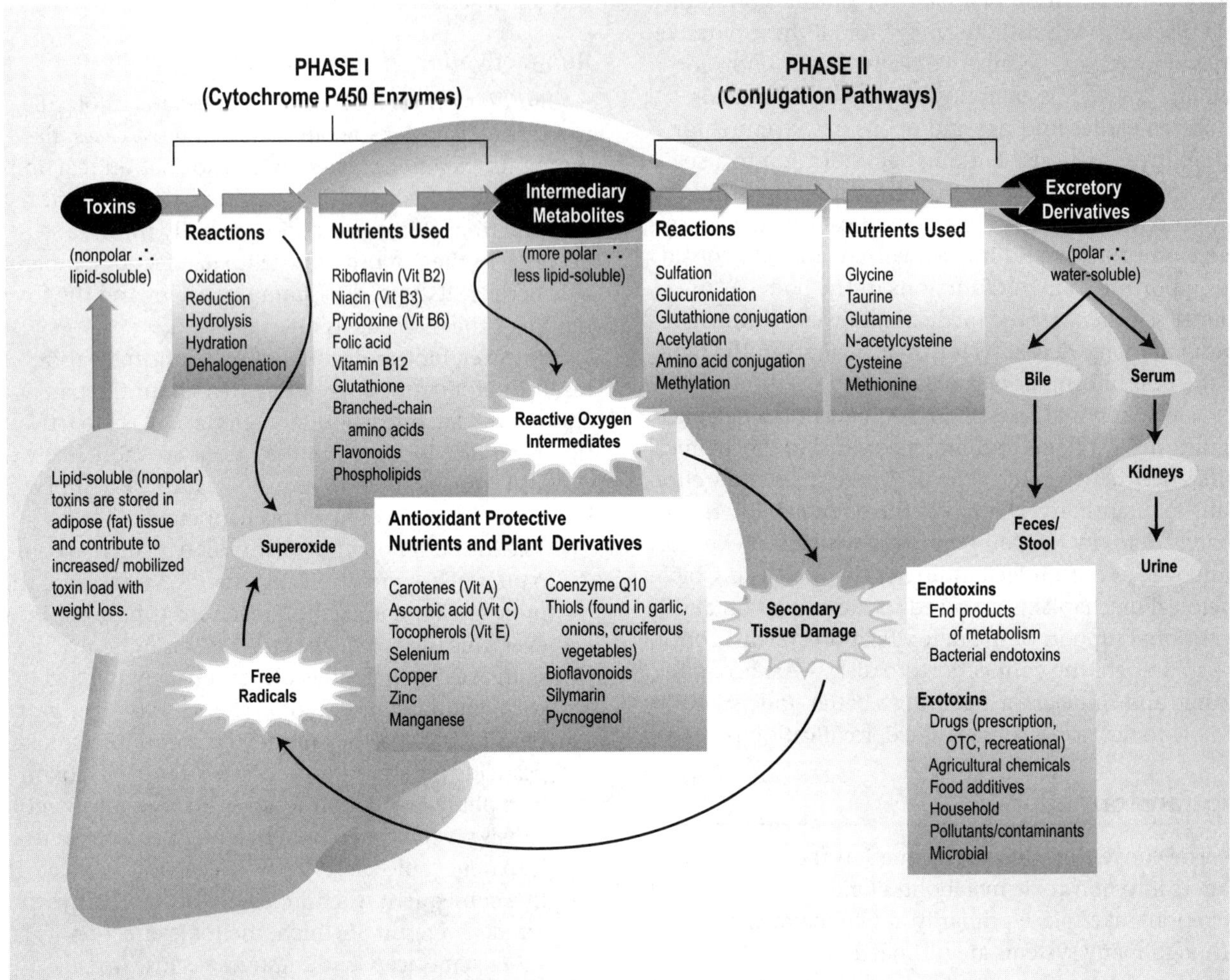

Figure 22.1 **Liver detoxification pathways and supportive nutrients**

Those highly lipophilic xenobiotics tend to readily penetrate lipid cell membranes and accumulate in fatty tissues. This is particularly true for lipophilic xenobiotics that are resistant to biotransformation (e.g., PCBs, DDT). Figure 22.2 demonstrates the process and sequencing of absorption, biotransformation, and excretion.

Phase I Reactions

Phase I detoxification is generally the first enzymatic defense against foreign compounds. In phase I, oxidation, reduction, and/or hydrolysis reactions are used to either expose or add a functional group, usually a hydroxyl (-OH), a carboxyl (-COOH), or an amino (-NH_2) group (see Figure 22.3). The structure of the molecule determines which of these reactions takes place. They are responsible for beginning the transformation process of detoxifying xenobiotics such as petrochemical hydrocarbons, many medications, and some endogenous substances (including steroid hormones and other end products of metabolism that would also be toxic if allowed to accumulate). In most cases, this biotransformation allows the phase I compound to undergo phase II conjugation reactions. In some cases, the compound may be eliminated directly after the phase I reaction.[23]

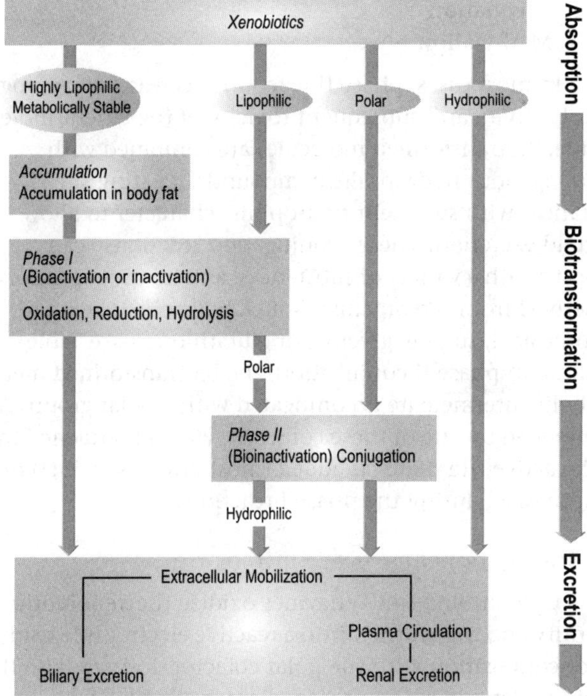

Figure 22.2 **Absorption, biotransformation, excretion**

The phase I system is actually a group of many isoenzymes (several hundred variations have been identified) that have affinities for different substrates. Although several types of phase I detoxification enzymes exist, the most common are the cytochrome P450 superfamily of mixed function oxidases.[24] P450s are responsible for metabolism of most xenobiotics[25] and have an extremely broad range of substrate specificities. The mammalian P450 enzymes are found predominantly in the endoplasmic reticulum and mitochondria in most cells.[26,27] The greatest abundance is in the liver; however, significant cytochrome P450 activity occurs in the gut wall, kidneys, lungs, and even the brain. Many forms of P450 enzymes have been isolated and their DNA sequences determined, providing evidence that these P450 enzymes are distinct gene products.[28] They are "involved in the metabolic oxidation, peroxidation, and reduction of many endogenous and exogenous compounds including xenobiotics, steroids, bile acids, fatty acids, eicosanoids, environmental pollutants, and carcinogens" and have been linked to the "development of numerous diseases and disorders including cancer and cardiovascular and endocrine dysfunction ... ."[29]

Type of Reaction	Substrate	Metabolite(s)
A. Oxidations		
I. Mixed-function oxidase-dependent reactions		
aromatic hydroxylation	R–C_6H_5 (benzene ring)	R–C_6H_4–OH
aliphatic hydroxylation	$R - CH_3$	$R - CH_2OH$
epoxidation	$R-C(H)=C(H)-R'$	$R-C(H)-C(H)-R'$ (O bridge)
N-hydroxylation	$C_6H_5-NH_2$	C_6H_5-NHOH
O-dealkylation	$R-O-CH_3$	$ROH + CH_2O$
N-dealkylation	$R-NHCH_3$	$R-NH_2 + CH_2O$
S-dealkylation	$R-S-CH_3$	$R-SH + CH_2O$
deamination	$R-CH(NH_2)-CH_3$	$R-C(=O)-CH_3 + NH_3$
S-oxidation	$R-S-R'$	$R-S(\rightarrow O)-R'$
dechlorination	CCl_4	$[CCl_3\bullet] \rightarrow CHCl_3$
oxidative desulfuration	$(R_1-O)(R_2-O)P(=S)-O-R_3$	$(R_1-O)(R_2-O)P(=O)-O-R_3$
II. Amine oxidation	$R-CH_2-NH_2$	$R-CHO + NH_3$
III. Dehydrogenation	CH_3-CH_2-OH	CH_3CHO CH_3COOH
B. Reductions		
azoreduction	$R-N=N-R'$	$R-NH_2 + R'-NH_2$
nitroreduction	$R-NO_2$	$R-NH_2$
carbonyl reduction	$R-C(=O)-R'$	$R-CH(OH)-R'$
C. Hydrolyses		
esters	$R-C(=O)-O-R'$	$R-C(=O)-OH - R'-OH$
amides	$R-CONH_2$	$R-COOH + NH_3$

Figure 22.3 **Overview of possible types of phase I biotransformation reactions**

The cytochrome P450 enzymes use oxygen and cofactor NADH (reduced nicotinamide adenine dinucleotide, which is the active form of niacin) to add a reactive hydroxyl radical. As a consequence of this step in detoxification, reactive molecules (which may be more toxic than the parent molecule) are produced. If these reactive molecules are not further metabolized by phase II conjugation, they may cause damage to proteins, RNA, and DNA within the cell. Several studies have shown evidence of associations between induced phase I cytochrome P450 activities and/or decreased phase II activities and an increased risk of diseases such as cancer[30] and Parkinson's disease.[31,32]

Although phase I activities detoxify both endogenous and exogenous molecules, most information on them has been derived from studies of drug metabolism. (Understanding and assessing the metabolism of endogenous molecules is a more difficult research pursuit.) Thanks to the rapid progress of technology, ongoing data collection is helping to elucidate the specific roles of many of these P450s in drug metabolism. Since environmental xenobiotics are detoxified by the same enzymes as drugs, there may be much we can learn from this research about where we might detect the effects of environmental xenobiotics on detoxification. Figure 22.4 shows the predominant interactions of drugs with nine P450 enzymes; these percentages represent the number of interactions of the substances with the enzymes, from data collected as of June 2001.[33] (This figure represents only a very small subset of the data published; the report is 365 pages long and identifies substrates, inducers, inhibitors, reactions, and other information for an amazing number of drugs and drug types.)

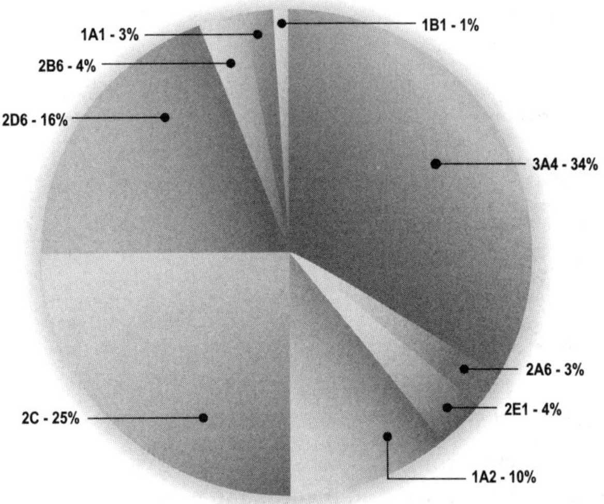

Figure 22.4 **Percentages of cytochrome P450s involved in drug interactions**

Phase II Reactions

The major phase II detoxification activities in humans include:

- Glucuronide conjugation (proceeds via enzymatic reactions in which active glucuronic acid is used)
- Sulfate conjugation (proceeds via enzymatic reactions in which active sulfate is used)
- Glutathione conjugation or mercapturic acid formation (an enzymatic process resulting from the conjugation of reactive intermediates with glutathione; the conjugated product is then converted into mercapturic acid and excreted)
- Amino acid conjugation
- Acetylation
- Methylation

In most cases, phase II reactions decrease the biological activity and subsequent toxicity of the parent molecule. Biotransformed molecules are combined with endogenous hydrophilic compounds, creating substances with sufficient hydrophilic character to allow rapid excretion. These "conjugation reactions" can occur with a variety of substances, and involve cofactors derived from the organism's metabolism (e.g., glucuronic acid, sulfate, glycine, or glutathione—see Table 22.2). In phase II conjugation, the biotransformed metabolic intermediate is conjugated with a polar group provided by one of these cofactors, which is attached to the active site that was added (most often as an OH) or unmasked during the phase I reactions.

Clinical Implications of Biotransformation

Cytochrome P450 enzymes oxidize the xenobiotic entity and transform it into a reactive electrophile ready for conjugation with the polar cofactor during phase II of the detoxification process. Because the biotransformed xenobiotics most often are more reactive than their parent molecules, this process plays a significant role in establishing or increasing the toxic nature of a xenobiotic. This reactive biotransformed intermediate may exert toxic effects within the liver (or systemically, if it escapes from the hepatocyte) if not immediately transformed further by one of the several conjugating enzymes (phase II detoxification). These effects may include one or more of the following reactions:

1. **Covalent binding of the reactive metabolite to:**
   - Proteins (e.g., cross linking of structural proteins; change in conformation of receptors, membrane pumps, enzyme carrier proteins, or peptide hormones).
   - Lipids (e.g., cell membrane phospholipid binds to reactive intermediate forming lipid-soluble xenobiotic and initiating lipid peroxidation).
   - Nucleic acids (e.g., irreversible binding to DNA, initiating carcinogenesis).

Table 22.2 **Major Phase II Detoxification Activities in Humans**

Reaction	Enzyme	Localization[a]	Substrates
H_2O	Epoxide hydrolase	Microsomes	Epoxides Cytosol
Glutathione	Glutathione transferases	Microsomes	Electrophiles
Glucuronic acid (UDPGA)[b]	Glucuronyl transferases	Microsomes	Phenols, thiols, amines Carboxylic acids
Sulfuric acid	Sulfotransferase	Cytosol	Phenols, thiols, amines (PAPS)[b]
Methyl group (SAM)[b]	N- and O-methyl transferases	Cytosol Microsomes	Phenols, amines
Acetic acid (Acetyl-CoA)[b]	N-acetyl transferases	Cytosol	Amines
Amino acids (Acetyl-CoA, taurine, glycine)	Amino acid transferases	Microsomes	Carboxylic acids

[a] Microsome refers to membrane-associated activities, but these activities may be localized to the cellular membrane or to internal membranes; cytosol refers to soluble activities present in the cytosolic portion of the cell.
[b] Abbreviations in parentheses are co-substrates: UDPGA = urindine-3,5′-diphosphoglucuronic acid; PAPS = 3′-phosphoadenosine 5′-phosphosulfate; SAM = S-adenosylmethionine; CoA = coenzyme A.

2. **Creating (or increasing) oxidative stress:**
   - Cytochrome P450 enzymes are oxidases which, in the process of xenobiotic biotransformation, generate reactive oxygen species (superoxide, peroxide, or hydroxyl radicals) in excess of the normal flux of reactive oxygen species generated by mitochondrial respiratory activity.
   - Xenobiotics, once biotransformed, are reactive electrophiles which are quenched by cellular antioxidant defenses (superoxide dismutase, catalase, glutathione peroxidase). This excess demand for antioxidant activity can lead to depletion of cellular antioxidant defenses, thus increasing oxidative stress.

Phase I detoxification requires little nutritional support to be fully active. In fact, during fasting or starvation, phase I activity may increase substantially while circulating xenobiotics are freed from both adipose and lean tissue, resulting in a significant increase in toxic stress. Therefore, traditional approaches to fasting or detoxification involving minimal nutritional support for an extended period of time may have negative clinical consequences in chronically ill patients. For excretion of xenobiotics to be effective, phase I activity requires antioxidant support and phase II activity requires specific nutritional support.

Importance of Balancing Phase I and Phase II Detoxification

Proper functioning of both phases is essential because the reactive intermediate metabolites produced during phase I may be more harmful or toxic than the original substance. The two phases must be functioning in balance to successfully complete the detoxification process. The amounts and types of steroids, fatty acids, and other endogenous molecules involved in cellular communication can also be greatly influenced by altered or compromised detoxification status of an individual. Therefore, the balance of activities between the phase I and phase II processes is of fundamental important in detoxification and, as shown in Figure 22.1, less tissue damage from oxidant stress and free radical generation occurs when these reactive intermediates are promptly and efficiently acted upon by a phase II reaction. If phase II reactions are inhibited in some way, or if phase I has been upregulated without a concomitant increase in phase II, the optimal balance may be compromised (imbalanced detoxification). Furthermore, the phase II reactions require cofactors that are consumed during the process and must be replenished through dietary sources and energy in the form of ATP.[34]

The Role of the Intestine in Detoxification

Most literature on detoxification refers to liver enzymes and to the liver as the site of the majority of detoxification activity for both endogenous and exogenous compounds. However, the gastrointestinal lining is the first point of contact for the majority of xenobiotics. Over the course of a lifetime, the gastrointestinal tract processes more than 25 tons of food, which represents the largest load of antigens and xenobiotics confronting the human body.[35] Furthermore, because most drugs are consumed orally, the gastrointestinal tract is also the body's first contact with many drugs. It is not surprising, then, that the gastrointestinal tract has developed a complex set of physical and biochemical systems to manage this load of exogenous compounds. Several factors influence how much of a chemical ends up in the systemic circulation, thus requiring detoxification by the liver.

The gastrointestinal tract initially provides a physical barrier to exogenous components, but it also influences detoxification in several other ways.[36,37] (An extended discussion of this subject can be found in Chapter 31.) Gut microflora can produce compounds that either induce or inhibit detoxification activities. Pathogenic bacteria can produce toxins that enter the circulation and increase toxic load (more information about toxic load can be found further along in this chapter). Moreover, in a process called enterohepatic recirculation, the gut microflora also has the ability to remove some of the conjugation moieties. Once moieties such as glucuronyl side chains are removed, the xenobiotic may revert to its original form and re-enter the circulation, leading to an increased toxic load.

Detoxification enzymes such as CYP3A4 and the antiporter activities (Figure 22.5) have been found in high concentrations at the tip of villi in the intestine.[38,39] Adequate first-pass metabolism of xenobiotics by the gastrointestinal tract requires integrity of the gut mucosa. Compromised barrier function of the mucosa will more easily allow xenobiotics to transit into circulation without an opportunity for detoxification. Support for healthy gut mucosa is instrumental in decreasing toxic load.

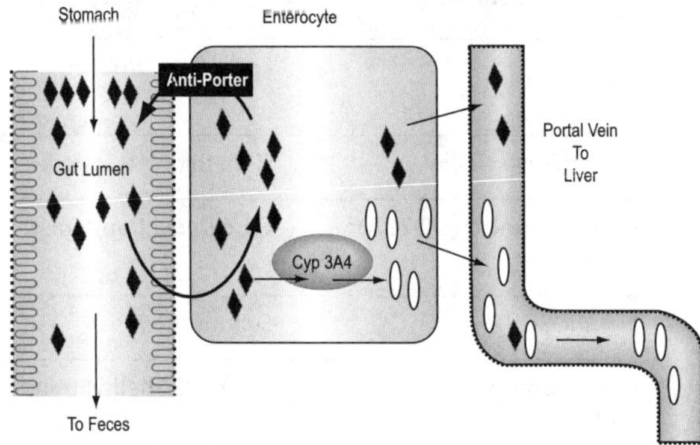

The antiporter acts as a pump to transport the xenobiotic back into the gut lumen, allowing another opportunity for metabolism by CYP3A4 in the enterocyte.

Figure 22.5 **Phase III metabolism: The antiporter**

Recently, antiporter activity (p-glycoprotein or multidrug resistance) was re-defined as the phase III detoxification system in some literature, although the term has not caught on with everyone in the scientific field.[40] Antiporter activity is an important factor in the first-pass metabolism of pharmaceuticals and other xenobiotics. The antiporter process is an energy-dependent efflux pump that pumps xenobiotics out of a cell, thereby decreasing the intracellular concentration of such substances.[41] Since many of the detoxification enzymes are located at or near the cell membrane barrier, if a xenobiotic is not metabolized the first time it is taken into a cell, the process of pumping it out of the cell and back into the intestinal lumen and then taking it into the cell again (a recirculation process) affords the cell another opportunity to metabolize the substance before it gets too far within the cytosol, where it can do damage. Antiporter activity in the intestine appears to be co-regulated with the intestinal phase I CYP3A4 enzyme, providing further support for its role in detoxification.

Two genes encoding antiporter activity have been described: multidrug resistance gene 1 (MDR1) and multidrug resistance gene 2 (MDR2). The MDR1 gene product is responsible for drug resistance of many cancer cells and is normally found in epithelial cells in liver, kidney, pancreas, small and large intestine, brain, and testes. MDR2 activity is expressed primarily in the liver and may play a role similar to that of intestinal MDR1 for liver detoxification enzymes; however, its function is currently undefined. One downside to the antiporters has been the observation that they are sometimes overexpressed in cancer cells, allowing those cells a protection against chemotherapy. For this reason, clinical trials are underway to evaluate the use of inhibitors of antiporter activity in cancer cells to enhance the activity of chemotherapeutic agents in resistant cancers.[42,43,44] A third, similar gene has also been described (MDR3), but its role in detoxification has not been elucidated.[45,46]

Regulation of Detoxification Activities

Detoxification systems help manage exposure to exogenous compounds, and a number of factors influence the activity of the enzymes involved in this process. Specific detoxification pathways may be induced or inhibited, depending on the presence of various dietary or xenobiotic compounds, the age and sex of the individual, lifestyle habits such as smoking, and genetics. Furthermore, disease can also influence activity of the enzymes. In some disease states, detoxification activities appear to be induced or upregulated, but in other conditions these activities may be inhibited from acting or not produced at high levels.

Factors influencing detoxification:
Diet and lifestyle
Environment (xenobiotic exposure)
Genetic polymorphisms
Age and gender
Disease
Medications (competitive inhibition)

Induction Activities

Several situations can cause induction of phase I and phase II enzyme activities. When the body is faced with a high xenobiotic load, the phase I and/or phase II enzymes involved in detoxifying the compound(s) can be induced, leading to a greater amount of enzyme and a faster rate of detoxification. Inducers can upregulate selectively, affecting only one enzyme or one phase of detoxification, or broadly, affecting multiple activities.[47]

For example, polycyclic hydrocarbons from cigarette smoke and aryl amines from charbroiled meats result in dramatic induction of the CYP1A1 and CYP1A2 enzymes. This leads to a substantial increase in phase I activity, with little or no induction of phase II enzymes.[48,49,50] Also, taking phenobarbitol for epilepsy can eventually lead to chronic induction of phase I. Induction of some phase I activities without co-induction of phase II may lead to an uncoupling of the phase I and phase II balance and, therefore, a higher level of reactive intermediates that can cause damage to DNA, RNA, and proteins.

Many compounds in the flavonoid family (found in fruits and vegetables) are capable of inducing multiple phase II activities. For example, ellagic acid in red grape skin has been shown to induce several of the phase II enzymes while decreasing phase I activity.[51,52] Cruciferous vegetables (the Brassica family, such as cabbage, bok choy, broccoli, and Brussels sprouts), garlic oil, rosemary, and soy all contain compounds that can induce several phase II enzyme activities.[53,54,55,56] Commonly, the glutathione S-transferase and glucuronyl transferases are co-induced by these multifunctional inducers. In general, this increase in phase II supports better detoxification in an individual and helps promote and maintain a healthy balance between phase I and phase II activities. This enhancement of phase II activity has been proposed to explain, at least in part, the ability of fruits and vegetables to protect against many cancers.[57,58,59,60]

Inhibition Activities

Both phase I and phase II enzyme activities can also be inhibited. Inhibition can occur by competition between two or more compounds for the same detoxifying enzyme. Increased toxic load can lead to inhibition of a number of compounds by simply overwhelming the systems and competing for multiple detoxification enzyme activities—a process called competitive inhibition. Some compounds selectively inhibit only one detoxifying activity, such as quinidine, which competitively inhibits CYP2D6 activity. Cimetidine is an example of a compound that can bind directly to the heme iron of the cytochrome P450 reactive site to inhibit phase I metabolism. Much has been written about grapefruit juice, which contains high amounts of the flavonoid naringenin, and its ability to inhibit first-pass metabolism of many drugs that are detoxified through the CYP3A4 enzyme-antiporter system in the intestine.[61,62] Table 22.3 lists some pharmaceutical inhibitors of phase I cytochrome P450 enzymes; a more complete list of inhibitors and inducers of P450 enzymes can be found in the Appendix.

Table 22.3 **Some Pharmaceutical Inhibitors of Phase I Cytochrome P450 Enzymes**

Pharmaceutical	P450 Enzyme Inhibited
H2-Receptor Blockers	
Cimetidine	All Cytochrome P450s
Antiarrhythmics	
Quinidine	CYP2D6
Propafenone	CYP2D6
Antibiotics	
Erythromycin	CYP3A4
Clarithromycin	CYP3A4
Troleandomycin	CYP3A4
Fluoroquinolones	CYP1A2
Antidepressants	
Nefazodone	CYP3A4
Fluoxetine	CYP2D6, CYP2C19, CYP3A4
Norfluoxetine	CYP2D6, CYP1A2
Paroxetine	CYP2D6
Sertraline	CYP2D6
Antifungals	
Itraconazole	CYP3A4
Fluconazole	CYP3A4
Ketoconazole	CYP3A4

A common mechanism of inhibition for some of the phase II enzymes is depletion of necessary cofactors. In humans, sulfation is particularly susceptible to inhibition due to compromised cofactor status. The serum sulfate concentration is a balance between (1) absorption of inorganic sulfate and its production from cysteine, and (2) elimination of sulfate by urinary excretion and sulfation of low molecular weight substrates. In humans, the serum sulfate level varies dramatically over 24 hours, and is decreased in individuals who are fasting or ingesting high levels of substances that are metabolized by sulfation (such as acetaminophen). Humans excrete approximately 20 to 25 millimoles of sulfate in 24 hours; therefore, sulfate reserves must be maintained through dietary intake of sulfur-containing amino acids or inorganic sulfate, both of which have been shown to support increased serum sulfate levels.[63]

Detoxifying Enzymes and Genetic Polymorphism

A significant amount of data has now accumulated demonstrating that widespread genetic polymorphisms for the expression of cytochrome P450 enzymes exist within the human species.[64,65] Population studies have shown great variations in individual metabolizing ability for all detoxification pathways, including both cytochrome P450 systems and conjugating pathways.[66,67] A well-described polymorphism in this category is a low activity form of CYP2D6, an enzyme that is an important metabolizer of many narrow-spectrum drugs, including antiarrhythmics, antidepressants, and antipsychotics. Individuals with this polymorphism comprise 5–10% of Caucasian populations and are referred to as poor metabolizers (PMs). This impairment may affect the metabolism of more than 25 therapeutic drugs and a wide range of xenobiotics, to different degrees within different individuals.[68] Because each of us has two alleles (two genes encoding a specific gene), it is possible to have one gene that encodes the wild type (average activity) and another one with a SNP that encodes lower activity. Individuals who receive two versions of the gene encoding a slower CYP2D6 activity have a severely limited ability to metabolize xenobiotics that require this enzyme.[69] Research has suggested that adverse side effects occurring from drugs that need CYP2D6 activity for elimination may be reduced by decreasing dosages in those individuals who are slow metabolizers of CYP2D6.[70]

On the other end of the spectrum are individuals described as extensive metabolizers (EMs). Such individuals require a higher dose of certain drugs to achieve therapeutic effects and may have a more robust capability to handle certain environmental toxins. Although apparently less common than PMs, EMs have been identified for CYP2D6. Heritable polymorphisms are also known for several conjugating enzymes (phase II detoxification) that are extensively involved in the metabolism of exogenous chemicals.[71] For example, genetic polymorphisms of the glutathione-S-transferase (phase II, glutathione conjugation) enzyme family are known to occur,[72] and are regarded as a significant factor conferring susceptibility to environmental toxins. The role of these genotypic variants in the development of functional illnesses such as chronic fatigue syndrome or fibromyalgia may be significant, but the subject has not been well studied.

Distinguishing phenotypic variability from polymorphic genetic variability adds to the complexity of understanding human individuality. "Genotypic variability is easy to identify by means of polymerase chain reaction-based or DNA chip-based methods, whereas phenotypic variability requires direct measurement of enzyme activities in liver, or, indirectly, measurement of the rate of metabolism of a given compound *in vivo*. There is a great deal of phenotypic variability in human beings, only a minor part being attributable to gene polymorphisms."[73,74]

Metallothioneins and Genetic Polymorphism

One of the most important detoxification systems in all species, from bacteria to humans, depends upon the production of a family of at least four different proteins known as metallothioneins (MT). MTs are highly unusual proteins composed of about 30% cysteine. They are responsible for storage, transfer, and detoxification of intracellular metal ions.[75] The primary role of MT in the absence of toxic metals is the transport and short-term storage of zinc and copper. However, the importance of MT in protection against and elimination of toxic metals is also well described. MT is known to efficiently bind several toxic metals (particularly cadmium and mercury) and act as a transporter of the toxic metal to the liver or kidneys where glutathione conjugation and subsequent excretion of the toxic metal may then take place. Because MT forms high affinity complexes with several metals, it may prevent toxic metals from reacting with other biomolecules, or acting as free radical catalysts, thus attenuating their toxicity.[76]

There is a wide variation in the concentration of MTs between species. Humans, for example, have about ten times the concentration of MT in their organs as do rats or mice. Additionally, genotypic polymorphisms for expression of certain MTs within a species have been demonstrated. Mutant mice and rat models have been identified with complete absence of the genes for one out of four MT isoforms. In these MT-deficient animals, susceptibility to the toxic effects of heavy metals is increased by 60 to 100-fold. In contrast to this, it has been shown in animal models that resistance to heavy metal toxicity may be conferred in mutants possessing multiple copies of MT genes in their chromosomes. These animals may be capable of more prolific upregulation of MT production.[77]

Genetic polymorphisms for MT expression also exist in humans.[78] Human cancer cell lines are known to be highly polymorphic in their ability to express MT genes. This is a primary reason that cancer patients vary in their resistance to metal cancer chemotherapeutic drugs.[79] Some laboratories have begun to offer test panels to assess MT function. These assays may provide clinically significant means to screen an individual's susceptibility to metal intoxication. Importantly, gene expression for MT production is highly inducible (e.g., through zinc supplementation, fasting, and exercise).[80,81,82,83] Because of this, working with factors that induce optimal production of MT may be important during a heavy metal detoxification regimen.

The emerging field of toxicogenomics will undoubtedly revolutionize medicine and pharmacology on several fronts.[84] Assessing a patient's genetic susceptibility to environmental toxins or adverse drug reactions will enable clinicians to tailor their interventions and will likely lead to more effective treatments for patients with a variety of complex disorders.

Age, Gender, and Disease Influences

Several other factors also influence expression and the resultant activity of many detoxification enzymes. For example, similar to many other proteins, detoxification activities are under strict developmental control. The phase I CYP3A enzymes and the phase II enzymes catalyzing glucuronidation, sulfation, and glutathione conjugation are present in the human fetus. At birth, these enzymes are capable of catalyzing most biotransformation reactions, but the rate of these reactions is generally slower than in adults. Within the first two weeks of life, phase I and phase II detoxification systems become more fully expressed.[85] However, as the body ages, the phase I and II detoxification pathways decline in efficiency and effectiveness, likely contributing to many of the health effects associated with aging.[86,87]

Gender also affects the type, amount, and activity of various detoxification enzymes. The CYP3A family of detoxification enzymes is particularly sensitive to hormones. The CYP3A4 enzyme appears to be regulated, at least in part, by progesterone or the ratio of progesterone to estrogen. For example, premenopausal women generally show 30% to 40% more CYP3A4 activity than men or postmenopausal women.[88] Pregnant women also appear to have increased levels of CYP3A activity as well. CYP3A4 is the major phase I detoxification pathway for the anti-epileptic agents phenobarbital and phenytoin. Researchers have suggested this hormone regulation of CYP3A explains why many women require a higher dose of antiepileptic medications during their pregnancy.[89]

Disease and health status of the individual also affect detoxification activities. Because the majority of detoxification occurs in the liver, it is not surprising that impairment of normal liver function due to alcoholic disease, fatty liver disease, biliary cirrhosis, and hepatocarcinomas can lead to lower detoxification activity in general. The phase I and phase II enzyme activities are localized differently within a cell. Phase I activities are associated with membrane, but the majority of phase II activity occurs in the cytosol (fluid component of the cytoplasm). Different types of phase I and phase II activities may be localized differently in the organ systems as well, which is the case in the liver. This compartmentalization means that a disease that influences one region of the liver may affect some activities more than others. Moreover, influences on cell membrane integrity (for example, from dietary lipids or oxidation of membrane lipids) could influence phase I activity more than phase II. Therefore, the amount of decrease in detoxification activity resulting from disease or loss of integrity of the tissue may vary from one isozyme to another.

Some conditions can actually increase or induce detoxification system function. The phase I activity of CYP2E1 is a good example of this. CYP2E1 catalyzes oxidation of ethyl alcohol to acetaldehyde, and also detoxifies many of the small carbon-chain molecules, including ketone bodies, that result from gluconeogenesis and the breakdown of fatty acids. CYP2E1 is increased in insulin-dependent diabetes, in morbidly obese individuals, and, conversely, during starvation.[90,91] The reason CYP2E1 is induced in morbidly obese individuals and during starvation is not fully understood; however, it may have to do with the role CYP2E1 plays in metabolism of products from gluconeogenesis and energy metabolism and may influence how these pathways become imbalanced during altered metabolism. The full range of changes in other detoxification systems in response to health status is not fully understood.

Induction of various P450 isoenzymes can be detrimental when carcinogens are not capable of causing genetic damage until they undergo activation to a reactive (electrophilic) intermediate.[92] For example, it has been shown that the risk for hepatic carcinoma is associated with the degree or activity of a particular isoenzyme of the cytochrome P450 system.[93] Another example is seen in individuals with a high inducibility phenotype for phase I CYP1A1. These individuals appear to have a higher risk for cancer, regardless of exposure to smoking or other known carcinogens.[94] As many cancers can be related to environmental exposure or dietary intake, it is apparent that individual detoxification ability can be an important factor in their development.[95]

Effects of Medications

The consequences of defective drug metabolizing enzymes and pathways in a patient are varied:

- Inefficient elimination of an active drug or toxic substance may cause a functional overdose.
- Inefficient activation or increased elimination of a drug may result in a lack of efficacy.
- Symptoms of toxicity, with idiosyncracies unrelated to the substance, may appear.
- Exacerbation of symptoms in chronic conditions may occur.
- Association with an apparently spontaneous disease has been noted.[96]

Various medications such as SSRIs, macrolide antibiotics, and H2 blockers (e.g., cimetidine) may inhibit one or more of the phase I enzyme systems (Table 22.3).[97] When this occurs, endogenous and exogenous toxicants may remain in the body untransformed, thus causing toxic reactions. In 1998, using a meta-analysis procedure, researchers from the University of Toronto reported that fatal adverse drug events from correctly prescribed medications are much more common than previously identified and may be between the fourth and sixth leading cause of death in hospitals in the United States.[98] These researchers attempted to exclude adverse events associated with errors in drug administration, drug abuse, and accidental poisoning. The authors of the study suggest that these adverse drug events may result from factors such as age, gender, and multiple drug exposure. Unfortunately, no data exist to correlate adverse drug events with detoxification profiles. However, accumulated data suggest that individuals with inhibited or compromised detoxification pathways would be more susceptible to adverse drug events.[99] There is considerable discussion in the research literature of ways to integrate into clinical practice genotyping for the purposes of enhancing drug safety and maximizing drug efficacy.[100] Gene expression profiling for anticancer drugs,[101,102] antidepressants and antipsychotics,[103] and many others is now available in research settings; the challenge will be to bring the technology—and the expert interpretation of the data—into the clinical setting.

Functional Assessment of Phase I and II Detoxification and Toxic Load

The detoxification system in humans is extensive, highly complex, and under myriad regulatory mechanisms. Until recently, science has had difficulty calculating and objectively analyzing the individual response to toxic compounds. In any large population exposed to the same low levels of carcinogens, some individuals will develop cancer while others will not. The variability that one finds here and in other diseases appears to be associated, in part, with the individual's ability to detoxify various pro-carcinogens and other xenobiotics. Therefore, it is not only the level of the toxin in the environment, but also the total amount of toxin in the individual—and his or her response to that load—that is significant.

Toxic Load[ii]

Understanding how xenobiotics affect human health is germane to the concept of *total load*. Total load describes the total of all exposures and influences that bear on human physiology. Since these factors often determine the efficiency of the body's detoxification system, nutrient status and organ reserve, they are central to any question of how xenobiotics affect humans. The concept of total load suggests that the totality of factors can seriously affect an individual's system of metabolic management.

For many years, efforts to understand how xenobiotics affect human health focused on determining whether or not a substance produced cancer in laboratory animals. Once studies confirmed this finding for animals, researchers applied these studies to humans. While these efforts provided much insight into detoxification, metabolism, and cell biology, in many ways they now detract from more pertinent questions, such as: What is the capacity of xenobiotics to alter the *function* of biological systems, and how does this contribute to illness? According to the latter perspective, cancer, as an end-stage manifestation of chemical exposure, seems to be only a second-order issue, since so many physiological events precede its development.

In the early 1990s, two seminal volumes published by the National Academy of Sciences raised concerns about the *functional* changes induced by exposure to low levels of xenobiotics. These volumes, *Environmental Neurotoxicology*[104] and *Biologic Markers in Immunotoxicology*,[105] highlight two important issues—functional changes result from low-level chemical exposure, and their effects can multiply when an individual is exposed to more than one agent.

An animal study about the lethal dose of lead and mercury dramatically illustrates this latter point—the multiplicity of toxic effects. In this study, scientists administered LD1 of mercury *combined* with the LD1 of lead to animals. (LD1 is the acute dose leading to death of 1% of a test population. LD50 refers to the dose that produces a fatal response in 50% of the animals and is a typical measure used in toxicology.) Remarkably, the LD1 of mercury + LD1 of lead resulted in LD100, or 100% mortality, within five days.[106] This study demonstrated a profound difference in outcome between low-toxicity substances administered in combination and low-toxicity substances administered alone.

Given the ubiquitous nature of chemicals in the environment, it is likely that *single* exposure is more the exception than the rule. It is also likely that, despite considerable research, we actually know very little about the true effects of chemicals on human function, because so little research is done on chemical synergy. More important, considering the little we know about factors that influence physiologic function and their synergistic effect on chemical function, determining the effect of chemicals on human function is extremely difficult.

However, working within the concept of total load, it is clear that assessing both the sources of foreign substances and the patient's ability to deal with and process those foreign substances is central to the question of how toxicants and xenobiotics differentially affect humans. Rea[107,108] has succinctly outlined the following factors that influence the total load phenomenon:

- Xenobiotics (insecticides, herbicides, drugs, solvents, metals, etc.)

[ii] Excerpted from *Clinical Nutrition: A Functional Approach* (2nd Ed). Institute for Functional Medicine, Gig Harbor, WA: 2004.

- Infections (streptococcus, pseudomonas, parasites, etc.)
- Toxins (aflatoxin, fusarium, penicillium toxins, ergot toxins, etc.)
- Biological inhalants (molds, algae, pollens, foods, etc.)
- Physical phenomena (electromagnetic fields, ionizing radiation)
- Lifestyle (drinking, smoking, etc.)
- Mechanical problems (biomechanical dysfunction, such as nasal, intestinal, or other obstruction)
- Hormonal aberration (DHEA, cortisol, estrogen, progesterone, testosterone, etc.)
- Psychosocial factors (stress, coping skills, belief systems, psychological trauma)

While nutritional status is not a direct part of the total load, the factors noted above are widespread and influenced by nutritional status. Rea, who has followed more than 20,000 patients with chemical sensitivity, reported laboratory evidence that nutrient abnormalities are widespread among these patients. He noted that nutrient supplementation was central to restoring physiologic balance; however, reducing total load was also essential to patient recovery. His findings suggest that total load *and* nutrient metabolism are inseparable components of any program designed to manage the physiological alteration associated with chemicals.

Challenge Testing

In assessing an individual's detoxification ability, one evaluates the functional capacity of his or her detoxification systems. The complexity of those systems (and the biochemical uniqueness of each individual) suggests that a single test or type of assay to fully assess detoxification status may not be possible. For some enzyme activities, such as CYP2D6, which is primarily influenced by genetics, determination of slow or fast metabolism is possible with one gene analysis. However, to understand the detoxification profile of a particular individual at a moment in time, other approaches are necessary.

Measuring functional capacity and performance of an organ system or biochemical pathway is not new. Exercise EKG and the oral glucose tolerance tests are two common challenge tests in which functional capacity and, therefore, organ reserve are appraised. A challenge test differs substantially from the more commonly used clinical assessments, such as the liver tests found in most serology panels.

The standard liver tests SGOT, GGPT, and SGPT measure liver pathology—not liver metabolic function.[109] Elevation of these enzymes in the serum occurs as a consequence of hepatocyte damage. Because the majority of detoxification occurs in the liver, a clinician may make the assumption that elevated liver enzymes may also mean compromised detoxification ability. However, because the different detoxification activities are compartmentalized and detoxification occurs in other tissues as well, establishing a definitive link between elevated liver markers and altered detoxification is not always possible; altered detoxification can be demonstrated without any changes in these liver enzyme markers and, conversely, these markers may be altered and some detoxification functions may be performing adequately.

Challenge tests measure the detoxifying ability of an individual when challenged with a test substance. These tests allow assessment of the metabolic capacity of the detoxification systems, and thus provide a functional view of an individual's ability to adequately deal with his or her environment.

To evaluate the various metabolic pathways of detoxification discussed above, probe substances (see Table 22.4), whose detoxification pathways are well established, are ingested. Their metabolites are measured in the urine, blood, or saliva. This type of test takes into account the myriad factors influencing detoxification capacity, and remains the standard today. [110,111,112,113]

Probe substances. Many environmental toxins, such as those in polyaromatic hydrocarbons used as pesticides, several carcinogens in cigarette smoke, and the polyaromatic amines found in charbroiled beef, are detoxified by CYP1A2 activity. Genetics, nutrition, medications, and environmental factors (including alcohol, heavy metals, and smoking) can all influence the inducibility of this enzyme system. [114,115,116,117,118,119,120]

Research over the past 20 years has shown that the caffeine challenge test is a useful, non-invasive way to assess CYP1A2 detoxification activity.[121] Elevation or depression of the rate of caffeine clearance suggests upregulation or downregulation, respectively, of the phase I system. For this challenge test, a defined amount of caffeine is ingested, after which two to three saliva samples are obtained at specified times. Caffeine is almost completely absorbed by the intestine, and its rate of clearance is measured in saliva.[122,123] Dietary elimination of caffeine-containing foods and medications should be instituted 24 hours before the test.

Table 22.4 **Examples of *in vivo* Probes for Drug Metabolizing Enzymes**

Enzyme	Probe Drug(s)
CYP1A2	Caffeine
CyP2C9	Tolbutamide
CYP2C19	Mephenytoin, Proguanil
CYP2D6	Sparteine, Dextromethorphan, Debrisoquine
CYP2E1	Chlorzoxazone
CYP3A4	Erythromycin (breath test), Midazolam, 6β-Hydroxycortisol
N-acetyl transferase	Sulphadimidine, Isoniazid, Caffeine
Glucuronyl transferase	Oxazepam, Acetaminophen
Sulfation	Acetaminophen
Glycination	Benzoic acid, Salicylate

As previously mentioned, phase II reactions involve a number of distinct conjugating substances. The most important appear to be amino acid conjugation, glutathione conjugation, glucuronidation, and sulfation. Acetaminophen has been used as a probe substance to assess glucuronidation and sulfation. Acetaminophen is primarily metabolized directly through the phase II sulfation and glucuronidation pathways to form urinary acetaminophen sulfate and acetaminophen glucuronide, respectively.[124] (Figure 22.6 depicts acetaminophen detoxification in humans.) If these pathways are inhibited or compromised due to depleted cofactor status, the acetaminophen is metabolized through an alternate pathway requiring a phase I biotransformation followed by conjugation with glutathione and conversion to acetaminophen mercapturate. The biotransformed intermediate, N-acetyl-p-benzoquinoneimine (NAPQI), is a highly neurotoxic substance and, if not rapidly cleared by glutathione conjugation, can result in severe toxicity.[125] The standard emergency treatment for acetaminophen overdose is to use high levels of N-acetylcysteine to detoxify NAPQI.

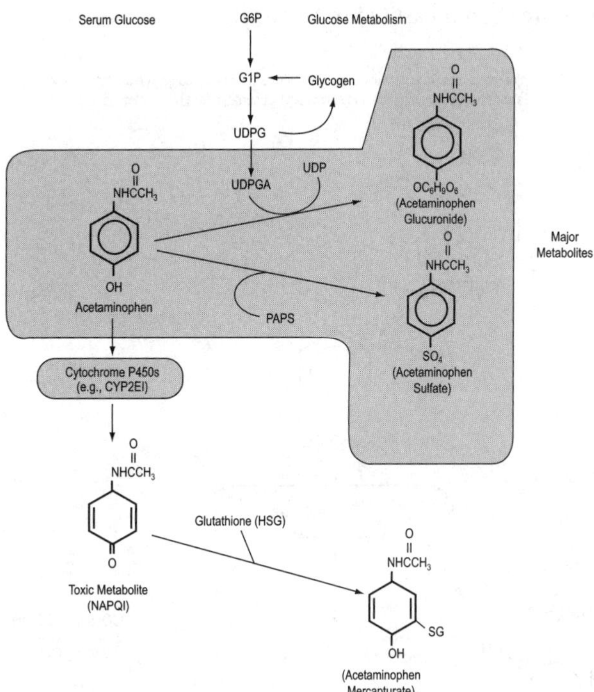

Figure 22.6 **The detoxification of acetaminophen in humans**

The major metabolites from the detoxification of acetaminophen are acetaminophen glucuronide and acetaminophen sulfate. Acetaminophen mercapturate is a minor metabolite and N-acetyl-p-benzoquinoneimine (NAPQI) is a hepatotoxic intermediate that may accumulate if phase I activity is induced and/or the phase II glutathione conjugation pathway is unable to further metabolize NAPQI to the mercapturate for excretion.

Several amino acids are used as conjugation moieties for amino acid conjugation, including glycine, taurine, arginine, and ornithine. The glycine conjugation pathway appears to be a major amino acid conjugation pathway in humans and, therefore, can be a means of evaluating amino acid conjugation activity. The glycine conjugation pathway can be assessed using either aspirin or sodium benzoate as probe substances. Aspirin is readily degraded into salicylic acid, which is eventually conjugated and metabolized through glycine conjugation and glucuronidation to form salicyluric acid (the major metabolite) and salicyl glucuronides (minor metabolites), respectively (Figure 22.7).[126] Alternatively, in individuals with salicylate sensitivities, the common food preservative sodium benzoate can be used to assess phase II glycine conjugation.[127] Either way, the metabolites are then measured in the urine.

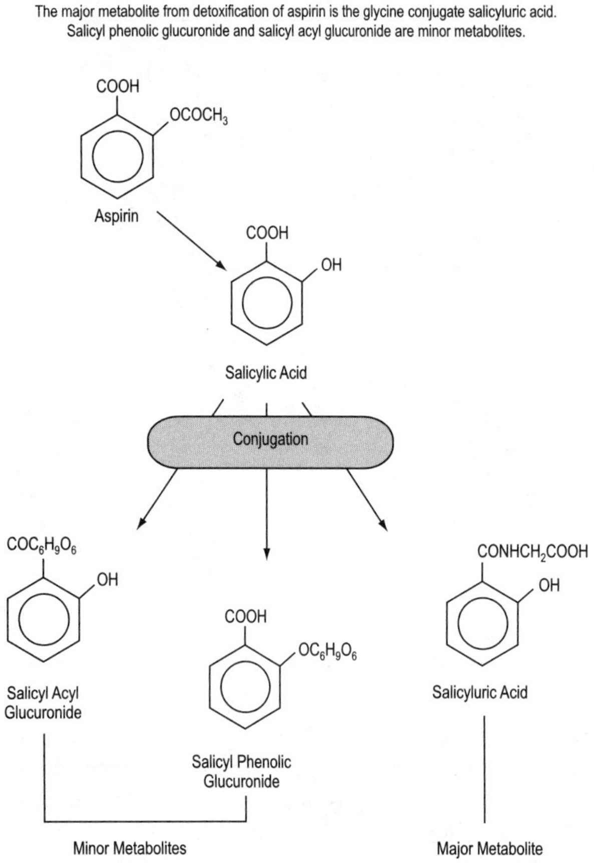

The major metabolite from detoxification of aspirin is the glycine conjugate salicyluric acid. Salicyl phenolic glucuronide and salicyl acyl glucuronide are minor metabolites.

COOH
$OCOCH_3$
Aspirin
COOH
OH
Salicylic Acid
Conjugation
$COC_6H_9O_6$
OH
Salicyl Acyl Glucuronide
COOH
$OC_6H_9O_6$
Salicyl Phenolic Glucuronide
$CONHCH_2COOH$
OH
Salicyluric Acid
Minor Metabolites
Major Metabolite

Figure 22.7 **The detoxification of aspirin in humans**

These probe markers serve as useful, well-researched challenge substances for functional evaluation of four important phase II detoxification pathways.[128] As with the caffeine challenge, foods and medications containing aspirin, acetaminophen, and sodium benzoate are eliminated 24 hours prior to challenge tests utilizing those substances. Using a combination of probe substances to measure sulfation, glucuronidation, glycination, and activation of phase I activity, a clinician is provided with an assessment of an individual's detoxification capacity that offers insight into the unique response and possible sensitivity the patient may display to his or her environment.

For most toxins in need of detoxification, multiple pathways are involved. Under optimal conditions, there is a particular affinity of a xenobiotic for a particular pathway. The body may compensate for an underdeveloped, or bottlenecked, pathway. Alternative pathways may be less desirable because of incomplete detoxification or accumulation of toxic intermediates, as described above. Not only are the sufficiencies of the various individual pathways important, but the relative balance of phase I and phase II detoxification is critical, as it determines the longevity of the biotransformed intermediates.

Testing for the Presence of Toxic Elements

Testing for the presence of the most common toxic elements, mercury (Hg), lead (Pb), arsenic (As), cadmium (Cd), aluminum (Al), and nickel (Ni), can be an integral part of the overall assessment.[129] These toxic elements are largely undetected by standard laboratory analyses. Furthermore, toxic symptoms may occur due to low-level but chronic exposure.[130] In addition to subtle (but cumulative) metabolic toxicity, these heavy metals may impair other detoxification pathways so that negative effects of xenobiotics are intensified. For example, antimony exposure depletes hepatic glutathione in rat models, resulting in impaired phase II glutathione conjugation activity, which affects the ability of the body to detoxify other toxic compounds that require conjugation with glutathione.[131]

Elemental analysis of hair and provocative urine testing (e.g., DMSA oral) provide the most reliable measures of presence of toxic metals.[132] Serum testing can also be valuable for lead, mercury, aluminum, and cadmium, as well as other toxic metals. Identification and removal of toxic elements such as these may result in a positive clinical outcome for patients experiencing fatigue and cognitive disorders. Excretion of the elements can be monitored in urine.

A Clinical Perspective on Detoxification

Several decades of extensive research into detoxification of xenobiotics has resulted in an evolution of our clinical understanding of detoxification.[133,134] Chapter 31 presents a discussion of the clinical approach to improving detoxification. Before approaching the question of intervention, however, a solid understanding of the metabolic systems involved in detoxification—and the common influences upon them—is vital. Although the research is far from mature, there are many indicators that clinicians should be aware of.

Substances that induce or upregulate phase I, such as alcohol, smoking, coffee, and certain medications, can have a deleterious effect upon the balance of phase I to phase II activity, because the phase II pathways may be unable to keep up with the increased demand. The result would be an increase in activated intermediates and free radicals, which can react with and damage proteins, RNA, and DNA, further promoting a cycle of imbalanced detoxification in the individual.

The phase II conjugation enzyme systems are dependent on the presence of adequate amounts of cofactors and conjugation moieties, such as glutathione, sulfate, and glycine. Therefore, nutritional insufficiency of these cofactors could be deleterious to adequate balance between phase I and phase II activity. Moreover, the phase II activities are highly dependent on the presence of adequate energy in the form of ATP to carry out the conjugation reactions, so depletion of ATP reserves can also influence the balance of phase I to phase II activities.

Clinical Presentation

There are a number of common warning signs indicating that toxicity may be a factor for patients:

- A history of increasing sensitivity to exogenous exposures (toxic xenobiotics)
- Abundant use of medications
- Significant use of potentially toxic chemicals in the home or work environment
- Sensitivity to odors
- Musculoskeletal symptoms (similar to fibromyalgia)
- Cognitive dysfunction
- Unilateral paresthesia
- Autonomic dysfunction and recurrent patterns of edema
- Worsening of symptoms after anesthesia or pregnancy
- Paradoxical responses or sensitivity to medications or supplements[135]

Several specific clinical examples are summarized below.

Gilbert's syndrome. Gilbert's syndrome (GS), thought to be a condition with little morbidity, is a genetically-induced, nutritionally-exacerbated metabolic disorder that affects the way bilirubin is processed by the liver, causing jaundice. GS is caused by an alteration of activity in one of the glucuronyl transferase enzyme that catalyzes the phase II conjugation step of glucuronidation.[136] A study published in 1992 suggested that GS can predispose people to bioactivation and potential toxicity of drugs for which glucuronidation constitutes a major, alternate pathway of elimination.[137] Unfortunately, other than one study of zinc sulfate in 2002,[138] a recent PubMed search on Gilbert's syndrome brings up no significant recent follow-up on those early findings. Further research would be highly desirable, especially since there are at least 10 versions of glucuronyl transferase, and it is not known what effect each has on the other.

Chronic fatigue syndrome. Research reported in the mid-1990s on the etiology of chronic fatigue syndrome (CFS) suggested that there might be a relationship between impairment of detoxification pathways and symptomatology, partly as a result of toxic exposure.[139,140] Correction of these imbalances and deficiencies has been of significant benefit to some patients.[141] A clinical trial published in 1995 used a food elimination diet and nutritional modulation to support detoxifying pathways; significant improvement in subjective symptomatology as well as phase I and II activities was reported.[142] Unfortunately, the research base on this issue is still sparse and unconvincing; interest in the investigation of toxicity as a cause and improved detoxification as a therapeutic response appears to have waned of late. Both the etiology of the condition and the nature of effective treatments are as yet unclear. Many researchers have hypothesized that multiple causes may require that treatment approaches be adapted to the various sub-group characteristics, once they can be clearly defined.[143,144,145]

Encephalopathy and pancreatitis. These two conditions provide examples of how xenobiotics can influence the clinical picture. Exposure to various solvents is correlated with development of chronic toxic encephalopathy, which may present as diverse neuropsychiatric disorders. A genetic defect in one of the glutathione transferase enzymes (and therefore GSH-conjugation deficiencies) results in lowered detoxification capacity and greater likelihood of encephalopathy.[146,147] Idiopathic pancreatitis can be associated with upregulation of the cytochrome P450 enzymes in many patients.

Patient histories often include exposure to diesel fumes, paint solvents, and trichloroethylene. This type of xenobiotic exposure also seems to accentuate the susceptibility to ethanol-related pancreatitis.[148]

Chronic degenerative diseases. Detoxification has clinical implications for chronic degenerative diseases as well. Research on the etiology of Parkinson's disease has shown defects in the ability of patients to adequately metabolize sulfur-containing xenobiotics.[149] This altered detoxification may then render susceptible individuals at higher risk for neurotoxicity when exposed to sulfur-containing compounds.[150] The combination of genetic susceptibility, reduced detoxification capacity, and increased exposure to neurotoxins creates an increased risk of damage that may lead to clinical disease over the course of time. Connections to Alzheimer's, Parkinson's, and other motor neuron diseases have also been made.[151,152] Genetic makeup is certainly a major factor, but strong support for nutritional and environmental factors is vital.[153] Research has supported the relationship between compromised detoxification ability, lupus erythematosus, and rheumatoid arthritis.[154]

Detoxification and hormone-related conditions. It is clear that the modern abundance of chemicals in our environment results in the eventual exposure of nearly everyone to toxic compounds via water, air, and food. Many xenobiotics that show toxic effects are lipophilic. These substances can accumulate in the body and are found stored in the highest concentrations in reproductive, liver, and adipose tissues. For example, human seminal fluid may contain compounds such as pentachlorophenol, hexachlorobenzene, DDT metabolites, and PCBs. Adipose tissue also can contain PCBs, DDT metabolites, and chlordane.[155] In one study of hexachlorobenzene content in adipose tissue, it was shown that the median levels actually increased by 50% over levels determined five years previously.

The functional changes resulting from these xenobiotic accumulations can be profound. The compounds naphthalene, anthracene, and biphenyl have strong affinities for glucocorticoid and androgen receptors after being acted upon by hepatic conjugation reactions.[156] Combinations of xenobiotics may have effects on hormonal activity far beyond the sum of their individual activities.[157]

Since various drugs or chemicals may have an inhibitory or stimulatory effect on detoxification capacity, detoxification of other molecules through the same pathway(s) may be slowed down or speeded up, as in the case of cigarette smoking inducing certain phase I P450 isoenzymes. These same enzymes are involved in the detoxification of estrogen. As a consequence, it has been noted that serum estrogen levels are lower in women who smoke. This fact may in part explain the increased incidence of osteoporosis and menopausal symptoms in women smokers as compared to non-smokers.[158]

Supporting the Detoxification Systems

Chapter 31 will provide more guidance on the clinical approach to detoxification. In general, a program that supports healthy detoxification processes should do the following:

- Remove foods and beverages that are likely to contain toxins, food allergens, or antigenic challenge. (Antigens, as well as other endogenously produced and exogenous agents, increase the total xenobiotic load that must be handled by the detoxification pathways or other systems.)
- Eliminate or reduce ongoing toxic exposures in home and/or workplace.
- Meet basic daily nutritional needs, including adequate, high-biological-value protein content.
- Possibly provide increased amounts of the nutrients that function as cofactors for, or are otherwise required in, the enzymatic steps that occur in the biotransformation of toxic substances.
- Provide adequate hydration with clean water to promote elimination of biotransformed molecules.
- Consider interventions such as sauna or chelation, when specifically indicated, to reduce toxic load.

Nutrients critical to effective phase I and II detoxification include:

- Efficient sulfation reactions require (among other things) vitamin A, adequate protein in the diet, and adequate sources of dietary sulfur (sulfur-containing amino acids, and foods such as garlic and onions).
- Glucuronidation reactions require magnesium and may be inhibited by smoking, fasting, and possibly high fructose intake. As this is a membrane-bound enzyme system, the integrity of the lipid bilayer is important for efficient glucuronidation.
- Glutathione reactions are some of the most crucial in the deactivation of xenobiotics. Synthesis of the glutathione cofactor requires adequate vitamins B6 and B12, magnesium, and folate. Glutathione trans-

ferases may be inhibited by a number of dietary constituents, including alcohol and plant phenols, or induced by Brassica family compounds. Amino acid conjugation may be enhanced by administration of the cofactor amino acids (e.g., glycine or taurine).

Table 22.5 provides a list of plant compounds that influence detoxification.

Needs for additional nutrients or enhanced amounts of cofactors may be assessed by laboratory analyses such as determination of the amount of a nutrient or metabolite, assay of an activity dependent on the nutrient, and/or challenge testing. Individuals with increased phase-I-to-phase-II ratios and/or low urinary or serum sulfate may require nutritional antioxidant support as well as enhanced conjugating nutrient support. Glycine, taurine, and sulfhydryl donors (e.g., glutathione, N-acetylcysteine, methionine, cystine, and cysteine) should be considered in planning a detoxification regime for those individuals. In the absence of testing availability, certain circumstances discovered through the history and physical exam may also serve as general indicators of an individual's nutritional insufficiencies.

Table 22.5 **Plant-derived Compounds that Influence Detoxification**

Flavonoids	The flavonoid class of plant compounds contains a wide range of biologically active components. Examples include naringenin, which is found in grapefruit and inhibits the activity of CYP1A2 and CYP3A4. Naringenin is a very powerful inhibitor; a single glass of grapefruit juice has been shown to contain enough inhibitory activity to decrease up to 30% of CYP3A4 activity for 12–24 hours.[a] Pharmaceutical companies have promoted the use of this inhibitory activity to enhance the availability and clinical activity of some drugs. Unfortunately, this activity may also increase the toxicity of other compounds that are metabolized by these cytochrome P450 enzymes. Rutin and quercetin have been shown to act synergistically with ascorbic acid and tocopherol, and protect against oxidation injury induced by glutathione deficiency.[b,c] Rutin and its aglycone, quercetin, are flavonoids found in tea, onions, and some citrus foods that also inhibit cytochrome P450 activity.[d] Conversely, the flavonoids tangeretin and nobiletin, found in orange juice, have been shown to induce CYP3A4.[e] *Rosmarinus officinalis* (rosemary) contains the flavonoids carnosol, carnosic acid, rosmanol, and ursolic acid, which possess high antioxidant activity. These polyphenols have been shown to scavenge inflammation-induced nitric oxide and peroxynitrite radicals.[f] Carnosol and carnosic acid stimulate the phase II detoxification enzymes glutathione-S-transferase and quinone reductase, and suppress DNA damage from xenobiotics.[g]
Monoterpenoids	Monoterpenoids such as d-limonene are derived from citrus foods, in particular lemon, and have a number of interesting effects on the detoxification systems. In animal models, limonene increases levels of CYP2C; however, it inhibits the activity of CYP2E1.[h] These monoterpenoids induce the phase II detoxification glutathione and glucuronidation activities, which may account for their ability to improve resistance to glutathione depletion by chronic acetaminophen administration and inhibit tumorigenesis in animal models.[i,j]
Curcumin	Curcumin is the yellow pigment and an active component in the spice turmeric (*Curcuma longa*). Curcumin has a wide range of biological activities that include acting as a potent antioxidant, antiinflammatory agent, and antimutagen.[k,l] Curcumin has also been shown to induce glutathione production and glutathione-S-transferase activity, and may inhibit some cytochrome P450 activities.[m,n]
Forskolin	As many xenobiotics are stored in the adipose tissue, enhancement of lipolysis during a detoxification regimen can be of significant benefit. This natural product, derived from *Coleus forskohlii*, may be useful in increasing the cAMP levels, which can indirectly assist (via adenylcyclase) with lipolysis.[o,p]
Indole-3-carbinol	Indole-3-carbinol is found in the Brassica family of vegetables (cabbage, Brussels sprouts, broccoli). Metabolites of indole-3-carbinol are readily formed after its ingestion, and they inhibit the activity of the CYP1A1 and CYP1A2 isoforms in humans.[q] Indole-3-carbinol metabolites also have the capacity to enhance the phase II glutathione pathways, thereby providing a means to clear xenobiotics more efficiently.[r]

[a] Yee GC, Stanley DL, Pessa LJ, et al. Effect of grapefruit juice on blood cyclosporine concentration. Lancet. 1995;345:955-56.
[b] Negre-Salvayre A, Affany A, Hariton C, Salvayre R. Additional antilipoperoxidant activities of alpha-tocopherol and ascorbic acid on membrane-like systems are potentiated by rutin. Pharmacol. 1991;42:262-72.
[c] Skaper SD, Fabris M, Ferrari V, et al. Quercetin protects cutaneous tissue-associated cell types including sensory neurons from oxidative stress induced by glutathione depletion: cooperative effects of ascorbic acid. Free Rad Biol Med. 1997;22:669-78.
[d] Hollman PCH, deVries JHM, van Leeuwen SD, et al. Absorption of dietary quercetin glycosides and quercitin in healthy ileostomy volunteers. Am J Clin Nutr. 1995;62:1276-82.

[e] Li Y, Wang E, Patten CJ, et al. Effects of flavonoids on cytochrome P450-dependent acetaminophen metabolism in rats and human liver microsomes. Drug Metab Dispos. 1994;22:566-71.
[f] Lo AH, Liang YC, Lin-Shiau SY, et al. Carnosol, an antioxidant in rosemary, suppresses inducible nitric oxide synthase through down-regulating nuclear factor-kappaB in mouse macrophages. Carcinogenesis. 2002;23(6):983-91.
[g] Sotelo-Felix JI, Martinez-Fong D, Muriel P, et al. Evaluation of the effectiveness of Rosmarinus officinalis (Lamiaceae) in the alleviation of carbon tetrachloride-induced acute hepatotoxicity in the rat. J Ethnopharmacol. 2002;81(2):145-54.
[h] Maltzman TH, Christou M, Gould MN, Jefeoate CR. Effects of monoterpenoids on *in vivo* DMBA-DNA adduct formation and on phase I hepatic metabolizing enzymes. Carcinogenesis. 1991;12:2081-87.
[i] Lam LKT, Zhang J. Hasegawa S. Citrus limonoid reduction of chemically induced tumorigenesis. Food Tech. 1994;Nov:104-8.
[j] Reicks MM, Crankshaw D. Effects of d-limonene on hepatic microsomal mono-oxygenase activity and paracetamol-induced glutathione depletion in mouse. Xenobiotica. 1993;23:809-19.
[k] Ringman JM, Frautschy SA, Cole GM, et al. A potential role of the curry spice curcumin in Alzheimer's disease. Curr Alzheimer Res. 2005;2(2):131-6.
[l] Polasa K, Raghuram TC, Krishna TP, Krishnaswamy K. Effect of turmeric on urinary mutagens in smokers. Mutagenesis. 1992;7(2):107-9.
[m] Van Erk MJ, Teuling E, Stall YC, et al. Time- and dose-dependent effects of curcumin on gene expression in human colon cancer cells. J Carcinog. 2004;3(1):8.
[n] Leu TH, Maa MC. The molecular mechanisms for the antitumorigenic effect of curcumin. Curr Med Chem Anti-Canc Agents. 2002;2(3):357-70
[o] Kasai A, Yao J, Yamauchi K, et al. Influence of cAMP on reporter bioassays for dioxin and dioxin-like compounds. Toxicol Appl Pharmacol. 2006;211(1):11-19
[p] Reynisdottir S, Ellerfeldt K, Wahrenburg H, et al. Multiple lipolysis defects in the insulin resistance (metabolic) syndrome. J Clin Invest. 1994;93(6):2590-9.
[q] Gerhauser C, Klimo K, Heiss E, et al. Mechanism-based *in vitro* screening of potential cancer chemopreventive agents. Mutat Res. 2003;523-524:163-72.
[r] Shukla Y, Kalra N, Katiyar S, et al. Chemopreventive effect of indole-3-carbinol on induction of preneoplastic altered hepatic foci. Nutr Cancer. 2004;50(2):214-20.

Summary

We are inevitably exposed to higher levels of xenobiotics in food, water, and air; many of us also bear an increased endogenous toxic load from faulty digestion, poor dietary habits, and metabolism of many medications (competitive inhibition). Thus, our individual detoxification profiles may be highly relevant to our risk of disease and dysfunction. Research is opening up an extremely important field of inquiry into the identification and proper counseling of individuals with various genetic susceptibilities or inadequacies that may require dietary, environmental, or supplemental modification to accommodate their biochemical individuality.

Studies of detoxification function show that the enzymes that control the various phase I and phase II processes vary significantly from person to person, even in healthy people.[159,160] There are numerous pharmacogenetic variants affecting detoxification disposition that are manifested only upon drug or environmental challenge. This new understanding of detoxification brings us to a greater appreciation of Roger Williams's mid-20th century work and his popularization of the term and concept of "biochemical individuality."[161] Differences in detoxification capacities based upon individual genetic predispositions, environmental exposures, and nutritional insufficiencies can have a profound effect upon susceptibility to a wide variety of diseases (and upon our ability to respond to interventions, whether pharmaceutical, nutritional, or botanical). Xenobiotics may act as immunotoxic agents, suggesting a biochemical connection between the immune, nervous, and hepatic detoxification systems.[162] A very intriguing question is how many of the diseases we now consider idiopathic—of unknown origin—might be linked to atypical detoxification reactions? Disordered detoxification may have wide-ranging impact upon hepatic, renal, cardiovascular, neurological, endocrine, and immune system function. It certainly feels safe to say that the complicated interrelationships involved in exposure to various substances, genetically determined detoxification pathways, alteration of the pathways by foods, drugs, and chemicals, and sensitivity of tissues to secondary metabolites from toxic substances, play an under-recognized role in contributing to the development and perpetuation of many health problems.

Identifying slow, fast, or otherwise imbalanced individual detoxification pathways can be extremely important. Laboratory assessment of detoxification gives the health professional more precise and definitive tools for assessment, a better understanding of an individual's unique metabolic detoxification capacity, and the opportunity to tailor nutritional support and environmental factors to reduce symptoms associated with metabolic toxicity.

References

1. U.S. Environmental Protection Agency, 1987-1994. Toxics Release Inventory National Report, Washington, D.C.: Office of Toxic Substances.
2. The EPA website: http://www.epa.gov/All+chemicals&industry. Last visited 5-09-2005.
3. Pizzorno JE, Murray MT. Detoxification: A naturopathic perspective. Nat Med J. 1998;1:6-17.
4. Estabrook RW. Cytochrome P450: From a single protein to a family of proteins - with some personal reflections. In: Ioannides C, ed. Cytochromes P450: Metabolic and toxicological aspects. Boca Raton, FL: CRC Press, Inc; 1996:3-28.
5. Omura T. Forty years of cytochrome P450. Biochem Biophys Res Commun. 1999;266(3):690-8.
6. Estabrook RW. A passion for P450s (remembrances of the early history of research on cytochrome P450). Drug Metab Disp. 2003;31:1461-73.

7. Smith RL, Williams RT. History of the discovery of the conjugation mechanisms. In: Fishman WH, ed. Metabolic Conjugation and Metabolic Hydrolysis. New York: Academic Press, 1970.
8. Levsen K, et al. Structure elucidation of phase II metabolites by tandem mass spectrometry: an overview. J Chromatogr A. 2005;1067(1-2):55-72.
9. Dorne JL, Walton K, Renwick AG. Human variability in xenobiotic metabolism and pathway-related uncertainty factors for chemical risk assessment: a review. Food Chem Toxicol. 2005;43(2):203-16.
10. Daly AK. Pharmacogenetics of the cytochromes P450. Curr Top Med Chem. 2004;4(16):1733-44.
11. Guengerich FP. Cytochromes P450, drugs, and diseases. Mol Interv. 2003;3(4):194-204.
12. Bland J, Barrager E, Reedy R, Bland K. A medical food-supplemented detoxification program in the management of chronic health problems. Altern Ther Health Med. 1995 Nov 1;1(5):62-71.
13. Steventon G, Heafield M, Waring R, Williams A. Xenobiotic metabolism in Parkinson's disease. Neurology. 1989;39:883-887.
14. Huang Y, et al. Genetic contributions to Parkinson's disease. Brain Res Brain Res Rev. 2004;46(1):44-70.
15. Dawson TM, Dawson VL. Molecular pathways of neurodegeneration in Parkinson's disease. Science. 2003;302(5646):819-22.
16. Ning B, Wang C, Morel F, et al. Human glutathione S-transferase A2 polymorphisms: variant expression, distribution in prostate cancer cases/controls and a novel form. Pharmacogenetics. 2004;14(1):35-44.
17. Mohrenweiser HW. Genetic variation and exposure related risk estimate: will toxicology enter a new era? DNA repair and cancer as a paradigm. Toxicol Pathol. 2004;32(Suppl 1):136-45.
18. Chacko P, Joseph T, Mathew BS, et al. Role of xenobiotic metabolizing gene polymorphisms in breast cancer susceptibility and treatment outcome. Mutat Res. 2005;581(1-2):153-63.
19. Pizzorno JE, Murray MT. Detoxification: A naturopathic perspective. Nat Med J. 1998;1:6-17.
20. Hoffman D, Lavoie E, Hecht S. Nicotine: A precursor for carcinogens. Cancer Letts. 1985;26:67-75.
21. Weisburger JH. Prevention of cancer and other chronic diseases worldwide based on sound mechanisms. Biofactors. 2000;12 (1-4):73-81.
22. Casarett & Doull's Toxicology - The Basic Science of Poisons (6th Edition); McGraw-Hill, 2004; Edited by: Klaassen CD;1236.
23. Timbrell J. In: Principles of Biochemical Toxicology. 2nd Ed. London: Taylor and Francis; 1991.
24. Grant D. Detoxification pathways in the liver. J Inher Metab Dis. 1991;14:421-30.
25. Gonzalez FJ. Role of cytochrome P450 in chemical toxicity and oxidative stress: studies with CYP2E1. Mutat Res. 2005;569 (1-2):101-10.
26. Ryan DE, Lu AYH, Kawalek J, et al. Highly purified cytochrome P448 and P450 from rat liver microsomes. Biochem Biophys Res Commun. 1975;64:1134.
27. Poulos TL, Finzel BC, Gunsalus IC, et al. The 2.6-A crystal structure of Pseudomonas putida cytochrome P-450. J Biol Chem. 1985;260:16122-130.
28. Gonzalez FJ, Idle JR. Pharmacogenetic phenotyping and genotyping. Present status and future potential. Clin Pharmacokinet. 1994;26:59-70.
29. Aguiar M, Masse R, Gibbs BF. Regulation of cytochrome P450 by posttranslational modification. Drug Metab Rev. 2005;37(2):379-404.
30. Norppa H. Cytogenetic biomarkers and genetic polymorphisms. Toxicol Lett. 2004;149(1-3):309-34.
31. LeCouteur DG, Muller M, Yang MC, et al. Age-environment and gene-environment interactions in the pathogenesis of Parkinson's disease. Rev Environ Health. 2002;17(1):51-64.
32. Bonneh-Barkay D, Langston WJ, DiMonte DA. Toxicity of redox cycling pesticides in primary mesencephalic cultures. Antioxid Redox Signal. 2005;7(5-6);649-53.
33. Rendic S. Summary of information on human CYP enzymes: Human P450 metabolism data. Drug Metab Rev. 2002;34:83-448.
34. Grant D. Detoxification pathways in the liver. J Inher Metab Dis. 1991;14:421-30.
35. Sampson HA. Food hypersensitivity: manifestations, diagnosis, and natural history. Food Tech. 1992;May:141-44.
36. Scheline RR. Metabolism of foreign compounds by gastrointestinal microorganisms. Pharmacol Rev. 1973;25:451-523.
37. Cumings JH, Englyst HN. Fermentation in the human large intestine: Evidence and implications for health. Lancet. 1983;45 (5 Suppl):1206-8.
38. McKinnon RA, McManus ME. Localization of cytochromes P450 in human tissues: Implications for chemical toxicity. Pathology. 1996;28:148-55.
39. McKinnon RA, Burgess WM, Hall PM, et al. Characterization of CYP3A gene subfamily expression in human gastrointestinal tissues. Gut. 1995;36:259-67.
40. Benet L. 27th Gordon research conference on drug metabolism. July 6-13, 1997, personal communication.
41. Chin KV, Pastan I, Gottesman MM. Function and regulation of the multidrug resistance gene. Adv Cancer Res. 1993;60:157-80.
42. Bauer KS, Karp JE, Garimella TS, et al. A phase I and pharmacologic study of idarubicin, cytarabine, etoposide, and the multidrug resistance protein (MDR1/Pgp) inhibitor PSC-833 in patients with refractory leukemia. Leuk Res. 2005;29(3):263-71.
43. Planting AS, Sonneveld P, van der Gaast A, et al. A phase I and pharmacologic study of the MDR converter GF120918 in combination with doxorubicin in patients with advanced solid tumors. Cancer Chemother Pharmacol. 2005;55(1):91-99.
44. Kolitz JE, George SL, Dodge RK, et al. Dose escalation studies of cytarabine, daunorubicin, and etoposide with and without multidrug resistance modulation with PSC-833 in untreated adults with acute myeloid leukemia younger than 60 years: final induction results of Cancer and Leukemia Group B Study 9621. J Clin Oncol. 2004;22(21):4290-301.
45. Larkin A, Moran E, Alexander D, Clynes M. Preliminary immunocytochemical studies of MDR-1 and MDR-3 Pgp expression in B-cell leukaemias. Adv Exp Med Biol. 1999;457:65-70.
46. Larkin A, Moran E, Alexander D, et al. A new monoclonal antibody that specifically recognises the MDR-3-encoded gene product. Int J Cancer. 1999;80(2):265-71.
47. Park BK, Kitteringham NR, Pirmohamed M, Tucker GT. Relevance of induction of human drug-metabolizing enzymes: pharmacological and toxicological implications. Br J Clin Pharmacol. 1996;41:477-91.
48. Kall MA, Clausen J. Dietary effect on mixed function P450 1A2 activity assayed by estimation of cafffeine metabolism in man. Hum Exp Toxicol. 1995;14:801-7.
49. Parsons WD, Neims AH. Effect of smoking on caffeine clearance. Clin Pharmacol Ther. 1978;24:40-45.
50. Guengerich FP. Effects of nutritive factors on metabolic processes involving bioactivation and detoxification of chemicals. Ann Rev Nutr. 1984;4:207-31.
51. Manson MM, Ball HW, Barrett MC, et al. Mechanism of action of dietary chemoprotective agents in rat liver: induction of phase I and II drug metabolizing enzymes and aflatoxin B1 metabolism. Carcinogenesis. 1997;18:1729-38.
52. Barch DH, Rundhaugen LM, Pillay NS. Ellagic acid induces transcription of the rat glutathione S-transferase-Ya gene. Carcinogenesis. 1995;16:665-8.

53. Pantuck EJ, Pantuck CB, Garland WA, et al. Stimulatory effect of Brussels sprouts and cabbage on human drug metabolism. Clin Pharm Ther. 1979;25:88-95.
54. Offord EA, Mace K, Ruffieux C, et al. Rosemary components inhibit benzo[a]pyrene- induced genotoxicity in human bronchial cells. Carcinogenesis. 1995;16:2057-62.
55. Ip C, Lisk DJ. Modulation of phase I and phase II xenobiotic-metabolizing enzymes by selenium-enriched garlic in rats. Nutr Cancer. 1997;28:184-88.
56. Appelt LC, Reicks MM. Soy feeding induces phase II enzymes in rat tissues. Nutr Cancer. 1997;28:270-75.
57. Van Breda SG, van Agen E, Engels LG, et al. Altered vegetable intake affects pivotal carcinogenesis pathways in colon mucosa from adenoma patients and controls. Carcinogenesis. 2004;25(11):2207-16.
58. Lhoste EF, Gloux K, De Waziers I, et al. The activities of several detoxication enzymes are differentially induced by juices of garden cress, water cress and mustard in human HepG2 cells. Chem Biol Interact. 2004;150(3):211-19.
59. Elangovan V, Sekar N, Govindasamy S. Chemopreventive potential of dietary bioflavonoids against 20-methylcholanthrene-induced tumorigenesis. Cancer Lett. 1994;87:107-13.
60. Smith TJ, Yang CS. Effects of food phytochemicals on xenobiotic metabolism and tumorigenesis. In: Food Phytochemicals I: Fruits and Vegetables. Washington, DC: American Chemical Society Press. 1994:17-48.
61. Feldman EB. How grapefruit juice potentiates drug availability. Nutr Rev. 1997;55:398-400.
62. Weber A, Jager R, Borner A, et al. Can grapefruit juice influence ethinylestradiol bioavailability? Contraception. 1996;53:41-47.
63. Mulder GJ. Sulfate availability *in vivo*. In: Mulder GJ, ed. Sulfation of drugs and related compounds. Boca Raton, FL: CRC Press, Inc; pp. 31-52.
64. Gonzalez F, Gelboin H. Role of human cytochrome P450s in risk assessment and susceptibility to environmentally based disease. J Toxicol Environ Health 1993;40:289-308.
65. Dervieux T, Meshkin B, Neri B. Pharmacogenetic testing: proofs of principle and pharmacoeconomic implications. Mutat Res. 2005 Jun 3;573(1-2):180-94.
66. Allorge D, Loriot MA. Pharmacogenetics or the promise of a personalized medicine: variability in drug metabolism and transport. Ann Biol Clin (Paris). 2004;62(5):499-511.[Article in French]
67. Waring R, Emery P. The genetic origin of responses to drugs. Br Med Bull. 1995;51:449-61.
68. Gaedigk A, Blum M, Gaedigk R, et al. Deletion of the entire cytochrome P450 CYP2D6 gene as a cause of impaired drug metabolism in poor metabolizers of the debrisoquine/sparteine polymorphism. Am J Hum Genet. 1991;48:943-50.
69. Meyer UA, Zanger UM, Skoda RC, et al. Genetic polymorphisms of drug metabolism. Prog Liver Dis. 1990;9:307-23.
70. Iarbovici D. Single blood test might predict drugs' effects on patients. J NIH Res. 1997;9:34-45.
71. Weber W. Influence of heredity on human sensitivity to environmental chemicals. Environ Mol Mutagen. 1995;25 Suppl 26:102-14.
72. Hayes JD, Strange RC. Glutathione S-transferase polymorphisms and their biological consequences. Pharmacology. 2000;61:154-66.
73. Ponsoda X, Donato MT, Perez-Cataldo G, et al. Drug metabolism by cultured human hepatocytes: how far are we from the *in vivo* reality? Altern Lab Anim. 2004;32(2):101-10.
74. Guengerich FP. Cytochrome P450: what have we learned and what are the future issues? Drug Metab Rev. 2004;36(2):159-97.
75. Vallee B. The function of metallothionein. Neurochem Int. 1995;27:23-33.
76. Aschner M, Cherian M, Klaassen C, et al. Metallothioneins in brain—the role in physiology and pathology. Toxicol Appl Pharmacol. 1997;142:229-42.
77. Chopra A, Thibordeau J, Tam Y, et al. New mouse somatic cell mutants resistant to cadmium affected in the expression of their metallothionein genes. J Cell Physiol. 1990;142:316-24.
78. Sato M, Kondoh M. Recent studies on metallothionein: protection against toxicity of heavy metals and oxygen free radicals., Tohoku J Exp Med 2002;196:9-22.
79. Kondo Y, Woo E, Michalska A, et al. Metallothionein null cells have increased sensitivity to anticancer drugs. Cancer Res. 1995;55:2021-23.
80. Brewer GJ. Zinc therapy induction of intestinal metallothionein in Wilson's disease. Am J Gastroenterol. 1999;94: 301-2.
81. Sullivan VK, Burnett FR, Cousins RJ. Metallothionein expression is increased in monocytes and erythrocytes of young men during zinc supplementation. J Nutr 1998;128:707-13.
82. Bobillier Chaumont S, Maupoil V, Jacques Lahet J, Berthelot A. Effect of exercise training on metallothionein levels of hypertensive rats. Med Sci Sports Exerc. 2001;33:724-28.
83. Kondoh M, Kamada K, Kuronaga M, et al. Antioxidant property of metallothionein in fasted mice. Toxicol Lett. 2003;143: 301-6.
84. Pennie WD, Tugwood JD, Oliver GJ, Kimber I. The principles and practice of toxigenomics: applications and opportunities. Toxicol Sci. 2000;54(2):277-83.
85. Benet LZ, Kroetz DL, Sheiner LB. Pharmacokinetics: The dynamics of drug absorption, distribution, and elimination. In: Milinoff PB, Ruddon RW, Goodman Gilman A, eds. The Pharmacological Basis of Therapeutics. 9th ed. New York, NY: McGraw-Hill. 1996:3-27.
86. Burzynski SR. Aging: gene silencing or gene activation? Med Hypotheses. 2005;64(1):201-8.
87. Gems D, McElwee JJ. Broad spectrum detoxification: the major longevity assurance process regulated by insulin/IGF-1 signaling? Mech Ageing Dev. 2005;126(3):381-87.
88. Gustavson LE, Benet LZ. Menopause: Pharmacodynamics and pharmacokinetics. Exp Gerontol. 1994;29:437-444.
89. Benet LZ. 27th Gordon research conference on drug metabolism. July 6-13, 1997, personal communication.
90. Rannug A, Alexandrie AK, Persson I, Ingelman-Sundberg M. Genetic polymorphism of cytochromes P450 1A1, 2D6, and 2E1: Regulation and toxicological significance. J Occupational Environ Med. 1995;37:25-36.
91. Ronis MJJ, Lindros KO, Ingelman-Sundberg M. The CYP2E subfamily. In: Ioannides C, ed. Cytochromes P450: Metabolic and Toxicological Aspects. Boca Raton, FL: CRC Press, Inc; 1996:211-239.
92. Miller E, Miller J. Searches for ultimate chemical carcinogens and their reactions with cellular macromolecules. Cancer. 1981;47:2327.
93. Agundez JA, Ledesma MC, Benitiz J. CYP2D6 genes and risk of liver cancer. Lancet. 1995;345(8953):830-1.
94. Kawajiri K, Nakaji K, Imai K, et al. Identification of genetically high risk individuals to lung cancer by DNA polymorphisms of the cytochrome P4501A1 gene. FEBS Lett. 1990;263:131.
95. Ketterer B, Harris JM, Talaska G, et al. The human glutathione S-transferase supergene family, its polymorphism, and low level environmental exposure to carcinogens. Nature. 1994;369:154-156.
96. Meyer U, Zanger U, Grant D, et al. Genetic polymorphisms of drug metabolism. Adv Drug Res. 1990;19:197-241.
97. Goldberg RJ. The P450 system. Arch Fam Med. 1996;5:406-12.
98. Lazarou J, Pomeranz BH, Corey PN. Incidence of adverse drug reactions in hospitalized patients. JAMA. 1998;279:1200-17.
99. Iarbovici D. Single blood test might predict drugs' effects on patients. J NIH Res. 1997;9:34-45.
100. Phillips KA, Van Bebber SL. Measuring the value of pharmacogenomics. Nat Rev Drug Discov. 2005;4(6):500-9.

101. Breaux JK, Los G. Gene expression profiling to characterize anticancer drug sensitivity. Methods Mol Med. 2005;111:197-231.
102. Efferth T, Volm M. Pharmacogenetics for individualized cancer chemotherapy. Pharmacol Ther. 2005;107(2):155-76.
103. Kirchheiner J, Nickchen K, Bauer M, et al. Pharmacogenetics of antidepressants and antipsychotics: the contribution of allelic variations to the phenotype of drug response. Mol Psychiatry. 2004;9(5):442-73.
104. Environmental Neurotoxicology. National Research Council. Washington, D.C. National Academy Press; 1992.
105. Biologic Markers in Immunotoxicology. National Research Council. Washington, D.C. National Academy Press; 1992.
106. Schubert J, Riley EJ, Tyler SA. Combined effects of toxicology—a rapid systematic testing procedure: cadmium, mercury, and lead. J Toxicol Environ Health. 1978;4:763-776.
107. Rea WJ. Chemical Sensitivity. Vol. 4. Boca Raton, Fla: CRC Press, Inc. 1997:1011-1067.
108. Rea WJ, Didriksen N, Simon TR, et al. Effects of toxic exposure to molds and mycotoxins in building-related illnesses. Arch Environ Health. 2003;58(7):399-405.
109. Neuschwander-Tetri BA. Common blood tests for liver disease. Which ones are most useful? Postgrad Med. 1995;98(1):49-63.
110. Quick AJ. The synthesis of hippuric acid: a new test of liver function, Am J Med Sci. 1933;185:630-37.
111. Park BK, Kitteringham NR, Pirmohamed M, Tucker GT. Relevance of induction of human drug-metabolizing enzymes: pharmacological and toxicological implications. Br J Clin Pharmacol. 1996;41:477-491.
112. Patel M, Tang BK, Kalow W. Variability of acetaminophen metabolism in Caucasians and Orientals. Pharmacogenetics. 1992;2:38-45.
113. Levy G. Pharmacokinetics of salicylate elimination in man. J Pharmaceutical Sci. 1965; 54:959-967.
114. Fulton B, Jeffery E. The temporal relationship between hepatic GSH loss, heme oxygenase induction, and cytochrome P450 loss following intraperitoneal aluminum administration to mice. Toxicol Appl Pharmacol. 1994;127:291-97.
115. Lieber C. Alcohol, liver, and nutrition. J Am Coll Nutr. 1991;10(6):602-32.
116. Guengerich F. Effects of nutritive factors on metabolic processes involving bioactivation and detoxication of chemicals. Ann Rev Nutr. 1984;4:207-31.
117. Kall M, Clausen J. Dietary effect on mixed function P450 1A2 activity assayed by estimation of caffeine metabolism in man. Human Exp Toxicol. 1995;14(10):801-7.
118. Anderson K. Dietary regulation of cytochrome P450. Annu Rev Nutr. 1991;11;141-67.
119. Jaw S, Jeffery E. Interaction of caffeine with acetaminophen. Biochem Pharmacol. 1993;46(3)493-501.
120. Parsons W, Neims AH. Effect of smoking on caffeine clearance. Clin Pharmacol Ther. 1978;24:40-45.
121. Setchel K, Welsh M, Klooster M, et al. Rapid high-performance liquid chromatography assay for salivary and serum caffeine following an oral load-an indicator of liver function. J Chromatogr. 1987;385:267-74.
122. Brockmoller J, Roots I. Assessment of liver metabolic function. Clin Pharmacokinet Concepts. 1994;27(3):216-47.
123. Jost G, Wahllander A, Von Mandach R, Preisig R. Overnight salivary caffeine clearance: a liver function test suitable for routine use. Hepatology. 1987;7(2):338-44.
124. Patel M, Tang B, Kalow W. Variability of acetaminophen metabolism in Caucasians and Orientals. Pharmacogenetics 1992;2:38-45.
125. Whitcomb DC, Block G. Association of acetaminophen hepatotoxicity with fasting and ethanol use. JAMA. 1994;272(23):845-509.
126. Hutt A, Caldwell J, Smith R. The metabolism of aspirin in man: a population study. Xenobiotica. 1986;16(3):239-249.
127. Quick AJ. The synthesis of hippuric acid: A new test of liver function. Am J Med Sci. 1933;185:630-37.
128. Patel M, Tang B, Kalow W. Variability of acetaminophen metabolism in Caucasians and Orientals. Pharmacogenetics. 1992;2:38-45.
129. Pizzorno JE, Murray MT. Detoxification: A naturopathic perspective. Nat Med J. 1998;1:6-17.
130. Shukla GS, Singhal RL. The present status of biological effects of toxic metals in the environment: lead, cadmium, and manganese. Can J Physiol Pharmacol. 1984;62:1015-31.
131. Gyurasics A, et al. Increased biliary excretion of glutathione is generated by the glutathione-depletion hepatobiliary transport of antimony and bismuth. Biochem Pharmacol. 1992;44:1275-81.
132. Foo S, et al. Metals in hair as biological indices for exposure. Int Arch Occup Environ Health. 1993;65:S83-S86.
133. Davies M. Sulphoxidation and sulphation capacity in patients with primary biliary cirrhosis, J Hepatol. 1995; May,22(5):551-60.
134. Bradley H. Sulfate metabolism is abnormal in patients with rheumatoid arthritis: Confirmation by *in vivo* biochemical findings. J Rheumatol. 1994 Jul;21(7):1192-96.
135. Rea W. Chemical Sensitivity, vol. 4. Boca Raton, FL: CRC Press, 1997:2052-2060.
136. Black M, Billings B. Hepatic bilirubin UDP-glucuronyl transferase activity in liver disease and Gilbert's syndrome. New Engl J Med. 1969;280:1266-71.
137. De Morais S, Uetecht J, Wells P. Decreased glucuronidation and increased bioactivation of acetaminophen in Gilbert's syndrome. Gastroenterology. 1992;102:577-86.
138. Mendez-Sanchez N, Martinez M, Gonzalez V, et al. Zinc sulfate inhibits the enterohepatic cycling of unconjugated bilirubin in subjects with Gilbert's syndrome. Ann Hepatol. 2002;1(1):40-3.
139. Rigden D, Bralley JA, Bland J. Nutritional upregulation of hepatic detoxification enzymes. J Appl Nutr 1992;44(3&4):2-15.
140. Buist RA. Chronic fatigue syndrome and chemical overload. Int Clin Nutr Rev. 1988;8(4):173-5.
141. Rigden S. Entero-Hepatic resuscitation program for CFIDS. The CFIDS Chronicle Spring, 1995 pp. 46-49.
142. Bland J, Barrager E, Reedy RG, Bland K. A medical food supplemented detoxification program in the management of chronic health problems. Altern Ther Health Med. 1995 Nov 1;1(5):62-71
143. Hamilton WT, Gallagher AM, Thomas JM, White PD. The prognosis of different fatigue diagnostic labels: a longitudinal survey. Fam Pract. 2005;22(4):383-8.
144. Rimes KA, Chalder T. Treatments for chronic fatigue syndrome. Occup Med (London):2005;55(1):32-9.
145. Huibers MJ, Bleijenberg G, van Amelsvoort LG, et al. Predictors of outcome in fatigued employees on sick leave: results from a randomised trial. J Psychosom Res. 2004;57(5):443-49.
146. Burim RV, et al. Polymorphisms in glutathione S-transferases GSTM1, GSTT1 and GSTP1 and cytochromes P450 CYP2E1 and CYP1A1 and susceptibility to cirrhosis or pancreatitis in alcoholics. Mutagenesis. 2004;19(4):291-98.
147. Soderkvist P, Ahmadi A. Glutathione S-transferase M1 null genotype as a risk modifier for solvent-induced chronic toxic encephalopathy. Scand J Work Environ Health. 1996;22:360-63.
148. Braganza JM, Jolley JE, et sl. Occupational chemicals and pancreatitis: a link? Int J Pancreatol. 1986;1:9-19.
149. Steventon GB, Heafield MT, Waring RH, Williams AC. Xenobiotic metabolism in Parkinson's disease. Neurology. 1989;39:883-87.
150. Heafield MT, Fearn S, Steventon GB, et al. Plasma cysteine and sulphate levels in patients with motor neurone, Parkinson's and Alzheimer's disease. Neurosci Lett. 1990;110:216-20.

151. Perlmutter D. Parkinson's diseases—new perspectives. Townsend Newslett. Jan 1997:48-50.
152. Steventon GB, Heafield MT, Waring RH, Williams AC. Xenobiotic metabolism in Parkinson's disease. Neurology. 1989;39:883-87.
153. Wi, JM. Carcinogen hemoglobin adducts, urinary mutagenicity, and metabolic phenotype in active and passive cigarette smokers. J Natl Cancer Inst. 1991;83(13):963.
154. McKinnon RA, Nebert DW. Possible role of cytochromes P450 in lupus erythematosus and related disorders. Lupus. 1994;3:473-478.
155. Dougherty RC, et al. Negative chemical ionization studies of human and food chain contamination with xenobiotic chemicals. Environ Health Perspect. 1980;36:103-17.
156. Chang CS, Liao SS. Topographic recognition of cyclic hydrocarbons and related compounds by receptors for androgens, estrogens, and glucocorticoids. J Steroid Biochem. 1987;27:123-31.
157. Calabrese EJ. Toxicological consequences of multiple chemical interactions: a primer. Toxicology. 1995;105:121-35.
158. Michnovicz J. Environmental modulation of oestrogen metabolism in humans. Int Clin Nutr Rev. 1987;7(4):169-73.
159. Temelli A, Mogavero S, Giulianotti PC, et al. Conjugation of benzoic acid with glycine in human liver and kidney: a study on the interindividual variability. Xenobiotica 1993;23(12):1427-33.
160. Meyer U, Zanger U, Grant D, et al. Genetic polymorphisms of drug metabolism. Adv Drug Res. 1990;19:197-241.
161. Williams RJ. Biochemical individuality: The basis of the genetotrophic concept. New York: John Wiley, 1956.
162. Goldin FE, Tatnayaka ID. Acetaminophen and macrophage activation. Int Hepato Comms. 1995;4:16-18.

Chapter 23
Immune Imbalances and Inflammation

Robert Rountree, MD

Teach thy tongue to say 'I do not know' and thou shalt progress.
—Moses Maimonides, ca 1200 A.D.

Discovery consists in seeing what everyone else has seen and thinking what no one else has thought.
—Albert Szent-Gyorgyi, MD, PhD
Nobel Laureate (Physiology or Medicine), 1937

Introduction

The Inflammatory Response

One of the most enduring clinical observations made by the physicians of antiquity was that the human body responds to trauma or infection in a predictable manner, a phenomenon called inflammation. Written descriptions of this phenomenon date as far back as the Ebers papyrus (1550 BC), but the first concise, empirical definition has been attributed to Cornelius Celsus, circa 30–40 AD, who described its cardinal signs as redness and swelling with heat and pain (*rubor et tumor cum calore et dolore*). Galen of Pergamum (ca. 129–199 AD) later added a fifth sign: disturbed function (*et functio laesa*). Two centuries later, it was proposed that excessive secretion (*fluor*), should also be added to this group.[1]

Whether the stimulus is a laceration, a burn, or an inhaled speck of pollen by a person with atopic syndrome, a remarkably similar combination of signs is elicited. These similarities imply that only a limited number of physiological pathways are required to produce this pattern, but superficial appearances can be deceptive. It is true that there is considerable overlap in effector mechanisms, but the machinery that runs those effector mechanisms is extremely complex. In fact, we cannot fully comprehend how this machinery works—much less how to gracefully manipulate it—without first making some significant revisions in the scientific paradigm used to interpret its actions.

Even though it lacks an identifiable single conductor, inflammation is nevertheless a highly-orchestrated event that utilizes an intricate reciprocity between the innate and acquired/adaptive branches of the immune system.[2] It relies on the basic process of signal transduction to convert information that specialized molecular sensors perceive as constituting foreignness, danger, or damage into a series of enzymatically-catalyzed biochemical cascades.[3] In turn, the downstream metabolites unleashed by these cascades activate the transcription of messenger proteins that are then dispatched to inform and instruct the larger cellular community of the host regarding the nature of the impending threat. What follows is a veritable symphony of intercellular dialogue, consisting of the enlistment and coordination of an integrated network of cell types whose mission is to defend their host and repair the damage caused by intrusions from pathogenic microbes or toxic biologic substances resulting from thermal, electromagnetic, mechanical, or chemical injury.[4,5,6]

Immune Imbalance, Inflammation and Chronic Disease

It has become increasingly evident that the process described by Celsus is a sword with two very sharp edges. The immune system's ability to mount an adequate inflammatory response is critical to survival—its absence is tantamount to a death sentence. When the immune system operates in a balanced fashion, the process is self-limited and largely beneficial. But the dysfunction that results from a wide variety of systemic imbalances can lead to a loss of regulatory control, in which case the process becomes perpetual and destructive to the host.[7] The most obvious examples of this outcome can be found in chronic inflammatory disorders such as rheumatoid arthritis, inflammatory bowel disease, and eczema, or the granulomatous response to tuberculosis and other intracellular infections.

As it turns out, however, these conditions are only the tip of the iceberg and the consequences of imbalanced immune function are much more pervasive than previously appreciated.[8,9] Inflammation is now understood to be a central aspect of the pathophysiology of a wide range of conditions from obesity,[10] diabetes mellitus,[11] atherosclerosis,[12,13] and hypertension, to Alzheimer's and Parkinson's diseases, cancer,[14,15] depression,[16,17,18,19] and autism. Support is increasingly growing for the contention that ALL chronic illness has a significant inflammatory component. Even the frailty associated with biological aging (and perhaps aging itself) appears to result from the cumulative effects of inflammation.[20,21,22]

All of this tells us that the physiology of inflammation is not a locally isolated phenomenon, but instead is a process that is closely intertwined with the overall health of the individual.[23,24,25] Consequently, the revelations that emerge from investigating how these mechanisms operate under normal and abnormal conditions are proving to have profound implications for every branch of medicine. Before we can adequately and intelligently assume the task of safely and effectively influencing the course of chronic inflammatory disorders, it is essential for us to fully understand the underlying mechanisms at work. Since the tenor of the interaction between immune cells and foreign substances determines whether the outcome will be quiescent tolerance or the initiation of an inflammatory cascade,[26] it is critical that we understand what influences this interaction on a structural and biochemical level. It has become increasingly clear to researchers in the life sciences that structure and function are inextricably interrelated. Consequently, we must have a working knowledge of the normal molecular biology of inflammatory triggers, effector cells, and their mediators before we can truly understand how this process goes awry.

The Cellular and Molecular Biology of Immunity and Inflammation

Knowing how specific three-dimensional structures interact with immune and other effector cells to activate the inflammatory response, and how various mediators act on a molecular level to amplify or dampen that response, will help us find precise ways to modify the body's reactions when interventions are needed. Such interventions could involve prevention, modulation, or augmentation of immune function; whatever the strategy, the overriding principle—according to the tenets of functional medicine—is to achieve a positive outcome without causing additional harm in the process. To better appreciate the critical role that triggers and mediators play in this process, it is essential to understand the overall context in which the immune system operates.

Innate and Acquired Immunity: Development and Function

The primary roles of a healthy, balanced immune system are:

1. identify potentially infectious or injurious substances (e.g., necrotic cellular debris),
2. distinguish self antigens (i.e., non-threatening) from non-self (i.e., threatening),
3. assess the potential level of threat posed by infectious, toxic or non-self antigens,
4. mount a response that is appropriate to the level of threat, and
5. repair any damage that ensues from adversarial encounters.

The primary responsibility for identifying infectious or injurious substances is assigned to the innate arm of the immune system.[27,28] For this reason, the sentinel agents of innate immunity, including macrophages, dendritic cells, and related antigen-presenting cells (APCs), are widely distributed throughout mucosal surfaces, connective tissues, and organs.[29] Natural killer cells, which constitute between 5 and 15% of peripheral circulating lymphocytes, are also involved in innate immunity.[30,31,32]

Rather than identifying every possible antigen, APCs express cell surface receptors for patterns unique to microorganisms, allowing for rapid identification of pathogens without the need for prior exposure to them. APCs are typically activated and are able to initiate an inflammatory response within minutes to a few hours after injury.[33] An important skill possessed by dendritic cells is their ability to migrate (under the influence of chemokines, TNF-α, IL-1β and other inflammatory cytokines) from epithelial and mucosal surfaces to draining lymph nodes or to far-flung systemic sites, which gives them access to increasingly large venues for broadcasting warning messages about locally generated infractions.[34,35]

In contrast, the tasks of the acquired/adaptive arm are to provide an expandable army of clones that can (1) amplify the cascade initiated by activated APCs, and/or (2) functionally recognize pathogens missed by the innate system.[36] Accomplishing the second task relies on an exquisite sensitivity for distinguishing between self- and non-self antigens. This requires a high level of refinement and training, enabling the lymphocytes to become efficient but extremely obedient killing machines. Without this training, they could attack their host (which is exactly what happens in autoimmune disorders). The early phases of training are under control of the thymus. This training has been referred to as "self-referential," in that it exclusively relies on *internal* cues for preparing the lymphocytes to recognize a potentially vast array of *external* cues that it may encounter throughout the life of the host. Lymphocytes that fail in their early training and react to self antigens are rapidly eliminated.

The later phases of training involve "mentoring" by APCs and regulatory lymphocytes. Exposure to a pathogen allows APCs to capture it and subsequently process and display its peptide fragments in the MHC II (major histocompatibility complex) sites on their surface membranes. Contact with these MHC-peptide complexes on mature dendritic cells acts to prime lymphocytes so that they will be able to recognize the pathogen during subsequent exposure. Because of its reliance on clonal expansion, the acquired immune system may take days or even weeks before its reaction to infectious and other non-self triggers becomes apparent. Rejection of a transplanted organ or delayed hypersensitivity reactions are typical examples, while IgE-mediated, type I allergic reactions are an obvious exception to this generalization.[37]

Innate immunity and chronic inflammation. For many years it was thought that the innate system was mostly involved in the *acute* inflammatory response, and that the primary mediator of *chronic* inflammation was the acquired immune system (i.e., B and T lymphocytes). However, new evidence indicates that an overstimulated or dysfunctional innate system—acting in conjunction with affected vascular and connective tissues—plays at least as prominent a role in instigating and perpetuating chronic conditions.[38,39,40] For example, dendritic cells can function both as initiators *and* active modulators of the immune response by ongoing induction of lymphocytes.[41] Although increased numbers of activated B and T lymphocytes are typically found wherever there is chronic inflammation (e.g., the synovitis associated with rheumatoid arthritis or the persistent dermatitis with eczema), both cell types are under the *direct control* of dendritic cells.[42]

Dendritic cells can also actively participate in the ongoing tolerization of T lymphocytes against self-antigens. This suggests that the loss of tolerance that appears in autoimmunity or transplant rejection, or the increased tolerance that occurs with cancer, could—paradoxically—both be manifestations of dysregulation by dendritic cells.[43,44,45] Recognizing this has led to renewed interest in the specific pathways involved in the activation, maturation, and subsequent deactivation of dendritic cells and other APCs.

Molecular Triggers of the Immune Response and their Receptors

As previously noted, one of the primary triggers for the innate immunologic reaction is a group of specific microscopic structures. These structures have been termed pathogen-associated molecular patterns (PAMPs). PAMPs are highly conserved, "generic" motifs that are abundant in many different microorganisms, including viruses, bacteria, and fungi. Since they are *not* normally found in vertebrates, their presence serves as a major warning signal to APCs and phagocytes. PAMPs include bacterial lipopolysaccharides (LPS, aka endotoxin) from gram-negative cell walls; teichoic and lipoteichoic acids (LTA) predominantly from gram-positive bacteria; flagellin, pilin, and N-formyl-methionine found in bacterial proteins; peptidoglycan, mannans, glucans, glycolipids, and zymosan from fungal cell walls; double-stranded RNA from viruses; unmethylated cytosine-guanine dinucleotide sequences (CpG DNA) found in bacterial and viral genomes.

APCs and other innate immune cells recognize PAMPs through a variety of transmembrane and intracellular glycoprotein receptors. While these receptors can identify over 1,000 different structures, they have no capacity for recognizing self-associated antigens. In other words, they are incapable of reacting to host tissues. There are two main classes of pattern-recognition receptors, signaling and endocytic. In addition, a series of soluble pattern-recognition receptors circulate in the bloodstream, where they function as opsonins that can bind to microbes, initiating the complement cascade and phagocytosis.[46]

Toll-like receptors (TLRs) are the primary signaling pattern-recognition receptors.[47,48] At least nine different TLRs have been identified. Typically appearing in pairs, different cell types express different TLR combinations, translating into varying abilities of an APC to respond to a particular bacteria, virus, fungus, etc. A significant feature of the TLR system is its presence in all multicellular organisms, indicating the ancient and fundamental role it has played throughout evolution. (In contrast, specific antigen recognition by antibodies—acquired/adaptive immunity—occurred much later in the course of evolution and is only found in vertebrate species.) TLRs are members of the larger superfamily of interleukin-1 receptors, with which they share the same intracellular subunit and many of the same downstream signaling molecules.[49,50,51,52,53]

Intracellular Signaling Pathways and their Gene Products

These highly specialized pathogen sensors transduce the warning signals conveyed by foreign macromolecules into a flurry of activity by intracellular protein kinases and related enzymes that employ phosphorylation and similar catalytic processes to turn on a network of intracellular biochemical pathways.[54,55,56,57] In most cases, this leads to the activation in the cytosol of nuclear-factor kappa B (NFκB) by uncoupling it from I-kappa B inhibitor proteins, which are subsequently degraded.[58] This allows the translocation of NFκB to the nucleus, where it binds to specific gene-promoter regions on DNA, resulting in the increased transcription and translation of proinflammatory cytokines, type II inducible cyclooxygenases, inducible nitric oxide synthases, various adhesion molecules (VCAM, ICAM, etc.), and metalloproteinases.[59,60,61]

Interestingly, even though activation of the NFκB family of transcription factors is a constant feature of this process, ligand binding to different pairs of TLRs results in the synthesis of different types and mixtures of cytokines. For example, TLRs that bind to viral components (e.g., TLR-3 and TLR-8) lead to increased production of interferons.[62] Zymosan from fungal cell walls will bind to a different combination of TLRs (TLR-2/TLR-6) than bacterial endotoxins (TLR-4/TLR-4).[63] Both lead to increased production of proinflammatory cytokines, including IL-2, TNF-α and IL-8, but the specific profile will be slightly different depending on the initial trigger. Since NFκB is upregulated in all these situations, this indicates the collateral involvement of a large network of additional receptors, transcription factors and co-regulatory molecules that determine the specific gene promoter regions to which NFκBs are able to bind. For example, endotoxin's effects are also mediated through LPS binding protein and CD14, both of which collaborate with TLR4 to stimulate the synthesis of proinflammatory cytokines.[64] Similarly, the effects of fungal beta-glucans are also mediated through binding to dectin-1, a recently identified transmembrane lectin APC receptor that collaboratively promotes the activation of TLR2 signaling.[65]

Additional Innate Receptors: Endocytic Receptors, Scavenger Receptors, and RAGEs

In addition to signaling pattern-recognition receptors, endocytic receptors also play a critical role in the innate inflammatory response. Located on the surface of macrophages and other phagocytes, these multiligand receptors facilitate the binding, engulfment and degradation of pathogens and cellular debris. The predominant members of this class include a superfamily of macrophage scavenger receptors and receptors for advanced glycosylation end products (RAGEs). Macrophage scavenger receptors, like toll-like receptors, are also glycoproteins that bind to many of the same PAMPS, including endotoxin from gram-negative and lipoteichoic acid from gram-positive bacteria. However, they also "scavenge" negatively-charged endogenous substances that have been chemically altered or modified, such as oxidized LDL, HDL, and other lipids, glyco-oxidized adducts (i.e., advanced glycosylation end products), and amyloid E-protein.[66] RAGEs differ from scavenger receptors in that they bind exclusively to endogenously generated molecules, including AGEs, amyloid fibrils, and prion-derived peptides.[67]

Like TLRs, scavenger receptors and RAGEs utilize activated NFκB as the central conduit for increasing transcription and translation of proinflammatory cytokines and enzymes. The normal role of signaling and endocytic scavenger receptors is to assist with host defense, cell adhesion, and removal of debris from systemic circulation. However, considering that they are activated by many of the same triggers associated with *chronic* inflammation, it is not surprising to find that genetic variants, resulting in an upregulation of their expression, have been linked to a seemingly disparate group of conditions, including atherosclerosis, Alzheimer's disease, and cancer (e.g., prostate).[68,69] This is consistent with the converse observation—for example, polymorphisms in toll-like receptor 4 that *downregulate* its response to LPS are associated with decreased production of proinflammatory cytokines and an increased risk of contracting severe bacterial infections, but a *decreased risk* of developing atherosclerosis.[70] Similarly, a person with increased expression of macrophage scavenger receptors and RAGEs would be more vulnerable to the inflammatory effects of a diet high in free radicals, oxidized fat, and refined carbohydrates.[71]

NFκB-mediated Gene Activation: Final Common Pathway for Inflammatory Responses

In summary, the innate immune system depends heavily on signals provided by all of these receptors to determine the need for possible defensive action. Consequently, this signal transduction network and its downstream cascades of enzymatic activation are increasingly being recognized as a major crossroads that links inflammatory triggers with the effector cells and mediators that achieve their effects.[72] Directly in the center of this crossroads is the NFκB protein family, which appears to be upregulated in almost every acute *and* chronic inflammatory disorder, whether it is appendicitis, pancreatitis, periodontitis, tuberculosis, cancer, diabetes, inflammatory bowel disease, rheumatoid arthritis, neurodegenerative disease, COPD, osteolytic bone disease, or muscular dystrophy.[73,74,75,76,77,78,79]

NFκB proteins can be activated by a variety of physiologic and nonphysiologic stimuli, including exposure of cells to PAMPs,[80] reactive oxygen species (particularly oxidized lipids),[81] reactive nitrogen species, glycated proteins,[82] homocysteine, gliadin, arsenic, lead, iron or nickel, polycyclic aromatic hydrocarbons,[83] polychlorinated biphenyls (PCBs), cigarette smoke,[84] TNF-α, IL-1, IL-18, interferon and other inflammatory cytokines, activated B and T lymphocytes, adenosine, bradykinin,[85] angiotensin II, ionizing radiation, mechanical lung ventilation, and even simple mechanical stretching of muscle fibers.[86] Although the acute activation of NFκB plays a central role in both innate and acquired defenses against infection, it can become constitutively activated with chronic oxidative stress or with aging (in which case, constitutive expression does not just appear in hematopoietic cells, but in a wide range of tissues).[87,88,89] Although this constitutive activation would appear to be invariably detrimental, the discovery that it can also occur in healthy lymphoid tissue raises the possibility that low-level gene promotion by NFκB may exert a beneficial influence in maintaining immunologic homeostasis.[90]

The issue of NFκB's beneficial effects is extremely significant in light of current efforts to synthesize pharmaceutical agents to inactivate NFκB.[91,92,93] Glucocorticoids are the best known example of such agents.[94] One of the main therapeutic effects of glucocorticoids is to increase the intracellular synthesis of I-kappa B, which binds to and inhibits NFκB.[95] The potent anti-inflammatory effects of glucocorticoids are well known, as are their side effects. A designer pharmaceutical agent that is even more effective than glucocorticoids at inhibiting NFκB would be predicted to have even more negative consequences. In contrast, a large number of naturally occurring phytochemicals derived from foods and botanical medicines have been found to downregulate NFκB without completely inhibiting it. These substances include alpha lipoic acid,[96] vitamin C, vitamin E, N-acetylcysteine,[97] cat's claw extract,[98] silymarin from milk thistle, flavonoids from citrus,[99] resveratrol from purple grape skin,[100,101] curcumin from turmeric,[102,103] green and black tea polyphenols,[104] ginkgolides from Ginkgo biloba, parthenolide from feverfew,[105] boswellic acid from Boswellia serrata,[106] and baicalin from Chinese skullcap.[107] Even *simple caloric restriction* (which reduces oxidative stress), can reduce NFκB activation. Considering that many of these foods or herbs have been safely consumed for long periods of time—in some cases over a thousand years—without reports of significant adverse efforts, exploring their therapeutic potential as immunomodulators should be an extremely high priority for immunologists, pharmacologists, and *clinicians*.)

Depending on the type of cell involved, reactive oxygen species, heavy metals, and other toxins can activate numerous other transcription factors besides NFκB, such as AP-1, a collective term for a group of dimeric proteins with varying subunits (e.g., Jun, Fos, or Activating Transcription Factor) found in endothelial cells that regulate many of the same genes as NFκB, including cytokines, chemokines, matrix metalloproteinases, adhesion molecules, and inducible nitric oxide synthase. Also expressed in endothelial cells are hypoxia-inducible transcription factors (HIF-1, HIF-1β, and HIF-2), which strongly influence transcription of numerous proinflammatory vascular genes.[108]

The Role of Danger Signals in Immune Activation

It is important to point out that simple exposure to PAMPs is often insufficient for activating an immune response. This is especially important with regard to commensal bacteria in the intestines. Most of these bacteria possess macromolecules that are theoretically capable of binding numerous receptors on antigen-presenting cells. Although many of these potential triggers are masked by secretory IgA or mucin glycoproteins, a significant level of interaction with dendritic cells and macrophages still occurs on a regular basis.[109] However, in healthy individuals, the inflammatory response to these bacteria is kept under control and tolerance is the rule.[110,111] What accounts for this ongoing truce between immune cells and their mortal enemies that allows a lifetime of relatively quiet cohabitation?

Inhibition of toll-like receptor signaling by intracellular proteins like interleukin-1 receptor-associated kinase-M (IRAK-M) and regulatory effects of suppressor lymphocytes and their associated cytokines (e.g., TGF-β, IL-4 and IL-10) clearly play a role in keeping the peace and maintaining homeostasis in the innate system.[112,113,114,115,116] Intestinal macrophages—the largest such reservoir in the body—have been found to display profound inflammatory anergy without limitations in their phagocytic or bacteriocidal activity.[117] This appears to result from downregulation of their ability to produce proinflammatory cytokines by TGF-β and other non-specific suppressor factors, all of which may be induced by exposure to high concentrations of soluble dietary antigens.

Even though tolerance is the norm, the state of calm is relatively fragile and can easily be disrupted, a situation that most likely occurs on a frequent and regular basis.[118,119,120] While most of those disruptions are not clinically evident, they can manifest as transient autoimmune phenomena sometimes associated with bacterial and viral infections, such as rashes and arthralgias. A breach in tolerance can also lead to persistent post-infection problems like rheumatic valvular disease, post-streptococcal glomerulonephritis, or immune-mediated behavioral problems like tics and obsessive-compulsive disorder associated with PANDAS syndrome (Pediatric Autoimmune Neuropsychiatric Disorder associated with Streptococcal Infections).[121]

It may be that the source of disruption leading to activation or intolerance is not just a stranger, but a stranger combined with molecular indications of threat: "stranger plus danger." A theory championed by the immunologists Charles Janeway and Polly Matzinger (among others) is that when the message of foreignness transmitted by PAMPs is accompanied by specific danger signals, the result is robust activation of APCs.[122,123] Without the presence of these additional signals, innate immune cells might be less likely to respond to a potential inflammatory trigger.[124] To use an analogy, consider a street cop in a rough neighborhood, who has become inured to the minor thefts of petty criminals. However, he doesn't hesitate to swing into action when alerted by alarms from a bank being robbed.

Sources of danger signals. Injured or dying cells—a sequelae of trauma, post-ischemic reperfusion, or accelerated apoptosis—release a wide variety of substances that might communicate danger messages.[125,126] Crystalline uric acid (monosodium urate), a degradation product of DNA and RNA, is a strong candidate to be one of the principal endogenous danger signals. Well known for its role in the excruciatingly painful inflammation of acute gouty arthritis, uric acid has been shown to stimulate the maturation of dendritic cells and enhance their ability to present foreign antigens to T lymphocytes.[127] Mammalian DNA is immunologically "cloaked" by methyl groups, but *undermethylated* DNA (found in systemic lupus erythematosus and other autoimmune disorders) is also thought to act as a danger signal in certain contexts.[128] Other candidates for communicating danger are heat shock proteins (HSPs), pluripotential molecular chaperones that are elaborated by cells subjected to a wide variety of physical and emotional stressors.[129] Among many other actions, HSPs have been found to stimulate the maturation of dendritic cells and also to initiate an acute inflammatory response by binding directly to toll-like receptors.[130]

Individuals who are less physically fit tend to be less adept at producing HSPs; as a consequence, their immune systems are less effective at mounting an appropriate inflammatory response to bacterial or viral invasion. This may offer a partial explanation for why people who exercise more are often more resistant to infection. Another implication of these findings is that the biochemical events set in motion by non-pathogenic stressors—such as severe or persistent emotional turmoil—could result in the loss of tolerance to normal intestinal flora, thus paving the way for inflammatory bowel disease or possibly even atherosclerosis.[131]

Loss of Tolerance, Th1/Th2 Imbalance, and the Role of Normal Gut Flora

Despite the growing body of data illuminating the phenomenon, it is clear that much remains to be understood about oral tolerance. Of equal importance to the factors that can disrupt the peace and lead to a loss of tolerance are those that can help to restore and maintain it. The latter is a concept that is just starting to be exploited through the use of probiotic bacteria, which have been shown to enhance the tolerizing effects of suppressor T cells, but undoubtedly work through numerous other mechanisms as well.[132,133] Certain species of lactobacilli have even been shown to produce IL-10, which exerts similar immunomodulatory and anti-inflammatory effects as regulatory lymphocytes. Research on the tolerizing effects of very low doses of specific orally-administered antigens such as type II collagen (in rheumatoid arthritis) and myelin basic protein (multiple sclerosis) has also been promising, although there are many unknowns about the most effective dosage and length of administration required to achieve a clinical effect.[134]

An emerging body of literature postulates that one reason for the rising tide of atopic syndrome, inflammatory bowel disease, and autoimmune disease (e.g., type 1 diabetes, multiple sclerosis) in modern societies is the lack of exposure to tolerizing amounts of antigens in the first year of life.[135,136,137,138,139] Numerous studies show that children who are raised on farms, have multiple siblings, spend time in day-care centers, or live with cats or dogs in the first 6 to 12 months of life are less likely to develop allergies than children from relatively sterile urban environments.[140] In contrast, offspring of mothers who took antibiotics during pregnancy are more likely to be atopic.[141] The "hygiene hypothesis" suggests that an infant's immature immune system requires a certain level of inoculation by dietary antigens to become fully competent.[142,143] In this case, competence is defined as the balanced expression of cell-mediated immunity, driven by Th1 cytokines (INF-γ, IL-2, and IL-12), with that of humoral immunity, driven by Th2 cytokines (IL-4, 5, 6, and 10). Since Th1 cytokines exert counter-regulatory effects on Th2 lymphocytes and vice versa, it is critical that both subsets are equally active (or equally suppressed) to achieve balanced immune functioning.[144,145,146,147]

Under normal circumstances, the neonatal immune system is somewhat biased towards Th2 dominance. After birth, the intestinal flora develops in conjunction with growth factors present in colostrum and breast milk.[148,149] Exposing the gut to small amounts of antigens from helminths or "friendly" microbes, including saprophytic mycobacteria and lactobacilli, results in interactions between the normal flora, dendritic cells, and macrophages in the gastrointestinal-associated lymphoid tract.[150,151,152,153,154,155] This serves to program and mature the APCs, which induce CD4+CD25+ regulatory lymphocytes (Tr1 and Th3 cells) to secrete IL-10, TGF-β and other regulatory cytokines; they, in turn, exert a modulatory effect on both Th1 and Th2 lymphocytes along with enhanced production of secretory IgA.[156,157] The net effect of activating regulatory lymphocytes is suppressed immune responses to ingested antigens.[158,159,160,161] In the absence of such regulatory programming, a subset of children with polymorphisms in innate receptors such as TLR2 or NOD2 have a higher risk of developing atopic syndrome or inflammatory bowel disease. Interestingly, even though regulatory lymphocytes appear to be activated by specific antigens, they *respond* in a "generic" non-antigen specific manner—a phenomenon referred to as bystander suppression.

The obvious question is whether Th1/Th2 imbalances or similar dysregulated immune function can be prevented *in utero* or during the neonatal period. While no one is recommending feeding dirt to children, administration of probiotic bacteria to both pregnant women and neonates decreased the incidence of atopic syndrome in several clinical trials.[162,163] The apparent success of this approach has led to increased interest in the possibility that restoring immune tolerance in the gut could also reverse disorders of immune dysregulation, such as inflammatory bowel disease, autoimmune arthritis, or asthma, even after they have become firmly established.[164,165,166] In addition to the use of specific strains of probiotic bacteria, trials are also underway with the use of helminth-derived antigens. While some of the findings are mixed and many questions remain about the specifics of this strategy, early results do suggest sufficient beneficial effects to warrant further study.

Acquired/Adaptive Immune Responses and Inflammation

As previously discussed, repeated exposure to specific pathogens or other antigens can also activate the acquired, antigen-specific immune response primarily mediated by B and T lymphocytes. This type of response is familiar as the etiology of the Gell and Coombs schema of hypersensitivity reactions, including type I, IgE-mediated, immediate allergic reactions; type II antibody/complement mediated cytotoxic reactions; type III immune complex/complement reactions; and type IV cell-mediated (T-cell, macrophage) delayed reactions.[167] Each category of unbalanced or excessive immune responses is associated with a specific group of inflammatory disorders, such as atopic syndrome and anaphylaxis (type I), hemolytic transfusion reactions (type II), serum sickness and connective tissue disorders with associated vasculitis, synovitis, endocarditis, and glomerulonephritis (type III), and contact dermatitis or thyroiditis (type IV).[168]

Although innate responses are usually distinguished by their immediacy of onset relative to the acquired response—type I reactions excepted—their ultimate manifestations often share many overlapping features with acquired responses and can have almost identical signs and symptoms. For example, the dermatitis caused by exposing a sensitized individual to the Rhus antigen from a poison ivy plant can appear very similar to a localized sunburn. Even though the specific constellation of physiologic and biochemical pathways that are activated may vary considerably depending on the specific type of injury, the portal of entry and the region or system of the body that is affected, the overall process maintains a recognizable thematic consistency. This unifying theme is the restoration of health and homeostasis by defending tissues against invasion by pathogens and repairing the damage incurred by that invasion.

Endogenous Inflammatory Mediators and their Physiologic Effects

Since it is designed to defend and repair the body against pathogens and trauma, the inflammatory response could accurately be defined as *a process with a purpose*. Whether initiated by the release of debris from injured or necrotic cells, the activation of macrophages and monocytes by PAMPs, AGEs or oxidized LDL, or the exposure to environmental or autologous antigens, a set of common pathways will be invoked, leading ultimately to the increased production of proinflammatory cytokines. As key players in this process, these messenger molecules transmit alarm signals that activate numerous cell types, including additional leukocytes, platelets, local endothelial cells, and fibroblasts. Activation of phospholipase A2 in membranes of leukocytes and platelets liberates arachidonic acid, which then undergoes rapid enzymatic conversion into prostaglandins, thromboxanes, and leukotrienes.[169,170] Mast cells, basophils, and other leukocytes degranulate, releasing histamine and proteolytic enzymes. Activated endothelial cells release pro-coagulant factors. The complement cascade is activated and bradykinin is liberated from high molecular-weight kininogen.

The net effect of all these events is hypersensitization of sensory nerve fibers to noxious stimuli, an increase in local vascular perfusion, hyperpermeability of post-capillary venules, an increase in coagulability, smooth muscle relaxation (vasodilatation) or contraction (bronchoconstriction), and mobilization of additional leukocytes. Once mobilized by chemokines, leukocytes become sticky and attach to endothelial adhesion molecules (VCAM-1, etc.) on the vascular wall, roll (under the influence of selectins), become superadherent (under the influence of ICAM-1), and extravasate into the injured area. Activated platelets release thromboxanes, become sticky, clump together and adhere to rough surfaces of the extracellular matrix exposed by injury to the endothelium.

As noted previously, these complex and diverse physiologic shifts are united by common goals. Increased blood flow allows the rapid removal of debris and pathogens. Increased capillary permeability permits the migration of leukocytes to the site of injury. Shifting fluids into the extravascular compartment results in dilution of toxins and pathogens. Increased coagulation causes the formation of microthrombi, which assist in walling off the injured area. Complement split products bind to pathogens, thereby increasing their susceptibility to phagocytosis (i.e., opsonization). Pain activates a withdrawal reflex, preventing additional trauma. Increased temperature has an antiseptic effect.

The acute phase response: systemic effects of local inflammation. In addition to the local consequences of an inflammatory reaction, there are additional systemic effects known as the acute phase response. As previously discussed, activation of TLRs on tissue macrophages and other leukocytes by pathogens results in increased production of IL-6, IL-1-β and TNF-α. These proinflammatory cytokines then travel via the systemic circulation to the liver, where they induce synthesis of a group of proteins called acute phase reactants.[171] Increased levels of glucocorticoids work synergistically with IL-6 and IL-1-β to further stimulate hepatic protein synthesis. During an acute inflammatory response, collective production of these proteins is dramatically elevated, and can range up to 45 grams per day.[172]

There is an initial, rapid increase in C-reactive protein (from 100 to 1000 fold in 24-48 hours) and mannan-binding protein (MBP), both of which function as soluble pattern-recognition receptors, adding further to the body's ability to recognize PAMP structures on foreign invaders. C-reactive protein acts as an opsonin by binding to phospholipids in microbial membranes. This increases phagocytosis along with activation of the classic complement cascade. Similarly MBP participates in opsonization by binding to mannose found in bacterial and fungal cell walls. There is also a rapid increase in serum amyloid A, which influences leukocyte adhesion, migration, proliferation, and aggregation.[173]

Over time, these rapidly released proteins are joined by a slower increase in hepatic production of proteins involved in coagulation (fibrinogen, prothrombin, plasminogen-activator inhibitor-1), transport proteins (ferritin, ceruloplasmin, and haptoglobin), hepcidin, antiproteolytic proteins (α-1-antitrypsin, α-2-macroglobulin), complement (CH50, CH100), and complement components (C3 and C4). Elevations in the erythrocyte sedimentation rate, a commonly used clinical marker for the presence of an acute phase response, are primarily a reflection of elevated plasma fibrinogen, and tend to change relatively slowly. In contrast, C-reactive protein levels can change rapidly and tend to be a much more precise marker of the overall degree of inflammation.[174]

The liver's need for the raw materials to synthesize these proteins contributes to an overall state of catabolism, exemplified by the diversion from plasma of amino acids that are normally used for skeletal muscle. The endocrine system in turn, releases a host of hormones that induce catabolism and gluconeogenesis, including adrenocorticotropic hormone, cortisol, catecholamines, growth hormone, insulin, glucagons, and thyroxin. In addition to myalgias, muscle wasting, and cachexia, other systemic consequences of this acute phase response include anorexia, lethargy, dysthymia, anemia (inhibition of erythropoietin), leukocytosis, thrombocytosis, hypoalbuminemia, hyperglycemia, hyperlipidemia (primarily hypertriglyceridemia), increased plasma glutathione, increased inducible nitric oxide synthase, hypercupremia, hypozincemia, and hypoferremia. Activation of toll-like receptors and/or systemic elevations of pyrogenic cytokines (primarily IL-6 but also IL-1-β and TNF-α) raise prostaglandin E2 in the hypothalamic thermal control center, which responds by increasing body temperature.[175] It has been of great clinical interest to recognize that surgical trauma creates a scenario identical to this acute phase reaction (with all of its attendant morbidity), and that the intensity of the response corresponds to the extent of the trauma. Strenuous exercise and childbirth can also produce mild acute-phase reactions.

Counter-regulatory Control Mechanisms

Although the intrinsic goal of this process is to restore homeostasis by fighting off infection and repairing tissue, it is obvious that the acute-phase reaction can quickly become detrimental if it continues unabated. As with oral tolerance, the immune system provides numerous checks and balances to keep the acute-phase response from getting out of control. One of the most extensive anti-inflammatory counter-regulatory mechanisms is mediated by two peroxisome proliferator-activated receptors, PPARα and PPARγ. These nuclear receptor transcription factors were first discovered as ligands for lipid- and glucose-regulating pharmaceutical agents—PPARα for fibrates, and PPARγ for thiazolidinediones—and were therefore thought to primarily be involved in control of metabolism. It was then determined that fatty acids and eicosanoids were natural PPAR ligands; for example, leukotriene B4 (LTB4) activates PPARα, while prostaglandin J2 binds to PPARγ. When these mediators are released during the inflammatory cascade, they bind to and activate effector cells, but also bind to PPARs, which then negatively interfere with NFκB-driven production of multiple inflammatory gene products. Research now shows that increased activity of PPARs can lower overall oxidative stress and reduce the inflammation found with asthma, cardiovascular disease, and cancer.[176,177,178,179,180,181,182,183,184]

(As with NFκB, significant efforts are being made to find potent pharmaceutical agents that stimulate PPAR activity; however, as evidenced by the severe hepatoxicity exhibited by some of these agents, such an approach is fraught with difficulties. Part of the problem may be that the effects of activating PPARs are not exclusively anti-inflammatory—in certain contexts, they can exert inflammatory effects as well. However, for reasons that are not completely understood, dietary essential fatty acids, including fish oil (EPA/DHA)[185] and 9,11 isomers of conjugated linoleic acid (CLA) have also been found to activate PPARs without any associated toxicity. DHEA, an endogenous androgenic steroid that is widely used as a dietary supplement, has been shown to upregulate PPARα without evidence of hepatotoxicity in normal therapeutic doses, which may explain some of DHEA's purported "anti-aging" effects. Similarly, diindolylmethane, a glucosinolate derivate from cruciferous vegetables, appears to be a specific ligand for PPARγ, and may exert influence on lipid and glucose metabolism.)

Other critical counter-regulatory control points involve:

1. downregulation of TLR activation by IRAK-M;[186,187]
2. modulation of cytokine activity, by increased production of lipoxins,[188,189,190] resolvins, transforming growth factor-beta, and/or other anti-inflammatory cytokines (IL-4, IL-10);[191]
3. neutralizing effects of circulating cytokine receptors (e.g., IL-1 receptor antagonist, soluble TNF-α receptor); and
4. dampening of the intracellular signaling pathways induced by eicosanoids or cytokines (e.g., inhibition of phospholipase A2 by uteroglobin and other endogenous mediators).[192]

Obviously, the scales that hold inflammatory mediators in one tray and anti-inflammatory mediators in the other must be extremely precise in their measurements.[193] All it takes is a slight tip in the balance and the entire system can become disrupted. Hence, the great care that must be taken when one attempts to manipulate this system with pharmaceutical agents.

Loss of Regulatory Control: A Maladaptive State Resulting in Chronic Inflammation

While the overall trend is similar, different people who have the same illness (or undergo similar degrees of trauma) can experience wide variations in their production of acute-phase reactants. This indicates that each component of the inflammatory response is subject to individual regulatory control, which is a reflection of the interplay between genetic predisposition and environmental influences. It follows then that one of the predominant factors in determining the overall health of an individual is whether the person's immune system is operating in a fundamentally balanced or imbalanced fashion.[194] When the immune system is acting in a balanced and appropriate way, the vast majority of inflammatory reactions to ongoing insults do not create significant or noticeable perturbations in a person's overall state of health. These reactions are adaptive in the sense that they are part of a self-regulating cybernetic loop.[195] In other words, they are in a continuous state of readjustment based on feedback about current conditions in the internal and external environment.[196]

Inflammatory reactions become problematic when they are (1) extreme, as in the case of sepsis, disseminated intravascular coagulation, anaphylaxis, and anaphylactic shock; (2) progressively destructive, as in the deleterious sequelae of reperfusion after myocardial or neural ischemia, certain chemical injuries, sunburn, or frostbite; or (3) persistent or recurrent, as in the case of allergy or autoimmune disease. In these scenarios, the largely beneficial response to acute injury transforms into a detrimental pattern that injures the very same tissues that it was designed to heal. Simply put, the damage caused by an inflammatory response to injury can sometimes be equivalent to—or greater than—than the original injury.

Many chronic inflammatory diseases are characterized by elevated levels of C-reactive protein,[197] INF-γ, IL-1, IL-6,[198] and TNF-α, i.e., the very same mediators expressed during the acute phase reaction.[199,200,201] Although the elevations may not be as high as they are in the acute phase, they are distinct and reproducible. It's as if the acute-phase reaction has been dampened, but never adequately extinguished. Instead of an inferno, a better analogy would be a slow, smoldering fire with intermittent eruptions. A wealth of evidence has now accumulated showing this is the case for a wide range of conditions, including asthma, eczema, osteoarthritis, rheumatoid arthritis, systemic lupus erythematosus, thyroiditis, neurodegenerative disorders, diabetes mellitus, and cardiovascular disease.[202,203,204,205,206,207]

In the examples given above, the pattern of reaction may not serve any overtly useful purpose at all. Consequently, this situation can be described as maladaptive. No longer part of a carefully orchestrated cybernetic feedback system, the pattern operates without the self-regulating constraints that normally prevent it from being harmful. This shift from a balanced state of dynamic immunologic activity that is oriented toward maintaining homeostasis, to a state of chronic imbalance, can be likened to a planned, controlled burn in a dry forest that leaps past strategically placed barriers and becomes an expanding conflagration. A particularly deleterious aspect of a maladaptive inflammatory reaction is that it can become stuck in a recursive, "feed-forward" cycle, independent of the triggers that initially set it in motion. In addition to intracellular protein kinase-based cascades, a host of extracellular cascades can also be activated, including complement, kininogen-bradykinin, and coagulation (fibrinogen), all of which serve to amplify the inflammatory response.

Anaphylaxis, self-amplifying cascades, and the butterfly effect. Anaphylaxis is perhaps the most dramatic example of how remarkably efficient this self-amplification process can be. Initial exposure to antigenic epitopes present in hymenoptera venom, certain foods, latex, drugs, etc. leads to activation of T-helper 2 lymphocytes, which utilize IL-4 and related cytokines to transform B lymphocytes into plasma cells that secrete IgE antibodies specific to the epitope. These IgE antibodies bind to Fc receptors on the surface of mast cells found in the respiratory mucosa, gastric mucosa, skin, and connective tissue.[208]

In susceptible (e.g., atopic) individuals, re-exposure from ingestion or inhalation of the epitope results in binding to ligand recognition sites on the IgE antibodies. When two or more IgE antibodies are bound, this cross-linking aggregation activates membrane-linked G proteins, which in turn activate tyrosine kinases. This initiates a cascade of phosphorylation reactions involving numerous intracellular proteins, resulting in increased intracellular levels of cGMP, an influx of Ca++ into the cell, and—within minutes of the initial exposure—subsequent degranulation, which liberates an array of vasoactive and smooth muscle-constricting mediators including histamine, heparin, TNF-α, and adenosine, followed by *de novo* synthesis of additional proinflammatory cytokines, prostaglandins, and leukotrienes.[209] Once released into the extracellular environment, these mediators then activate additional mast cells through "non-antigenic" pathways, a process of recruitment that allows a local phenomenon to rapidly escalate until it involves multiple organ systems.[210]

As mentioned earlier in this discussion, the linear cause-and-effect paradigm that has long dominated conventional medicine does not fully encompass the complex network of physiologic reactions that occur in situations like anaphylaxis, sepsis, or disseminated intravascular coagulation, or the mechanisms by which streptococcal pharyngitis leads to rheumatic valvular disease. A linear model would liken anaphylaxis to a "domino effect," in which an initial trigger sets into motion a series of sequential events. But this model falls short in its ability to predict when the reaction will occur and what the speed of onset and severity—the overall trend—will be once it develops. For example, it is well known that anaphylaxis is not a dose-response phenomenon: the relative severity of anaphylactic reactions is independent of the amount of antigen involved. In some situations, extremely minute quantities of antigen (e.g., a sudden whiff of peanuts from the package opened by a passenger in the next row on an airplane) are sufficient to activate a fatal response within minutes.

But why does a person have different reactions to the same food at different times? And why does the reaction self-attenuate in some situations but not others? A more sophisticated explanatory model might approach these questions by exploring in great detail every aspect of the initial conditions in which the reaction was triggered. In other words, seemingly peripheral information such as the person's mood, the temperature of the room, or the time of day when the reaction occurred might be given equal weight to the level of antigenic exposure. This emphasis on having a thorough knowledge about the context in which a problem developed is based on a concept called the "butterfly effect," which describes the tendency of a complex system to be highly sensitive to initial conditions.

Inflammation: a complex response to simple phenomena. Complex systems like the human body are prone to acting in unpredictable ways. The butterfly effect suggests that—in the right context—a butterfly flapping its wings could set off a series of events that result in a tornado in some other part of the world. In other words, when the right force is applied at the right time to a susceptible object, this tiny shift in initial conditions leads to a disturbance in the overall balance of the system that results in a series of interconnected, self-amplifying, exponentially expanding reactions that become dramatically more powerful and on a much larger scale than the original shift in energy.

This concept is the essence of chaos theory, and it provides a potential framework that can encompass all of the complex physiological pathways described in this chapter, without pretending to fully comprehend the specific ways in which these pathways work in every conceivable situation.[211,212,213,214,215] As will be discussed later, the scientific paradigm represented by chaos theory is not limited to the study of inflammation and immune disorders, but applies to the entire discipline of functional medicine. The important point here is that a minuscule disruptive event can be sufficient to create a severe or chronic inflammatory condition.[216] But it is also true that a relatively minor intervention—if carefully conceived—can sometimes create a positive perturbation that leads to a restoration of balance. For example, simply taking a probiotic supplement can cause major changes in the gut flora, resulting in a series of physiologic events that ultimately decreases the person's systemic allergic symptoms.

Returning to the example at hand, after considering how destructive mast cell degranulation can be—not just in the case of anaphylaxis but also because of its major role in a wide range of immunologic reactions—it is tempting to perceive this entire system as nothing more than a dangerous remnant from a less hygienic past. Perhaps IgE and the weapons it unleashes were useful when humans were under continuous assault by helminths and other parasitic infections, but it's hard to believe that they are necessary in the age of modernity. Or are they? Again, it's important to point out that the inflammatory process has a purpose: to maintain the overall health of the individual. In fact, several studies have shown that mast cells play a critical role in the innate immune response against bacterial infection. They also help modulate Th1 delayed hypersensitivity reactions. And, considering the diverse range of cytokine receptors they display, and their ubiquity in the body, it is likely that they interact with other cell types in essential ways that we do not yet understand. The ultimate conclusion is that no single aspect of the inflammatory process—no single cell type, no individual eicosanoid, cytokine, adhesion molecule, or transcription factor—is inherently bad. This concept strongly challenges interventions derived from a monocular perspective focusing on the elimination of individual mediators without recognition of the potential for "collateral" damage in such a process.

The Drug-Disease Model of Inflammation: History and Current Issues

Clearly, determining the myriad exogenous and endogenous factors involved in catalyzing and perpetuating the transformation from acute to chronic inflammation is one of the most pressing issues in medicine today. The answers to the questions about what factors allow the inflammatory process to get out of control and stay out of control, and what interventions are the most effective, safest, and most easily implemented to prevent and treat chronic inflammation, have major ramifications for every branch of medicine, from pathology to public health policy. One of the defining features of functional medicine is the unique perspective it provides for exploring these issues. By reviewing how the disease-centered model came to dominate the diagnosis and treatment of chronic inflammatory disorders, we can analyze the shortcomings inherent in that approach, and clinicians can achieve a better understanding of how the functional medicine perspective differs and what it has to offer.

Value Systems and the Goals of Scientific Research

Consider the implications of the following statement, "Many of the key enzymes and proteins in the arachidonic acid signaling cascade were identified, and rational drug design is in progress to interact with these targets."[217] Implicit in the quotation is an intimate reciprocity long shared by the disciplines of immunology and pharmacology (and, by implication, the pharmaceutical industry).[218] For example, an immunologist might start the discovery process by investigating specific inflammatory mediators (e.g., leukotrienes), then explore upstream to find the biochemical pathways involved in their production (metabolic conversion from arachidonic acid precursors), followed by the enzymes that catalyze the rate-limiting, regulatory steps in those pathways (e.g., 5′ lipo-oxygenase). This information is shared with pharmacologists, who then develop synthetic agents that inhibit the activity of those regulatory enzymes (e.g., zileuton, a 5′ lipo-oxygenase inhibitor) or block the receptors activated by the mediators (e.g., montelukast). Reports regarding the clinical effects of those drugs then serve as feedback for further refining the immunologists' understanding of how exogenous and endogenous factors modify the inflammatory cascade. In turn, this information is used to develop anti-inflammatory agents with a higher degree of specificity for their targets, with the expectation that this specificity will translate into improved efficacy.

An alternate version of this process might begin with identification of a plant extract or synthetic drug that appears to have anti-inflammatory or immunomodulatory properties. Working downstream, pharmacologists attempt to elucidate the mechanisms by which the extract or drug exerts its effects. Eventually, this leads to a greater understanding of which endogenous mediators are being affected, what specific pathways are involved, and what factors influence the activity of those pathways. The ultimate goal of this process is to develop a patentable substance that can be extracted and isolated from the plant or synthesized in the laboratory.

Contrast the strategies described above to the following goals:

- identify anti-inflammatory substances in commonly eaten foods or inexpensive, readily obtainable supplements and herbs;
- disseminate that information widely so that it can be used to improve the overall health of the population; and
- search for common dietary and environmental triggers that are contributing to our epidemic of inflammatory disease and then use that information to shape public policy.

Unfortunately, achieving these latter goals requires heavily funded research and education initiatives. Because natural products, dietary interventions, and lifestyle changes do not involve patentable drugs, they don't attract the same kind of support that pharmaceutical research does. The challenge is to find ways to achieve these goals, to ease the burden of chronic disease on our population, and thereby to help ease the cost burden of health care as it is practiced today.

NSAIDs and the Development of the Pharmaceutical Industry

The development of nonsteroidal anti-inflammatory drugs (NSAIDs) can serve as a model for how the pharmaceutical industry originated in, but then moved away from, access to therapeutic natural products. The narrative stretches back approximately 2500 years to the time of Hippocrates of Cos (460–377 BC). Even as he was attempting to understand the mechanisms behind the various diseases of his day (many of which later turned out to be immune system disorders), Hippocrates engaged in empirical medicine by prescribing an extract made from a popular folk remedy of his day to alleviate pain (*dolor*) and fever (*calor*) in his patients. One of the main ingredients in this extract was willow bark (*Salix alba*), an herb that had already been used for over a thousand years. In the 1820s, after another two millennia of popular use, a glycoside called salicin was isolated from the bark. In 1839, Karl Löwig mixed salicin with hydrochloric acid (similar to the gastric environment) and produced salicylic acid. Later identified in many other plants, salicylates were determined to be the active constituent responsible for the herb's anti-inflammatory properties. Salicylic acid quickly came into widespread use as a panacea for a wide range of illnesses.

In 1853, the French chemist Charles Gerhardt was able to synthesize a crude version of acetyl-salicylic acid (ASA) by adding an acetyl group to salicylic acid. Several years later, Carl Kraut managed to refine the process and produce a pure form of ASA. However, the clinical significance of this compound was not appreciated until 1897, when Arthür Eichengrun, a chemist with the German dye production company Friedrich Bayer, instructed his colleague, Felix Hoffman, to repeat Gerhardt's acetylation experiments with the hope that a pure version of ASA might provide a more tolerable alternative to salicylic acid. Eichengrun then tried the drug on himself, after which he conducted clinical trials that showed it caused much less gastric discomfort and nausea than its precursor. In 1899, he subsequently renamed this drug aspirin, to denote an acetylated form of salicylic acid obtained from *Spiraea*, the Latin genus for meadowsweet, which—like willow bark—is a rich source of the parent compound. (Unfortunately, when the Nazis came into power, Eichengrun—a Jew—was sent to a concentration camp, and the credit for discovering aspirin went to the "Aryan" Hoffman and his superior, Heinrich Dreser. However, the true story eventually emerged and Eichengrun's role was reinstated.)[219,220]

Aspirin achieved distinction as the first major synthetic drug ever sold in tablet form—an event which spawned the modern pharmaceutical era. Aggressively marketed around the world, aspirin quickly became extremely popular and has continued to be one of the most successful synthetic medicines in history: over 100 billion aspirin tablets are now taken each year all over the planet.[221] Salicylates in willow bark, meadowsweet, and numerous other plants were eventually found to work by inhibiting cyclooxygenase (originally called prostaglandin H2 synthase), the rate-limiting enzyme involved in the conversion of arachidonic acid into proinflammatory prostaglandins and thromboxanes.[222]

Indomethacin, one of aspirin's first commercially viable successors, was synthesized in 1963. Although it was a very potent drug, its usefulness was limited by significant GI toxicity. In 1969, after 15 years of evaluating a host of potential competitors through an extensive trial and error process, ibuprofen was introduced as an effective and well-tolerated aspirin alternative. In 1971, not long after ibuprofen's release, Dr. John Vane discovered that the mode of action of aspirin, ibuprofen, and indomethacin was to block the production of *prostaglandins*: short-lived, locally-acting chemical mediators (also called autocoids) that are now known to be present in all inflamed tissue.[223] He later determined that the specific enzyme blocked by all of these drugs was cyclooxygenase—a feat for which he shared the Nobel Prize in 1982 and was knighted in 1984. The desire to find ever-safer and more potent alternatives led to a detailed study of structure-function relationships between cyclooxygenase, salicylates, and ibuprofen. Out of this research emerged a plethora of related cyclooxygenase inhibitors that came to be referred to as NSAIDs.

Within a few short years, NSAIDs became the treatment of choice for many manifestations of the inflammatory response, particularly fever and pain. They also became, and remain, the standard of care for treating inflammatory arthritides and many types of nociceptive pain (i.e., pain caused by injury to tissues). In addition, some of them have been shown to play a role in preventive medicine. Because of its antiplatelet properties, low-dose aspirin has proved to be particularly effective at preventing myocardial infarctions and other thrombotic disease. More recently, it has been shown to help prevent neoplasms of the colon and breast.

Despite these advantages, NSAIDs also have significant limitations. They have no discernible impact on many inflammatory manifestations, including allergic reactions, urticaria, asthma, and atopic syndromes. In fact, NSAIDs are frequently implicated in allergic drug reactions. They are minimally effective for neuropathic pain, fasciitis, or tendonitis (even though they are often prescribed for these problems). They also commonly produce side effects, including gastrointestinal hemorrhage, edema, and renal damage. Less appreciated by mainstream practitioners—despite extensive documentation in the medical literature—is the fact that NSAIDs can increase small intestine permeability and create a chronic inflammatory enteropathy. By accelerating the translocation of macromolecules and pathogenic microbes from the GI tract into the systemic circulation, NSAIDs inadvertently increase the total antigenic load. This, in turn, leads to the increased formation of antigen-antibody complexes that can initiate inflammatory reactions, either in the bloodstream or after their deposition in connective tissues or basement membranes.

Concerns about the limitations of NSAIDs resulted in a push for safer and more effective alternatives. Laboratory research in the 1980s and early 1990s at Washington University, St. Louis, conducted by Needleman, Siebert, Fu and Masferrer, and at the University of Rochester, led by Donald Young and his colleagues, led to the discovery that there were two isoforms of cyclooxygenase with distinctly different functions. According to the model developed by these researchers, COX-1 is a ubiquitous, constitutively expressed intracellular enzyme located in the endoplasmic reticulum that plays a primary "housekeeping" role in maintaining healthy gastric mucosa and renal blood flow. It is the only COX isoform expressed in platelets, where it catalyzes production of precursors to thromboxane A2, a potent proaggregatory agent.[224]

COX-2 shares a 60% sequence homology with COX-1. Under normal conditions it is barely detectable. However, after exposure to certain inflammatory triggers—including trauma, free radicals, cytokines, growth factors, and endotoxins from pathogenic microbes—it is rapidly induced, appearing in the endoplasmic reticulum and nuclear membrane of macrophages, synoviocytes, and many other cells.[225] An important distinction is that COX-2 expression is readily blocked by glucocorticoids, which generally do not affect COX-1 activity.

The working model postulated that COX-1 is a "good" enzyme and that COX-2 is primarily—perhaps exclusively—responsible for producing the mediators responsible for pain and inflammation. Since both isoforms catalyze the same biochemical reactions and produce the same end products, the presumption is that the difference in their biologic effects results from the site of action and the level of mediators produced—i.e., COX-1 produces a constant but low level of prostanoids, in contrast to COX-2, which, after induction, produces much higher levels.[226]

Since drugs like aspirin and ibuprofen nonselectively inhibit both COX-1 and COX-2, it is axiomatic that their anti-inflammatory properties are accompanied by the undesirable side effects previously mentioned, including gastric ulceration and renal toxicity. Young and Needleman's model implied that an ideal anti-inflammatory drug could bypass these effects, provided that it specifically inhibited COX-2 when used at normal therapeutic doses. This concept was utilized to synthesize celecoxib, the first of the selective COX-2 inhibitors, which was introduced to the market in 1998. Rofecoxib followed soon after in 1999, and later valdecoxib. Bolstered by the initial positive results of the CLASS and VIGOR trials, and heavily promoted as safe and effective alternatives to nonselective NSAIDs, within a few years of their release these agents became some of the top-selling drugs in the world, each generating $2.5–3 billion in annual sales.

The popularity of COX-2 inhibitors provided more evidence for the successful strategies used to market them than evidence of their clinical effectiveness. The reality was that they never lived up to their promise. Serious questions have been raised about the hypothesis that prostanoids involved in inflammation are exclusively produced by COX-2, and that COX-1 is exclusively responsible for producing the prostanoids that protect renal function and the gastric mucosa. In point of fact, COX-1 has been found to be inducible in certain inflammatory states and COX-2 appears to participate in several beneficial housekeeping roles throughout the body, especially in the CNS and the renal cortex, where its constitutive expression is widespread.[227]

A major concern has been that, even though COX-2 inhibitors are 10–20 times more expensive than nonselective NSAIDs, they have never been found to be any better at relieving pain or inflammation. Furthermore, when used in higher doses or for long periods of time, they can still cause GI injury, and are associated with an increased risk of myocardial infarction and other thrombotic events.[228] (The mechanism for this effect is not fully understood, but is most likely related to the preferential blockade of prostacyclin production by endothelial COX-2, without the concomitant inhibition of thromboxane by COX-1. This leads to a relative increase in thromboxane activity compared to prostacyclin—the exact opposite of the effect that is achieved by low-dose aspirin.[229,230]) It was no surprise to many informed observers when, in September 2004, Merck and Company suddenly withdrew rofecoxib from the world market after a clinical trial testing its potential to prevent recurrence of colonic polyps showed a significant increase in heart attacks and strokes in study participants after 18 months of use.

Linear Thinking, Magic Bullets, and Limitations of the Disease-Specific Paradigm

This story about a fundamental pathophysiologic process and the evolution of a class of drugs used to modify that process reveals how a conglomeration of personalities, empirical knowledge, scientific discoveries, and economic incentives all mesh together to create a consensus based on what appears to be a logically-derived, evidence-based standard of care that may, in reality, turn out to be deeply flawed. The rapid rise and fall in popularity of COX-2 inhibitors and the ongoing, aggressive search for similar pharmaceutical agents show how easy it is for a kind of mass delusion to develop, both within the medical community and among the general public. It illustrates the limitations inherent in the conventional paradigm, which continues to focus on overly simplistic solutions for complex problems—solutions that, unfortunately, continue to be disproportionately influenced by the profit motive.[231]

The ongoing wish to discover therapeutic "magic bullets" is a direct consequence of thinking about disease as a linear process. (A line with branches, perhaps, but still a line.) It presupposes that the best way to control a pathologic process is to figure out which physiologic pathways have become dysfunctional, identify the most influential steps in those pathways, and then control, shut down or eliminate those steps. In most cases, this control is achieved with potent synthetic pharmaceutical agents. A consequence of this way of thinking is that every disease tends to get paired with the specific drug used to treat it. In some cases the pairing is very useful, but in others it is misleading or even counterproductive. It *might* be useful to consider type 1 diabetes mellitus a primary insulin deficiency, even though its pathophysiology is more complex than that. (Consider that, before the discovery of insulin, salicylates were commonly used as a relatively successful treatment for hyperglycemia.) However, despite being cast in the same mold as type 1, type 2 diabetes mellitus is not simply a matter of insulin deficiency. Similarly, rheumatoid arthritis is no more a methotrexate deficiency than eczema is a corticosteroid deficiency, even though such relationships are frequently implied in the medical literature.

This model is based on a Newtonian view of the world in which diseases are classified as discrete, self-contained entities for which the *differences* between each disease are more important than the similarities. For example, it would be extremely unlikely for a conventional practitioner to consider the similarities between seemingly disparate diseases like rheumatoid arthritis, ulcerative colitis, and multiple sclerosis, even though all three conditions could be seen as different manifestations of the chronic inflammatory response. Studies showing that people with psoriasis are predisposed to the metabolic syndrome might appear anomalous until one considers that the chronic inflammation associated with psoriasis can exacerbate insulin resistance.

Even though parallels may exist, each disease is thought to develop and progress on its own linear pathway of cause and effect. This perspective is exemplified by the ascendance of specialty (and subspecialty) medicine, where physicians work with one bodily system (or perhaps one organ or even one disease), as though each disease could somehow be extracted from the surrounding ocean of physiological processes in which it formed. According to this model, an individual is born with a set of genes that determine the risk of developing a specific disease. Although that risk can be modified by environmental factors, the person's genetic predisposition plays the dominant role. Once the genes have been fully expressed and a disease has developed, the pathologic process cannot be reversed, only controlled.

The War against Inflammation: Negative Consequences of Treating Symptoms instead of Correcting Underlying Dysfunction

In metaphoric terms, inflammatory diseases are viewed as a kind of war that needs to be fought with the most powerful weapons available. The most desired outcome is to win that war by shutting off the inflammatory process as quickly as possible. Since the end justifies the means, one should be prepared to accept a certain degree of collateral damage. In this case, collateral damage translates into side effects from the treatment being administered. So long as the side effects are not immediately debilitating (based on the practitioner's assessment, not the patient's), they should be considered a necessary evil in the fight against disease.

For example, disease-modifying, anti-rheumatic drugs (DMARDs) such as methotrexate or leflunomide are being recommended increasingly early in the course of rheumatoid arthritis, even in cases of relatively mild severity. The effectiveness of these drugs for providing relief of inflammatory signs and symptoms is heavily emphasized to justify their use as first line therapies. However, another fact that receives much less attention is that both of these drugs have a very narrow therapeutic window because of their severe toxicity. Among other things, they are potent immunosuppressive agents associated with a significantly increased risk of developing malignant neoplasms.

Similarly, monoclonal antibodies against various cytokines, such as TNF-α and its receptors, are increasingly being used as a therapeutic target for rheumatoid arthritis and other autoimmune disorders. The dramatic clinical successes associated with these drugs obscures three important facts: (1) cytokines are multifunctional—they are not inherently good or bad; (2) cytokines rarely act alone—they act in concert, as integral parts of a large, complex signaling network; (3) different combinations of cytokines can have very different effects, depending on the specific receptor cells they are activating. Understanding this leads to the conclusion that any attempt to block a single aberrant message without changing the imbalanced system that created it in the first place will inevitably lead to untoward long-term consequences.

For example, infliximab, a TNF-α blocker used to treat RA, Crohn's disease, and psoriasis, increases the risk of developing tuberculosis, sepsis, and pneumonia, indicating that TNF-α is a critical part of the host defense against certain pathogens.[232,233] Similarly, natalizumab is a monoclonal antibody that binds to and inhibits α-4-β-1 integrin, an adhesion molecule that is expressed by activated lymphocytes and monocytes. Blocking this adhesion molecule prevents the migration of leukocytes across the blood-brain barrier—a process that is thought to be an essential step in the inflammatory demyelination found in multiple sclerosis. Although the drug initially showed great promise in decreasing the number of relapses and new lesions in people with MS, it had to be given intravenously once a month and was extraordinarily expensive. However, soon after its introduction to the market, it was voluntarily withdrawn by the manufacturer and further clinical trials were stopped following reports of three confirmed cases (including one fatality) of progressive multifocal leukoencephalopathy that developed in patients after taking the drug.[234] These problems clearly illustrate the potentially dire consequences that can result from isolated approaches to interfering with the inflammatory cascade that do not consider the impact of the intervention on the entire system.[235]

Interventions for Chronic Endothelial Inflammation: Statins vs. Diet and Lifestyle Changes

Another current example of thinking inside the box is the use of statin drugs to prevent cardiovascular disease. For many years, it has been assumed that the primary therapeutic action of statins results from their ability to lower serum cholesterol by competitively inhibiting the 3-hydroxy-3-methylglutaryl coenzyme-A reductase enzyme responsible for catalyzing the reduction of HMG-CoA into CoA and mevalonate, a cholesterol precursor. However, there is an increasingly large body of evidence that the lipid-lowering properties of statins are actually secondary to their anti-inflammatory effects, which appear to be at least partially achieved through the downregulation of NFκB. Statins are now being increasingly repositioned as anti-inflammatory drugs with the potential to treat cancer, multiple sclerosis, or Alzheimer's disease.[236,237]

This begs the obvious question: if cardiovascular disease is primarily a chronic inflammatory disorder[238,239] (see Chapters 18 and 27, for a focused discussion of the inflammatory basis of CVD), why do we continue to utilize a class of expensive, prescription drugs based on a concept of pathophysiology that is flawed and outdated? From a public health standpoint, wouldn't it be more cost effective (not to mention logical) to investigate the benefits of carefully designed diets that are rich in phytochemicals with known anti-inflammatory effects, and lower in inflammatory triggers such as *trans* fatty acids and refined carbohydrates?[240,241,242] The benefits of such an approach would appear to be illustrated by numerous studies showing that a Mediterranean diet can decrease mortality to a much greater extent than statins, and at a fraction of the cost.[243,244] However, despite these major challenges to their title as the standard of care for prevention of cardiovascular disease, statins continue to be prescribed to larger and larger percentages of the population, thus discounting the value of diet and nutrition. (The many benefits of diet and nutrition as therapeutic strategies for both prevention and management of chronic disease are thoroughly explored in Chapter 26.)

Compartmentalized Thinking and the Suppression of Innovation

One of the biggest problems that emerges from this kind of compartmentalized thinking is that it stifles innovation and discourages the use of interventions that require stepping out of the box to get a broad overview.[245] Dr. David Horrobin, a pioneer in the use of dietary essential fatty acids as biological response modifiers for psychiatric disorders and chronic inflammatory diseases, addressed this issue in an elegant essay titled, "The Philosophical Basis of Peer Review and the Suppression of Innovation."[246] In his article, Horrobin described the potentially detrimental effects of the peer review process, which can become so focused on maintaining acceptable standards of research methodology that it loses sight of the larger goal of medicine, which is to find, in his words, "improved ways of curing, relieving, and comforting patients." In another editorial, Horrobin says that our current system of research inhibits progress and discourages research into the potential benefits of natural substances:

> No drug that does not have the support of a substantial company is likely to be funded. No drug can attract such corporate support unless it is fully patent protected. In this climate, there can be few trials of nutrients or biochemical intermediates, of novel uses for old drugs, and of natural products, which were all major sources of past therapeutic success. We have taken drug discovery procedures from patient-orientated clinicians and handed them over to large bureaucracies who will work only with patent-protected products that give an adequate financial return. No wonder that real progress is so slow.[247]

An open and prepared mind is needed to recognize valuable information that may not fit neatly into any of the prevailing ideas in health care today. It is, in part, the goal of this book to prepare the way for new thinking.

Cookbook Medicine: Behaviorism, Practice Guidelines, and Diagnosis-based Protocols

Several decades ago, similar issues about the most effective strategies for solving problems were confronted in the field of cognitive psychology. For many years a "stimulus-response" model was thought to be the basic unit of behavior. The stimulus-response unit assumes that similar stimuli will elicit similar behavioral responses. Despite its popularity, this model proved to have many limitations in predicting how humans might react to various situations. In 1960, Miller, Galanter and Pribram challenged the paradigm by proposing an alternate unit called the TOTE model (Test-Operate-Test-Exit).[248] The obvious flexibility and widespread applicability of the TOTE unit led to its adoption as a fundamental concept in information-processing theory. Instead of organizing around fixed *response patterns*, the TOTE model emphasizes the importance of having a fixed *goal* as the desired outcome. A range of different behaviors can be employed as a "test" to see if they achieve the goal. If they do not, the behavior is immediately "exited" (without applying a value judgment) and another attempt is instituted, repeating the process until the goal is ultimately achieved. In essence, the stimulus-response model is organized around a fixed methodology, which implies a variable outcome, in contrast to the TOTE model, which maintains a fixed goal, but allows a variable range of behaviors to achieve that goal.

The stimulus-response unit has many parallels with the protocol model that has increasingly come to dominate clinical care. In the protocol model, the "stimulus" is a diagnosis, which is linked to a set of algorithms or "behaviors" that are recommended interventions based on a standard of care called practice guidelines. These practice guidelines are derived from an expert consensus regarding current evidence. In reality, they represent a fixed methodology (often pejoratively referred to as a "cookbook" approach) to a given stimulus. The problem with such an approach is self-evident: if every individual with a problem is treated the same way, then the outcomes are likely to be highly variable. For example, if every individual with a blood pressure of 140/90 is treated with a thiazide diuretic—per current practice guidelines—some will improve, some will have no response at all, others will have allergic reactions, others will develop severe hypokalemia, and a few will have idiosyncratic reactions that cannot be explained by the known mechanism of action of the drug.

Patient-centered Functional Medicine: Teleology Replaces Dogma

The patient-centered approach espoused by functional medicine is very different from the protocol model. The validity of clinical protocols based on a predetermined generalized standard of care is not a given. Instead, the assumption is that each patient is an individual who may require a unique set of interventions for solving the problem(s) at hand. If the goal of solving the problem is paramount, then the practitioner does not have to be bound to a specific methodology. In other words, functional medicine emphasizes teleology over dogma. Rather than pursuing increasingly regimented and standardized treatments for specific diseases, functional medicine clinicians seek to identify the underlying patterns and processes that led to the development of disease or dysfunction in the first place. This model gives the practitioner much more leeway in designing interventions that are tailored for a specific patient. It also makes a considerable demand on the practitioner to stay current with emerging knowledge in many fields: biochemistry and physiology, genetics and genomics, behavioral change and environmental medicine, to name some of the most important ones. Interventions based on improving function can draw on an expanded database that includes information from diverse sources—bench science *and* clinical research, drugs *and* diet, nutritional supplements *and* botanical medicines. Suddenly, the therapeutic armamentarium is much larger and much more flexible.

The functional medicine matrix provides a tool for information gathering and clustering that can help to sift and sort the larger volume of data that comes to the clinician's attention in this model. (See the final section of the book, *Putting It All Together*, for a discussion on using the matrix.) Potential imbalances in various bodily systems and environmental inputs are identified and used to construct a web-like map that illustrates a person's overall condition and helps to pinpoint general areas where interventions may be most needed and most widely effective. A rich and colorful picture of a person's life emerges. The matrix tool makes it abundantly clear that it is, indeed, more important to know what kind of person has a disease than what kind of disease a person has (to paraphrase William Osler). Gathering information in this manner allows the practitioner to maintain an open mind about what is happening in the life of the patient, and a high degree of flexibility about how to work with any conditions that may be present. The assumption is that one can always reach for a deeper understanding of how an individual's health has gone awry—there will always be other questions to ask.

While it is respectful of the full range of therapeutic options and possibilities, functional medicine is not complementary and alternative medicine (CAM)—a very broad field containing numerous systems, disciplines, and modalities with specialized and often quite distinct beliefs and practices. Rather, functional medicine creates a shared arena, based in Western medical science, that is available to conventional and CAM practitioners alike. Clinicians take from functional medicine concepts and approaches that can be applied within their scope of practice, whatever it may be. Functional medicine includes diagnostic techniques and interventions that are science based at minimum and evidence based whenever possible; many of those practices have been validated in clinical trials, and others are extrapolated from current research findings about the potential underlying mechanisms involved in a particular disease process. Functional medicine does not eschew a conventional understanding of the pathological basis of disease, since the clinical utility of these concepts—especially for treatment of acute conditions—is undeniable. In fact, as illustrated by the discussion of basic concepts of inflammation, a thorough understanding of pathophysiology is a prerequisite to mastery of this material. However, it is understood that the lack of placebo-controlled, double-blind studies to support an intervention does not constitute a *prima facie* rationale for automatically discounting that intervention if the underlying science is strong. (See Chapters 5 and 6 for a full discussion of how functional medicine uses science and the research base.)

Functional Medicine Applied to Immune Imbalances

An example will help illustrate these concepts. Rather than immediately reaching for the prescription pad for patients with hypertension, a functional medicine practitioner will ask an array of questions geared toward identifying any underlying imbalances that might be contributing to the person's elevated blood pressure. The informed practitioner will be particularly cognizant of current research that strongly suggests hypertension is actually a chronic inflammatory disorder, for which oxidative stress is one of the primary triggers. Consequently, very important questions include:

- What kind of diet does the person have? Particularly, what is the intake of refined carbohydrates, and is there exposure to rancid fats?
- What kind of exercise does the patient engage in? For how long and how often?
- Has there been any exposure to heavy metals, pesticides, or other environmental toxins that might be an ongoing source of oxidative stress?[249]
- What is the intake of antioxidants and essential fatty acids (that might have a mitigating effect on the disorder)?[250,251,252,253]
- What about electrolytes and trace elements, especially magnesium?
- Are there any unresolved stresses in the person's life that might be causing hypothalamic-pituitary adrenal imbalances that, in turn, could be adversely affecting the renin-angiotensin system, which could be upregulating NFκB-mediated transcription of inflammatory mediators?[254,255,256,257]
- What coping strategies are utilized?
- How well does the patient sleep at night?
- Are there any symptoms suggestive of sleep apnea?

Similarly, a patient might present with an initial complaint of recurrent, painful, and swollen joints in the hands, knees, and/or feet, accompanied by redness and warmth. The traditional medical model would steer a practitioner to order a blood test for rheumatoid factor and start the person on a non-steroidal anti-inflammatory drug. What then, should the practitioner do if the NSAID is ineffective and/or the blood test comes back negative? The conventional choice would most likely involve switching to a more potent pharmaceutical agent and expanding the array of immunological tests performed in search of an alternate diagnosis to rheumatoid arthritis—in other words, looking for another box in which to place the person.

A functional medicine practitioner, on the other hand, will likely seek more detailed information about the person's lifestyle and dietary habits. An extensive history would be taken to look for any stressful events (both emotional and physical) that might have occurred before the symptoms first appeared.[258] Potential exposures to environmental toxins would be explored.[259] A review of systems would be performed with particular attention paid to issues such as gastrointestinal symptoms or reactions to food.[260,261,262] The search for previous medical problems might extend even as far back as infancy with questions regarding the presence of colic, frequent ear infections, heavy use of antibiotics, or NSAIDs.

Functional Medicine's Origins in Systems Biology, Complexity Theory, and Cybernetics

In contrast to a mechanistic, Newtonian model, this kind of approach is modeled on current theories about systems biology, quantum mechanics, and nonlinear dynamics (also called chaos or complexity theory).[263,264,265,266,267,268] According to Hiroaki Kitano, in his article, "Systems Biology: A Brief Overview,"

> System-level understanding, the approach advocated in systems biology, requires a shift in our notion of "what to look for" in biology. While an understanding of genes and proteins continues to be important, the focus is on understanding a system's structure and dynamics. Because a system is not just an assembly of genes and proteins, its properties cannot be fully understood merely by drawing diagrams of their interconnections.[269]

After closely examining the constellation of physiologic events involved in inflammation (both acute and chronic), one cannot help but agree with Maimonides' adage that there is much more that we don't know than what we do know about the way this process with a purpose works—about how all the different parts and pathways manage to interact in an effective manner. Despite its extreme degree of complexity, it does follow recognizable and predictable trends.[270] One of those trends is the tendency for the situation to recur if the underlying conditions that set it off in the first place are still present. This suggests the ultimate futility of chasing down one enzyme or inflammatory mediator at a time to extinguish an aberrant inflammatory response. One is reminded of the hydra, a mythological beast from Argolis with many heads from which it spewed a deadly venom. When one head was severed, it would simply grow another one.

By examining the concatenation of events involved in inflammation, one can conclude that not just the immune system, but the entire human organism is a complex adaptive system, composed of multiple interacting and self-regulating cybernetic loops.[271,272,273] The neurologic, endocrine, and immune systems each have their internal feedback loops, and these dynamically interact with all the other systems. Dr. Albert Szent-Gyorgyi, the noted Hungarian biochemist who first isolated ascorbic acid and flavonoids, postulated that living systems possess a kind of organizing force called *syntropy*, that acts as a counterbalance to the disintegrative force called entropy. Somewhat controversial at the time, his concept of syntropy now appears to be a prescient forerunner of complexity theory.

When humans develop a disease, it is not random occurrence, but rather a behavioral pattern that emerges as a result of an underlying imbalance in one or more of these systems. It is a fallacy to think of a disease as an object that can be placed in a container. The measles virus can be placed in a test tube, but the infectious disease we call measles cannot. Measles is not a thing; it is a behavioral process, the result of a complex interaction between a person's immunologic genotype and their external and internal environments. Unfortunately, by nominalizing disease processes, our current system of medical nomenclature ends up limiting our concepts—and therefore our choices—about the most effective way to approach those processes. It is much more difficult to find a single, effective, safe cure for a disease than it is to look for ways to modify the disease process.

Functional medicine draws from complexity theory by focusing on the recognition of repeating patterns that might be influencing the person's condition. These patterns are more accurately described as an interconnecting web rather than a series of crisscrossing lines. In the same way a tree branches out into complex, but repeating "holographic" patterns called fractals, an inflammatory disorder can also be expressed in repeating patterns that may appear random on initial evaluation, but with closer examination can be found to possess a consistent internal coherence.[274,275] The most useful strategy in such a situation is to analyze the overall trend of the pattern—in which direction is it headed? Is it slowing down, stabilizing, or accelerating? What external or internal factors could be responsible for this trend? And, most important, what can be done to influence the trend without causing major disruptions in the person's physiology?

Supporting Homeostasis/Homeodynamics and Self-healing

Similar to Szent-Gyorgyi's notion of syntropy, an American physiologist, Walter Cannon, PhD, recognized in the 1930s that the human body possesses a certain "wisdom" that continuously returns it to a state of internal equilibrium. He called this state "homeostasis," from the Greek words meaning "to remain the same." Homeostasis is achieved by a series of behavioral adjustments based on information about the body's internal and external environments. As described in Chapter 9, we propose using the more accurate term "homeodynamics," to indicate that most bodily processes actually fluctuate continually within a certain viable range in order to respond to environmental influences. This process of information feedback was termed "cybernetics" by Dr. Norbert Weiner, the mathematician/philosopher. Homeodynamics coupled with cybernetics provides a rational, scientific underpinning for the notion that each patient possesses an inherent ability for self-healing, for returning to a state of healthy balance.[276,277,278] Placing a stronger emphasis on the patient's role in the healing process creates a partnership between patient and practitioner. In this model, the practitioner's role is both healer and educator, helping patients make appropriate decisions regarding their goals for emotional, mental, and physical health—and identifying appropriate means for achieving them.

Modifying Processes Rather than Curing Diseases

Consider the example of celiac disease, also called gluten enteropathy. According to the linear disease model, it results from a genetic intolerance to low molecular weight lectins (gliadins) found in wheat, barley, and rye. Exposure to these proteins results in chronic inflammation of the small intestine villi, leading to malabsorption, often accompanied by diarrhea, malaise, and weight loss. Additional complications can include anemia, osteoporosis, and gastrointestinal lymphoma. Theoretically, all one needs to do is eliminate gluten and the condition will eventually resolve.

This information is accurate, but it is not an adequate description of the phenomenon. It does not explain the high degree of phenotypic variability of the condition for which many people can be asymptomatic, despite regular ingestion of gluten-containing foods.[279] A significant percentage of people who have the MHC class II "celiac genes" (i.e., HLA DQ2 and HLA DQ8) won't develop the disorder, and not everyone with the disorder can be found to have the genes. It also does not fully address the wide range of extraintestinal inflammatory manifestations associated with gluten-sensitivity, including dermatitis herpetiformis, thyroiditis, type 1 diabetes, and neurologic dysfunction such as cerebellar ataxia. When these conditions are associated with celiac disease, they are referred to as manifestations of an autoimmune process, which clearly involves more than a simple inflammatory reaction to gluten.[280,281,282]

A closer look at the pathophysiology reveals that the condition we call celiac disease results from a complex interaction between not one but several HLA and non-HLA genes, in combination with dietary gluten and other environmental factors that are not yet fully understood. One of those "environmental factors" may be the microbial ecology in the person's intestines. A person with a healthy balance of normal flora relative to pathogens may be less susceptible to developing overt reactions to gluten. Or, it could be that a person who is exposed to a lot of environmental toxins or has a high baseline level of oxidative stress may be more prone to becoming symptomatic or developing autoimmune manifestations.[283] These are hypotheses that are well worth investigating.

By thinking of this problem as a disorder *process* rather than a *disease*, the possibilities for working with it begin to expand beyond a simple elimination of gluten. For example, a practitioner of functional medicine might recommend that a person with celiac disease go beyond simple elimination of gluten and undergo a bowel restoration program designed to remove potential pathogens, replace deficient digestive enzymes, repair inflamed intestinal mucosa, and reinoculate the microflora with probiotics.[284] (This is the 4R program, described fully in Chapter 28.) In addition, a program might be instituted for modifying the inflammatory process. Omega-3 fatty acids,[285,286] antioxidants,[287] and anti-inflammatory phytochemicals such as bioflavonoids could be used.

As mentioned in the earlier discussion on oral tolerance, this kind of intervention was illustrated by several studies conducted in Finland in which children with intractable eczema were given a course of probiotic bacteria (lactobacillus GG). The children who received the probiotics showed a significant improvement in their skin condition.[288] Why would a product designed to improve bowel health be considered a therapeutic intervention for a skin disorder? Now that we have explored the complex underlying patterns of inflammatory and immune imbalance, we can perceive the body as an interconnecting web of cybernetic loops, wherein it is perfectly logical to think of the gastrointestinal tract as a potential trigger or mediator (or modulator) for inflammatory reactions that could appear anywhere else in the body.

Summary

Acute inflammation is the body's normal physiologic response to injury or invasion by pathogens. Chronic inflammation is a maladaptive immunologic process responsible for a wide variety of seemingly disparate diseases. A close examination of the molecular biology of inflammation reveals an extraordinarily complex process that utilizes signal transduction networks linked to a series of intricately regulated enzymatic cascades and intercellular messenger molecules that is best understood through the lens of complexity theory and non-linear dynamics. Inflammatory diseases result from imbalances in this network and are not isolated phenomena that can be separated from the context in which they developed.

The butterfly effect tells us that the same trigger can have vastly different results depending on the context in which that trigger appears. Similarly, the same intervention can have vastly different effects depending on the individual who receives that intervention. Consequently, the problem of excessive or chronic inflammation is not adequately addressed by isolating individual inflammatory autacoids and using potent pharmacologic agents to inhibit the production or actions of those substances. Instead, a wider lens is needed to view the entire landscape of an individual's life.

Within that landscape can be recognized (1) antecedents such as genetic polymorphisms and epigenetic factors that could increase the person's predisposition to a immunologic dysregulation and imbalances, (2) acute or recurrent exogenous triggers resulting from a person's lifestyle or environmental exposures that might be responsible for activating an inappropriate inflammatory response, and (3) endogenous mediators that are being overexpressed in response to those triggers. It is appreciated that the ongoing presence of these triggers and mediators fuels the fire and perpetuates the pathology of inflammatory disease.

The functional medicine practitioner's role is to become a conductor of the client's metabolic symphony, someone who relies on the individual's inherent syntropic ability to help restore homeodynamic balance. The most direct and practical ways to accomplish this are:

1. help the client to make dietary and lifestyle changes that will reduce exposure to harmful inflammatory triggers, and
2. employ a rational mixture of antioxidants, biological response modifiers, or/and other therapeutic nutrients and supplements (including enzymes, prebiotics, and probiotics) to assist the person's immune system in moving back toward balance.

References

1. Mitchinson MJ. Fluor: another cardinal sign of inflammation. Lancet. 1989; 2:1520.
2. Parslow, TG, Stites DP, Terr AI (Ed), Imboden JB. Medical Immunology, 10th edition. McGraw-Hill/Appleton and Lange, 2001.
3. Pahl HL. Signal transduction from the endoplasmic reticulum to the cell nucleus. Physiol Rev. 1999;79: 683-701.
4. Aller, MA, Arias, JL, Nava, MP. Posttraumatic inflammation is a complex response based on the pathological expression of the nervous, immune, and endocrine functional systems. Exp Biol and Med. 2004;229:170-81.
5. Jerne NK. Towards a network theory of the immune system. Ann Immunol (Paris). 1974;125C(1–2):373–89.
6. Parslow, TG, Stites DP, Terr AI (Ed), Imboden JB. Medical Immunology, 10th edition. McGraw-Hill/Appleton and Lange, 2001.
7. Dent LA. For better or worse: common determinants influencing health and disease in parasitic infections, asthma and reproductive biology. J Reprod Immunol. 2002;57(1-2):255-72.
8. Lucey DR, Clerici M, Shearer GM. Type 1 and type 2 cytokine dysregulation in human infectious, neoplastic, and inflammatory diseases. Clin Microbiol Rev. 1996;9(4):532-562.
9. McCarty MF. Interleukin-6 as a central mediator of cardiovascular risk associated with chronic inflammation, smoking, diabetes, and visceral obesity: down-regulation with essential fatty acids, ethanol and pentoxifylline. Med Hypotheses. 1999 May;52(5):465-77.
10. Invitti C. Obesity and low-grade systemic inflammation. Minerva Endocrinol. 2002;27(3):209-14.
11. Devaraj S, Jialal I. Alpha tocopherol supplementation decreases serum C-reactive protein and monocyte interleukin-6 levels in normal volunteers and type 2 diabetic patients. Free Radic Biol Med. 2000;29(8):790-92.
12. Benagiano M, Azzurri A, Ciervo A, et al. T helper type 1 lymphocytes drive inflammation in human atherosclerotic lesions. Proc Natl Acad Sci U S A. 2003;100(11):6658–63.
13. Dwyer JH, Allayee H, Dwyer KM, et al. Arachidonate 5-lipoxygenase promoter genotype, dietary arachidonic acid, and atherosclerosis. N Eng J Med. 2004;350(1):29-37.
14. Lucey DR, Clerici, M and Shearer, GM. Type 1 and type 2 cytokine dysregulation in human infectious, neoplastic, and inflammatory diseases. Clin Microbiol Rev. 1996;9(4):532-62.
15. Subbaramaiah K, Zakim D, Weksler BB, et al. Inhibition of cyclooxygenase: a novel approach to cancer prevention. Proc Soc Exp Biol Med. 1997;216:201-10.
16. Frank AK, Frank MM, Atkinson JP, Cantor H. Samter's Immunological Diseases, 6th Edition. Lippincott, Williams, Wilkins, 2001.
17. Glaser R. Mild depressive symptoms are associated with amplified and prolonged inflammatory responses after influenza virus vaccination in older adults. Arch Gen Psychiatry. 2003;60(10):1009-14.
18. Licinio J, Wong ML. The role of inflammatory mediators in the biology of major depression: central nervous system cytokines modulate the biological substrate of depressive symptoms, regulate stress-responsive systems, and contribute to neurotoxicity and neuroprotection. Mol Psychiatry. 1999;4(4):317-27.
19. Schwarz MJ. T-helper-1 and T-helper-2 responses in psychiatric disorders. Brain Behav Immun. 2001;15:340-70.

20. Brod SA. Unregulated inflammation shortens human functional longevity. Inflamm Res. 2000;49(11):561-70.
21. Harris TB, Ferrucci L, Tracy RP, et al. Associations of elevated interleukin-6 and C-reactive protein levels with mortality in the elderly. Am J Med. 1999;106(5):506-12.
22. Walston J, et al. Frailty and activation of the inflammation and coagulation systems with and without clinical comorbidities: results from the Cardiovascular Health Study. Arch Intern Med. 2002;162(20):2333-41.
23. Aller MA, Arias JL, Nava MP. Posttraumatic Inflammation Is a Complex Response Based on the Pathological Expression of the Nervous, Immune, and Endocrine Functional Systems. Exp Biol Med. 2004; 229:170-81.
24. Black PH. Immune system-central nervous system interactions: effect and immunomodulatory consequences of immune system mediators on the brain. Antimicrobial Agents Chemother. 1994;38(1):7-12.
25. Dent LA. For better or worse: common determinants influencing health and disease in parasitic infections, asthma and reproductive biology. J Reprod Immunol. 2002 Oct-Nov;57(1-2):255-72.
26. Stagg AJ, Hart AL, Knight SC, Kamm MA. Microbial-gut interactions in health and disease. Interactions between dendritic cells and bacteria in the regulation of intestinal immunity. Best Pract Res Clin Gastroenterol. 2004 Apr;18(2):255-70.
27. Medzhitov R, Janeway CA Jr. Decoding the patterns of self and nonself by the innate immune system. Science. 2002;296(5566):298-300.
28. Parslow TG, Stites DP, Terr AI (Editor), Imboden JB. Medical Immunology, 10th edition. McGraw-Hill/Appleton, Lange 2001.
29. Medzhitov R, Janeway CA Jr. Innate immunity. N Engl J Med. 2000;343(5):338-44.
30. Janeway CA, Medzhitov R. Innate immune recognition. Annu Rev Immunol. 2002;20:197-216.
31. Janeway CA. How the immune system works to protect the host from infection: a personal view. Proc Nat Acad Sci U S A, 2001;98(13):7461-68.
32. Parslow TG, Stites DP, Terr AI (Editor), Imboden JB. Medical Immunology, 10th edition. McGraw-Hill/Appleton, Lange 2001.
33. Ibid.
34. Janeway CA, Medzhitov R. Innate immune recognition. Annu Rev Immunol. 2002;20:197-216.
35. Janeway CA. How the immune system works to protect the host from infection: a personal view. Proc Nat Acad Sci U S A, 2001;98(13):7461-68.
36. Parslow TG, Stites DP, Terr AI (Editor), Imboden JB. Medical Immunology, 10th edition. McGraw-Hill/Appleton, Lange 2001.
37. Ibid.
38. Janeway CA, Medzhitov R. Innate immune recognition. Annu Rev Immunol. 2002;20:197-216.
39. Janeway CA. How the immune system works to protect the host from infection: a personal view. Proc Nat Acad Sci U S A, 2001;98(13):7461-68.
40. Nguyen MD, D'Aigle T, Gowing G, et al. Exacerbation of motor neuron disease by chronic stimulation of innate immunity in a mouse model of amyotrophic lateral sclerosis. J Neurosci. 2004:24(6):1340-1349.
41. Stagg AJ, Hart AL, Knight SC, Kamm MA. Microbial-gut interactions in health and disease. Interactions between dendritic cells and bacteria in the regulation of intestinal immunity. Best Pract Res Clin Gastroenterol. 2004 Apr;18(2):255-70.
42. Banchereau J, Steinman RM. Dendritic cells and the control of immunity. Nature. 1998;392:245-52.
43. Bach JF. The effect of infections on susceptibility to autoimmune and allergic diseases. N Engl J Med. 2002;347 (12):911-20.
44. Georgiev M, Agle LM, Chu JL. Mature dendritic cells readily break tolerance in normal mice but do not lead to disease expression. Arthritis Rheum. 2005;52(1):225-38.
45. Shlomchik MJ, Craft JE, Mamula MJ. From T to B and back again: positive feedback in systemic autoimmune disease. Nat Rev Immunol. 2001;1(2):147-53.
46. Fujita T. Evolution of the lectin-complement pathway and its role in innate immunity. Nat Rev Immunol. 2002;2(5):346-53.
47. Medzhitov R, Preston-Hurlburt P, Janeway CA Jr. A human homologue of the Drosophila Toll protein signals activation of adaptive immunity. Nature. 1997;388(6640):394-97.
48. Palsson-McDermott EM, O'Neill LA. Signal transduction by the lipopolysaccharide receptor, Toll-like receptor-4. Immunology, 2004;13:153-62.
49. Abreu MT. Immunologic regulation of toll-like receptors in gut epithelium. Curr Opin Gastroenterol. 2003;19(6):559-64.
50. Iwasaki A, Medzhitov R. Toll-like receptor control of the adaptive immune responses. Nat Immunol. 2004;5(10):987-95.
51. O'Neill LA. Immunity's early-warning system. Sci Am. 2005 Jan;292(1):24-31.
52. Underhill DM. Toll-like receptors: networking for success. Eur J Immunol. 2003;33(7):1767-75.
53. Reuter BK, Pizarro TT. Commentary: the role of the IL-18 system and other members of the IL-1R/TLR superfamily in innate mucosal immunity and the pathogenesis of inflammatory bowel disease: friend or foe? Eur J Immunol. 2004;34(9):2347-55.
54. Akira S. Toll-like receptor signaling. J Biol Chem. 2003;278(40):38105-108.
55. Iwasaki A, Medzhitov R. Toll-like receptor control of the adaptive immune responses. Nat Immunol. 2004;5(10):987-95.
56. O'Neill LA. Immunity's early-warning system. Sci Am. 2005 Jan;292(1):24-31.
57. Palsson-McDermott EM, O'Neill LA. Signal transduction by the lipopolysaccharide receptor, Toll-like receptor-4. Immunol, 2004;13:153-62.
58. Baldwin AS Jr. The NF-kappa B and I kappa B proteins: new discoveries and insights. Annu Rev Immunol. 1996;14:649-83.
59. Pahl HL. Activators and target genes of Rel/NF-kB transcription factors. Oncogene. 1999;18:6853-66.
60. Pahl HL. Signal transduction from the endoplasmic reticulum to the cell nucleus. Physiol Rev. 1999;79:683-701.
61. Paik J, Lee JY, Hwang D (2002) Signaling pathways for TNFα-induced COX-2 expression: mediation through MAP kinases and NFκB, and inhibition by certain nonsteroidal anti-inflammatory drugs. Adv Exp Med Biol. 2002;50:503-08.
62. Sato A, Iwasaki A. Induction of antiviral immunity requires Toll-like receptor signaling in both stromal and dendritic cell compartments. Proc Natl Acad Sci U S A. 2004(46):16274-79.
63. Palsson-McDermott EM, O'Neill LA. Signal transduction by the lipopolysaccharide receptor, Toll-like receptor-4. Immunol. 2004;13:153-162.
64. Rodriguez D, Keller AC, Faquim-Mauro EL, et al. Bacterial lipopolysaccharide signaling through Toll-like receptor 4 suppresses asthma-like responses via nitric oxide synthase 2 activity. J Immunol. 2003;171:1001-08.
65. Brown GD, Herre J, Williams DL, et al. Dectin-1 mediates the biological effects of beta-glucans. J Exp Med. 2003;197(9):1119-24.
66. Platt N, Gordon S. Is the class A macrophage scavenger receptor (SR-A) multifunctional?—The mouse's tale. J Clin Invest. 2001. 108:649–54.
67. Schmidt AM, Shi DY, Shi FY, Stern DM. The multiligand receptor RAGE as a progression factor amplifying immune and inflammatory responses. J Clin Invest. 2001;108:949–55.
68. Ibid.

69. Zheng SL, Augustsson-Balter K, Chang B, et al. Sequence variants of toll-like receptor 4 are associated with prostate cancer risk: results from the Cancer Prostate in Sweden Study. Cancer Res. 2004;64(8):2918-22.
70. Kiechl S, Lorenz E, Reindl M, et al. Toll-like receptor 4 polymorphisms and atherogenesis. N Eng J Med. 2002;347(3):185-92.
71. Conner EM, Grisham MB. Inflammation, free radicals and antioxidants. Nutrition. 1996;12(4):272-77.
72. Pahl HL. Signal transduction from the endoplasmic reticulum to the cell nucleus. Physiol Rev. 1999;79:683-701.
73. Baldwin AS Jr. The NF-kappa B and I kappa B proteins: new discoveries and insights. Annu Rev Immunol. 1996;14:649-83.
74. Kumar A, Takada Y, Boriek AM, Aggarwal BB. Nuclear factor-kappaB: its role in health and disease. J Mol Med. 2004;82(7):434-48.
75. Paik J, Lee JY, Hwang D (2002) Signaling pathways for TNFα-induced COX-2 expression: mediation through MAP kinases and NFκB, and inhibition by certain nonsteroidal anti-inflammatory drugs. Adv Exp Med Biol. 2002;50:503-08.
76. Pande V, Ramos MJ. Nuclear factor kB: a potential target for anti-HIV chemotherapy. Curr Med Chem. 2003;10:1603-15.
77. Panwalkar A, Verstovsek S, Giles F. Nuclear factor-kB modulation as a therapeutic approach in hematologic malignancies. Cancer. 2004;100:1578-89.
78. Peng SL. Transcription factors in the pathogenesis of autoimmunity. Clin Immunol. 2004;110:112-23.
79. Pikarsky E, Porat RM, Stein I, et al. NF-kB functions as a tumour promoter in inflammation-associated cancer. Nature. 2004;431:461-66.
80. Ghosh S, May MJ, Kopp EB. NF-kappa B and Rel proteins: evolutionarily conserved mediators of immune responses. Annu Rev Immunol. 1998;16:225-60.
81. Kutuk O, Basaga H. Inflammation meets oxidation: NF-kB as a mediator of initial lesion development in atherosclerosis. Trends Mol Med. 2003;9:549-57.
82. Peiro C, Matesanz N, Nevado J, et al. Glycosylated human oxyhaemoglobin activates nuclear factor-kB and activator protein-1 in cultured human aortic smooth muscle. Br J Pharmacol. 2003;140:681-90.
83. Pei XH, Nakanishi Y, Inoue H, et al. Polycyclic aromatic hydrocarbons induce IL-8 expression through nuclear factor kB activation in A549 cell line. Cytokine. 2002;19:236-41.
84. Pei XH, Nakanishi Y, Takayama K, Bai F and Hara N. Benzo[a]pyrene activates the human p53 gene through induction of nuclear factor kB activity. J Biol Chem. 1999;274:35240-46.
85. Pan ZK, Christiansen SC, Ptasznik A, Zuraw BL. Requirement of phosphatidylinositol 3-kinase activity for bradykinin stimulation of NF-kB activation in cultured human epithelial cells. J Biol Chem. 1999;274:9918-22.
86. Pande V, Ramos MJ. NF-kappaB in human disease: current inhibitors and prospects for de novo structure based design of inhibitors. Curr Chem Chem. 2005;12(3):357-74.
87. Kumar A, Takada Y, Boriek AM, Aggarwal BB. Nuclear factor-kappaB: its role in health and disease. J Mol Med. 2004;82(7):434-48.
88. Kutuk O, Basaga H. Inflammation meets oxidation: NF-kB as a mediator of initial lesion development in atherosclerosis. Trends Molecular Med. 2003;9:549-57.
89. Stuhlmeier KM, Kao, JJ, Back FH. Arachidonic acid influences proinflammatory gene induction by stabilizing the Inhibitor-B/Nuclear Factor-B (NF-B) complex, thus suppressing the nuclear translocation of NF-B. J Biol Chem. 1997;272(39):24679-83.
90. Perkins ND. NF-kB: tumor promoter or suppressor? Trends Cell Biol. 2004;14:64-69.
91. Palanki MS, Erdman PE, Ren M, et al. The design and synthesis of novel orally active inhibitors of AP-1 and NF-kappaB mediated transcriptional activation. SAR of *in vitro* and *in vivo* studies. Bioorg Med Chem Lett. 2003;13(22):4077-80.
92. Pande V, Ramos MJ. Nuclear Factor kB: a potential target for anti HIV chemotherapy. Curr Med Chem. 2003;10:1603-15.
93. Panwalkar A, Verstovsek S, Giles F. Nuclear factor-kB modulation as a therapeutic approach in hematologic malignancies. Cancer. 2004;100:1578-89.
94. Payne DN, Adcock IM. Molecular mechanisms of corticosteroid actions. Paediatr Respir Rev. 2001;2:145-50.
95. Auphan N, DiDonato JA, Rosette C, et al. Immunosuppression by glucocorticoids: inhibition of NF-kappa-B activity through induction of I-kappa-B synthesis. Science. 1995;270:286-90.
96. Packer L. A-lipoic acid: a metabolic antioxidant which regulates NF-kB signal transduction and protects against oxidative injury. Drug Metab Rev. 1998;30:245-75.
97. Pajonk F, Riess K, Sommer A, McBride WH. N-acetyl-L-cysteine inhibits 26S proteasome function: implications for effects on NF-kB activation. Free Radic Biol Med. 2002;32:536-43.
98. Akesson C, Lindgren H, Pero RW, et al. An extract of Uncaria tomentosa inhibiting cell division and NF-kappa B activity without inducing cell death. Int Immunopharmacol. 2003;3(13-14):1889-900.
99. Chen CC, Chow MP, Huang WC, et al. Flavonoids inhibit tumor necrosis factor-alpha-induced up-regulation of intercellular adhesion molecule-1 (ICAM-1) in respiratory epithelial cells through activator protein-1 and nuclear factor-kappaB: structure-activity relationships. Mol Pharmacol. 2004;66(3):683-93.
100. Kundu JK, Surh YJ. Molecular basis of chemoprevention by resveratrol: NF-kB and AP-1 as potential targets. Mutat Res. 2004;555:65-80.
101. Pellegatta F, Bertelli AA, Staels B, et al. Different short- and long-term effects of resveratrol on nuclear factor-kB phosphorylation and nuclear appearance in human endothelial cells. Am J Clin Nutr. 2003;77:1220-28.
102. Kumar A, Dhawan S, Hardegen NJ, Aggarawal BB. Curcumin (Diferuloylmethane) inhibition of tumor necrosis factor (TNF)-mediated adhesion of monocytes to endothelial cells by suppression of cell surface expression of adhesion molecules and of Nuclear Factor-kB activation. Biochem Pharmacol. 1998;55:775-83.
103. Plummer SM, Holloway KA, Manson MM, et al. Inhibition of cyclo-oxygenase 2 gene expression in colon cells by the chemopreventative agent curcumin involves inhibition of NF-kB activation via the NIK/IKK signalling complex. Oncogene. 1999;18:6013-20.
104. Pan MH, Lin-Shiau SY, Ho CT, Lin JH, Lin JK. Suppression of lipopolysaccharide-induced nuclear factor-kappaB activity by theaflavin-3,3'-digallate from black tea and other polyphenols through down-regulation of IkB kinase activity in macrophages. Biochem Pharmacol. 2000;59:357-67.
105. Kwok BHB, Koh B, Ndubuisi MI, Elofsson M, Crews CM. The anti-inflammatory natural product parthenolide from the medicinal herb Feverfew directly binds to and inhibits IkB kinase. Chem Biol. 2001;8:759-66.
106. Syrovets T, Buchele B, Krauss C. Acetyl-boswellic acids inhibit lipopolysaccharide-mediated TNF- induction in monocytes by direct interaction with IkappaB kinases. J Immunol. 2005;174(1):498-506.
107. Bremner P, Heinrich M. Natural products as targeted modulators of the nuclear factor-kappaB pathway. J Pharm Pharmacol. 2002 Apr;54(4):453-72.
108. Semenza GL. Hypoxia-inducible factor-1: master of O2 homeostasis. Curr Opin Genet Dev. 1998;8:588–94.
109. Shanahan F. Nutrient tasting and signaling mechanisms in the gut V. Mechanisms of immunologic sensation of intestinal contents. Am J Physiol Gastrointest Liver Physiol. 2000;278:G191–96.

110. Jump RL, Levine AD. Mechanisms of natural tolerance in the intestine: implications for inflammatory bowel disease. Inflamm Bowel Dis. 2004;10(4):462-78.
111. Strachan DP. Hay fever, hygiene, and household size. BMJ. 1989;299(6710):1259-60.
112. Kobayashi K, Hernandez LD, Galan JE, et al. IRAK-M is a negative regulator of Toll-like receptor signaling. Cell. 2002;110(2):191-202.
113. Nakayama K, Okugawa S, Yanagimoto S, et al. Involvement of IRAK-M in peptidoglycan-induced tolerance in macrophages. J Biol Chem. 2004 Feb 20;279(8):6629-34.
114. Parijs LV, Abbas AK. Homeostasis and self-tolerance in the immune system: turning lymphocytes off. Science. 1998;280:243-48.
115. Wahl SM, Costa GL, Mizel DE, et al. Role of transforming growth factor beta in the pathophysiology of chronic inflammation. J Periodontol. 1993;64(5 Suppl):450-55.
116. Weiner HL. Oral tolerance: immune mechanisms and the generation of Th3-type TGF-beta-secreting regulatory cells. Microbes Infect. 2001;3(11):947-54.
117. Smythies LE, Sellers M, Clements RH, et al. Human intestinal macrophages display profound inflammatory anergy despite avid phagocytic and bacteriocidal activity. J Clin Invest. 2005;115(1):66-75.
118. Jump RL, Levine AD. Mechanisms of natural tolerance in the intestine: implications for inflammatory bowel disease. Inflamm Bowel Dis. 2004;10(4):462-78.
119. Shanahan F. Nutrient tasting and signaling mechanisms in the gut V. Mechanisms of immunologic sensation of intestinal contents. Am J Physiol Gastrointest Liver Physiol. 2000;278:G191–96.
120. Strachan DP. Hay fever, hygiene, and household size. BMJ. 1989;299(6710):1259-60.
121. Bach JF. The effect of infections on susceptibility to autoimmune and allergic diseases. N Engl J Med. 2002;347 (12):911-20.
122. Matzinger P. The danger model: a renewed sense of self. Science. 2002;296(5566):301-5.
123. Pulendran B. Immune activation: death, danger and dendritic cells. Curr Biol. 2004;14(1):R30-32.
124. Jerome KR, Corey L. The danger within. N Eng J Med. 2004;350(4):411-12.
125. Pulendran B. Immune activation: death, danger and dendritic cells. Curr Biol. 2004 Jan 6;14(1):R30-32.
126. Shi Y, Evans JE, Rock KL. Molecular identification of a danger signal that alerts the immune system to dying cells. Nature. 2003;425:516-21.
127. Jerome KR, Corey L. The danger within. N Eng J Med. 2004;350(4):411-12.
128. Richardson B. DNA methylation and autoimmune disease. Clin Immunol. 2003;109(1):72-79.
129. Moseley PL. Heat shock proteins and the inflammatory response. Ann N Y Acad Sci. 1998;856:206-13.
130. Campisi J, Leem TH, Fleshner M. Stress-induced extracellular Hsp72 is a functionally significant danger signal to the immune system. Cell Stress Chaperones. 2003;8(3):272-86.
131. Xu Q. Role of heat shock proteins in atherosclerosis. Arterioscler Thromb Vasc Biol. 2002;22:1547-59.
132. Drakes M, Blanchard T, Czinn S. Bacterial probiotic modulation of dendritic cells. Infect Immun. 2004;72(6):3299-3309.
133. Kanauchi O. Modification of intestinal flora in the treatment of inflammatory bowel disease. Curr Pharm Des. 2003;9(4):333-46.
134. Barinaga, M. Treating arthritis with tolerance. Science. 1993;261:1669-70.
135. Feillet H, Bach JF. Increased incidence of inflammatory bowel disease: the price of the decline of infectious burden? Curr Opin Gastroenterol. 2004;20(6):560-64.
136. Perzanowski MS, Ronmark E, Platts-Mills TA, Lundback B. Effect of cat and dog ownership on sensitization and development of asthma among preteenage children. Am J Respir Crit Care Med. 2002;166(5):696-702.
137. Rook GA, Adams V, Hunt J, et al. Mycobacteria and other environmental organisms as immunomodulators for immunoregulatory disorders. Springer Semin Immunopathol. 2004;25(3-4):237-55.
138. Rook GA, Stanford JL. Give us this day, our daily germs. Immunol Today. 1998;19(3):113-16.
139. Watts G. The defense of dirt. BMJ. 2004;328:1226.
140. Strachan DP. Hay fever, hygiene, and household size. BMJ. 1989;299(6710):1259-60.
141. Benn CS, Melbye M, Wohlfahrt J, et al. Cohort study of sibling effect, infectious diseases, and risk of atopic dermatitis during first 18 months of life. BMJ. 2004;328:1223-27.
142. Strachen DP. Family size, infection and atopy: the first decade of the "hygiene hypothesis." Thorax. 2000;55(suppl 1):S2-10.
143. Weiss ST. Eat dirt–The hygiene hypothesis and allergic diseases. N Engl J Med. 2002;347:930-31.
144. Benagiano M, Azzurri A, Ciervo A, et al. T helper type 1 lymphocytes drive inflammation in human atherosclerotic lesions. Proc Natl Acad Sci U S A. 2003;100(11):6658–63.
145. Kidd P. Th1/Th2 balance: The hypothesis, its limitations, and implications for health and disease. Alt Med Rev. 2003;8(3):223-46.
146. Kiely PD. The Th1-Th2 model—what relevance to inflammatory arthritis? Ann Rheum Dis. 1998;57:328-30.
147. Prescott SL. New concepts of cytokines in asthma: is the Th1/Th2 paradigm out the window? J Paediatr Child Health. 2003;39(8):575-79.
148. Adkins B, Leclerc C, Marshall-Clarke S. Neonatal adaptive immunity comes of age. Nature Rev Immunol. 2004;4:553-64.
149. Field CJ. The immunological components of human milk and their effect on immune development in infants. J Nutr. 2005;135(1):1-4.
150. Chin J. Intestinal microflora: negotiating health outcomes with the warring community within us. Asia Pac J Clin Nutr. 2004;13(Suppl):S24-25.
151. Kirjavainen PV, Arvola T, Salminen SJ, Isolauri E. Aberrant composition of gut microbiota of allergic infants: a target of bifidobacterial therapy at weaning? Gut. 2002;51:51-55.
152. Ridge JP, Fuchs E, Matzinger P. Neonatal tolerance revisited: turning on newborn T cells with dendritic cells. Science. 1996;271(5256):1723-26.
153. Ibid.
154. Rook GA, Adams V, Hunt J, et al. Mycobacteria and other environmental organisms as immunomodulators for immunoregulatory disorders. Springer Semin Immunopathol. 2004;25(3-4):237-55.
155. Yan F, Polk DB. Commensal bacteria in the gut: learning who our friends are. Curr Opin Gastroenterol. 2004;20(6):565-71.
156. Wahl SM, Costa GL, Mizel DE et al. Role of transforming growth factor beta in the pathophysiology of chronic inflammation. J Periodontol. 1993;64(5 Suppl):450-55.
157. Weiner HL. Oral tolerance: immune mechanisms and the generation of Th3-type TGF-beta-secreting regulatory cells. Microbes Infect. 2001;3(11):947-54.
158. Björkstén B, Sepp E, Julge K, et al. Allergy development and the intestinal microflora during the first year of life. J Allergy Clin Immunol. 2001;108(4):516-20.
159. Bluestone JA, Tang Q. Therapeutic vaccination using CD4+CD25+ antigen-specific regulatory T cells. Proc Natl Acad Sci U S A. 2004;101(Suppl 2):14622–26.
160. Dieckmann D, Plottner H, Berchtold S. Ex vivo isolation and characterization of CD4+CD25+ T Cells with regulatory properties from human blood. J Exper Med. 2001;193(11):1303-10.

161. Perdigon G, Vintini E, Alvarez S. Study of the possible mechanisms involved in the mucosal immune system activation by lactic acid bacteria. J Dairy Sci. 1999;82(6):1108-14.
162. Björkstén B, Sepp E, Julge K, et al. Allergy development and the intestinal microflora during the first year of life. J Allergy Clin Immunol. 2001;108(4):516-20.
163. Kalliomaki M, Salminen S, Arvilommi H, et al. Probiotics in primary prevention of atopic disease: a randomised placebo-controlled trial. Lancet. 2001;357:1076-79.
164. Barinaga, M. Treating arthritis with tolerance. Science. 1993;261:1669-70.
165. Kanauchi O. Modification of intestinal flora in the treatment of inflammatory bowel disease. Curr Pharm Des. 2003;9(4):333-46.
166. Strachan DP. Hay fever, hygiene, and household size. BMJ. 1989;299(6710):1259-60.
167. Parslow TG, Stites DP, Terr AI (Editor), Imboden JB. Medical Immunology, 10th edition. McGraw-Hill/Appleton, Lange 2001.
168. Ibid.
169. Fitzpatrick FA, Soberman R. Regulated formation of eicosanoids. J Clin Invest. 2001;107(11):1347-51.
170. Funk CD. Prostaglandins and leukotrienes: advances in eicosanoid biology. Science. 2001;294:1871-75.
171. Moshage H. Cytokines and the hepatic acute phase response. J Pathol. 1997;181:257-66.
172. Gabay C, Kushner I. Acute-phase proteins and other systemic responses to inflammation. N Eng J Med. 1999;340(6):448-54.
173. Ibid.
174. Ibid.
175. Dinarello CA. Infection, fever, and exogenous and endogenous pyrogens: some concepts have changed. J Endotoxin Res. 2004;10(4):201-22.
176. Angeli V, Hammad H, Staels B. Peroxisome proliferator-activated receptor gamma inhibits the migration of dendritic cells: consequences for the immune response. J Immunol. 2003;170:5295-301.
177. Chinetti G, Fruchart JC, Staels B. Peroxisome proliferator-activated receptors (PPARs): nuclear receptors at the crossroads between lipid metabolism and inflammation. Inflamm Res. 2000;49(10):497-505.
178. Clark RB. The role of PPARs in inflammation and immunity. J Leukoc Biol. 2002;71:388-400.
179. Delerive P, Gervois P, Fruchart JC, Staels B. Induction of IkappaBalpha expression as a mechanism contributing to the anti-inflammatory activities of peroxisome proliferator-activated receptor-alpha activators. J Biol Chem. 2000;275(47):36703-07.
180. Kleemann R, Verschuren L, de Rooij BJ, et al. Evidence for anti-inflammatory activity of statins and PPARalpha activators in human C-reactive protein transgenic mice *in vivo* and in cultured human hepatocytes *in vitro*. Blood. 2004;103(11):4188-94.
181. Poynter ME, Daynes RA. Peroxisome proliferator-activated receptor activation modulates cellular redox status, represses nuclear factor-B signaling, and reduces inflammatory cytokine production in aging. J Biol Chem. 1998; 273:32833-41.
182. Ricote M, Huang JT, Welch JS, Glass CK. The peroxisome proliferator-activated receptor gamma (PPARgamma) as a regulator of monocyte/macrophage function. J Leukoc Biol. 1999;66:733-39.
183. Woerly G, Honda K, Loyens M. Peroxisome proliferator–activated receptors alpha and gamma down-regulate allergic inflammation and eosinophil activation. J Exper Med. 2003;198(3):411-21.
184. Pang L, Nie M, Corbett L, Knox AJ. Cyclooxygenase-2 expression by nonsteroidal anti-inflammatory drugs in human airway smooth muscle cells: role of peroxisome proliferator-activated receptors. J Immunol. 2003;170:1043-51.
185. Mishra A, Chaudhary A, Sethi, S. Oxidized omega-3 fatty acids inhibit nf-b activation via a PPAR-alpha dependent pathway. Arterioscler Thromb Vasc Biol. 2004;24(9):1621-27.
186. Kobayashi K, Hernandez LD, Galan JE, et al. IRAK-M is a negative regulator of toll-like receptor signaling. Cell. 2002 Jul 26;110(2):191-202.
187. Nakayama K, Okugawa S, Yanagimoto S, et al. Involvement of IRAK-M in peptidoglycan-induced tolerance in macrophages. J Biol Chem. J Biol Chem. 2004 Feb 20;279(8):6629-34.
188. Fierro IM, Serhan CN. Mechanisms in anti-inflammation and resolution: the role of lipoxins and aspirin-triggered lipoxins. Braz J Med Biol Res. 2001;34:555-66.
189. Kantarci A, Van Dyke TE. Lipoxins in chronic inflammation. Crit Rev Oral Biol Med. 2003;14(1):4-12.
190. McMahon B, Godson C. Lipoxins: endogenous regulators of inflammation. Am J Physiol Renal Physiol. 2004;286:F189-F201.
191. Opal SM, DePalo VA. Anti-inflammatory cytokines. Chest. 2000;117:1162-72.
192. Fitzpatrick FA, Soberman R. Regulated formation of eicosanoids. J Clin Invest. 2001;107(11):1347-51.
193. Serhan CN. Endogenous chemical mediators in anti-inflammation and pro-resolution. Curr Med Chem. 2002;1(3):177-92.
194. Dent LA. For better or worse: common determinants influencing health and disease in parasitic infections, asthma and reproductive biology. J Reprod Immunol. 2002;57(1-2):255-72.
195. Gibbs WW. Cybernetic cell. Sci Am. 2001;285(2):52-57.
196. Segel LA, Bar-Or RL. On the role of feedback in promoting conflicting goals of the adaptive immune system. J Immunol. 1999;163:1342-49.
197. Danesh J. C-reactive protein and other circulating markers of inflammation in the prediction of coronary heart disease. N Engl J Med. 2004;350(14):1387-97.
198. Harris TB, Ferrucci L, Tracy RP, et al. Associations of elevated interleukin-6 and C-reactive protein levels with mortality in the elderly. Am J Med. 1999;106(5):506-12.
199. McCarty MF. Interleukin-6 as a central mediator of cardiovascular risk associated with chronic inflammation, smoking, diabetes, and visceral obesity: down-regulation with essential fatty acids, ethanol and pentoxifylline. Med Hypotheses. 1999 May;52(5):465-77.
200. Pradhan AD, Manson JE, Rifai N, et al. C-reactive protein, interleukin 6, and risk of developing type 2 diabetes mellitus. JAMA. 2001;286(3):327-34.
201. Rader DJ. Inflammatory markers of coronary risk. N Engl J Med. 2000;343(16):1179-82.
202. Devaraj S, Jialal I. Alpha tocopherol supplementation decreases serum C-reactive protein and monocyte interleukin-6 levels in normal volunteers and type 2 diabetic patients. Free Radic Biol Med. 2000;29(8):790-92.
203. McCarty MF. Interleukin-6 as a central mediator of cardiovascular risk associated with chronic inflammation, smoking, diabetes, and visceral obesity: down-regulation with essential fatty acids, ethanol and pentoxifylline. Med Hypotheses. 1999;52(5):465-77.
204. Pradhan AD, Manson JE, Rifai N, et al. C-reactive protein, interleukin 6, and risk of developing type 2 diabetes mellitus. JAMA. 2001;286(3):327-34.
205. Rader DJ. Inflammatory markers of coronary risk. N Engl J Med. 2000;343(16):1179-82.
206. Vlassara H, Cai W, Crandall J, et al. Inflammatory mediators are induced by dietary glycotoxins, a major risk factor for diabetic angiopathy. Proc Natl Acad Sci USA. 2002;99(24):15596-601.
207. Wright RJ, Cohen RT, Cohen S. The impact of stress on the development and expression of atopy. Curr Opin Allergy Clin Immunol. 2005;5:23-29.
208. Parslow TG, Stites DP, Terr AI (Editor), Imboden JB. Medical Immunology, 10th edition. McGraw-Hill/Appleton, Lange 2001.
209. Funk CD. Prostaglandins and leukotrienes: advances in eicosanoid biology. Science. 2001;294:1871-75.

210. Parslow TG, Stites DP, Terr AI (Editor), Imboden JB. Medical Immunology, 10th edition. McGraw-Hill/Appleton, Lange 2001.
211. Bernardes AT, dos Santos RM. Immune network at the edge of chaos. J Theor Biol. 1997;186(2):173-87.
212. Coffey DS. Self-organization, complexity and chaos: the new biology for medicine. Nat Med. 1998;4(8):882-85.
213. Dalgleish A. The relevance of non-linear mathematics (chaos theory) to the treatment of cancer, the role of the immune response and the potential for vaccines. Q J Med. 1999;92:347-59.
214. Jerne NK. Towards a network theory of the immune system. Ann Immunol (Paris). 1974;125C(1–2):373–89.
215. Weng G, Bhalla US, Iyengar R. Complexity in biological signaling systems. Science. 1999;284(5411):92-96.
216. Bernardes AT, dos Santos RM. Immune network at the edge of chaos. J Theor Biol. 1997 May 21;186(2):173-87.
217. Serhan CN. Eicosanoids in leukocyte function. Curr Opin Hematol. 1994;1(1):69-77.
218. Kassirer JP. On the Take: How Medicine's Complicity with Big Business Can Endanger Your Health. NY, Oxford University Press, 2004.
219. Jack DB. One hundred years of aspirin. Lancet. 1997;350(9075):437-39.
220. Jeffreys D. Aspirin: The Remarkable Story of a Wonder Drug. Bloomsbury USA, 2004.
221. Jack DB. One hundred years of aspirin. Lancet. 1997;350(9075):437-39.
222. Awry EH, Loscalzo J. Aspirin. Circulation. 2000;101:1206-18.
223. Vane JR. Inhibition of prostaglandin synthesis as a mechanism of action for aspirin-like drugs. Nat New Biol. 1971;231:232-235.
224. Markenson J. Clinical Implications of Cyclooxygenase Enzymes: COX-1/COX-2 Role of the New NSAIDs. Cancer Control. 1999;6(2 Suppl 1):22-25.
225. Bhattacharyya J, Biswas S, Datta AG. Mode of action of endotoxin: role of free radicals and antioxidants. Curr Med Chem. 2004;11(3):359-368.
226. Mitchell JA, Akarasereenont P, Thiemermann C, et al. Selectivity of nonsteroidal antiinflammatory drugs as inhibitors of constitutive and inducible cyclooxygenase. Proc Natl Acad Sci U S A. 1993;90:11693-97.
227. Lipsky PE, Brooks P, Crofford LJ, et al. Unresolved issues in the role of cyclooxygenase-2 in normal physiologic processes and disease. Arch Intern Med. 2000;160:913-20.
228. Bertolini A, Ottani A, Sandrini M. Selective COX-2 inhibitors and dual acting anti-inflammatory drugs: critical remarks. Frontiers in Medicinal Chemistry. 2004;1(1):85-95.
229. Clarke RJ, Mayo G, Price P, FitzGerald GA. Suppression of thromboxane A2 but not of systemic prostacyclin by controlled-release aspirin. N Engl J Med. 199;325 (16):1137-41.
230. McAdam BF, Catella-Lawson F, Mardini IA. Systemic biosynthesis of prostacyclin by cyclooxygenase (COX)-2: The human pharmacology of a selective inhibitor of COX-2. Proc Natl Acad Sci U S A. 1999;96:272–77.
231. Kassirer JP. On the Take: How Medicine's Complicity with Big Business Can Endanger Your Health. NY, Oxford University Press, 2004.
232. Anon. Tuberculosis associated with blocking agents against tumor necrosis factor-alpha. California, 2002-2003. MMWR Morb Mortal Wkly Rep. 2004;53:683-86.
233. Cominelli F. Cytokine-based therapies for Crohn's Disease—new paradigms. N Engl J Med. 2004;351(20):2045-48.
234. Berger JR, Koralnik IJ. Progressive multifocal leukoencephalopathy and natalizumab—Unforeseen consequences. N Engl J Med. 2005;353(4):414-16.
235. Dent LA. For better or worse: common determinants influencing health and disease in parasitic infections, asthma and reproductive biology. J Reprod Immunol. 2002 Oct-Nov;57(1-2):255-72.
236. Kleemann R, Verschuren L, de Rooij BJ, et al. Evidence for anti-inflammatory activity of statins and PPARalpha activators in human C-reactive protein transgenic mice *in vivo* and in cultured human hepatocytes *in vitro*. Blood. 2004;103(11):4188-94.
237. Kluft C, Kleemann R, de Maat MPM. How best to counteract the enemies? By controlling inflammation in the coronary circulation. Eur Heart J Suppl. 2002;4:G53-65.
238. Rader DJ. Inflammatory markers of coronary risk. N Engl J Med. 2000;343(16):1179-82.
239. Ridker PM, Cushman M, Stampfer MJ, et al. Inflammation, aspirin, and the risk of cardiovascular disease in apparently healthy men. N Engl J Med. 1997;336(14):973-79.
240. Dwyer JH, Allayee H, Dwyer KM, et al. Arachidonate 5-lipoxygenase promoter genotype, dietary arachidonic acid, and atherosclerosis. N Eng J Med. 2004;350(1):29-37.
241. Jenkins DJ, Kendall CW, Marchie A, et al. Direct comparison of a dietary portfolio of cholesterol-lowering foods with a statin in hypercholesterolemic participants. Am J Clin Nutr. 2005;81(2):380-87.
242. Mozaffarian D. Dietary intake of *trans* fatty acids and systemic inflammation in women. Am J Clin Nutr. 2004;79(4):606-12.
243. Jenkins DJ, Kendall CW, Marchie A, et al. Direct comparison of a dietary portfolio of cholesterol-lowering foods with a statin in hypercholesterolemic participants. Am J Clin Nutr. 2005;81(2):380-87.
244. Knoops, et al. Mediterranean diet, lifestyle factors, and 10-year mortality in elderly European men and women. The HALE Project. JAMA. 2004;292:1433-39.
245. Horrobin DF. Innovation in the pharmaceutical industry. J R Soc Med. 2000;93:341–45.
246. Horrobin DF. The philosophical basis of peer review and the suppression of innovation. JAMA. 1990;263:1438-41.
247. Horrobin DF. Evidence-based medicine and the need for non-commercial clinical research directed towards therapeutic innovation. Exp Biol Med. 2002; 227:435-37.
248. Miller GA, Galanter E, Pribram KH. Plans and the Structure of Behavior. Holt, Rinehart, Winston, NY, 1960.
249. Perseghin G, Petersen K, Shulman GI. Cellular mechanism of insulin resistance: potential links with inflammation. Int J Obes Relat Metab Disord. 2003;27:S6-11.
250. Conner EM, Grisham MB. Inflammation, free radicals and antioxidants. Nutrition, 1996;12(4):272-77.
251. Devaraj S, Jialal I. Alpha tocopherol supplementation decreases serum C-reactive protein and monocyte interleukin-6 levels in normal volunteers and type 2 diabetic patients. Free Radic Biol Med. 2000;29(8):790-92.
252. Pischon T, Hankinson SE, Hotamisligil GS, et al. Habitual dietary intake of n-3 and n-6 fatty acids in relation to inflammatory markers among us men and women. Circulation. 2003;108:155-60.
253. Plat J, Mensink RP. Food components and immune function. Curr Opin Lipidol. 2005;16:31-37.
254. Aller MA, Arias JL, Nava MP. Posttraumatic inflammation is a complex response based on the pathological expression of the nervous, immune, and endocrine functional systems. Exp Biol Med. 2004;229:170-81.
255. Black PH. Immune system-central nervous system interactions: effect and immunomodulatory consequences of immune system mediators on the brain. Antimicrobial Agents Chemother. 1994;38(1):7-12.
256. Padgett DA, Glaser R. How stress influences the immune response. Trends Immunol. 2003;24:444-48.
257. Perseghin G, Petersen K, Shulman GI. Cellular mechanism of insulin resistance: potential links with inflammation. Int J Obes Relat Metab Disord. 2003;27:S6-11.

258. Wright RJ, Cohen RT, Cohen S. The impact of stress on the development and expression of atopy. Curr Opin Allergy Clin Immunol. 2005;5:23-29.
259. Powell JJ, Van de Water J, Gershwin ME. Evidence for the role of environmental agents in the initiation or progression of autoimmune conditions. Environ Health Perspect. 1999;107 (Suppl 5):667-72.
260. Cordain L, Toohey L, Smith MJ, Hickey MS. Modulation of immune function by dietary lectins in rheumatoid arthritis. Br J Nutr. 2000;83:207-17.
261. Freed DLJ. Do dietary lectins cause disease? BMJ. 1999;318:1023-24.
262. Newberry RD, Stenson WF, Lorenz RG. Prostaglandins and the induction of food sensitive enteropathy. Gut. 2000;46:154–55.
263. Bottiger LE. Integrative biology (physiology)—a necessity! J Intern Med. 1995;237(4):345-47.
264. Coffey DS. Self-organization, complexity and chaos: the new biology for medicine. Nat Med. 1998;4(8):882-85.
265. Dalgleish A. The relevance of non-linear mathematics (chaos theory) to the treatment of cancer, the role of the immune response and the potential for vaccines. Q J Med. 1999;92:347-59.
266. Gibbs WW. Cybernetic cell. Sci Am. 2001;285(2):52-57.
267. Jerne NK. Towards a network theory of the immune system. Ann Immunol (Paris). 1974;125C(1–2):373–89.
268. Weng G, Bhalla US, Iyengar R. Complexity in biological signaling systems. Science. 1999;284(5411):92-96.
269. Kitano H. Systems biology: a brief overview. Science. 2002;295(5560):1662-64.
270. Coffey DS. Self-organization, complexity and chaos: the new biology for medicine. Nat Med. 1998;4(8):882-85.
271. Bernardes AT, dos Santos RM. Immune network at the edge of chaos. J Theor Biol. 1997;186(2):173-87.
272. Coffey DS. Self-organization, complexity and chaos: the new biology for medicine. Nat Med. 1998;4(8):882-85.
273. Weng G, Bhalla US, Iyengar R. Complexity in biological signaling systems. Science. 1999;284(5411):92-96.
274. Bernardes AT, dos Santos RM. Immune network at the edge of chaos. J Theor Biol. 1997;186(2):173-87.
275. Dalgleish A. The relevance of non-linear mathematics (chaos theory) to the treatment of cancer, the role of the immune response and the potential for vaccines. Q J Med. 1999;92:347-359.
276. Coffey DS. Self-organization, complexity and chaos: the new biology for medicine. Nat Med. 1998;4(8):882-85.
277. Segel LA, Bar-Or RL. On the role of feedback in promoting conflicting goals of the adaptive immune system. J Immunol. 1999;163:1342-49.
278. Parijs, LV, Abbas, AK. Homeostasis and self-tolerance in the immune system: turning lymphocytes off. Science. 1998;280:243-48.
279. Tiberti C, Bao F, Bonamico M. Celiac disease-associated transglutaminase autoantibody target domains at diagnosis are age and sex dependent. Clin Immunol. 2003;109(3):318-24.
280. Bizzaro N, Villalta D, Tonutti E, et al. IgA and IgG tissue transglutaminase antibody prevalence and clinical significance in connective tissue diseases, inflammatory bowel disease, and primary biliary cirrhosis. Dig Dis Sci. 2003;48(12):2360-65.
281. Pena AS, Crusius JB. Food allergy, coeliac disease and chronic inflammatory bowel disease in man. Vet Q. 1998;20:S49-52.
282. Ventura A, Neri E, Ughi C et al. Gluten-dependent diabetes-related and thyroid-related autoantibodies in patients with celiac disease. J Pediatrics. 2000;137(2):263-65.
283. Peng SL. Transcription factors in the pathogenesis of autoimmunity. Clin Immunol. 2004;110:112-23.
284. Kanauchi O. Modification of intestinal flora in the treatment of inflammatory bowel disease. Curr Pharm Des. 2003;9(4):333-46.
285. Alexander JW. Immunonutrition: the role of omega-3 fatty acids. Nutrition. 1998;14(7-8):627-33.
286. James MJ, Gibson RA, Cleland LG. Dietary polyunsaturated fatty acids and inflammatory mediator production. Am J Clin Nutr. 2000 Jan;71:343S-48S.
287. Devaraj S, Jialal I. Alpha tocopherol supplementation decreases serum C-reactive protein and monocyte interleukin-6 levels in normal volunteers and type 2 diabetic patients. Free Radic Biol Med. 2000;29(8):790-92.
288. Kalliomaki M, Salminen S, Arvilommi H, et al. Probiotics in primary prevention of atopic disease: a randomised placebo-controlled trial. Lancet. 2001;357:1076-79.

Chapter 24
Digestive, Absorptive, and Microbiological Imbalances

Thomas Sult, MD

Introduction

Imbalances in the gastrointestinal system are vital to understand and detect, as visits for GI distress of one kind or another account for a very significant number of healthcare visits.[1] Further along in the book (see Chapter 28), we will explore the functional medicine approach to clinical care for these disorders. Here, we want to review and analyze the role that each element of the GI system plays in achieving health, so that we can understand where imbalances arise and how they manifest in the patient. We'll begin with a brief review of the basic structures and functions involved in digestion and absorption.

Structures of the Digestive System

The digestive or alimentary tract starts at the mouth and ends at the anus. It is composed primarily of the tubular structures: the mouth, esophagus, stomach, three parts of the small intestine (duodenum, jejunum, ileum), and four parts of the large intestine (cecum, ascending, transverse and descending colon). With the ancillary organs included (salivary glands, liver, gall bladder, and pancreas), the digestive system is formed. While not considered integral parts of the digestive system structures, the nervous, endocrine, and immune systems have considerable input to and receive output from that system.

As we will see, there are many opportunities for missteps and malfunctions in this complex, multi-stage process. Although space precludes an exhaustive discussion of all the activities involved in digestion, we will discuss some of the most clinically pertinent areas of interest.

The Brain

It may seem odd to list the brain as being one of the structures involved in the digestive process, but we learned long ago from Pavlov and his dogs that the brain can start the digestive process.

The "Second Brain"

Michael Gershon, MD, in his book, *The Second Brain*, writes, "We now know that there is a brain in the bowel, however inappropriate that concept might seem to be. The ugly gut is more intellectual than the heart and may have a greater capacity for feeling." This second brain is the enteric nervous system (ENS). While the brain "exerts considerable neuroregulatory influence," reports Gershon, it is often trumped by the ENS.[2] Chapter 28 contains a detailed discussion of the ENS by Dr. Gershon.

The Mouth

Mastication, or chewing, is the process of cutting, grinding, and mixing the food bolus with saliva. Saliva is a complex mix of lubricants, enzymes, and antimicrobials. An under-recognized and very important function of the saliva is the antimicrobial component. Saliva contains several anti-infective agents including thiocyanate, lactoferrin, secretory IgA (sIgA), and lysozyme. These agents help prevent infective agents from hitchhiking with the food bolus into the lower GI tract, thus preventing infection and dysbiosis. Salivary sIgA is the primary immunoglobulin of the mucosal immune system; its levels are improved by pleasant emotions.[3] Interestingly, overtraining in athletes will lower sIgA, resulting in upper respiratory infection (URI).[4] It appears that this effect can be muted with the use of acupuncture.[5] In the elderly, moderate exercise has been shown to improve sIgA, possibly reducing the age-associated lowered resistance to URI.[6] Pathogen-specific sIgA has been reported in response to bacteria and fungal species.[7,8]

Connecting the mouth to the stomach is the esophagus. Dysmotility disorders of the esophagus are common. The origin of these phenomena is not known, but evidence exists to suggest that ENS autoimmunity is partly responsible; however, controversy still exists.[9]

The Stomach

The stomach holds food in storage and further mixes the food bolus with HCl and gastric digestive enzymes. These enzymes continue the process of digestion that was begun in the mouth. Proteins are broken down into peptides. Lipids are broken down into free fatty acids. This prepares the food bolus, or chyme, for delivery to the small intestine.

The stomach produces HCl in the parietal cells via an ATP-dependent process. (This is the site of action of the proton pump inhibitors or PPIs.) This acid environment favors the unfolding, or denaturation, of proteins to facilitate enzymatic breakdown. Pepsinogen is converted to pepsin and many microorganisms are destroyed by the low pH.

These processes are under both neural and hormonal control. The primary central nervous system (CNS) influence on gastric secretion and motility is the vagus nerve. The primary hormonal influence is gastrin. The vagus nerve is the dominant CNS input, but is still a minority influence on the GI system. The ENS has inputs to the GI system that are orders of magnitude larger.[10]

Gastrin is produced in the antrum of the stomach in G cells. Its secretion is stimulated by the presence of protein in the gastric lumen. It is inhibited by a pH lower than 3. Gastrin stimulates gastric motility and the release of gastric acid and pepsinogen. It also plays a role in the proliferation of gastric mucosal cells, especially the acid-secreting cells. One is left to wonder what the long-term implications of chronic acid suppression might be on the total number of acid-secreting cells and gastric motility.

The Small Intestine

The stomach, which is both adapted to and secretes acid, differs substantially from the duodenum, which is adapted to a neutral pH environment. The chyme that is deposited into the duodenum from the stomach has a very low pH that must be neutralized. A sophisticated feedback system exists to perform this function. Within the duodenum is a set of sensing cells that communicate with the hormonal system, the nervous system, and the ENS.[11] When acid is sensed within the duodenum, S-cells release secretin. Secretin then stimulates the pancreas to release bicarbonate. Secretin also slows gastric empting until the pH is in a neutral range. At that point, secretin is no longer released and the stomach begins to empty again. In this way, the rise and fall of pH in the duodenum regulates the ebb and flow of chyme from the stomach into the duodenum.

I-enteroendocrine cells of the duodenum and jejunum secrete cholecystokinin. This hormone, released in response to protein and fat, is responsible for the flow of pancreatic enzymes and gallbladder contraction.[12,13] Excessive cholecystokinin can stimulate hypertrophy and hyperplasia of the pancreas.[14] The regulation of pH, motility, and enzyme secretion is likely too complicated for a simple hormone system. A complex network of nerves and ganglia exists to provide control and feedback for duodenal, hepatic, and pancreatic function. In fact, the distal stomach seems to be involved in these neuro loops as well. They function in concert with, and independently from, the CNS. In addition, they appear to be able to override the effects of the CNS in many circumstances.[15,16,17,18]

It now appears that the endocrine release serves as a backup system to the ENS, which is the primary minute-to-minute control system.[19] In addition, it appears that most of the neurotransmitters recovered in blood are derived from the enteric-nervous system rather than the central nervous system. Not surprisingly, common side effects of many neuro/psychoactive drugs, including antidepressants, are GI related[20,21] and may even have therapeutic GI effects.[22]

Small intestine motility. The motility of the gut involves a complex and highly organized set of events. Each segment of the gut shows coordinated and independent activity that propels the chyme from the duodenum to the large intestine, and mixes the chyme with the digestive "juices" within the gut lumen. The "slow" waves of the small intestine range from 10–12 cycles per minute at the proximal (duodenal) end to 6–9 cycles per minute at the ileum. It is highly likely that this activity is coordinated by the ENS.[23,24,25,26] This control is likely related to functional heterogeneity in the myenteric plexus that corresponds to the anatomical heterogeneity of the gut.[27] In part, this is accomplished via Hox genes and their regulation by intercellular signals. This pathway organizes the gut structure by utilizing cell autonomous programs, directed by transcription factors, allowing cells of the embryonic gut to affect the developmental fate of their neighbor cells. Both temporal and spatial expressions of relevant genes are orchestrated in this way. The result is the establishment of major structural components of the gut such as sphincters and muscle layers.[28] It is likely that differences in enzyme and transporter protein distribution are similarly regulated.

It is now recognized that many disorders of motility are in reality an inflammatory process of the ENS. A partial list of such disorders includes: paraneoplastic, infectious and achalasia disorders; congenital hypertrophic pyloric stenosis; chronic intestinal pseudo-obstruction; Hirschsprung's disease and chronic idiopathic constipation; neurological disorders; and probably irritable bowel syndrome. Several causes have been identified, including viral antigen expression in the enteric neural environment, molecular mimicry (onconeural antigens), and the role exerted by cellular and humeral autoimmunity.[29] Inflammatory bowel disease (IBS) and infection are associated with disordered smooth muscle and secretory function. Inflammation-induced changes of the ENS have been reported in IBS and chronic infectious colitis, and are responsible for the dysmotility of these conditions.[30] Gall bladder function is a complex and coordinated event, with implications for motility. Cholesterol has a direct inhibitory effect on gall bladder smooth muscle cell membrane causing impaired contraction. Inflammation within the gall bladder wall has a similar effect.[31]

The Large Intestine

From the terminal ileum, the chyme moves through the ileocecal valve and into the large intestine. This segment of the gut has two primary responsibilities: fermentation (ascending colon) and absorption (descending colon). Gut organisms in the ascending colon act on carbohydrate fractions (resistant starch) left in the chyme. They produce short-chain fatty acids that are used as fuel for the enterocyte. A fraction of the short-chain fatty acids is absorbed by diffusion, transported via the portal vein, and utilized by other tissues for energy. While the importance of short-chain fatty acids to humans is not yet fully mapped out, it may be that absorption of these fatty acids accounts for some of the cardiac and anti-cancer benefits of fiber.[32] Consumption of fibers may influence changes in the microflora of the gut. These changes may mediate immune interactions in several ways. First, the bacteria may influence immunity through direct contact with immune cells. Second, the production of short-chain fatty acids may play a role. And third, enhanced mucin production may alter immunity.[33] The primary functions of the descending colon are the absorption of water and electrolytes, and the formation of the stool.

The Guardian of the Interior

There are two routes of entry into the body from the intestines. The first is the portal system. Blood from the splanchnic arteries is enriched with nutrients at the small intestine. It then collects in the portal vein and is delivered to the liver. This is the major entry for water-soluble nutrients, such as amino acids, short-chain fatty acids, and water-soluble vitamins. The second route is via the lymph system: the nutrients (or other substances) collect at the basolateral membrane and move into the lymph channels, entering the blood circulation at the thoracic duct. This mechanism bypasses the liver, its first pass effect, and therefore its detoxification ability. The lymph is the primary entry method for lipid-soluble substances.

About 70% of lymph tissue in the body is associated with the gut, which is logical since the gut is the major portal of entry to the body. Antigens that have survived acidification, enzymatic breakdown, and microbial defenses are examined by the gut-associated lymphoid tissue (GALT). Development of the GALT is dependent upon intestinal microbes. The development of the GALT is not, however, an antigen-specific process. Various types of intestinal microbes under certain types of stress conditions guide GALT development,[34] thus blurring even further the line between the bacteria and the human, and lending more support to the notion of the "undiscovered organ" (see Chapter 28 for more discussion on gut flora and GALT).

The GALT is comprised of a network of uniquely arranged B cells, T cells, and phagocytes, which sample the luminal antigens. This activity takes place at specialized epithelia which are called follicle-associated epithelia (FAE). These FAE coordinate responses between the immune cells and other mucosal barrier components. The primary "sampling" cell is the M-cell. Recently, non-Peyer's patches-associated M-cells, termed villous

M-cells, have been discovered. These villous M-cells are able to process antigens from a variety of bacteria and mount an antigen-specific immune response. This seems to be an independent component of mucosal immune integrity.[35] The GALT is composed of organ-specific, tissue-homing T cells. These T cells are induced in mesenteric or Peyer's lymph nodes but not in peripheral lymph nodes. The GALT dendritic cells gain their ability to confer gut-homing capacity on the T cells from the intestinal mucosal microenvironment. Additionally, these same dendritic cells seem to be involved in immunogenic vs. tolerogenic responses and Th1 vs. Th2 subpopulation selection.[36] At least in part, chemokines are responsible for lymphocyte trafficking within the GALT. They also play a role in intestinal segmental specialization and lymphocyte subset selective localization. The result is direction and differentiation of intestinal effector and memory lymphocytes within the GALT, along with homeostatic and inflammatory localization of lymphocytes to the intestines.[37]

Antigens not recognized as beneficial will be processed by the GALT. Through constant vigilance, the GALT differentiates food and commensal bacterial antigens from pathogenic antigens. The mucosal barrier microenvironment heavily influences the immune response that results from antigen interaction.[38] Generally, the GALT will inhibit the development of allergy and autoimmunity. The GALT reaction to enteric antigens is to induce both mucosal and systemic immunity. It has been shown that oral antigens from bacterial lysates may reduce the frequency and seriousness of diarrhea, mucosal infection, and diverticulitis. This is accomplished by increasing IgA and cytokines at the mucosa and luminal level.[39] But the response to food or pathogenic antigens starts out the same. It is the microenvironment that determines whether the final response will be tolerogenic or immunogenic. Food antigens, when presented with an adjuvant, will induce an immunogenic response. More disconcerting is that a chronic intestinal infection or inflammation may in itself be an adjuvant.[40] This may lead to multiple food allergies or sensitivities. Whether it is the adjuvant nature of chronic inflammation or some other mechanism that results in auto-antibodies to mucin in ulcerative colitis (UC) is unclear. In any event, once present, they serve to differentiate UC from Crohn's disease. Additionally, they perpetuate chronic mucosal inflammation in UC.[41] The pathogenesis of ulcerative colitis is related to a disturbance in immune regulatory T cells. A serum factor from a UC patient was shown to be interleukin-7, which has been shown to induce T cell proliferation in the thymus.[42]

Nutritional elements have been shown to enhance the function of the GALT. A combination of arginine, n-3 fatty acids, and nucleotides was able to significantly reduce sepsis and multi-organ failure in trauma patients. One paper suggested that "Immunonutrition [as a] ... strategy available to clinicians caring for trauma patients ... should be strongly considered ... ."[43] At least in parenterally fed mice, glutamine supplementation may improve GALT volume and function. Arginine may improve CD4 cell percentages but not volume of the GALT.[44] Recent studies have shed some light on these issues. Specific nutrients may be able to enhance enteral blood flow in a site-specific manner. In rats, an immune-enhanced enteral diet, enriched with arginine, fish oil, and RNA fragments, was able to increase blood flow to the ileum. Because the GALT is located primarily in the terminal jejunum and ileum, this may affect GALT activity.[45]

Unfortunately some pathogens have developed strategies to take advantage of these GALT features and are able to penetrate the defenses.[46] Translocation is the process of a large molecule moving through a biologic barrier. This is also known as leaky gut.[47] In the presence of a leaky gut, translocation may result in allergy, autoimmunity, or high levels of inflammatory immune complexes delivered to the liver, resulting in detoxification pathway stress. This process has been linked to arthritic conditions. Some of these symptoms and diseases are related to immune interactions between gut luminal microbes and HLA tissue types.[48,49,50] Alternatively, this leakiness may overwhelm the liver detoxification systems and allow the escape of toxic substances into the systemic circulation, resulting in distant effects such as encephalitis.[51]

Digestion and Absorption

Digestion is largely an intraluminal, extracellular process. Primary functions of the digestive system are:

- Breakdown of complex foods and absorption of nutrients (monosaccharides, monoacylglycerols, fatty acids, amino acids, vitamins, minerals, water, and phytonutrients).

- Barrier to keep out unwanted substances and organisms (bacteria and toxins).
- Site for specialized cells that produce mucus, fluids, digestive enzymes, intrinsic factor, peptide hormones, and other "neurotransmitters."
- Production of other cells that have sensing functions.
- Communication of information about the environment to the endocrine and immune systems.

The control of pancreatic and gall bladder function by the ENS and hormonal system has been described above. The structural aspects of the small intestine also contribute to digestion and absorption. Due to the circular folds of the mucosa, the villi and the microvilli, the area of the cylindrical intestine, is increased about 600 times to a total area of 200 square meters. This provides for greater concentrations of epithelial-derived enzymes and greater surface area for absorption.[52]

Absorption occurs by four general mechanisms:

- The first mechanism is passive diffusion, which is the primary absorption route for water, short-chain fatty acids, and gases such as H2 and CO2. Passive diffusion can be bi-directional, moving down the concentration gradient in an energy-independent manner.
- The second mechanism is mediated transport, both passive and active, involving specific carrier or transport proteins at the cell membrane. Frequently, the transport protein on the luminal or brush border membrane (BBM) side of the enterocyte differs from the transport protein on the basolateral membrane (BLM) side of the enterocyte.[53] The simplest mediated transport is facilitated diffusion. The transport protein can be regulated, but the transport is down an established electrochemical gradient. The active mediated transport mechanisms involve energy expenditure. They may involve uniport pumping of one item, symport pumping of two items in the same direction, or antiport exchange of items in and out of the cell. These systems may use primary or secondary energies to accomplish the task. An example of primary energy use is the Na/K ATPase pump. This system pumps Na out and K into cells at the expense of ATP, where 1 mol of ATP pumps 3 mol of Na and 2 mol of K (an antiport). In the secondary energy utilization system, an established electrochemical gradient is used to power the system. An example of this is the SGLT1 transporter. In this system, glucose is transported against its concentration gradient by co-transporting Na out of the cell with its concentration gradient (a symport).[54] By using the "stored" energy from the Na/K ATPase pump, the cell can concentrate glucose without the use of additional ATP. Single nucleotide polymorphisms (SNPs) at the level of the transport protein gene, or proteomic problems with regulation of these sites may lead to various diseases.[55] Additionally, SNPs, proteomic, or other problems with the brush border enzymes or their regulation may involve defects in enzyme synthesis, alterations in intracellular transport, and catalytically-altered apoenzyme.[56]
- A third mechanism of absorption is pinocytosis. This is a receptor-mediated process. It is the general route of absorption for intact proteins and other large molecules. Smaller molecules may "hitchhike" with these larger molecules in the solution of the involuted vacuole. Pinocytosis is subject to all of the genomic, proteomic and metabolomic processes, and is affected by SNPs and errors of receptor-mediated processes.
- The last route of absorption is paracellular, involving the absorption of substances between the enterocytes at the "tight junctions." It is normal for water to be absorbed in this way, and electrolytes go with the water via "solvent drag." Epithelial cells possess the capacity to alter the permeability of the tight junction. This process is controlled by cytoplasm factors.[57] It now appears that the cytoskeleton is in direct communication with the tight junction and helps to control its function.[58] Unfortunately, it is possible that a loss of integrity of the tight junctions, through inflammation or infection, will allow the absorption of substances in an unregulated manner. These substances, when present at the basolateral membrane, may be immunogenic, create a toxic burden, or both.

Increased permeability has been observed in several disorders and may be both an effect and a mediator of disease. One study reported the sensitivity of intestinal permeability for prediction of relapse in Crohn's disease at 81%.[59] Bowel disorders with increased permeability include inflammatory bowel disease, Crohn's disease, food allergy, and celiac disease. Systemic diseases with increased permeability include inflammatory joint disease, rheumatoid arthritis, ankylosing spondylitis, Reiter's syndrome, chronic dermatological conditions, schizophrenia, and allergic disorders.[60,61]

The small intestine is able to respond to environmental changes with significant alterations in brush border enzymes and enterocyte transporter and receptor proteins. When hibernating hamsters were examined, these proteins were optimized to deal with the extremes of hibernation vs. feeding in an energy-efficient manner.[62] When rats are challenged with various dietary compositions, the expression of villous enzymes, transporters, and receptor proteins changes rapidly to optimize utilization of the foods available.[63] The distribution of enzymes and transporter and receptor proteins is not random.[64] The small intestine is a regionally task-specific organ, with longitudinal controls in place to insure correct mixing and digestion of chyme. If a significant bolus of undigested food reaches the ileum, the "ileal brake" will stop the progression of food until adequate breakdown has occurred (another function of the ENS). The expression of transporter and receptor proteins is also region specific.

The enterohepatic circulation of bile acids is an example of such a process. Bile is produced in the liver and stored in the gall bladder. With proper stimulation, it is released into the duodenum to aid in digestion. While it is reabsorbed by passive diffusion throughout the entire length of the intestine, there are receptor-mediated transport mechanisms found only in the distal ileum.[65,66] This insures an ample supply of bile acids throughout the colon during digestion. This system is very efficient and results in the loss of only about 1% of the bile to the feces. Liver organ reserve may be taxed by any situation that increases transit time in excess of bile salt reabsorption. The average liver synthesis of bile acids is 0.5 grams per day, yet some 50 grams flow though the gut each day. Essentially, the same 4 grams of bile acids are recirculated through the gut some 12 times per day. If the gut were to lose a larger percentage of bile to the fecal mass, the digestion of fats would be impaired. The major excretory pathway of cholesterol out of the body is via the 1% of unrecirculated bile. Bile acid sequestrant medication, used to lower cholesterol, may contribute to liver stress and poor digestion of fats due to excess bile acid loss to the fecal mass.

Organisms of the Gut

Within the gut is a population of about 400 different microbial species; however, 30 to 40 species account for about 99% of the intestinal load. The absolute numbers of these microorganisms is vast; they outnumber our own human cells by at least an order of magnitude.[67,68] It is estimated that the total weight of these microbes is in the vicinity of six pounds, placing it among the body's largest "organs." These microbes have several functions and seem to be truly symbiotic and mutualistic. At least one species has the ability to bind to specific receptors on the enterocyte.[69] It is interesting that the population of genetic subgroups, within a species of bacteria, varies with its position within the colon. This suggests significant sub-specialization by sites within the gut.[70] This population of microbes may be termed the "undiscovered organ."[71]

The traditional view of these microorganisms is that they are single living and not cooperative; however, recent advances in microbiology tell us that they are cooperative, not only within a species but among various species.[72,73] They also exhibit complex life cycles.[74] They live in single cell or planktonic forms and colonial forms known as biofilms. Biofilms are highly ordered, often multi-species films exhibiting cooperation and specialization within the film.[75] They exhibit complex structures that are achieved by poorly understood mechanisms that appear to involve bacteriophage-induced cell death. These bacteriophages appear to live within the bacterial genome as prophages. Some evidence suggests these phages are controlled in a manner that creates reproducible three-dimensional structures including microcolonies, channels, and matrix.[76] The structure is protective and forms nutrient flow channels.

The expressed genetic heterogeneity of two forms of the same species is often significant.[77] The interactions of various microorganisms is dependent on their planktonic vs. biofilm states. In one example, when *Candida* is in its filamentous form, Pseudomonas was able to attach, therefore forming a dense biofilm, and killing the *Candida*. When *Candida* was in its yeast form, no binding, biofilm, or kill occurred.[78] The expression of certain genes, or lack thereof, has been reported to be involved in both virulence and drug resistance.[79,80,81] The biofilm was originally thought to be a simple diffusion barrier to antibiotics.[82] It is now clear that specific components of the biofilm interact with antibiotics in a neutralizing way. [83] These interactions are not mediated by beta-lactamase. Pathogenic microbes have been shown to preferentially increase the thickness of their biofilm matrix layer when exposed to antibiotics.[84] Biofilm formation is now recognized as the major reason for resistance to pathogenic and opportunistic bacterial and fungal strains.[85]

While not confirmed, it is likely that the probiotic species within the gut live in a mix of individual planktonic forms and complex multispecies biofilms, which are thought to play a key role in the protective functions of probiotics. Probiotic species that are able to produce biofilms have been studied.[86,87,88] The mechanism of biofilm formation involves brakes in the peptidoglycan cell wall through an autolysin mechanism, resulting in colony formation and biofilm production.[89] In addition to forming biofilms, probiotic species seem to inhibit the formation of invasive biofilms. Lactobacillus demonstrates a significant ability to inhibit biofilms of undesirable species.[90]

Several other naturally occurring biofilm inhibitors are now recognized. They seem to work by inhibiting a set of "quorum sensing" signaling molecules.[91] Several components of the innate immune system, including lactoferrin, are able to prevent biofilm formation.[92] Lactoferrin is active against a broad spectrum of bacteria, fungi, and protozoa. The effects are both direct cidal activity, due to its binding to specific receptors, and iron binding and sequestration.[93] Specific fractions of human milk have anti-biofilm activity that works by blocking microorganism lectins that are active in biofilm formation.[94] Cellulase has been used as a biofilm inhibitor. Investigators believe it may be effectively used in combination with other agents to treat biofilm contamination of medical devices.[95] Several extracts from marine algae have been shown to significantly inhibit several species of biofilm forming organisms.[96] Salicylates are also potent inhibitors of biofilm formation.[97] Other prostaglandin inhibitors have shown promise as biofilm inhibitors. Several NSAIDs were able to inhibit biofilm formation in *C. albicans*, with aspirin showing the greatest effect. It is well known that prostaglandins are produced in *C. albicans* and they play a key role in colony formation. Now it seems prostaglandins play an important role in fungal biofilm formation.[98]

It has been pointed out that nature has been doing "biological warfare" for millennia.[99] The more rapidly evolving probiotic species may be better adapted to fighting off invading species than our own more slowly changing immune systems. Components of probiotic biofilm have significant anti-infective, anti-adherent qualities, and possibly anti-tumor activity. The morphogenetic autoregulatory substance farnesol inhibits biofilm formation in *C. albicans*. In the case of the anti-tumor activity, at least one component appears to be a conserved transduction pathway, the same farnesol pathway. Inhibition of this pathway induced apoptosis in epidermoid cancers with reduction of ras oncogene expression and lowered PPAR activity.[100]

Clinical Implications of GI Imbalance

Probiotics

Both prevention and management of some human diseases may be addressed with the use of probiotic bacteria. Preliminary findings of several recent human trials suggest probiotics may help both gastrointestinal and systemic conditions.[101] When this protective probiotic biofilm is disrupted by any number of perturbing factors, it may be replaced with a dysbiotic set of organisms that create their own biofilm. Because biofilms often exhibit unique forms of antibiotic resistance, it is often difficult to eradicate these invading species.[102,103] This construct of biofilm formation lends new insight into a complex problem and suggests new ways of intervening, including the use of biofilm inhibitors or probiotics capable of defeating the biofilms of the dysbiotic species. Perhaps both these interventions will be coupled with antimicrobial and prebiotic techniques.

With the complexity of the microorganism interactions and the high order of both microorganism-to-microorganism, as well as microorganism-to-human symbiosis, what else are these probiotics able to do? They have a large number of functions:

- They produce cytochrome P450-like enzymes and help with detoxification.
- The presence of increased numbers of P450-like enzymes from bacterial origin may induce the expression of liver P450 enzymes.[104] How might bacteria communicate with the human liver to induce genetic expression of P450? It appears that conserved communication pathways are common to both prokaryotes and eukaryotes. Signal molecules from prokaryotes are able to affect pathways within the eukaryotes, even in complex

organisms.[105] The discovery of these conserved pathways may explain a great deal of the symbiotic nature of these relationships.

- Probiotics have also been shown to produce some B vitamins and vitamin K.
- They aid in digestion, enhance absorption of nutrients, combat diarrhea, and interact with immune system components to improve resistance.[106,107]
- Additionally, probiotics exert antimutagenic, antitumor, and immunomodulation effects. Probiotics have shown antitumor activity in several transplantable tumors in mice.[108]
- They may also modulate the leakiness of the gut.[109] This could help practitioners with the task of treating inflammatory ENS neuropathies.

The Gut-Brain Axis

The distinction between pure inflammation and ENS interaction is blurring. The gut contains the greatest concentration of immune tissue in the body. These immune cells are intertwined with the greatest concentration of nerves outside of the CNS. Both the immune cells and the nerves seem to be in intimate communication with the mucosal epithelia via a large array of signaling molecules. These interactions control both physiologic and pathophysiologic features of gut function.[110,111] It is now known that bi-directional ENS and CNS communication is commonplace, occurring via neuronal, immunological, and endocrinological pathways. This has been termed the brain-gut axis. Disturbances of immune, endocrine, CNS, or ENS inputs can have significant bi-directional consequences. The same neurotransmitters influence gastrointestinal, endocrine, immune, behavioral, and emotional function.[112] While psychological stress has been shown to induce relapse of established intestinal disease, new evidence suggests that psychological stress can induce intestinal inflammation in a previously healthy host.[113] These new findings suggest, for instance, a component of depression may be in the gut, and a component of IBS may be in the head.

Inflammatory Enteric Neuropathy

It may be that serum anti-ENS antibodies to detect the early stages of inflammatory degenerative enteric neuropathy may be helpful.[114] ENS inflammatory neuropathy exhibits dense infiltrates of inflammatory immune cells. These inflammatory reactions are located at the neural microenvironment. It appears that symptoms of inflammatory ENS neuritis may develop acutely or indolently. An example of the acute form may be the development of IBS after an acute illness, while the indolent form may be the slow, progressive development of paraneoplastic syndromes.[115] Degenerative and genetic mechanisms also play a critical role in ENS pathology underlying gut dysmotility. It is highly likely that the same or similar neurotoxic events that occur in the CNS are at work in the ENS. This has been demonstrated for glutamate. Excessive stimulation by glutamate has resulted in both acute and delayed cell death by both necrosis and apoptosis. This may be an important mechanism of gut damage from anoxia, ischemia, and excitotoxins present in food.[116]

Controlling the Inflammatory Environment

Control of the inflammatory environment plays a critical role in GI health. While exhaustive lists of inflammatory mediators and excitotoxins have been developed, simpler strategies for the management of inflammation may be available. Control of leakiness of the gut and antigen presentation at the lamina propria within the gut may help balance T-helper cell population distribution and thus control inflammation.[117] Additionally, control of leakiness of the gut wall may reduce inappropriate gut luminal content/immune interactions, thus reducing immune-mediated inflammation, both locally and at a distance.[118] Clinically, if we are able to improve gut leakiness and improve T-helper cell populations to a more tolerogenic form, this may lead to improved inflammatory mediators within the gut. This may be accomplished by using oligo-antigenic diets, anti-inflammatory agents, and factors that improve microbial balance.

References

1. Lacy B, Lee R. Irritable bowel syndrome: a syndrome in evolution. J Clin Gastroenterology. 2005;39(5) Supplement 3:S230-S42.
2. Gershon MD. The enteric nervous system now. Chapter in The Second Brain. 1st ed. New York: HarperCollins, 1998. 190-235.
3. Watanuki S, Kim YK. Physiological responses induced by pleasant stimuli. J Physiol Anthropol Appl Human Sci. 2005;24(1):125-8.
4. Mackinnon LT, Hooper S. Mucosal (secretory) immune system responses to exercise of varying intensity and during overtraining. Int J Sports Med. 1994;15 Suppl 3:S179-83.
5. Akimoto T, Nakahori C, Aizawa K, et al. Acupuncture and responses of immunologic and endocrine markers during competition. Med Sci Sports Exerc. 2003;35(8):1296-302.

6. Akimoto T, Kumai Y, Akama T, et al. Effects of 12 months of exercise training on salivary secretory IgA levels in elderly subjects. Br J Sports Med. 2003;37:76-79.
7. El Hamshary EM, Arafa WA. Detection of IgA anti-Entamoeba histolytica in the patients' saliva. J Egypt Soc Parasitol. 2004;34(3 Suppl):1095-104.
8. Chirigos MA, Jirillo E. Saliva secretory IgA antibodies against molds and mycotoxins in patients exposed to toxigenic fungi. Immunopharmacol Immunotoxicol. 2005;27(1):185.
9. Moses PL, Ellis LM, Anees MR, et al. Antineuronal antibodies in idiopathic achalasia and gastro-oesophageal reflux disease. Gut. 2003;52(5):629-36.
10. Gershon MD. The enteric nervous system now. Chapter in The Second Brain. 1st ed. New York: HarperCollins, 1998. 190-235.
11. Kirchgessner AL, Gershon MD. Innervation and regulation of the pancreas by neurons in the gut. Z Gastroenterol Verh. 1991;26:230-33.
12. Liddle RA, Goldfine ID, Rosen MS, et al. Cholecystokinin bioactivity in human plasma. Molecular forms, responses to feeding, and relationship to gallbladder contraction. J Clin Invest. 1985;75(4):1144-52.
13. O'Rourke MF, Reidelberger RD, Solomon TE. Effect of CCK antagonist L 364718 on meal-induced pancreatic secretion in rats. Am J Physiol. 1990;258(2 Pt 1):G179-G184.
14. Peterson H, Solomon T, Grossman M. Effect of chronic pentagastrin, cholecystokinin, and secretin on pancreas of rats. Am J Physiol. 1978;234:E286-E293.
15. Tiscornia OM, Dreiling DA, Yacomotti J, et al. Neural control of the exocrine pancreas: an analysis of the cholinergic, adrenergic, and peptidergic pathways and their positive and negative components. 1: Neural mechanisms. Mt Sinai J Med. 1987;54(5):366-83.
16. Tiscornia OM, Dreiling DA, Yacomotti J, et al. Neural control of the exocrine pancreas: an analysis of the cholinergic, adrenergic, and peptidergic pathways and their positive and negative components. 2. Integration of neural and hormonal mechanisms. Mt Sinai J Med. 1988;55(2):126-31.
17. Mawe GM. Nerves and hormones interact to control gallbladder function. News Physiol Sci. 1998;13:84-90.
18. Kirchgessner AL, Gershon MD. Innervation and regulation of the pancreas by neurons in the gut. Z Gastroenterol Verh. 1991;26:230-33.
19. Mawe GM, Collins SM, Shea-Donohue T. Changes in enteric neural circuitry and smooth muscle in the inflamed and infected gut. Neurogastroenterol Motil. 2004;16(Suppl 1):133-36.
20. Dalton SO, Johansen C, Mellemkjaer L, et al. Use of selective serotonin reuptake inhibitors and risk of upper gastrointestinal tract bleeding: a population-based cohort study. Arch intern Med. 2003;163(1):59-64.
21. Lim DK, Mahendran R. Risperidone and megacolon. Singapore Med J. 2002;43(10):530-32.
22. Halpert A, Dalton CB, Diamant NE, et al. Clinical response to tricyclic antidepressants in functional bowel disorders is not related to dosage. Am J. Gastroenterol. 2005;100(3):664-71.
23. Gershon MD. The enteric nervous system: a second brain. Hosp Pract (Off Ed). 1999;34(7):31-8, 41.
24. Coates MD, Mahoney CR, Linden DR, et al. Molecular defects in mucosal serotonin content and decreased serotonin reuptake transporter in ulcerative colitis and irritable bowel syndrome. Gastroenterology. 2004;126(7): 1657-64.
25. Kapur RP, Gershon MD, Milla PJ, Pachnis V. The influence of Hox genes and three intercellular signalling pathways on enteric neuromuscular development. Neurogastroenterol Motil. 2004;16(Suppl 1): 8-13.
26. De Giorgio R, Guerrini S, Barbara G, et al. New insights into human enteric neuropathies. Neurogastroenterol Motil. 2004;16(Suppl 1):143-47.
27. Mawe GM, Gershon MD. Functional heterogeneity in the myenteric plexus: demonstration using cytochrome oxidase as a verified cytochemical probe of the activity of individual enteric neurons. J Comp Neurol. 1986;249(3): 381-91.
28. Kapur RP, Gershon MD, Milla PJ, Pachnis V. The influence of Hox genes and three intercellular signalling pathways on enteric neuromuscular development. Neurogastroenterol Motil. 2004;16(Suppl 1): 8-13.
29. Camilleri M. Diagnosis and treatment of enteric neuromuscular diseases. Clin Auton Res. 2003;13(1):10-15.
30. Mawe GM, Collins SM, Shea-Donohue T. Changes in enteric neural circuitry and smooth muscle in the inflamed and infected gut. Neurogastroenterol Motil. 2004;16(Suppl 1):133-36.
31. Ibid.
32. Kendall CW, Emam A, Augustin LS, Jenkins DJ. Resistant starches and health. J AOAC Int. 2004;87(3):769-74.
33. Schley PD, Field CJ. The immune-enhancing effects of dietary fibres and prebiotics. Br J Nutr. 2002;87(Suppl 2):S221-S230.
34. Rhee KJ, Sethupathi P, Driks A, et al. Role of commensal bacteria in development of gut-associated lymphoid tissues and preimmune antibody repertoire. J Immunol. 2004;172(2):1118-24.
35. Jang MH, Kweon MN, Iwatani K, et al. Intestinal villous M cells: an antigen entry site in the mucosal epithelium. Proc Natl Acad Sci USA. 2004;101(16):6110-15.
36. Johansson-Lindbom B, Svensson M, Wurbel MA, et al. Selective generation of gut tropic T cells in gut-associated lymphoid tissue (GALT): requirement for GALT dendritic cells and adjuvant. J Exp Med. 2003;198(6):963-69.
37. Kunkel EJ, Campbell DJ, Butcher EC. Chemokines in lymphocyte trafficking and intestinal immunity. Microcirculation. 2003;10(3-4):313-23.
38. Nagler-Anderson C. Man the barrier! Strategic defences in the intestinal mucosa. Nat Rev Immunol. 2001;1(1):59-67.
39. Aiuti F, Iebba F. [Intestinal mucosa immunity and oral vaccines especially regarding E. coli vaccines: a review]. Infez Med. 2002;10(4):191-203.
40. Nagler-Anderson C, Shi HN. Peripheral nonresponsiveness to orally administered soluble protein antigens. Crit Rev Immunol. 2001;21(1-3):121-31.
41. Takaishi H, Ohara S, Hotta K, et al. Circulating autoantibodies against purified colonic mucin in ulcerative colitis. J Gastroenterol. 2000;35(1):20-27.
42. Watanabe M, Watanabe N, Iwao Y, et al. The serum factor from patients with ulcerative colitis that induces T cell proliferation in the mouse thymus is interleukin-7. J Clin Immunol. 1997;17(4):282-92.
43. Bastian L, Weimann A. Immunonutrition in patients after multiple trauma. Br J Nutr. 2002;87(Suppl 1):S133-S134.
44. Fukatsu K. Ueno C, Maeshima Y, et al. L-arginine-enriched parenteral nutrition affects lymphocyte phenotypes of gut-associated lymphoid tissue. JPEN J Parenter Enteral Nutr. 2004;28(4):246-50.
45. Rhoden D, Matheson PJ, Carricato ND, et al. Immune-enhancing enteral diet selectively augments ileal blood flow in the rat. J Surg Res. 2002;106(1) 25-30.
46. Acheson DW, Luccioli S. Microbial-gut interactions in health and disease. Mucosal immune responses. Best Pract Res Clin Gastroenterol. 2004;18(2):387-404.
47. Krantz BA, Melnyk RA, Zhang S, et al. A phenylalanine clamp catalyzes protein translocation through the anthrax toxin pore. Science. 2005;309(5735):777-81.

48. Darlington LG, Ramsey NW. Review of dietary therapy for rheumatoid arthritis. Br J Rheumatol. 1993;32(6):507-14.
49. McGonagle D, Gibbon W, Emery P. Classification of inflammatory arthritis by enthesitis. Lancet. 1998;352(9134):1137-40.
50. Rooney PJ, Jenkins RT, Buchanan WW. A short review of the relationship between intestinal permeability and inflammatory joint disease. Clin Exp Rheumatol. 1990;8(1):75-83.
51. Hunter JO. Food allergy—or enterometabolic disorder? Lancet. 1991;338(8765):495-96.
52. Waldeck F. Functions of the Gastrointestinal Canal. In Human Physiology. Schmidt RF, Lang F, Thews G (Eds.). New York: Springer-Verlag, 2004, p 602.
53. Thomson AB, Wild G. Adaptation of intestinal nutrient transport in health and disease. Part I. Dig Dis Sci. 1997;42(3):453-69.
54. Levin RJ. Digestion and absorption of carbohydrates—from molecules and membranes to humans. Am J Clin Nutr. 1994;59(3 Suppl):690S-8S.
55. Ibid.
56. Lentze MJ. Molecular and cellular aspects of hydrolysis and absorption. Am J Clin Nutr. 1995;61(4 Suppl):946S-51S.
57. Madara JL, Marcial MA. Structural correlates of intestinal tight-junction permeability. Kroc Found Ser. 1984;17:77-100.
58. Madara JL. Intestinal absorptive cell tight junctions are linked to cytoskeleton. Am J Physiol. 1987;253(1 Pt 1):C171-C175.
59. Wyatt J, Vogelsang H, Hubl W, et al. Intestinal permeability and the prediction of relapse in Crohn's disease. Lancet. 1993;341(8858):1437-39.
60. Holden W, Orchard T, Wordsworth P. Enteropathic arthritis. Rheum Dis Clin North Am. 2003;29(3):513-30.
61. Fink MP. Intestinal epithelial hyperpermeability: update on the pathogenesis of gut mucosal barrier dysfunction in critical illness. Curr Opin Crit Care. 2003;9(2):143-51.
62. Galluser M, Raul F, Canguilhem B. Adaptation of intestinal enzymes to seasonal and dietary changes in a hibernator: the European hamster (Cricetus cricetus). J Comp Physiol [B]. 1988;158(2):143-49.
63. Raul F, Goda T, Gosse F, Koldovsky O. Short-term effect of a high-protein/low-carbohydrate diet on aminopeptidase in adult rat jejunoileum. Site of aminopeptidase response. Biochem J. 1987;247(2):401-05.
64. Raul F, Lacroix B, Aprahamian M. Longitudinal distribution of brush border hydrolases and morphological maturation in the intestine of the preterm infant. Early Hum Dev. 1986;13(2):225-34.
65. Lester R, Smallwood RA, Little JM, et al. Fetal bile salt metabolism. The intestinal absorption of bile salt. J Clin Invest. 1977;59(6):1009-16.
66. Lester R, Zimniak P. True transport: one or more sodium-dependent bile acid transporters? Hepatology. 1992;18(5):1279-82.
67. Tannock GW (Ed). Probiotics: A Critical Review. Horizon Scientific Press: England, 1999.
68. Lee Y-K, Nomoto K, Salminen S, Gorbach SL. Handbook of Probiotics. Wiley-Interscience, 1999.
69. Kailasapathy K, Chin J. Survival and therapeutic potential of probiotic organisms with reference to Lactobacillus acidophilus and Bifidobacterium spp. Immunol Cell Biol. 2000;78(1):80-88.
70. Dixit SM, Gordon DM, Wu XY, et al. Diversity analysis of commensal porcine Escherichia coli - associations between genotypes and habitat in the porcine gastrointestinal tract. Microbiology. 2004;150(Pt 6):1735-40.
71. Sult T. The Undiscovered Organ: Intestinal Microbes in Health and Disease. AHMA Review Course in Holistic Medicine Minneapolis, MN: AHMA, 1999.
72. Chen X, Schauder S, Potier N, et al. Structural identification of a bacterial quorum-sensing signal containing boron. Nature. 2002;415(6871):545-49.
73. Schauder S, Shokat K, Surette MG, Bassler BL. The LuxS family of bacterial autoinducers: biosynthesis of a novel quorum-sensing signal molecule. Mol Microbiol. 2001;41(2):463-76.
74. Agladze K, Jackson D, Romeo T. Periodicity of cell attachment patterns during Escherichia coli biofilm development. J Bacteriol. 2003;185(18):5632-38.
75. Al-Bakri AG, Gilbert P, Allison DG. Immigration and emigration of Burkholderia cepacia and Pseudomonas aeruginosa between and within mixed biofilm communities. J Appl Microbiol. 2004;96(3):455-63.
76. Webb JS, Thompson LS, James S, et al. Cell death in Pseudomonas aeruginosa biofilm development. J Bacteriol. 2003;185(15):4585-92.
77. Schembri MA, Kjaergaard K, Klemm P. Global gene expression in Escherichia coli biofilms. Mol Microbiol. 2003;48(1):253-67.
78. Hogan DA, Kolter R. Pseudomonas-Candida interactions: an ecological role for virulence factors. Science. 2002;296(5576):2229-32.
79. Singh PK, Schaefer AL, Parsek MR, et al. Quorum-sensing signals indicate that cystic fibrosis lungs are infected with bacterial biofilms. Nature. 2000;407(6805):762-64.
80. Mah TF, Pitts B, Pellock B, et al. A genetic basis for Pseudomonas aeruginosa biofilm antibiotic resistance. Nature. 2003;426(6964):306-10.
81. Hogan DA, Kolter R. Pseudomonas-Candida interactions: an ecological role for virulence factors. Science. 2002;296(5576):2229-32.
82. Roberts ME, Stewart PS. Modeling antibiotic tolerance in biofilms by accounting for nutrient limitation. Antimicrob Agents Chemother. 2004;48(1):48-52.
83. Mah TF, Pitts B, Pellock B, et al. A genetic basis for Pseudomonas aeruginosa biofilm antibiotic resistance. Nature. 2003;426(6964):306-10.
84. Bagge N, Schuster M, Hentzer M, et al. Pseudomonas aeruginosa biofilms exposed to imipenem exhibit changes in global gene expression and beta-lactamase and alginate production. Antimicrob Agents Chemother. 2004;48(4):1175-87.
85. Donlan RM, Costerton JW. Biofilms: survival mechanisms of clinically relevant microorganisms. Clin Microbiol Rev. 2002;15(2):167-93.
86. Mercier C, Durrieu C, Briandet R, et al. Positive role of peptidoglycan breaks in lactococcal biofilm formation. Mol Microbiol. 2002;46(1):235-43.
87. Agladze K, Jackson D, Romeo T. Periodicity of cell attachment patterns during Escherichia coli biofilm development. J Bacteriol. 2003;185(18):5632-38.
88. Martino PD, Fursy R, Bret L, et al. Indole can act as an extracellular signal to regulate biofilm formation of Escherichia coli and other indole-producing bacteria. Can J Microbiol. 2003;49(7):443-49.
89. Mercier C, Durrieu C, Briandet R, et al. Positive role of peptidoglycan breaks in lactococcal biofilm formation. Mol Microbiol. 2002;46(1):235-43.
90. Chung J, Ha ES, Park HR, Kim S. Isolation and characterization of Lactobacillus species inhibiting the formation of Streptococcus mutans biofilm. Oral Microbiol Immunol. 2004;19(3):214-16.
91. McLean RJ, Pierson LS, Fuqua C. A simple screening protocol for the identification of quorum signal antagonists. J Microbiol Methods. 2004;58(3):351-60.
92. Singh PK, Parsek MR, Greenberg EP, Welsh MJ. A component of innate immunity prevents bacterial biofilm development. Nature. 2002;417(6888):552-5.
93. Orsi N. The antimicrobial activity of lactoferrin: current status and perspectives. Biometals. 2004;17(3):189-96.

94. Lesman-Movshovich E, Lerrer B, Gilboa-Garber N. Blocking of Pseudomonas aeruginosa lectins by human milk glycans. Can J Microbiol. 2003;49(3):230-35.
95. Loiselle M, Anderson KW. The use of cellulase in inhibiting biofilm formation from organisms commonly found on medical implants. Biofouling. 2003;19(2):77-85.
96. Hellio C, Bremer G, Pons AM, et al. Inhibition of the development of microorganisms (bacteria and fungi) by extracts of marine algae from Brittany, France. Appl Microbiol Biotechnol. 2000;54(4):543-49.
97. Farber BF, Hsieh HC, Donnenfeld ED, et al. A novel antibiofilm technology for contact lens solutions. Ophthalmology. 1995;102(5):831-36.
98. Alem MA, Douglas LJ. Effects of aspirin and other nonsteroidal anti-inflammatory drugs on biofilms and planktonic cells of Candida albicans. Antimicrob Agents Chemother. 2004;48(1):41-47.
99. Plotkin MJ. Tales of a Shaman's Apprentice. 1st ed. New York: Penguin Books, 1993.
100. Caraglia M, D'Alessandro AM, Marra M, et al. The farnesyl transferase inhibitor R115777 (Zarnestra) synergistically enhances growth inhibition and apoptosis induced on epidermoid cancer cells by Zoledronic acid (Zometa) and Pamidronate. Oncogene. 2004. 23(41):6900-13.
101. Saavedra JM, Tschernia A. Human studies with probiotics and prebiotics: clinical implications. Br J Nutr. 2002;87(Suppl 2):S241-S246.
102. Bagge N, Schuster M, Hentzer M, et al. Pseudomonas aeruginosa biofilms exposed to imipenem exhibit changes in global gene expression and beta-lactamase and alginate production. Antimicrob Agents Chemother. 2004;48(4):1175-87.
103. Mah TF, Pitts B, Pellock B, et al. A genetic basis for Pseudomonas aeruginosa biofilm antibiotic resistance. Nature. 2003;426(6964):306-10.
104. John GH, et al. The presence of cytochrome p450-like protein in the human intestinal microflora eubacterium aerofaciens. Microbial Ecology in Health & Disease. 2001;13:3-8.
105. Gallio M, Sturgill G, Rather P, Kylsten P. A conserved mechanism for extracellular signaling in eukaryotes and prokaryotes. Proc Natl Acad Sci USA. 2002;99(19):12208-13.
106. Probiotics a Critical Review. Tannock GW, Ed. Wymondham, Norfolk, England: Horizon Scientific Press, 2004.
107. Handbook of Probiotics. Lee Y, et al., Eds. New York: John Wiley and Sons, Inc, 1999.
108. Probiotics 2. Fuller R, Ed. Boston: Chapman and Hall, 1997.
109. Probiotics 3. Fuller R, Perdigon G, Eds. Boston: Kluwer Academic Publishers, 1997.
110. Sharkey KA, Mawe GM. Neuroimmune and epithelial interactions in intestinal inflammation. Curr Opin Pharmacol. 2002;2(6):669-77.
111. Mulak A, Bonaz B. Irritable bowel syndrome: a model of the brain-gut interactions. Med Sci Monit. 2004;10(4):RA55-RA62.
112. Ibid.
113. Soderholm JD, Yang PC, Ceponis P, et al. Chronic stress induces mast cell-dependent bacterial adherence and initiates mucosal inflammation in rat intestine. Gastroenterology. 2002;123.4:1099-108.
114. Wood JD. Neuropathy in the brain-in-the-gut. Eur J Gastroenterol Hepatol. 2000;12(6):597-600.
115. De Giorgio R, Guerrini S, Barbara G, et al. Inflammatory neuropathies of the enteric nervous system. Gastroenterology. 2004;126(7):1872-83.
116. Kirchgessner AL, Liu MT, Alcantara F. Excitotoxicity in the enteric nervous system. J Neurosci. 1997;17(22):8804-16.
117. Constant SL, Bottomly K. Induction of Th1 and Th2 CD4+ T cell responses: the alternative approaches. Annu Rev Immunol. 1997;15:297-322.
118. Rooney PJ, Jenkins RT, Buchanan WW. A short review of the relationship between intestinal permeability and inflammatory joint disease. Clin Exp Rheumatol. 1990;8(1):75-83.

Chapter 25
Structural Imbalances

Alex Vasquez, DC, ND

Introduction

When discussing the "structural" aspect of the functional medicine matrix, we commonly think of the musculoskeletal system; this is appropriate since the majority of the body is comprised of the bones, muscles, and interconnecting joints that form our limbs, torso, neck, and craniomandibular complex. Structural considerations are also relevant for several nonmusculoskeletal conditions. In some patients, aspects of their "structural imbalances" or "structural dysfunction" may be readily apparent and obviously relevant to their primary health concern. In other patients, structural imbalance may be more subtle and/or less obviously relevant to their clinical situation. It is important to distinguish subtle from unimportant; many structural imbalances and dysfunctions may go undetected, or may be categorized as "not relevant," if they lie outside the practitioner's awareness or scope of training and specialty. Examples of these important subtleties and breaches of structural integrity include the slight increases in intestinal permeability associated with eczema, inflammatory bowel disease, and several types of arthritis,[1] and the proprioceptive defects and subtle aberrations of joint motion that may contribute to chronic back and neck pain and predispose to recurrent injury and therapeutic recalcitrance.[2,3]

The more we know about micro- and macrophysiology, the more we are challenged when attempting to draw clear boundaries between organ systems and biochemical vs. nutritional vs. structural vs. neurologic processes. It is increasingly clear that all musculoskeletal conditions involve numerous overlaps with other elements of the matrix. The best way to convey the interconnectedness of the structural aspect of the matrix with these other elements is simply to discuss and give examples of each with an appreciation of the bi-directional linkage whereby one aspect affects the other. The sections that follow provide a brief review of those aspects of the matrix that most strongly affect and are affected by structural imbalances. A graphic representation of these interconnections is provided in Figure 25.1. (In a sense, this whole book provides the underlying evidence for these multifaceted and multidirectional interconnections, but Chapter 10 addresses the issue directly.)

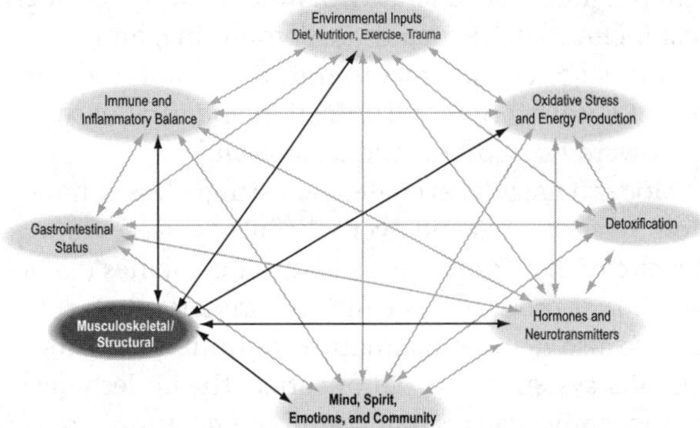

Figure 25.1 **Interconnectedness of structural aspects of the matrix with other elements**

Environmental Inputs

Our use of the phrase "environmental inputs" implies our appreciation of the roles of diet, nutrition, exercise, and trauma in human health and disease. We should add the importance of sun exposure as an environmental factor with relevance for a wide range of clinical problems, since insufficient sun exposure generally leads to a deficiency of vitamin D, which can exacerbate inflammation,[4] musculoskeletal pain,[5,6] and increase the risk of inflammatory diseases such as rheumatoid arthritis.[7] (To compensate in part for lack of sun exposure, administration of vitamin D in doses of 4,000 IU per day for adults can reduce inflammation, alleviate musculoskeletal pain, and ameliorate a wide range of health problems.[8]) Other environmental and lifestyle factors, such as repetitive overuse, can promote tissue inflammation and trauma to articular tissues, thus accelerating joint degeneration by inducing chondrocyte senescence via oxidative mechanisms.[9] As an intangible environmental input, exposure to psychoemotional stressors is consistently associated with an increased propensity toward allergic and inflammatory diseases.[10]

The American/Western style of eating (commonly referred to as SAD, for the standard American diet) is characterized by foods with an excess of linoleic and arachidonic acids, an overabundance of foods with high glycemic loads and indices, and a deficiency of phytonutrients. Since arachidonic and linoleic acids and high-sugar foods are proinflammatory, the American diet can be described as inherently proinflammatory and thus contributory to the scourge of painful musculoskeletal conditions that plagues Westerners.[11] Therefore, treatment programs for patients with inflammatory disorders must include advice for a health-promoting, anti-inflammatory diet in order to shift the balance of their physiology away from inflammation and catabolism and toward homeostasis and anabolism.[12]

Moderate regular exercise, increasingly less common in our over-stressed and over-scheduled times, stimulates the release from muscle tissue of cytokines ("myokines") that produce a net anti-inflammatory effect.[13] Exercise also helps to maintain a coordinated neuromuscular system and avoid or correct the underlying proprioceptive defects that contribute to chronic musculoskeletal pain, particularly in the low back, knees, and ankles.[14] As an external therapeutic intervention, spinal manipulation can also be placed in this category of environmental inputs; it is noteworthy that spinal manipulation has also been shown to benefit non-musculoskeletal systems, particularly pulmonary and gastrointestinal.[15] Environmental inputs can help shift the balance toward—or away from—a localized or systemic inflammatory response. In summary, the environment can be therapeutically manipulated to reduce the prevalence and severity of painful inflammatory musculoskeletal disorders.

Gastrointestinal Status

On a microscopic level, the integrity of the intestinal mucosa deserves attention, since increased intestinal permeability can promote macromolecule absorption, which can lead to immune complex deposition and systemic immune dysfunction that can exacerbate musculoskeletal inflammation.[16] In this way, the status of the gut influences the status of the musculoskeletal system, and the converse is also true. From a therapeutic standpoint, some patients note a subjective improvement in gastrointestinal function following chiropractic-type spinal manipulation,[17] and this exemplifies how the status of the musculoskeletal system can influence the status of the GI system. It is increasingly clear that the gut shares a bi-directional linkage with the nervous system, and therefore the nervous system, via the musculoskeletal system, can be used as a modulator of gastrointestinal function. A full discussion of these issues from the clinical perspective can be found in Chapter 28, including a detailed discussion of the enteric nervous system (the gut-brain connection).

Mind, Spirit, Emotions, and Community

Musculoskeletal pain and inflammation can cause at least three types of secondary depression. First, inflammatory mediators released from degenerative tissues and systemic inflammation have psychoactive effects that can contribute to fatigue, somnolence, anxiety, depression, dementia, and psychosis.[18,19] Second, patients with acute or chronic musculoskeletal disorders are, of course, frequently in pain and are commonly less able to pursue hobbies and activities that would otherwise give them pleasure. Third, decreased mobility can contribute to a reduction in social contact, and the sense of social isolation that results can lead to mental and emotional distress.[20] In these ways, musculoskeletal dysfunction can adversely affect mental and social health.

Treatments aimed at improving musculoskeletal health can have positive emotional, mental, and social benefits. Exercise helps alleviate depression, and group exercises can provide a valuable source of social contact, which may further alleviate depression and promote social health.[21] High-dose vitamin D supplementation corrects the vitamin D deficiency that is common in patients with musculoskeletal pain,[22] provides an important anti-inflammatory benefit,[23] and alleviates musculoskeletal pain.[24] Other effects of vitamin D repletion include lessening the severity of depression[25] and enhancing mood, sociability, and overall sense of well-being.[26] The proteolytic enzyme bromelain provides anti-inflammatory benefits, helps to alleviate the pain of osteoarthrtitis, and enhances an overall sense of well-being.[27] Full-body soft tissue massage and myofascial manipulation can help to alleviate depression and insomnia, enhance mood, and lessen the severity of premenstrual syndrome for women.[28] Similarly, EPA and DHA from fish oil can ease joint pain and inflammation while also providing an antidepressant benefit.[29] Meditative relaxation appears capable of reducing inflammatory responses by neurogenic mechanisms,[30] and it is reasonable for orthopedic patients to regularly practice meditation and relaxation techniques.

Immune and Inflammatory Imbalances

The muscles and joints that comprise the bulk of the structural aspect of the matrix are commonly affected by inflammatory and immune imbalances. Musculoskeletal rheumatic diseases such as rheumatoid arthritis and the enteropathic spondyloarthropathies clearly exemplify the effects of a dysregulated immune system upon the structures of the peripheral joints and spine, respectively. In patients with inflammatory musculo-skeletal disorders, emphasis should be placed first on normalizing and then on optimizing immune function by addressing the underlying factors that have synergized to affect immunodysregulation and create or intensify autoimmunity. Suppressing immune response with immunosuppressants such as prednisone, anti-inflammatory drugs such as NSAIDs (which promote joint destruction and chondrolysis[31,32]), or selective COX-2-inhibiting drugs (which consistently elevate the risk of cardiovascular death[33,34,35]) should not be the first treatment approach. Rather, addressing the underlying causes of proinflammatory imbalance is a more reasonable clinical approach for immune-mediated pain and inflammation than simply suppressing the inflammatory consequences that result. Many (and perhaps most) diseases categorized under "immune and inflammatory imbalance" will have a propensity to affect the structural/musculoskeletal systems, since inflammatory conditions generally exacerbate joint inflammation and degeneration.

Hormones and Neurotransmitters

Endocrine disturbances can contribute to immune dysfunction, which can then contribute to a systemic inflammatory response that leads to structural imbalances in the gastrointestinal tract and musculoskeletal systems. Absolute or relative excesses of estrogen and insufficiencies of testosterone, cortisol, and DHEA are common in patients with inflammatory/rheumatic disorders.[36,37,38,39,40] Detection and correction of thyroid autoimmunity may alleviate inflammatory musculoskeletal disorders, such as adhesive capsulitis.[41] As an endocrine disease, diabetes mellitus can contribute to carpal tunnel syndrome and adhesive capsulitis, and the elaboration of proinflammatory mediators from adipose tissue (adipokines) underscores the importance of weight optimization as part of the treatment for patients with inflammatory disorders.[42] Massage therapy has been shown to have "neuroendocrine" effects by raising levels of dopamine and serotonin and by alleviating depression, anxiety, and insomnia.[43] Any discussion of the effects of the nervous system on the musculoskeletal system must emphasize the importance of neurogenic inflammation as a major contributor to joint inflammation and cartilage degeneration. Indeed, sensory nerves exacerbate local tissue catabolism via the direct release of inflammatory and degeneration-inducing signals, including cytokines and prostaglandins.[44] Thus the neuroendocrine and musculoskeletal systems can affect each other in a bi-directional manner, and this interaction allows for the establishment of a feed-forward cycle wherein trauma-induced tissue injury results in immunogenic inflammation and associated pain, the latter of which then triggers neurogenic inflammation, which then amplifies the ongoing immunogenic inflammation.

Detoxification

The link connecting musculoskeletal pain with impaired detoxification has not been fully characterized. However, detoxification programs are empirically beneficial for relieving aches and pains and many other specific and nonspecific complaints.[45] Many dietary, lifestyle, and interventional modalities can facilitate the removal of endogenous and exogenously acquired toxicants and can therefore be thought of as promoting detoxification of these substances; many of these same modalities are beneficial for patients suffering from musculoskeletal pain and inflammation. Health-promoting vegetarian diets have been shown to alleviate the pain and inflammation of rheumatoid arthritis,[46] and such diets can also promote urinary alkalinization,[47] which enhances the excretion of toxic xenobiotics and poisons.[48] Moderate exercise can help alleviate the pain of and disability caused by conditions such as fibromyalgia and osteoarthritis,[49] and exercise promotes the lymphatic flow and lipolysis that are generally considered essential for the mobilization of fat-stored xenobiotics. Detoxification programs are discussed in greater detail elsewhere in this text (see Chapters 22 and 31).

Oxidative Stress and Energy Production

Inflammatory musculoskeletal disorders are commonly associated with increased oxidative stress,[50] which can impair mitochondrial function, leading to expedited chondrocyte senescence and an overall reduced synthesis of the proteoglycans that form cartilage.[51,52] This supports the rationale for using dietary and supplemental antioxidant therapy in the treatment and prevention of degenerative or symptomatic musculoskeletal conditions. More specifically, nutrients that support mitochondrial function may be of value in reducing oxidative stress resulting from impaired energy metabolism.[53] An excellent example of this concept and its clinical application is the use of niacinamide in the treatment of osteoarthritis; niacinamide is known to support mitochondrial function, and it is safe and effective in the treatment of osteoarthritis.[54]

Structural Interconnections

Subtle structural dysfunction can lead to clinical conditions of sufficient severity that intervention is warranted. In addition to deficits in proprioceptive function that contribute to low-back and lower-extremity pain and injury,[55,56] subtle restrictions in or excesses of joint mobility, particularly of the spinal column, may lead to chronic pain. Clinically, the technique of motion palpation is a validated method of joint assessment and can be used to quantify and qualify subtle abnormalities in axial and peripheral joint function.[57,58] Restrictions in motion can be ameliorated with manual manipulative therapy,[59] and excesses in motion can be addressed by therapeutic exercise and ergonomic modifications.[60] This approach is particularly relevant for patients with, for example, chronic back and neck pain wherein deficits in proprioception and imbalances in muscle strength and tension can be alleviated with a multicomponent intervention that includes spinal manipulation, proprioceptive retraining, targeted muscle strengthening, and post-isometric stretching.[61] Intra-articular adhesions and entrapment of synovial folds and intra-articular menisci are anatomical contributors to localized pain that call for a physical rather than pharmacologic intervention, and these can be alleviated with manipulative therapy,[62] although some cases of entrapped synovial folds may be treated surgically.[63]

Summary

Several important considerations are relevant to the prevention or alleviation of musculoskeletal pain, the most common reason for considering the structural aspect of the matrix. Frequently overlooked causes of musculoskeletal pain and/or overt or subclinical inflammation include vitamin D deficiency, consumption of a proinflammatory diet, lack of exercise, excess adipose tissue and resultant elaboration of adipokines, proprioceptive deficits, subtle joint dysfunction, including intraarticular adhesions, and entrapment of intraarticular menisci and synovial folds. All of these are correctible with nonpharmacologic and nonsurgical means; addressing them successfully will help improve the patient's overall health and reduce the impact of these problems on other aspects of the functional medicine matrix. (See Chapter 29 for further discussion of clinical approaches to structural imbalances.)

References

1. Miller AL. The pathogenesis, clinical implications, and treatment of intestinal hyperpermeability. Alt Med Rev. 1997:2(5):330-345.
2. Revel M, Minguet M, Gregoy P, et al. Changes in cervicocephalic kinesthesia after a proprioceptive rehabilitation program in patients with neck pain: a randomized controlled study. Arch Phys Med Rehabil. 1994;75(8):895-9.
3. Rogers RG. The effects of spinal manipulation on cervical kinesthesia in patients with chronic neck pain: a pilot study. J Manipulative Physiol Ther. 1997;20(2):80-5.
4. Timms PM, Mannan N, et al. Circulating MMP9, vitamin D and variation in the TIMP-1 response with VDR genotype: mechanisms for inflammatory damage in chronic disorders? QJM. 2002;95:787-96.
5. Al Faraj S, Al Mutairi K. Vitamin D deficiency and chronic low-back pain in Saudi Arabia. Spine. 2003;28:177-9.
6. Plotnikoff GA, Quigley JM. Prevalence of severe hypovitaminosis D in patients with persistent, nonspecific musculoskeletal pain. Mayo Clin Proc. 2003;78(12):1463-70.

7. Cantorna MT. Vitamin D and autoimmunity: is vitamin D status an environmental factor affecting autoimmune disease prevalence? Proc Soc Exp Biol Med. 2000 Mar;223(3):230-3.
8. Vasquez A, Manso G, Cannell J. The clinical importance of vitamin d (cholecalciferol): a paradigm shift with implications for all healthcare providers. Alternative Therapies in Health and Medicine 2004; 10: 28-37.
9. Martin JA, Brown T, Heiner A, Buckwalter JA. Post-traumatic osteoarthritis: the role of accelerated chondrocyte senescence. Biorheology. 2004;41(3-4):479-91.
10. Wright RJ, Cohen RT, Cohen S. The impact of stress on the development and expression of atopy. Curr Opin Allergy Clin Immunol 2005;5(1):23-9.
11. Aljada A, Mohanty P, Ghanim H, et al. Increase in intranuclear nuclear factor kappaB and decrease in inhibitor kappaB in mononuclear cells after a mixed meal: evidence for a proinflammatory effect. Am J Clin Nutr. 2004;79(4):682-9.
12. Seaman DR. The diet-induced proinflammatory state: a cause of chronic pain and other degenerative diseases? J Manipulative Physiol Ther. 2002 Mar-Apr;25(3):168-79.
13. Petersen AM, Pedersen BK. The anti-inflammatory effect of exercise. J Appl Physiol. 2005 Apr;98(4):1154-62
14. Willems T, Witvrouw E, Verstuyft J, Vaes P, De Clercq D. Proprioception and muscle strength in subjects with a history of ankle sprains and chronic instability. J Athl Train. 2002 Dec;37(4):487-493.
15. Leboeuf-Yde C, Axen I, Ahlefeldt G, et al. The types and frequencies of improved nonmusculoskeletal symptoms reported after chiropractic spinal manipulative therapy. J Manipulative Physiol Ther. 1999 Nov-Dec;22(9):559-64.
16. Inman RD. Antigens, the gastrointestinal tract, and arthritis. Rheum Dis Clin North Am. 1991 May;17(2):309-21.
17. Leboeuf-Yde C, Axen I, Ahlefeldt G, et al. The types and frequencies of improved nonmusculoskeletal symptoms reported after chiropractic spinal manipulative therapy. J Manipulative Physiol Ther. 1999 Nov-Dec;22(9):559-64.
18. Wilson CJ, Finch CE, Cohen HJ. Cytokines and cognition--the case for a head-to-toe inflammatory paradigm. J Am Geriatr Soc. 2002 Dec;50(12):2041-56.
19. Kronfol Z, Remick DG. Cytokines and the brain: implications for clinical psychiatry. Am J Psychiatry. 2000;157(5):683-94.
20. Bradley LA. Psychosocial factors. In: Klippel JH (ed). Primer on the Rheumatic Diseases. 11th edition. Atlanta: Arthritis Foundation; 1997: 413-415.
21. Harold Elrick, MD. Exercise is Medicine. The Physician and Sportsmedicine - Volume 24 - No. 2 - February 1996.
22. Plotnikoff GA, Quigley JM. Prevalence of severe hypovitaminosis D in patients with persistent, nonspecific musculoskeletal pain. Mayo Clin Proc. 2003;78(12):1463-70.
23. Timms PM, Mannan et al. Circulating MMP9, vitamin D and variation in the TIMP-1 response with VDR genotype: mechanisms for inflammatory damage in chronic disorders? QJM. 2002;95:787-96.
24. Al Faraj S, Al Mutairi K. Vitamin D deficiency and chronic low-back pain in Saudi Arabia. Spine. 2003;28:177-9.
25. Lansdowne AT, Provost SC. Vitamin D3 enhances mood in healthy subjects during winter. Psychopharmacology (Berl). 1998;135:319-23.
26. Vieth R, Kimball S, Hu A, Walfish PG. Randomized comparison of the effects of the vitamin D3 adequate intake versus 100 mcg (4000 IU) per day on biochemical responses and the wellbeing of patients. Nutr J. 2004;3(1):8.
27. Walker AF, Bundy R, Hicks SM, Middleton RW. Bromelain reduces mild acute knee pain and improves well-being in a dose-dependent fashion in an open study of otherwise healthy adults. Phytomedicine. 2002;9:681-6.
28. Hernandez-Reif M, Martinez A, Field T, et al. Premenstrual symptoms are relieved by massage therapy. J Psychosom Obstet Gynaecol. 2000 Mar;21(1):9-15.
29. Covington MB. Omega-3 fatty acids. Am Fam Physician. 2004;70(1):133-40.
30. Lutgendorf S, Logan H, Kirchner HL, et al. Effects of relaxation and stress on the capsaicin-induced local inflammatory response. Psychosom Med. 2000 Jul-Aug;62(4):524-34.
31. Vidal y Plana RR, Bizzarri D, Rovati AL. Articular cartilage pharmacology: I. *In vitro* studies on glucosamine and non steroidal antiinflammatory drugs. Pharmacol Res Commun. 1978 Jun;10(6):557-69.
32. Newman NM, Ling RS. Acetabular bone destruction related to nonsteroidal anti-inflammatory drugs. Lancet. 1985; 2(8445): 11-4.
33. Mukherjee D, Nissen SE, Topol EJ. Risk of cardiovascular events associated with selective COX-2 inhibitors. JAMA. 2001 Aug 22-29;286(8):954-9.
34. Topol EJ. Failing the public health—rofecoxib, Merck, and the FDA. N Engl J Med. 2004;351(17):1707-9.
35. Ray WA, Griffin MR, Stein CM. Cardiovascular toxicity of valdecoxib. N Engl J Med. 2004;351(26):276.
36. Jefferies WM. Mild adrenocortical deficiency, chronic allergies, autoimmune disorders and the chronic fatigue syndrome: a continuation of the cortisone story. Med Hypotheses. 1994 Mar;42(a3):183-9.
37. Jefferies WMcK. Safe Uses of Cortisol. Second Edition. Springfield, CC Thomas, 1996.
38. Tengstrand B, Carlstrom K, Hafstrom I. Bioavailable testosterone in men with rheumatoid arthritis-high frequency of hypogonadism. Rheumatology (Oxford). 2002 Mar;41(3):285-9.
39. Tengstrand B, Carlstrom K, Fellander-Tsai L, Hafstrom I. Abnormal levels of serum dehydroepiandrosterone, estrone, and estradiol in men with rheumatoid arthritis: high correlation between serum estradiol and current degree of inflammation. J Rheumatol. 2003 Nov;30(11):2338-43.
40. Booji A, Biewenga-Booji CM, Huber-Bruning O, et al. Androgens as adjuvant treatment in postmenopausal female patients with rheumatoid arthritis. Ann Rheum Dis. 1996 Nov;55(11):811-5.
41. Bowman CA, Jeffcoate WJ, Pattrick M, Doherty M. Bilateral adhesive capsulitis, oligoarthritis and proximal myopathy as presentation of hypothyroidism. Br J Rheumatol. 1988 Feb;27(1):62-4.
42. Vasquez A. Integrative Orthopedics: The Art of Creating Wellness While Managing Acute and Chronic Musculoskeletal Disorders. Houston; Natural Health Consulting Corporation. (www.OptimalHealthResearch.com): 2004.
43. Hernandez-Reif M, Field T, Krasnegor J, Theakston H. Lower back pain is reduced and range of motion increased after massage therapy. Int J Neurosci. 2001;106(3-4):131-45.
44. Gouze-Decaris E, Philippe L, Minn A, et al. Neurophysiological basis for neurogenic-mediated articular cartilage anabolism alteration. Am J Physiol Regul Integr Comp Physiol. 2001 Jan;280(1):R115-22.
45. Bland JS, Barrager E, Reedy RG, Bland K. Medical food-supplemented detoxification program in the management of chronic health problems. Altern Ther Health Med. 1995 Nov 1;1(5):62-71.
46. Hafstrom I, Ringertz B, Spangberg A, et al. A vegan diet free of gluten improves the signs and symptoms of rheumatoid arthritis: the effects on arthritis correlate with a reduction in antibodies to food antigens. Rheumatology (Oxford) 2001;40(10):1175-9.
47. Sebastian A, Frassetto LA, Sellmeyer DE, et al. Estimation of the net acid load of the diet of ancestral preagricultural Homo sapiens and their hominid ancestors. Am J Clin Nutr. 2002 Dec;76(6):1308-16.
48. Proudfoot AT, Krenzelok EP, Vale JA. Position Paper on urine alkalinization. J Toxicol Clin Toxicol. 2004;42(1):1-26.

49. Goldenberg DL, Burckhardt C, Crofford L. Management of fibromyalgia syndrome. JAMA 2004;292:2388-9.
50. Basu S, Whiteman M, Mattey DL, Halliwell B. Raised levels of F(2)-isoprostanes and prostaglandin F(2alpha) in different rheumatic diseases. Ann Rheum Dis. 2001 Jun;60(6):627-31.
51. Yudoh K, Nguyen T, Nakamura H, et al. Potential involvement of oxidative stress in cartilage senescence and development of osteoarthritis: oxidative stress induces chondrocyte telomere instability and downregulation of chondrocyte function. Arthritis Res Ther. 2005;7(2):R380-91.
52. Martin JA, Buckwalter JA. Aging, articular cartilage chondrocyte senescence and osteoarthritis. Biogerontology. 2002;3(5):257-64.
53. Martin JA, Buckwalter JA. The role of chondrocyte senescence in the pathogenesis of osteoarthritis and in limiting cartilage repair. J Bone Joint Surg Am. 2003;85-A Suppl 2:106-10.
54. Kaufman W. Niacinamide therapy for joint mobility. Therapeutic reversal of a common clinical manifestation of the "normal" aging process. Conn State Med J 1953;17:584-591.
55. Willems T, Witvrouw E, Verstuyft J, et al. Proprioception and Muscle Strength in Subjects With a History of Ankle Sprains and Chronic Instability. J Athl Train. 2002 Dec;37(4):487-493.
56. Bullock-Saxton JE, Janda V, Bullock MI. Reflex activation of gluteal muscles in walking. An approach to restoration of muscle function for patients with low-back pain. Spine. 1993 May;18(6):704-8.
57. Humphreys BK, Delahaye M, Peterson CK. An investigation into the validity of cervical spine motion palpation using subjects with congenital block vertebrae as a 'gold standard'. BMC Musculoskelet Disord. 2004 Jun 15;5(1):19.
58. Bergmann T, Peterson D, Lawrence D. Chiropractic Technique, Principles and Procedures. Churchill Livingstone, 1993.
59. Maigne JY, Vautravers P. Mechanism of action of spinal manipulative therapy. Joint Bone Spine. 2003;70(5):336-41.
60. BenEliyahu DJ. Conservative management of posttraumatic cervical intersegmental hypermobility and anterior subluxation. J Manipulative Physiol Ther. 1995;18(5):315-21.
61. Vasquez A. Integrative Orthopedics: The Art of Creating Wellness While Managing Acute and Chronic Musculoskeletal Disorders. Houston; Natural Health Consulting Corporation. (www.OptimalHealthResearch.com): 2004.
62. Bergmann T, Peterson D, Lawrence D. Chiropractic Technique, Principles and Procedures. Churchill Livingstone, 1993.
63. Duparc F, Putz R, Michot C, Muller JM, Freger P. The synovial fold of the humeroradial joint: anatomical and histological features, and clinical relevance in lateral epicondylalgia of the elbow. Surg Radiol Anat. 2002 Dec;24(5):302-7.

Section VI

A Practical Clinical Approach

Chapter 26
Clinical Approaches to Environmental Inputs

- ***Diet and Nutrition***
- ***Micronutrient Insufficiency Leads to DNA and Mitochondrial Damage***

Diet and Nutrition

Mark Hyman, MD

Introduction

Functional medicine is neither a new healthcare discipline nor a new subspecialty of medicine; it does not fundamentally alter our current understanding of the biomedical sciences. Rather, it applies what we have learned from the scientific literature—and from clinical medicine—through a different model, interpreting the findings in the context of both genetics and environment, and looking at functionality from the deepest levels of physiology and biochemistry to the most obvious psychosocial influences on health.

Guided by the organizing framework or *matrix* of functional medicine, clinicians are empowered to offer effective solutions for difficult and complex clinical problems. Space travel was not based on belief or superstition, but on physics. The first man to venture into space did so based on scientific theory, and he did so successfully, using established scientific principles, despite the fact that it had never been done before. Analogously, medicine, as we know it, is poised at the edge of a new frontier. Scientific inquiry has taken us deep into the realm of biology, and new principles and concepts have emerged. These new principles and concepts will set the stage and provide the tools for navigating *inner space*, where the complex interplay of genes, molecules, and environment promotes health and creates disease. While we await future research to unify and weave together diverse strands of scientific discovery and undoubtedly shed new light on this matrix, the weight of current evidence already provides a roadmap and some extremely useful tools.

The matrix of functional medicine (discussed in Chapter 34) is an evolving prism or lens for understanding medicine, but we must not confuse the lens with the object of perception. The profound complexity of biologic systems, and their interplay with the environment, is far too vast to be encompassed by any one theory. However, the matrix—the principles, the environmental inputs, the fundamental physiological processes and the core clinical imbalances—is a remarkably robust model for addressing the epidemic of chronic degenerative diseases, the myriad chronic syndromes, and the environmental, lifestyle, and immune disorders that are the plagues of the 21st century. By applying these principles to the everyday problems that affect our patients, we enter uncharted territory with respectful caution, an attitude of open inquiry, free of dogma, and ready for discovery.

Understanding the intersection of diet and disease, and the role of nutrition in both the creation and amelioration of disease, is both practical and instructive. It is practical because nutrition is the single most powerful clinical tool in preventing and treating disease. It is instructive because food (along with oxygen) is the key substrate for life and influences every biologic process and every core clinical imbalance. The duality of nutritional influences on health is striking. On one hand, our current diet is the principal agent of chronic degenerative disease in our time. On the other hand, when the current science of clinical nutrition is applied artfully, it has the power to prevent, reverse, and even cure many of our chronic diseases.

Dietary Influences on Health: Creating Imbalance or Balance

A one-size-fits-all approach to nutritional advice has proved problematic. Likewise, popular interest in nutrition and the vast market for dietary "cure-alls" and "quick fixes" has led to a confusing, often contradictory, array of "expert" advice. Even in the clinical setting, practical application of nutrition must take into account diversity of nutritional needs across the genetic and chronological spectrum, food preferences of individuals from different cultural backgrounds, the complex psychological aspects of food, and the lack of effective tools for matching dietary recommendations to the individual. Despite those limitations, there are some basic nutritional principles upon which most scientists and nutritional experts agree. There are also a number of therapeutic nutritional strategies that can be applied widely and successfully in the treatment of chronic disease. Understanding the role of nutrition in creating *and* correcting the core clinical imbalances is essential for knowing how to influence the basic biologic functions of health and disease.

Food plays a dual role—it can help and it can harm. A standard American diet (SAD) contributes to degenerative and immune disorders. It is a diet rich in refined sugars such as high fructose corn syrup, saturated fat, and trans-fatty acids, and low in fiber, legumes, nuts, fruits and vegetables, essential fatty acids, essential nutrients, and phytonutrients. The pH of our modern diet is low (acidic), and the sodium:potassium ratio is very high. This dietary pattern has been very clearly and strongly linked to chronic disease. Conversely, a diet that is better adapted to our evolutionary needs can ameliorate dysfunction and improve health. A healthful diet is primarily plant based; rich in fruits, vegetables, nuts, seeds, and legumes; high in fiber, essential fatty acids and nutrients; and low in saturated fat, *trans* fats, refined sugars, and carbohydrates. It should have an alkaline pH and a low sodium-to-potassium ratio.[1]

Frankly, we could stop right there. Changing dietary patterns in the manner just described would go a long way toward reversing our epidemic of chronic disease. However, most of us live in the real world, where our patients are seldom able to so completely alter their dietary habits. Most of our patients already have many of the dysfunctions and diseases of contemporary life, and we must treat them with all the skill at our command. Therefore, we will take this opportunity to delve deeply into clinically relevant issues surrounding food and nutrients, so that we can equip ourselves with knowledge and practical clinical approaches for managing our patients (and ourselves) more effectively.

Genetic and Evolutionary Influences on Dietary Choices

Food and its components (including macronutrients, micronutrients, phytonutrients, food additives, and contaminants) can act directly or indirectly to affect gene expression and consequently influence health and disease. This is the new field of *nutrigenomics*. Food, then, must be recognized to contain *information* as well as energy. Nutrients impact cell signaling and other informational processes. Critical aspects include the influence of nutrients on second messenger balances (cGMP:cAMP); their role in information processing; regulation of growth factors; production of cytokines; and apoptosis, particularly in relation to cancer.

Individual genetic predispositions will often dictate unique dietary requirements. Although foundational principles can be applied to nearly all individuals, refinement of dietary inputs is necessary to accommodate specific individual needs (influenced not only by genes, but also by environment and age). Two of the clearest examples of the links between genetics and diet in the cause and cure of disease are celiac disease and metabolic syndrome. Both have a genetic connection; both are strongly linked to multiple dysfunctions and diseases across organ systems; and both can produce a vast array of presenting complaints.

Gluten. Numerous immune and inflammatory disorders occur as a result of exposure to gliadin, a unique protein found in wheat and other grains. Up to 30% of Northern Europeans carry the HLA DQ8 or DQ2 gene and 1% express the syndrome of celiac disease.[2] Wheat protein is a relatively new food in European populations and may explain the development of an immune response in reaction to gluten in the diet. Avoidance of gluten alleviates the symptoms and frequently reverses the immune dysregulation, systemic inflammation, and autoimmunity associated with its ingestion. In addition to a direct upregulation of the inflammatory response, gluten may trigger a cascade of other imbalances leading to increased oxidative stress, thyroid dysfunction, infertility, and menstrual disorders. Further, it has been shown to initiate the formation of neuroactive peptides or gluten exorphins,[3] which affect cognitive function and contribute to morbidity in the autistic spectrum disorders.

Metabolic syndrome. The effects of a shift away from our evolutionary diet are dramatically manifested in the transition from a wild, omega-3 fatty acid-rich diet, abundant in vitamins, minerals, phytonutrients (from whole foods), and fiber to a diet high in processed foods, refined sugars and flours, and nearly absent of phytonutrients, vitamins, and minerals. Current research suggests that this shift in our dietary pattern has led to the current pandemic of obesity, metabolic syndrome, and diabetes,[4,5] as well as to associated imbalances in nearly every core physiologic system, contributing to cardiovascular disease, cancer, and dementia. Today's modern diet not only lacks many essential components of healthful nutrition, required by our genetic and evolutionary development, but it also contains substances never before ingested by humans, notably high fructose corn syrup and trans-fatty acids. Both of these common substances further enhance the tendency toward insulin resistance and a cascade of hormonal dysfunctions (including pancreatic, thyroid, adrenal, and sex steroid imbalances) that, in turn, lead to increased inflammation, oxidative stress, hepatic congestion, impaired detoxification, and structural imbalances of the cell membranes. A daunting litany, and one that will be echoed throughout this chapter as we examine our subject from many different perspectives. The good news, however, is that shifting from a processed and refined diet to a whole-foods, plant-based diet, devoid of refined sugars and carbohydrates, trans-fatty acids, and processed foods, directly influences and reverses the cascade of hormonal dysregulation central to the metabolic syndrome. Additionally, such dietary patterns have been shown to reduce oxidative stress and inflammation, while improving detoxification and membrane structural integrity.

Clinical Nutrition: A Young Science

Nutrition is a young science, poised to provide answers to aid practicing physicians in preventing, controlling, and treating the exploding global burden of chronic disease. The view of nutrition as simply a source of energy or calories to prevent malnutrition, and micronutrients to prevent deficiency diseases, is being supplanted by a new conception of nutrition in health and disease. Macro- and micronutrients and other non-nutritive substances in food are integral to understanding the causes, prevention, and treatment of disease. Nutrients are the fundamental substrates for our physiology and biochemistry; they are both etiologic factors and corrective tools. Translating basic science, epidemiological research, and small randomized trials into practical nutritional policy and advice remains challenging. However, when the data are viewed collectively, an important set of guiding concepts emerges that help us organize our interpretation and clinical utilization of the data.

While on a foundational level, the first law of thermodynamics holds, further investigation has revealed the "calories-in, calories-out" model of energy balance to be overly simplistic. Nutrients play a key role in bioenergetics beyond calorie content. A deeper understanding of bioenergetics illustrates that caloric content of food is only part of the story. Macronutrient composition of the diet asserts influence on thermoregulation, with variable effects on obesity, challenging the simple calorie-counting approach. In addition, the upregulated metabolism of detoxification and toxic overload creates significant energy costs.

The functional medicine practitioner's core questions. While the concept of fundamental clinical imbalances is a useful navigational tool for assessing and treating common clinical problems, it is, at best, an approximate description of a very complex biologic system—the human organism. An input or intervention designed to affect one organ or function may subsequently affect the entire interrelated and interdependent system—the whole human being. The practitioner must be skilled at interpreting the complex array of symptoms, tests results, and responses to treatment. While such complexity presents a challenge to the clinician, it is important to keep in mind that the essence of functional medicine is contained within two very simple questions: What harms us? What makes us thrive?

These key questions facilitate thinking about every clinical problem and provide access to the whole functional medicine matrix. They underlie the principles, the environmental inputs, the fundamental physiologic processes, and the core clinical imbalances. These two questions can be applied to every inquiry, for every illness, and for the promotion and creation of optimal health. And they are of paramount interest when considering clinical nutrition.

Exploring the first question, what harms or disturbs a person, may identify problems such as poor diet, chronic stress, toxic exposures, allergies, and/or infections. Delving into this question requires careful historical inquiry, focused testing, and environmental assessments, all of which we will explore as our discussion proceeds. The second question—what is currently missing and ultimately necessary for the full and vital expression of life—concerns food, water, air, vitamins, minerals, conditionally essential nutrients, light, sleep, rest, rhythm, and love.

The amount and particular balance of these "ingredients" differs for each individual. Wherever there is an imbalance, it is the result of something creating harm, or of some essential life-sustaining ingredient that is missing. In this context, understanding both what is present and what is missing in your patient's diet must be understood. (To borrow a turn of phrase from Kenneth Pelletier, PhD, "food as slayer and food as healer" are both likely roles.) Keeping these concepts in mind will help the practitioner filter new data and understand the context of this emerging research and information in the field of nutrition.

An exhaustive review of nutrition and its effects on health and disease is beyond the scope of the chapter. However, by using the model of chronic disease to illustrate the role nutrition plays in disease causation and in each of the fundamental processes that underlie our physiological, biochemical, and genomic functioning, we can glimpse the potential of nutritional intervention to influence the global burden of chronic disease. Fortunately, even before we begin our journey, we can summarize (see Table 26.1) the most important general nutritional advice that clinicians can give to their patients. If we do nothing more than guide patients in these directions, we will have accomplished a great deal.

The Global Burden of Chronic Disease: The Role of Diet and Lifestyle

Chronic disease has replaced infectious and acute illnesses as the leading cause of death in the world, both in developed and developing countries.[6] In 2002, the leading chronic diseases, including heart disease (17 million), cancer (7 million), chronic lung diseases (4 million), and diabetes (1 million), caused 29 million deaths worldwide. These ailments are almost entirely attributable to lifestyle risk factors such as poor diet, sedentary lifestyle, tobacco, and alcohol use. The misperception that these diseases affect primarily developed and affluent societies has led to a misappropriation of resources, which fails to deal with the exponential growth of chronic lifestyle- and diet-related disease. The major global health policy makers and agencies do not allocate appropriate resources to prevention of lifestyle problems because they have yet to fully acknowledge the extent of the problem, or perhaps because perceived or real economic concerns govern their actions. Heads of state, health ministries, the World Health Organization, academic and research institutions, non-governmental organizations, private donors, the World Bank, and the United Nations allocate only a fraction of their resources to chronic disease prevention, despite a rich evidence base for the role of lifestyle and diet in the prevention of the major chronic diseases. An examination of the nutritional literature and direct comparison to other efforts at prevention (pharmacologic) is needed to highlight the powerful, cost-effective, and critical role nutrition plays in causation, prevention, and treatment of chronic disease.

Table 26.1 **General Nutritional Advice**

Eat More of:	Eat Less (or None) of:	Beneficial Dietary Habits
• Anti-inflammatory foods • Detoxifying foods • Fiber • Food you love that makes you feel nourished • High quality, healthy protein • Omega-3 fats • Real, organic food • Vegetables and fruit • Nuts and seeds • Legumes • Whole grains	• High fructose corn syrup • High glycemic-index foods • High glycemic-load meals • *Trans* or hydrogenated fats	• Eat breakfast • Eat protein and fat with every meal (especially breakfast) • Eat something every 3–4 hours • Finish last meal at least 2–3 hours before bedtime • Improve pH balance through intake of alkaline (plant-based) foods • Lower the dietary sodium: potassium ratio • Take a multivitamin and other nutrients as needed

Diet, Lifestyle, and Chronic Disease—the Emerging Research

An emerging body of literature provides a firm foundation for practice and public policy in nutritional and lifestyle interventions for chronic disease.[7] A single nutrient, food, or lifestyle habit when studied as an isolated intervention—while helpful—may not show significant effect but, when assessed collectively, the power of lifestyle over pharmacologic approaches for primary and secondary prevention is clear. Adherence to healthful lifestyle practices in an elderly population (specifically, a Mediterranean diet pattern, moderate physical activity, non-smoking status, and moderate alcohol consumption) was associated with nearly a 70% reduction in all-cause and cause-specific mortality.[8] Other observational studies[9] showed similar data including an 83% reduction in coronary artery disease,[10] 91% reduction in diabetes in women,[11] and a 71% reduction in colon cancer in men.[12] While more difficult in design and execution, a few randomized trials have confirmed the effectiveness of diet and lifestyle in disease prevention. The Lyon Diet Heart Study[13] showed a 79% reduction in heart disease in patients with established heart disease after a few years of following a Mediterranean diet. The PREMIER group used an intervention of increased activity, weight loss, and Dietary Approaches to Stop Hypertension (DASH), which reduced blood pressure over six months.[14] In a secondary prevention trial, an integrated lifestyle approach of a plant-based diet, exercise, smoking cessation, and stress reduction demonstrated a 50% reduction in cardiac events.[15] A large systematic review of all pharmacologic and dietary interventions on total and cardiovascular mortality analyzed 97 studies with 137,140 patients in the intervention groups and 138,976 in the control groups. The largest reductions in all-cause and cardiovascular mortality resulted from fish oil, followed by statins.[16]

Long-term assessment of outcomes in dietary trials is difficult; determining the precise effects of trans-fat intake, carbohydrate quantity and quality, and alcohol consumption on chronic disease burden can be particularly challenging. Yet randomized trials of a healthful lifestyle can be (and already have been) used to assess shorter-term effects on clinical outcomes, biochemical markers of risk, and intermediate end-points. Where these are not possible, a careful analysis of basic science research, along with available clinical and epidemiological research, should be used to help form a picture of the overall role of dietary influences on disease. A randomized trial comparing a Mediterranean diet (whole grains, vegetables, fruits, nuts, olive oil, fish) vs. a control group following a "cardiac healthy" diet primarily focused on achieving less than 30% fat, exemplified the importance of intermediate markers of disease. Even after controlling for weight loss and physical activity, the authors found that inflammatory markers, insulin resistance, and endothelial function improved in the treatment group.[17]

The evidence is already undeniable that healthful dietary patterns such as those we have been discussing are associated with a decrease in chronic disease burden and all-cause mortality. The harmful effects of trans and certain saturated fats, refined carbohydrates, and other food additives or toxins are also well supported in the medical literature. The effects of diet can be viewed through their impact on processes such as gene expression, cell-signaling and informational systems, and bioenergetics. Our understanding of the many complex effects of these processes is being expanded continuously as the research base evolves. For the clinician, the concepts of nutritional imbalances, inflammation, oxidative stress, hormone imbalance, digestive function, impaired detoxification, mitochondrial function, and energy balance serve to focus our analysis of the dietary influences on health, and provide a context and method for interpreting and integrating new data into the practice of functional medicine.

Dietary Influences on Cardiovascular Disease: A Unified Theory of Causation

Cardiovascular disease (CVD) is a recurring theme in this book; it serves as a measure of our chronic disease burden (see the *Introduction* section) and as a primary example of the inflammation model of disease (Chapters 18 and 27). It is a central condition in the detailed functional medicine case study that wraps up our *Putting It All Together* section (Chapter 37). Here, we will discuss the profound causative influence of diet and nutrients on CVD. This thematic emphasis seems appropriate, because CVD is the leading killer in the United States today.

The effects of diet on health can be viewed in two ways:

- First, understanding the effects of diet on conditions such as cardiovascular disease can provide a more effective approach to assessment and therapy. This view also helps to illustrate the limitations of our current disease classification system, which does little to provide a unifying concept for the underlying dysfunctional biochemistry and physiology in any particular condition.
- Second, the effects of diet on each of the core clinical imbalances of the functional medicine matrix can provide a unique and novel prism through which to see both the common underlying causes and also many new therapeutic opportunities for chronic diseases that cross many organ systems.

Cardiovascular disease, both because of its high prevalence and its intimate connection to diet, is the model used here to describe the relation between particular foods and clinical imbalances. The effect of diet as both etiologic agent and therapeutic agent will then be explored. There are many gateways to using the functional medicine matrix in clinical practice. The old classification of disease should not be discarded, but rather seen within the context of a patient-centered, function-oriented model. Functional medicine provides a useful meta-framework for interpretation of the relevant data leading to new and unique understanding and treatments.

Historically, cardiovascular disease has been described as predominately an arterial pathology, with focus placed on the health and disease of the vascular tree, and the treatment on opening or bypassing the arterial blockage. However, the origins of cardiovascular disease are now seen predominantly as nutritional, neuroendocrine, oxidative, and inflammatory. The development and rupture of plaque in the arterial wall are processes related to a cascade of events that occurs over decades; these processes are primarily endocrine and immune in nature. The hallmarks of cardiovascular disease (hypertension, coagulopathy, and endothelial dysfunction) are secondary to upstream inputs controlled, in the main, by diet. The diet directly influences insulin sensitivity, oxidative stress, inflammation, lipid status, methylation, cardiocyte cellular energetics, membrane stability, and electrophysiologic dysfunction; these are the root functions that are imbalanced in all chronic degenerative diseases and cardiovascular disease in particular.

CVD and Diet: The Evidence for Causation and Reversal

Willett and Hu, in "Optimal Diets for the Prevention of Coronary Disease,"[18] reviewed the extensive literature of the last two decades on the dietary influences on cardiovascular disease. They looked at dietary fats, carbohydrates, micronutrients, and phytonutrients. Their conclusions were summarized in three practical strategies:

1. substitute non-hydrogenated unsaturated fats for saturated and trans-fats,
2. increase the consumption of omega-3 fatty acids from fish, fish oil supplements, or plant sources, and
3. consume a diet high in fruit, vegetables, nuts, whole grains, and low in refined grain products.

Further, they predicted that such a diet, together with regular physical activity, avoidance of smoking, and maintenance of a healthy body weight can prevent the majority of cardiovascular diseases in Western populations.

While these conclusions are relatively simple, the science behind them is complex. Both observational and interventional studies confirm links between diet and insulin resistance. Primary genetic lipid disorders are rare and the majority of cardiovascular disease in our society is linked to metabolic syndrome, which is propagated by a diet high in refined sugar, carbohydrates, saturated and trans-fats, and low in fiber and phytonutrients. This leads to insulin resistance at the membrane level, hyperinsulinemia, impairment of fatty acid oxidation, upregulation of inflammatory cytokines such as interleukin 6 (IL-6) and tumor necrosis factor-α (TNF-α), coagulopathy, reduction in adiponectin, and endocrine dysfunction in adrenal, thyroid, and sex steroid hormones. In a prospective study of 181 consecutive patients presenting to the emergency room with myocardial infarction, two-thirds had either undiagnosed diabetes or impaired glucose tolerance after a 2-hour glucose tolerance test.[19] In a cross-sectional study of 234 men, a direct correlation was seen between the glycemic milieu and cardiovascular risk, even in those with normal glucose tolerance. Likewise, even within the current definition of normal glucose tolerance, the degree of stenosis on the angiogram was shown to be directly related to the level of glucose and insulin after a glucose load.[20] A high glycemic-index and glycemic-load diet is clearly associated with atherothrombotic risk.[21,22] Trans-fatty acids have well-documented, specific atherogenic, inflammatory, and pro-thrombotic effects.[23,24] Though diet is the predominant influence on the key processes of glucose metabolism, lipid balance, inflammation, methylation, and oxidative stress, any trigger that affects these functions can lead to cardiovascular disease (see Figure 26.1). Examples of other important influences include infections, environmental toxins, stress, smoking, and allergens.

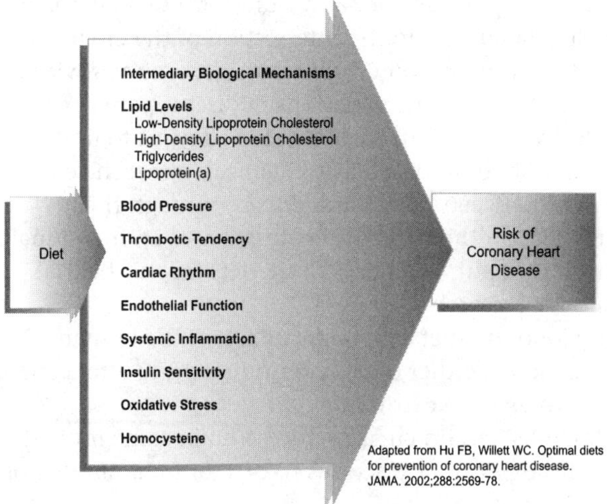

Figure 26.1 **Influence of diet on risk of coronary heart disease**

Diet is both the agent of dysfunction and the agent of healing in cardiovascular disease. With the exception of smoking and lack of exercise, nearly all the modifiable risk factors for coronary heart disease in the INTERHEART[25] study of 52 countries (a case-control study with 15,152 cases and 14,820 controls) were caused by and remediable through diet, including abnormal lipids, hypertension, diabetes, and abdominal obesity. Many clinical trials have demonstrated the benefits of diet in improving either clear endpoints such as myocardial infarction and death, or intermediate endpoints such as lipid levels, inflammatory markers, oxidative stress, and glucose metabolism.

Eating the right fats is key to prevention and treatment of coronary artery disease. Dietary n-6 and n-3 fatty acid balance plays a critical role in cardiovascular health.[26] Linoleic acid downregulates LDL-C production and enhances its clearance. Eicosapentaenoic acid (EPA) and docosahexaenoic acid (DHA) improve vascular endothelial function, lower blood pressure and triglycerides, improve insulin sensitivity, activate PPAR receptors, stabilize cardiac membranes (thus reducing cardiac arrhythmias),[27] and reduce inflammation and platelet sensitivity. A Mediterranean-style, low glycemic-load diet[28] (whole grains, fruits, vegetables, nuts, higher fiber foods, olive oil, and a lower ratio of n-6 to n-3 fatty acids) improved endothelial function and vascular inflammatory markers in patients with metabolic syndrome. After two years' adherence to the diet, there was global improvement in the endothelial function score, as a measure of blood pressure and platelet aggregation response to L-arginine; lipid and glucose parameters; insulin sensitivity; and circulating levels of high-sensitivity C-reactive protein (hs-CRP) and interleukins 6 (IL-6), 7 (IL-7), and 18 (IL-18). A lipid-lowering dietary portfolio of soy, almonds, plant sterols, and viscous fiber was equivalent to a low-fat diet plus a statin (lovastatin) in lowering lipids, and was *more* effective in lowering C-reactive protein and homocysteine.[29] A dietary and lifestyle intervention in women with android obesity demonstrated reductions in markers of inflammation, oxidative stress, and platelet aggregation, which can be indicators of insulin resistance.[30]

The DASH and PREMIER[31] trials clearly established the beneficial effects of a plant-based diet on reduction in cardiac risk factors. Consumption of a diet high in fruits and vegetables, whole grains, fish, poultry, and low-fat dairy products had a significant inverse association with the risk of cardiovascular disease.[32] Conversely, eating a diet high in red and processed meats, refined grains, high-fat dairy products, sweets, and desserts had a significant positive association with coronary artery disease (CAD).[33] Ornish's 10% fat atherosclerosis-reversal diet may have been effective more for its plant based, fiber, vitamin, mineral and phytonutrient-rich food, than because of any absolute effect from reduction of fat. The total fat content of the diet is less important than the type of fat; risks increase with higher levels of saturated and trans-fats, and decrease with high levels of omega-3 and monounsaturated fats.[34] Increasing dietary protein from plant foods (soy, nuts, legumes, and seeds) and low-fat animal sources may have additional beneficial effects on the reduction of cardiovascular risk.[35] Homocysteine and impaired methylation have been linked to cardiovascular disease,[36] and plant-based diets rich in whole grains, fruits, and vegetables reduce homocysteine and its adverse effects. Not only does the composition of the diet affect cardiac risk factors, the timing and frequency of meals is also important.[37] The specific ideal amounts or ratios of protein, fat and carbohydrate are not entirely clear, nor are they crucial to health, so long as the basic concepts of a healthful diet outlined above are maintained. The effects of this diet are multiple and support the normalization of function and restoration of balance. This dietary pattern improves insulin sensitivity, reduces inflammation and oxidative stress, lowers homocysteine, LDL-C and triglycerides, raises HDL-C, improves endothelial function, lowers blood pressure, is anti-coagulant, anti-arrhythmic, and improves mitochondrial function and cardiocyte energetics. Cardiovascular disease is perhaps the clearest example where diet is both the cause and the cure. It reminds us of Hippocrates' ancient admonition, *"Leave your potions in the chemist's crucible if you can heal your patient with food."*

Practical Dietary Guidelines for the Reduction of Cardiovascular Disease

- Replace saturated and trans-fats with mono-unsaturated and polyunsaturated fats.
- Increase intake of omega-3 fatty acids from fish or plant sources.
- Increase intake of fruits, vegetables, whole grains, legumes, nuts and seeds.
- Increase intake of fiber.
- Reduce glycemic load of diet by reducing or eliminating refined sugars and flours.
- Eat regular meals and snacks.
- Eat real, unprocessed food low in added sodium.
- Use low-fat animal products in moderation (low-fat dairy and poultry).

The Role of Diet-Gene Interactions in Health and Disease

Nutrigenomics

Having established the incontrovertible link between diet and disease, using CVD as the example, let's return to the link between diet and genetic expression in general. The genomic era in medicine will mark a turning point in our understanding of the etiology and treatment of disease. The human genome consists of approximately 30,000 genes, which in turn contain approximately 5 million single-nucleotide polymorphisms (SNPs). Over 1,000 human disease genes have been identified, 97% of which cause monogenic diseases. Unfortunately, the illnesses that plague humans in the 21st century are not monogenic diseases. The chronic illnesses that cause the most significant mortality and morbidity in the world, including cardiovascular disease, diabetes, obesity, cancer, and neurodegenerative diseases, are polygenic and result from the complex interaction between multiple genes and multiple environmental factors. The most important factor, one that influences gene expression multiple times every day, is our diet.

Nutrigenomics is an integrative field of science where the questions of nature and nurture may finally be elucidated. It is in the intersection of the environment with the genome where nutrigenomics provides key insights into the variations in disease patterns within a population. Such insights allow us to understand how common dietary chemicals affect the equilibrium between health and disease through their influence on the structure or function of an individual genome. Kaput[38] proposes five tenets for this field of genomic research:

1. Common dietary chemicals act on the human genome, either directly or indirectly, to alter gene expression or structure.
2. Under certain circumstances and in some individuals, diet can be a serious risk factor for a number of diseases.
3. Some diet-regulated genes (and their normal, common variants) are likely to play a role in the onset, incidence, progression, and/or severity of chronic diseases.
4. The degree to which diet influences the balance between healthy and disease states may depend on an individual's genetic makeup.
5. Dietary intervention should be based on knowledge of nutritional requirement, nutritional status, and genotype.

Regulation of Post-translational Gene Expression

Multiple mechanisms exist through which diet influences gene function, or expression, and structure. These include direct effects on gene expression, transcription, translation, post-translational influence on gene products, epigenetic effects, and DNA repair. Indirect effects include selective alteration of gene expression through transcription factor systems that regulate the activation of sets of genes under different environmental conditions. Some nutrients can bind to or activate specific transcription factors, while other nutrients affect redox balance to indirectly affect transcription factor activity.

Key examples can illustrate the clinical utility of understanding these SNPs and the role of nutrients in gene expression. Vitamins act as powerful regulators of post-translational gene expression through their actions as coenzymes in many common diseases (for example, the effects of folate on methylenetetrahydrofolate reductase or MTHFR). Dietary fat and carbohydrate can regulate expression of the LDL phenotype (effects of *trans* fatty acids and insulin resistance on LDL particle size). Dietary fat and antioxidants regulate inflammation through their effect on a class of nuclear receptors involved in gene transcription (for example, the effects of omega-3 fatty acids, trans-fats, and antioxidants on the family of nuclear receptors called peroxisome proliferation activation receptors, or PPARs).

Bruce Ames, in a landmark paper on nutrients and gene expression stated that, "the molecular basis of disease arising from as many as one-third of the mutations in a gene is an **increased** Michaelis constant, or K_m (decreased binding affinity) of an enzyme for the vitamin-derived coenzyme or substrate, which in turn lowers the rate of the reaction."[39] The implication is that many diseases arising from SNPs may be treated through the intake of high doses of substrates (nutrients) for particular reactions by accommodating for variant enzymes. He describes over 50 diseases where high-dose vitamin therapy can reduce the incidence of disease from variant enzymes. (This chapter concludes with a contribution from Dr. Ames discussing the potential genotoxicity of micronutrient insufficiency.)

An abundance of research surrounds the methylenetetrahydrofolate 677C→T (MTHFR) polymorphism. The variant enzyme results in a smaller pool of 5-methyltetrahydrofolate and an accumulation of homocysteine, which has been associated with an elevated risk of cardiovascular disease. A higher frequency of the 677C→T polymorphism has been associated with cardiovascular disease, neural tube defects, Down syndrome, migraines, diabetic nephropathy, congenital cardiac malformations, dementia, male infertility, cervical dysplasia[40] and other conditions. Paradoxically, in colon cancer, the 677C→T (MTHFR) polymorphism reduces colon cancer risk, but only in the presence of adequate folate.[41]

Another common polymorphism, ALDH2 or mitochondrial aldehyde dehydrogenase (NAD^+) has been associated with intolerance to alcohol and an increased risk of vasospastic angina, dementia, oral, and esophageal and stomach cancer.[42] The enzyme catalyzes the NAD-dependent oxidation of ethanol. The Glu487-to-lysine variant has a 150-fold increase in the K_m for its NAD cofactor. This leads to high blood acetaldehyde levels in alcohol consumption and in the absence of adequate niacin, and increases the risk for carcinogenesis and neurotoxicity. Multiple genes may interact to increase risk. In the presence of the ALDH2 variant and the Apo E 4 variant allele, the age of Alzheimer's onset is significantly reduced. Long-term niacin use may have the potential to reduce this risk. This underscores the importance of multiple polymorphisms of low-penetrance combining in any one individual to affect risk. It is the interplay with the environment (diet, exercise, stress, environmental toxins) that affects the outcome in the individual. Most polymorphisms have a relative risk for the related disease of < 2. Therefore, an integrated approach using nutrition, exercise,[43] and stress management tools is more likely to optimize gene expression and reduce the risk of chronic disease.

A major challenge in nutrigenomics-focused research on human disease prevention is that randomized trials are often not easy or feasible due to practical or ethical considerations. Combining gene analysis of polymorphisms with observational studies can help strengthen causal connections between dietary factors and disease prevention.[44] For example, higher urinary levels of isothiocyanates from cruciferous vegetables have been associated with lower risks of lung cancer. The strongest risk reduction was found in those with polymorphisms for glutathione S-transferase genes that delayed the elimination of the isothiocyanates, perhaps increasing their benefit.[45]

Diet and the Fundamental Physiological Processes: Enhancing Optimal Function and Reducing Disease

Human life, particularly, in health and disease, is the result of countless independent forces impinging simultaneously on the total organism and setting in motion a multitude of inter-related responses.

—René Dubos

An exhaustive review of the dietary influences on human biology would require a separate volume entirely, but much of the background and scientific support for this approach to patient care has been outlined earlier in this textbook. We will now examine some specific instances where food creates imbalance and where a change in diet can promote healing. The fundamental role of food in health and disease can be appreciated, and a context for its application in diagnosis and therapy can be understood through the exploration of examples within each of the core physiologic dysfunctions of the functional medicine matrix. Each subsequent section will end with clinical suggestions for assessment and therapy. These recommendations are not exhaustive, but rather demonstrative of an approach to translating the science into clinical practice.

A common theme will appear—that very similar interventions will address the causes and become the treatment for most of the chronic diseases of the 21st century. Modifications, adjustments, inclusions, and exclusions will always be required, depending on the genetics, history, and stage of dysfunction of your patient, but the basic principles of a diet that supports health will be the same: an organic whole-foods diet, rich in a variety of fruits and vegetables, fiber, whole grains, legumes, nuts and seeds, lean animal protein, and monounsaturated and omega-3 fatty acids; and low in processed foods, sugar, high fructose corn syrup, *trans* fatty acids, caffeine, and alcohol. (Clinicians cannot ignore the need for exercise and stress management, of course, but those are covered elsewhere in the book.) Even when delineation of "ideal" percentages of macronutrients or micronutrient doses for an individual patient is not possible, following the guiding principles of providing the basic nutritional substrates for optimal function will yield remarkable clinical results. Controversies do exist about the specific components of a healthy diet (for example, whether soy is helpful or harmful, or whether all saturated fats are harmful). However, the science of nutrition and nutrigenomics provides a firm foundation upon which to create improved clinical outcomes in chronic disease.

Functional Medicine and Nutrition: A Natural Partnership

The principles, processes, and imbalances of functional medicine are best understood as a didactic tool that helps clinicians better explain the mystery of biology and human function using a lens that is more refined and developed, but nonetheless only an approximation of reality. The web-like physiology and biochemistry of the human being is complex and densely interconnected. Any input, harmful or helpful, enters the system and creates a multitude of interrelated responses. A single input, such as gluten, in a susceptible individual can trigger damage to the intestinal mucosa, impairing nutrient absorption and creating B12, mineral, and vitamin D deficiencies, in addition to upregulating the gut-associated lymphoid tissue (GALT) and activating a systemic immune response that can, in turn, lead to oxidative stress and imbalances in thyroid and sex hormones. Inflammation may in turn affect nuclear PPAR receptors through TNF-α, increasing insulin resistance, impairing fatty acid oxidation, and leading to changes in body composition. What an extraordinary outcome from the ingestion of a single component of some very common foods!

This is only one example of what occurs repeatedly in living systems, where there is an infinite array of macroscopic and microscopic, physical and meta-physical inputs, both beneficial and harmful. Humility in the face of the vast mystery of human life and function must be our guide.

We cannot fully master the practice of medicine and healing, but we can be guided by three simple principles that make the challenge less daunting:

1. One input (environmental or genetic) may cause many diseases, and one disease may be caused by many inputs.
2. Always consider the two key questions of functional medicine: What harms this patient? What makes this patient thrive?
3. The science behind functional medicine can be difficult to understand, but it can also be relatively simple to practice.

The functional medicine matrix provides a way to sift and sort data obtained from the medical literature, the patient history, and the biochemical and physiologic assessments of laboratory work and physical examination. It is a framework that helps to organize our thinking and our approach to patients. It is a fundamentally new and refreshing way of providing innovative and effective solutions for what ails our patients in the 21st century.

The Matrix: Dietary Influences on Hormonal Balance

The influence of diet on hormone balance is vast and includes the differential effects of specific types of carbohydrates and fats, amino acids, fiber and gut flora, as well as micronutrient effects on hormone synthesis, receptor function, metabolism, and detoxification. Anti-nutrients—harmful foods and non-nutritive substances in our food supply, including xenobiotics, exogenous hormones, and antibiotics—have powerful effects on hormone function. The most striking and useful clinical examples of dietary influences on hormonal balance will be reviewed, including effects on the master hormones (insulin, cortisol, and adrenlin), on thyroid function, and on sex hormone balance. We will also review the ways in which diet can create imbalance or restore optimal function. Specific diagnostic and therapeutic strategies will be presented.

The master hormones. Hormonal signals act both as a symphony of endocrine signals governing diverse functions throughout the organism, and as a hierarchical system where dysfunction in the "governing" hormones leads to dysfunction throughout the system. The key governing hormones regulated by dietary inputs, which interact in an immediate and direct feedback system, are insulin, cortisol, and adrenalin. These, in turn, influence sex steroid hormones, thyroid hormones, growth hormone, and others. (See Sidebar for common symptoms of HPA axis dysfunction.)

Perhaps the most visible intersection of diet and hormones is the influence of diet on glucose metabolism in the metabolic syndrome. To review briefly what has been thoroughly discussed elsewhere in this book, in the context of genetic predisposition or in the face of overwhelming exposure to refined carbohydrates (180 pounds of sugar consumed per person per year in the United States), a chronic state of hyperinsulinemia, hypercortisolemia, and hyperadrenalism is induced, with its cascade of adverse biologic effects. A high glycemic-load diet increases central adiposity, elevates triglycerides and LDL-C, and reduces HDL-C. It also upregulates inflammatory cytokines such as IL-6 and TNF-α, increases advanced glycation end products, oxidative stress, and elevates PAI-1 and fibrinogen. Other problems include non-alcoholic steatohepatitis and impaired detoxification; PCOS in various presentations (including anovulation, infertility and hirsutism); endothelial dysfunction leading to cardiovascular disease; dementia and cancer (including hormonal cancers); and other chronic morbidities resulting from obesity. Dietary factors[46] other than high glycemic load carbohydrates that contribute to the epidemic of metabolic syndrome include lack of dietary fiber, essential fatty acid deficiency, caffeine, excess saturated and trans-fatty acids, protein insufficiency,[47] micronutrient deficiencies (vitamin E, biotin, the B vitamins, zinc, bioflavonoids, alpha lipoic acid, arginine, carnitine, and inositol), and deficiency of antioxidants.[48] High glycemic-load diets not only increase insulin resistance but shift the hypothalamic-pituitary-adrenal (HPA) axis toward sympathetic overactivity, with increases in cortisol, ACTH, and norepinephrine, and decreased heart rate variability.[49,50] Table 26.2 provides some therapeutic strategies for managing insulin resistance, and Table 26.3 provides a list of laboratory tests for assessing indicators of the condition.

Symptoms of Adrenal and HPA Axis Dysfunction

- Cravings for salt and/or sweets
- Dark circles under the eyes
- Dizziness upon standing
- Fatigue
- Feeling stressed
- Feeling tired but wired
- Feeling weak and shaky
- Frequent infections (catching cold easily)
- Headaches
- Heart palpitations
- Hypoglycemia
- Impaired ability to tolerate exercise
- Low blood pressure
- Mental fogginess or trouble concentrating
- Need to start the day with caffeine
- Non-restorative sleep
- Panic attacks or being easily startled
- Poor tolerance for alcohol, caffeine, and other drugs
- Sleep problems—difficulty either falling asleep or staying asleep
- Sweaty palms and feet when nervous
- Water retention
- Weak muscles

Table 26.2 **Therapeutic Strategies: Insulin Resistance**

Dietary Recommendations: To Minimize the Causes of IR	Dietary Recommendations: To Improve Insulin Sensitivity	Nutrient Supplementation	Lifestyle Changes
Eliminate refined flours and sugars	Increase fiber to 50 g/day	Increase levels of magnesium, chromium, vanadium, vitamin E, biotin, B complex	Engage in regular stress management practices such as yoga, deep breathing, meditation, guided imagery, etc.
Eliminate sodas and sweetened drinks	Use predominantly soluble fiber**	Take a high-potency multivitamin and mineral daily	Engage in regular exercise: cardiovascular exercise for 30–45 minutes, 5–6 days/week; and strength training 10–30 minutes, 3 days/week.
Eliminate artificial sweeteners*	Reduce the glycemic load of meals	Alpha lipoic acid, 200 mg, twice a day	
Eliminate junk food and processed foods	Eat beans or legumes daily	Supplement EFAs: EPA, DHA (fish oil), ALA (flax seeds or oil), GLA (borage or evening primrose oil)	Eat smaller, more frequent meals (3 meals and 2–3 snacks).
Eliminate trans or hydrogenated fats	Have protein and fat with every meal or snack	Ginseng may help regulate insulin, blood sugar, and adrenal function	Eat no later than 2–3 hours before bedtime.
Limit alcohol to 3 drinks per week	Have lean protein for breakfast	Arginine may improve insulin resistance	
Limit caffeine	Eat omega-3 fats daily Have 2 tbsp ground flax seeds daily Reduce saturated fat from animal foods (meat, poultry, dairy)	Other herbal or nutritional supplements may be helpful: green tea, fenugreek, cinnamon, gymnena sylvestre, bitter melon, and garlic	

*Artificial sweeteners can trigger insulin response from brain signals and can fuel cravings for sweets.

**Soluble fiber slows sugar absorption from the gut, and is found in legumes, nuts, seeds, whole grains, vegetables, and fruit.

Other secondary hormones and neuropeptides[51] are influenced by dietary macronutrient quality and balance, stress, and physical activity, all of which also influence appetite and energy balance. There exists an intricate and dynamic cross talk between the gut endocrine system (ghrelin, peptide YY, cholecystokinin (CCK), proglucagon products), the adipocytokines, adipo-hormones (leptin, adiponectin, resistin), and the hypothalamic neuropeptides (neuropeptide Y (NPY), α melanocyte stimulating hormone (αMSH), agouti-related protein (AgRP), cocaine and amphetamine-regulated transcript (CART), orexin). In summary, these cell-signaling molecules act either directly or indirectly to inhibit or stimulate food intake, and in turn are influenced by meal composition, food quantity, and timing.

Influences on hormonal signaling from food go beyond their caloric aspects. A low glycemic-load diet over two years with a 10% weight loss caused less reduction in resting energy expenditure or metabolic rate than a low-fat diet with an identical 10% weight loss, as well as greater reductions in insulin resistance, serum triglycerides, C-reactive protein, blood pressure, and self-reported hunger. This demonstrates that changes in dietary composition can affect the physiologic adaptations that defend body weight.[52] Regular meal frequency (5–6 small meals a day) results in lower total energy intake, greater post-prandial thermogenesis, lower fasting total and LDL cholesterol, and post-prandial insulin profiles.[53]

Table 26.3 **Laboratory Testing for Insulin Resistance Indicators**

Test to be Performed	Results to be Concerned About
75 gram glucose tolerance test with insulin levels	FBS > 90; fasting insulin > 8; 2 hour BS > 140; 2 hour insulin > 40
Ferritin	> 200
Fibrinogen	> 350
High sensitivity-C-reactive protein	> 1.0
Homocysteine	> 8.0
Liver function tests	Elevated AST, ALT, GGT
Low serum magnesium	< 2.0
NMR lipid profile (assessment of lipid particle size)	Small LDL and HDL particles and large VLDL particles
Total cholesterol, HDL-C, LDL-C, triglycerides	HDL levels < 50 for men, < 60 for women; triglycerides > 100; triglyceride/HDL ratio > 5
Uric acid	> 7.0

The sex hormones. Sex hormones are influenced by diet in many ways. One prime example is estrogen, and conditions related to estrogen/progesterone imbalance, including hormonal cancers, endometriosis, premenstrual syndrome, uterine fibroid tumors, fibrocystic breasts, cervical dysplasia, and infertility. Improving hormonal balance can be accomplished by nutritional and lifestyle interventions such as increasing fiber, reducing fat, increasing intake of phytoestrogens, weight loss, and exercise. Certain nutrients and phytonutrients may enhance specific pathways of estrogen metabolism and detoxification (e.g., isoflavones, essential fatty acids, indole-3-carbinol, B vitamins, magnesium, limonene, and antioxidants). While diet can lead to suppression of hormones in diseases like anorexia nervosa, the focus here will be on modulation of excess endogenous and exogenous estrogens through diet. Table 26.4 provides a summary of symptoms, risk factors, and therapeutic strategies for hormonal imbalance in women.

Symptoms and Signs of Insulin Resistance

- Sugar cravings
- Hypoglycemia (night sweats, irritability, palpitations, dizziness, fatigue relieved by eating)
- Post-prandial fatigue after carbohydrate meals
- Chronic fungal infections
- Fatigue
- Central obesity (waist to hip ratio > 0.8 in women and 0.9 in men)
- Polycystic ovary syndrome or infertility
- Hypertension
- Family history of diabetes, hypoglycemia, or alcoholism

These interventions affect many of the underlying physiological causes for hormonal imbalance, primarily the following:

- Diet can modulate estrogen synthesis, receptor activity, and detoxification and metabolism of estrogens. Briefly, estrogen is detoxified and metabolized predominantly through phase I (hydroxylation) and phase II (methylation and glucuronidation). Hydroxylation produces either 2-hydroxyestrone (2-OH), 4-OH or 16α-OH. 2-OH is a weak estrogen and may have anti-cancer properties. 16α-OH and 4-OH metabolites have estrogenic and carcinogenic properties. Methylation renders the metabolites more inert, and glucuronidation is the major excretory pathway. All these detoxification pathways are influenced by diet. [A comprehensive review of women's hormones can be found in Chapter 19 (Part I) and Chapter 32 (Part II).]
- Dietary causes of hormonal imbalance include excess energy intake and obesity, leading to increased conversion of androgens to estrogen by aromatase.
- Hyperinsulinemia increases ovarian testosterone production and reduces sex hormone binding globulin (SHBG), increasing free estrogen levels.

Table 26.4 **Hormone Imbalance in Women: Symptoms, Risk Factors, and Therapeutic Strategies**

Common Symptoms	Risk Factors	Therapeutic Strategies: Dietary Recommendations	Therapeutic Strategies: Nutrient Supplementation	Therapeutic Strategies: Lifestyle Changes
Premenstrual Syndrome: • Backache, joint or muscle pain • Depression • Edema, swelling, puffiness, or water retention • Feeling bloated • Feeling unable to cope with ordinary demands • Headaches • Monthly weight fluctuation • Mood swings • Premenstrual food cravings (sugar or salt) • Tender, enlarged breasts • Irregular cycles, heavy bleeding, light bleeding • Infertility • Premenstrual migraines • Breast cysts or lumps or fibrocystic breasts • Uterine fibroids **Perimenopause or Menopause:** • Bloating or weight gain around the middle, facial hair • Dry skin, hair and vagina • Hot flashes • Insomnia • Joint pains • Loss of libido or sex drive • Mood swings or depression or anxiety • Night sweats • Palpitations • Trouble with memory or concentration	• Use of birth control pill or other hormones • Family history of breast, ovarian or uterine cancer • Exposure to pesticides (food, water, air) • Obesity	**Eliminate or reduce:** • Alcohol consumption at no more than 3 glasses a week • Artificial sweeteners • Minimize dairy products • Processed foods • Refined sugars and carbohydrates • Saturated/*trans* fats • Xenobiotics, antibiotics and hormones in food **Increase or emphasize:** • 1–2 cups/day of cruciferous vegetables (broccoli, collards, kale, etc.) • Fiber, up to 25–50 g/day; include legumes, whole grains, vegetables, nuts, seed, fruits) • Filtered water (reverse osmosis) to eliminate xenoestrogens • Garlic for sulfur and to help with detoxification • Intake of omega-3 fatty acids (wild salmon, sardines, herring, flax seeds) • Organic foods to minimize intake of xenoestrogens, hormone and antibiotics • Phytoestrogen consumption (soy, flax) ***Follow guidelines for balancing glucose metabolism (Table 26.2).**	• Antioxidants and phytonutrients (vitamin E, resveratrol, curcumin, NAC, green tea, selenium, etc.) • Calcium, magnesium and vitamin D • Indole-3-carbinol • Methylation cofactors (folate, B6, B12) • Multivitamin and mineral • Omega-3 fatty acids • Probiotics	• Regular exercise • Stress management • Weight reduction

- High-fat diets promote C-16α hydroxylation over C-2 hydroxylation.
- Antioxidant-deficient diets may promote the oxidation of catechol estrogens (2-OH and 4-OH) yielding toxic reactive molecules called quinones.
- Alcohol interferes with estrogen detoxification, increasing estradiol levels and the risk of breast cancer.[54]
- Environmental toxins are a significant source of exogenous estrogen exposure (xenoestrogens), many of which find their way into our food supply through pesticides and herbicides. Hormones used in commercial livestock and milk production also increase exposure to environmental estrogens.[55] Even antibiotics found in the food supply may be associated with increased breast cancer risk by altering gut flora involved in enterohepatic circulation of estrogens.[56]

Fortunately, diet can also promote normalization of estrogen metabolism through diverse mechanisms:

- Dietary fiber and lignins (found in flax seeds, the bran layer of grains, beans, and seeds) reduce the enterohepatic circulation of estrogen by binding unconjugated estrogens and enhancing fecal excretion. They also increase serum levels of SHBG and improve the balance of intestinal flora, reducing intestinal β glucuronidase and deconjugation of estrogens.
- Reducing glycemic load can diminish adverse effects on sex hormones.
- Essential fatty acids (EPA) increase C-2 hydroxylation and decrease C-16α hydroxylation in breast cancer cells.
- Probiotics found in food (yogurt and fermented products) and in supplements may help normalize estrogen metabolism by reducing β glucuronidase, producing bacteria, and promoting the formation of anti-carcinogenic enterolactones from lignins.
- Indole-3-carbinol, a compound found in cruciferous vegetables such as broccoli, Brussels sprouts and cabbage, increases the protective 2-OH estrogens. Clinically, it may help in the prevention and treatment of estrogen-related cancers and has been shown to reverse cervical dysplasia.
- Phytonutrients, often mislabelled phytohormones, modulate hormonal response through multiple mechanisms, including competitive inhibition at the receptor sites, increasing plasma SHBG levels, decreasing aromatase activity, and shifting estrogen metabolism from the C-16α to the C-2 pathway. The main dietary sources are isoflavones from soy,[i] kudzu root, legumes, and clover, and lignans from flaxseeds, other seed oils, whole grains, legumes and vegetables.
- Other beneficial phytonutrients include curcumin, which can increase hepatic glutathione, and glutathione-S-transferase, hence facilitating the detoxification of quinones from the oxidation of catechol estrogens. Antioxidants in food and supplements may also help reduce the oxidation of catechol estrogens into quinones.
- Multiple plant compounds may inhibit or modulate NFκB: soy isoflavones have been shown to have anti-tumor and health-promoting effects[57] that may be a function of their effects on NFκB. NFκB is a critical gene transcription factor, the activation of which induces the expression of IL-6. Interleukin 6 (IL-6) is an inflammatory cytokine controlled in part by hormonal feedback mechanisms. Excess IL-6 production stimulates tumorigenesis (breast, prostate, colon, lung, and ovary) and accelerates aging in general.

Other dietary factors promote hormonal balance, including methylation cofactors, folate, pyridoxine, and cobalamin. Elevated intracellular levels of B6 decrease gene transcription responses when estrogen binds to the estrogen receptor. Methylation cofactors are also critical in DNA synthesis, repair, and methylation.

Testing hormonal function is a complicated subject, and is discussed in depth by Dr. Bethany Hays in her contributions to this book (Chapters 19 and 32). In terms of basic assessment approaches, the following are useful laboratory tests:

- 24-hour urine for estrogen metabolism
- 2:16α OH estrogen ratios
- FSH, LH, estradiol, progesterone, free testosterone, SHBG
- Homocysteine

---

[i] Basic science and clinical data on soy are varied, yet both epidemiological and experimental data in animals and humans, with historically consumed levels of isoflavones, demonstrate protective effects through modification of estrogen receptor activity, increases in SHBG, and lower rates of hormone-dependent cancers. Soy isoflavones may help to restore balance by integrating hormonal ligand activities and by interfering with signaling cascades.

- TSH, free T_4, free T_3, thyroid peroxidase antibodies
- SNPs involved in hormone metabolism and detoxification, such as MTHFR, CYP 1B1, COMT, and GSTM1

The Matrix: Dietary Influences on Oxidative Stress, Mitochondrial Function, and Energy Metabolism

Oxidative stress, with its resultant mitochondrial injury, is a vital common pathway in the pathophysiology of disease. Thousands of peer-reviewed papers delineate the role of oxidative stress in nearly every disease, acute and chronic. Exhaustive epidemiologic evidence suggests that dietary antioxidants are protective against most of the age-related diseases, including cardiovascular diseases, neurodegenerative diseases, cancers, and inflammatory disorders. Interventional studies of antioxidants in the prevention of disease are mixed,[58] often because of design flaws and confounding factors. Regardless of the current controversies surrounding antioxidant supplementation, recognizing clinical and laboratory manifestations of oxidative stress and mitochondrial dysfunction is essential. Specific dietary and nutraceutical interventions can reduce oxidative stress and enhance mitochondrial function and bioenergetics (see Tables 26.5, 26.6 and 26.7 for detailed information on common symptoms, associated conditions, dietary, nutritional supplementation, and lifestyle/environment recommendations).

Oxidation and reduction (redox) are basic biochemical reactions that exist throughout nature. In humans, this process is controlled through the exogenous and endogenous exposure or production of oxidants and antioxidants. Redox balance is intimately involved in the control of cell signaling and gene transcription, apoptosis, and aging in each cell and for the total organism. Dietary, environmental, and even psychological factors influence redox status. The biology of aging (and hence all age-related degenerative disease) is intimately connected to uncontrolled oxidation, mitochondrial injury, DNA mutations, and cell death. Oxidants cause damage to biomolecules, including DNA, organelles, cell membranes, lipids, and proteins.

Table 26.5 **Oxidative Stress and Mitochondrial Dysfunction: Symptoms, Associated Conditions, and Contributing Factors**

Common Symptoms of Oxidative Stress	Common Conditions Associated with Oxidative Stress	Consequences of Free Radical Attack	Dietary Sources of Oxidative Stress and Mitochondrial Injury
• Allergies • Anxiety • Depression • Digestive problems • Dizziness • Fatigue • Headaches • Hypoglycemia • Irritability • Lowered resistance to infection • Muscle and joint pains • Muscle weakness • Poor mental function and cognition	• ALS • Alzheimer's disease • Asthma • Cancer • Cardiovascular disease • Chronic Fatigue Syndrome • Diabetes • Fibromyalgia • Iron overload (or hemochromatosis) • Multiple chemical sensitivity • Multiple sclerosis • Occupational exposures • Osteoarthritis • Parkinson's disease • Rheumatoid arthritis	• Breaking apart and clumping together of proteins • Breaking off proteins from cell membranes, destroying the integrity of the cell • Changes in immune function • Damage and disruption of organelles and the nuclear membrane • Damage to DNA and mutations • Fusion of proteins and fats in cell membranes causing damage to cell communication • Inactivation of enzymes • Increased permeability of cell membrane	• Charbroiled foods and polycyclic aromatic hydrocarbons • Excess sugar/glucose • Excess alcohol that can lead to an increase in cytokines • Exposure to petrochemicals and heavy metals in the diet • Overeating; excess caloric intake • Processed and nutrient-poor foods in the diet • Rancid fats from the diet • Under-nutrition and nutritional deficiencies

Table 26.6 **Oxidative Stress: Therapeutic and Protective Strategies**

Lifestyle and Environment Changes	Nutritional Supplementation	Botanical Antioxidants
• Minimize environmental toxin exposures • Minimize ionizing radiation (ultraviolet, x-rays, radon) • Reduce exposure to tobacco smoke (first or second hand) • Reduce air pollutants with HEPA or ULPA filters (carbon monoxide and nitrogen dioxide) • Avoid excessive or insufficient exercise • Improve inadequate sleep/wake rhythms/cycles • Treat chronic infections • Reduce internal sources of oxidative stress, i.e., gut ecology imbalances • Improve liver and gut detoxification • Reduce exposure to fungal toxins from environmental and internal molds and fungi • Reduce stress; cortisol and stress both increase inflammation • Deep breathing to increase oxygenation of tissues and cells	• Mixed carotenoids including beta and alpha carotene, lutein, lycopene and zeaxanthin • Mixed tocopherols 400 to 800 IU/day—including d-alpha, gamma and delta tocopherols • Proanthocyanidins 50–100 mg/day • Selenium 100–200 mcg/day • Vitamin A 5,000 to 10,000 IU/day • Vitamin B complex • Vitamin C 500–2000 mg/day • Vitamin D 400 IU to 1200 IU/day • Zinc 15–75 mg/day	**Botanical antioxidant pigments:** • Carotenoids (lycopene, beta, alpha and gamma carotene, lutein, astaxanthin, zeaxanthin, phytoene, phytofluene) in orange and yellow vegetables • Green tea polyphenols • Anthocyanidins (berries, beets, grapes) • Quercitin (fruit and vegetable rind) • Curcuminoids (turmeric) • Trans-resveratrol (phytoalexin from grapes) **Herbal antioxidants:** • Ashwagandha (*Withania somnifera*), ancient Ayurvedic adaptogen • Blueberry and bilberry (*Vaccinium myrtillus*) • Chocolate (*Theobroma cacao*) • Cranberry (*Vaccinium macrocarpon*) • Garlic (*Allium sativum*) • Ginger (*Zingiber officinales*) • Ginkgo (*Ginkgo biloba*) • Grape seed (*Vitus vinifera*) • Green tea (*Camellia sinensis*) • Hawthorne (*Crataegus oxyacantha*) • Horse chestnut (*Aesculus hippocastanum*) • Milk thistle (*Silybum marianum*) • Purple grape (*Vitis labrusca*) • Rosemary (*Rosmarinus officinalis*) • Spinach • Turmeric (*Curcuma longa*)

The single most important factor regulating the redox balance is diet. Reactive oxygen species (ROS) are generated in the mitochondria as a by-product of the conversion of calories and oxygen into the body's usable energy source—ATP or adenosine triphosphate. Our cells contain 100,000 trillion mitochondria. They consume 90% of our oxygen intake. Forty percent of each cardiocyte is filled by mitochondria. Fatigue is a central component of most diseases, a phenomenon directly related to oxidative stress and mitochondropathy. Endogenous antioxidant mechanisms such as SOD, catalases, and GSHPx are also dependent on essential dietary nutrients as cofactors (Zn, Cu, Mn, vitamin C and Se). Exogenous antioxidants (dietary antioxidants, polyphenols, phytonutrients, and conditionally essential nutrients) protect DNA, molecules, mitochondria, and cells from excess oxidative damage. Endogenous oxidant production is directly tied to caloric intake—hence, the reduction in age-promoting cell signaling and gene transcription found in caloric restriction.[59] (Caloric restriction is the only clearly established method to enhance longevity in animal models.)

Table 26.7 **Supplements to Enhance Mitochondrial Function**

Basic Mitochondrial Support	Enhanced Mitochondrial Support
• Amino acids: arginine, aspartic acid, cysteine • B complex vitamins • Biotin 1000–2000 mcg/day • Calcium 800–1200 mg/day • Magnesium 400–600 mg/day • Pantothenic acid 50–500 mg/day • Riboflavin 10–100 mg/day • Thiamine 10–100 mg/day • Zinc 20–50 mg/day	• Acetyl-L-Carnitine 500 to 4000 mg/day • Alpha lipoic acid 100 to 600 mg/day • Coenzyme Q10, 50 to 1200 mg/day • Creatine 2–4 g/day • N-acetylcysteine (or NAC) 500 to 2000 mg/day • NADH 5 to 20 mg/day • Reduced Glutathione 300 to 600 mg/day

A nutrient-poor, calorie-rich, high glycemic-load, antioxidant-deficient, refined diet (generally, the standard American diet, or SAD) increases ROS and all of their downstream biologic effects. Exogenous food additives, petrochemicals, heavy metals, and iron excess or deficiency also increase oxidative stress. Dietary factors (or any factors) that increase inflammation (trans and saturated fats, deficiencies of essential fatty acids, high glycemic load, lack of fiber, etc.) also increase oxidative stress through cell-signaling pathways involving NFκB and other key transcription factors.[60]

In susceptible individuals, dietary antigens (gluten, dairy, eggs, etc.) trigger imbalances in Th1 and Th2 cytokines, thus increasing oxidative stress. Cell membrane and mitochondrial membrane function, critical in cell signaling and signal transduction, are determined in part by the quality of membrane fatty acids. Fluid monounsaturated and polyunsaturated (omega-3) fatty acids support normal membrane function and help to balance the inflammatory prostaglandin cascade. ROS can also trigger cell signals that increase inflammation through regulation of gene transcription factors such as NFκB, and modulation of the PPAR family of nuclear receptors leading to a feed-forward cycle of inflammation, oxidative stress, mitochondrial injury, and accelerated disease processes and aging.

Dietary interventions to reduce oxidative stress and mitochondrial damage must take into consideration the way in which the redox system functions. By design, it is dependent on multiple antioxidants from the diet, endogenous antioxidants and their cofactors, as well as relatively higher levels of dietary phytonutrients such as polyphenols. Each antioxidant becomes oxidized in the process of reducing ROS. In turn, it is reduced down the chain, thereby preventing uncontrolled oxidative stress reactions. This occurs in every cell and tissue and is dependent on an adequate supply of the basic dietary antioxidants such as vitamin C, the tocopherols, carotenoids, and the proper substrates for synthesis and recycling of glutathione (glutamine, glycine, cysteine, selenium, and phytonutrients) and lipoic acid. Glutathione is the final common pathway for the reduction of oxidants, and also plays a critical role in detoxification. Glutathione is depleted and oxidative stress increased in most chronic disease.[61]

It must be remembered, however, that reduction *and* oxidation together are involved in cell signaling. Quenching all ROS is not the objective. Creating redox balance is central to the prevention and treatment of disease, however difficult to clinically assess or measure. Diagnosing oxidative stress and acquired mitochondrial dysfunction is both difficult and important as a target for therapy. (Table 26.8 contains a list of tests that can be used to detect problems in these areas.) Further, it is difficult to determine whether oxidative stress is the cause or consequence of age-related disease.[62] Indeed, it is both, and modulation of redox status through dietary macronutrients, micronutrients, and phytonutrients is an important clinical therapeutic tool.

Dietary strategies to balance redox status must begin by increasing intake of a variety of antioxidant-rich foods,[63] as well as foods that provide phytonutrients such as flavonoids and polyphenols (found in teas, red wine, cocoa).[64,65] The concept of a "metabolic tune-up" was introduced by Bruce Ames, PhD. This important strategy focuses on the use of supplements to optimize function by reducing DNA damage and mitochondrial oxidative decay, and improving the K_m of enzymes by providing higher doses of the corresponding micronutrient co-enzyme.[66] While evidence in large controlled human clinical trials is limited, the intelligent use of nutraceuticals in modulating redox status and optimizing function is safe and can be clinically effective.

Table 26.8 **Testing for Oxidative Stress and Mitochondrial Dysfunction**

Testing for Oxidative Stress	Testing for Mitochondrial Dysfunction
• 4-hydroxy-2(E)-nonenal (4-HNE) • Antioxidant enzyme assays of super oxide dismutase (SOD), glutathione peroxidase (GSHPx), and catalase • Assessment of iron overload: transferrin saturation, ferritin, serum iron and total iron binding capacity • Assessment of antioxidants (blood levels) can occasionally be helpful (e.g., vitamin A, vitamin E, CoQ10, and beta-carotene) • F2-isoprostanes • Lipid peroxides (TBARS) in urine or serum • Malondialdehyde (MDA) • Myeloperoxidase • Serum lactoferrin • Urinary 8 hydroxy-2-deoxyguanosine (8-OH-2DG) • Urinary hydroxyl markers, including catechol and 2,3-dihydroxybenzoate measured after an aspirin and acetaminophen challenge • Whole blood or intracellular glutathione and reduced glutathione	• Cardio metabolic stress testing: VO2max • Muscle biopsy (rarely) • Organic acids

The Matrix: Dietary Influences on Detoxification

Diet and detoxification intersect in two important ways. Diet is a source of many environmental and natural toxins. Diet also is the source of amino acids, fiber, nutrients, and phytonutrients critical for facilitating elimination of both metabolic and environmental toxins through phase 1 and phase 2 detoxification, as well as through gastrointestinal and renal excretion. Diet interacts with many phase 1 and phase 2 genes regulating detoxification and can be used as an aid in coping with the increased burden of environmental and dietary toxins. A number of degenerative and chronic diseases have been linked to toxic overload, or impaired detoxification; these include the neurodegenerative diseases, cancers, chronic fatigue, fibromyalgia, and endocrine, autoimmune, and inflammatory disorders. (Analysis of these topics and the evidence behind them can be found in Chapters 22 and 31.)

The major sources of food toxins include the petrochemical residues in our food and water from certain farming practices, mercury from industrial waste (often found in predatory fish), lead in our water supply, advanced glycation end-products from food preparation, polycyclic aromatic hydrocarbons from charbroiled meats, trans-fats, and naturally-occurring plant toxins such as aflatoxins. Minimizing the exposure to these toxin sources is important; however, the most important role for diet is providing the substrates and cofactors for optimal detoxification through cellular, hepatic, gastrointestinal, and renal mechanisms.

With the advent of four million synthetic compounds, heavy metals, and the metabolic/digestive waste from the planet's billions of people (not to mention the commercially raised livestock), our innate detoxification-coping capacities have been exceeded. All humans in the 21st century store chemical toxins, and about 25% store heavy metals in our tissues. Managing this toxic burden is metabolically expensive, and requires adequate nutrients and cofactors that support detoxification pathways. The major categories of toxins are chemical toxins, heavy metals, microbial compounds (from bacteria, yeast, or other organisms), and the breakdown products of normal protein metabolism. The heavy metals most implicated in disease are lead, mercury, cadmium, arsenic, nickel, and aluminum. The chemical toxins include toxic chemicals and volatile organic compounds (VOCs), solvents (cleaning materials, formaldehyde, toluene, benzene), drugs, alcohol, pesticides, herbicides, and food additives. Bacteria and yeast in the gut produce waste products, metabolic products, and cellular debris that can interfere with many body functions and lead to increased inflammation and autoimmune diseases. These include endotoxins, toxic amines, toxic derivatives of bile, and various carcinogenic substances such as putrescine and cadaverine. Last, the body must rid itself of the by-products of normal protein metabolism, including urea and ammonia.

The detoxification system is comprised of the skin, liver, kidneys, intestines, and lungs. It relies on the right balance of macronutrients, fiber, micronutrients, and phytochemicals to be effective. For example, methylation cofactors are essential for phase II detoxification. Adequate protein nutrition is required to supply the amino acids used in phase II reactions such as glutathione and glycine conjugation and sulfation. Phytochemicals (including, for example, the glucosinolates in cruciferous vegetables and the catechins in green tea) increase the activity of glutathione-S-transferases. Teas may have other benefits such as binding metals in the diet.[67] Polyphenols[68] (flavonoids in berries and other plant foods with deeply-colored pigments) enhance the expression of γ glutamylcysteine synthetase, increasing intracellular glutathione concentration, which is depleted in many chronic diseases. Catechol-O-methyltransferase (COMT) and cytochrome enzymes, including 1B1, detoxify toxic estrogen metabolites. These enzymes can be facilitated through dietary intervention with methylation cofactors and indole-3-carbinol from cruciferous vegetables. These gene-environment interactions influence the risks of cancer, osteoporosis, cardiovascular disease, neurodegenerative disease, depression, and more.[69]

The functional capacity to metabolize and excrete toxins varies from person to person and determines the rate and amount of toxin accumulation. The total load—all the exposures and influences that tax an individual's physiology—need to be considered when trying to create optimal health. Even low-level toxins have a profound effect on cells, biological systems, and their proper functioning, so efforts at limiting exposure are important, and maximizing the effectiveness of our detoxification capacity and elimination organs is critical. The clinical approach to detoxification must be individualized, based on biochemical and genetic variations from patient to patient (as well as differences in their environmental exposures). However, there are some basic principles that encourage mobilization of toxins, maximize their excretion, and minimize their redistribution in other sites in the body. It is important to ensure these aspects of healthy detoxification are working well together. They depend on the right food, exercise, adequate sweating, vitamins, minerals, accessory (or conditionally essential) nutrients, hyperthermic or heat treatments like saunas or steam baths, stress management, and occasionally heavy metal chelation treatments with medications like DMSA for removal of accumulated mercury, arsenic, and lead.

The translation of the science of detoxification into clinical practices is not mature; however, the application of that science to common health problems can be a remarkably effective tool for the clinician. (Please refer to Chapter 31 on Detoxification and Biotransformation for a more comprehensive discussion of these and additional relevant issues.) Assessment of exposures, testing endogenous detoxification capacity, identifying a patient's detoxification-related SNPs, and performing provocation tests for heavy metals are all useful evaluation approaches. Table 26.9 contains a list of tests by which toxic load and detoxification capacity can be assessed, and the suggestions provided in Table 26.10 can help to correct impaired detoxification systems, maximize endogenous detoxification capacity, and safely eliminate stored toxins. Treatment choices need to be individualized for each patient, depending on symptoms, genetic predispositions, environmental exposures, functional capacity, dietary habits, concomitant illnesses, and medications.

Table 26.9 **Assessing Toxic Burden and Detoxification Capacity**

- Detoxification SNPs can be evaluated: phase 1 (CYP 1A1, 1B1, etc.) and phase 2 (COMT, NAT, GSTM1, GSTP1, etc.)
- Detoxification challenge tests can assess functionality (provocations with caffeine, aspirin, acetaminophen).
- Detoxification enzymes can be measured:
  - Reduced glutathione
  - Glutathione peroxidase
  - SOD (super oxide dismutase)
- Heavy metal toxicity can be assessed:
  - RBC or whole blood
  - Hair analysis
  - Chelation challenge with DMSA
- Chemical antibodies to various toxins and metals can occasionally be useful.
- Organophosphates can be identified through a 24-hour urine collection.
- Organochlorine residues can be identified through a fat biopsy. This is used mostly for research purposes, but certain labs process clinical specimens.
- Urinary d-glucarate can be used to assess exposure to industrial toxins or xenobiotics.
- Urinary organic acids—specific compounds can be measured:
  - Sulfates
  - Pyroglutamate
  - Orotate
- Urinary porphyrins, by-products of damaged hemoglobin, can be clues to damage done by chemical or heavy metal toxins.
- Urinary trimellitic anhydrides (TMA) can be used to assess exposure to volatile organic compounds (VOCs).

Table 26.10 **Detoxification Strategies: Dietary, Environmental, and Lifestyle Approaches**

Avoiding and Removing Toxins	Dietary Support for Detoxification	Nutritional Supplementation
• Avoid excess exposure to environmental petrochemicals (garden chemicals, dry cleaning, car exhaust, secondhand smoke) • Clean and monitor heating systems for release of carbon monoxide, the most common cause of death by poisoning in America • Drink filtered water (reverse osmosis or carbon filter) • Enhance lymphatic flow with regular exercise, yoga, or lymphatic massage • Facilitate excretory functions: 1–2 bowel movements a day; 6–8 glasses of water a day; sweat regularly and profusely with exercise and the use of steam baths or saunas • HEPA/ULPA filters and ionizers to reduce dust, molds, volatile organic compounds, and other sources of indoor air pollution • House plants • Minimize EMR (electromagnetic radiation) and ionizing radiation • Organic food and animal products to avoid petrochemical pesticides, herbicides, fumigants, hormones, and antibiotics • Reduce heavy metal exposure (predatory and river fish, water, lead paint, thimerosol-containing products, etc.) • Reduce or eliminate the use of toxic household and personal care products (aluminium-containing underarm deodorant, antacids, and pots and pans) • Remove allergens from the diet and the environment • Treat gut infections and imbalanced gut ecology—often a source of endotoxins	• Bioflavonoids in grapes, berries, and citrus fruits • Burdock root for liver detoxification and increasing the production of urine and sweat • Celery increases urine flow • Chlorophyll in dark green leafy vegetables and in wheat grass • Cilantro can help remove heavy metals • Cruciferous vegetables (cabbage, broccoli, collards, kale, Brussels sprouts) 1 cup daily • Curcuminoids (turmeric and curry) • Dandelion greens help liver detoxification, improve the flow of bile, and increase urine flow • Foods that contain the monoterpene limonene (citrus peel, caraway, and dill weed oil) can also boost glucuronidation used for hormones and many medications • Fresh vegetable juices (carrots, celery, cilantro, beets, parsley, ginger) • Garlic (a few cloves a day) • Green tea boosts liver detoxification (increases GST enzymes) • High-quality, sulfur-containing proteins—eggs, whey protein, garlic, onions • Increase fiber intake through use of beans, whole grains, vegetables, fruits, nuts and seeds • Pycnogenol in grape seeds is a powerful antioxidant that can protect against toxic by-products of detoxification • Rosemary has carnosol, a potent booster of detoxification enzymes • Try decaffeinated green tea in the morning • Try herbal detoxification teas containing a mixture of burdock root, dandelion root, ginger root, licorice root, sarsaparilla root, cardamom seed, cinnamon bark, and other herbs	• Alpha lipoic acid 100–600 mg/day • Amino acids (taurine 500 mg 2x/day, glycine 500 mg 2x/day) • B-complex vitamins • Bioflavonoids • Carnitine 1000–3000 mg/day in divided doses • Daily high potency multi-vitamin and mineral formula • Essential fatty acids to facilitate glucuronidation • Extra-buffered vitamin C with mineral ascorbates in powder, capsule, or tablets during periods of increased detoxification • Milk thistle (silymarin) 70 to 210 mg/day • Mixed carotenoids 15,000 to 25,000 U/day • Molybdenum 50 to 200 mcg/day • N-acetylcysteine 500 to 1000 mg/day • Probiotics to help normalize gut flora and reduce endotoxins • Selenium 200 mcg/day • Zinc 30 to 50 mg/day

The Matrix: Dietary Influences on Inflammation

Inflammation and immune dysfunction are both cause and manifestation of core physiologic disturbances that are intimately associated with accelerated aging and chronic disease. The inflammatory response cuts across all organ systems and medical specialties, and wears many different guises. For that reason, the subject is addressed frequently in this book, from a number of different perspectives. For in-depth discussions of the underlying physiology, as well as the assessment and management of the inflammatory process, see Chapters 18, 23, and 27. In this chapter, we draw many of those threads together to examine the role of diet as an underlying common influence on the inflammatory process.

Inflammation can function both as a systemic trigger for, and as a mediator in, all the major degenerative diseases, including cardiovascular disease, neurodegenerative disease, and the increasingly prevalent allergic and autoimmune disorders. Diet and exercise are the two major modulators of the inflammatory response. Other inflammatory triggers include infections, gut dysbiosis, toxins, stress, environmental allergens, and trauma. Cytokines (interferon, interleukins, tumor necrosis factor, etc.) and eicosanoids (prostaglandins, prostacyclins, leukotrienes, thromboxanes) are the messenger molecules of the immune system. They upregulate or downregulate inflammation, depending on the needs of the organism. A maladaptive shift toward inflammation occurs in the face of specific inputs (high glycemic-load diet, intake of food allergens, inflammatory fats) and in the absence of other inputs (omega-3 fatty acids, exercise, etc.).

While inflammation has many causes, two factors stand out in our 21st century epidemic of chronic disease:

- first, the increase in inflammatory response secondary to a high glycemic-load diet, and the resultant metabolic syndrome;
- second, and closely related, is our sedentary lifestyle.

A host of other autoimmune, allergic, and inflammatory disorders are related to diet in two major ways: genetic or acquired food sensitivities or allergies, and macronutrient, micronutrient, and phytonutrient modulation of the inflammatory response.

Chronic, age-related degenerative diseases. Inflammation is central to all of the degenerative diseases that represent the leading causes of death in the 21st century. Elevations of inflammatory markers such as C-reactive protein and IL-6 have been found to increase all-cause mortality,[70] cardiovascular and neurodegenerative diseases, many cancers, macular degeneration, diabetes, and hypertension. Identifying all the proximal triggers of inflammation in patients is important. Often, dietary factors are the most significant modulators of inflammation. A high glycemic-load diet,[71] metabolic syndrome,[72] and a sedentary lifestyle are responsible for the majority of inflammation and degenerative disease. Additional dietary factors that contribute to inflammation include saturated and trans-fatty acids,[73] caffeine,[74] alcohol in excess,[75] deficiency of antioxidants, micronutrient deficiencies, and a low-fiber diet (which adversely affects gut flora and increases exposure to metabolic and environmental toxins). Pharmacologic modulators of inflammation have been proposed, including aspirin, non-steroidal anti-inflammatories (NSAIDs), and non-traditional anti-inflammatories such as statins, thiazolidinediones, and fibrates. However, a comprehensive lifestyle approach—including the modulation of diet by reduction in saturated[76] and trans-fats and glycemic load; use of multivitamins,[77] supplemental antioxidants[78] (key cell-signaling factors in gene transcription of inflammatory mediators), omega-3 fatty acids,[79] fiber,[80] and probiotics;[81] and the addition of regular exercise[82]—can collectively reduce systemic inflammatory mediators to a greater degree than pharmacologic interventions. Interventions that reduce inflammation reduce overall morbidity and mortality across the disease spectrum.

Testing for indicators of inflammation. A general assessment of inflammation is provided by C-reactive protein and sedimentation rate. Since those will not localize the source of inflammation, other approaches are used to further clarify the clinical picture; these include testing for celiac disease (discussed below) and antibody testing for both autoimmune conditions (thyroid, anti-thyroglobulin, anti-nuclear, and other antibodies) and chronic infections (including polymerase chain reaction, or PCR, testing and assessment of yeast overgrowth and fungal organisms). Stool and vaginal cultures can be done, as well as urinary organic acids for yeast metabolites (which are all inhibitors of metabolic function). Indicators of gut inflammation can be assessed through urinary organic acids and stool analysis (dysbiosis), hydrogen breath testing (small bowel bacterial overgrowth), and lactulose-mannitol challenge (intestinal permeability).

Food allergy, GALT, and immunity: Relationships to chronic disease. In addition to the factors discussed above, two other diet-inflammation relationships have important clinical relevance: food sensitivities of various types, and the role of diet in gut microecology and GALT activation.

Food allergy is not a single disease, nor is it caused by one pathophysiologic disturbance. Food allergy (or sensitivity) can be defined as an adverse immunological or hypersensitivity response to food. This response may be antibody or cell mediated. There are also many food reactions that are not immunologically mediated, including food intolerances (e.g., lactose) and food sensitivities (e.g., preservatives, additives, MSG, sweeteners such as aspartame, sulfites, etc.). Classic food allergy[83] has been recognized as IgE-dependent and is acute in onset (urticaria, asthma or anaphylaxis); food sensitivities tend to be either IgE-associated and delayed in onset (atopic dermatitis), or cell-mediated and both delayed and chronic (celiac disease).

Some recognition has been given to the role of IgG-mediated immune response and chronic disease,[84] but the research has been sparse and inconclusive, due to the pleiomorphic nature of individual responses to foods. Using elimination/provocation diets and, to some degree, IgG food antibody testing,[85] clinicians have identified inflammatory triggers responsible for a wide array of chronic symptoms not mediated by the classic IgE food allergy pathway. Conditions responsive to elimination diets include: headaches, IBS, fatigue, autoimmune disorders, chronic sinusitis, arthritis, inflammatory skin disorders, fibromyalgia, and CFIDS. While these disorders are often multifactorial, persistent immune activation of the GALT by foods can be a perpetuating factor. Food sensitivities or chronic GALT activation can be primary or secondary, cell-mediated responses, antibody-mediated responses, or both. However, in most cases, some precipitating event disturbs the gut mucosal integrity, leading to GALT activation that is then mediated by genes, food proteins, and microbial antigens. This initiates either a Th2 allergic response or a Th1 autoimmune response. Systemic inflammation then ensues, along with a wide host of common and often difficult-to-treat ailments. Elimination diet is one of the most powerful and underutilized tools available to the clinician for addressing chronic symptoms. (Elimination diet as a clinical tool is discussed in Chapter 35.)

Oral tolerance to common food antigens is impaired when the gut mucosal barrier is disturbed. This barrier must achieve a fine balance among very different and vitally important functions: fending off microbial antigens from gut flora, mounting a rapid response to pathogens, allowing assimilation of innocuous food antigens, and facilitating (or suppressing) inflammatory responses. Changes in diet to promote normalization of gut flora and to reestablish normal gut mucosal barrier integrity are critical in addressing the morbidity of chronic allergic and inflammatory diseases. Because health and disease function in a web-like manner, discerning cause or effect in any particular disease may be difficult (or even irrelevant). An approach that removes offending agents and restores balance within the core systems will yield remarkable clinical results. Food allergy or sensitivity may be the cause or the result of disturbed gut mucosal integrity. To resolve the clinical problem at hand, attention must be paid to both removing the offending allergens (forever, in the case of a genetically programmed immune response such as in celiac disease, or temporarily, in the case of an acquired IgG food sensitivity because of an intestinal insult), *and* restoring normal gut microecology and mucosal integrity.

Gluten—a pervasive influence. The relationship between gluten and chronic disease represents a classic food-disease connection. Unfortunately, the variable nature of clinical response to this single food antigen can obscure the diagnosis. Genetic susceptibility to gluten is found in up to 30% of those of European descent, yet in only 1% of the population is the disease fully expressed. There appears to be a graded response to gluten from mild to life threatening. The list of conditions associated with celiac disease is long.[86] (See Table 26.11.)

Screening for celiac disease is important in the face of *any* inflammatory, autoimmune, or chronic disease. Typical screening is done for IgA and IgG antigliadin antibodies and IgA antiendomysial antibodies; tissue transglutaminase (tTG) antibodies can be tested for in questionable cases. Total IgA should always be measured to rule out IgA deficiency. If IgA deficiency is present, tTG IgG can be helpful. These tests lack 100% sensitivity (or specificity). Intestinal biopsy for villous atrophy is the gold standard,[87] but lesions can be patchy and there is evidence that clinical symptoms and non-local manifestations can be independent of mucosal pathology. Occasionally useful is testing for HLA DQ2 and HLA DQ8 genotypes (which are present in 95% of celiac cases), especially in the face of IgA deficiency.[88] Stool testing for local IgA anti-gliadin antibodies or tTG can be confirmatory in suspicious cases where serum IgA or IgG and tTG are negative. A 12-week trial of elimination/provocation is, however, the most useful diagnostic approach.

The intersection of inflammation and clinical disease, and the opportunities for disease management, are, perhaps, the most fruitful, effective, and satisfying areas of functional medicine. The increasing prevalence of two major clinical problems—chronic degenerative diseases, and chronic inflammatory and immune diseases—are both intimately tied to diet and lifestyle, and those tools promise the greatest clinical effect when applied intelligently. Tables 26.12 and 26.13 summarize some of the most common conditions associated with inflammation, the major causes of inflammation, and provide suggestions for nutrient supplementation, botanical anti-inflammatory agents, and lifestyle changes.

Table 26.11 **Clinical Presentations of Celiac Sprue**

Common Features	Less Common Features	Associated Conditions	Complications
Adults • Iron-deficiency anemia • Diarrhea **Children** • Diarrhea • Failure to thrive • Abdominal distention	**General** • Short stature • Delayed puberty **Gastrointestinal** • Recurrent aphthous stomatitis • Recurrent abdominal pain • Steatorrhea **Extraintestinal** • Folate-deficiency anemia • Osteopenia or osteoporosis • Dental-enamel hypoplasia • Vitamin K deficiency • Hypertransaminasemia • Thrombocytosis (hyposplenism) • Arthralgia or arthropathy • Polyneuropathy • Ataxia • Epilepsy (with or without cerebral calcification) • Infertility • Recurrent abortions • Anxiety and depression • Follicular keratosis • Alopecia	**Definite associations** • Dermatitis herpetiformis • IgA deficiency • Type 1 diabetes • Autoimmune thyroid disease • Sjögren's syndrome • Microscopic colitis • Rheumatoid arthritis • Down syndrome • IgA nephropathy **Possible associations** • Congenital heart disease • Recurrent pericarditis • Sarcoidosis • Cystic fibrosis • Fibrosing alveolitis • Lung cavities • Pulmonary hemosiderosis • Inflammatory bowel disease • Autoimmune hepatitis • Primary biliary cirrhosis • Addison's disease • Systemic lupus erythematosus • Vasculitis • Polymyositis • Myasthenia gravis • Schizophrenia	• Refractory sprue • Enteropathy-associated T-cell lymphoma • Carcinoma of the oropharynx, esophagus, and small bowel • Ulcerative jejunoileitis • Collagenous sprue

Information from Farrell RJ, Kelly CP. Celiac sprue. N Engl J Med. 2002;346:180-88.

Table 26.12 **Inflammation: Major Causes and Associated Conditions**

Some Common Conditions Associated with Inflammation	Major Causes of Inflammation
• Allergies • Asthma • Attention deficit disorder (ADD) • Autism • Autoimmune diseases (lupus, rheumatoid arthritis, autoimmune thyroiditis) • Cancer • Cardiovascular disease • Chronic fatigue syndrome (CFS) • Cystitis • Dementia • Dermatitis (eczema, psoriasis, acne) • Diabetes • Emphysema and bronchitis • Fibromyalgia • Glomerulonephritis • Inflammatory bowel diseases (IBD) • Inflammatory liver disease (hepatitis from alcohol, sugar, viruses) • Irritable bowel syndrome (IBS) • Neurodegenerative disease (Alzheimer's, Parkinson's, MS, ALS) • Obesity • Osteoarthritis • Prostatitis • Reflux (GERD) • Sinusitis	• Allergens – Environmental allergens (dust, animal dander, pollens, etc.) – Common food allergens and sensitivities: Citrus Corn and corn products Dairy products—milk, cheese, yogurt Gluten grains—wheat, barley, oats, rye, spelt, kamut Yeast Eggs • Dysglycemia and insulin resistance (the major dietary causes of inflammation) • Environmental allergy (pollens, dust, molds, animals) • External (exogenous) toxins – Synthetic compounds (air pollution, water pollution, food additives, pesticides – Prescription drugs, drugs of abuses, cosmetics, household chemicals – Naturally occurring compounds (microbial toxins, mycotoxins) – Plant toxins – Heavy metals (e.g., lead, mercury, arsenic, cadmium) • Infection—acute or chronic • Internal (endogenous) toxins, gut-derived: – Ammonia – Nitrites – Amines such as cadaverine and putrescine • Lack of blood flow • Malnutrition • Nutrient deficiencies (e.g., omega-3 fatty acids, zinc, vitamin C, folate) • Oxidative stress • Physical injury or trauma • Psychological stress

Table 26.13 **Managing Inflammation: Dietary Suggestions, Anti-inflammatory Phytonutrients, and Lifestyle Recommendations**

Dietary and Nutrient Suggestions	Anti-Inflammatory Phytonutrients	Lifestyle Recommendations
• **Elimination Diet** for assessment (to identify inflammatory triggers) and treatment (to relieve the inflammatory burden)* • Balanced B complex • Essential fatty acids (flax, fish, and evening primrose oil) • Mixed carotenoids 15,000–25,000 IU/day • Multimineral supplement • Vitamin A 5000 to 10,000 IU/day • Vitamin C 500 to 2000 mg/day • Vitamin E mixed tocopherols 400 to 800 IU/day	**Bioflavonoids** • *Ginkgo biloba* • Pycnogenol or grape seed extract • Quercetin • Rutin **Immune tonic herbs** • Astragalus • Garlic • Licorice • Siberian ginseng (*Eleutherococcus senticosus*) **Tonic immune-boosting mushrooms** • Hakumokuji (*Tremella fuciformis*) • Kawaratake (*Coriolus versicolor*) • Maitake (*Frifola frondosa*) • Reishi (*Ganoderma lucidum*) • Shitake (*Lentius edodes*) • Tochukaso (*Cordyceps sinensis*) **Other anti-inflammatory and immune-boosting herbs and compounds** • Aloe vera • Boswellia (*Boswellia serrata*) • Capsaicin • Enzymes (bromelain and other proteolytic enzymes) • Ginger (*Zingiber officinalis*) • Glucosamine and chondroitin sulfate • Green tea (*Camellia sinensis*) • Immune active whey proteins with immunoglobulins and natural antibody complexes • Niacinamide • Probiotics • Turmeric (*Curcuma longa*)	• **Correct insulin resistance**—see recommendations under Hormonal Imbalances • Exercise • Reduce obesity • Relaxation, meditation, laughter: experiment and explore – Autogenic training – Breathing techniques – Chukra therapy (group laughing session) – Guided Imagery – Hypnosis – Journaling – Laughter—what makes you laugh? – Meditation – Mindfulness – Prayer – Psychotherapy – Relaxation techniques – Support groups – Yoga

*Please see the Appendix for a comprehensive elimination diet protocol.

The Matrix: Dietary Influences on Digestive Function

The health of the gut determines what nutrients are absorbed and therefore it is directly linked to the health of the total organism. It is often said that we are what we eat, but it is more accurate to say we are what we absorb. Chronic intestinal inflammation may lead to nutrient malabsorption and the resultant effects of chronic micronutrient deficiencies. Regardless of the illness, the role of gut health is critical. Gut imbalances can create, or fuel, an upregulated immune system, and nutritional imbalances from improper absorption can adversely affect the entire organism. This makes the gut a primary target for clinical intervention in the treatment of disease and the creation of health.

Intestinal health can be defined as the optimal digestion, absorption, and assimilation of food in the context of a balanced microecology, and an intact intestinal barrier function. These processes are continuously influenced by dietary and environmental inputs. The well-recognized inflammatory disorders—asthma, allergic rhinitis, inflammatory bowel disease, arthritis, autoimmune diseases—and the recently-recognized inflammatory disorders—cardiovascular disease, diabetes, obesity, neurodegenerative disease, and cancer—can often be traced back to the gut. When a clinician thinks "inflammation," the next thought must be "the gut."

Causes of gut dysfunction. Over 100 million Americans have digestive disorders. There are more than 200 over-the-counter (OTC) remedies for digestive disorders, many of which—most unfortunately—can create additional digestive problems. Visits for intestinal disorders are among the most common to primary care physicians. Rampant intestinal ill health is *not* a normal condition of human beings. It is the result of major changes in our evolutionary diet and the effect on the balance of the intestinal ecosystem. Cordain and colleagues, in "Origins and Evolution of the Western Diet: Health Implications for the 21st Century,"[89] outline the data that connect changes in our food patterns since the agricultural revolution to the diseases of today. The collision of our ancient genome with a modern diet is a significant causal factor in modern diseases. Cordain claims that seven fundamental nutritional characteristics of our diet have changed, and that these explain the dramatic rise in chronic and degenerative diseases:

1. glycemic load,
2. fatty acid composition,
3. macronutrient composition,
4. micronutrient density,
5. acid-base balance,
6. sodium-potassium ratio, and
7. fiber content.

Among many other adverse influences on health, these changes have affected the gut by changing the microenvironment of the intestinal tract. Problems can arise from inadequate stomach acid, poor digestive enzyme function, inadequate nutrient absorption, destruction of healthy bacteria, overgrowth of abnormal bacteria or yeasts, fermentation of starches, and disturbed signals to the enteric nervous system[90] of the gut, secondary to stress, various toxins, and antigens. Recent research has connected gut problems to symptoms and diseases far outside the gut: allergies, asthma, eczema, arthritis, headaches, autism, fibromyalgia, chronic fatigue and more.

The intestine is an "intelligent" organ. In addition to its role in digestion, absorption, and assimilation of nutrients, it interacts directly with the environment and protects the host from external threats through the microflora, the mucosal intestinal barrier, and the local immune system.[91] It is a complex ecosystem, much like the rainforest; if its balance is disturbed, its problems can create a ripple effect throughout the entire system. The forces that disturb the equilibrium are rampant: poor diet, food allergens, toxic food components, viruses, bacteria, parasites, overgrowth of yeast, use of medications (especially antibiotics, anti-inflammatories, and acid blocking drugs), various illnesses, and stress.

Investigating gut dysfunction. We must ask some key questions to understand why the gut may be malfunctioning; the answers will help the clinician design a program to correct underlying dysfunctions:

- Are digestive enzymes and acid production adequate to break food down to its component parts and make the food particles small enough for absorption?
- Is the gut mucosal barrier working properly, selectively absorbing the right things (amino acids, sugars, fats, vitamins, and minerals, etc.), and keeping out the harmful things (undigested food particles, microbial particles, or toxins)?

- Does the microflora have the right kind and amount of good healthy bacteria, located in the right places along the digestive tract?
- Are the components of the microflora in proper balance, without undue competition from potentially harmful bacteria, yeasts, and parasites?
- Is the microflora getting the right kind and amount of fiber (both insoluble and soluble) and nutrients to stay healthy and flourishing?
- Are problems in the gut causing stress on the liver and immune system because toxins or allergens are being absorbed through a leaky gut or disturbed intestinal barrier?

The process of answering these questions will identify the starting point(s) to help the patient restore intestinal health and treat the host of disorders that manifest as direct intestinal symptoms or symptoms from more distant sites.

Therapeutic options for digestive imbalances. The term "functional foods" has entered the nutritional and popular lexicon to indicate a food that "is shown to beneficially affect one or more target functions in the body beyond adequate nutritional effects in a way that is relevant to either the state of well-being and health, or to a reduction in disease incidence."[92] This paradigm—that there are foods *and nutrients* that impair gut function and others that enhance it—is a useful lever to impact chronic health complaints that exist across multiple organ systems.

A number of these foods and nutrients have been studied and found to repair and heal the intestinal mucosal barrier, improve microflora balance, and modulate the proinflammatory state of the GALT.[93,94] Important examples include:

- Glutamine improves gut and systemic immune function, especially in patients in prolonged states of parenteral nutrition; helps heal GI mucosa after damage from radiation or chemotherapy; and reduces episodes of bacterial translocation and clinical sepsis.
- Arginine is a precursor for nitric oxide, and has demonstrated benefits in inflammatory bowel diseases, as well as intestinal diseases resulting from trauma, critical illness, or cancer.
- Zinc leads to improvements in children with GI diseases; prevents childhood mortality; and corrects deficiencies linked to anorexia, hypogeusia, poor growth, alopecia, delayed sexual maturation, skin diseases, and severe diarrhea.
- Vitamin A plays an important role in epithelial cell integrity, immune function, and retinal function. Deficiencies are implicated in the risk of diarrhea, respiratory infections, impaired gut function, and death in children.
- Probiotics enhance mucosal immune defense, protect against microbial translocation and colonization, and improve inflammatory bowel disease and atopic disease.
- Prebiotics (fermentable starches such as inulin and fructose oligosaccharides) have many potential health benefits, such as improved bowel function, increased mineral absorption, and lowered risk of colon cancer, though human studies are limited.
- Gamma linolenic acid leads to progressive improvement in rheumatoid arthritis with long-term use; suppresses human T-cell proliferation, tumor growth, and metastasis; normalizes nerve conduction and sciatic endoneurial blood flow; and suppresses oxidative damage associated with diabetes (when administered with vitamin C).

Clinically, functional medicine finds some of its most powerful applications with inflammatory diseases mediated by gut dysfunction and improved by repairing gut function. Applying basic principles of functional medicine such as the 4R program (see Chapter 28 for an in-depth presentation of this gut repair approach) can correct many conditions related to food allergy and gut dysbiosis (often synergistically related). While many types of interventions to restore gut balance may be necessary—including elimination of food allergens and heavy metals, use of herbs, medications, enzymes, probiotics, essential fatty acids, amino acids and various nutrients, and the addition of stress management and exercise to the patient's lifestyle—improving diet is a critical. By restoring our dietary patterns to correct the adverse evolutionary shifts discussed above, many of the dietary causes of gut dysfunction and related illnesses can be corrected.

A number of clinical tools can be extremely useful in improving gut function. While more clinical research is needed, these interventions are based on the most fundamental principle of functional medicine: remove what harms and provide what heals. The details may be different from person to person, but the concept will guide diagnosis and therapy. This is an area of medicine where some clinical applications that are logical extensions of the underlying science have outpaced the clinical research literature; fortunately, the positive clinical outcomes from this approach warrant its application where conventional approaches routinely fail.

Elimination diet. One of the most powerful tools for identification of problems and for beginning a GI repair program is the elimination diet (discussed more fully in Chapter 35). This is typically a trial of an oligoantigenic diet (elimination of a number of the most common dietary triggers, to reduce intake to those foods least likely to cause or mediate any ongoing inflammatory reaction). A well-structured elimination diet, besides getting rid of possible triggers of inflammation and immune irritation, offers the patient the opportunity to experience a much healthier approach to eating. It is usually a mostly plant-based diet that includes organic and unprocessed foods that are high in vitamins, minerals, antioxidants, anti-inflammatory phytochemicals, fiber, and essential fatty acids, and excludes saturated and trans-fats, sugar, empty calories, and the 4,000 food additives, hormones, antibiotics, and xenobiotics (foreign toxic chemicals) that are everyday fare for most Americans. Many common ailments will resolve with a brief (2–6 week) elimination diet. Even in those patients without particular symptoms or obvious allergies, an elimination diet can give the immune system a rest and allow for deeper healing and repair throughout the body.

Other dietary approaches to improving digestive function include replacing hydrochloric acid and digestive enzymes, where needed; increasing fiber; adding both probiotics and prebiotics; treating infections and dysbiosis; using nutrients that help heal the gut; and changing lifestyle and eating habits. Interestingly, HOW we eat can be just as important as WHAT we eat. If we are stressed, or eat in a hurry, or eat too much at the wrong time of day, our "gut brain" gets confused. This "second brain" (as the gut is often called) turns on signals that make us gain weight, and that impair digestion and absorption of nutrients, relax gut muscles that prevent reflux (the lower esophageal sphincter), and tighten muscles that should relax to let the food pass from the stomach (the pylorus), increasing reflux. By following a few simple guidelines, digestion can improve significantly and patients can even lose weight. Table 26.14 provides suggestions for increasing fiber and making dietary and lifestyle changes; Table 26.15 presents information on the use of probiotics and prebiotics; Table 26.16 addresses yeast infections; Table 26.17 addresses parasitic infections; Table 26.18 addresses bacterial infections; and Table 26.19 provides information on gut-healing nutrients.

Restoring the integrity of the digestive ecosystem can be fairly straightforward for many patients, but steps should be taken in the proper sequence and therapeutic strategies should be initiated and evaluated systematically. The following are useful guidelines in planning your patient's gut healing program:

- Day 1: Start the elimination diet first; have the patient follow it one or two weeks to assess the effect on digestive function. It may be continued for four weeks or longer, depending on the response.
- Day 3: Start digestive enzymes and a trial of hydrochloric acid (HCl) *if appropriate* (see symptoms) after two days on the elimination diet.
- Day 7: Start probiotics to reintroduce healthy bacteria back into the digestive system.
- Day 14: Attempt to identify the source of dysbiosis—yeast overgrowth, small bowel bacterial overgrowth, parasites, H. pylori, etc. (through testing or further analysis of symptom patterns and history). Testing prior to initiating a program may be indicated in some patients, although often an elimination diet is effective in identifying the problems and further testing is not needed.
- If indicated by findings in the previous step, initiate non-prescription or prescription medications for identified sources of infection at least two weeks before beginning the next step.
- Day 28 (or later, depending on whether any medications have been introduced): Start the "repair phase" of gut healing by adding healing nutrients, essential fatty acids, and any other components that you have determined are necessary for restoration of the integrity of the gut lining. Continue on this phase for at least two months. Use probiotics for at least three months and consider a long-term reduced maintenance dose.

Table 26.14 **Therapeutic Strategies for Healing the Gut: Adding Fiber, Changing Dietary and Lifestyle Habits**

Suggestions for Increasing Fiber	Dietary and Lifestyle Changes
• 2 tbsp/day of ground **flax seeds**. Use a coffee grinder just for the flax seeds. Grind 1/2 cup at a time and keep tightly sealed in a glass jar in the fridge or freezer. Sprinkle on salads, on grain or vegetable dishes, or mix in a little unsweetened applesauce. • **Beans** (all forms of legumes) are the highest sources of dietary fiber. • Increase **vegetable** intake—with few calories, high levels of antioxidants, and protective phytochemicals, these are excellent fiber sources. • Use **whole grains** such as brown rice or quinoa. • Include a few servings of **low glycemic-index fruits** to the diet daily (berries are the highest in fiber and other protective phytochemicals). • Include handful of **nuts** each day: almonds, walnuts, pecans or hazelnuts. • Consider a good **fiber supplement** containing soluble and insoluble fibers and no sweeteners or additives, if necessary. • **Start slowly.** Switching abruptly to a high-fiber diet can cause gas and bloating. Increase the total amount gradually, up to 50 g/day.	• Chew each mouthful 25 to 50 times, or at least try! This releases EGF (epithelial growth factor), needed for repair and healing of the digestive lining. • Eat slowly and do not do anything else while eating. Remember, it takes 20 minutes for the brain to get the message that the stomach is full. • Take pleasure in meals; take time to enjoy eating with friends or family; create simple meal time rituals such as a blessing, or soothing environment. • Pick beautiful and attractive foods that please all the senses. • Eat regularly, at least every 3–5 hours. Studies have shown that people overeat if they are extremely hungry. Hypoglycemia can cause swings in blood sugar and carbohydrate cravings. • Mix it up—try to avoid mono-meals. Have a variety of fruits and vegetables, protein-rich foods, whole grains, and small amounts of healthy oils and fats in each meal. • Never eat standing up. • Stop eating three hours before bedtime. Late evening eating can increase reflux and promote weight gain. • BREATHE! Activate the parasympathetic "gut brain" by taking 5 deep breaths before eating—5 seconds in and 5 seconds out for 5 breaths. • Get a water filter (reverse osmosis is the best) to avoid intake of pathogenic microbes. Portable carbon filters in water bottles are available for those on the move. • Wash all fruits and vegetables thoroughly and peel all fruits and vegetables that are not going to be thoroughly cooked. • Wash hands after being outside, and always before and after handling food. • Wash hands after handling raw food and soak utensils and cutting boards if they were used for slicing raw fish, meat, or poultry to reduce exposure to Salmonella. **Stress Reduction** Dealing with stress is critical to repairing the digestive system. The connections between the brain and the gut are powerful. **The enteric nervous system or the "gut brain" has more neurotransmitters than the brain.** These chemical messengers play a critical role in proper GI function, or malfunction. Tools such as meditation, yoga, or other relaxation therapies can retrain the "automatic" nervous system and overcome the dangers of excessive stress, and its effect on our digestion and feeding behavior.

Table 26.15 **Using Probiotics and Prebiotics**

Role of Healthy Flora	Probiotics	Prebiotics
• The microflora of the human adult consists of >100,000 billion bacteria and >400 different species. • The microflora synthesizes vitamins and nutrients (biotin, B12, folic acid, pantothenic acid, pyridoxine, riboflavin, vitamin K, butyric acid and amino acids). • These microbes produce short-chain fatty acids (SCFAs), the substrate fuel for intestinal epithelial cells. • They improve digestion and absorption of nutrients by producing digestive enzymes. • The microflora metabolizes environmental and internal toxins; for example, they convert mercury into less toxic forms. • They prevent other microbes from colonizing the gut (which is what happens with traveler's diarrhea), and they can metabolize bacterial toxins. • They make it difficult for potential invaders by competing for nutrients. • They stimulate immune function by increasing antibody production (including producing natural antibiotics to kill pathogenic microbes), and by producing anti-cancer compounds like n-butyrate. • The microflora converts food phytochemicals into protective compounds (e.g., flax seed lignans are converted into enterolactones that have anti-cancer properties). • Charbroiled foods containing polycyclic aromatic hydrocarbons, and aflatoxin (the toxic mold on peanuts) can be neutralized by the microflora.	Therapeutically, probiotics have been found useful in diarrhea, in controlling asthma, allergies and eczema, and in reducing leaky gut and inflammatory molecules (cytokines). Supplementing pregnant women and then their infants for six months with a Lactobacillus GG resulted in a 50% reduction in asthma, eczema and allergy in the children at 2 years of age.* Start a 6- to 12-week course of a probiotic to restore normal symbiosis or ecological balance: • Take 5–10 billion organisms a day on an empty stomach in divided doses (twice a day). Preparations include freeze-dried bacteria packaged in powders, tablet, or capsule form. • In treatment of more severe GI dysfunction, daily doses of 50 billion or more organisms have been used. • Look for reputable, refrigerated brands of mixed flora including *Lactobacillus acidophilus*, *Lactobacillus rhamnosis* or GG and B. bifidum. • Some products contain no live flora because they are very susceptible to damage from heat, processing, or improper storage. • Some strains do not colonize the gut well. • Try some strains backed by research such as Lactobacillus GG (Culturelle), and the DDS-1 strain of *Lactobacillus acidophilus*. * Kalliomaki, M. Probiotics in primary prevention of atopic disease: a randomized placebo-controlled trial. Lancet. 2001;357:1076-79.	In addition to supplementing with healthy bacteria (probiotics), studies have shown that providing good food for the flora can improve outcomes. The food for probiotics is called prebiotics and includes mostly non-digestible plant components that are used by the flora for their nourishment. Some common foods that fill these criteria include fructose-containing oligosaccharides, which occur naturally in a variety of plants such as onion, asparagus, burdock root, Jerusalem artichoke, chicory, and banana.** Or, consider supplements of fructose-containing oligosaccharides such as inulin or chicory root. ** Roberfroid MB. Prebiotics: preferential substrates for specific germs? Am J Clin Nutr. 2001;73(2 Suppl):406S-9S.

Table 26.16 **Identifying and Treating GI Yeast Infections**

Predisposing Factors and Associated Conditions	Symptoms of Yeast Infection	Therapeutic Strategies
Predisposing factors: • Altered bowel flora • Decreased digestive secretions • Dietary factors including a high-sugar, high-fat, low-fiber diet • Impaired immunity • Impaired liver function • Nutrient deficiency • Prolonged antibiotic use • Psychological stress **Past history:** • Chronic antibiotic use for infections or acne • Chronic vaginal yeast infections • Oral birth control pills • Oral steroid hormones **Demographics:** • Female • Age 15–50 years **Associated conditions:** • Eczema • Irritable bowel syndrome • Psoriasis • Sensitivity to foods, chemicals, or other allergens	**General symptoms:** • Craving for foods rich in carbohydrates or yeast • Chronic fatigue • Loss of energy • General malaise • Decreased libido **Gastrointestinal symptoms:** • Thrush • Bloating and gas • Intestinal cramps • Rectal itching • Altered bowel function **Genitourinary symptoms:** • Vaginal yeast infections • Frequent bladder infections • Interstitial cystitis **Hormonal symptoms:** • Menstrual irregularities, pain, bleeding, etc. • Premenstrual syndrome • Thyroid dysfunction **Nervous system symptoms:** • Depression • Irritability • Inability to concentrate **Immune symptoms:** • Allergies • Chemical sensitivities • Suppressed immune function	• Deal with predisposing factors (such as chronic use of antibiotics, steroids, hormones—stop unless absolutely medically necessary). • Trial of yeast-control diet: elimination of refined carbohydrates, sugar, and fermented foods. • Test for yeast overgrowth. • Non-prescription antifungals include oregano, garlic, citrus seed extract, berberine, tannins, undecylenate, isatis tinctoria, caprylic acid. • Antifungal prescription medications include nystatin, fluconazole, itraconazole, terbinafine. • Immunotherapy • Identify potential environmental toxic fungi (Stachybotrys, strains of Aspergillus, Chaetomium and Penicillium). • Utilize the 4R Program (Chapter 28) and institute stress reduction and stress management practices (addressed in previous tables in this chapter).

Adapted from the *Textbook of Natural Medicine*, Pizzorno and Murray, Churchill Livingstone, 1999.

Table 26.17 **Identifying and Treating GI Parasitic Infections**

Signs and Symptoms of Parasitic Infections	Common Parasites	Therapeutic Strategies
• Abdominal pain and cramps • Constipation • Diarrhea • Excessive flatulence • Fatigue • Fever • Food allergy • Foul-smelling stools • Gastritis • Greasy stools • Headaches • Hives • Increased intestinal permeability • Indigestion • Irritable bowel syndrome and irregular bowel movements • Low back pain • Low levels of secretory IgA • Malabsorption • Poor appetite • Weight loss	• ***Giardia lamblia**** • *Entamoeba coli and Endolimax nana* • *Blastocystis hominis* • ***Entamoeba histolytica**** • ***Cryptosporidium species**** • *Dientamoeba fragilis* • *Entamoeba hartmani* ***Bold-faced parasites are considered more dangerous**, but other minor parasites can often be the cause of symptoms.	**General approaches:** • Drink filtered water. • Wash and/or peel fruits and vegetables, especially if eaten raw, or consider soaking them in a dilute hydrogen peroxide solution of 1 teaspoon of 3% hydrogen peroxide and 2 quarts of water, then rinse with filtered water. • Avoid salad bars and street vendors. • Wash hands carefully with soap and water before eating and after coming in from outdoors, especially if working in the garden or dirt. • If eating out, eat only freshly prepared foods, not things that have been sitting out for a while or microwaved. • Wash sponges in the dishwasher daily. • Thoroughly wash all cutting boards and kitchen surfaces after use. **Non-prescription approaches:** • Take digestive enzymes for a few months— parasites often cause malabsorption and maldigestion. • Avoid vitamins during treatment because vitamins help the parasites flourish. • Herbal therapies include *Artemesia annua*, oregano, and berberine-containing plants (*Hydrastis canadensis*, *Berberis vulgaris*, *Berberis aquifolium*, and *Coptis chinesis*). **Prescription medications:** • Humatin (paromomycin) in adult doses of 250 mg 3x/day for 14 days and Bactrim DS or Septra DS (trimethoprim and sulfamethoxazole) every 12 hours for 14 days. • Yodoxin (iodoquinol) 650 mg 3x/day for 14 days. Yodoxin is antifungal as well as being anti-parasitic. • Flagyl (metronidazole) 500 mg 3x/day for 10 days with meals.

Table 26.18 **Identifying and Treating GI Bacterial Infections**

Small Bowel Overgrowth

The upper portion of the intestine is generally sterile. Small bowel overgrowth of bacteria or other organisms can lead to irritable bowel syndrome, food allergies, inflammatory diseases and autonomic dysfunction.* Symptoms can be similar to low stomach acid and ineffective digestive enzymes (indigestion, bloating, and fullness after eating), but can also include signs associated with yeast overgrowth, nausea, diarrhea, arthritis, and autoimmune diseases.

Testing

- Hydrogen breath testing for small bowel bacterial overgrowth
- Organic acids: indican, D-lactate

Treatment

Repair the digestive system:

- Follow general guidelines for improving gut function (see previous tables).
- Avoid easily fermentable foods, including sugars, starches, and soluble fiber (until the problem is corrected).
- No wheat or sucrose; no lactose (milk sugar)
- Additional restrictions depend on symptoms and response and may include: no gluten grains, no cereal grains, no potatoes, no fruit, juices and honey, no legumes; cook all vegetables.

Non-prescription preparations:

- Oregano, citrus seed extract, isatis, or berberine compounds
- Special spices for the gut include garlic, onions, turmeric, ginger, cinnamon, sage, rosemary, oregano, and thyme. All these can be added to the diet to support healthy digestive functioning.

Prescription medications:

Occasionally prescription medication may be needed. Some of the useful compounds include:

- Rifaximin 200–400 mg 3/day** (non-absorbed antibiotic)
- Metronidazole 250 mg 3x/ day for 7 days (for anaerobes or bacteria that don't like oxygen, like Bacteroides or Clostridia species)
- Tetracycline 500 mg 2x/day for 7 days (also for anaerobes)
- Ciprofloxacin 500 mg 2/day for 3 days (for aerobes)
- Bismuth (as in Pepto-Bismol®)
- Antifungal preparations (as above)

Helicobacter Pylori

The role of this bacterium as the cause of stomach ulcers has been clarified. It is found in 90–100% of people with duodenal ulcers, 70% of people with gastric ulcers, and in about 50% of people over the age of 50. It may be associated with stomach cancer, inflammation throughout the body, and possibly with heart disease. It is often acquired in childhood and can be the cause of lifelong gastritis or stomach inflammation. For many patients, it is also implicated in reflux and heartburn, although studies have been inconclusive. Genetic and nutritional differences among individuals can affect whether or not H. pylori causes gut symptoms or cancer. For those with elevated C-reactive protein, chronic digestive symptoms, or a family history of gastric cancer, treatment is advisable. Currently, most physicians treat only documented ulcers, possibly overlooking many people who could benefit from treatment.

Low stomach acid predisposes to the growth of H. Pylori, as do low antioxidant defense systems. Low levels of vitamin C and E in gastric fluids promote the growth of H. Pylori.

Testing

- Breath testing
- CLO test or intestinal biopsy
- H. Pylori antibodies
- Stool antigen test

Treatment

Non-prescription preparations:

- Bismuth subcitrate 240 mg 2x/day before meals for 2 weeks. It can cause a temporary harmless blackening of the tongue and stool.
- DGL or deglycyrrhizinated licorice can help eradicate the organism and relieve symptoms.
- Myrrh gum resin

Prescription medications:

- Amoxicillin 1 gram 2x/day, Clarithromycin 500 mg 2x/day, omeprazole 20 mg 2x/day for 10 days
- Prevpac (Lansoprazole-Amoxicillin-Clarithromycin combination) one 2x/day for 14 days
- Helidac (Bismuth-Metronidazole-Tetracycline combination) one 4x/day with meals for 2 weeks
- Tritec (ranitidine bismuth citrate) 400mg 2x/day for 28 days

*Lin HC. Small intestinal bacterial overgrowth: a framework for understanding irritable bowel syndrome. JAMA. 2004;292(7):852-58. Pimentel et al. Eradication of small intestinal bacterial overgrowth reduces symptoms of irritable bowel syndrome. Am J Gastroenterol. 2001;96(8):2505-6.

** Baker DE. Rifaximin: a nonabsorbed oral antibiotic. Rev Gastroenterol Disord. 2005;5(1):19-30.

Table 26.19 **Testing for Gut Function; Gut-Healing Nutrients**

Testing for Gut Function	Gut-Healing Nutrients
Comprehensive digestive stool analysis Hydrogen breath testing for small bowel overgrowth Intestinal permeability (lactulose-mannitol challenge) Organic acid urine testing for dysbiosis Parasitology analysis **Complete blood count:** This common test can give many clues to underlying infection. It shows the different types of white blood cells and their responses to different organisms. Useful indicators include the following: • Anemia with an elevated mean corpuscular volume (MCV) can be sign of B12 or folate deficiency. B12 is absorbed in the small intestine and if there is chronic inflammation, bacterial overgrowth, or a parasite, it is often poorly absorbed resulting in an elevated MCV. Anything over 95 may indicate B12 malabsorption or folate deficiency. Anemia with a low MCV may indicate iron deficiency from intestinal blood loss or malabsorption as found in celiac disease. • A low neutrophil and high lymphocyte count can be a sign of chronic yeast or viral infections. A low total white blood cell count can also be a sign of stress to the immune system. • Eosinophils are elevated in parasitic infections or from exposure to allergens. Further testing for parasites or allergies should follow. Homocysteine and methylmalonic acid—these can help pick up B12 or folate deficiency secondary to malabsorption or inadequate intake. 25-OH vitamin D is an important fat-soluble vitamin that is deficient in malabsorption states.	Specialized gut support products and nutrients are often necessary for gut healing and repair. These are the final tools for correcting digestive problems, healing a leaky gut, and reducing relapse or recurrence of digestive and immune problems. These should be taken for 1-3 months, depending on the severity of symptoms and response to treatment. These compounds needed for gut repair can be divided into four main categories: **Gut food:** Glutamine 1,000–10,000 mg a day. This is a nonessential amino acid that is the preferred fuel for the lining of the small intestine and can greatly facilitate healing. It can be taken for one to two months. It generally comes in powder form and is often combined with other compounds that facilitate gut repair. **Nutrients and antioxidants:** • Zinc 20–50 mg • Vitamin A 5,000–10,000 U/day • Vitamin B5 pantothenic acid 100–500 mg/day • Vitamin E 400 to 800 IU/day in the form of mixed tocopherols These can be taken separately, or as part of a good high-potency multivitamin. **Essential fats and oils:** • GLA (gamma linolenic acid) 2-6 grams/day • Gamma-oryzanol (rice brain or rice brain oil) 100 mg three times a day • Omega-3 fatty acids 3 to 6 grams a day of EPA/DHA **Anti-inflammatories and gut detoxifiers:** • N-acetylcysteine 500 mg twice a day • Reduced Glutathione 300 mg twice a day • Quercetin 500 mg twice a day and other bioflavonoids These potent anti-inflammatories and detoxifiers are key to restoring balance in the gut lining by protecting it from oxidant damage and helping with detoxification within the gut.

Not following all of these steps, and/or not following them in order, can lead to more digestive upset in the short term, and may not allow full healing, even if the patient feels better initially. This approach is designed to move systematically through a gut repair program and to prevent relapse.

Dietary Influences on Sarcopenia

Sarcopenia,[95] or "poverty of the flesh," is the term we use to describe the decline in muscle mass and strength seen in "healthy aging." Sarcopenia differs from wasting (an involuntary weight loss due to inadequate caloric intake), or cachexia (general physical wasting and malnutrition usually associated with chronic disease), or a cytokine-driven loss of lean body mass with the maintenance of weight. Conventionally, sarcopenia is perceived as a loss of muscle solely related to decreased activity, common in the aging population, and it is associated with a progressive increase in dysfunction and disability. The economic costs of sarcopenia have been estimated to be between $11.8 and $26.2 billion per year, or approximately 1.5% of total health care expenditures.[96]

While physical activity and strength training are central to reversing sarcopenia and its related dysfunction (see the Exercise sections of Chapters 13 and 29), nutritional, hormonal, immune, and metabolic factors play a large role in as well, so it is a good example of a condition that involves multiple areas of the functional medicine matrix. Understanding these relationships opens the door to interventions other than increased activity that correct underlying causes of sarcopenia.

The dynamics of the aging muscle are regulated by factors influenced by dietary intake—insulin resistance, oxidative stress, inflammation, protein nutrition, sex hormone balance, and mitochondrial function. Any input that influences these metabolic and hormonal factors will have an effect on sarcopenia. Old concepts of decreased protein synthesis in aging have been challenged. Older men were found to have higher rates of protein synthesis than younger men, dispelling the notion that sarcopenia is due to inadequate basal or fasting protein synthesis.[97] Therefore, other factors that shift the balance from anabolism to catabolism must be considered.

Protein intake, digestion, absorption, assimilation, and utilization (and hence muscle protein synthesis) are affected by the amount and quality of protein intake, as well as by age. One-third of women and men over 60 years of age eat less than 0.8 g/kg of protein per day (the RDA) and approximately 15% eat less than 75% of the RDA for protein. Factors that influence protein digestion and absorption include hypochlorhydria,[98] use of acid-blocking medications, zinc deficiency, food allergies, celiac disease, and dysbiosis. Supplementation with essential amino acids may enhance protein synthesis in healthy elderly adults. However, consumption of these amino acids, along with non-essential amino acids and carbohydrates (as frequently found in protein drinks), impairs the anabolic response of muscle proteins to the positive effects of amino acids.[99] Ensuring adequate digestion, protein intake, and availability of essential amino acids is important for maintaining normal muscle mass with aging.

Sarcopenia is related to a reduction in anabolic stimuli (physical activity, CNS activity, reductions in estrogens, androgens, growth hormone, and insulin sensitivity) and an increase in catabolic stimuli (subclinical inflammation and oxidative stress).[100] Hormonal changes with age are affected by diet and environment, and include decreases in estrogen, testosterone, and growth hormone. Estrogen and testosterone are anabolic, and they inhibit catabolic cytokines (including IL-1 and IL-6). Insulin inhibits protein breakdown. Insulin resistance, which increases with age, high glycemic-load diets, visceral fat mass, and inactivity, impairs the protective effect of insulin. Inflammation has also been linked to catabolism and sarcopenia through increases in IL-6, IL-1, and TNF-α in healthy aging adults. This may be mediated through direct catabolic effects, anorexia of aging triggered by inflammation, inducing insulin resistance or lowering growth hormone and insulin-like growth factor-1 concentrations, and increasing apoptosis.[101] Oxidative stress contributes to sarcopenia through damage to cellular components, including DNA, proteins, lipids, cell membranes, and the sarcoplasmic reticulum.[102]

Interventions that improve protein intake and digestion, reduce insulin resistance, inflammation and oxidative stress, and improve hormonal balance can reduce age-related sarcopenia and loss of function, particularly when combined with physical activity and stress management.[103] The web-like nature of our physiology is clearly evident in the pathophysiology of sarcopenia. This understanding can be used to design a comprehensive approach to normalize function. Each patient should, of course, have a personalized assessment and plan, but the following suggestions indicate some dietary and lifestyle strategies for preventing and reversing sarcopenia:

- Ensure adequate protein intake (0.8 gm/kg to 1.2 gm/kg depending on activity level).
- Consider essential amino acid supplementation without non-essential amino acids or carbohydrates.
- Improve insulin sensitivity.
- Reduce inflammation.
- Reduce oxidative stress.
- Improve hormonal balance.
- Initiate resistance and aerobic conditioning.
- Initiate stress management to mitigate the catabolic effects of chronic cortisol exposure.

The Risks in our Food Supply

Harmful Foods: Dietary Components as a Causative Factor in Disease

A number of foods and non-nutritive substances in our diet adversely affect our health and need to be reduced or eliminated. Some have well-documented risks, such as *trans* fatty acids, while others pose potential risks. Other components of our diet have also been shown to cause (or have the potential to cause) harm, including refined polyunsaturated oils, fake fats (Olestra, Simplesse®), refined sugars, high fructose corn syrup, refined carbohydrates, artificial sweeteners, food toxins, and genetically engineered foods.

Trans fatty acids (trans-fats). In many controlled metabolic studies, *trans* fatty acids[104] (found in stick margarine, vegetable shortening, commercially baked goods, deep-fried foods, fast foods, and many restaurant foods) raise LDL-C and lower HDL-C compared to *cis* fatty acids,[105] and raise the total cholesterol-to-HDL ratio (TC/HDL) twice as much as saturated fat. Trans-fats also increase plasma lipoprotein(a) and triglycerides, and impair endothelial function by their inhibition of the enzyme delta-6-desaturase, which may adversely affect essential fatty acid metabolism and prostaglandin balance. High intakes of trans-fats can promote insulin resistance and increase the risk of type 2 diabetes.[106] *Trans* fatty acids may also increase the risk of colon and breast cancer,[107,108] allergic diseases in children,[109] and neurodegenerative diseases.[110] *Trans* fatty acids adversely affect plasma markers of inflammation in healthy men including elevations in C-reactive protein, interleukin-6, tumor necrosis factor-alpha, and E-selectin.[111,112] Elimination of *trans* fatty acids from our diet may help to reduce the incidence of cardiovascular disease, neurodegenerative diseases, obesity, diabetes, cancers, and inflammatory disorders.

Fake fats. Olestra and Simplesse may have adverse health effects by reducing availability of fat-soluble vitamins, including serum retinol, 25-hydroxyvitamin D, alpha-tocopherol, phylloquinone, and carotenoid concentrations,[113] in addition to the risk of stool incontinence.

High fructose corn syrup. High fructose corn syrup (HFCS) consumption increased >1,000% (0.292kg/person/year to 33.4kg/person/year) from 1970 to 1990 and now represents >40% of caloric sweeteners added to foods and beverages.[114] The introduction of HFCS into the food supply is associated with the beginning of the obesity epidemic. While other factors for this epidemic (including reduced levels of physical activity, increased portion sizes, eating outside the home and at fast-food restaurants) certainly play a very important role, changes in the types of foods eaten, and the overall "toxic food environment,"[115] including the effect of HFCS in soft drinks and other sweetened beverages, merit serious consideration as an etiologic factor in the obesity epidemic.

The digestion, absorption, and metabolism of fructose differ in significant ways from glucose. Fructose is absorbed through a non-sodium dependent process and enters the cell in an insulin-independent manner. In high doses, it becomes an unregulated source of carbon precursors (acetyl-CoA) for hepatic lipogenesis, specifically triacylglycerol (triglyceride) synthesis. This is associated with reductions in HDL and increases in the more atherogenic LDL-B particles. It is important to note that reductions in LDL-C with high-carbohydrate diets are often associated with conversion from LDL-A to LDL-B, and that change is associated with increased cardiovascular risk. Increased consumption of HFCS may be a cause of increasing dyslipidemias that may be better treated by reducing HFCS than by statin therapy.

Fructose does not stimulate insulin secretion or the consequent increase in leptin, which serves as a counter-regulatory afferent signal for reductions in appetite. While glucose is transported into the brain, affecting neuroregulatory appetite signals, fructose is not. Ghrelin, a gastric peptide that stimulates appetite, is not reduced with fructose consumption. Fructose may also decrease adiponectin levels, the adipocyte peptide. Adiponectin improves insulin sensitivity independent of obesity. Thus, the normal regulatory mechanisms associated with carbohydrate (as well as fat or protein) consumption do not function optimally in a diet high in HFCS, leading to increased appetite, energy intake, and weight gain. This effect is seen predominately in liquid vs. solid foods. Fructose consumption is associated with insulin resistance, increased energy intake, impaired metabolism, weight gain, dyslipidemias, and hypertension.[116] Though more research is needed to further clarify the metabolic and endocrine effects of fructose consumption, sufficient data exist on the adverse consequences of fructose on body weight, adiposity, and the metabolic indexes associated with insulin resistance to recommend dramatic reductions HFCS in our food supply. (It is important to note that the quantities of fructose consumed in fruit are significantly lower than in sweetened beverages, and the metabolic effects of fructose in fruit are modified by increased intake of fiber, micronutrients, phytonutrients, and antioxidants.)

Refined carbohydrates and sugars. High glycemic index (GI) or glycemic load (GL) foods lead to obesity,[117] heart disease,[118] diabetes, cognitive impairment,[119] dementia, and cancer (colon, breast, prostate, pancreas).[120] Insulin resistance or metabolic syndrome affects 80 million Americans.[ii,121] In 1997, the average American "consumed a record average 154 pounds of caloric sweeteners. That amounted to more than two-fifths of a pound—or 53 teaspoonfuls—of added sugars per person per day … ."[122] This is a sharp contrast to the estimated 20 teaspoons *per year* eaten by our genetically similar Paleolithic ancestors. This pattern of eating carries with it multiple adverse effects, including weight gain, increased caloric consumption, increased hunger, decrease in the efficiency of energy utilization,[123] and adverse effects on the mesolimbic dopaminergic system, which links sugar consumption and drug addiction through stimulation of similar neural reward pathways.[124] These foods also increase catecholamines, cortisol, inflammatory markers such as C-reactive protein, interleukin-6 and tumor necrosis factor-α, and markers of coagulopathy such as PAI-1 and fibrinogen. High GI foods or GL meals lead to hyperinsulinemia, elevated triglycerides, low HDL, hypertension, elevated waist-to-hip ratio or visceral obesity, decreased adiponectin, autonomic dysfunction, non-alcoholic steatohepatitis, hyperuricemia, hormonal disorders such as polycystic ovary syndrome in women and infertility and low testosterone in men, as well as mood swings, anxiety, depression, and fatigue.

Unfortunately, despite this litany of adverse effects, refined carbohydrates and sugars are ever present in our diet. White bread, sugar, pasta, white rice, and white potatoes are quickly absorbed starches with a high glycemic index.[125] Consumption of these foods has increased dramatically since the introduction of the food pyramid that advises us to eat 6–11 servings of rice, bread, cereal, and pasta a day. Soft drinks or sugar-sweetened beverages and alcohol in excess contribute to the problem as well. Care should be taken in reading food labels to identify sugar in other guises, such as high-fructose corn syrup, sucrose, glucose, maltose, dextrose, lactose, fructose, corn syrup, or white grape juice concentrate. Sugar is sugar by any other name; this includes honey, barley malt, maple sugar, sucanat, natural cane sugar, or dehydrated cane juice. Food processors do not have to state if there is added sugar in their products. They are required only to list the total grams of sugar. It is best to avoid or reduce hidden sugars in all foods, including (but not limited to) ketchup, salad dressings, luncheon meats, canned fruits, bread, peanut butter, crackers, soups, sausage, yogurt, relish, cheese dips, chewing gum, and breakfast cereals, and to choose foods with a low glycemic index or meals with a low glycemic load.[126]

Harmful Non-Nutritive Food Additives: Intentional and Unintentional

Artificial sweeteners. Aspartame (NutraSweet®),[127] neotame, acesulfame potassium, saccharin, sucralose, and dihydrochalcones are consumed by two-thirds of adults and are significant components of our diets. Questions remain about their safety, including both short- and long-term risks. The manufacturers of these products largely publish the safety data;[iii] and post-market surveillance and monitoring are limited. Aspartame, an excitotoxin,[128] provides an example of the potential problems of non-nutritive sweeteners in our diet. Some studies suggest adverse effects,[129,130,131] including toxicity from methanol and formaldehyde[132] derived from the amino acids in aspartame. Methanol, a toxic alcohol, is present in small quantities in aspartame; however, when heated (in a soda can on a hot day, or in a hot truck during transport, for example) more methanol is created, leading to the possibility of more serious toxic effects. Other effects include stimulation of hunger through the cephalic phase insulin response; a number of studies have shown that aspartame ingestion may actually lead to increased food/calorie intake.[133,134] Animal and human studies show that aspartame may disrupt brain chemistry[135] and induce neurophysiological changes that might increase seizure risk,[136] depres-

[ii] Estimates range from 47 million to over 100 million, depending on the criteria used. Recent data suggest that even those who do not meet the current criteria for glucose intolerance (2 hour sugar >140mg/dl) have a graded increase for cardiovascular risk and angiographic lesions. It is likely that over 90% of the 65% of Americans who are overweight (figure from U.S. population data) have some degree of insulin resistance, making the prevalence much greater.

[iii] Of 166 studies, 74 had at least partial industry-related funding and 92 were independently funded. While 100% of industry-funded studies conclude aspartame is safe, 92% of independently funded research identified aspartame as a potential cause of adverse effects.

sion,[137] and headaches.[138,139] While conclusions have yet to be reached with regard to the specific outcomes in humans or safe dosage effects, the existing evidence warrants vigilance. Until better data on long-term risks of non-nutritive sweeteners are available, physicians should caution their patients about the use of such substances, in light of the conflicting safety data.

Sorbitol, malitol, and xylitol are common non-absorbed sugar alcohol sweeteners found in food; they can be responsible for increased intestinal gas production, bloating, and abdominal pain.

Intentional food additives. The FDA has approved the use of almost 4,000 food additives. Most of these are studied as single agents in animal models to determine risk, but it is humans who consume them, in large quantities and in multiple combinations that have never been studied. A 1985 study reported that the average American consumes 13–15 grams of these per day—nearly three teaspoons full or about five pounds of additives a year. The main types of food additives include coloring agents, antioxidants, emulsifiers, stabilizers, stimulants, flavorings, preservatives, and artificial sweeteners. Specific additives that can cause symptoms include tartrazine (FD&C yellow #5), sulfites, nitrates and nitrites, BHT, BHA, and aspartame.

Tartrazine is banned in Sweden because of adverse reactions, including hives, asthma, eczema, and other allergic conditions. This is a common coloring in foods and many drugs, including some antihistamines, antibiotics, steroids, and sedatives. Sulfites are common in wine and dried fruits, and are sprayed on fresh foods such as salad bars and shrimp; they often cause allergic reactions, including hives, asthma, and even death. Detoxification of sulfites is impaired with molybdenum deficiency. Nitrates and nitrites are known gastric carcinogens. BHT (butylated hydroxytoluene) and BHA (butylated hydroxyanisole) are the most common antioxidants in prepared and packaged foods; they can cause hives.

MSG, a common flavor enhancer found in many commercially prepared foods, is responsible for the "Chinese restaurant syndrome," and can cause other symptoms and reactions, including headaches, trouble thinking, memory loss, and fainting spells. This additive is especially dangerous, as it often lurks covertly.

Petrochemical pesticides, herbicides, fumigants, hormones, and antibiotics. The Environmental Protection Agency (EPA) has been monitoring human exposure to toxic environmental chemicals since 1972, when they began the National Human Adipose Tissue Survey (NHATS). This endeavor involves the analysis of levels of various toxins in fat tissues from cadavers and elective surgeries (ever wonder what happens to fat removed during liposuction?). Five of the most toxic chemicals were found in 100% of samples: OCDD, a dioxin, styrene, 1,4-dichlorobenzene, xylene, and ethylphenol. Nine additional chemicals were found in 91–98% of samples: benzene, toluene, ethylbenzene, DDE (a breakdown product of DDT, banned in the US since 1972), three dioxins, and one furan. Polychlorinated biphenyls (PCBs) were found in 83% of the population. A Michigan study found DDT in over 70% of four year olds, probably received through breast milk. In the context of our global economy, it's possible to eat food that was picked a day before in Guatemala, Indonesia, or Asia, where the use of pesticides is much less regulated. Many of these chemicals are stored in fat tissue, making animal products concentrated sources. One hundred percent of beef, as well as 93% of processed cheese, hot dogs, bologna, turkey, and ice cream are all contaminated with DDT. Children fed an organic diet have significantly lower pesticide levels in urine samples than children fed a conventional diet.[140]

Beyond chemicals, other potential hazards in foods include hormones and resistant microorganisms, or bacteria. Dairy products contain various growth hormones (BGH) and residues of synthetic estrogens, such as diethylstilbestrol (DES), used to stimulate growth. Antibiotic-resistant bacteria that originated from animal sources have been isolated in humans. We now have trans-species (chicken to human) resistance of bacteria. "The Union of Concerned Scientists recently estimated that, each year, 24.6 million lb (11.2 million kg) of antimicrobials are given to animals for non-therapeutic purposes and 2 million lb (900,000 kg) are given for therapy; in contrast, 3 million lb (1.3 million kg) are given to humans."[141]

The potential health risks of these substances include problems with immunity, such as decreased resistance to infection and increased autoimmunity, toxin-associated cancers, neurologic damage and neurodegenerative diseases such as Parkinson's disease,[142,143] and hormonal disruptions such as infertility and thyroid disorders.[144,145]

Mercury. Predatory fish (swordfish, shark, tile fish, king fish, tuna) consumption is a significant source of mercury exposure in our diet and has been associated with toxic effects on the immune, nervous, cardiovascular, renal, gastrointestinal, and dermatologic systems.[146] Mechanisms of toxicity include damage to DNA, RNA, mitochondria, enzymes, immunopathology, and autoimmunity. Mercury can act as a metabolic uncoupler, hapten or immune-sensitizing small molecule, and enzyme inhibitor by binding irreversibly to the sulfhydryl-containing proteins. Avoidance of mercury-containing fish is an important way to reduce risk. The Environmental Protection Agency (EPA) has established guidelines for safe fish consumption; these are provided on their website.[147]

Genetically engineered foods. The scientific literature documenting the benefits and risks of genetically modified (GM) foods is replete with opinion and weak on science.[148] There are many claims for potential benefits and few published studies about potential risks. Unfortunately, there are no clear conclusions on harm or benefit.

Proposed benefits include: improvement in fruit and vegetable shelf-life and organoleptic quality; improved nutritional quality and health benefits in foods; improved protein and carbohydrate content of foods; improved fat quality; improved quality and quantity of meat, milk and livestock; the use of GM livestock to grow organs for transplant into humans; increased crop yields; improvement in agriculture through breeding insect-, pest-, disease-, and weather-resistant and herbicide-tolerant crops; use of GM plants as bio-factories to yield raw materials for industrial uses; use of GM organisms in drug manufacture, in recycling and/or removal of toxic industrial wastes.

Controversies and risks proposed include: alteration in nutritional quality of foods, potential toxicity, possible antibiotic resistance from GM crops, potential allergenicity and carcinogenicity from consuming GM foods, environmental pollution, unintentional gene transfer to wild plants, possible creation of new viruses and toxins, limited access to seeds due to patenting of GM food plants, threat to crop genetic diversity, and religious, cultural and ethical concerns.[149] Unfortunately, financial and political interests cloud open scientific inquiry, and fear of harm interferes with honest evaluation of potential benefits. Prudence suggests caution until further, and more long-term, studies are completed to evaluate the risks to human health. We can hope that a significant portion of those studies will be funded by a completely disinterested source.

In addition to guidelines provided throughout this chapter, the following suggestions can help all of us minimize the risks in our food supply:

1. Eliminate *trans* fats.
2. Eliminate artificial sweeteners and HFCS.
3. Eat organic plant and animal foods to minimize risk of ingesting petrochemicals, hormones, and antibiotics.
4. Eliminate large predatory fish such as tuna, swordfish, tile fish, and shark (see EPA fish advisory for mercury content of food to reduce intake of mercury).
5. Minimize intake of GMO or genetically modified foods until further data clarify the safety profile.

We can also become more aware of preserving the healing components of food through proper storage and preparation. Nutrients are highest in fresh, local, and organic foods. Food handling may damage nutrients through excessive exposure to heat, light, air and water. For example, essential oils are damaged by high heat and exposure to light; nuts and seeds oxidize if left at room temperature. Phytonutrients are delicate and may need special preparation to maximize their healing potential. Microwaving foods increases the advanced glycation end products (AGEs), thereby increasing oxidative stress and inflammation when microwaved foods are consumed. Here are a few guidelines for maintaining maximum healing properties of foods:

- Choose fresh, whole, unprocessed foods.
- Choose foods that are organic and locally grown when possible.
- Include a wide diversity of colorful plant foods to maximize the intake of phytonutrients, vitamins, and minerals.
- Avoid high heat preparation of fruits and vegetables and overcooking.
- Do not microwave food.
- Store food in airtight, dark containers to reduce oxidation.
- Keep oils and oil-containing foods (nuts and seeds) in dark, airtight containers in cool or cold storage to prevent oxidation.

Summary

Diet and Nutrition in the Clinical Setting: The Clinician's Role

The clinician provides treatment. The skilled therapeutic use of diet and nutrition, while powerful, can be a challenging tool to apply in the management of disease. Despite the fact that specific dietary programs or interventions may not have been thoroughly studied, a collective view of the current body of literature provides a rich and solid foundation for dietary recommendations that address the underlying causes of disease and restore normal physiologic functions. When analyzed from an evolutionary perspective, diet can be understood, not just as a source of energy, but also as *the* central way in which our genes interact with our environment. Part of the clinician's job is to communicate this clearly to patients, along with basic knowledge about the risks in our common dietary patterns and in our food supply.

The known and unknown components in our diet influence, in a moment-to-moment way, the biologic mediators and cellular communication that determine health or disease. Understanding this unique quality of food gives the practitioner a sharp tool with which to attack chronic disease. Food, and the amino acids, fatty acids, carbohydrates, fibers, vitamins, minerals, and phytonutrients contained within it, directly influence hormone and neurotransmitter functioning, including the HPA axis, insulin, adrenal, thyroid, and sex hormones; redox status and mitochondrial bioenergetics; inflammatory and immune mediators; detoxification enzyme functions, digestive function and gut ecology; as well as cell membrane status, sarcopenia, and structural health. In short, diet provides the clinician with an effective point of access to the entire functional medicine matrix.

Understanding these processes gives the practitioner a new way to assess and treat common clinical problems. The process of finding the "right diet" for an individual patient can be daunting; however, a careful medical and family history, physical examination, and focused testing can help clarify a patient's unique needs. Those needs may also change over the course of the patient's life, or the course of an illness. What might agree with them at one moment, might not at another, and then might again later. This is the art of applied nutritional science.

The clinician educates. Most people accept that too many calories, or too much fat, or too much sugar is bad for them, and they are aware that reducing their intake of those foods may prevent obesity and cancer. However, the deeper relationship between food and health and disease is still a surprise to many patients. The role of the clinician is to delineate for the patient the ways in which diet creates imbalance, and can also be used to create balance, reverse dysfunction, and restore health. Clinicians can use food to resolve many of their patients' difficult chronic conditions. From a practical perspective, the most powerful and pervasive therapeutic tools a clinician has are diet and nutrition. These have a greater effect in the prevention and treatment of chronic disease than any medication or therapy, except perhaps exercise.

The clinician helps patients change behavior. The prevailing belief is that patients want easy answers and are unwilling to change dietary or lifestyle habits. My assertion is that we, as clinicians, have too often abdicated the role of mentor in helping patients change. (A vital piece of the puzzle is provided in Chapter 36, where information is presented on one very successful method of helping patients to change unhealthy behaviors.) Patients are often willing to change or adjust their diet if they are given the right information, are taught to shop, choose, and prepare healing foods, and to understand how to balance their metabolism through food. If both patients and practitioners are empowered with the belief that changing dietary habits can help to resolve their symptoms and create good health, then change becomes simpler. Admonishing the patient to lose weight and exercise, without translating that advice into practical information adapted to the patient's environment, resources, and psychological readiness, is not helpful and is often strikingly unsuccessful. Clinicians may need to "reinvent" their clinical practices to become more effective at achieving these goals. The anachronistic model of an eight-minute office visit is neither effective, nor cost-effective, in helping patients to change. New models must be explored, including group-delivered care, group-delivered education, nutritionist referrals, cooking classes, collective guided experiences with elimination or detoxification diets, and networking with community resources for exercise and stress management. The days of therapeutic nihilism in nutritional therapy have come to a close. A new opportunity is available to use nutritional science and its clinical application to empower patients, enhance clinical outcomes, reduce costs, and transform our healthcare system.

Training Programs

- Applying Functional Medicine in Clinical Practice (AFMCP), The Institute for Functional Medicine (www.functionalmedicine.org)
- Rosenthal Center for Complementary and Alternative Medicine, Columbia University (www.rosenthal.hs.columbia.edu)
- The Program in Integrative Medicine, University of Arizona http://integrativemedicine.arizona.edu
- Continuum Center for Health and Healing, Albert Einstein College of Medicine (www.healthandhealingny.org)

A listing of internet-based resources for healthcare practitioners is available in the Appendix.

Micronutrient Insufficiency Leads to DNA and Mitochondrial Damage

Bruce N. Ames, PhD[iv]

Introduction

An optimum intake of micronutrients and metabolites, which varies with age and genetic constitution, would tune up metabolism and contribute to a marked increase in health, particularly for the poor, young, obese, and elderly, at little cost. The focus for this tune up would be in three areas:

- Preventing DNA damage. Deficiency of vitamins B12, folic acid, B6, C or E, or iron or zinc appears to mimic radiation in damaging DNA by causing single- and double-strand breaks, oxidative lesions or both. Half of the population may be deficient in at least one of these micronutrients.
- Preventing other problems associated with common micronutrient deficiencies of, for example, iron, zinc or biotin, which can cause mitochondrial decay with oxidant leakage leading to accelerated aging, DNA damage, and neural decay.
- Repairing mitochondrial oxidative decay, which is a major contributor to aging and increased mutagenic oxidants, can be ameliorated by feeding old rats the normal mitochondrial metabolites acetyl carnitine and lipoic acid at high levels.

Intake of the 40 essential micronutrients (vitamins, minerals, and other biochemicals that humans require) is commonly thought to be adequate. Classic deficiency diseases such as scurvy, beriberi, and pernicious anemia are rare. The evidence suggests, however, that much chronic metabolic damage occurs between the level that causes acute micronutrient deficiency disease and the recommended dietary allowances (RDAs). In addition, the prevention of more subtle metabolic damage may not be addressed by current RDAs. When one input in the metabolic network is inadequate, repercussions are felt on a large number of systems and can lead to degenerative deficiency disease. This may, for example, result in an increase in DNA damage (and cancer), or neuron decay (and cognitive dysfunction) or mitochondrial decay (and accelerated aging and degenerative diseases). The optimum amount of folic acid or zinc that is truly "required" is the amount that maximizes a healthy lifespan; that amount is likely to be higher than the amount needed to prevent acute deficiency disease. The requirements of the elderly for vitamins and metabolites are likely to be different from those of the young, but this issue has not been seriously examined. An optimal intake of micronutrients and metabolites also varies with genetic constitution. A tune-up of micronutrient metabolism should give a marked increase in health at little cost. It is a distortion of priorities for much of the world's population to have an inadequate intake of a vitamin or mineral, at great cost to individual health and to the economy, when a year's supply of a daily multivitamin/mineral pill as insurance against deficiencies costs less than a few packs of cigarettes. The poor, and the obese, in general, eat the worst diets and have the most to gain from multivitamin/mineral supplementation and improvement in diet.

[iv] This study was supported by the National Foundation for Cancer Research Grant M2661, The National Center for Minority Health and Health Disparities Grant P60 MD00222, The Department of Defense Prostate Cancer Research Program W81XWH-05-1-0106 and The National Center for Complementary and Alternative Medicine R21 AT001918 and Research Scientist Award K05 AT001323. This paper has been adapted in part from Ames, BN. A role for supplements in optimizing health: the metabolic tune-up. Arch Biochem Biophys. 2004;423:227-34.

The Calorie-Rich, Micronutrient-Poor Diet

For most of human evolution, calorie shortage was likely to have limited population growth, and as food was mostly calorie-poor and unprocessed, micronutrients may have been fairly adequate. The advent of agriculture changed that, and diets became less varied. The introduction of the potato to Europe from South America in the late 1500s markedly increased the European population over the next few centuries, as the cultivation of potatoes spread and as cultivars were selected that thrived in each climate. "In 1845 close to 40% of the population of Ireland lived chiefly on potatoes. The emergence of the 'potato people' occurred against the background of the quadrupling of the population after 1700 … ."[150] Rice was clearly the main factor enabling high population density in Asia. The introduction of the sweet potato from the New World to New Guinea also was associated with a marked increase in the population.[151,152] Now, carbohydrate and fat calories come with few micronutrients and are remarkably inexpensive, soft drinks with a high content of sugar are consumed instead of water, and the U.S. and other countries have an obesity epidemic associated with micronutrient malnutrition.[153]

Why Micronutrients?

Although optimal nutrition will benefit many degenerative diseases, and although optimal nutrition clearly involves more than micronutrients (e.g., fiber), there are important reasons for focusing on micronutrients and health, particularly DNA damage and mitochondrial damage:[154,155]

- More than 20 years of effort to improve the American diet have not been notably successful, particularly for the poor, although the effort should continue. A parallel approach that focuses on micronutrient malnutrition is overdue and might be more successful, because it should be easier to convince people to take a multivitamin/mineral pill as insurance against ill health than to change their diet appreciably.
- A multivitamin/mineral pill is inexpensive, recognized as safe, and supplies the range of vitamins and minerals that a person requires, although not the essential omega-3 fatty acids. Inadequate intakes of omega-3 fatty acids are widespread and are important for brain function.[156] Fish oil supplements with these essential fatty acids are available and inexpensive. Inadequate fiber intakes, both soluble and insoluble, are widespread.[157] Fiber supplementation is also inexpensive.

Fortification of food is another approach that is useful, e.g., the recent U.S. folate fortification. However, fortification of food does not allow for differences between individuals. For example, menstruating women need more iron than men or older women, who may be getting too much. That is why two types of vitamin pills are marketed: one with iron and one without. With more knowledge, it seems likely that a variety of multivitamin pills will be developed reflecting more specific knowledge about needs that vary with age, sex, genetics, etc.

DNA Damage from Vitamin and Mineral Deficiencies

DNA damage, which is a cause of cancer (although not the only one), is recognized as deleterious and can be assayed easily and relatively inexpensively in human white cells during intervention studies, in contrast to cancer. Our strategy in the laboratory has been to use a variety of human cell lines in culture, to cause growth limitation by deficiency of a particular micronutrient and then to measure DNA damage by a variety of assays, followed by human intervention studies. We are also developing improved assays for measuring DNA damage in humans. Deficiency of vitamins B12, folic acid, B6, niacin, C or E, and iron or zinc appears to mimic radiation in damaging DNA by causing single- and double-strand breaks, oxidative lesions, or both. Half of the population may be deficient in at least one of these micronutrients.[158,159] Micronutrient deficiency may contribute to some of the increased cancer in the quarter of the population that eats the fewest fruits and vegetables (five to nine portions a day is advised), when compared to the quarter with the highest intake. Eighty percent of American children and adolescents and 68% of adults do not eat five portions a day.[160] A major source of some vitamins such as folate is fruits and vegetables. Low folate intake has been associated with several types of cancer (see below). Heart disease is also associated with low fruit and vegetable intake and some of this effect appears due to micronutrient content.[161]

Folate

Folate deficiency causes disruption of DNA synthesis, repair, and methylation, which leads to chromosome breaks due to massive incorporation of uracil in human DNA.[162] Subsequent single-strand breaks in DNA form during base-excision repair; two nearby single-strand breaks on opposite strands cause the chromosome to break. The level of folate at which we see high uracil and breaks was, before the recent flour supplementation, the level that 25% of the U.S. population and close to 50% of poor urban minorities experienced due to poor diets.

Our current understanding of folate deficiency and its relationship to cancer illustrates the importance of considering the findings of all types of research—epidemiological, molecular, clinical, and interventional—when investigating the link between diet and cancer. There is much epidemiological evidence indicating that low folate intake increases the risk of many types of cancer.[163] As shown in Table 26.20, reduced folate intake has been associated with a higher risk of colon cancer,[164,165] and long-term use of a folate-containing supplement has been shown to lower the risk of colon cancer by 75%.[166] There is also some evidence that low folate intake increases the risk of breast cancer,[167,168] pancreatic cancer in smokers,[169,170] and gastric, ovarian, and oesophageal cancers.[171,172]

In vitro studies have shown that folic-acid deficiency causes a dose-dependent increase in uracil incorporation into human lymphocyte DNA.[173] Folate administration reduces both DNA uracil incorporation and the occurrence of chromosome breaks in human cells.[174] *Ex vivo* experiments have shown that all the markers of chromosome damage in human lymphocytes are minimized at folic-acid concentrations that are higher than the RDA.[175,176,177] Folate supplementation above the RDA has also been shown to reduce chromosome breakage in humans.[178,179] In other studies, chromosome breaks have been linked to cancer.[180]

A clue to the folate-cancer connection was the discovery of a polymorphism (C677T) in the gene that encodes methylene-THF reductase (MTHFR)—the enzyme that reduces methylene-tetrahydrofolate (CH2=THF) to methyl THF. This polymorphism decreases the activity of MTHFR, which increases the methylene-THF pool at the expense of the methyl-THF pool, resulting in decreased incorporation of uracil into DNA and a decreased number of chromosome breaks. It is a common polymorphism in populations of people who live in northern regions of the world, with 5–25% of individuals being homozygous for this polymorphism and up to 50% being heterozygous.

Several studies have shown a two- to four-fold lower risk of colon cancer in individuals who are homozygous for the 677T allele of methylene-THF reductase (MTHFR-TT), compared with individuals who are homozygous for the C677 allele and have a high folate intake.[181,182,183,184,185,186,187] At low folate levels, however, the MTHFR-TT genotype does not seem to be protective and might even be a risk factor. Other studies on adenomatous polyps show an increased risk for developing the MTHFR-TT genotype.[188,189,190] Adult acute lymphocytic leukemia (ALL)[191] and childhood ALL[192] have also been inversely associated with the MTHFR-TT genotype, indicating that folate deficiency might promote ALL. (See Table 26.20.)

Unfortunately, the MTHFR-TT genotype is not all good news. As the lower level of MTHFR decreases the methyl-THF pool, it increases serum levels of homocysteine—a risk factor for endothelial-cell damage and cardiovascular disease.[193] Individuals who are homozygous for this allele have a two-fold increase in plasma homocysteine levels.

Low dietary intake of folate, B12, or B6 has been associated with a higher risk for developing cervical squamous epithelial lesions in a case-control study.[194] In contrast to studies mentioned above, individuals with the MTHFR-TT genotype also had a higher incidence of cervical cancer. The authors suggest this is due to a lack of inhibitory methylation—that results from a decreased methyl-THF pool—of human papillomavirus (HPV), which is a significant cause of cervical cancer.[195]

Why is this polymorphism so frequent in populations in northern Europe? Although it is credible that these populations were, historically, chronically folate deficient because of their diet, cancer and heart disease come too late in life to select for individuals with a lower risk. The MTHFR-TT genotype might be selected for based on its ability to reduce uracil incorporation into sperm DNA, which consequently results in less DNA damage in offspring.[196,197] Levels of non-methyl THFs are positively associated with sperm count and density.[198] Folate levels are therefore also important for male reproductive function, and further support the

Table 26.20 **Evidence for Folate, B6, and B12 Deficiency and Cancer Risk**

Type of Cancer	Comments	References
Colorectal cancer, adenomas	Lower intake of folate was associated with higher risk of colon cancer; long-term use of folate supplement lowers the risk of colon cancer by 75%.	165, 166, 316
	No association was seen between folate, B6, and B12 and risk of colorectal hyperplastic polyps.	*See below.
Breast cancer	Strong inverse association was seen between folate intake and risk of breast cancer among women who drink alcohol, which interferes with folate absorption.	167, 168
	No association was seen between folate and B6 and breast cancer.	214
Pancreatic cancer	Risk of pancreatic cancer in smokers was inversely associated with dietary folate.	169, 170
Oesophageal and gastric cancers	Folate and vitamin B6 were inversely associated, and vitamin B12 was positively associated, with these cancers in a case–control study.	172
Acute lymphoblastic leukemia—children	Acute lymphoblastic leukemia (ALL) was inversely associated with the variant MTHFR genotypes, indicating a role for folate in the development of ALL.	192
Acute lymphocytic leukemia—adults	A significant reduction in risk of ALL was found in those with the MTHFR 677TT genotype, indicating that folate deficiency might be a risk factor.	187
Cervical cancer	Risk of invasive cervical cancer was elevated for women with higher serum homocysteine.	217
	Dietary intakes of folate, B6, and B12 were inversely related to the risk of developing cervical dysplasia.	194
	No statistically significant association between folate, B12, and cervical cancer was found.	213
Prostate cancer	Lower intake of B6 was associated with prostate cancer.	215
Lung cancer	Lower intake of B6 (higher B6 serum level) was associated with lung cancer.	216
Ovarian cancer	Low dietary folate intake was associated with ovarian cancer, especially among woman who consumed alcohol (2 drinks/day).	171

*Ulrich CM, Kampman E, Bigler J, et al. Lack of association between the C677T MTHFR polymorphism and colorectal hyperplastic polyps. Cancer Epidemiology, Biomarkers and Prevention. 2000;9:427-433.

concept that folate deficiency can cause DNA damage. Germ-line damage to the sperm has also been linked to childhood cancers.[199] Further studies are required to determine if ALL is higher in children whose fathers have a poor diet.[200]

Vitamins B12 and B6

Vitamin B12 deficiency would be expected to cause chromosome breaks by the same uracil-misincorporation mechanism that is found with folate deficiency.[201] Both B12 and methyl-THF are required for the methylation of homocysteine to methionine. If cells are deficient in either folate or B12, homocysteine accumulates. When B12 is deficient, tetrahydrofolate is trapped as methyl-THF, reducing the methylene-THF pool, which is required for methylation of deoxyuridine monophosphate (dUMP) to deoxythymidine monophosphate (dTMP). B12 deficiency, like folate deficiency, therefore causes uracil to accumulate in DNA (author's unpublished observations). In a study of healthy elderly men[202] and young adults, increased chromosome breakage was associated with low dietary intake of either B12 or folate, or with elevated levels of homocysteine.[203,204,205] B12 supplementation above the RDA was necessary to minimize chromosome breakage.[206,207]

Vitamin B6 deficiency would also be expected to result in uracil misincorporation. B6 deficiency causes a decrease in the enzyme activity of serine hydroxymethyl transferase, which supplies the methylene group for methylene-THF.[208] Several studies have shown that, in individuals with the MTHFR-TT genotype, vitamin B6 intake is associated with protection against colon cancer and/or adenomas.[209,210,211]

Recent epidemiological studies have indicated an association between B6 or B12 deficiency and cancer prevention, but results are mixed.[212,213,214] In one case–control study of diet and cancer, vitamin B6 deficiency was associated with prostate cancer.[215] A significantly lower risk of lung cancer was found in men with higher serum B6 levels.[216] Compared to men with the lowest vitamin B6 concentrations, men in the highest quintile had about one-half the risk of lung cancer. No associations were made between B12, folate, or homocysteine and lung cancer. Serum homocysteine levels were found to predict the risk of developing invasive cervical cancer in a large case-control study.[217]

Oxidation, Micronutrients, and Cancer Risk

Oxidants are mutagens and are produced as byproducts of normal mitochondrial energy production.[218] Radiation is a known oxidative mutagen. Antioxidant micronutrients, such as vitamins C and E, might function as anti-mutagens and anti-carcinogens.[219,220] The evidence that supplementation with these vitamins lowers cancer risk is inconclusive.

Both experimental and epidemiological data indicate that vitamin C protects against stomach cancer.[221,222,223] This is a plausible conclusion, as oxidative damage from inflammation caused by *Helicobacter pylori* infection is a risk factor for stomach cancer.[224] Fruit and vegetable intake—the main dietary source of vitamin C—is also inversely associated with stomach cancer. Mayne and colleagues have also reported an inverse association between vitamin C and oesophageal adenocarcinoma.[225] Many other studies, however, have reported no effect of vitamin C on cancer risk. A thorough review of intervention studies showed both positive[226] and negative[227] studies, and so the evidence is inconclusive.[228] There are several reasons why a positive effect might not have been observed. The blood cell saturation of vitamin C occurs at about 100 mg/day in humans.[229] Evidence indicates that this level minimizes DNA damage.[230,231,232,233] Perhaps the differing results from various studies were caused by differences in whether vitamin C reached tissue saturation levels in the population that was studied. If only a small proportion of the population had inadequate tissue saturation by vitamin C intake, a real effect would be missed. Other factors that might explain the difference in results include failure to adequately assess vitamin C intake, failure to assess whether people were using vitamin supplements or failure to take into account the effect of modifiers such as body-mass index or smoking (which decreases plasma vitamin C levels).[234]

Many studies have investigated the effects of vitamin C supplementation in humans using biomarkers of oxidative damage to DNA, lipids (lipid oxidation releases mutagenic aldehydes), and protein.[235,236,237,238,239] For example, intervention studies with antioxidant supplements (100 mg per day of vitamin C, 28 mg per day of vitamin E, and 25 mg per day of β-carotene) were found to decrease DNA strand breaks in lymphocytes, as measured by the comet assay.[240] Subsequent studies showed β-carotene by itself was ineffective at reducing the number of DNA breaks,[241] but that vitamin C was effective alone.[242]

Studies in rats have shown that spontaneous oxidative damage occurs at a rate of about 66,000 DNA adducts per diploid cell[243,244] and, unlike uracil misincorporation, is likely to occur with equal frequency on both strands. Repair of oxidative adducts by glycosylase results in transient single-strand breaks in DNA. Increased oxidative damage is therefore associated with low vitamin C intake.[245] Individuals who are deficient in both folate and antioxidant intake would have higher levels of both oxidative damage and uracil incorporation in their DNA, and be expected to have a high level of double-strand DNA breakage. Radiation (an oxidative mutagen) and folate deficiency have been shown to act synergistically in causing chromosome breakage in tissue-culture cells.[246]

Smoking is another producer of oxidative stress. A smoker needs to consume 40% more vitamin C than a non-smoker in order to maintain a comparable blood-plasma level of vitamin C.[247] Several studies have examined the associations between paternal smoking, vitamin C intake, oxidative damage to sperm DNA, and childhood cancer in the offspring. Smoking depletes vitamin C, which is required to protect DNA in sperm against oxidative damage.[248,249,250] Smokers, or men with low ascorbate intake, have lower seminal-plasma ascorbic-acid levels and higher levels of oxidative DNA damage in their sperm than either nonsmokers or men with adequate ascorbate intake.[251,252]

Unfortunately, there have been few studies that have rigorously examined the effect of paternal vitamin C level by itself on cancer in offspring. Nevertheless, there is evidence that children with fathers who smoke have an increased rate of childhood cancer.[253,254,255,256] An epidemiological study from China makes a particularly strong case that ALL, lymphoma, and brain cancer are each increased three- to four-fold in children of male smokers.[257] The associations were strongest in men with the highest number of pack years of smoking. It seems likely, given the available evidence, that the cancer risk to offspring of male smokers would be higher when dietary antioxidant intake is low.

Inadequate Heme Synthesis Causes Mitochondrial Decay and Oxidative DNA Damage

Heme biosynthesis is predominantly in the mitochondria. Interfering with heme synthesis causes specific loss of heme-a, a component of complex IV, with consequent release of oxidants.[258,259] Iron deficiency (25% of menstruating women in the U.S. ingest < 50% of the RDA) also causes release of oxidants and mitochondrial decay,[260] presumably through lack of heme-a.[261] The poor tend to have the lowest levels and intake.[262,263] Biotin deficiency, which is quite common in the population[264,265] also causes defective mitochondrial complex IV and oxidant leakage (Atamna et al., in preparation). There is evidence that deficiency of copper,[266,267] a component of complex IV, or pantothenate[268] (Atamna et al., in preparation) leads to a decrease in complex IV. Zinc deficiency causes marked release of oxidants with marked oxidative damage to DNA,[269,270] due to the inactivation of δ-aminolevulinate dehydratase, an enzyme of heme biosynthesis containing eight zinc atoms (Atamna et al., in preparation). Zinc deficiency is associated with cancer in both humans and rodent models.[271] Zinc intake inadequacy (10% of people in the U.S. ingest < 50% of the RDA) in human cells in culture causes oxidative DNA damage, inactivation of copper, zinc-superoxide dismutase, inactivation of tumor suppressor protein p53 (a zinc protein) and inactivation of oxidative DNA repair; these effects can multiply to cause severe genetic damage.[272,273] The consequences of these various deficiencies are likely to be accelerated aging, neural decay, and cancer.[274,275]

Common micronutrient deficiencies are likely to damage DNA by the same mechanism as radiation and many chemicals, and appear to be orders of magnitude more important.[276,277,278] The need to set micronutrient requirements to minimize DNA damage has been reviewed by Fenech.[279] We have compared radiation with folate deficiency to try to put risks in perspective.[280] The poor and others at risk are not served if huge resources are put into minor hypothetical risks[281] and major risks are not addressed.

Dark Skin, Vitamin D, and Calcium Deficiency

The hormone vitamin D is formed in the skin with the aid of ultraviolet (UV) light from sunlight; however, too much exposure to UV light is dangerous. Humans who originate from northern areas with little UV radiation have light skin to maximize their exposure to UV rays, whereas people from southern areas have dark skin to minimize their UV light exposure. Northern populations in the U.S. are exposed to insufficient sunlight and individuals are often chronically vitamin-D deficient unless they drink vitamin D-fortified milk or take a supplement. Dark-skinned people who don't drink fortified milk and who live in northern cities, such as Boston, Detroit, Cleveland, Chicago, and Seattle, are the people most at risk unless they take a supplement. "Although both dark- and light-skinned individuals can produce vitamin D in response to UV light, this response is much more limited in dark-skinned individuals. The 25-hydroxyvitamin D, or 25(OH)D, levels in African-Americans and Hispanics are, therefore, lower than Caucasians in the U.S."[282] In a study in Boston, 80% of African-Americans and 60% of Hispanics were vitamin D deficient[283] (and M. F. Holick, personal communication). Vitamin D is necessary for calcium mobilization for bone formation, and brittle bones are a consequence of vitamin D deficiency. In addition, there is an inverse relationship between vitamin D intake or levels and several types of cancer, primarily colorectal cancer and colorectal adenomas; there is also evidence for a connection with prostate cancer.[284,285,286,287,288] A higher intake of calcium has been shown to lower risk for colorectal adenoma recurrence.[289] A plausible mechanism by which vitamin D deficiency could increase cancer is the known inhibitory effect of vitamin D metabolites on cell proliferation, an essential component of carcinogenesis.[290] African-Americans have almost double the prostate cancer rate of whites and also have lower levels of the vitamin D metabolite 25(OH)D in their blood.[291] Recent epidemiological studies suggest that much of the increased cancer rate in African Americans is due to vitamin D deficiency.[292]

Dark-skinned people such as African-Americans and some Hispanics tend not to drink milk as adults, because of lactose intolerance. Europeans and other northern people domesticated cows thousands of years ago and developed the ability as adults to metabolize lactose, which is a major sugar in cow's milk. Most of the rest of the world cannot use lactose as adults and therefore show lactose intolerance when they drink cow's milk and tend to avoid it; 70% of African-Americans, 53% of Mexican-Americans and 90% of Asians are lactose intolerant compared to 15% of northern Europeans and their descendants. As African-Americans and Hispanics also tend not to take vitamin supplements, these individuals are all the more likely to be calcium and vitamin D deficient.[293] Most nutrient deficiencies also correlate well with poverty and low education. However, in some cases, such as vitamin D or calcium, it is clear that genetics is an important contributor. African-Americans have lower calcium, magnesium, potassium, and folate intakes than whites.[294] The vitamin D/calcium story illustrates why understanding genetics is important in some cases to develop appropriate interventions for the populations and individuals at risk.

Multivitamins in Humans

Evidence is accumulating that a multivitamin/mineral supplement is good insurance, and would markedly improve health (e.g., heart disease, cancer, immune function, and cataracts), particularly for the poor, the young, the obese, and the elderly.[295,296,297,298,299,300,301,302,303,304,305,306,307] The caveat is, of course, that too much of many of the minerals (e.g., iron, zinc, copper, selenium) and some of the vitamins (e.g., vitamin A, β-carotene) are toxic, though taking a multivitamin/mineral as insurance is not of concern. Mae West's dictum about sex, "Too much of a good thing is wonderful," doesn't apply to micronutrients. Advice to take a multivitamin should always be coupled with advice to eat a good diet, as we also need fiber, omega-3 fatty acids, and other ingredients in a balanced diet.[308] It is also good to keep in mind Mark Twain's caution: "The main distinguishing characteristic between man and the lower animals is the desire to take pills."

Delaying the Mitochondrial Decay of Aging

Oxidative mitochondrial decay is a major contributor to aging.[309,310,311,312,313] We are making progress in reversing some of this decay in old rats by feeding them the normal mitochondrial metabolites acetylcarnitine (ALC) and R-lipoic acid (LA) at high levels. The principle behind this effect appears to be that, with age, increased oxidative damage to protein causes a deformation of the structure of key enzymes with a consequent lessening of affinity (K_m) for the enzyme substrate.[314] The effect of age on decreasing the binding affinity of carnitine acyltransferase for ALC or acetyl CoA can be mimicked by reacting it with malondialdehyde (a lipid-peroxidation product that increases with age). Feeding the substrate ALC with LA, a mitochondrial antioxidant, restores the velocity of the reaction (K_m) for ALC transferase and mitochondrial function.[315] LA is an effective inducer of phase II antioxidant enzymes, including glutathione synthesis, as well as being a potent antioxidant.[316,317,318]

In old rats (vs. young rats), mitochondrial membrane potential, cardiolipin level, respiratory control ratio, and cellular O2 uptake are lower; oxidants/O2, neuron RNA oxidation, and mutagenic aldehydes from lipid peroxidation are higher.[319,320,321,322,323,324,325,326,327] Ambulatory activity and cognition decline with age.[328,329] Feeding old rats ALC with LA for a few weeks restores mitochondrial function; lowers oxidants, neuron RNA oxidation and mutagenic aldehydes; and increases rat ambulatory activity and cognition (as assayed with the Skinner box and Morris water maze).[v,330,331,332] ALC and LA are also effective in improving the aging rat heart.[333] A recent meta-analysis of 21 double-blind clinical trials of acetylcarnitine in the treatment of mild cognitive impairment and mild Alzheimer's disease showed a modest efficacy vs. placebo.[334] A meta-analysis of four clinical trials of lipoic acid for treatment of neuropathic deficits in diabetes showed significant efficacy vs. placebo.[335] One should keep in mind, however, that a micronutrient-poor diet, as pointed out above, accelerates mitochondrial decay.

[v] Dr. Ames is one of the founders of Juvenon (www.juvenon.com), a company that has licensed the University of California patent on acetyl carnitine + lipoic acid for rejuvenating old mitochondria (Ames and T. Hagen, inventors), sells acetyl carnitine + lipoic acid supplements, and does clinical trials on them. Ames's founder's stock was put in a non-profit foundation at the founding in 1999. He is the director of Juvenon's Scientific Advisory Board, but has no stock in the company and has not taken, and will not take, any reimbursement from them.

Public Health

A metabolic tune-up via micronutrient supplementation is likely to have great health benefits, particularly for those with inadequate diets, such as many of the poor, young, obese, and elderly, who are most vulnerable to micronutrient insufficiency. Unfortunately, these needs are not being addressed adequately by the medical community. The issues discussed here highlight the need to educate the public about the crucial importance of optimal nutrition and the potential health benefits of a simple and affordable daily multivitamin/multi-mineral supplement. Tuning up metabolism to maximize the human health span will require scientists, clinicians, and educators to abandon the outdated paradigm of seeing micronutrients as merely preventing deficiency disease, and explore more meaningful ways to prevent chronic disease and achieve optimal health through better nutrition. It is becoming clear that unbalanced diets will be the major contributor to ill health in the population, with smoking following close behind.

References

1. Cordain L, Eaton SB, Sebastian A, et al. Origins and evolution of the Western diet: health implications for the 21st century. Am J Clin Nutr. 2005 Feb;81(2):341-54.
2. Farrell RJ, Kelly CP. Current concepts: celiac sprue. N Engl J Med. 2002; 346:180-88.
3. Fukudome S, Yoshikawa M. Opioid peptides derived from wheat gluten: their isolation and characterization. FEBS Lett. 1992 Jan 13;296(1):107-11.
4. Salmeron J, Manson JE, Stampfer MJ, et al. Dietary fiber, glycemic load, and risk of non–insulin-dependent diabetes mellitus in women. JAMA. 1997;277:472-77.
5. Liu S, Willett WC. Dietary glycemic load and atherothrombotic risk. Curr Atheroscler Rep. 2002;4:454-61.
6. Yach D, Hawkes C, Gould CL, Hofman KJ. Global burden of chronic diseases: overcoming impediments to prevention and control. JAMA. 2004;291(21):26.
7. Rimm EB, Stampfer MJ. Diet, lifestyle, and longevity—the next steps? JAMA. 2004;292(12):1490-92.
8. Knoops KT, de Groot LC, Kromhout D, et al. Mediterranean diet, lifestyle factors, and 10-year mortality in elderly European men and women: the HALE project. JAMA. 2004;292(12):1433-39.
9. Trichopoulou A, Costacou T, Bamia C, Trichopoulos D. Adherence to a Mediterranean diet and survival in a Greek population. N Engl J Med. 2003;348(26):2599-608.
10. Stampfer MJ, Hu FB, Manson JE, et al. Primary prevention of coronary heart disease in women through diet and lifestyle. N Engl J Med. 2000;343:16-22.
11. Hu FB, Manson JE, Stampfer MJ, et al. Diet, lifestyle, and the risk of type 2 diabetes mellitus in women. N Engl J Med. 2001;345:790-97.
12. Platz EA, Willett WC, Colditz GA, et al. Proportion of colon cancer risk that might be preventable in a cohort of middle-aged US men. Cancer Causes Control. 2000;11:579-88.
13. de Lorgeril M, Renaud S, Mamelle N, et al. Mediterranean alpha-linolenic acid-rich diet in secondary prevention of coronary heart disease. Lancet. 1994;343:1454-59. [Published correction appears in: Lancet. 1995;345:738.]
14. Writing Group of the PREMIER Collaborative Research Group. Effects of comprehensive lifestyle modification on blood pressure control: main results of the PREMIER Clinical Trial. JAMA. 2003;289:2083-93.
15. Ornish D, Scherwitz LW, Billings JH, et al. Intensive lifestyle changes for reversal of coronary heart disease. JAMA. 1998;280:2001-7.
16. Studer M, Briel M, Leimenstoll B, et al. Effect of different antilipidemic agents and diet on mortality: a systematic review. Arch Intern Med. 2005;165(7):725-30.
17. Esposito K, Marfella R, Ciotola M, et al. Effect of a Mediterranean-style diet on endothelial dysfunction and markers of vascular inflammation in the metabolic syndrome: a randomized trial. JAMA. 2004;292(12):1440-46.
18. Hu FB, Willett WC. Optimal diets for prevention of coronary heart disease. JAMA. 2002;288:2569-78.
19. Norhammar N, Tenerz Å, Nilsson G, et al. Glucose metabolism in patients with acute myocardial infarction and no previous diagnosis of diabetes mellitus: a prospective study. Lancet. 2002;359:2140-44.
20. Sasso FC, Carbonara C, Nasti R, et al. Glucose metabolism and coronary heart disease in patients with normal glucose tolerance, JAMA, 2004;291:1857-63.
21. Liu S, Willett W. Dietary glycemic load and atherothrombotic risk. Curr Atheroscler Rep. 2002;4:454-61.
22. Liu S, Willett WC, Stampfer MJ, et al. A prospective study of dietary glycemic load, carbohydrate intake, and risk of coronary heart disease in US women. Am J Clin Nutr. 2000;71(6):1455-61.
23. Stachowska E. Dietary trans-fatty acids and composition of human atheromatous plaques. Eur J Nutri. 2004;43:313-18.
24. Mozaffarian D, Pischon T, Hankinson SE, et al. Dietary intake of trans-fatty acids and systemic inflammation in women, Am J Clin Nutr. 2004;79(4):606-12.
25. Yusuf S. Effect of potentially modifiable risk factors associated with myocardial infarction in 52 countries (the INTERHEART study): case-control study. Lancet. 2004;364:937-52.
26. Wijendran V. Dietary n-6 and n-3 fatty acid balance and cardiovascular health. Annu Rev Nutr. 2004;24:597-615.
27. Marchioli R, Barzi F, Bomba E, et al. GISSI-Prevenzione Investigators. Early protection against sudden death by n-3 polyunsaturated fatty acids after myocardial infarction: time-course analysis of the results of the Gruppo Italiano per lo Studio della Sopravvivenza nell'Infarto Miocardico (GISSI)-Prevenzione. Circulation. 2002;105(16):1897-903.
28. Esposito K, Marfella R, Ciotola M, et al. Effect of a Mediterranean-style diet on endothelial dysfunction and markers of vascular inflammation in the metabolic syndrome: a randomized trial. JAMA. 2004;292(12):1440-46.
29. Jenkins DJ, Kendall CW, Marchie A, et al. Effects of a dietary portfolio of cholesterol-lowering foods vs lovastatin on serum lipids and C-reactive protein, JAMA. 2003;290(4):502-10.
30. Davi G, Guagnano MT, Ciabattoni G, et al. Platelet activation in obese women: role of inflammation and oxidant stress. JAMA. 2002;288(16):2008-14.
31. Appel LJ, Champagne CM, Harsha DW, et al. Writing Group of the PREMIER Collaborative Research Group. Effects of comprehensive lifestyle modification on blood pressure control: main results of the PREMIER clinical trial. JAMA. 2003;289(16):2083-93.

32. Steffen LM, Jacobs DR Jr, Stevens J, et al. Associations of whole-grain, refined-grain, and fruit and vegetable consumption with risks of all-cause mortality and incident coronary artery disease and ischemic stroke: the Atherosclerosis Risk in Communities (ARIC) Study. Am J Clin Nutr. 2003;78(3):383-90.
33. Fung TT, Willet WC, Stampfer MJ, et al. Dietary patterns and the risks of coronary heart disease in women. Arch Intern Med. 2001;161:187-62.
34. Hu FB, Stampfer MJ, Manson JE, et al. Dietary fat intake and the risk of coronary heart disease in women. N Engl J Med. 1997;337:1491-99.
35. Appel LJ. The effects of protein intake on blood pressure and cardiovascular disease. Curr Opin Lipidol. 2003;14(1):55-59.
36. Toole JF, Malinow MR, Chambless LE, et al. Lowering homocysteine in patients with ischemic stroke to prevent recurrent stroke, myocardial infarction, and death: The Vitamin Intervention for Stroke Prevention (VISP) randomized controlled trial. JAMA.2004;291:565-57.
37. Farshchi HR, Taylor MA, Macdonald IA. Beneficial metabolic effects of regular meal frequency on dietary thermogenesis, insulin sensitivity, and fasting lipid profiles in healthy obese women. Am J Clin Nutr. 2005;81(1):16-24.
38. Kaput J, Rodriguez RL. Nutritional genomics: the next frontier in the postgenomic era. Physiol Genomics. 2004;16(2):166-77.
39. Ames BN, Elson-Schwab I, Silver EA. High-dose vitamin therapy stimulates variant enzymes with decreased coenzyme binding affinity (increased K(m)): relevance to genetic disease and polymorphisms. Am J Clin Nutr. 2002;75(4):616-58.
40. Piyathilake CJ, Macaluso M, Johanning GL, et al. Methylenetetrahydrofolate reductase (MTHFR) polymorphism increases the risk of cervical intraepithelial neoplasia. Anticancer Res. 2000;20(3A):1751-57.
41. Yin G, Kono S, Toyomura K, et al. Methylenetetrahydrofolate reductase C677T and A1298C polymorphisms and colorectal cancer: The Fukuoka Colorectal Cancer Study. Cancer Sci. 2004;95(11):908-13.
42. Ames BN, Elson-Schwab I, Silver EA. High-dose vitamin therapy stimulates variant enzymes with decreased coenzyme binding affinity (increased K(m)): relevance to genetic disease and polymorphisms. Am J Clin Nutr. 2002;75(4):616-58.
43. Paffenbarger RS. Chair summary and comments. Med Sci Sports Exerc. 2001;3:S493-94.
44. Willett WC. Balancing life-style and genomics research for disease prevention. Science. 2002;296(5568):695-98.
45. London SJ, Yuan JM, Chung FL, et al. Isothiocyanates, glutathione S-transferase M1 and T1 polymorphisms, and lung-cancer risk: a prospective study of men in Shanghai, China. Lancet. 2000;356(9231):724-29.
46. Kelly, G. Insulin resistance: lifestyle and nutritional interventions. Altern Med Rev. 2000;5(2):109-32.
47. Appel LJ. The effects of protein intake on blood pressure and cardiovascular disease. Curr Opin Lipidol. 2003;14(1):55-59.
48. Evans, J, Goldfine, I, Maddux, B. Oxidative stress and stress-activated signaling pathways: a unifying hypothesis of type 2 diabetes. Endocr Rev. 2002;23: 599–622.
49. Tentolouris N, Tsigos C, Perea D, et al. Differential effects of high-fat and high-carbohydrate isoenergetic meals on cardiac autonomic nervous system activity in lean and obese women. Metabolism. 2003;52(11):1426-32.
50. Vicennati V, Ceroni L, Gagliardi L, et al. Comment: response of the hypothalamic-pituitary-adrenocortical axis to high-protein/fat and high-carbohydrate meals in women with different obesity phenotypes. J Clin Endocrinol Metab. 2002;87(8):3984-88.
51. Wynne K, Stanley S, McGowan B, Bloom S. Appetite control. J Endocrinol. 2005;184:291-318.
52. Pereira MA, Swain J, Goldfine AB, et al. Effects of a low-glycemic-load diet on resting energy expenditure and heart disease risk factors during weight loss. JAMA. 2004;292(20):2482-90.
53. Farshchi HR, Taylor MA, Macdonald IA. Beneficial metabolic effects of regular meal frequency on dietary thermogenesis, insulin sensitivity, and fasting lipid profiles in healthy obese women. Am J Clin Nutr. 2005;81(1):16-24.
54. Singletary KW, Gapstur SM. Alcohol and breast cancer: review of epidemiologic and experimental evidence and potential mechanisms JAMA. 2001;286(17):2143-51.
55. Steingraber, S. Living Downstream, Reading (MA): Addison-Wesley, 1997.
56. Velicer CM, Heckbert SR, Lampe JW, et al. Antibiotic use in relation to the risk of breast cancer. JAMA. 2004;291:827.
57. Dijsselbloem N, Vanden Berghe W, De Naeyer A, Haegeman G. Soy isoflavone phyto-pharmaceuticals in interleukin-6 affections. Multi-purpose nutraceuticals at the crossroad of hormone replacement, anti-cancer and anti-inflammatory therapy. Biochem Pharmacol. 2004;68(6):1171-85.
58. Hyman M, Pizzorno J, Weil A. A rational approach to antioxidant therapy and vitamin E. Altern Ther Health Med. 2005;11(1):14.
59. Mattson MP, Wan R. Beneficial effects of intermittent fasting and caloric restriction on the cardiovascular and cerebrovascular systems. J Nutr Biochem. 2005;16(3):129-37.
60. Evans, J, Goldfine, I, Maddux, B. Oxidative stress and stress-activated signaling pathways: a unifying hypothesis of type 2 diabetes. Endocr Rev. 2002;23: 599–622.
61. Trevisan M, Browne R, Ram M, et al. Correlates of markers of oxidative status in the general population. Am J Epidemiol. 2001;154(4):348-56.
62. Anderson, J. Oxidative stress in neurodegeneration: cause or consequence? Nat Rev Neurosci. 2004;5;518-25.
63. Engelhart M, et al. Dietary intake of antioxidants and risk of Alzheimer disease. JAMA. 2002;287(24):3223–29.
64. Sies H, Schewe T, Heiss C, Kelm M. Cocoa polyphenols and inflammatory mediators. Am J Clin Nutr. 2005;81(1);304S-12S.
65. Scalbert A, Johnson IT, Saltmarsh M. Polyphenols: antioxidants and beyond. Am J Clin Nutr. 2005;81(1);215S-17S.
66. Ames B. A role of supplements in optimizing health: the metabolic tune-up. Arch Biochem Biophys. 2004;423:227-34.
67. Samman S, Sandstrom B, Toft MB, et al. Green tea or rosemary extract added to foods reduces nonheme-iron absorption. Am J Clin Nutr. 2001;73(3):607-12.
68. Moskaug JO, Carlsen H, Myhrstad MC, Blomhoff R. Polyphenols and glutathione synthesis regulation Am J Clin Nutr. 2005;81(1 Suppl):277S-83S.
69. Vogler GP, Kozlowski LT. Differential influence of maternal smoking on infant birth weight: gene-environment interaction and targeted intervention. JAMA. 2002;287:241-42.
70. Harris TB. Associations of elevated interleukin-6 and C-reactive protein levels with mortality in the elderly. Am J Med. 1999;106(5):506-12.
71. Liu S, Manson JE, Buring JE, et al. Relation between a diet with a high glycemic load and plasma concentrations of high-sensitivity C-reactive protein in middle-aged women. Am J Clin Nutr. 2002;75(3):492-98.
72. Ridker PM, Buring JE, Cook NR, Rifai N. C-reactive protein, the metabolic syndrome, and risk of incident cardiovascular events: an 8-year follow-up of 14,719 initially healthy American women. Circulation. 2003;107(3):391.

73. Lopez-Garcia E, Schulze MB, Meigs JB, et al. Consumption of trans-fatty acids is related to plasma biomarkers of inflammation and endothelial dysfunction. J Nutr. 2005;135(3):562-66.
74. Zampelas A, Panagiotakos DB, Pitsavos C, et al. Associations between coffee consumption and inflammatory markers in healthy persons: the ATTICA study. Am J Clin Nutr. 2004;80(4):862-67.
75. Tilg H., Diehl AM. Mechanisms of disease: cytokines in alcoholic and nonalcoholic steatohepatitis. N Engl J Med. 2000; 343:1467-76.
76. Adam O, Beringer C, Kless T, et al. Anti-inflammatory effects of a low arachidonic acid diet and fish oil in patients with rheumatoid arthritis. Rheumatol Int. 2003;23(1):27-36.
77. Church TS, Earnest CP, Wood KA, Kampert JB. Reduction of C-reactive protein levels through use of a multivitamin. Am J Med. 2003;115(9):702-7.
78. van Herpen-Broekmans WM, Klopping-Ketelaars IA, Bots ML, et al. Serum carotenoids and vitamins in relation to markers of endothelial function and inflammation. Eur J Epidemiol. 2004;19(10):915-21.
79. Mori TA, Beilin LJ. Omega-3 fatty acids and inflammation. Curr Atheroscler Rep. 2004;6(6):461-67.
80. Ajani UA, Ford ES, Mokdad AH. Dietary fiber and C-reactive protein: findings from national health and nutrition examination survey data. J Nutr. 2004;134(5):1181-85.
81. Kalliomaki M, Salminen S, Arvilommi H, et al. Probiotics in primary prevention of atopic disease: a randomised placebo-controlled trial. Lancet. 2001;357(9262):1076-79.
82. Kohut ML, Senchina DS. Reversing age-associated immunosenescence via exercise. Exerc Immunol Rev. 2004;10:6-41.
83. Sicherer SH. Food allergy. Lancet. 2002;360(9334):701-10.
84. Isolauri E, Rautava S, Kalliomaki M. Food allergy in irritable bowel syndrome: new facts and old fallacies. Gut. 2004;53(10):1391-93.
85. Atkinson W, Sheldon TA, Shaath N, Whorwell PJ. Food elimination based on IgG antibodies in irritable bowel syndrome: a randomised controlled trial. Gut. 2004;53(10):1459-64.
86. Farrell RJ, Kelly CP. Current concepts: celiac sprue. N Engl J Med. 2002; 346:180-188.
87. Lee SK, Green PH. Endoscopy in celiac disease. Curr Opin Gastroenterol. 2005;21(5):589-94.
88. Alaedini A, Green PH.Narrative review: Celiac disease: Understanding a complex autoimmune disorder. Ann Intern Med. 2005;142(4):289-98.
89. Cordain L, Eaton SB, Sebastian A, et al. Origins and evolution of the Western diet: health implications for the 21st century. Am J Clin Nutr. 2005;81(2):341-54.
90. Gershon M. The Second Brain. Perennial Currents, 1999.
91. Bourlioux P, Koletzko B, Guarner F, Braesco V. The intestine and its microflora are partners for the protection of the host: report on the Danone Symposium "The Intelligent Intestine," held in Paris, June 14, 2002. Am J Clin Nutr. 2003;78(4):675-83.
92. Isolauri, E. Probiotics in human disease, Am J Clin Nutr. 2001;73(suppl):1142S-46S.
93. Duggan C, Gannon J, Walker WA. Protective nutrients and functional foods for the gastrointestinal tract. Am J Clin Nutr. 2002;75(5):789-808.
94. Bourlioux P, Koletzko B, Guarner F, Braesco V. The intestine and its microflora are partners for the protection of the host: report on the Danone Symposium "The Intelligent Intestine," held in Paris, June 14, 2002. Am J Clin Nutr. 2003;78(4):675-83.
95. Roubenoff R, Hughes VA. Sarcopenia: current concepts. J Gerontol A Biol Sci Med Sci. 2000;55(12):M716-24.
96. Janssen I, Shepard DS, Katzmarzyk PT, Roubenoff R. The healthcare costs of sarcopenia in the United States. J Am Geriatr Soc. 2004;52(1):80-85.
97. Volpi E, Sheffield-Moore M, Rasmussen BB, Wolfe RR. Basal muscle amino acid kinetics and protein synthesis in healthy young and older men. JAMA. 2001;286(10):1206-12.
98. Russell RM. Changes in gastrointestinal function attributed to aging. Am J Clin Nutr. 1992;55(6 Suppl):1203S-07S.
99. Volpi E, Kobayashi H, Sheffield-Moore M, et al. Essential amino acids are primarily responsible for the amino acid stimulation of muscle protein anabolism in healthy elderly adults. Am J Clin Nutr. 2003;78(2):250-58.
100. Roubenoff R, Hughes VA. Sarcopenia: current concepts. J Gerontol A Biol Sci Med Sci. 2000;55(12):M716-24.
101. Roubenoff R. Catabolism of aging: is it an inflammatory process? Curr Opin Clin Nutr Metab Care. 2003;6(3):295-99.
102. Fulle S, Protasi F, Di Tano G, et al. The contribution of reactive oxygen species to sarcopenia and muscle ageing. Exp Gerontol. 2004;39(1):17-24.
103. Salehian B, Kejriwal K. Glucocorticoid-induced muscle atrophy: mechanisms and therapeutic strategies. Endocr Pract. 1999;5(5):277-81.
104. Ascherio A, Willett WC. Health effects of trans-fatty acids Am J Clin Nutr. 1997;66:1006-10.
105. Willett WC. Balancing life-style and genomics research for disease prevention. Science. 2002;296(5568):695-98.
106. Bray GA, Lovejoy JC, Smith SR, et al. The influence of different fats and fatty acids on obesity, insulin resistance and inflammation. J Nutr. 2002;132(9):2488-91.
107. Kohlmeier L, Simonsen N, van 't Veer P, et al. Adipose tissue trans-fatty acids and breast cancer in the European Community Multi-center study on antioxidants, myocardial infarction, and breast cancer. Cancer Epidemiol Biomarkers Prev. 1997;6(9):705-10.
108. Bakker N, van't Veer P, Zock PL. Adipose fatty acids and cancers of the breast, prostate and colon: an ecological study. EURAMIC Study Group. Int J Cancer. 1997 7;72(4):587-91.
109. Stendera S, Dyerbergb J. Influence of trans-fatty acids on health. Ann Nutr Metab. 2004;48:61-66.
110. Morris MC, Evans DA, Bienias JL, et al. Dietary fats and the risk of incident Alzheimer disease. Arch Neurol. 2003;60(2):194-200.
111. Baer DJ, Judd JT, Clevidence BA, Tracy RP. Dietary fatty acids affect plasma markers of inflammation in healthy men fed controlled diets: a randomized crossover study. Am J Clin Nutr. 2004;79(6):969-73.
112. Mozaffarian D, Pischon T, Hankinson SE, et al. Dietary intake of trans-fatty acids and systemic inflammation in women. Am J Clin Nutr. 2004;79:606-12.
113. Rock CL, Thornquist M. Demographic, dietary and lifestyle factors differentially explain variability in serum carotenoids and fat-soluble vitamins: baseline results from the sentinel site of the olestra post-marketing surveillance study. J Nutr. 1999;129:855–64.
114. Bray GA, Nielsen SJ, Popkin BM. Consumption of high-fructose corn syrup in beverages may play a role in the epidemic of obesity. Am J Clin Nutr. 2004;79(4):537-43.
115. Brownell KD, Horgen KB. Food Fight: The Inside Story of America's Obesity Crisis - and What We Can Do about It. McGraw-Hill Companies. 2003.
116. Elliott SS, Kim NL, Stern JS, Tiff K, Havel PJ. Fructose, weight gain, and the insulin resistance syndrome. Am J Clin Nutr. 2002;76(5):911-22.

117. Schulze MB, Manson JE, Ludwig DS, et al. Sugar-sweetened beverages, weight gain, and incidence of type 2 diabetes in young and middle-aged women. JAMA. 2004;292(8):927-34.
118. Lakka HM, Laaksonen DE, Lakka TA, et al. The metabolic syndrome and total and cardiovascular disease mortality in middle-aged men. JAMA. 2002;288(21):2709-16.
119. Yaffe K, Kanaya A, Lindquist K, et al. The metabolic syndrome, inflammation, and risk of cognitive decline. JAMA. 2004;292(18):2237-42.
120. Calle EE, Rodriguez C, Walker-Thurmond K, Thun M. Overweight, obesity, and mortality from cancer in a prospectively studied cohort of U.S. adults. N Engl J Med. 2003;348:1625-38.
121. Ford ES, Giles WH, Dietz WH. Prevalence of the metabolic syndrome among US adults: findings from the third National Health and Nutrition Examination Survey. JAMA. 2002;287(3):356-59.
122. Food Consumption, Prices, and Expenditures, 1970-1997. Economic Research Service, USDA. Statistical Bulletin No. 965. April 1999. Accessed at: http://www.ers.usda.gov/publications/sb565/.
123. Pereira MA, Swain J, Goldfine AB, et al. Effects of a low-glycemic-load diet on resting energy expenditure and heart disease risk factors during weight loss. JAMA. 2004;292(20):2482-90.
124. Levine AS, Kotz CM, Gosnell BA. Sugars: hedonic aspects, neuroregulation, and energy balance. Am J Clin Nutr. 2003;78(4):834S-42S.
125. Ludwig DS. The glycemic index: physiological mechanisms relating to obesity, diabetes, and cardiovascular disease. JAMA. 2002;287(18):2414.
126. Foster-Powell K , Holt SHA, Brand-Miller JC. International table of glycemic index and glycemic load values: Am J Clin Nutr. 2002;76:5-56.
127. Smith JD, Terpening CM, Schmidt SO, Gums JG. Relief of fibromyalgia symptoms following discontinuation of dietary excitotoxins. Ann Pharmacother. 2001;35(6):702-6.
128. Blaylock R. Excitoxins, University of Mississippi Medical Center
129. Uribe M. Potential toxicity of a new sugar substitute in patients with liver disease. N Engl J Med. 1982;306(3):173-74.
130. Olney JW. Excitotoxic food additives--relevance of animal studies to human safety. Neurobehav Toxicol Teratol. 1984;6(6):455-62.
131. Garriga MM, Metcalfe DD. Aspartame intolerance. Ann Allergy. 1988 Dec;61(6 Pt 2):63-9.
132. Trocho C, et al. Formaldehyde derived from dietary aspartame binds to tissue components *in vivo*. Life Sci. 1998;63(5):337.
133. Lavin JH, et al. The effect of sucrose- and aspartame-sweetened drinks on energy intake, hunger and food choice of female, moderately restrained eaters Int J Obes. 1997;21:37-42.
134. Tordoff MG, Alleva AM. Oral stimulation with aspartame increases hunger. Physiol Behav. 1990;47:555–59.
135. Sharma RP, Coulombe RA Jr. Effects of repeated doses of aspartame on serotonin and its metabolite in various regions of the mouse brain. Food Chem Toxicol. 1987;25(8):565-68.
136. Camfield, PR, et al., Aspartame exacerbates EEG spike-wave discharge in children with generalized absence epilepsy: a double-blind controlled study. Neurology. 1992;42:1000-3.
137. Walton RG, et al. Adverse reactions to aspartame: double-blind challenge in patients from a vulnerable population. Biol Psychiatry. 1993;34(1-2):13-17.
138. Van Den Eeden SK, et al. Aspartame ingestion and headaches: a randomized, crossover trial. Neurology. 1994;44:1787-93.
139. Lipton RB, et al. Aspartame as a dietary trigger of headache. Headache. 1989;29(2):90-92. http://www.dorway.com/peerrev.html.
140. Curl CL, Fenske RA, Elgethun K. Organophosphorus pesticide exposure of urban and suburban preschool children with organic and conventional diets. Environ Health Perspect. 2003;111(3):377-82.
141. Gorbach SL. Antimicrobial use in animal feed—time to stop. N Engl J Med. 2001;345:1202-3.
142. Cory-Slechta DA, Thiruchelvam M, Richfield EK, et al. Developmental pesticide exposures and the Parkinson's disease phenotype. Birth Defects Res A Clin Mol Teratol. 2005;73(3):136-39.
143. Allam MF, Del Castillo AS, Navajas RF. Parkinson's disease risk factors: genetic, environmental, or both? Neurol Res. 2005;27(2):206-8.
144. Colborn T. Neurodevelopment and endocrine disruption. Environ Health Perspect. 2004;112(9):944-49.
145. Koppe JG. Are maternal thyroid autoantibodies generated by PCBs the missing link to the impaired development of the brain? Environ Health Perspect. 2004;112(15):A862.
146. Hyman MH. The impact of mercury on human health and the environment. Altern Ther Health Med. 2004;10(6):70-75.
147. http://www.epa.gov/waterscience/fishadvice/advice.html - Joint Federal Advisory for Fish.
148. Pusztai A. Can science give us the tools for recognizing possible health risks of GM food? Nutr Health. 2002;16(2):73-84.
149. Uzogara SG. The impact of genetic modification of human foods in the 21st century: a review. Biotechnol Adv. 2000;18(3):179-206.
150. Clarkston LA, Crawford ME. Feast and famine: a history of food and nutrition in Ireland 1500-1920. Oxford University Press New York. 2001.
151. Watson JB. Pigs, fodder, and the Jones effect in postipomoean New Guinea. Ethnology. 1977;16:57-70.
152. Worsley AT, Oldfield F. Palaeoecological studies of three lakes in the highlands of Papua New Guinea. II. Vegetational history over the last 1600 years. J Ecology. 1988;76:1-18.
153. Kant AK. Consumption of energy-dense, nutrient-poor foods by adult Americans: nutritional and health implications. The third national health and nutrition examination survey, 1988-1994. Am J Clin Nutr. 2000;72:929-36.
154. Ames BN, Wakimoto P. Are vitamin and mineral deficiencies a major cancer risk? Nat. Rev. Cancer. 2002;2:694-704.
155. Walter PW, Knutson MD, Paler-Martinez A, et al. Iron deficiency and iron excess damage mitochondria and mitochondrial DNA in rats. Proc Natl Acad Sci U S A. 2002;99:2264-69.
156. Simopoulos AP. n-3 fatty acids and human health: defining strategies for public policy. Lipids. 2001;36 Suppl:S83-9.
157. Dietary Reference Intakes for Energy, Carbohydrate, Fiber, Fat, Fatty Acids, Cholesterol, Protein, and Amino Acids. National Academies Press Washington, DC. 2004.
158. Ames BN, Wakimoto P. Are vitamin and mineral deficiencies a major cancer risk? Nat Rev Cancer. 2002;2:694-704.
159. Ames, BN. DNA damage from micronutrient deficiencies is likely to be a major cause of cancer. Mutat Res. 2001;475:7-20.
160. Ibid.
161. Hung HC, Joshipura KJ, Jiang R, et al. Fruit and vegetable intake and risk of major chronic disease. J Natl Cancer Inst. 2004;96:1577-84.
162. Blount BC, Mack MM, Wehr C, et al. Folate deficiency causes uracil misincorporation into human DNA and chromosome breakage: implications for cancer and neuronal damage. Proc Natl Acad Sci U S A. 1997;94:3290-95.
163. Kim, YI. Folate and carcinogenesis: evidence, mechanisms, and implications. J Nutr Biochem. 1999;10:66-88.
164. Kim, YI. Carcinogenesis, in Present Knowledge in Nutrition. ILSI Press: Washington, DC. 2001;573-589.
165. Giovannucci E, Rimm EB, Ascherio A, et al. Alcohol, methyl-deficient diets and risk of colon cancer in men. J. Natl Cancer Inst. 1995;87:265-273.
166. Giovannucci E, Stampfer MJ, Colditz GA, et al. Multivitamin use, folate, and colon cancer in women in the nurses' health study. Ann Intern Med. 1998;129:517-24.
167. Rohan TE, Jain MG, Howe GR, Miller AB. Dietary folate consumption and breast cancer risk. J Natl Cancer Inst. 2000;92:266-69.

168. Zhang S, Hunter DJ, Hankinson SE, et al. A prospective study of folate intake and the risk of breast cancer. JAMA. 1999;281:1632-37.
169. Stolzenberg-Solomon RZ, Pietinen P, Barrett MJ, et al. Dietary and other methyl-group availability factors and pancreatic cancer risk in a cohort of male smokers. Am J Epidemiol. 2001;153:680-87.
170. Stolzenberg-Solomon RZ, Albanes D, Nieto FJ, et al. Pancreatic cancer risk and nutrition-related methyl-group availability indicators in male smokers. J Natl Cancer Inst. 1999;91:535-41.
171. Larsson SC, Giovannucci E, Wolk A. Dietary folate intake and incidence of ovarian cancer: the Swedish mammography cohort. J Natl Cancer Inst. 2004;96:396-402.
172. Mayne ST, Risch HA, Dubrow R, et al. Nutrient intake and risk of subtypes of esophageal and gastric cancer. Cancer Epidemiol Biomarkers Prev. 2001;10:1055-62.
173. Crott JW, Mashiyama ST, Ames BN, Fenech MF. Methylenetetrahydrofolate reductase C677T polymorphism does not alter folic acid deficiency-induced uracil incorporation into primary human lymphocyte DNA *in vitro*. Carcinogenesis. 2001;22:1019-25.
174. Blount BC, Mack MM, Wehr C, et al. Folate deficiency causes uracil misincorporation into human DNA and chromosome breakage: implications for cancer and neuronal damage. Proc Natl Acad Sci U S A. 1997;94:3290-95.
175. Crott JW, Mashiyama ST, Ames BN, Fenech MF. Methylenetetrahydrofolate reductase C677T polymorphism does not alter folic acid deficiency-induced uracil incorporation into primary human lymphocyte DNA *in vitro*. Carcinogenesis. 2001;22:1019-25.
176. Fenech M, Aitken C, Rinaldi J. Folate, vitamin B12, homocysteine status and DNA damage in young Australian adults. Carcinogenesis. 1998;19:1163-71.
177. Fenech, M. Micronutrients and genomic stability: a new paradigm for recommended dietary allowances (RDAs). Food Chem Toxicol. 2002;40:1113-17.
178. Fenech M, Aitken C, Rinaldi J. Folate, vitamin B12, homocysteine status and DNA damage in young Australian adults. Carcinogenesis. 1998;19:1163-1171.
179. Fenech, M. Micronutrients and genomic stability: a new paradigm for recommended dietary allowances (RDAs). Food Chem Toxicol. 2002;40:1113-17.
180. Hagmar L, Bonassi S, Stromberg U, et al. Chromosomal aberrations in lymphocytes predict human cancer: a report from the European Study Group on Cytogenetic Biomarkers and Health (ESCH). Cancer Res. 1998;58:4117-21.
181. Chen J, Giovannucci E, Kelsey K, et al. A methylenetetrahydrofolate reductase polymorphism and the risk of colorectal cancer. Cancer Res.1996;56:4862-64.
182. Le Marchand L, Donlon T, Hankin JH, et al. B-vitamin intake, metabolic genes, and colorectal cancer risk (United States). Cancer Causes Control. 2002;13:239-48.
183. Ma J, Stampfer MJ, Giovannucci E, et al. Methylenetetrahydrofolate reductase polymorphism, dietary interactions, and risk of colorectal cancer. Cancer Res. 1997;57:1098-1102.
184. Slattery ML, Potter JD, Samowitz W, et al. Methylenetetrahydrofolate reductase, diet, and risk of colon cancer. Cancer Epidemiol Biomarkers Prev. 1999;8:513-18.
185. Levine AJ, Siegmund KD, Ervin CM, et al. The methylenetetrahydrofolate reductase 677CÆT polymorphism and distal colorectal adenoma risk. Cancer Epidemiol Biomarkers Prev. 2000;9:657-63.
186. Ulrich CM, Kampman E, Bigler J, et al. Colorectal adenomas and the C677T MTHFR polymorphism: Evidence for gene-environment interaction. Cancer Epidemiol Biomarkers Prev.1999;8:659-68.
187. Skibola CF, Smith MT, Kane E, et al. Polymorphisms in the methylenetetrahydrofolate reductase gene are associated with susceptibility to acute leukemia in adults. Proc Natl Acad Sci U S A. 1999;96:12810-15.
188. Le Marchand L, Donlon T, Hankin JH, et al. B-vitamin intake, metabolic genes, and colorectal cancer risk (United States). Cancer Causes Control. 2002;13:239-48.
189. Levine AJ, Siegmund KD, Ervin CM, et al. The methylenetetrahydrofolate reductase 677CÆT polymorphism and distal colorectal adenoma risk. Cancer Epidemiol Biomarkers Prev. 2000;9:657-63.
190. Ulrich CM, Kampman E, Bigler J, et al. Colorectal adenomas and the C677T MTHFR polymorphism: Evidence for gene-environment interaction. Cancer Epidemiol. Biomarkers Prev.1999;8:659-68.
191. Skibola CF, Smith MT, Kane E, et al. Polymorphisms in the methylenetetrahydrofolate reductase gene are associated with susceptibility to acute leukemia in adults. Proc Natl Acad Sci U S A. 1999;96:12810-15.
192. Wiemels JL, Smith RN, Taylor GM, et al.. Methylenetetrahydrofolate reductase (MTHFR) polymorphisms and risk of molecularly defined subtypes of childhood acute leukemia. Proc Natl Acad Sci U S A. 2001;98:4004-9.
193. Ames BN. Cancer prevention and diet: Help from single nucleotide polymorphisms. Proc Natl Acad Sci U S A. 1999;96:12216-18.
194. Goodman MT, McDuffie K, Hernandez B, et al. Association of methylenetetrahydrofolate reductase polymorphism C677T and dietary folate with the risk of cervical dysplasia. Cancer Epidemiol Biomarkers Prev. 2001;10:1275-80.
195. Ibid.
196. Ames BN. DNA Damage from micronutrient deficiencies is likely to be a major cause of cancer. Mutat. Res.2001;475:7-20.
197. Wallock LM, Tamura T, Mayr CA, et al. Low seminal plasma folate concentrations are associated with low sperm density and count in male smokers and nonsmokers. Fertil Steril. 2001;75:252-59.
198. Ibid.
199. Mayr CA, Woodall AA, Ames BN. DNA damage to sperm from micronutrient deficiency may increase the risk of birth defects and cancer in offspring, in Preventive Nutrition: The Comprehensive Guide for Health Professionals, A Bendich and RJ Deckelbaum, Editors. 2001, Humana Press, Inc.: Totowa, NJ. p. 373-386.
200. Wiemels JL, Smith RN, Taylor GM, et al. Methylenetetrahydrofolate reductase (MTHFR) polymorphisms and risk of molecularly defined subtypes of childhood acute leukemia. Proc Natl Acad Sci U S A. 2001;98:4004-9.
201. Ames BN. Cancer prevention and diet: Help from single nucleotide polymorphisms. Proc Natl Acad Sci U S A. 1999;96:12216-218.
202. Fenech MF, Dreosti IE, Rinaldi JR. Folate, vitamin B12, homocysteine status and chromosome damage rate in lymphocytes of older men. Carcinogenesis. 1997;18:1329-36.
203. Fenech M, Aitken C, Rinaldi J. Folate, vitamin B12, homocysteine status and DNA damage in young Australian adults. Carcinogenesis. 1998;19:1163-71.
204. Fenech MF, Dreosti IE, Rinaldi JR. Folate, vitamin B12, homocysteine status and chromosome damage rate in lymphocytes of older men. Carcinogenesis. 1997;18:1329-36.
205. Fenech M. Micronucleus frequency in human lymphocytes is related to plasma vitamin B12 and homocysteine. Mutat Res. 1999;428:299-304.
206. Fenech M, Aitken C, and Rinaldi J. Folate, vitamin B12, homocysteine status and DNA damage in young Australian adults. Carcinogenesis. 1998;19:1163-71.
207. Fenech M. Micronutrients and genomic stability: a new paradigm for recommended dietary allowances (RDAs). Food Chem Toxicol. 2002;40:1113-17.
208. Stabler SP, Sampson DA, Wang LP, Allen RH. Elevations of serum cystathionine and total homocysteine in pyridoxine-, folate-, and cobalamin-deficient rats. J Nutr Biochem. 1997; 8:279-89.

209. Le Marchand L, Donlon T, Hankin JH, et al. B-vitamin intake, metabolic genes, and colorectal cancer risk (United States). Cancer Causes Control. 2002;13:239-48.
210. Slattery ML, Potter JD, Samowitz W, et al. Methylenetetrahydrofolate reductase, diet, and risk of colon cancer. Cancer Epidemiol Biomarkers Prev. 1999;8:513-18.
211. Ulrich CM, Kampman E, Bigler J, et al. Colorectal adenomas and the C677T MTHFR polymorphism: evidence for gene-environment interaction. Cancer Epidemiol Biomarkers Prev.1999;8:659-68.
212. Mayne ST, Risch HA, Dubrow R, et al. Nutrient intake and risk of subtypes of esophageal and gastric cancer. Cancer Epidemiol Biomarkers Prev. 2001;10:1055-62.
213. Alberg AJ, Selhub J, Shah KV, et al. The risk of cervical cancer in relation to serum concentrations of folate, vitamin B12, and homocysteine. Cancer Epidemiol Biomarkers Prev. 2000;9:761-64.
214. Wu K, Helzlsouer KJ, Comstock GW, et al. A prospective study on folate, B12, and pyridoxal 5'-phosphate (B6) and breast cancer. Cancer Epidemiol Biomarkers Prev. 1999;8:209-17.
215. Key TJ, Silcocks PB, Davey GK, et al. A case-control study of diet and prostate cancer. Br J Cancer. 1997;76:678-87.
216. Hartman TJ, Woodson K, Stolzenberg-Solomon R, et al. Association of the B-vitamins pyridoxal 5'-phosphate (B(6)), B(12), and folate with lung cancer risk in older men. Am J Epidemiol. 2001;153:688-94.
217. Weinstein SJ, Ziegler RG, Selhub J, et al. Elevated serum homocysteine levels and increased risk of invasive cervical cancer in US women. Cancer Causes Control. 2001;12:317-24.
218. Hagen TM, Liu J, Lykkesfeldt J, et al. Feeding acetyl-L-carnitine and lipoic acid to old rats significantly improves metabolic function while decreasing oxidative stress. Proc Natl Acad Sci U S A. 2002;99:1870-75.
219. Jacob RA, Vitamin C, in Modern Nutrition and Health and Disease, ME Shils, et al., Editors. 1999, Williams & Wilkins: Baltimore. p. 467-484.
220. Ames BN, Shigenaga MK, Hagen TM. Oxidants, antioxidants, and the degenerative diseases of aging. Proc Natl Acad Sci U S A. 1996;90:7915-22.
221. Mayne ST, Risch HA, Dubrow R, et al. Nutrient intake and risk of subtypes of esophageal and gastric cancer. Cancer Epidemiol Biomarkers Prev. 2001;10:1055-62.
222. Jacob RA, Vitamin C, in Modern Nutrition and Health and Disease, ME Shils, et al., Editors. 1999, Williams & Wilkins: Baltimore. p. 467-484.
223. Kono S, Hirohata T. Nutrition and stomach cancer. Cancer Causes Control. 1996;7:41-55.
224. Zhang ZW, Abdullahi M, Farthing MJ. Effect of physiological concentrations of vitamin C on gastric cancer cells and Helicobacter pylori. Gut. 2002;50:165-69.
225. Mayne ST, Risch HA, Dubrow R, et al. Nutrient intake and risk of subtypes of esophageal and gastric cancer. Cancer Epidemiol Biomarkers Prev. 2001;10:1055-62.
226. Kim YI. Carcinogenesis, in Present Knowledge in Nutrition. ILSI Press: Washington, DC. 2001;573-589.
227. Willett WC. Diet and cancer: one view at the start of the millennium. Cancer Epidemiol Biomarkers Prev. 2001;10:3-8.
228. Moller P, Loft S. Oxidative DNA damage in human white blood cells in dietary antioxidant intervention studies. Am J Clin Nutr. 2002;76:303-10.
229. Levine M, Conry-Cantilena C, Wang Y, et al.. Vitamin C pharmacokinetics in healthy volunteers: evidence for a recommended dietary allowance. Proc Natl Acad Sci U S A. 1996;93:3704-9.
230. Fraga CG, Motchnik PA, Shigenaga MK, et al. Ascorbic acid protects against endogenous oxidative damage in human sperm. Proc Natl Acad Sci U S A. 1991;88:11003-6.
231. Duthie SJ, Ma A, Ross MA, Collins AR. Antioxidant supplementation decreases oxidative DNA damage in human lymphocytes. Cancer Res. 1996;56:1291-95.
232. Harats D, Chevion S, Nahir M, et al. Citrus fruit supplementation reduces lipoprotein oxidation in young men ingesting a diet high in saturated fat: presumptive evidence for an interaction between vitamins C and E *in vivo*. Am J Clin Nutr. 1998;67:240-45.
233. McCall MR, Frei B. Can antioxidant vitamins materially reduce oxidative damage in humans? Free Radic Biol Med. 1999;26:1034-53.
234. Block G, in Vitamin C: The State of the Art in Disease Prevention Sixty Years after the Nobel Prize, R Paoletti, et al., Editors. 1998, Springer-Verlag: Milano. p. 51-58.
235. Byers T, Guerrero N. Epidemiologic evidence for vitamin C and vitamin E in cancer prevention. Am J Clin Nutr. 1995;62:13855-925.
236. Chan SWY, Reade PC. The role of ascorbic acid in oral cancer and carcinogenesis. Oral Dis. 1998;4:120-29.
237. Jacobs EJ, Connell CJ, McCullough ML, et al. Vitamin C, vitamin E, and multivitamin supplement use and stomach cancer mortality in the Cancer Prevention Study II cohort. Cancer Epidemiol Biomarkers Prev. 2002;11:35-41.
238. Jacobs EJ, Connell CJ, Patel AV, et al. Vitamin C and vitamin E supplement use and colorectal cancer mortality in a large American Cancer Society cohort. Cancer Epidemiol Biomarkers Prev. 2001;10:17-23.
239. Dietrich M, Block G, Hudes M, et al. Antioxidant supplementation decreases lipid peroxidation biomarker F(2)-isoprostanes in plasma of smokers. Cancer Epidemiol Biomarkers Prev. 2002;11:7-13.
240. Duthie SJ, Ma A, Ross MA, Collins, AR. Antioxidant supplementation decreases oxidative DNA damage in human lymphocytes. Cancer Res. 1996;56:1291-95.
241. Collins AR, Olmedilla B, Southon S, et al. Serum carotenoids and oxidative DNA damage in human lymphocytes. Carcinogenesis. 1998;19:2159-62.
242. Panayiotidis M and Collins AR. Ex vivo assessment of lymphocyte antioxidant status using the comet assay. Free Radic Res. 1997;27:533-37.
243. Beckman KB, Saljoughi S, Mashiyama S, Ames BN. A simpler, more robust method for the analysis of 8-oxoguanine in DNA. Free Radic Biol Med. 2000;29:357-67.
244. Helbock HJ, Beckman KB, Shigenaga MK, et al. DNA oxidation matters: The HPLC-EC assay of 8-oxo-deoxyguanosine and 8-oxoguanine. Proc Natl Acad Sci U S A. 1998;95:288-93.
245. Fraga CG, Motchnik PA, Shigenaga MK, et al. Ascorbic acid protects against endogenous oxidative damage in human sperm. Proc Natl Acad Sci U S A. 1991;88:11003-6.
246. Branda RF, Blickensderfer DB. Folate deficiency increases genetic damage caused by alkylating agents and gamma-irradiation in Chinese hamster ovary cells. Cancer Research. 1993;53:5401-8.
247. Institute of Medicine Food and Nutrition Board Dietary Reference Intakes for Vitamin C, Vitamin E, Selenium and Carotenoids. National Academy Press Washington, DC. 2001.
248. Fraga CG, Motchnik PA, Shigenaga MK, et al. Ascorbic acid protects against endogenous oxidative damage in human sperm. Proc Natl Acad Sci U S A. 1991;88:11003-6.
249. Fraga CG, Motchnik PA, Wyrobek AJ, et al. Smoking and low antioxidant levels increase oxidative damage to sperm DNA. Mutat Res. 1996; 351:199-203.
250. Lykkesfeldt J, Christen S, Wallock LM, et al. Ascorbate is depleted by smoking and repleted by moderate supplementation: a study in male smokers and nonsmokers with matched dietary antioxidant intakes. Am J Clin Nutr. 2000;71:530-36.
251. Fraga CG, Motchnik PA, Shigenaga MK, et al. Ascorbic acid protects against endogenous oxidative damage in human sperm. Proc Natl Acad Sci U S A. 1991;88:11003-6.

252. Fraga CG, Motchnik PA, Wyrobek AJ, et al. Smoking and low antioxidant levels increase oxidative damage to sperm DNA. Mutat Res. 1996;351:199-203.
253. Sorahan T, Prior P, Lancashire RJ, et al. Childhood cancer and parental use of tobacco: deaths from 1971 to 1976. Br J Cancer. 1997;76:1525-31.
254. Sorahan T, Lancashire RJ, Prior P, et al.. Childhood cancer and parental use of alcohol and tobacco. Ann Epidemiol. 1995;5:354-59.
255. Sorahan T, Lancashire RJ, Hulten MA, et al. Childhood cancer and parental use of tobacco - deaths from 1953 to 1955. Br J Cancer. 1997;75:134-38.
256. Ji BT, Shu XO, Linet MS, et al. Paternal cigarette smoking and the risk of childhood cancer among offspring of nonsmoking mothers. J Natl Cancer Inst. 1997;89:238-44.
257. Ibid.
258. Atamna H, Walter PW, and Ames BN. The role of heme and iron-sulfur clusters in mitochondrial biogenesis, maintenance, and decay with age. Arch Biochem Biophys. 2002;397:345-53.
259. Atamna H, Killilea DW, Killilea AN, Ames BN. Heme deficiency may be a factor in the mitochondrial and neuronal decay of aging. Proc Natl Acad Sci U S A. 2002;99:14807-12.
260. Walter PW, Knutson MD, Paler-Martinez A, et al. Iron deficiency and iron excess damage mitochondria and mitochondrial DNA in rats. Proc Natl Acad Sci U S A. 2002;99:2264-69.
261. Atamna H, Walter PW, Ames BN. The role of heme and iron-sulfur clusters in mitochondrial biogenesis, maintenance, and decay with age. Arch Biochem Biophys. 2002;397:345-53.
262. Frith-Terhune AL, Cogswell ME, Khan LK, et al. Iron deficiency anemia: higher prevalence in Mexican American than in non-Hispanic white females in the third National Health and Nutrition Examination Survey, 1988-1994. Am J Clin Nutr. 2000;72:963-68.
263. Kumanyika SK and Krebs-Smith SM. Preventive nutrition issues in ethnic and socioeconomic groups in the United States, in Primary and Secondary Preventive Nutrition. 2000, Humana Press: Totowa, NJ. p. 325-356.
264. Mock DM, Henrich CL, Carnell N, Mock NI. Indicators of marginal biotin deficiency and repletion in humans: validation of 3-hydroxyisovaleric acid excretion and a leucine challenge. Am J Clin Nutr. 2002;76:1061-68.
265. Mock DM, Quirk JG, Mock NI. Marginal biotin deficiency during normal pregnancy. Am J Clin Nutr. 2002;75:295-99.
266. Ibid.
267. Rossi L, Lippe G, Marchese E, et al. Decrease of cytochrome c oxidase protein in heart mitochondria of copper-deficient rats. Biometals. 1998;11:207-12.
268. Brambl R, Plesofsky-Vig N. Pantothenate is required in Neurospora crassa for assembly of subunit peptides of cytochrome c oxidase and ATPase/ATP synthase. Proc Natl Acad Sci U S A. 1986;83:3644-48.
269. Ho E, Ames BN. Low intracellular zinc induces oxidative DNA damage, disrupts p53, NFκB, and AP1 DNA-binding, and affects DNA repair in a rat glioma cell line. Proc Natl Acad Sci U S A. 2002;99:16770-75.
270. Ho E, Courtemanche C, Ames BN. Zinc deficiency induces oxidative DNA damage and increases P53 expression in human lung fibroblasts. J Nutr. 2003;133:2543-48.
271. Fong LY, Zhang L, Jiang Y, Farber JL. Dietary zinc modulation of COX-2 expression and lingual and esophageal carcinogenesis in rats. J Natl Cancer Inst. 2005;97:40-50.
272. Ho E, Ames BN. Low intracellular zinc induces oxidative DNA damage, disrupts p53, NFκB, and AP1 DNA-binding, and affects DNA repair in a rat glioma cell line. Proc Natl Acad Sci U S A. 2002;99:16770-75.
273. Ho E, Courtemanche C, Ames BN. Zinc deficiency induces oxidative DNA damage and increases P53 expression in human lung fibroblasts. J Nutr. 2003;133:2543-48.
274. Atamna H, Killilea DW, Killilea AN, Ames BN. Heme deficiency may be a factor in the mitochondrial and neuronal decay of aging. Proc Natl Acad Sci U S A. 2002;99:14807-12.
275. Atamna H, Frey WH 2nd. A role for heme in Alzheimer's disease: heme binds amyloid beta and has altered metabolism. Proc Natl Acad Sci U S A. 2004;101:11153-58.
276. Ames BN. DNA Damage from micronutrient deficiencies is likely to be a major cause of cancer. Mutat. Res.2001;475:7-20.
277. Gold LS, Slone TH, Manley NB, Ames BN Misconceptions about the Causes of Cancer. The Fraser Institute Vancouver, BC, Canada 2002.
278. Courtemanche C, Huang AC, Elson-Schwab I, et al. Folate deficiency and ionizing radiation cause DNA breaks in primary human lymphocytes: a comparison. FASEB J. 2004;18:209-11.
279. Fenech M. Nutritional treatment of genome instability: a paradigm shift in disease prevention and in the setting of recommended dietary allowances. Nutr Research Rev. 2003;16:109-22.
280. Courtemanche C, Huang AC, Elson-Schwab I, et al. Folate deficiency and ionizing radiation cause DNA breaks in primary human lymphocytes: a comparison. FASEB J. 2004;18:209-11.
281. Gold LS, Slone TH, Manley NB, Ames BN Misconceptions About the Causes of Cancer. The Fraser Institute Vancouver, BC, Canada 2002.
282. Abrams SA. Nutritional rickets: an old disease returns. Nutr Rev. 2005;60:111-15.
283. Holick MF. McCollum Award Lecture, 1994: vitamin D—new horizons for the 21st century. Am J Clin Nutr. 1994;60:619-30.
284. Levine AJ, Harper JM, Ervin CM, et al. Serum 25-hydroxyvitamin D, dietary calcium intake, and distal colorectal adenoma risk. Nutr Cancer. 2001;39:35-41.
285. Platz EA, Hankinson SE, Hollis BW, et al. Plasma 1,25-dihydroxy- and 25-hydroxyvitamin D and adenomatous polyps of the distal colorectum. Cancer Epidemiol Biomarkers Prev. 2000; 9:1059-65.
286. Platz EA, Rimm EB, Willett WC, et al. Racial variation in prostate cancer incidence and in hormonal system markers among male health professionals. J Natl Cancer Inst. 2000;92:2009-17.
287. Holt PR, Arber N, Halmos B, et al. Colonic epithelial cell proliferation decreases with increasing levels of serum 25-hydroxy vitamin D. Cancer Epidemiol Biomarkers Prev. 2002;11:113-19.
288. Feskanich D, Ma J, Fuchs CS, et al. Plasma vitamin D metabolites and risk of colorectal cancer in women. Cancer Epidemiol Biomarkers Prev. 2004;13:1502-8.
289. Martinez ME, Marshall JR, Sampliner R, et al. Calcium, vitamin D, and risk of adenoma recurrence (United States). Cancer Causes Control. 2002;13:213-20.
290. Holt PR, Arber N, Halmos B, et al. Colonic epithelial cell proliferation decreases with increasing levels of serum 25-hydroxy vitamin D. Cancer Epidemiol Biomarkers Prev. 2002;11:113-19.
291. Platz EA, Rimm EB, Willett WC, et al. Racial variation in prostate cancer incidence and in hormonal system markers among male health professionals. J Natl Cancer Inst. 2000;92:2009-17.
292. Giovannucci E, Willett WC. Vitamin D intake and total cancer mortality. J Natl Cancer Inst, in press. 2005.
293. Kumanyika SK, Krebs-Smith SM. Preventive nutrition issues in ethnic and socioeconomic groups in the United States, in Primary and Secondary Preventive Nutrition. 2000, Humana Press: Totowa, NJ. p. 325-356.
294. Ibid.
295. Ames BN, Wakimoto P. Are vitamin and mineral deficiencies a major cancer risk? Nat Rev Cancer. 2002;2:694-704.

296. Giovannucci E, Stampfer MJ, Colditz GA, et al. Multivitamin use, folate, and colon cancer in women in the nurses' health study. Ann Intern Med. 1998;129:517-24.
297. Olshan AF, Smith JC, Bondy ML, et al. Maternal vitamin use and reduced risk of neuroblastoma. Epidemiology. 2002;13:575-80.
298. Oakley Jr. GP. Eat right and take a multivitamin. N Engl J Med. 1998;338:1060-1.
299. Bendich A, Mallick R, Leader S. Potential health economic benefits of vitamin supplementation. West J Med. 1997;166:306-12.
300. Scholl TO, Hediger ML, Bendich A, et al. Use of multivitamin/mineral prenatal supplements: influence on the outcome of pregnancy. Am J Epidemiol. 1997;146:134-41.
301. Willett WC, Stampfer MJ. Clinical practice. What vitamins should I be taking, doctor? N Engl J Med. 2001;345:1819-24.
302. Barringer TA, Kirk JK, Santaniello AC, et al. Effect of a multivitamin and mineral supplement on infection and quality of life. A randomized, double-blind, placebo-controlled trial. Ann Intern Med. 2003;138:365-71.
303. Fairfield KM, Fletcher RH. Vitamins for chronic disease prevention in adults: scientific review. JAMA. 2002;287:3116-26.
304. Holmquist C, Larsson S, Wolk A, de Faire U. Multivitamin supplements are inversely associated with risk of myocardial infarction in men and women—Stockholm Heart Epidemiology Program (SHEEP). J Nutr. 2003;133:2650-54.
305. Jacobs EJ, Connell CJ, Chao A, et al. Multivitamin use and colorectal cancer incidence in a US cohort: does timing matter? Am J Epidemiol. 2003;158: 621-28.
306. Aisen PS, Egelko S, Andrews H, et al. A pilot study of vitamins to lower plasma homocysteine levels in Alzheimer disease. Am J Geriatr Psychiatry. 2003;11:246-49.
307. Church TS, Earnest CP, Wood KA, Kampert JB. Reduction of C-reactive protein levels through use of a multivitamin. Am J Med. 2003;115:702-7.
308. Willett WC. Eat, Drink and be Healthy. Simon and Schuster New York. 2001.
309. Helbock HJ, Beckman KB, Shigenaga MK, et al. DNA oxidation matters: The HPLC-EC assay of 8-oxo-deoxyguanosine and 8-oxoguanine. Proc Natl Acad Sci U S A. 1998; 95:288-93.
310. Shigenaga MK, Hagen TM, Ames BN. Oxidative damage and mitochondrial decay in aging. Proc Natl Acad Sci U S A. 1994; 1:10771-78.
311. Beckman KB, Ames BN. The free radical theory of aging matures. Physiol Rev. 1998; 78:547-81.
312. Beckman KB, Ames BN. Mitochondrial aging: open questions. Ann N Y Acad Sci 1998;854:118-27.
313. Hagen TM, Yowe DL, Bartholomew JC, et al. Mitochondrial decay in hepatocytes from old rats: Membrane potential declines, heterogeneity and oxidants increase. Proc Natl Acad Sci U S A. 1997;94:3064-69.
314. Liu J, Killilea D, Ames BN. Age-associated mitochondrial oxidative decay: improvement of carnitine acetyltransferase substrate binding affinity and activity in brain by feeding old rats acetyl-L-carnitine and/or R-a-lipoic acid. Proc Natl Acad Sci U S A. 2002;99:1876-81.
315. Ibid.
316. Suh JH, Shenvi SV, Dixon BM, et al. Decline in transcriptional activity of Nrf2 causes age-related loss of glutathione synthesis, which is reversible with lipoic acid. Proc Natl Acad Sci U S A. 2004;101:3381-86.
317. Smith AR, Shenvi SV, Widlansky M, et al. Lipoic acid as a potential therapy for chronic diseases associated with oxidative stress. Curr Med Chem. 2004;11:1135-46.
318. Suh JH, Wang H, Liu RM, et al. (R)-alpha-lipoic acid reverses the age-related loss in GSH redox status in post-mitotic tissues: evidence for increased cysteine requirement for GSH synthesis. Arch Biochem Biophys. 2004;423:126-35.
319. Hagen TM, Liu J, Lykkesfeldt J, et al. Feeding acetyl-L-carnitine and lipoic acid to old rats significantly improves metabolic function while decreasing oxidative stress. Proc Natl Acad Sci U S A. 2002;99:1870-75.
320. Hagen TM, Yowe DL, Bartholomew JC, et al. Mitochondrial decay in hepatocytes from old rats: Membrane potential declines, heterogeneity and oxidants increase. Proc Natl Acad Sci U S A. 1997; 94:3064-69.
321. Liu J, Killilea D, Ames, BN. Age-associated mitochondrial oxidative decay: improvement of carnitine acetyltransferase substrate binding affinity and activity in brain by feeding old rats acetyl-L-carnitine and/or R-a-lipoic acid. Proc Natl Acad Sci U S A. 2002;99:1876-81.
322. Liu J, Head E, Gharib AM, et al. Memory loss in old rats is associated with brain mitochondrial decay and RNA/DNA oxidation: partial reversal by feeding acetyl-L-carnitine and/or R-a-lipoic acid. Proc Natl Acad Sci U S A. 2002;99:2356-61.
323. Hagen TM, Wehr CM, and Ames BN. Mitochondrial decay in aging. Reversal through dietary supplementation of acetyl-L-carnitine and N-tert-butyl-a-phenylnitrone. Ann N Y Acad Sci 1998; 854: 214-23.
324. Hagen TM, Ingersoll RT, Wehr CM, et al. Acetyl-L-carnitine fed to old rats partially restores mitochondrial function and ambulatory activity. Proc Natl Acad Sci U S A. 1998;95:9562-66.
325. Hagen TM, Ingersoll RT, Liu J, et al. (R)-a-Lipoic acid-supplemented old rats have improved mitochondrial function, decreased oxidative damage, and increased metabolic rate. FASEB J. 1999;13:411-18.
326. Hagen TM, Vinarsky V, Wehr CM, Ames BN. (R)-a-Lipoic acid reverses the age-associated increase in susceptibility of hepatocytes to tert-butylhydroperoxide both *in vitro* and *in vivo*. Antiox Redox Signal. 2000;2:473-83.
327. Lykkesfeldt J, Hagen TM, Vinarsky V, Ames BN. Age-associated decline in ascorbic acid concentration, recycling and biosynthesis in rat hepatocytes—reversal with (R)-a-Lipoic acid supplementation. FASEB J. 1998; 12:1183-89.
328. Hagen TM, Liu J, Lykkesfeldt J, et al. Feeding acetyl-L-carnitine and lipoic acid to old rats significantly improves metabolic function while decreasing oxidative stress. Proc Natl Acad Sci U S A. 2002;99:1870-75.
329. Liu J, Head E, Gharib AM, et al. Memory loss in old rats is associated with brain mitochondrial decay and RNA/DNA oxidation: partial reversal by feeding acetyl-L-carnitine and/or R-a-lipoic acid. Proc Natl Acad Sci U S A. 2002;99:2356-61.
330. Hagen TM, Liu J, Lykkesfeldt J, et al. Feeding acetyl-L-carnitine and lipoic acid to old rats significantly improves metabolic function while decreasing oxidative stress. Proc Natl Acad Sci U S A. 2002;99:1870-75.
331. Liu J, Killilea D, Ames BN. Age-associated mitochondrial oxidative decay: improvement of carnitine acetyltransferase substrate binding affinity and activity in brain by feeding old rats acetyl-L-carnitine and/or R-a-lipoic acid. Proc. Natl Acad Sci U S A. 2002;99:1876-81.
332. Liu J, Head E, Gharib AM, et al. Memory loss in old rats is associated with brain mitochondrial decay and RNA/DNA oxidation: partial reversal by feeding acetyl-L-carnitine and/or R-a-lipoic acid. Proc Natl Acad Sci U S A. 2002;99:2356-61.

333. Hagen TM, Moreau R, Suh JH, Visioli F. Mitochondrial decay in the aging rat heart: evidence for improvement by dietary supplementation with acetyl-L-carnitine and/or lipoic acid. Ann N Y Acad Sci. 2002;959:491-507.
334. Montgomery SA, Thal LJ, Amrein, R. Meta-analysis of double blind randomized controlled clinical trials of acetyl-L-carnitine versus placebo in the treatment of mild cognitive impairment and mild Alzheimer's disease. Int Clin Psychopharmacol. 2003;18:61-71.
335. Ziegler D. The Terrible Twins: Neuropathy and Diabetes. Diabetes Monitor. 2002;1-6.

Chapter 27
Clinical Approaches to Immune Imbalance and Inflammation

- ***The Biology of Inflammation: A Common Pathway in Cardiovascular Diseases, Part II***
- ***Inflammation and Autoimmunity: A Functional Medicine Approach***
- ***Essential Fatty Acids***

The Biology of Inflammation: A Common Pathway in Cardiovascular Diseases, Part II

Peter Libby, MD

Introduction[i]

Recognition that inflammatory pathways play a central role in circulatory pathophysiology furnishes a new dimension to understanding even the most familiar and clinically compelling cardiovascular diseases, notably atherosclerosis and acute myocardial infarction, both of which are discussed in detail. In addition, these inflammatory aspects of cardiovascular diseases may provide, in some cases, new therapeutic opportunities to forestall the development or the consequences of various cardiovascular conditions. Seemingly far afield at the outset, contemporary inflammation biology has concrete clinical ramifications for the practitioner. Learning to redirect inappropriate inflammatory responses may help us to improve patient outcomes in years to come. This essay will illustrate how inflammatory pathways contribute to two common and clinically compelling cardiovascular diseases. The first example, atherosclerosis, affects the blood vessels. The second, acute myocardial infarction, affects the heart itself.

[i] Adapted, with permission, from: Libby P. Inflammation: a common pathway in cardiovascular diseases. Dialogues in Cardiovascular Medicine. 2003;8(2):59-73. The original article has been divided into two parts for this book; part I can be found in Section IV: Fundamental Physiological Processes, as Chapter 18. **Acknowledgement:** Supported in part by a grant from the National Heart, Lung, and Blood Institute (HL-34636).

Atherosclerosis: A Chronic Cardiovascular Inflammatory Disease

In the past, most considered atherosclerosis a type of lipid storage disease caused by excessive cholesterol accumulating in arteries in bland pools of extracellular lipid. Recent work, however, has heightened interest in inflammatory aspects of atherosclerosis, not only at a fundamental level, but also in relation to the clinic. Actually, atherosclerosis involves inflammation at all stages, ranging from the earliest steps in atheroma formation, straight through to the ultimate clinical complications of this common affliction.

Inflammation and the Initiation of Atherosclerosis

The first steps in atherogenesis recapitulate host defenses against microbial pathogens, as explicated in Part I of this discussion (see Chapter 18). However, in this caricature of a normal host defense pathway, lipids appear to play an important role as a trigger. Lipoproteins enter the arterial intima, where they can undergo modification by oxidation, creating oxidized forms of lipids that can incite inflammation.[1] Another type of modification of lipoproteins arises by chemical condensation with glucose residues and subsequent chemical reactions that yield advanced glycation end products (AGEs).[2] Hyperglycemia such as that encountered in diabetics accelerates formation of AGEs. AGE-modified proteins can also stimulate inflammation. Recent evidence has renewed interest in the possibility that infectious agents themselves may participate in atherogenesis.[3] Viral or bacterial pathogens may trigger the localized inflammatory response inculpated in the initiation of atherosclerosis. Modified lipids, glycated proteins, and infectious agents and their products alike can elicit the expression of proinflammatory cytokines from cells resident in the arterial wall, including endothelium and vascular smooth muscle cells.[4] The proinflammatory cytokines thus produced can elicit on the endothelial surface the expression of adhesion molecules, such as VCAM-1, specialized in the recruitment of mononuclear cells. VCAM-1 binds just the sub-classes of leukocytes found in early atheroma, monocyte/macrophages, and T-lymphocytes. Experiments in animals with defective VCAM-1 molecules show reduced atherosclerosis in response to hypercholesterolemia, supporting a role for this adhesion molecule in lesion formation.[5]

Once adherent, the mononuclear cell enters the artery wall in response to chemoattractant stimuli. In the case of tissue microbial invasion, postcapillary venules typically serve as the portal for entry of the leukocyte into the affected tissue. In the case of atherosclerosis, the artery wall itself being the site of the inflammatory response, the chemoattractants such as MCP-1 cause the leukocyte to enter the arterial intima. Once resident within the intimal layer, the monocyte undergoes differentiation into a macrophage. In the context of atherogenesis, the macrophage takes on a special phenotype, the lipid-laden foam cell. Engorgement with lipid cannot occur by binding of LDL particles to the classic LDL-receptor. Cholesterol loading rapidly reduces the expression of the LDL-receptor. This autoregulation mechanism prevents foam cell formation. In atheroma, macrophages express a variety of "scavenger receptors" that evade this regulatory step, continue to be expressed despite cellular lipid accumulation, and permit foam cell formation by facilitating entry of modified lipoprotein particles into the phagocyte.[6] While resting monocytes express only low levels of scavenger receptors, after exposure to certain inflammatory mediators found in atheroma, such as M-CSF, macrophages express higher levels of these receptors that facilitate foam cell formation.[7] Mutations in various scavenger receptors limit evolution of fatty lesions in hypercholesterolemic mice.[8,9] Leukocyte adhesion, chemoattraction, and activation thus occur within the nascent atheroma, replicating the steps in a typical inflammatory response. The foam cell-rich fatty streak represents the first stage of atheroma formation.

Inflammation and Evolution of Atheromatous Plaque

If inflammatory stimulation persists, fatty streaks can progress to more complicated forms of atherosclerosis, such as the fibro-fatty plaque. Fibrogenesis results from elaboration by arterial smooth muscle cells of extracellular matrix macromolecules, including collagens, elastin, and various proteoglycan molecules. Smooth muscle cells in the plaque arise from precursors resident in the intima in humans. Lesional smooth muscle cells may also arise by migration of medial smooth muscle cells into the intima, across the demarcating internal elastic lamina. In some types of arterial pathology, bone marrow-derived precursors may also give rise to smooth muscle cells involved in fibrous lesion formation.[10] A variety of peptide growth factors can stimulate smooth muscle migration and proliferation, as well as regulate their biosynthesis of extracellular matrix macromolecules that form the fibrous part of complex atherosclerotic plaques. Protein mediators that stimulate smooth muscle migration and division include platelet-derived growth factor and basic fibroblast growth factor (bFGF).[11] Although named growth factors, in practical terms, these proteins could just as well be called cytokines, as no strict difference separates these two categories of biological mediators.

Cytokines such as IL-1 or TNF can augment the production of growth factors such as PDGF or bFGF by smooth muscle cells, providing a direct link between inflammation and the control of growth of vascular smooth muscle cells. PDGF *in vivo* probably promotes smooth muscle migration to a greater extent than proliferation. PDGF can also augment collagen production by vascular smooth muscle cells, consistent with its role in lesion evolution.

Atherosclerotic lesions also contain considerable numbers of T-lymphocytes.[12] These T cells bear markers of activation. Atherosclerotic lesions contain IFN-γ, a typical product of activated T cells. Smooth muscle cells and macrophages in human lesions also express class II histocompatibility antigens, an indicator of stimulation by IFN-γ. The reader can surmise from the foregoing summary of the cellular immune response that the atherosclerotic lesion thus contains all of the cells involved in acquired immunity. Antigens found in atherosclerotic plaques, such as modified lipoproteins and heat shock proteins (produced by cells in the atherosclerotic lesion), can act as antigens, stimulating an ongoing cellular immune response in the atheroma. In addition to innate immunity (activated macrophages) and the afferent limb of cellular immunity mediated by helper T cells, cell death mediated by Fas ligation and/or cytolytic T cells may also contribute to apoptosis of smooth muscle cells and macrophages, now clearly demonstrated in advanced human atherosclerotic lesions.[13] In illustrating the basic biology of chronic immune responses, this essay invoked the example of the granuloma engendered by infection with the tubercle bacillus. In many ways, the atheroma resembles a specialized form of granuloma, non-caseating, but with a lipid core. Many of the cellular biology and pathophysiological responses in the atheroma resemble those in the infectious granuloma. In addition, many of the molecular mediators, the cytokines and growth factors, participate in both processes. Thus, the atheroma, far from being a bland accumulation of lipids, rather resembles a smoldering chronic inflammatory response, another example of host defenses gone awry.

Inflammation and the Acute Complications of Atherosclerosis

Atheromata seldom cause acute clinical manifestations because of their obstructive, space-occupying properties. Such substantial stenoses may cause stable angina pectoris, but most acute coronary syndromes result from thrombosis-complicating plaques. In fact, many acute coronary syndromes result not from highly stenotic lesions, but from lesions that may cause lesser degrees of stenosis. Clinical data supporting this view have emerged from angiograms performed following lysis of the culprit clot by thrombolytic therapy. A substantial minority of lesions that precipitate acute myocardial infarction produces stenoses of less than 50% once the occlusive thrombus has undergone lysis. Serial angiographic studies have also shown that the culprit lesion of acute myocardial infarction often showed modest degrees of stenosis on antecedent angiograms. Other serial angiographic studies have shown that a substantial number of human atherosclerotic plaques in coronary arteries evolve rapidly and discontinuously, rather than slowly and smoothly in time.

We now recognize that most thrombotic complications of atherosclerosis that cause acute events result from the physical disruption in the atherosclerotic plaque. One form of disruption, superficial erosion, may involve concomitant inflammation, although opinions on this point differ. However, all observers agree that a fracture of the fibrous cap, the most common cause of fatal acute myocardial infarction in humans, arises at sites of heightened inflammatory responses.[14,15] Analysis of 20 culprit lesions of fatal acute myocardial infarctions showed that T-lymphocytes and macrophages predominated at sites of clinical plaque rupture, causing fatal thrombi. Smooth muscle cells and macrophages in these zones of fatal plaque disruption showed expression of the class II histocompatibility antigen HLA-DR. This result supports a role for activated T cells and macrophages in clinically significant plaque disruption. Interruption in collagen synthesis by smooth muscle cells caused by the T cell product IFN-γ (the inducer of class II histocompatibility molecules) may account for weakness and fragility of the plaque's fibrous cap at places of rupture. Autopsy studies have shown that the presence of T lymphocytes correlates inversely with indices of the synthesis of fibrillar forms of collagen, the extracellular matrix macromolecule that lends strength to the plaque's fibrous cap.

Weakening the fibrous cap results not only from decreased collagen synthesis, but from augmented collagen degradation as well. Activated macrophages secrete several types of proteinases that can attack the extracellular matrix molecules responsible for the integrity of the plaque's fibrous cap. Macrophages exposed to inflammatory cytokines step up their production of collagenases of the matrix metalloproteinase (MMP) family and lysosomal enzymes capable of dissolving arterial extracellular matrix macromolecules. These findings provide a firm foundation for involvement of inflammation in weakening of the plaque's fibrous cap and plaque disruption and thrombosis.

Once the fibrous cap fails, blood coagulation factors undergo activation by contact with tissue factor expressed by macrophages in the plaque's lipid core.[16] The expression of the tissue factor gene requires activation by inflammatory mediators. As discussed in the context of gram-negative sepsis, bacterial lipopolysaccharide can induce tissue factor expression in human monocyte/macrophages. T cells, found adjacent to macrophages in fatally disrupted human atherosclerotic plaques, can activate tissue factor expression on macrophages by producing CD154 (CD40 ligand).[17] Once again, pathways first unraveled in the context of cellular immune responses appear to participate importantly in aspects of atherogenesis, this time regulating the thrombogenicity of the plaque's lipid core.

Atherosclerosis and Inflammation: Therapeutic Implications

The foregoing discussion has illustrated the pivotal role of inflammation in all phases of atherosclerosis, lesion initiation, progression, and complication. This central role of inflammation and immunity in atherogenesis suggests that anti-inflammatory therapies might have a role in the management of this ubiquitous disease. Indeed, we have advanced the notion that lipid-lowering therapy exerts its benefit in atherosclerosis in part by acting as a specific anti-inflammatory intervention directed at the relevant instigation stimulus in this disease. Experimental studies have validated the concept that lipid lowering causes inflammation associated with atherosclerosis to subside.[18] Human observations have shown decreases in inflammatory markers such as CRP with lipid lowering. While much of this benefit probably accrues due to lipid lowering itself, some of the pharmacologic agents used in lipid management may have direct effects independent of their hypolipidemic actions. For example, statins may possess so-called "pleiotropic" effects. By interfering with intracellular signaling pathways, statins may interrupt certain inflammatory pathways. However, many *in vitro* studies of pleiotropic actions of statins employ concentrations not likely achievable under clinical circumstances. Other classes of agents used to manage atherosclerotic risk factors, including the fibric acid derivatives and thiazolidinediones (such as the insulin-sensitizing "glitazone" drugs), may have direct anti-inflammatory effects mediated by binding to nuclear receptors known as peroxisomal proliferation activating receptors (PPARs).[19] Once again, although based on substantial *in vitro* evidence, the clinical relevance of these nonlipid-dependent effects of PPAR agonists remains speculative at a clinical level.

Acute Myocardial Infarction: An Inflammatory Cardiac Disease

The previous section discussed how inflammation can set the stage for acute coronary syndromes in concluding myocardial infarction. However, myocardial infarction itself unleashes an inflammatory response at the level of the ventricular myocardium. Tissue injury can stimulate the innate immune response. Tissue necrosis elicits recruitment of the leukocyte emblematic of the acute inflammatory response, the granulocyte. The inflammatory response mediated by granulocytes in infarcting myocardium may actually extend the injury. These specific granules of neutrophils contain a form of collagenase (MMP-8) that can cleave interstitial collagen in the myocardium, favoring expansion of the infarct zone, the first step in myocardial remodeling. Such infarct expansion correlates with worsened clinical outcome. The reactive oxygen species released by the activated neutrophil can heighten local tissue injury in the infarcting myocardium. In addition, endothelial damage following on neutrophil activation can contribute to the "no-reflow" phenomenon and microvascular dysfunction that currently represents an obstacle to reperfusion therapies. Strategies that limit neutrophil accumulation following coronary ligation can alleviate some of the consequences of reperfusion injury.

Within days after acute myocardial infarction, the acute inflammatory response gives way to a more chronic reaction. Macrophages supplant polymorphonuclear leukocytes as the principal inflammatory cell type. The macrophages also contribute to tissue remodeling. Production of interstitial collagenases and other proteolytic enzymes can accentuate tissue remodeling initiated by granulocyte-derived proteinases. Administration of inhibitors of matrix metalloproteinases can limit left ventricular remodeling following experimental coronary ligation. Targeted disruption of the gene encoding MMP-9 can likewise limit infarct expansion.

The macrophage in the infarct can phagocytize dead cardiac myocytes and their debris. The macrophage also releases fibrogenic mediators that elicit tissue repair. Granulation tissue, comprised of stromal cells proliferating in response to protein growth factors migrating into the infarcted zone in response to these mediators, leads to scar formation replacing zones of coagulation necrosis of cardiac myocytes.

Angiogenesis also characterizes granulation tissue, replacing infarcted myocardium. Inflammatory mediators released by leukocytes infiltrating the infarcted zone may promote the production of angiogenic peptides such as acidic fibroblast growth factor (aFGF), bFGF, and vascular endothelial growth factor (VEGF). Thus, the "mopping up" operation affected by the chronic inflammatory cells may also promote collateral growth as part of the normal reparative mechanism in the aftermath of an acute myocardial infarction.

The tissue injury of acute myocardial infarction elicits an acute-phase response. CRP and serum amyloid-A levels in peripheral blood in the throes of an acute coronary event correlate with prognosis. Thus, the degree of the inflammatory response mounted in response to an ischemic insult to the myocardium can have considerable clinical consequence.

The exposure to immune cells of antigens usually contained within cells due to acute ischemic injury can elicit immune responses as well. Antimyosin antibodies can instigate autoimmune myocarditis in experimental models. The postpericardiotomy syndrome (Dressler's) may represent an autoimmune response engendered by myocardial injury. The above examples illustrate how inflammatory responses participate in many aspects of acute myocardial infarction and its clinical complications.

Summary

The general pathway of inflammation plays out in most cardiovascular diseases of clinical import. The recognition of the role of inflammatory processes in cardiovascular diseases furnishes a new dimension to the understanding of their pathophysiology; it also provides us with a model for understanding the inflammatory and innate immunity responses in other conditions. The inflammatory aspects of cardiovascular diseases may provide, in some cases, new therapeutic opportunities to forestall the development or the consequences of various cardiovascular conditions (see, for example, the discussion on essential fatty acids that concludes this chapter). Contemporary inflammation biology has concrete clinical ramifications for the practitioner. Learning to redirect inappropriate inflammatory responses may help us to improve patient outcomes in years to come.

Inflammation and Autoimmunity: A Functional Medicine Approach

Alex Vasquez, DC, ND

Introduction

Numerous diseases and clinical entities can be categorized under the headings of "allergy," "autoimmune diseases," and "inflammatory imbalances," and these conditions can range from mild allergies such as seasonal rhinitis to acute inflammatory emergencies such as vision-threatening temporal arteritis or neuropsychiatric lupus. Whether we call these conditions "allergic" or "autoimmune" is somewhat irrelevant; what is more important is recognizing that these conditions represent mild or severe forms of *immune system dysfunction*, wherein the immune system has begun over-responding to normally benign immunogens, whether environmental or endogenous. From this perspective, we can approach the evaluation and treatment of immune dysfunction patients with a unique set of questions. After determining the nature of the immune dysfunction, its severity, and target immunogen(s)—and once we have ruled out or appropriately managed acute emergencies—we can ask: *What factors have contributed to the genesis and perpetuation of the immune dysfunction?* Rather than merely suppressing the manifestations of ongoing immune dysfunction with the use, for example, of corticosteroids and antihistamines, *what interventions are appropriate to help normalize/optimize immune function?* Beginning the clinical assessment and therapeutic intervention with these questions leads us in a much different direction than does the prescription pad and consideration of which dose of which drug to administer.[20]

Very much like the nervous system and the gastrointestinal tract, the immune system represents an interface between a complex, ever-changing external environment and an internal system that is striving to maintain homoeostasis and defend its boundaries from potentially harmful foreign substances. Influences from within and without may alter the status of this immunologic interface and result in dysfunction to which we then affix various labels: allergic, inflammatory, or autoimmune. Restoration of health may be attained by pursuing higher levels of concordance between the internal and external milieus, such as better matching of environmental conditions and nutritional intake to basic physiological needs.[21] Previous conceptualizations of allergic and rheumatic disorders failed to appreciate the interconnectedness of various body systems and thus relied on pharmacologic interventions to suppress manifestations of underlying dysfunction. Treating all allergic disorders with "antihistamine" monotherapy and treating rheumatic disorders with immunosuppressants are two common examples of standard approaches that mask but do not normalize underlying immune dysfunction. In order to integrate new data and intervene more effectively, we must appreciate the complex interconnectedness of body systems and their relationship to the external environment. In functional medicine, we work to remediate dysfunction whenever possible, rather than relying on pharmacologic symptom suppression.

Multiple Manifestations of Immune and Inflammatory Imbalance

As discussed in other sections of this book, inflammation is a complex process with numerous complications and implications, the final details of which have yet to be elucidated. The section of this chapter on essential fatty acids (EFAs) examines many of the common underlying processes that link a number of disparate conditions that all have an inflammatory cause or mediator. Here, we will consider this topic from a number of points on the functional medicine matrix, because complex patients with inflammation and immune problems may present with widely varying clinical pictures.

Where do we begin? When faced with complex patients who seem to be "hypersensitive to everything"—including common foods and their own body tissues—we are faced with a daunting task. We have all seen patients in clinical practice who have some evidence for multiple food allergies along with evidence of autoimmunity, most commonly thyroiditis. Other patients may present with inflammatory neuropathy or atopy, along with a history of environmental exposure (e.g., mold or mercury), particularly following a series of stressful life events. With patients such as these, there is generally no single "right" place to begin; rather, the treatment plan must be multifaceted to address numerous aspects contributing to immune dysregulation. With the necessity of a multifaceted approach in mind, we begin with a detailed history to listen for which areas are a high priority. In any group of patients with the same diagnostic label (e.g., multiple sclerosis or rheumatoid arthritis), the etiologies of their *individual* diseases might be quite different. By starting with an appreciation of the major influences in mind, we can better listen to our patients and therefore intervene more accurately. However, before the patient interview begins, we must already have an appreciation of the factors that can adversely affect immune regulation, so that we can ask appropriate questions during the interview.

What factors influence immune function and, when adversely altered, might predispose to immune dysfunction? What are the history, signs, and symptoms of each? What are the appropriate methods of assessment and intervention? How might these factors interact synergistically, such that a few minor perturbations might result in disastrous health consequences? An attempt to articulate answers to these questions is provided below; emphasis is placed on the areas considered most relevant for this discussion in general, though considerations beyond this list may be relevant for individual patients.

Psychoemotional Influences

That emotional and mental forms of stress can influence immune function is well established in the research literature and in our practical life experiences. We've all seen and experienced the sequential onset of infectious illness following acute or chronic stress. A few pertinent examples will serve to make the point:

- Military cadets in intensive training characterized by acute mental stress, sleep deprivation, and physical exertion show a greatly increased susceptibility to infectious disease, particularly cellulitis and pneumonia.[22]
- Mental-emotional factors can also play a role in the development of allergy. In a prospective case-control study, children exposed to the stress of international relocation were more likely to develop atopic sensitization.[23]
- Stress may promote the development and exacerbation of inflammatory bowel diseases by effecting reductions in protective mucus and secretory IgA and by increasing mucosal permeability; the subsequent reduction in mucosal defense increases antigen absorption, promotes sensitization to subthreshold exposure to immunogens, and results in clinical relapse.[24] Loss of sIgA leaves the respira-

tory, gastrointestinal, and genitourinary tracts less defended and more vulnerable to microbial colonization and antigen absorption.

- Mild emotional stress appears to increase bacterial and yeast adherence to mucosal surfaces, potentially leading to overgrowth, infection, and clinical manifestations associated with *Helicobacter pylori*, *Candida albicans*, *Escherichia coli*, *Haemophilus influenzae*, and others. The primary mechanism appears to be the stress-induced increase in salivary adhesion molecule sulfo-Lewis-a, which links microbes to mucosal glycoprotein MUC5B.[25]
- Mental-emotional stress commonly leads to sleep disturbance and insomnia, both of which exacerbate the body's inherent inflammatory tendency, as evidenced by increases in the inflammatory marker CRP in sleep-disturbed patients.[26]

Conversely, relaxing, pleasant experiences appear to reduce inflammatory responses, promote normalization of neuroendocrine status, and allow humoral and cellular elements of the immune system to function competently. Music therapy has been shown to increase salivary secretory IgA, decrease plasma cortisol, decrease symptoms in patients with bronchial asthma, and to reduce latex-induced wheal in patients with latex sensitization.[27] In a controlled clinical trial with 50 human subjects, stress reduction was shown to reduce experimental neurogenic inflammation.[28]

In sum, a shift in the balance of emotional experience away from relaxation and toward stress appears to increase susceptibility to allergy, infection, and neurogenic inflammatory responses. Clinically, we see that many immune-mediated disorders are exacerbated by stressful events, and that some patients must adopt a less stressful lifestyle if healing of their ailment is to be attained. Optimization of the patient's psychoemotional environment, frequent implementation of stress-reduction and meditative techniques, and the establishment and preservation of restorative sleep are important to shift the inherent tendency of the body away from inflammation and in the direction of health and homeostasis.

Endocrinologic Influences

Several hormones have immune-modulating effects and show characteristic patterns of imbalance in patients with inflammatory and atopic disease. Clinically, we observe that many patients with immune dysfunction have relatively lower levels of cortisol, dehydroepiandrosterone (DHEA), and testosterone, and more rarely, "subclinical" deficiencies of progesterone may be seen. Relative elevations in estradiol and/or exposure to estrogen-like compounds (xenoestrogens) are also common among patients with autoimmune disorders. Proof of principle is found in clinical trials and case reports demonstrating successful treatment of various allergic and autoimmune disorders when patients are treated with hormones such as testosterone, DHEA, and cortisol. Cortisol is a well-known immunoregulatory hormone, and it becomes immunosuppressive when administered or produced in supraphysiologic amounts or as a potentiated analog such as prednisone. Given that cortisol is immunoregulatory, and that chronic mental-emotional stress suppresses endogenous cortisol production,[29] a possible mechanism by which mental-emotional stress leads to the exacerbation of immune dysfunction is immediately apparent. Low endogenous production of cortisol appears to exacerbate many inflammatory, allergic, and autoimmune disorders, and administration of bioidentical cortisol in physiologic doses can lead to clinical improvement.[30,31]

DHEA levels are low in patients with systemic lupus erythematosus and the inflammatory bowel diseases (Crohn's disease and ulcerative colitis[32]); DHEA administration can lead to clinical improvement.[33,34] Compared to disease-free control groups, men with rheumatic/autoimmune diseases show lower levels of testosterone[35] and higher levels of estradiol,[36] thus leading to a significant reduction in the testosterone/estradiol ratio; reversal of this trend is clinically desirable. A clinical trial involving postmenopausal women with rheumatoid arthritis showed that androgen administration led to significant subjective and objective improvements.[37] The clinical significance of progesterone's role in immune function is much less clear, particularly since paradoxical responses to progesterone are seen in certain patient groups.[38] Hormonal assessment and appropriate intervention are valuable considerations in patients with allergic and rheumatic diseases.

Environmental and Xenobiotic Influences

Environmental contributions to autoimmune and inflammatory disorders deserve high priority in the evaluation and treatment of all patients with rheumatic diseases, which, again, are manifestations of immune dysfunction. The major considerations under the heading of "environment" include diet, nutrition, ultraviolet and ionizing radiation, exogenous microbial products (i.e., inhaled mycotoxins and bioaerosols), xenobiotics such as mercury, herbicides, pesticides, and the plethora of industrial, military, and petrochemical toxicants.[39]

- "Food allergies" (within which, for ease of discussion, we include intolerances and sensitivities as well as classic allergies) can precipitate a wide range of inflammatory disorders, including arthritis and inflammatory bowel disease.[40] In particular, sensitivity to wheat gluten can trigger lupus,[41,42] thyroid autoimmunity,[43,44] and several other autoimmune endocrinopathies.[45] Given that food allergies can damage the mucosa of the small intestine and thus promote macromolecular absorption, these reactions can also promote the development of additional food allergies via enhancement of antigen absorption, which promotes immune sensitization.
- Mercury is a type-1 sensitizing agent associated with autoimmune diseases[46] such as multiple sclerosis[47] and with atopic disease such as eczema.[48] Occupational exposure to the insecticide DDT is associated with reductions in serum IgG (suggesting immune suppression), as well as increases in serum antinuclear antibodies (suggesting immune dysregulation).[49] Indeed, the paradox of immunosuppression and concomitant autoimmunity is the classic manifestation of xenobiotic-induced immunotoxicity.
- Chronic exposure to mold from water-damaged buildings can induce neuronal autoimmunity and systemic inflammation, resulting in a clinical picture that may be labeled "multiple sclerosis" or "idiopathic peripheral neuropathy."[50]
- Vitamin D insufficiency is epidemic in the United States and is extremely prevalent (> 90%) among patients with chronic musculoskeletal pain;[51] this condition induces a systemic inflammatory response and causes skeletal pain by promoting the development of an unmineralized collagen matrix which hydrates, swells, and compresses sensory nerves in the periosteum. Insufficient sun exposure—whether from indoor living, sunscreen use, or nonequatorial latitudes—can result in a vitamin D deficiency that is easily correctible with oral supplementation in the range of 4,000 IU per day for adults.[52]

Thus, when evaluating patients with inflammatory, allergic, and autoimmune disorders, attention must be given to the environment in which the patient exists—including xenobiotic and dietary exposures, as well as the sufficiency or insufficiency of sun exposure and vitamin D intake.

Gastrointestinal and Mucosal Influences: Occult Infections

As discussed in depth in Chapter 28, impaired digestion and increased mucosal permeability can alter the intestinal milieu and promote macromolecule absorption, and these alterations may precipitate systemic inflammatory imbalance. More specifically, intestinal colonization with either pathogenic or immunogenic microbes such as yeast, gram-negative bacteria, protozoa, and amoebas may provoke an immune response that cross-reacts with human body tissues, inducing a systemic inflammatory disease.[53] Additional details are abundant in the research literature, strongly implicating altered bowel microflora, "dysbiosis," as the genesis for many chronic health problems.[54]

While most of this research is specifically relevant for the gastrointestinal tract, the mucosal surfaces of the nasopharynx, sinuses, lower respiratory tract, and the genitourinary mucosa must be considered, along with the patient's domestic, occupational, and recreational environments as sources of microbe-induced immune dysfunction. More recently, occult dental infections have become recognized as a source of proinflammatory immunogenic stimulation that contributes to a wide range of chronic health problems.[55,56,57,58] Regardless of their origin—whether endogenous (i.e., mucosal or dental) or exogenous (e.g., mold bioaerosols from water-damaged buildings)—many microbial products are clearly capable of initiating clinical disease and immune dysfunction in humans.[59]

In situations where further investigation is indicated, most practitioners begin searching for occult infections by assessing the gastrointestinal tract with comprehensive stool and parasitology analysis performed by a specialty laboratory (three stool samples from three days, analyzed separately). Abnormal microbes are then eliminated and health-promoting microbes are replaced with probiotics (see the 4R program discussion in Chapter 28). Empiric antimicrobial therapy against bacteria, amoebas, protozoas, and yeast may be implemented if test results are negative and clinical suspicion of occult infection or gastrointestinal colonization remains high. Thereafter, consideration of and assessment for occult dental infections by dental specialists ("biologic dentists"), occult infections in the respiratory and genitourinary tracts, and toxic microbial exposures from the patient's occupational, residential, and recreational environments can be pursued. Mucosal integrity of the small intestine can be assessed easily and accurately with the lactulose-mannitol assay.

Nutritional Influences

While it is true that consumption of foods to which a person is reactive can precipitate and exacerbate a wide range of inflammatory disorders, it is also true that certain foods and cultural styles of eating can either promote or retard the development of inflammatory and autoimmune disorders. The standard American diet, commonly referred to as SAD, is inherently proinflammatory due to its excess of sugars and arachidonic acid and its insufficiency of omega-3 fatty acids and phytonutrients.[60] *In vitro* evidence shows that corn oil, a rich source of the omega-6 fatty acid linoleic acid, induces an inflammatory response in hepatic Kupffer cells and an upregulation in inflammatory gene transcription that is consistent with data in humans linking vegetable oil consumption with inflammatory and malignant diseases.[61] Supplied in high amounts in dairy products, beef, pork, and other foods of land-animal origin, arachidonic acid is the precursor to the proinflammatory prostaglandins and leukotrienes that participate in the genesis and progression of essentially all inflammatory conditions; diets low in arachidonate tend to have a relative anti-inflammatory effect.

Consumption of meals with a high glycemic load and foods with a high glycemic index induces an inflammatory response demonstrated by elevations in C-reactive protein and other markers of inflammation. Whole, natural foods such as fruits, vegetables, nuts, seeds, and berries are generally rich sources of phytonutrients that have antioxidant and anti-inflammatory properties.[62] Certain dietary components, such as vitamin D, green tea, rosemary, grape seed extract, resveratrol, selenium, and zinc are also inhibitors of the NFκB proinflammatory cascade.

Modern diets are characteristically deficient in omega-3 fatty acids, and thus most of our patients are likewise deficient in these fatty acids that have anti-inflammatory benefits mediated by inhibiting proinflammatory prostaglandin production, increasing production of anti-inflammatory prostaglandins, and modulating genetic expression.[63] Harmonization of human physiology with a nutritional environment of whole natural foods, abundant exercise, and sufficient vitamin D is an important goal in the promotion of health and alleviation of disease.[64] Within the framework of a health-promoting diet, customization will be necessary for patients who are allergic to otherwise "healthy foods" such as citrus fruits and shellfish.

Neurogenic Influences

Neurogenic inflammation may play a major role in many allergic and autoimmune/inflammatory disorders, yet the importance of addressing the nervous system in the treatment of inflammatory conditions seems to be underappreciated by many healthcare practitioners. Neurogenic inflammation, the release of proinflammatory mediators by sensory terminals of the peripheral nervous system,[65] appears to play a role in diverse allergic and rheumatic diseases, including asthma[66] and rheumatoid arthritis.[67] Since neurogenic inflammation can be inhibited by interference with nociceptive input transmitted via afferent C fibers, and since intense mechanoreceptor stimulation by spinal manipulation interferes with nociceptive input transmitted via afferent C fibers,[68] it appears possible that spinal manipulation could help produce a neurogenically mediated anti-inflammatory benefit. Similarly, the overall benefits and anti-inflammatory effects of relaxation and stress reduction are partly mediated by reductions in neurogenically mediated inflammation.[69]

Additional evidence reviewed by Meggs[70] shows that neurogenic inflammation is a contributing factor in several common clinical entities, including migraine, rhinitis, and the multiple chemical sensitivity syndromes. The phenomenon of "neurogenic switching" as described by Meggs[71] is the mechanism by which sensory input, chemical exposure, or tissue damage in "location A" can be transmitted neurologically to produce pain, inflammation, and tissue degeneration in "location B," and the occurrence of this phenomenon has been demonstrated *in vivo*.[72] Indeed, neurogenic inflammation and its transmission to distant sites may be a significant factor in many inflammatory disorders encountered in clinical practice, and its amelioration via mechanoreceptor stimulation and stress-reduction techniques is worthy of consideration and additional research.

Therapeutic Interventions and Alternatives to NSAIDs

In late 2004 and early 2005, we witnessed the end of what can be referred to as the "cyclooxygenase paradigm" of inflammation. The specific targeting of the inflammation-induced cyclooxygenase-2 isoenzyme (COX-2) by selective pharmaceutical drugs rose and fell, leaving behind a legacy of human tragedy, exorbitant expenses, and suggestions of collusion between the pharmaceutical industry and the U.S. FDA, both of which failed to protect the public from medications that were well established as hazardous soon after their release onto the healthcare market.[73,74,75] By demonizing and targeting COX-2, the pharmaceutical industry overlooked the beneficial roles of one of this enzyme's major products—prostacyclin, which reduces both blood pressure and platelet aggregation. The widespread cardiovascular catastrophe that ensued due to the chronic administration of these COX-2 inhibitors injured at least 160,000 patients and killed an estimated 26,000–55,000 patients.[76] Previous to the introduction of COX-2 inhibitors, it was estimated that nonsteroidal anti-inflammatory drugs killed at least 16,500 arthritis patients per year.[77] Likewise, many surgical treatments for musculoskeletal pain carry excess risk and insufficient efficacy. For example, Bernstein and Quach[78] concluded in their 2003 review, "Arthroscopy for degenerative conditions of the knee is among the most commonly employed orthopedic procedures, but its effectiveness (like the effectiveness of many surgical operations) has never been proven in prospective trials."

For all these reasons, it seems vital that clinicians consider options to some of these conventional interventions. Safe and effective natural interventions for the treatment of musculoskeletal pain are well substantiated in the biomedical research literature and have been recently reviewed elsewhere. [79,80,81,82] Manipulative, nutritional, and botanical interventions are briefly outlined in the sections that follow.

Manual Therapies

Spinal manipulation. Naturopathic, chiropractic, and osteopathic physicians receive training in manually applied manipulative therapies, the best known of which is spinal manipulation. The conclusion that chiropractic management of low-back pain is superior to pharmaceutical and surgical management in terms of greater safety, greater effectiveness, and reduced cost has been consistently documented for more than a decade.[83] In a randomized trial involving 741 patients, Meade et al.[84] reported, "Chiropractic treatment was more effective than hospital outpatient management, mainly for patients with chronic or severe back pain. ... Secondary outcome measures also showed that chiropractic was more beneficial." A three-year follow-up study by these same authors[85] in 1995 showed, "At three years the results confirm the findings of an earlier report that when chiropractic or hospital therapists treat patients with low-back pain as they would in day-to-day practice those treated by chiropractic derive more benefit and long term satisfaction than those treated by hospitals." In 2004, Legorreta et al.[86] reported that the availability of chiropractic care was associated with significant cost savings among 700,000 patients with chiropractic coverage, compared to 1 million patients whose insurance coverage was limited to medical treatments. A literature review by Dabbs and Lauretti[87] found that spinal manipulation is safer than the use of NSAIDs in the treatment of neck pain. Contrasting the rates of manipulation-associated cerebrovascular accidents to the adverse outcomes of pharmaceutical and surgical treatments for spinal pain, Rosner[88] noted, "These rates are 400 times lower than the death rates observed from gastrointestinal bleeding due to the use of nonsteroidal anti-inflammatory drugs and 700 times lower than the overall mortality rate for spinal surgery." Similarly, in his review of the literature comparing the safety of chiropractic manipulation in patients with low-back pain associated with lumbar disc herniation, Oliphant[89] stated that, "The apparent safety of spinal manipulation, especially when compared with other [medically] accepted treatments for [lumbar disk herniation], should stimulate its use in the conservative treatment plan of [lumbar disk herniation]."

Mechanisms of action of spinal manipulation include the following:

1. releasing entrapped intra-articular menisci and synovial folds;
2. acutely reducing intradiscal pressure, thus promoting replacement of decentralized disc material;
3. stretching of deep periarticular muscles to break the cycle of chronic autonomous muscle contraction by lengthening the muscles and thereby releasing excessive actin-myosin binding;

4. promoting restoration of proper kinesthesia and proprioception;
5. promoting relaxation of paraspinal muscles by stretching facet joint capsules;
6. promoting relaxation of paraspinal muscles via "postactivation depression," which is the temporary depletion of contractile neurotransmitters;
7. temporarily elevating plasma beta-endorphin;
8. temporarily enhancing phagocytic ability of neutrophils and monocytes; and
9. activation of the diffuse descending pain inhibitory system located in the periaqueductal gray matter.

While this list of mechanisms of action is certainly not complete, for purposes of this section it is sufficient to point out that joint manipulation in general and spinal manipulation in particular have objective mechanistic effects that correlate with their clinical benefits. Additional details are provided in numerous published reviews,[90] textbooks, and the unsurpassed treatise by Leach.[91] When evaluated by the parameters of safety, effectiveness, and cost effectiveness, spinal manipulation is clearly a valuable and rational primary therapy for the treatment of spine-related pain and inflammation, such as neck pain and low-back pain. Clinicians should provide timely referral for manipulative therapy for their patients with spinal pain, if those skills are not within their own repertoire.

Other manual therapies and physiotherapeutic interventions. There is a growing body of research on massage, hydrotherapy, and other physiotherapies for the effective treatment of pain and inflammation associated with aging[92] or overexertion,[93] or caused by physical injuries such as frozen shoulder[94,95] and by diseases such as rheumatoid arthritis,[96] osteoarthritis,[97] and asthma.[98] Massage can also be safe and effective in the treatment of low-back pain.[99] Regardless of the approach recommended, a referral to a skilled practitioner is vital.

Nutritional Supplementation

Glucosamine and chondroitin sulfate. Articular cartilage is produced endogenously from nutrients that are biochemically transformed into glucosamine and chondroitin—the "building blocks" from which cartilage is built. Oral supplementation with glucosamine and chondroitin is intended to enhance cartilage anabolism and counteract the cartilage catabolism seen in inflammatory and degenerative processes.[100] Clinical trials with glucosamine and chondroitin sulfates have shown consistently positive results with osteoarthritis of the hands, hips, knees, temporomandibular joint, and low back. For example, in a three-year, placebo-controlled clinical trial, glucosamine sulfate was superior to placebo for pain reduction and preservation of joint space in patients with knee osteoarthritis.[101] The adult dose of glucosamine sulfate is generally 1,500–2,000 mg per day in divided doses, and the dose of chondroitin sulfate is approximately 1,000 mg daily. Both treatments are safe for multi-year use. Rare adverse effects include allergy and nonpathologic gastrointestinal upset. Clinical benefit is generally significant following 4–6 weeks of treatment, and is maintained for the duration of treatment. Glucosamine does not adversely affect glucose metabolism or insulin resistance in diabetics.

Niacinamide. More than 50 years ago, pioneering clinical studies by Kaufman[102] showed that niacinamide was effective in the treatment of osteoarthritis. Confirmation of these results was recently provided in a double-blind, placebo-controlled study documenting that niacinamide therapy improved joint mobility, reduced objective inflammation as assessed by ESR, reduced the impact of the arthritis on the activities of daily living, and allowed a reduction in medication use.[103] Inhibition of joint-destroying nitric oxide appears to be an important mechanism of action in the antirheumatic effect of niacinamide; however, the nutrient may also provide an antiarthritic benefit via enhancement of mitochondrial function and reversal of aging phenotypes that characterize chondrocyte senescence. The standard dose of niacinamide for the treatment of joint pain is 500 mg given orally six times per day. Hepatic dysfunction is rare when daily doses are kept below 3,000 mg per day, yet Gaby[104] recommends measurement of liver enzymes after three months of treatment and yearly thereafter.

Proteolytic enzymes. Enzyme preparations containing pancreatin, bromelain, papain, amylase, lipase, trypsin, and alpha-chymotrypsin are well absorbed into systemic circulation following oral administration and provide numerous health benefits, particularly in the treatment of conditions associated with inflammation or infection (cellulitis, diabetic ulcers, sinusitis, and bronchitis).[105] For example, in a double-blind, placebo-controlled trial with 59 patients, Taub[106] documented that oral administration of bromelain significantly promoted the resolution of congestion, inflammation, and edema in patients with acute and chronic refractory sinusitis; no adverse effects were noted. Reporting from the Tulane University Health Service Center, Trickett[107] reported that a papain-containing preparation benefited 40 patients with various injuries (e.g., contusions, sprains, lacerations, strains, fracture, surgical repair, and muscle tears); no adverse effects were seen. In a recent open trial of patients with knee pain, Walker et al.[108] found a dose-dependent reduction in pain and disability, as well as a significant improvement in psychological well-being in patients consuming bromelain orally. Although administration of single enzymes may be appropriate for clinical use, enzyme therapy is generally delivered in the form of polyenzyme preparations containing pancreatin, bromelain, papain, amylase, lipase, trypsin, and alpha-chymotrypsin. Tablets are administered between meals to preserve enzymatic action and enhance absorption.

Botanical Anti-inflammatories

Devil's Claw (*Harpagophytum procumbens*). Supported by centuries of use and numerous clinical trials, *Harpagophytum* is a moderately effective botanical analgesic suitable for clinical utilization. Clinical trials showing that *Harpagophytum* does not alter eicosanoid metabolism in humans suggests that this botanical works centrally or peripherally on the nervous system, and a recent experimental study shows that components of *Harpagophytum* have an antinociceptive effect in the spinal cord.[109] In a recent meta-analysis of 12 clinical trials, *Harpagophytum* was found to be clinically valuable and with adverse effects comparable to placebo.[110] In patients with osteoarthritis of the hip and knee, *Harpagophytum* is just as effective yet safer and better tolerated than the drug diacerein. In a study involving 183 patients with low-back pain, *Harpagophytum* was found to be safe and moderately effective in patients with "severe and unbearable pain" and radiating pain with neurologic deficit.[111] Most recently, *Harpagophytum* was studied in a head-to-head clinical trial with the notorious selective COX-2 inhibitor Vioxx® (rofecoxib); the data indicate that *Harpagophytum* was safer and at least as effective.[112] About 8% of patients may experience diarrhea or other mild gastrointestinal effects, and fewer patients may experience dizziness; *Harpagophytum* may potentiate anticoagulants. Treatment should be continued for at least four weeks, and many patients will continue to improve after eight weeks from the initiation of treatment.[113] Products are generally standardized for the content of harpagosides, with a target dose of at least 30 and preferably up to 60 mg harpagosides per day. Chrubasik[114] noted that while *Harpagophytum* appears to be safe and moderately effective for the treatment of musculoskeletal pain, different proprietary products show significant variances in potency and clinical effectiveness. Overall, the data suggest that *Harpagophytum* is better than placebo and at least as good as commonly-used NSAIDs,[115] suggesting that *Harpagophytum* should be clinically preferred over NSAIDs due to the lower cost and greater safety.

Cat's Claw (*Uncaria spp*). Like many other botanicals, *Uncaria* species, including *Uncaria tomentosa* and *Uncaria guianensis*, have been used for centuries, and modern research is providing proof of safety and efficacy. *Uncaria* demonstrates multifunctional anti-inflammatory benefits by reducing inflammation mediated by NFκB, TNF-α, COX-2, and PGE-2. Thirty patients with osteoarthritis of the knees benefited from highly concentrated, freeze-dried aqueous extraction of *Uncaria guianensis* dosed at one capsule of 100 mg daily; reduction in pain was approximately 36% at four weeks.[116] A year-long study of patients with active rheumatoid arthritis (RA) treated with sulfasalazine or hydroxychloroquine showed "relative safety and modest benefit" of *Uncaria tomentosa* (UT).[117] No major adverse effects have been noted; however, headache and dizziness are more common in patients receiving *Uncaria* than in patients in placebo groups. Based on its historical use as a contraceptive, this herb should not be used during pregnancy or by women desiring to conceive. Commercially prepared products contain between 250 and 500 mg per dose and are standardized to 3.0% alkaloids and 15% total polyphenols and administered 1–3 times per day. Other studies with *Uncaria tomentosa* have shown enhancement of post-vaccination immunity and enhancement of DNA repair in humans.

Willow bark (*Salix* spp). Actions of willow bark are manifold, including antioxidative, anticytokine, along with cyclooxygenase- and lipoxygenase-inhibiting effects. In a double-blind, placebo-controlled clinical trial in 210 patients with moderate/severe low-back pain (20% of patients had positive straight-leg raising test), extract of willow bark showed a dose-dependent analgesic effect, with benefits beginning in the first week of treatment.[118] In a head-to-head study of 228 patients comparing willow bark (standardized for 240 mg salicin) with Vioxx (rofecoxib), treatments were equally effective yet willow bark was safer and 40% less expensive.[119] The daily dose ranges from 120 to 240 mg of salicin, and products should include other components of the whole plant for enhanced efficacy. Except for rare allergy, no adverse effects are known. Use during pregnancy and with anti-coagulant medication is discouraged.

Boswellia (*Boswellia serrata*). Boswellia shows anti-inflammatory action via inhibition of 5-lipoxygenase with no effect on cyclooxygenase. A recent clinical study showed that Boswellia was able to reduce pain and swelling while increasing joint flexion and walking distance in patients with osteoarthritis of the knees.[120] While reports from clinical trials published in English are relatively rare, a recent abstract from the German medical research[121] stated, "In clinical trials promising results were observed in patients with rheumatoid arthritis, chronic colitis, ulcerative colitis, Crohn's disease, bronchial asthma and peritumoral brain edemas." Minor gastrointestinal upset has been reported, but otherwise this botanical is very well tolerated. Products are generally standardized to contain 37.5–65% boswellic acids, which are currently considered the active constituents with clinical benefit. The target dose is approximately 150 mg of boswellic acids thrice daily; dose and number of capsules/tablets will vary depending upon the concentration found in differing products.

Ginger (*Zingiber officinale*). Ginger is a well-known spice and food with a long history of consumption and use as an anti-inflammatory and antinausea agent. Components of ginger inhibit 5-lipoxygenase as well as cyclooxygenase. With its dual action in the reduction of inflammation-promoting prostaglandins and leukotrienes, as well as its ability to inhibit nitric oxide production, ginger has been shown to safely reduce the pain and disability associated with osteoarthritis, rheumatoid arthritis, muscle aches, osteoarthritis of the knees, and migraine headaches. Doses up to 1 g of ginger per day have been safely used during pregnancy to reduce nausea and vomiting[122] and hyperemesis gravidarum.[123] Doses for the treatment of rheumatic conditions have ranged from 1 g (one-half teaspoon) of powdered ginger up to 50 g per day of fresh or lightly cooked root. The volatile principles of ginger often create a warm or burning sensation in the stomach that is mild and reducible with food consumption, and research suggests that ginger has a protective benefit against gastric ulceration. No significant adverse effects due to ginger are known; the presence of cholecystitis or the use of Coumadin/warfarin are relative contraindications due to ginger's mild cholagogic and anticoagulant actions, respectively.

Summary

The data surveyed in this section will provide most clinicians with an expanded perspective on the causes of and available treatments for clinical entities characterized by pain, inflammation, and immune dysregulation. While alternatives to NSAIDs were reviewed, their use as first-line therapy for pain and inflammation is of secondary importance to the larger and more comprehensive goal of attaining overall health improvement and a reduction in any systemic inflammatory tendency initiated and perpetuated by occult infections, food allergies, hormonal aberrations, hypovitaminosis D, xenobiotic exposure, and a proinflammatory dietary pattern.

Clinicians implementing the clinical approach outlined here can conceptualize the strategy as containing two specific arms that can be implemented simultaneously for optimal clinical improvement. First, the patient's overall health and environmental status must be evaluated and optimized to the greatest extent possible (common sense may lead us to question the use of anti-inflammatory drugs while the patient continues to consume a proinflammatory diet, for example). Second, while both patient and doctor are engaged in characterizing and optimizing the patient's overall health—e.g., searching for and eliminating occult infections and treating nutritional deficiencies (such as vitamin D) and nutritional excesses (such as iron overload[124])—specific nutritional and botanical anti-inflammatory and analgesic interventions can be employed to effect a more rapid resolution of swelling, discomfort, and tissue injury. This dual approach to restoring overall health and reducing symptoms is gratifying for both the doctor and the patient. A comprehensive approach, inclusive of the nutritional and botanical therapies described herein, can be supported by peer-reviewed research in the biomedical literature and is safe and cost-effective.[125]

Essential Fatty Acids

Robert H. Lerman MD, PhD

Introduction

Essential fatty acids (EFAs) are of critical importance for two basic reasons. First, they are essential constituents of all cell membranes and thus are determinants of membrane stability, receptor action, membrane-bound enzyme activity, hormone binding, cell fluidity, signal transduction, and ion channel function.[126] Second, they are precursors of eicosanoids, second-messenger mediators involved in inflammation. It is the latter aspect that will be emphasized in this chapter. Evidence will be presented indicating the role of fatty acids and their derivative compounds in several inflammatory disorders, including cardiovascular disease, inflammatory bowel disease, rheumatoid arthritis, bronchial asthma, psoriasis, and renal disease.

Whereas acute inflammatory reactions are usually protective and part of the normal innate immune response, uncontrolled chronic inflammatory processes are detrimental[127,128] and lead to disease. The functional medicine use of EFAs in these conditions is an important therapeutic tool; understanding the common pathophysiology involved in inflammation allows the functional medicine practitioner to manage seemingly disparate disorders in a consistent fashion. While the emphasis will be placed on fatty acids as precursors to eicosanoids, the value of these essential constituents via their membrane functions should not be overlooked. Nevertheless, it is important to understand that whereas supplementation with essential fats to suppress inflammation is of great value, such management should not be construed as definitive. Always, the clinician must search for and, when possible, determine and correct the underlying cause(s) of dysfunction in order to produce sustained reversal of illness.

Definitions and Pathways

PUFAs, Eicosanoids, Prostanoids, Isoprostanes, and Resolvins

Polyunsaturated fatty acids (PUFAs) include the essential fatty acids (EFAs) and their derivatives, collectively referred to as "essential fats" to emphasize the fact that many of these PUFAs are critical to life.[129] Linoleic acid (LA; 18:2ω6) and α-linolenic acid (ALA: 18:3ω3) are the EFAs, the precursors of the ω6 and ω3 fatty acid families, respectively. EFA derivatives include compounds with 20 or more carbon atoms and 3 to 6 double bonds. Eicosanoids (from *eicosa* meaning "20" in Greek) are local acting, hormone-like lipid mediators with brief half lives, produced by oxidation of the 20 carbon ω6 fatty acids, arachidonic acid (AA; 20:4ω6) and dihomo-gamma linolenic acid (DGLA; 20:3ω6), as well as by the 20 carbon ω3 fatty acid, eicosapentaenoic acid (EPA; *20:5*ω3). These fatty acids are acquired only by ingestion of essential fats from foods or supplements. (Figure 27.1 shows the arachidonic acid cascade.)

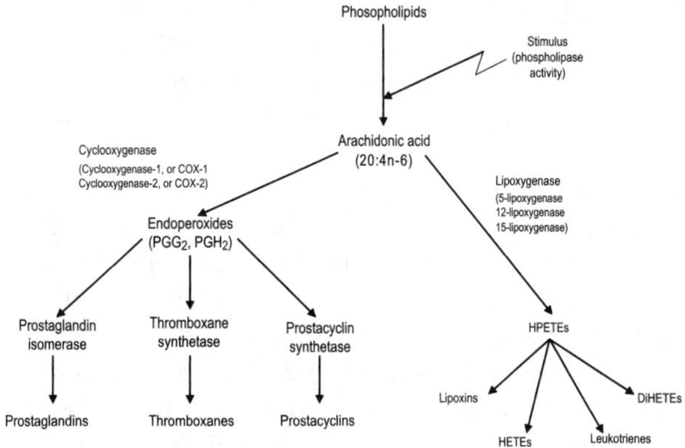

Figure 27.1 **Arachidonic acid (AA) cascade**

There are three main enzymatic pathways for synthesis of eicosanoids.[130] Some compounds are also formed non-enzymatically. Among the enzymatic pathways, cyclooxygenase (COX), also known as prostaglandin synthase, generates endoperoxides, which are converted into prostanoids: prostaglandins (PGs), thromboxanes (TXs), and prostacyclins (PGIs). The lipoxygenase (LOX) pathway leads to production of hydroperoxyeicosatetraenoic acids (HPETEs) and lipoxins. The so-called "third pathway" has drawn less attention and is mediated by cytochrome P450 enzymes to form a number of hydroxy fatty acids, HETEs, and epoxy acids. The main eicosanoids are the PGs, LTs (leukotrienes), and TXs. Most cells synthesize eicosanoids but the type of compound depends upon the particular cell. Platelets produce TXA_2, a potent platelet aggregator and vasoconstrictor, from AA, and TXA_3, a weaker platelet aggregator from EPA. Endothelial cells produce PGI_2, a potent vasodilator and platelet aggregation inhibitor, from AA, and PGI_3 with lesser vasodilatory and aggregation inhibitory effects, from EPA. Leukocytes produce LTB_4, a powerful chemotactic, vasoconstrictive, vascular permeability, and neutrophil aggregation factor, from AA, and LTB_5, with very weak chemotactic and vasoconstrictor activities, from EPA.[131]

Free radical-catalyzed peroxidation of AA leads to the formation of isoprostanes by the non-enzymatic pathway. Most of these eicosanoids are either biologically active or are converted into metabolites that have biological activities. F2-isoprostanes are potent vasoconstrictors. Measurement of F2-isoprostanes is one of the most reliable approaches for assessing oxidative stress status *in vivo*.[132] Neuroprostanes are similar compounds formed from free radical-mediated oxidation of DHA, which is highly enriched in neurons. F4-neuroprostanes appear valuable as a marker of oxidative stress in the brain in neurodegenerative diseases.[133] Isoprostanes are mediators of hypertension (HTN) and tissue ischemia.

Recently, resolvins, docosatrienes, and neuroprotectins have been identified in spontaneously resolving inflammatory exudates.[134] In initial studies, animals had been treated with aspirin, and the compounds isolated from the resolving exudates were termed aspirin-triggered resolvins. Subsequent studies indicated that these oxygenated products were also generated from EPA and DHA without aspirin. They possess potent anti-inflammatory, pro-resolving, protective, and immunoregulatory properties. They dampen inflammation and neutrophil-mediated injury and are considered self-protective mediators. Of note, DHA has been shown to be a substrate for human COX-2 in the formation of this class of compounds.[135] Expect to hear much more about them in the future.[136]

Eicosanoid Precursors

AA is the principal eicosanoid precursor, as the membranes of most cells contain substantially more AA than other eicosanoid precursors.[137] It is the precursor of proinflammatory and pro-aggregatory eicosanoids; EPA is the precursor of eicosanoids with antagonistic effects. (Figure 27.2 shows dietary influences on the EFA pathways.) DGLA is the precursor of 1-series eicosanoids with principally inflammatory modulating effects. DGLA may be converted to AA via the enzyme delta-5 desaturase (D5D), an enzyme that generally has low activity in humans. Thus, most AA is of dietary origin; its primary source in the U.S. diet is from animal products. DGLA comes mainly from dietary LA and requires conversion to gamma linolenic acid (GLA) by delta 6-desaturase (D6D), an enzyme whose activity may be impaired by a number of factors,[138] such as starvation, a very low-protein diet, high alcohol intake, smoking, stress-related hormones (corticosteroids and catecholamines), and intake of excessive saturated fat and/or *trans* fatty acids, as well as aging in males, ionizing radiation, some viral infections, atopic eczema, and type 1 diabetes. Vegetable and marine oils potently suppress both D6D and D5D, with effects of fish oils being greater.[139] A calorie-restricted intake may increase D6D activity three-fold and a very high-protein diet activates it.[140] When D6D is inhibited, bypassing that metabolic step by providing GLA from evening primrose oil or borage oil will allow substrate for DGLA with ultimate series-1 eicosanoid formation.

Enzymes and Inhibitors

Phospholipase A_2 (PLA_2) activation is responsible for the initial mobilization of AA from membrane phospholipids.[141] PLA_2 is located at the cell membrane and may be inhibited by drugs such as cortisone, and by natural agents such as licorice, vitamin E, and quercetin.[142] Two separate isoforms of COX, COX-1 and COX-2, catalyze the same reactions. COX-1 is a constitutive enzyme and its activity doesn't change much once the cell is mature. COX-2 is highly inducible in response to inflammatory stimuli[143] and is highly expressed in inflamed tissues. It is believed that eicosanoids produced by COX-1 activity are essential for physiological functions, while those produced by COX-2 lead to various pathological changes in body tissues. COX-2 is upregulated by cytokines, mitogens, and endotoxins and produces PGs involved in inflammatory processes. Non-steroidal anti-inflammatory drugs (NSAIDs) such as aspirin, indomethacin, and ibuprofen are non-selective COX inhibitors, inhibiting both COX-1 and COX-2 activities.[144,145,146] COX-1 derived eicosanoids are required for the protection of gastrointestinal mucosa, maintenance of renal function, and control of hemostasis. COX enzymes may be inhibited not only by medications but also by many natural agents including ginger,[147] turmeric (*Curcumin longa*),[148] melatonin,[149] green tea,[150] quercetin,[151] and cayenne.[152] Certain natural products (including hops fractions) act upstream, possibly at the level of NFκB, to reduce the production of COX-2.[153] 5-LOX is modulated by the EPA/AA ratio and inhibited by drugs such as colchicine,[154] as well as by

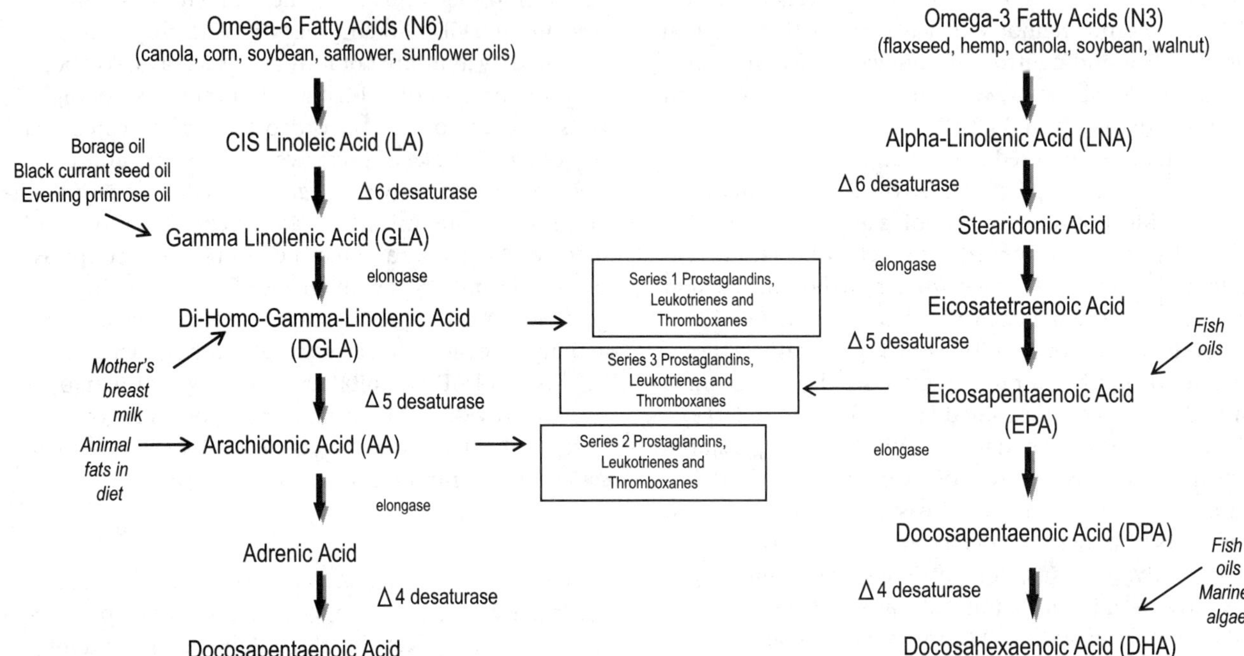

Figure 27.2 **Dietary sources and the AA cascade**

natural agents such as vitamin E,[155] onion (quercetin),[156] cloves (eugenol),[157] turmeric (curcumin),[158] resveratrol,[159] garlic (*Allium sativa*),[160] and *Boswellia serrata*.[161]

Recently, selective COX-2 inhibitors have come under fire, as they were found to increase myocardial infarction and stroke risk.[162] The proposed mechanism for this increased risk is as follows. Non-selective COX inhibitors, but not selective COX-2 inhibitors, significantly inhibit TXA_2-dependent platelet aggregation.[163] Unopposed COX-2 inhibition reduces biosynthesis of prostacyclins, which are vasodilators and potent systemic inhibitors of platelet aggregation in healthy humans. In addition, inhibition of PGI_2 and PGE_2 in the kidney leads to sodium and water retention, thus elevating blood pressure.[164]

Anti-inflammatory Effects of Dietary Omega-3 Fatty Acids

The first evidence of the importance of ω3s in inflammatory conditions arose from epidemiologic observations of the Inuit, indicating a low incidence of coronary heart disease, inflammatory bowel disease, asthma, and severe psoriasis. These people traditionally got their fat almost exclusively from marine mammals (primarily whale and seal meat) and fish. ALA suppresses the metabolic products of LA, a mechanism by which even the essential ω3 fatty acid (in flaxseed oil) has an anti-inflammatory effect. A more powerful anti-inflammatory effect is obtained by providing EPA (as in fish oil). As the conversion of ALA to EPA is slow and limited,[165] provision of EPA provides a more rapid and effective benefit in inflammatory conditions. Diets enriched with fish oil-derived fatty acids consistently raise plasma and membrane EPA levels.[166] EPA inhibits conversion of DGLA to AA and displaces AA in membrane phospholipids, thus decreasing AA availability for inflammatory eicosanoid formation. Omega-3 fatty acids have greater affinity for COX and LOX than ω6s. EPA also exerts anti-inflammatory effects by inhibiting the 5-LOX pathway in neutrophils and monocytes and inhibiting the LTB_4-mediated function of neutrophils.[167]

Not only do ω3 fatty acids reduce inflammation via the eicosanoid pathways, but they also suppress cytokines, the first messenger molecules. Flaxseed oil given over four weeks reduced TNF-α and mononuclear cell IL1-β production by 30%. Fish oil proved more effective over the same time period, reducing mononuclear cell TNF-α and IL1-β by 74% and 80%, respectively.[168]

Fish oils are also PPARγ agonists, similar to the thiazolidinedione class of drugs used in diabetes management.[169] Thiazolidinediones have anti-inflammatory effects.[170] As diabetes and metabolic syndrome are associated with inflammation, this activity of fish oils may also serve to dampen inflammation in genetically predisposed people. The interaction with genetic predisposition should not be forgotten, as the sensitivity to anti-inflammatory effects of fatty acids is influenced by individual genotypic characteristics.[171]

Despite the growing evidence of their importance, data are accumulating that as a nation we are consuming insufficient quantities of ω3 fatty acids.[172]

Anti-inflammatory Effects of GLA Alone and in Combination with EPA

Not only is DGLA the precursor to the 1-series eicosanoids with inflammatory modulating properties, but it is also the precursor to other molecules—15-hydroxyeicosatrienoic acid (15HETrE) and 15-OH-DGLA—that block synthesis of AA products via inhibition of 5-LOX and 12-LOX.[173,174] Neutrophils from subjects supplemented with GLA produce less of the inflammatory mediator LTB_4. In view of these effects, dietary supplements of GLA have been used to reduce the inflammatory response. Concern has been raised that GLA may increase AA in serum and lead to a proinflammatory response. By combining EPA with GLA (3.0 g/d of GLA and EPA over three weeks), proinflammatory AA metabolite synthesis was reduced, and potentially harmful increases in serum AA were not induced, while serum levels of EPA were significantly increased.[175] Pischon et al. found that ω6 fatty acids do not inhibit the anti-inflammatory effects of ω3 fatty acids and that the combination of both types of fatty acids may be associated with the lowest levels of inflammation.[176] Although more data are needed, the combination of GLA and EPA appears to be a reasonable approach in inflammatory conditions.

Effects of Fish Oils in Inflammatory Conditions

Rheumatoid arthritis. In rheumatoid arthritis (RA), joints are destroyed by abnormal multiplication of synoviocytes. COX-2 is induced in the synoviocytes and cartilage with release of PGE_2, PGF_2, PGI_2 and TXA_2 from the synoviocyte.[177] PGE_2 is involved in joint destruction by stimulating bone resorption. TXA_2 upregulates TNF-α and IL1-β synthesis. These cytokines, in turn, upregulate release of factors implicated in irreversible joint damage in RA, such as collagenase and stromelysin.[178] As described previously, fish oil inhibits TXA_2, thus inhibiting TNF-α and IL1-β synthesis, and thereby reducing destructive enzymes such as collagenase. In addition to the effects of fish oils on inflammation, as noted earlier, this mechanism provides an additional rationale for fish oil supplementation in patients with RA. There have been at least 13 randomized controlled trials in RA, using 2.6–7.1 g/d for 12–52 weeks, with improvement reported in all these studies.[179] The clinician and patient should be aware that these effects are generally delayed for 2–3 months. EPA + DHA, 90 mg/kg/day (3:2 ratio), is associated with a shorter period to response than 45 mg/kg/d. Thus, it is prudent to load initially with the higher dose, but use a lower dose for maintenance.[180]

Diet, as mentioned previously, is the major source of AA. Accordingly, Adam et al.[181] investigated the effects of a combination of fish oils with a diet low in AA. RA subjects were placed on either a Western diet (WD) with meat or meat products more than twice a week or an "anti-inflammatory diet" (AID) low in AA. Subjects were given menhaden oil (30 mg/kg) or corn oil, in a crossover design with 3-month treatments and a 2-month washout period. With AID during placebo treatment, there was a 14% decrease in the number of tender and swollen joints. The addition of fish oil led to a further reduction in number of tender (28% vs. 11%) and swollen (34% vs. 22%) joints in AID compared to WD groups. The authors concluded that "a diet low in AA ameliorates clinical signs of inflammation in patients with RA and augments the beneficial effect of fish oil supplementation."

Measurement of the fatty acid profile in RA may be helpful. Cleland et al.[182] reported that a peripheral blood mononuclear cell (PBMC) EPA ≥ 1.5% of total fatty acids is associated with suppression of TNF-α and IL-1β. This equates to a plasma phospholipid EPA ≥ 3.2%, an indicator of effective EPA fortification. The use of fish oil with pharmacologic management in RA has led to reduced NSAID use and dose reduction in potentially toxic medications. In RA patients not on medication, the PGI_2 level (assessed by measurement of urinary 2,3-dinor-6-keto-$PGF_{1\alpha}$) was approximately eight times higher than in a medicated group using NSAIDs, steroids, and disease-modifying antirheumatic drugs (DMARDs), and the TX/PGI_2 ratio was lower.[183] While not proven, fish oil could offset this TXA_2/PGI_2 imbalance from COX-2 inhibitors and potentially reduce cardiovascular disease risk.

There is moderate support for GLA in RA for reduction of pain, tender joint count, and stiffness.[184] GLA (2.8 g/d of GLA as FFA) was also used alone in a study of 56 active RA patients over six months and was well-tolerated and effective.[185] The dosages of fish oil and GLA are important. Anti-inflammatory effects have not been demonstrated at 1.0 g/d EPA+DHA. No significant change from baseline in tender joint count was found with 1.4 g EPA + 0.211 g DHA + 0.5 g GLA over four months in a double-blind, placebo-controlled trial.[186]

Inflammatory bowel disease. EFA supplementation in the management of patients with inflammatory bowel disease (IBD) is indicated to offset the effects of fat malabsorption, poor intake, and increased catabolism leading to EFA insufficiency or deficiency. We have documented evidence of plasma fatty acid abnormalities in 47 patients with chronic intestinal disorders, mostly Crohn's disease, compared with 56 controls.[187] On the whole, these patients exhibited indices of EFA status between those of patients with severe whole-body EFA deficiency and those of healthy subjects. More than 25% of the patients had biochemical evidence of EFA deficiency by at least one criterion. EFA supplementation is indicated not only to correct fatty acid insufficiency but also to provide anti-inflammatory support.[188] Fish oil use for immunomodulation is based on the hypothesis that IBD is due to an abnormal immunological response to altered antigen exposure, either viral or bacterial, involving T and B cells, cytokines, and complement, resulting in chronic, self-perpetuating inflammation. Early in the pathogenesis of IBD, multi-focal gastrointestinal infarctions may occur, suggesting a role for platelets and TXA_2. Thus, the rationale for the use of fish oil includes its effects on reducing TXA_2 production, with resultant inhibition of IL-1β and TNF-α production, as well as its effects on reducing LTB_4, and possibly its function as a free radical scavenger.[189]

There have been at least three double-blind studies in Crohn's disease using 2.7–5.1 g/d fish oil for periods of 12–52 weeks. In one study where the lowest dose was given, there was no benefit. In two studies, there were significant decreases in relapses.[190] The best form of fatty acids for maximal therapeutic effect is not clear. Evidence suggests that an enterically-coated free fatty acid (FFA) form of ω3s is preferable. Absorption studies of the triglyceride vs. ester vs. FFA forms indicated absorptions of 60%, 20%, and 95%, respectively. In addition, a study utilizing enterically-coated FFA capsules in patients with Crohn's disease, in remission, found that an enteric-coated fish-oil preparation containing 1.8 g EPA and 0.9 g DHA was effective in reducing the rate of relapse.[191] Fifty-nine percent of subjects in the fish oil group were still in remission after one year, vs. 26% in the placebo group.[192]

In seal oil, the ω3 fatty acids, EPA, docosapentaenoic acid (DPA; 22:5ω3), and DHA, are preferentially in the sn-1 or sn-3 positions on triglycerides, whereas in fish oil, EPA or DHA are preferentially in the sn-2 position. Fatty acids in the sn-2 position are not easily hydrolyzed in the intestine and are absorbed mainly as monoglycerides. However, fatty acids in the sn-1 and sn-3 positions are absorbed directly into the mucosa. DPA is the most potent inhibitor of platelet TXA_2 formation and platelet aggregation.[193] Seal oil providing 5.4 g/d EPA+DPA+DHA was instilled into the duodenum over 10 days in 10 IBD patients, nine with associated joint pain. Joint pain index, disease activity, and serum cholesterol decreased.[194] In a subsequent study, seal oil was compared with soy oil (10 mL three times daily over 10 days) via a nasoduodenal feeding tube in 19 patients with IBD. Follow-up of this short-term duodenal administration of ω3-rich seal oil over six months indicated significant, prolonged beneficial effects in IBD-related joint pain. The soy oil, on the other hand, led to a tendency to exacerbation.[195]

In ulcerative colitis patients, four double-blind studies have been reported using 1.8–5.4 g/d EPA+DHA for 12–52 weeks. One at the lowest dose had no benefit, one resulted in significant decrease in corticosteroids, and two led to benefit (histology, disease activity, decreased steroids). Also, two open studies reported benefit. The dose of fish oil is important, as indicated by the double-blind, placebo-controlled trial of Middleton et al.,[196] who provided 1.6 g GLA + 270 mg EPA + 45 mg DHA or placebo to 63 patients over 12 months. No differences were noted in sigmoidoscopic grades and relapse rates were similar (placebo 38%, EFAs 55%).

Renal disease. IgA nephropathy is an immune complex-mediated glomerulonephritis. It is the most common primary glomerulonephritis worldwide and leads to end-stage renal failure in 20–40% of patients. It is characterized by mesangial cell proliferation, matrix expansion, and IgA deposition in mesangial regions of the kidney. There is no definitive treatment for this condition. Omega-3 PUFAs, corticosteroids, and angiotensin-converting enzyme (ACE) inhibitors are under investigation. By mechanisms previously described above, fish oils exert anti-inflammatory effects in this condition. Other possible mechanisms for benefits in this condition include blood pressure lowering, reduction in serum lipids, and decreased vascular resistance. In addition, studies using an animal model of acute mesangial glomerulonephritis revealed that ω3 PUFAs are readily incorporated into renal cells and result in decreased glomerular cell proliferation *in vitro* and *in vivo*. Also, DHA inhibits cultured rat mesangial cell proliferation, suggesting that this fatty acid regulates proliferation in the absence of cytokines, growth factors, or inflammatory mediators from other cell types.[197] In IgA nephropathy, studies of the efficacy of ω3 PUFAs have led to varying results. However, the largest randomized clinical trial provided strong evidence that treatment for two years with 1.8 g of EPA and 1.2 g of DHA per day slowed the progression of renal disease in high-risk patients, with benefits persisting after 6.4 years of follow up.[198]

Animal studies and preliminary human studies have suggested a role for fish oil in the treatment of lupus nephritis. However, a double-blind, cross-over study in 26 patients with lupus nephritis followed for over two years indicated that fish oil dietary supplementation had no significant effect on proteinuria, glomerular filtration rate, disease activity index, or steroid consumption.[199] However, it did have a significant effect on lipid levels. There were methodologic difficulties in the study related to carryover effects and possible effects of the olive oil placebo.

In a double-blind clinical trial, 86 subjects randomly received either 6 g/d of fish oil or soy oil during the first three months after renal transplantation. Although lower lipid levels and a trend towards lower cytokine expression were found in the fish oil-treated group, treatment with fish oil did not influence acute rejection rate and had no beneficial effect on renal function or graft survival.[200] In another study, the use of combined treatment with a low-dose statin along with fish oil (1 g/d) was more effective than the statin treatment alone for changing the lipid profile after renal transplantation.[201]

Over 50% of all hemodialysis access grafts become thrombosed within a year after placement, and over 75% require a salvage procedure to maintain patency. The cost to maintain dialysis access for patients in the U.S. is over $1 billion per year. Fish oil supplementation appears to significantly enhance graft survival. In a study of 24 subjects, given either 4 g of fish oil (1.76 g of EPA and 0.96 g of DHA) or a placebo (4 g of corn oil), 75.6% of the grafts in the fish oil group were patent at one year vs. only 14.9% for the control group ($P<.03$).[202]

Psoriasis. Elevated levels of AA and its proinflammatory metabolites such as LTB_4 are found in psoriatic skin lesions, suggesting a therapeutic role for fish oils in this condition. Six of seven open studies using 1.1–13.5 g EPA + 1.7–3.6 g DHA over 6–27 weeks reported improvements. However, results of five double-blind studies using 1.6–3.1 g EPA + 1.0–1.9 g DHA/d over 8–17 weeks were mixed. Two led to improvement and three to no benefit. In an attempt to overcome methodologic issues of oral supplementation, EPA + DHA in triglyceride form were administered IV and compared with ω6 fatty acids given IV over 10–15 days in two studies. At ω3 doses of 4.7–9.4 g/day (2.1–4.2 g EPA+DHA/d), there was a significantly larger decrease in clinical symptoms, although some regression of psoriatic lesions occurred with ω6 fatty acids as well. In the larger (83 patients) of the two double-blind randomized trials, there was a higher response rate with ω3s than ω6s (37% vs. 23%).[203]

Bronchial asthma. Airway wall inflammation is present in mild asthma and is a prominent feature in fatal asthma attacks.[204] LTs have been implicated in the pathogenesis of bronchial asthma, with cysteinyl LTs (CysLT) considered the most important class of such molecules. CysLTs are 100–1,000 times more potent bronchoconstrictors than histamine, and CysLT receptor antagonists such as montelukasts are used therapeutically in asthma management.[205] LT production is increased with enhanced activity of key enzymes in CysLT synthesis, and markedly increased amounts of AA in eosinophils are recruited to areas of asthmatic inflammation. LTA_4 is the only LT synthesized and secreted by inflammatory cells. It is converted to LTC_4 in human mast cells, basophils, and eosinophils. LTC_4, in turn, is converted to LTD_4 and LTE_4 in the extracellular fluid. These latter three appear to be most important in asthma pathogenesis. Dysregulated production of CysLTs is often coupled with increased bronchial smooth muscle sensitivity to their bronchoconstrictor activity. Calabrese et al.[206] have found that the synthesis of CysLTs is increased in cells obtained by bronchial lavage from asthmatic patients. The expression of LTC_4 synthase is increased in eosinophils in these bronchial washings. Also, they report that these eosinophils from inflamed airways have increased AA content, some 4–10 times higher than that measured in peripheral blood cells. The elevated AA is related to high secretory phospholipase A_2 ($sPLA_2$), five times higher in patients with mild persistent asthma than from normal subjects. Secretory PLA_2 released in airways of asthmatics might function as a proinflammatory mediator. Thus, in asthmatics, large increases in the amount of AA occur in eosinophils recruited to an inflammatory area, and enhanced activity of key biosynthetic enzymes in CysLT synthesis leads to excessive CysLT production.[207]

In view of the effects of ω3 fatty acids and of GLA (as precursor to DGLA) on LT formation, supplementation of these fatty acids has been studied in asthmatic patients. In a randomized, double-blind parallel group study in 23 atopic subjects with mild to moderate asthma, patients received placebo (olive oil) and low-dose and high-dose combinations of GLA and EPA for four weeks. Both combinations significantly suppressed *ex vivo* LTB_4 and TNF-α biosynthesis when compared with placebo.[208] However, studies to date do not provide a definitive conclusion regarding the efficacy of ω3 fatty acid supplementation as a treatment for asthma in children and adults.[209] Omega-3 fatty acids have not consistently improved symptom severity, lung function, airway responsiveness, or medication use in asthmatic patients.[210] In a 12-month, double-blind, controlled trial of borage vs. corn oil in 54 subjects with stable asthma, increased generation of polymorphonuclear (PMN) 15-HETrE, decreased PMN AA, and decreased *ex vivo* LTB_4 generation by PMNs were seen.[211] Again, the study did not reveal statistically significant suppression of asthma scores. A promising controlled study[212] involved supplementation with ω3 fatty acids in the first 18 months of life in infants at high risk of developing asthma. The treatment group had a 9.8% absolute reduction in parent-reported wheeze-ever (P=0.02) and a 7.8% lower prevalence of wheeze for more than 1 week (P=0.04). Wheeze-ever, doctor visits for wheeze, bronchodilator use, and nocturnal coughing were significantly reduced in children in higher plasma ω3 fatty acid quintiles.[213] A five year follow-up study is underway.

Coronary artery disease (CAD). It is now well accepted that coronary artery disease is an inflammatory condition (see discussion above by Libby). Myocardial infarction occurs most often as a result of rupture of a vulnerable plaque with subsequent acute thrombosis, despite lack of severe coronary artery narrowing. Vulnerable plaque is characterized by a large lipid core, rich in inflammatory cells, and a thin fibrous cap with compromise of its structural integrity by matrix-degrading enzymes, such as metalloproteinases.[214] Eicosanoids are involved in various aspects of the atherosclerotic process. Their critical importance is seen in their involvement in platelet function, and is underscored by the benefits of approaches to block their activity, as with aspirin. The pathophysiological role of TXA_2 via the COX pathway is well established in the thrombotic process of acute coronary syndromes. Platelet activation occurs in acute ischemic syndromes and in stable angina with greatly increased TX production.[215] TXA_2 from AA in platelets produces platelet aggregation and vasoconstriction, whereas TXA_3 from EPA is almost biologically inactive. TXA_2 is one of the most potent vasoconstricting and platelet-aggregating substances known.[216] Both prostacyclin I_2 from AA and prostacyclin I_3 from EPA via the same pathway in endothelial cells are anti-aggregatory and vasodilatory. The AA product in leukocytes, LTB_4, is proinflammatory, chemotactic, promotes cell adhesion, and can amplify the inflammatory response. The EPA product from leukocytes, LTB_5, is anti-inflammatory, non-adhesive, and non-chemotactic.

PGs are vasoactive lipid mediators formed in response to stimulation of vascular smooth muscle cells by a variety of chemical agonists. Different receptor subtypes mediate the contractile and relaxing effects of PGs and TXA_2 on coronary vascular smooth muscle.[217]

Fish intake and CAD. Several studies have confirmed a relationship between fish intake and CAD mortality, including the Chicago Western Electric Study, which reported an inverse association between fish consumption and death from coronary heart disease, especially non-sudden death from myocardial infarction at year 30 in the follow-up of 1,822 men free of heart disease at the start of the study.[218] Many subsequent studies have found that the main cardiovascular benefit of fish intake was reduction in sudden cardiac deaths.

Fish intake does not have to be high to confer protection, according to several other studies. Ingestion of as little as one to two fish dishes per week has been found to reduce the incidence of CAD. In the 20-year prospective Zutphen Study of middle-aged men in the Netherlands, the consumption of about two fish meals weekly was associated with a 50% reduction in CAD mortality compared with men who ate no fish at all.[219] Protective effects were not noted until the fifth year of the study. However, not all studies have confirmed an inverse relationship between fish intake and CAD mortality.[220] A confounding factor in negative studies may have been smoking history. In the Honolulu Heart Program study of Japanese men, this was addressed. In the high-smoking group, the risk factor-adjusted relative risk for CAD mortality among those with intake of two or more servings of fish per week was half that of those with low fish consumption.[221] The Physicians Health Study of over 20,000 male physicians without evidence of prior cardiovascular disease found no association between dietary fish or ω3 intake and risk of MI or death from cardiovascular disease over a four-year follow-up. However, it did find a relationship between fish intake and sudden cardiac death at the 11 and 17 year follow-ups. Their prospective data at year 11 suggested that consumption of fish at least once per week may reduce the risk of sudden cardiac death in men by about 50%.[222] There was also a significantly reduced risk of total mortality with fish consumption. At the 17 year follow-up, baseline blood levels of long-chain ω3 fatty acids were inversely related to the risk of sudden death.[223] Compared with men whose blood levels of long-chain ω3 fatty acids were in the lowest quartile, the adjusted relative risk of sudden death was 0.28 among men with levels in the third quartile and 0.19 in the fourth quartile.

Not all studies confirm beneficial effects of fish oil in cardiovascular disease. The Diet and Reinfarction Trial (DART) included 2,033 men randomly assigned to receive or not receive advice to increase their intake of fatty fish. Those instructed to increase fish intake were told to consume 300 grams of fish (or equivalent fish oil capsules) per week (~ 3 fish meals/week). After two years, the group encouraged to eat fish had a 29% lower death rate than the control group.[224] However, there was an increased risk in all-cause mortality and stroke death over the next three years in those given fish advice.[225] In another study, 3,114 men under 70 with angina were randomly allocated to four groups, including one advised to eat two portions of oily fish each week or to take three fish oil capsules daily, and another given no specific dietary advice. After 3–9 years, men advised to eat oily fish, and particularly those supplied with fish oil capsules, had a higher risk of cardiac death.[226]

However, the large GISSI-Prevenzione clinical trial of 11,323 men and women with myocardial infarction provides convincing evidence of the benefits of fish oil supplementation. Dietary supplementation with ω3 PUFA (1 g/d), but not vitamin E, significantly lowered the risk of cardiovascular death by 17–30%, and the overall risk of death by 14–20%.[227] All subjects received advice to increase their consumption of fish, fruit, raw and cooked vegetables, and olive oil. Compared with people in the worst dietary score quartile, the odds ratio for those in the best score quartile was 0.51.[228] Total mortality was significantly lowered after three months of treatment (relative risk 0.59) and the reduction in risk of sudden death was statistically significant by four months (relative risk 0.47). The early effect of low-dose ω3s on total mortality and sudden death supports the hypothesis of an antiarrhythmic effect.[229]

ALA and CAD. The two populations with the world's lowest CAD mortality are the Japanese and the Cretans. Both have high ALA intake, the Japanese from canola and soybean oils, and the Cretans from walnuts and possibly purslane.[230] ALA supplementation was studied in the Lyon Heart Study, which compared the effects of a Mediterranean ALA-rich diet with a diet similar to the prudent American Heart Association guidelines. A total of 605 patients who survived a first MI were randomly assigned to an experimental or control group. In the experimental (Mediterranean diet) group, butter and cream were replaced by a canola oil-based margarine containing 5% ALA. They had significantly higher plasma ALA and EPA and lower LA and AA levels than controls. After 27 months of follow-up, there were 16 cardiac deaths in the controls and only three in the experimental group. There were 17 non-fatal MIs in controls and five in the treated group. Overall mortality was 20 in controls and eight in the experimental group. The study was terminated because the data were so compelling that it was deemed unethical to continue the investigation.[231] In an editorial, Alexander Leaf stated that "relatively simple dietary changes achieved greater reductions in risk of all-cause and coronary heart disease mortality in a secondary prevention trial than any of the cholesterol-lowering studies to date."[232]

Singh et al.[233] studied 1,000 patients with CAD in a randomized, single-blind trial, half assigned to an Indo-Mediterranean diet rich in whole grains, fruits, vegetables, walnuts, and almonds and the remainder to a step I National Cholesterol Education Program prudent diet. The mean intake of ALA was twice as high in the intervention group (1.8 g vs. 0.8 g per day) related to intake of mustard or soybean oil. There were significantly fewer total cardiac end points in the intervention group than the controls (39 vs. 76 events, $p<0.001$). Sudden cardiac deaths were also reduced (6 vs. 16, $p=0.015$), as were non-fatal myocardial infarctions (21 vs. 43, $p<0.001$).

Thus, the role of ω3s in the secondary prevention of CAD is clearly supported by randomized clinical trials. However, their role in primary prevention will need to await future clinical trials.[234]

Mechanisms of Omega-3 Fatty Acid Effects on Cardiac Risk Factors

Several mechanisms may be involved in the apparent favorable effect of ω3 fatty acids on risk and potential mortality from MI, in addition to the reduction in inflammation elucidated above: These include:

- reduction in platelet clumping,
- reduction in triglyceride levels,
- reduction in arrhythmias, and
- reduction in blood pressure.

In addition, ω3s may:

- increase LDL particle size, rendering them less likely to oxidize;
- retard growth of atherosclerotic plaque by inhibiting both cellular growth factors and the migration of monocytes;
- exert a direct cytoprotective effect against ischemia, free radical-induced damage, and lipid peroxidation;
- enhance insulin action;
- increase systemic arterial compliance; and
- help to reduce pulse pressure and total vascular resistance.[235]

Omega-3 fatty acids are incorporated into platelet membranes, leading to decreased platelet aggregation, probably due to inhibition of the synthesis of TXA_2. Also, there may be a minor decrease in platelet number and a slight prolongation of the bleeding time, an effect similar to and synergistic with that of aspirin. An intake of about 15 ml/d of marine oils causes anti-thrombotic changes in platelet membranes. Despite their effects on platelet function, standard doses of fish oil (3–4 g or 1.2 g of EPA + DHA) are unlikely to increase risk of hemorrhagic stroke.[236] Bleeding times have remained in the upper limit of normal with fish oil intakes as high as 9 g/d (EPA+DHA 6 g/d). Fish oil retards the growth of the atherosclerotic plaque by inhibiting both cellular growth factors and the migration of monocytes.[237]

Triglycerides are consistently lowered by 30% or more with ω3 fatty acid supplementation in subjects with elevated or normal triglyceride levels. Triglyceride synthesis may be inhibited, although enhanced breakdown may play a role.[238] Reductions in triglycerides have been achieved with a fish oil dose equivalent to 200 g of fatty fish or in response to ingestion of about three fish meals per week (300 g of fatty fish per week). Hypertriglyceridemia may contribute to atherosclerosis by increasing the expression of cell adhesion molecules (CAMs).[239] ICAMs mediate attachment of leukocytes and ICAM-1 is a predictor of risk for MI. Thus, fish oil may reduce high triglycerides and CAMs. HDL cholesterol does not change much in response to ω3 fatty acid supplementation, but there is suggestive evidence that the cardioprotective HDL_2 subfraction does.

Fish oil has been shown to exert a mild blood pressure-lowering effect in both normal and mildly hypertensive individuals, possibly related to promotion of beneficial nitric oxide synthesis in the endothelium.[240] As low a dose as 3 g of EPA and DHA was shown to be associated with a drop of 5 mm Hg systolic and 3 mm diastolic.[241] A 1% increase in blood ALA was associated with a 5 mm drop in blood pressure.[242] A meta-analysis of 1,356 subjects concluded that fish oils are associated with a small but significant lowering in blood pressure.[243] This appears to occur in patients with preexisting heart disease, lipid abnormalities or hypertension, but not in healthy subjects with normal blood pressure.

There is considerable evidence that ω3 fatty acids prevent cardiac arrhythmias, including inhibition of ventricular fibrillation and consequent cardiac arrest. Documentation comes from experiments in cultured myocytes, experiments in animals, epidemiologic correlations, and clinical trials.[244,245] Within minutes of the addition of ω3 fatty acids in tissue culture systems, susceptibility to arrhythmias is reduced. Also, heart rate variability, an independent risk factor of arrhythmic events and mortality, is increased by ω3 fatty acids. A significant increase in heart rate variability occurred when post-MI patients were given 5.2 g of ω3 fatty acids daily for 12 weeks.[246]

Effects of fish oils on restenosis after angioplasty or coronary artery bypass graft have been variable. An effect, if present, is considered weak.[247]

Optimal Fat Intake

How much fat should be consumed? Ornish has recommended 10% of calories as fat in a vegetarian diet.[248] Yet, the people of Crete eat a higher fat diet with 40% of calories as fat and have one-twentieth the mortality from CAD compared with Americans.[249] Furthermore, the Greenland Inuit rarely develop CAD, despite a diet high in fat and cholesterol. It must be concluded that it is the type of fat that is most important, not the amount.

Summary

An understanding of the common threads in the pathogenesis of CAD, RA, IBD, psoriasis, and asthma allows the practitioner to utilize fatty acid supplementation in these and other disparate inflammatory conditions. Such conditions may be approached with a consistent strategy, manipulating diet, fatty acids, and other supplements to safely lower inflammatory mediators, while attention is given to treating underlying factors in disease etiology.

References

1. Witztum JL, Berliner JA. Oxidized phospholipids and isoprostanes in atherosclerosis. Curr Opin Lipidol. 1998;9:441-448.
2. Schmidt AM, Yan SD, Wautier JL, Stern D. Activation of receptor for advanced glycation end products: a mechanism for chronic vascular dysfunction in diabetic vasculopathy and atherosclerosis. Circ Res. 1999;84:489-497.
3. Kol A, Libby P. The mechanisms by which infectious agents may contribute to atherosclerosis and its clinical manifestations. Trends Cardiovasc Med. 1998;8:191-199.
4. Clinton S, Underwood R, Sherman M, et al. Macrophage-colony stimulating factor gene expression in vascular cells and in experimental and human atherosclerosis. Am J Pathol. 1992;140:301-316.
5. Cybulsky MI, Iiyama K, Li H, et al. A major role for VCAM-1, but not ICAM-1, in early atherosclerosis. J Clin Invest. 2001;107:1255-1262.
6. Hajjar DP, Haberland ME. Lipoprotein trafficking in vascular cells. Molecular Trojan horses and cellular saboteurs. J Biol Chem. 1997;272:22975-22978.
7. Clinton S, Underwood R, Sherman M, et al. Macrophage-colony stimulating factor gene expression in vascular cells and in experimental and human atherosclerosis. Am J Pathol. 1992;140:301-316.
8. Suzuki H, Kurihara Y, Takeya M, et al. A role for macrophage scavenger receptors in atherosclerosis and susceptibility to infection. Nature. 1997;386:292-296.
9. Febbraio M, Podrez EA, Smith JD, et al. Targeted disruption of the class B scavenger receptor CD36 protects against atherosclerotic lesion development in mice. J Clin Invest. 2000;105:1049-1056.
10. Shimizu K, Sugiyama S, Aikawa M, et al. Host bone-marrow cells are a source of donor intimal smooth- muscle- like cells in murine aortic transplant arteriopathy. Nat Med. 2001;7:738-741.
11. Libby P, Ross R. Cytokines and growth regulatory molecules. In: Fuster V, Ross R, Topol E, eds. Atherosclerosis and Coronary Artery Disease. New York, NY: Lippincott-Raven; 1996:585-594.
12. Jonasson L, Holm J, Skalli O, et al. Regional accumulations of T cells, macrophages, and smooth muscle cells in the human atherosclerotic plaque. Arteriosclerosis. 1986;6:131-138.
13. Geng Y-J, Libby P. Evidence for apoptosis in advanced human atheroma. Co-localization with interleukin-1 b-converting enzyme. Am J Pathol. 1995;147:251-266.
14. Davies MJ. Stability and instability: the two faces of coronary atherosclerosis. The Paul Dudly White Lecture, 1995. Circulation. 1996;94:2013-2020.
15. Lee R, Libby P. The unstable atheroma. Arterioscler Thromb Vasc Biol. 1997;17:1859-1867.
16. Nemerson Y, Giesen PL. Some thoughts about localization and expression of tissue factor. Blood Coagulation Fibrinol. 1998;9:S45-47.
17. Mach F, Schoenbeck U, Bonnefoy J-Y, et al. Activation of monocyte/macrophage functions related to acute atheroma complication by ligation of CD40. Induction of collagenase, stromelysin, and tissue factor. Circulation. 1997;96:396-399.
18. Libby P, Aikawa M. Stabilization of atherosclerotic plaques: new mechanisms and clinical targets. Nat Med. 2002;8:1257-1262.
19. Marx N, Libby P, Plutzky J. Peroxisome proliferator-activated receptors (PPARs) and their role in the vessel wall: possible mediators of cardiovascular risk? J Cardiovasc Risk. 2001;8:203-210.
20. Ely JW, Osheroff JA, Ebell MH, et al. Analysis of questions asked by family doctors regarding patient care. BMJ. 1999 Aug 7;319(7206):358-61.
21. Heaney RP. Long-latency deficiency disease: insights from calcium and vitamin D. Am J Clin Nutr. 2003 Nov;78(5):912-9.
22. Biomedical studies of US Army ranger training. Military Operational Medicine Research Program. MOMRP Fact Sheet. 1999; August: Number 5, page 2.
23. Anderzen I, Arnetz BB, Soderstrom T, Soderman E. Stress and sensitization in children: a controlled prospective psychophysiological study of children exposed to international relocation. J Psychosom Res. 1997 Sep;43(3):259-69.
24. Collins SM. Stress and the Gastrointestinal Tract IV. Modulation of intestinal inflammation by stress: basic mechanisms and clinical relevance. Am J Physiol Gastrointest Liver Physiol. 2001;280:G315-8.
25. Bosch JA, de Geus EJ, Ligtenberg TJ, et al. Salivary MUC5B-mediated adherence (ex vivo) of Helicobacter pylori during acute stress. Psychosom Med. 2000 Jan-Feb;62(1):40-9.
26. Yokoe T, Minoguchi K, Matsuo H, et al. Elevated levels of C-reactive protein and interleukin-6 in patients with obstructive sleep apnea syndrome are decreased by nasal continuous positive airway pressure. Circulation. 2003 Mar 4;107(8):1129-34.
27. Kimata H. Listening to Mozart reduces allergic skin wheal responses and *in vitro* allergen-specific IgE production in atopic dermatitis patients with latex allergy. Behav Med. 2003 Spring;29(1):15-9.
28. Lutgendorf S, Logan H, Kirchner HL, et al. Effects of relaxation and stress on the capsaicin-induced local inflammatory response. Psychosom Med. 2000 Jul-Aug;62(4):524-34.

29. Zarkovic M, Stefanova E, Ciric J, et al. Prolonged psychological stress suppresses cortisol secretion. Clin Endocrinol (Oxf). 2003 Dec;59(6):811-6.
30. Jefferies WM. Mild adrenocortical deficiency, chronic allergies, autoimmune disorders and the chronic fatigue syndrome: a continuation of the cortisone story. Med Hypotheses. 1994 Mar;42(a3):183-9.
31. Jefferies WMcK. Safe Uses of Cortisol. Second Edition. Springfield, CC Thomas, 1996.
32. de la Torre B, Hedman M, Befrits R. Blood and tissue dehydroepiandrosterone sulphate levels and their relationship to chronic inflammatory bowel disease. Clin Exp Rheumatol. 1998 Sep-Oct;16(5):579-82.
33. Andus T, Klebl F, Rogler G, et al. Patients with refractory Crohn's disease or ulcerative colitis respond to dehydroepiandrosterone: a pilot study. Aliment Pharmacol Ther. 2003 Feb;17(3):409-14.
34. GL701 (DHEA, prasterone) for the Treatment of Systemic Lupus Erythematosus (SLE) in Women. Briefing Document. FDA Arthritis Advisory Committee. http://www.fda.gov/ohrms/dockets/ac/01/briefing/3740b1_01_gendlabs.pdf Accessed March 27, 2005
35. Tengstrand B, Carlstrom K, Hafstrom I. Bioavailable testosterone in men with rheumatoid arthritis-high frequency of hypogonadism. Rheumatology (Oxford). 2002 Mar;41(3):285-9.
36. Tengstrand B, Carlstrom K, Fellander-Tsai L, Hafstrom I. Abnormal levels of serum dehydroepiandrosterone, estrone, and estradiol in men with rheumatoid arthritis: high correlation between serum estradiol and current degree of inflammation. J Rheumatol. 2003 Nov;30(11):2338-43.
37. Booji A, Biewenga-Booji CM, Huber-Bruning O, et al. Androgens as adjuvant treatment in postmenopausal female patients with rheumatoid arthritis. Ann Rheum Dis. 1996 Nov;55(11):811-5.
38. Tan KS, McFarlane LC, Lipworth BJ. Paradoxical down-regulation and desensitization of beta2-adrenoceptors by exogenous progesterone in female asthmatics. Chest. 1997 Apr;111(4):847-51.
39. Environmental Working Group and Mount Sinai School of Medicine. "Body Burden." Accessed http://ewg.org/reports/bodyburden/ on March 27, 2005.
40. Gaby AR. The role of hidden food allergy/intolerance in chronic disease. Altern Med Rev. 1998 Apr;3(2):90-100
41. Zitouni M, Daoud W, Kallel M, Makni S. Systemic lupus erythematosus with celiac disease: a report of five cases. Joint Bone Spine. 2004 Jul;71(4):344-6.
42. Hadjivassiliou M, Sanders DS, Grunewald RA, Akil M. Gluten sensitivity masquerading as systemic lupus erythematosus. Ann Rheum Dis. 2004 Nov;63(11):1501-3.
43. Jiskra J, Limanova Z, Vanickova Z, Kocna P. IgA and IgG antigliadin, IgA anti-tissue transglutaminase and antiendomysial antibodies in patients with autoimmune thyroid diseases and their relationship to thyroidal replacement therapy. Physiol Res. 2003;52(1):79-88.
44. Collin P, Kaukinen K, Valimaki M, Salmi J. Endocrinological disorders and celiac disease. Endocr Rev. 2002 Aug;23(4):464-83.
45. Kumar V, Rajadhyaksha M, Wortsman J. Celiac disease-associated autoimmune endocrinopathies. Clin Diagn Lab Immunol. 2001 Jul;8(4):678-85.
46. Prochazkova J, Sterzl I, Kucerova H, Bartova J, Stejskal VD. The beneficial effect of amalgam replacement on health in patients with autoimmunity. Neuro Endocrinol Lett. 2004 Jun;25(3):211-8.
47. Huggins HA, Levy TE. Cerebrospinal fluid protein changes in multiple sclerosis after dental amalgam removal. Altern Med Rev. 1998 Aug;3(4):295-300.
48. Weidinger S, Kramer U, Dunemann L, et al. Body burden of mercury is associated with acute atopic eczema and total IgE in children from southern Germany. J Allergy Clin Immunol. 2004 Aug;114(2):457-9.
49. Cooper GS, Martin SA, Longnecker MP, et al. Associations between plasma DDE levels and immunologic measures in African-American farmers in North Carolina. Environ Health Perspect. 2004 Jul;112(10):1080-4.
50. Campbell AW, Thrasher JD, Madison RA, et al. Neural autoantibodies and neurophysiologic abnormalities in patients exposed to molds in water-damaged buildings. Arch Environ Health. 2003 Aug;58(8):464-74.
51. Holick MF. Vitamin D deficiency: what a pain it is. Mayo Clin Proc. 2003 Dec;78(12):1457-9.
52. Vasquez A, Manso G, Cannell J. The clinical importance of vitamin D (cholecalciferol): a paradigm shift with implications for all healthcare providers. Altern Ther Health Med 2004;10:28-37.
53. Wucherpfennig KW. Mechanisms for the induction of autoimmunity by infectious agents. J Clin Invest. 2001 Oct;108(8):1097-104.
54. Galland L. Intestinal protozoan infection is a common unsuspected cause of chronic illness. J Advancement Med. 1989;2: 539-552.
55. Amar S, Han X. The impact of periodontal infection on systemic diseases. Med Sci Monit. 2003 Dec;9(12):RA291-9.
56. Bermejo-Fenoll A, Sanchez-Perez A. Necrotising periodontal diseases. Med Oral Patol Oral Cir Bucal. 2004;9 Suppl:114-9; 108-14.
57. Li X, Kolltveit KM, Tronstad L, Olsen I. Systemic diseases caused by oral infection. Clin Microbiol Rev. 2000 Oct;13(4):547-58.
58. Jin LJ, Chiu GK, Corbet EF. Are periodontal diseases risk factors for certain systemic disorders--what matters to medical practitioners? Hong Kong Med J. 2003 Feb;9(1):31-7.
59. Gray MR, Thrasher JD, Crago R, et al. Mixed mold mycotoxicosis: immunological changes in humans following exposure in water-damaged buildings. Arch Environ Health. 2003 Jul;58(7):410-20.
60. Seaman DR. The diet-induced proinflammatory state: a cause of chronic pain and other degenerative diseases? J Manipulative Physiol Ther. 2002;25(3):168-79.
61. Rusyn I, Bradham CA, Cohn L, et al. Corn oil rapidly activates nuclear factor-kappaB in hepatic Kupffer cells by oxidant-dependent mechanisms. Carcinogenesis. 1999 Nov;20(11):2095-100.
62. Liu RH. Health benefits of fruit and vegetables are from additive and synergistic combinations of phytochemicals. Am J Clin Nutr. 2003 Sep;78(3 Suppl):517S-520S.
63. Vasquez A. Reducing pain and inflammation naturally. Part 2: New insights into fatty acid supplementation and its effect on eicosanoid production and genetic expression. Nutritional Perspectives 2005; January: 5-16.
64. O'Keefe JH Jr, Cordain L. Cardiovascular disease resulting from a diet and lifestyle at odds with our Paleolithic genome: how to become a 21st-century hunter-gatherer. Mayo Clin Proc 2004 Jan;79(1):101-8.
65. Richardson JD, Vasko MR. Cellular mechanisms of neurogenic inflammation. J Pharmacol Exp Ther. 2002 Sep;302(3):839-45.
66. Groneberg DA, Quarcoo D, Frossard N, Fischer A. Neurogenic mechanisms in bronchial inflammatory diseases. Allergy. 2004 Nov;59(11):1139-52.
67. Gouze-Decaris E, Philippe L, et al. Neurophysiological basis for neurogenic-mediated articular cartilage anabolism alteration. Am J Physiol Regul Integr Comp Physiol. 2001 Jan;280(1):R115-22.
68. Boal RW, Gillette RG. Central neuronal plasticity, low back pain and spinal manipulative therapy. J Manipulative Physiol Ther. 2004 Jun;27(5):314-26.
69. Lutgendorf S, Logan H, Kirchner HL, et al. Effects of relaxation and stress on the capsaicin-induced local inflammatory response. Psychosom Med. 2000 Jul-Aug;62(4):524-34.

70. Meggs WJ. Neurogenic inflammation and sensitivity to environmental chemicals. Environ Health Perspect. 1993 Aug;101(3):234-8.
71. Meggs WJ. Neurogenic switching: a hypothesis for a mechanism for shifting the site of inflammation in allergy and chemical sensitivity. Environ Health Perspect. 1995;103(1):54-6.
72. Decaris E, Guingamp C, Chat M, et al. Evidence for neurogenic transmission inducing degenerative cartilage damage distant from local inflammation. Arthritis Rheum. 1999;42(9):1951-60.
73. Topol EJ. Failing the public health--rofecoxib, Merck, and the FDA. N Engl J Med. 2004 Oct 21;351(17):1707-9.
74. Topol EJ. Arthritis medicines and cardiovascular events—"house of coxibs." JAMA. 2005 Jan 19;293(3):366-8.
75. Ray WA, Griffin MR, Stein CM. Cardiovascular toxicity of valdecoxib. N Engl J Med. 2004 Dec 23;351(26):2767.
76. Goldstein R. FDA Chooses Drug Industry Health Over Public Health. http://www.commondreams.org/views05/0223-35.htm Wednesday, February 23, 2005 and Memorandum from David J. Graham, MD, MPH, Associate Director for Science, Office of Drug Safety to Paul Seligman, MD, MPH, Acting Director, Office of Drug Safety entitled, "Risk of Acute Myocardial Infarction and Sudden Cardiac Death in Patients Treated with COX-2 Selective and Non-Selective NSAIDs," http://www.fda.gov/cder/drug/infopage/vioxx/vioxxgraham.pdf September 30, 2004.
77. Singh G. Recent considerations in nonsteroidal anti-inflammatory drug gastropathy. Am J Med. 1998 Jul 27;105(1B):31S-38S.
78. Bernstein J, Quach T. A perspective on the study of Moseley et al: questioning the value of arthroscopic knee surgery for osteoarthritis. Cleve Clin J Med. 2003;70(5):401, 405-6, 408-10.
79. Vasquez A. Integrative Orthopedics: Concepts, Algorithms, and Therapeutics. The art of creating wellness while effectively managing acute and chronic musculoskeletal disorders. Natural Health Consulting Corporation: www.WellBodyBook.com August 2004.
80. Vasquez A. Reducing pain and inflammation naturally. Part 1: New insights into fatty acid biochemistry and the influence of diet. Nutritional Perspectives 2004; October: 5, 7-10, 12, 14.
81. Vasquez A. Reducing pain and inflammation naturally. Part 2: New insights into fatty acid supplementation and its effect on eicosanoid production and genetic expression. Nutritional Perspectives 2005; January: 5-16.
82. Vasquez A. Reducing pain and inflammation naturally. Part 3: Improving overall health while safely and effectively treating musculoskeletal pain. Nutritional Perspectives 2005; in press.
83. Manga P, Angus D, Papadopoulos C, et al. The Effectiveness and Cost-Effectiveness of Chiropractic Management of Low-Back Pain. Richmond Hill, Ontario: Kenilworth Publishing; 1993.
84. Meade TW, Dyer S, Browne W, Townsend J, Frank AO. Low-back pain of mechanical origin: randomised comparison of chiropractic and hospital outpatient treatment. BMJ. 1990;300(6737):1431-7.
85. Meade TW, Dyer S, Browne W, Frank AO. Randomised comparison of chiropractic and hospital outpatient management for low-back pain: results from extended follow up. BMJ. 1995;311(7001):349-5.
86. Legorreta AP, Metz RD, Nelson CF, et al. Comparative analysis of individuals with and without chiropractic coverage: patient characteristics, utilization, and costs. Arch Intern Med. 2004;164:1985-92.
87. Dabbs V, Lauretti WJ. A risk assessment of cervical manipulation vs. NSAIDs for the treatment of neck pain. J Manipulative Physiol Ther. 1995;18:530-6.
88. Rosner AL. Evidence-based clinical guidelines for the management of acute low-back pain: response to the guidelines prepared for the Australian Medical Health and Research Council. J Manipulative Physiol Ther. 2001;24(3):214-20.
89. Oliphant D. Safety of spinal manipulation in the treatment of lumbar disk herniations: a systematic review and risk assessment. J Manipulative Physiol Ther. 2004;27:197-210.
90. Maigne JY, Vautravers P. Mechanism of action of spinal manipulative therapy. Joint Bone Spine. 2003;70(5):336-41.
91. Leach RA. (ed). The Chiropractic Theories: A Textbook of Scientific Research, Fourth Edition. Baltimore: Lippincott, Williams & Wilkins, 2004.
92. Hanks-Bell M, Halvey K, Paice JA. Pain assessment and management in aging. Online J Issues Nurs. 2004;9(3):8.
93. Cheung K, Hume P, Maxwell L. Delayed onset muscle soreness: treatment strategies and performance factors. Sports Med. 2003;33(2):145-64.
94. Jurgel J, Rannama L, Gapeyeva H, et al. Shoulder function in patients with frozen shoulder before and after 4-week rehabilitation. Medicina (Kaunas). 2005;41(1):30-8.
95. Guler-Uysal F, Kozanoglu E. Comparison of the early response to two methods of rehabilitation in adhesive capsulitis. Swiss Med Wkly. 2004;134(23-24):353-8.
96. Kavuncu V, Evcik D. Physiotherapy in rheumatoid arthritis. Medscape MedGenMed eJournal. May 17, 2004. Accessed online at http://www.medscape.com/viewarticle/474880_1.
97. Brousseau L, Yonge KA, Robinson V, et al. Thermotherapy for treatment of osteoarthritis. Cochrane Database Syst Rev. 2003;(4):CD004522.
98. Miller AL. The etiologies, pathophysiology, and alternative/complementary treatment of asthma. Altern Med Rev. 2001;6(1):20-47.
99. Dryden T, Baskwill A, Preyde M. Massage therapy for the orthopaedic patient: a review. Orthop Nurs. 2004;23(5):327-32.
100. Vidal y Plana RR, Bizzarri D, Rovati AL. Articular cartilage pharmacology: I. *In vitro* studies on glucosamine and non steroidal antiinflammatory drugs. Pharmacol Res Commun. 1978 Jun;10(6):557-69.
101. Reginster JY, Deroisy R, Rovati LC, et al. Long-term effects of glucosamine sulphate on osteoarthritis progression: a randomised, placebo-controlled clinical trial. Lancet. 2001;357(9252):251-6.
102. Kaufman W. Niacinamide therapy for joint mobility. Therapeutic reversal of a common clinical manifestation of the "normal" aging process. Conn State Med J. 1953;17:584-591.
103. Jonas WB, Rapoza CP, Blair WF. The effect of niacinamide on osteoarthritis: a pilot study. Inflamm Res 1996 Jul;45(7):330-4.
104. Gaby AR. Literature review and commentary: Niacinamide for osteoarthritis. Townsend Letter for Doctors and Patients. 2002: May; 32.
105. Taussig SJ, Yokoyama MM, Chinen A, et al. Bromelain: a proteolytic enzyme and its clinical application. A review. Hiroshima J Med Sci. 1975;24(2-3):185-93.
106. Taub SJ. The use of bromelains in sinusitis: a double-blind clinical evaluation. Eye Ear Nose Throat Mon. 1967 Mar;46(3):361-5.
107. Trickett P. Proteolytic enzymes in treatment of athletic injuries. Appl Ther. 1964;30:647-52.
108. Walker AF, Bundy R, Hicks SM, Middleton RW. Bromelain reduces mild acute knee pain and improves well-being in a dose-dependent fashion in an open study of otherwise healthy adults. Phytomedicine. 2002;9:681-6.
109. Shin MC, Chang HK, Jang MH, et al. Modulation of Harpagophytum procumbens on ion channels in acutely disassociated periaqueductal grey neurons of rats. Korean J Meridian Acupoint 2003; 20: 17-29.
110. Gagnier JJ, Chrubasik S, Manheimer E. Harpgophytum procumbens for osteoarthritis and low-back pain: a systematic review. BMC Complement Altern Med. 2004 Sep 15;4(1):13.

111. Chrubasik S, Junck H, Breitschwerdt H, et al. Effectiveness of Harpagophytum extract WS 1531 in the treatment of exacerbation of low-back pain: a randomized, placebo-controlled, double-blind study. Eur J Anaesthesiol 1999 Feb;16(2):118-29.
112. Chrubasik S, Model A, Black A, Pollak S. A randomized double-blind pilot study comparing Doloteffin and Vioxx in the treatment of low-back pain. Rheumatology (Oxford). 2003 Jan;42(1):141-8 See www.WellBodyBook.com/articles.htm for the full-text of this article.
113. Chrubasik S, Thanner J, Kunzel O, et al. Comparison of outcome measures during treatment with the proprietary Harpagophytum extract doloteffin in patients with pain in the lower back, knee or hip. Phytomedicine. 2002 Apr;9(3):181-94.
114. Chrubasik S, Conradt C, Roufogalis BD. Effectiveness of Harpagophytum extracts and clinical efficacy. Phytother Res. 2004 Feb;18(2):187-9.
115. Chrubasik S, Conradt C, Black A. The quality of clinical trials with Harpagophytum procumbens. Phytomedicine. 2003;10(6-7):613-23.
116. Piscoya J, Rodriguez Z, Bustamante SA, et al. Efficacy and safety of freeze-dried cat's claw in osteoarthritis of the knee: mechanisms of action of the species Uncaria guianensis. Inflamm Res. 2001 Sep;50(9):442-8 This article is available on-line at www.WellBodyBook.com/articles.htm.
117. Mur E, Hartig F, Eibl G, Schirmer M. Randomized double blind trial of an extract from the pentacyclic alkaloid-chemotype of Uncaria tomentosa for the treatment of rheumatoid arthritis. J Rheumatol. 2002 Apr;29(4):678-81.
118. Chrubasik S, Eisenberg E, Balan E, et al. Treatment of low-back pain exacerbations with willow bark extract: a randomized double-blind study. Am J Med. 2000;109:9-14.
119. Chrubasik S, Kunzel O, Model A, et al. Treatment of low-back pain with a herbal or synthetic anti-rheumatic: a randomized controlled study. Willow bark extract for low-back pain. Rheumatology (Oxford). 2001;40:1388-93.
120. Kimmatkar N, Thawani V, Hingorani L, Khiyani R. Efficacy and tolerability of Boswellia serrata extract in treatment of osteoarthritis of knee--a randomized double blind placebo controlled trial. Phytomedicine. 2003 Jan;10(1):3-7.
121. Ammon HP. [Boswellic acids (components of frankincense) as the active principle in treatment of chronic inflammatory diseases] [Article in German] Wien Med Wochenschr. 2002;152(15-16):373-8.
122. Vutyavanich T, Kraisarin T, Ruangsri R. Ginger for nausea and vomiting in pregnancy: randomized, double-masked, placebo-controlled trial. Obstet Gynecol 2001 Apr;97(4):577-82.
123. Fischer-Rasmussen W, Kjaer SK, Dahl C, Asping U. Ginger treatment of hyperemesis gravidarum. Eur J Obstet Gynecol Reprod Biol. 1991 Jan 4;38(1):19-24.
124. Vasquez A. Musculoskeletal disorders and iron overload disease: comment on the American College of Rheumatology guidelines for the initial evaluation of the adult patient with acute musculoskeletal symptoms. Arthritis & Rheumatism 1996; 39:1767-8.
125. Vasquez A. Integrative orthopedics: Concepts, Algoritims, and Therapeutics. The art of creating wellness while effectively managing acute and chronic musculoskeletal disorders. Natural Health Consulting Corp: Optimal ???. August 2004.
126. Zaloga GP, Marik P. Lipid modulation and systemic inflammation. Critical Care Clinics. 2001;17(1):201-17.
127. Gil A. Polyunsaturated fatty acids and inflammatory diseases. Biomed Pharmacother. 2002;56:388-96.
128. Calder PC. Dietary modification of inflammation with lipids. Proc Nutr Soc (2002), 61:345-58.
129. Siguel EN. Essential Fatty Acids in Health and Disease. First edition. Nutrek Press, Brookline, MA, 1994: 24.
130. Sharma S, Sharma SC. An update on eicosanoids and inhibitors of cyclooxygenase enzyme systems. Indian J Exp Biol. 1997;35(10):1025-31.
131. Gil A. Polyunsaturated fatty acids and inflammatory diseases. Biomed Pharmacother. 2002;56:388-96.
132. Montuschi P, Barnes PJ, Roberts LJ 2nd. Isoprostanes: markers and mediators of oxidative stress. FASEB J. 2004 Dec;18(15):1791-800.
133. Ibid.
134. Serhan CN. Novel omega - 3-derived local mediators in anti-inflammation and resolution. Pharmacol Ther. 2005;105(1):7-21.
135. Ibid.
136. Serhan CN, Gotlinger K, Hong S, Arita M. Resolvins, docosatrienes, and neuroprotectins, novel omega-3-derived mediators, and their aspirin-triggered endogenous epimers: an overview of their protective roles in catabasis. Prostaglandins Other Lipid Mediat. 2004;73(3-4):155-72.
137. Calder PC. Dietary modification of inflammation with lipids. Proc Nutr Soc. 2002;61:345-58.
138. Horrobin DF. Essential fatty acids: a review. In: Clinical Uses of Fatty Acids, edited by David F Horrobin, Eden Press, Inc, Montreal - London, pp 3-36, 1982.
139. Clarke SD. Personal communication. 2001.
140. Horrobin DF. Essential fatty acids: a review. In: Clinical Uses of Fatty Acids, edited by David F Horrobin, Eden Press, Inc, Montreal - London, pp 3-36, 1982.
141. Diaz BL, Arm JP. Phospholipase A2. Prostaglandins Leukot Essent Fatty Acids. 2003:69:87-97.
142. Lindahl M, Tagesson C. Selective inhibition of group II phospholipase A2 by quercetin. Inflammation. 1993;17(5):573-82.
143. Tapiero H, Nguyen Ba G, Couvreur P, Tew KD. Polyunsaturated fatty acids (PUFA) and eicosanoids in human health and pathologies. Biomed Pharmacother. 2002:56:215-22.
144. Tjendraputra E, Tran VH, Liu-Brennan D, et al. Effect of ginger constituents and synthetic analogues on cyclooxygenase-2 enzyme in intact cells. Bioorg Chem. 2001;29(3):156-63.
145. Goel A, Boland CR, Chauhan DP. Specific inhibition of cyclooxygenase-2 (COX-2) expression by dietary curcumin in HT-29 human colon cancer cells. Cancer Lett. 2001;172(2):111-18.
146. Vane JR. The mode of action of aspirin and similar compounds. J Allergy Clin Immunol. 1976;58(6):691-712.
147. Tjendraputra E, Tran VH, Liu-Brennan D, et al. Effect of ginger constituents and synthetic analogues on cyclooxygenase-2 enzyme in intact cells. Bioorg Chem. 2001;29(3):156-63.
148. Goel A, Boland CR, Chauhan DP. Specific inhibition of cyclooxygenase-2 (COX-2) expression by dietary curcumin in HT-29 human colon cancer cells. Cancer Lett. 2001;172(2):111-18.
149. Dong WG, Mei Q, Yu JP, et al. Effects of melatonin on the expression of iNOS and COX-2 in rat models of colitis. World J Gastroenterol. 2003;9(6):1307-11.
150. Kundu JK, Na HK, Chun KS, et al. Inhibition of phorbol ester-induced COX-2 expression by epigallocatechin gallate in mouse skin and cultured human mammary epithelial cells. J Nutr. 2003;133(11 Suppl 1):3805S-10S.
151. Cheong E, Ivory K, Doleman J, et al. Synthetic and naturally occurring COX-2 inhibitors suppress proliferation in a human oesophageal adenocarcinoma cell line (OE33) by inducing apoptosis and cell cycle arrest. Carcinogenesis. 2004;25(10):1945-52.
152. Vane JR. The mode of action of aspirin and similar compounds. J Allergy Clin Immunol. 1976;58(6):691-712.
153. Tripp M, Babish J, Darland G, et al. Hop and modified hop extracts have potent *in vitro* anti-inflammatory properties. Presentation. First International Humulus Symposium August 2, 2004, Corvallis, OR.

154. Peters-Golden M, McNish RW, Davis JA, et al. Colchicine inhibits arachidonate release and 5-lipoxygenase action in alveolar macrophages. Am J Physiol. 1996;271(6 Pt 1):L1004-13.
155. Zingg JM, Azzi A. Non-antioxidant activities of vitamin E. Curr Med Chem. 2004;11(9):1113-33.
156. Prasad NS, Raghavendra R, Lokesh BR, Naidu KA. Spice phenolics inhibit human PMNL 5-lipoxygenase. Prostaglandins Leukot Essent Fatty Acids. 2004;70(6):521-28.
157. Ibid.
158. Ibid.
159. MacCarrone M, Lorenzon T, Guerrieri P, Agro AF. Resveratrol prevents apoptosis in K562 cells by inhibiting lipoxygenase and cyclooxygenase activity. Eur J Biochem. 1999;265(1):27-34.
160. Sendl A, Elbl G, Steinke B, et al. Comparative pharmacological investigations of Allium ursinum and Allium sativum. Planta Med. 1992;58(1):1-7.
161. Safayhi H, Mack T, Sabieraj J, et al. Boswellic acids: novel, specific, nonredox inhibitors of 5-lipoxygenase. J Pharmacol Exp Ther. 1992;261(3):1143-46.
162. Juni P, Nartey L, Reichenbach S, et al. Risk of cardiovascular events and rofecoxib: cumulative meta-analysis. Lancet. 2004;364(9450):2021-29.
163. McAdam BF, Catella-Lawson F, Mardini IA, et al. Systemic biosynthesis of prostacyclin by cyclooxygenase (COX)-2: The human pharmacology of a selective inhibitor of COX-2. Proc Natl Acad Sci U S A. 1999;96(1):272-77.
164. Krum H, Liew D, Aw J, Jaas S. Cardiovascular effects of selective cyclooxygenase-2 inhibitors. Expert Rev Cardiovasc Ther. 2004;2(2):265-70.
165. Burdge G. Alpha-linolenic acid metabolism in men and women: nutritional and biological implications. Curr Opin Clin Nutr Metab Care. 2004;7(2):137-44.
166. Barham JB, et al. Addition of eicosapentaenoic acid to gamma-linolenic acid-supplemented diets prevents serum arachidonic acid accumulation in humans. J Nutr. 2000;130:1925-31.
167. Lee TH, Hoover RL, Williams JD, et al. Effect of dietary enrichment with eicosapentaenoic and docosahexaenoic acids on *in vitro* neutrophil and monocyte leukotriene generation and neutrophil function. N Engl J Med. 1985;312(19):1217-24.
168. Ibid.
169. Stoll BA. N-3 fatty acids and lipid peroxidation in breast cancer inhibition. Br J Nutr. 2002;87(3):193-98.
170. Dandona P, Aljada A, Chaudhuri A. Vascular reactivity and thiazolidinediones. Am J Med. 2003;115 Suppl 8A:81S-86S.
171. Zampelas A, Paschos G, Rallidis L, Yiannakouris N. Linoleic acid to alpha-linolenic acid ratio. From clinical trials to inflammatory markers of coronary artery disease. World Rev Nutr Diet. 2003;92:92-108.
172. Holman RT. The slow discovery of the importance of omega-3 essential fatty acids in human health. J Nutr. 1998;128:427S-33S.
173. Chilton-Lopez, Surette ME, Swan DD. Metabolism of gammalinolenic acid in human neutrophils. J Immunol. 1996;156(8):2941-47.
174. Belch JJF, Hill A. Evening primrose oil and borage oil in rheumatologic conditions. Am J Clin Nutr. 2000;71(suppl):352S-56S.
175. Barham JB, et al. Addition of eicosapentaenoic acid to gamma-linolenic acid-supplemented diets prevents serum arachidonic acid accumulation in humans. J Nutr. 2000;130:1925-31.
176. Pischon T, Hankinson SE, Hotamisligil GS, et al. Habitual dietary intake of n-3 and n-6 fatty acids in relation to inflammatory markers among US men and women. Circulation. 2003;108:155-60.
177. Hishinuma T, Nakamura H, Sawai T, et al. Analysis of urinary prostacyclin and thromboxane/prostacyclin ratio in patients with rheumatoid arthritis using gas chromatography/selected ion monitoring. Prostaglandins Leukot Essent Fatty Acids. 2001;65(2):85-90.
178. Cleland LG, James MJ, Proudman SM. The role of fish oils in the treatment of rheumatoid arthritis. Drugs. 2003;63(9):845-53.
179. Ibid.
180. Ibid.
181. Adam O, Beringer C, Kless T, et al. Anti-inflammatory effects of a low arachidonic acid diet and fish oil in patients with rheumatoid arthritis. Rheumatol Int. 2003;23:27-36.
182. Cleland LG, James MJ, Proudman SM. The role of fish oils in the treatment of rheumatoid arthritis. Drugs. 2003;63(9):845-53.
183. Hishinuma T, Nakamura H, Sawai T, et al. Analysis of urinary prostacyclin and thromboxane/prostacyclin ratio in patients with rheumatoid arthritis using gas chromatography/selected ion monitoring. Prostaglandins Leukot Essent Fatty Acids. 2001;65(2):85-90.
184. Soeken KL, Miller SA, Ernst E. Herbal medicines for the treatment of rheumatoid arthritis: a systematic review. Rheumatology (Oxford). 2003;42(5):652-59.
185. Zurier RB, Rossetti RG, Jacobson EW, et al. Gamma-linolenic acid treatment of rheumatoid arthritis. A randomized, placebo-controlled trial. Arthritis Rheum. 1996;39(11):1808-17.
186. Remans PH, Sont JK, Wagenaar LW, et al. Nutrient supplementation with polyunsaturated fatty acids and micronutrients in rheumatoid arthritis: clinical and biochemical effects. Eur J Clin Nutr. 2004;58(6):839-45.
187. Siguel EN, Lerman RH. Prevalence of essential fatty acid deficiency in patients with chronic gastrointestinal disorders. Metabolism. 1996;45(1):12-23.
188. Belluzzi A, Boschi S, Brignola C, et al. Polyunsaturated fatty acids and inflammatory bowel disease. Am J Clin Nutr. 2000;71(1):339S-42S.
189. Ibid.
190. Calder PC. Polyunsaturated fatty acids, inflammation, and immunity. Lipids. 2001;36(9):1007-24.
191. Belluzzi A, Brignola C, Campieri M, et al. Effect of an enteric-coated fish-oil preparation on relapses in Crohn's disease. N Engl J Med. 1996;334(24):1557-60.
192. Belluzzi A. N-3 fatty acids for the treatment of inflammatory bowel diseases. Proc Nutr Soc. 2002;61(3):391-95.
193. Arslan G, Brunborg LA, Froyland L. Effects of duodenal seal oil administration in patients with inflammatory bowel disease. Lipids. 2002;37(10):935-40.
194. Ibid.
195. Bjorkkjaer T, Brunborg LA, Arslan G, et al. Reduced joint pain after short-term duodenal administration of seal oil in patients with inflammatory bowel disease: comparison with soy oil. Scand J Gastroenterol. 2004;39(11):1088-94.
196. Middleton SJ, Naylor S, Woolner J, Hunter JO. A double-blind, randomized placebo-controlled trial of essential fatty acid supplementation in the maintenance of remission of ulcerative colitis. Aliment Pharmacol Ther. 2002;16:1131-35.
197. Donadio JV. The emerging role of omega-3 polyunsaturated fatty acids in the management of patients with IgA nephropathy. J Ren Nutr. 2001;11(3):122-28.
198. Donadio JV, Grande JP. The role of fish oil/omega-3 fatty acids in the treatment of IgA nephropathy. Semin Nephrol. 2004;24(3):225-43.
199. Clark WF, Parbtani A. Omega-3 fatty acid supplementation in clinical and experimental lupus nephritis. Am J Kidney Dis. 1994;23(5):644-47.
200. Hernandez D, Guerra R, Milena A, et al. Dietary fish oil does not influence acute rejection rate and graft survival after renal transplantation: a randomized placebo-controlled study. Nephrol Dial Transplant. 2002;17(5):897-904.

201. Grekas D, Kassimatis E, Makedou A, et al. Combined treatment with low-dose pravastatin and fish oil in post-renal transplantation dyslipidemia. Nephron. 2001;88(4):329-33.
202. Schmitz PG, McCloud LK, Reikes ST, et al. Prophylaxis of hemodialysis graft thrombosis with fish oil: double-blind, randomized, prospective trial. J Am Soc Nephrol. 2002,13(1):184-90.
203. Mayser P, Grimm H, Grimminger F. n-3 fatty acids in psoriasis. Br J Nutr. 2002;87(Suppl 1):S77-82.
204. Carey MA, Germolec DR, Langenbach R, Zeldin DC. Cyclooxygenase enzymes in allergic inflammation and asthma. Prostaglandins Leukot Essent Fatty Acids. 2003;69(2-3):157-62.
205. Calabrese C, Triggliaio M, Marone G, Mazzarella G. Arachidonic acid metabolism in inflammatory cells of patients with bronchial asthma. Allergy. 2000;55(Suppl 61):27-30.
206. Ibid.
207. Ibid.
208. Spector SL, Surette ME. Diet and asthma: has the role of dietary lipids been overlooked in the management of asthma? Ann Allergy Asthma Immunol. 2003;90(4):371-77.
209. Schacter HM, et al. Health Effects of Omega-3 Fatty Acids on Asthma. Summary, Evidence Report/Technology Assessment No. 9. 2004; AHRQ Publication No 04-E013-1.
210. Wong KW. Clinical efficacy of n-3 fatty acid supplementation in patients with asthma. J Am Diet Assoc. 2005;105(1):98-105.
211. Ziboh VA, Naguwa S, Vang K, et al. Suppression of leukotriene B4 generation by ex-vivo neutrophils isolated from asthma patients on dietary supplementation with gammalinolenic acid-containing borage oil: possible implication in asthma. Clin Dev Immunol. 2004;11(1):13-21.
212. Mihrshahi S, Peat JK, Marks GB, et al. Eighteen-month outcomes of house dust mite avoidance and dietary fatty acid modification in the Childhood Asthma Prevention Study (CAPS). J Allergy Clin Immunol. 2003;111(1):162-8.
213. Mihrshahi S, Peat JK, Webb K, et al. Effect of omega-3 fatty acid concentrations in plasma on symptoms of asthma at 18 months of age. Pediatr Allergy Immunol. 2004 Dec;15(6):517-22.
214. Corti R, Hutter R, Badimon JJ, Fuster V. Evolving concepts in the triad of atherosclerosis, inflammation and thrombosis. J Thromb Thrombolysis. 2004;17(1):35-44.
215. Montalescot G, Maclouf J, Drobinski G, et al. Eicosanoid biosynthesis in patients with stable angina: beneficial effects of very low dose aspirin. J Am Coll Cardiol. 1994;24(1):33-38.
216. Ross R. Atherosclerosis—an inflammatory disease. N Engl J Med. 1999;340(2):115-126.
217. Schror K. The effect of prostaglandins and thromboxane A2 on coronary vessel tone—mechanisms of action and therapeutic implications. Eur Heart J. 1993;14(Suppl I):34-41.
218. Daviglus ML, Stamler J, Orencia AJ. Fish consumption and the 30-year risk of fatal myocardial infarction. N Engl J Med. 1997;336(15):1046-53.
219. Kromhout D, Bosschieter EB, de Lezenne Coulander C. The inverse relation between fish consumption and 20-year mortality from coronary heart disease. N Engl J Med. 1985;312(19):1205-9.
220. Ibid.
221. Rodriguez BL, Sharp DS, Abbott RD, et al. Fish intake may limit the increase in risk of coronary heart disease morbidity and mortality among heavy smokers. Circulation. 1996;94(5):952-56.
222. Albert CM, Hennekens CH, O'Donnell CJ, et al. Fish consumption and risk of sudden cardiac death. JAMA. 1998;279(1):23-28.
223. Albert CM, Campos H, Stampfer MJ, et al. Blood levels of long-chain n-3 fatty acids and the risk of sudden death. N Engl J Med. 2002;346(15):1113-18.
224. Burr ML, Fehily AM, Gilbert JF, et al. Effects of changes in fat, fish, and fibre intakes on death and myocardial reinfarction: Diet and Reinfarction Trial (DART). Lancet. 1989;2(8666):757-61.
225. Ness AR, Hughes J, Elwood PC, et al. The long-term effect of dietary advice in men with coronary disease: follow-up of the Diet and Reinfarction trial (DART). Eur J Clin Nutr. 2002;56(6):512-18.
226. Burr ML, Ashfield-Watt PA, Dunstan FD, et al. Lack of benefit of dietary advice to men with angina: results of a controlled trial. Eur J Clin Nutr. 2003;57(2):193-200.
227. Dietary supplementation with n-3 polyunsaturated fatty acids and vitamin E after myocardial infarction: results of the GISSI-Prevenzione trial. Gruppo Italiano per lo Studio della Sopravvivenza nell'Infarto miocardico. Lancet. 1999;354(9177):447-55.
228. Barzi F, Woodward M, Marfisi RM, et al. Mediterranean diet and all-causes mortality after myocardial infarction: results from the GISSI-Prevenzione trial. Eur J Clin Nutr. 2003;57(4):604-11.
229. Marchioli R, Barzi F, Bomba E, et al. Early protection against sudden death by n-3 polyunsaturated fatty acids after myocardial infarction: time-course analysis of the results of the Gruppo Italiano per lo Studio della Sopravvivenza nell'Infarto Miocardico (GISSI)-Prevenzione. Circulation. 2002;105(16):1897-903.
230. de Lorgeril M, Renaud S, Mamelle N, et al. Mediterranean alpha-linolenic acid rich diet in secondary prevention of coronary heart disease. Lancet. 1994;343:1454-59.
231. Leaf A. Dietary prevention of coronary heart disease: the Lyon Diet Heart Study. Circulation. 1999;99(6):733-35.
232. Ibid.
233. Singh RB, Dubnov G, Niaz MA. Effect of an Indo-Mediterranean diet on progression of coronary artery disease in high risk patients (Indo-Mediterranean Diet Heart Study): a randomised single-blind trial. Lancet. 2002;360(9344):1455-61.
234. Harper CR, Jacobson TA. The fats of life: the role of omega-3 fatty acids in the prevention of coronary heart disease. Arch Intern Med. 2001;161(18):2185-92.
235. Nestel P, Shige H, Pomeroy S. The n-3 fatty acids eicosapentaenoic acid and docosahexaenoic acid increase systemic arterial compliance in humans. Am J Clin Nutr. 2002;76(2):326-30.
236. Harris W. Fish oils, omega-3 polyunsaturated fatty acids, and coronary heart disease. Backgrounder (Roche Vitamins Inc.) 1997;2(1):1-8.
237. Connor SL, Connor WE. Are fish oils beneficial in the prevention and treatment of coronary artery disease? Am J Clin Nutr. 1997;66(4 Suppl):1020S-31S.
238. Ibid.
239. Abe Y, El-Masri B, Kimball KT, et al. Soluble cell adhesion molecules in hypertriglyceridemia and potential significance on monocyte adhesion. Arterioscler Thromb Vasc Biol. 1998;18(5):723-31.
240. Connor SL, Connor WE. Are fish oils beneficial in the prevention and treatment of coronary artery disease? Am J Clin Nutr. 1997;66(4 Suppl):1020S-31S.
241. Howe PRC. Fish oil supplements and hypertension. ISSFAL newsletter. 1996;3(4):2-5.
242. Berry ME, Hirsch J. Does dietary linolenic acid influence blood pressure? Amer J Clin Nutr. 1986;44:336-40.
243. Harris W. Fish oils, omega-3 polyunsaturated fatty acids, and coronary heart disease. Backgrounder (Roche Vitamins Inc.) 1997;2(1):1-8.
244. Singh RB, Dubnov G, Niaz MA, et al. Effect of an Indo-Mediterranean diet on progression of coronary artery disease in high risk patients (Indo-Mediterranean Diet Heart Study): a randomised single-blind trial. Lancet. 2002;360(9344):1455-61.
245. Connor SL, Connor WE. Are fish oils beneficial in the prevention and treatment of coronary artery disease? Am J Clin Nutr. 1997;66(4 Suppl):1020S-31S.

246. Christensen JH. n-3 fatty acids and the risk of sudden cardiac death. Emphasis on heart rate variability. Dan Med Bull. 2003 Nov;50(4):347-67.
247. de Lorgeril M, Salen P. Dietary prevention of post-angioplasty restenosis. From illusion and disillusion to pragmatism. Nutr Metab Cardiovasc Dis. 2003;13(6):345-48.
248. Ornish D, Scherwitz LW, Billings JH, et al. Intensive lifestyle changes for reversal of coronary heart disease. JAMA. 1998;280(23):2001-2007.
249. Simopoulos AP, Robinson J. The Omega Plan: the medically proven diet that restores your body's essential nutritional balance. Harper Collins, New York, pp 7-12, 24-36, 49-60, 1998.

Chapter 28
Clinical Approaches to Gastrointestinal Imbalance

- ***Digestion and Absorption***
- ***Balance of Flora, GALT, and Mucosal Integrity***
- ***The Enteric Nervous System***
- ***The "4R" Program***

Digestion and Absorption

Thomas Sult, MD

Introduction

Functional medicine is a holographic approach to health care: the whole (the macrocosm) is contained within each of the parts (the microcosm). When any part is not functioning at an optimal level, the system as a whole is degraded. This is why we always address underlying functionality (the micro level)—there, we can see how system failure in one area affects the performance of other areas that may seem, at a macro level, to be unrelated. Using this approach, we often cross multiple conventional boundaries when discussing treatment. Here, we will explore digestion and absorption, what impairs the functionality of these vital processes, and what can be done to optimize them as part of an integrated approach to improving general physiologic function.

In this essay, we will briefly review some of the most important influences on digestion and absorption. Further on in the chapter, an in-depth discussion of microflora, mucosal integrity, and the gut-activated lymphoid tissue (GALT) will be provided. The chapter will close with a detailed presentation of the 4R program for gut restoration and repair. There will necessarily be some overlap as these topics are introduced and analyzed by different authors, but different perspectives help all of us to arrive at a comprehensive understanding of this complex system.

"As a group, functional gastrointestinal disorders are the most common gastrointestinal disorder seen by both generalists and specialists."[1] They account for a very significant number of healthcare visits. Many of the so called "idiopathic GI syndromes" such as IBS have been found, in many cases, to have treatable causes.[2] Many of these idiopathic GI syndromes have been found to be postinfectious or autoimmune.[3]

The GI system is the primary gateway by which the external environment interacts with the body. It serves as both portal and obstruction to the entry of substances into the human body, working continuously to distinguish beneficial from harmful influences, allowing entry to the former and denying entry to the latter. An undamaged esophagus is a potent barrier, but the selectively permeable membrane that lines the GI tract from stomach to anus is critical to the homeodynamic function of the body. Even small aberrations in its function can have problematic results.

Function and Dysfunction in Digestion and Absorption

Digestion and absorption are under tight regulatory control. Both the neuronal and hormonal systems are involved with this regulation. Most of the moment-to-moment control is provided by the neuronal system, with feedback and amplification from the hormonal system.[4] Problems of digestion and absorption may occur mechanically, in functions such as mastication, motility, or permeability, and often originate from genetic polymorphisms, post-translational errors, or enzyme kinetic issues. Most often, GI complaints are caused by multiple interdependent dysfunctions.[5]

Loss of digestion and absorption efficiency and integrity may lead to cascading multisystem failure. Maldigestion can lead to symptoms of gas, bloating, diarrhea, pain, and/or constipation—that is, general irritability of the system. Gut irritability, left untreated, may lead to leaky gut and the development of food allergies, bacterial or yeast overgrowth, and the production of toxins. Toxins may accelerate the irritation and leakiness, resulting in toxic molecules entering the portal and then systemic circulation. This creates stress on systemic defenses, leading to immune, hormonal, or inflammatory imbalance. If systemic stress is left unchecked, and eventually outstrips the body's general adaptation response, adrenal insufficiency may occur.

Complex inflammatory interactions have been implicated in dysmotility disorders and autoimmune phenomena of the gut.[6] Errors of enzymatic control or suboptimal genetic predisposition may lead to additional problems.[7] The distribution of enzymes and transporters within the gut is clearly purposeful.[8,9] Environmental changes[10] as well as food availability changes have a great influence on enzyme and transporter expression and distribution.[11] Additionally, this distribution changes with age, again in a seemingly purposeful manner.[12]

Antigen load at the level of the lamina propria within the gut is another area of great concern.[13] With increasing leakiness of the GI wall, more antigen/immune interactions occur.[14] This results in increasing recruitment and production of inflammatory mediators. These mediators place the systemic immune system at a higher level of "irritability," resulting in a lowered threshold for additional immune interactions.[15]

Symptoms and Conditions

Symptoms that may cause the clinician to suspect digestion and absorption as the focal problem include abdominal pain, gas, bloating, constipation, or diarrhea. GI disorders that should trigger the same suspicion include irritable bowel syndrome (IBS), infectious enterocolitis, celiac disease, Crohn's disease, and other irritable bowel diseases. Systemic disorders that should also raise red flags concerning digestion and absorption include allergy, arthralgias, acne, autism, anxiety, depression, fatigue, myalgias, palpitations, neurologic disorders, immune deficiency disorders, and certain cancers.

Complex Interactions

If there are a finite number of basic imbalances that affect the GI system, assessing for each and treating appropriately should have profound impact on digestion and absorption. Indeed, clinically, this is the case, but the permutations are complex. Some imbalances can be both cause and effect. Inflammation, for example, may be caused by and may also contribute to leaky gut, comorbid conditions (such as infection or systemic disease), food allergy, aberrations of the enteric nervous system (ENS), autoimmunity, or molecular mimicry. In turn, any of these conditions could be an expression of others from the same list. To help explain this complex interacting model, I use the analogy of the bike wheel. A typical wheel has 36 spokes. With even one spoke broken, the whole wheel will be thrown out of balance, making it likely that other spokes will break under the additional stress. In a short time, the wheel will be so out of true that it will no longer fit between the forks. At that point, the entire bike is useless. Similarly, our patients experience cascading multisystem failure.

Enzymatic Function

Digestion is the mechanism for extracellular (and essentially extra-organism, as the gut lumen is technically external to the body) enzymatic breakdown of food. To accomplish this requires sufficient basic resources. Enzymes, HCl, soaps, bile salts, and transport proteins are needed. Where do the enzymes come from? Salivary enzymes are produced in the mouth; the stomach also produces enzymes; and a significant source of digestive enzymes comes from the pancreas. However, the majority of enzymes actually originate from the small intestine microvilli. When assessing digestive function, these key components must be considered.

Gastric acid secretion. Common symptoms of low gastric acidity include bloating, belching, burning, and flatulence, within moments of ingesting a meal. Nausea after taking supplements, post-adolescent acne, iron deficiency, chronic intestinal infection, and undigested food in the stool are also possible symptoms. Gastric acidity is known to decrease with age; approximately 10% of people over 60 will have low levels.[16]

HCl has many functions within the gut, but two are of prime importance:

- HCl sterilizes the food bolus. The pH of the stomach can reach as low as 1. This level of acidity is capable of killing many hitchhiking microbes.
- The acid environment of the stomach favors the unfolding or denaturation of proteins. This opens sites of enzymatic action on the proteins and prepares them for degradation by gastric and pancreatic enzymes.

It is common in clinical practice to see patients on acid-suppression therapy. They frequently say they have not improved, despite taking their medication for long periods of time. The underlying mechanism of acid indigestion in the elderly is the loss of mucus-secreting protection out of proportion to the loss of acid secreting parietal cell function. This results in a back-diffusion of activated HCL without sufficient mucous-barrier function to protect the lining cells of the stomach. In the absence of overt ulcer disease, it is reasonable to consider HCl repletion therapy with meals, but to continue acid suppressors until functional improvement of the mucous secreting cells can be achieved. In many cases, symptoms will resolve and patients will feel better in a matter of days.

Gastric enzymes. The primary function of gastric pepsins is to degrade proteins into peptide fragments, preparing them for downstream enzymatic breakdown. Low gastric pepsin activity will delay protein breakdown and result in symptoms of protein maldigestion.

Small intestine phase. Pancreatic enzymes are released into the small intestine lumen by a complex regulatory mechanism. This mechanism involves elements of the ENS (enteric nervous system) and hormonal systems. Impaired regulation of these systems may result in poorly coordinated or insufficient release of enzymes. The result of either dysfunction may be complex protein, fat, and carbohydrate maldigestion, with symptoms of gas, bloating, abdominal pain, and diarrhea.

Under normal circumstances, the pancreatic enzymes break proteins into mono-, di-, and tri-peptides and oligopeptides. All but the oligopeptides are absorbed by specialized receptor/transporter sites within the gut. The oligopeptides must be further broken down at the level of the brush border of the small intestine. An insufficiency of brush-associated proteolytic enzymes will again result in protein maldigestion. This brush border enzyme concentration may be reduced due to polymorphic genetic inheritance, or by inflammatory or infectious causes. If there is a regulatory or polymorphic problem with the receptor/transporter sites within the gut, malabsorption will result. Therapeutic approaches to restoring enzymatic function include ensuring adequate provision of cofactors to improve "mass action," and reducing inflammation and treating infections to minimize the presence of perturbing factors.

While some digestion of fats does occur in the stomach, most is accomplished in the small intestine. Bile salts "saponify" the fats (i.e., make them into a "soap") and break them into smaller packets for enzymatic degradation; therefore, adequate bile acids are essential for fat digestion. Liver congestion or inflammation from toxic load or cholestasis may result in poor bile delivery. The common practice of cholecystectomy may also hinder fat digestion by leaving the patient with a constant trickle of bile rather than a bolus at appropriate times. This creates a relative bile insufficiency. Bile salt repletion may be very helpful in such patients. As with proteins, if the pancreas is unable to secrete sufficient enzymes, digestion will suffer. Fat maldigestion is an unpleasant syndrome characterized by gas, bloating, foul-smelling and floating stool. Digestive enzymes taken as supplements may be of benefit to patients with these problems. Enzymes are complex proteins and therefore are susceptible to the acidic and enzymatic breakdown that happens in the stomach. For that reason, one should consider enteric-coated or acid-resistant enzyme supplements.

Clinical Practice

Based on the fundamental mechanisms of pathogenesis outlined above and in prior sections of this book (see, for example, Chapters 17 and 24), the goals of treatment should be to place the patient on a therapeutic oligoantigenic elimination diet, reduce inflammation, improve gut permeability, improve digestive constituents, optimize absorption, modulate immune interactions, and improve GI microflora (discussed separately later in this chapter).

Foods as Triggers—Allergy and Sensitivity

The complex mechanisms of sorting out nutrients from non-nutrients at the level of the gut mucosa are not clearly understood. It is clear that many foods can become allergens. IgE-mediated food allergy is seen in about 5–7.5% of children and 1–2% of adults.[17] Food intolerances appear to be considerably more common.[18] Food intolerance has been linked to a number of conditions. While not an exhaustive list, we will discuss below a few examples of common food/illness interactions.

Asthma is a common medical problem responsible for many deaths and considerable disability, and with a disproportionate impact on the inner-city poor.[19] It has increased in prevalence and severity in recent years, with increasing levels of morbidity and mortality, thus driving the search for new treatment approaches.[20] Although most of the increase has been attributed to airborne, rather than food, allergens,[21] and to our increasingly artificial habitats,[22] the role of dietary factors has been investigated,[23] and several studies link foods to asthma. The mechanism underlying diet and asthma is not clear, but oligoantigenic diets help improve the condition.[24] In addition to the elimination of problem foods, the inclusion of certain beneficial foods has had favorable effects on the severity of asthma. Including more vegetables in the diet seems to reduce asthma,[25] and the incorporation of fish oils also reduces asthmatic symptoms.[26,27] The mechanism of fish oils appears to involve the inhibition of leukotriene biosynthesis.[28]

Atopic dermatitis is another common problem with abundant evidence that, at least in some individuals, the culprit is food intolerance. In one multicentered trial of 1,085 children with atopic dermatitis, an elimination diet was as effective as oral sodium cromoglycate in controlling symptoms.[29] A review of the literature on treatment of eczema/dermatitis syndrome (AEDS) with dietary approaches suggests that, for patients with IgE serum antibodies or multiple food sensitizations, food elimination is efficacious.[30] In fact, it is common for parents to use food elimination techniques on their children with dermatitis even before seeing a pediatric dermatologist. In one study, as many as 75% of children seen at a pediatric dermatology clinic had tried an elimination diet, and 39% of those reported a favorable response.[31] Not all food intolerances are immediate. Prolonged observation may be needed to reveal food sensitivity. When workups that include common tests such as skin prick or blood testing are not diagnostic, elimination-provocation food challenges with prolonged observation after re-introduction may be helpful.[32] Once again, it is not just the elimination of problem foods but also the inclusion of beneficial foods that seems important. In a dog model of dermatitis, fish oils were able to reduce the need for steroids to suppress symptoms,[33] although orally-administered essential fatty acids alone have not always been shown effective in the treatment of dermatitis.[34]

Childhood migraine,[35,36] migraine with epilepsy,[37] and migraine with hyperkinetic behavior[38] have all been studied and shown to respond to an oligoantigenic diet. In all of these studies, a significant proportion of the children improved. In one study, as an incidental finding, several of the children had enuresis, which also improved for about half of them.

Gluten. Many studies have linked foods and food components to neurologic conditions, with gluten as one of the most frequently implicated substances. Gluten ataxia accounts for as much as 40% of sporadic ataxia and responds to gluten elimination even in the absence of gluten enteropathy.[39] In another study, the investigators suggest that "Antigliadin antibody testing is essential at first presentation of patients with sporadic ataxia."[40]

Gluten is clearly a common problem in human illness.[41] In addition to ataxia, it has been implicated in neuropathy.[42] MRI changes within the brain have been seen in gluten sensitivity, including white matter lesion similar to MS.[43] Skin conditions such as dermatitis herpetiformis[44] and lupus[45] have been reported. All have responded to the elimination of gluten.

Dairy. Cow's milk proteins can cause allergic reactions in some people. In newborns, a syndrome similar to pyloric stenosis has been described.[46] In another study, cow's milk proteins were able to induce a significant immune response with the production of several inflammatory cytokines.[47] Of interest is that probiotic bacterial species are able to mute at least some of these responses.[48]

Elimination Diet

Clinically, the therapeutic importance of an adequate trial of an elimination diet cannot be overstated. With this one therapeutic modality, the practitioner can reduce food antigenicity and inflammatory reactions, improve gut permeability, rebalance Th1 and Th2 cytokines, rebuild the brush border, and improve digestion and absorption. This diet is designed to remove commonly offending foods, such as gluten, dairy, and other substances. Because reactions can be immediate or delayed, a careful observation period is essential. (More detailed discussions of the elimination diet can be found in Chapters 26 and 35 and the Appendix.) Implementation is simple but not necessarily easy for patients and their families. Patients are asked to eliminate a list of specific foods from their diets for a period of at least four weeks. This period of time is needed because some of the reactions are not due to simple allergy. Some improvements stem from the reduction of the antigenic load at the level of the gut, and the resultant T-helper cell Th1 vs. Th2 immune shifting. While the simple sensitivities may take hours to days to improve, the Th subtype rebalancing may take weeks to clear antigens from the gut and show improved symptoms on a clinical scale.

No one likes to change dietary habits, but it is an essential part of treating the chronically ill patient. It is imperative to stress the importance of complete adherence to the plan. When patients are prescribed an elimination diet, they will typically start "negotiating" the terms. They will want to have this food or that, or will want to eat "just a little" of another. I tell them a story about a friend of mine who is allergic to cats. He was having dinner in a home where there were cats. The cats had been removed the day before, and the house had been cleaned and dusted twice. Despite all of this effort, this person had watery eyes in five minutes, wheezes in 10, and a full-blown asthma attack in 20 minutes. He was forced to leave the dinner party. Food allergies and sensitivities can, of course, be more subtle and more distant from the trigger—thus decreasing that very obvious link between cause and effect that my friend experienced. But, as clinicians, we must remember, and we must teach our patients, that the allergy cascade is often an amplification process. The degree of allergic response is not always a result of total antigen load; exposure alone can trigger it. In the highly sensitized individual, very small quantities of an allergen will produce, in some cases, an anaphylactic reaction.

While we will not be able to remove every possible antigen from the diet, we should strive to reduce the total antigenic load as much as possible. Strict adherence to the elimination diet will help in this regard. After the exclusion period, foods should be reintroduced slowly and thoughtfully. The tendency of the patient is to jump back into a regular diet. The most important information-gathering part of the elimination diet is the reintroduction period. By introducing one new food every three or more days, patients can catalog any new or recurrent symptoms, whether they manifest immediately or over a period of several days. This systematic process allows the patient and the practitioner to build a list of problem foods. These should be avoided during the GI rebuilding period and, in some cases, permanently deleted from the diet.

Inflammation Reduction

Inflammation at the level of the gut mucosa plays a pivotal role in the development of GI diseases and other systemic diseases.[49,50,51] Therefore, it is prudent to optimize inflammatory balance within the gut. The gut inflammation regulatory system is complex but approachable. As has been described by Plotkin,[52] complex relationships often exist in nature; clinically, we can exploit them even without full understanding of their complex interdependence. Inflammation is regulated by multiple processes within the body. No single anti-inflammatory agent will suppress or inhibit the entire inflammatory spectrum. To that end, choosing complex food sources of anti-inflammatory agents often suits the functional practitioner best.

Many foods (and active constituents of foods) have been shown to have anti-inflammatory activity and, interestingly, many have a bi-functional role in the inflammatory cascade. That is, they are anti-inflammatory in one instance and proinflammatory in another. Such substances are called adaptogens. They may be advantageous to clinicians who are often working without full and accurate information at the level of the micro-milieu. Digestive enzymes can function in this manner. Several investigators have demonstrated anti-inflammatory effects of enzymes found in bromelain,[53,54,55] but pancreatic enzymes in the face of intestinal ischemia will cause an inflammatory response[56] (probably to protect the organism from invasion). The biliary system tends to blunt this response with cholecystokinin, especially in the face of acute pancreatitis.[57]

Other anti-inflammatory foods, herbs, and spices include:

- Essential fatty acids (thoroughly reviewed in Chapter 27) clearly play an important role in helping to reduce many forms of inflammation.

- Curcumin shows anti-inflammatory activities.[58]
- Several Chinese herbal extracts have anti-inflammatory activity.[59,60,61]
- Cat's claw appears to have anti-inflammatory activity.[62]
- Many other Western herbal extracts have also shown anti-inflammatory activity.[63]
- Green tea has also been studied extensively. Its anti-inflammatory activity appears robust.[64,65,66]
- Cruciferous vegetables show not only anti-inflammatory effect but also anti-mutagenic effects.[67,68]

Including foods and food substances rich in anti-inflammatory nutrients along with an elimination diet may help to create a synergistic response in controlling inflammation.

Gut Permeability

Leaky gut (LG), or intestinal hyperpermeability, is a common clinical syndrome, implicated in a wide array of conditions. Several lines of research suggest a significant role for LG in health and disease. One aspect is cytokine balance. Th1 vs. Th2 balance appears to be influenced by antigen presentation at the gut mucosal level.[69] While inflammation appears to play a role in the development of LG, NSAIDs have been shown to enhance rather than retard its development. Blockade of the COX-2 receptor has been associated with an upregulation of COX-2 receptor numbers and may be responsible for this. Complex nutraceutical approaches to inflammation reduction, as briefly mentioned above, may have the effect of reducing inflammation without upregulating COX receptors.

Arabinogalactans from a variety of sources, including kiwi and larch, have positive effects on cell growth and gut function. Kiwi has been shown to be a potent proliferant of epithelial cells and for that reason seems helpful in LG.[70] Larch has several important benefits to LG including immunologic, metabolic, and growth factors.[71] Soluble and insoluble fibers also exert a positive effect on LG; insoluble fiber helps with bulk formation and waste elimination, and soluble fiber improves short-chain fatty acid production, a key nutrient for enterocytes and promotion of probiotic growth. Glutamine and bioactive peptides have also been shown to help ameliorate LG. See Chapter 31 for an extensive discussion on leaky gut.

Heavy Metals

Heavy metal accumulation may also play a part in poor digestion, due to its association with degraded enzyme function, dysbiosis, and bacterial or fungal overgrowth. The primary site of heavy metal poisoning is at the level of the metalloenzyme, the site of catalytic function within the enzyme. In simplest terms, the heavy metal displaces the mineral at the metalloenzyme site, resulting in degraded or absent enzymatic function. These heavy metals also have antibiotic activity. (The historic use of mercury salts is an example of this.) The antibiotic function tends to alter the gut microflora and thus can lead to dysbiosis.

Detoxification is most commonly thought of as a biotransformation process for organic or immune complex clearance, but specific pathways exist for the detoxification of toxic metals. They appear to have the same polymorphic enzymatic functionality as other enzyme systems and the consequent SNP (single nucleotide polymorphism) variability. Unfavorable SNPs will commonly lead to an elevated burden of toxic metals without excessive exposure. For example, some autistic patients have elevated provoked urine toxic metals, while the rest of the family tests in the normal range.[72] These same children will often have dysbiosis that is very difficult to clear. Upon the discovery of the toxic load and treatment thereof, the dysbiosis can generally be treated more successfully.

Optimization of Absorption

Absorption is accomplished by several means. Most are under regulatory control. This would suggest that mass action and Le Chatelier's principle would dictate mitigation of absorption difficulties with presentation of adequate substrate for the receptor/transporter molecule and/or its cofactors. Also, some forms of absorption are energy dependent. There may be direct or indirect energy utilization. In any case, a metabolic disturbance that adversely affects energy balance will negatively affect absorption.

An important engine for absorption is the Na/K-ATPase pump. This pump powers many of the energy-dependent absorption pathways. Unfortunately, most of the work on Na/K-ATPase has been done on skeletal muscle and not on enterocytes. Nonetheless, regulation of Na/K-ATPase has been shown to be similar across tissue types. Magnesium, a commonly deficient mineral,[73] is required for active transport into the cell by Na/K-ATPase. Magnesium-deficient animals and humans have been found to have reduction in Na/K-ATPase activity.[74] Potassium, a key ion in the Na/K-ATPase pump, is frequently deficient, especially in the presence of certain diuretics. Deficiency of potassium has been associated with poor Na/K-ATPase activity.[75] Thyroid hormone is involved in the expression of genes that encode for Na/K-ATPase. Problems with thyroid function, whether low thyroid hormone or poor peripheral conversion of T_4 to T_3, may adversely affect activity of this critical absorption pathway. Insulin is a potent stimulator of Na/K-ATPase activity. The prevalence of insulin resistance in our culture may play an untoward role in nutrient absorption because of its regulation of the ATPase enzyme. Additionally, catecholamines play a significant role in the regulation of ATPase's activity.[76] It may be that, in the chronically unwell, adrenal insufficiency could lead to underactivity of Na/K-ATPase activity, leading to poor absorption. Adrenal insufficiency may play another role in absorption abnormality by altering glucocorticoid metabolism. Glucocorticoid steroids (GCS) are potent stimulators of Na/K-ATPase. In adrenal exhaustion, the low concentration of GCS may inhibit this enzyme.[77]

Even this very brief review of energy-dependent nutrient absorption makes it clear that optimization of all elements of the functional medicine web is critical to improving the performance of the digestion and absorption system.

Modulation of Immune Interactions

As we know, a majority of the lymphatic tissue in the body is closely associated with the gut. The gut associated lymphoid tissue or GALT (discussed further on in this chapter) is estimated to represent as much as 70% of the total body reserves of lymphoid tissue. Gut pathology has also been associated with dysregulation of the GALT.[78] Additionally, systemic symptoms and disease states have been associated with this same dysregulation.[79] Oral tolerance is an important mechanism of immune regulation and appears to be regulated by the development of a healthy GI microflora and proper timing of antigen presentation. (See Figure 28.1.) Breast feeding appears to optimize both of these variables. In the perinatal period, this appears to be an important mechanism for immune regulation.[80]

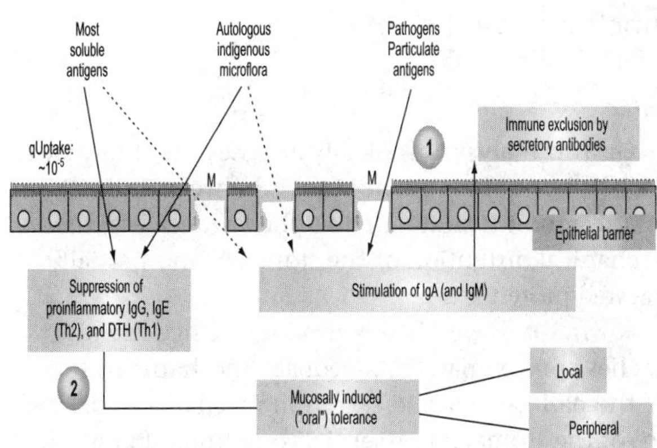

Figure 28.1 Developing oral tolerance

Source: Ann N Y Acad Sci. 2002 May;964:13-45. Figure 1. © 2002 New York Academy of Sciences, USA. Used with permission.

The events that lead to cell priming and Th1/Th2 development are complex. (A thorough discussion of issues surrounding immune and inflammatory balance can be found in Chapter 23.) It had been thought that the cytokine environment was the primary skewing agent. It is now recognized that the cytokine environment probably amplifies the skewing, but the antigen itself (and the way it is presented) is the primary skewing agent.[81] This suggests that an intact gut mucosa will have a role to play in Th skewing. If antigen concentration at the presentation site is controlling this balance, and if improving the barrier function of the gut will limit the type and quantity of antigen presentations, then Th development will be affected.

In fact, the part played by HLA antigens and their interaction with GI microflora has been explored.[82] *Klebsiella* has been implicated in the pathogenesis of ankylosing spondylitis (AS), but not all persons with *Klebsiella* have AS. HLA B-27 has also been implicated in the pathogenesis of AS, yet not all persons with HLA B-27 have AS. From a functional medicine perspective, it seems likely that—in those persons with HLA B-27 and GI colonization with *Klebsiella* and leaky gut—the environment for the development of AS is ripe. The increased interaction of *Klebsiella* and the GALT will intensify the likelihood of cross-reactive immune responses between *Klebsiella* and human determinate sites in the spine, thus resulting in the clinical features of AS.

Laboratory Testing in Gastrointestinal Functional Medicine

Gastric Analysis

Gastric analysis is basically an assessment of gastric pH. The normal pH of the stool is between 1 and 2.3. Acid secretion is stimulated by the vagus nerve, the mechanical distention of the stomach, and partially digested proteins.

Normally functioning stomach: Once the pH reaches approximately 2, feedback mechanisms turn off the parietal cell acid secretion mechanism. pH control of the stomach is essential to optimal digestion, as described in other sections of this text. Additionally, pepsin 1 and 2 function optimally at a pH between 2 and 3. Above 5, pepsin is essentially inactive.

Gastric analysis can be accomplished in several ways. The Heidelberg analysis is performed when the patient swallows a small capsule and the gastric acidity is tracked by radio telemetry.[83] Various protocols exist to challenge the acid-secreting capacity of the gastric mucosa during the test.

Another option for gastric analysis:

1. The patient is put on a food and liquid fast for approximately eight hours.
2. A small caliber nasogastric (NG) tube is placed via the nostril into the stomach.
3. In the case of an NG tube, an aspirate is collected and the pH is checked. Normal fasting pH should be between 1 and 2.3.
4. The patient is challenged with bicarb solution (various protocols exist). The pH should reach 7 within five minutes after ingestion.
5. Patient should be lying on the left side (in an effort to keep the bicarb solution in the stomach as long as possible).
6. The pH should be measured by aspiration every five minutes.
7. The pH should reach less than 2 within 20 minutes.
8. Repeat up to four times to measure reserve of parietal cell activity.

Fat Absorption Test

If secretions from the pancreas and liver are adequate, absorption of dietary fat is almost complete. To assess for adequacy of digestion and absorption of fats, a fecal fat analysis can be done. Excessive fecal fat is called steatorrhea. This condition should be suspected when the patient has large, "greasy," and foul smelling stool. Steatorrhea can be caused by digestive disorders, such as failure of the pancreas or biliary secretion system,[84] by absorption problems, or by transport of fat across the intestinal mucosal membrane. While this test will help with the diagnosis of gross or profound fat malabsorption, it is not sensitive to subtle problems of fat absorption.

Procedure:[85,86]

1. A diet consisting of approximately 100 g of fat per day should be started three days prior to collection of stool and should end on the last day of stool collection.
2. No ethanol should be consumed during this time.
3. Collect stool for 72 hours commencing on the third day of the high-fat diet.
4. Send stool for fat analysis.
5. Normal range is 5–7 g of fat per 24 hours.

Enzyme Function

Various schemes have been proposed for pancreatic enzyme testing. Recently, an enzyme known as pancreatic elastase 1 (PE1) has been shown to have a very high correlation with more invasive tests to determine pancreatic function. PE1 is unique to the human pancreatic secretion and is not affected by pancreatic enzyme supplements. For these reasons, PE1 is a good test of baseline pancreatic function.[87,88] Most healthy patients will have a PE1 greater than 500 mcg/g. A PE1 greater than 200 mcg/g is considered normal. A PE1 of 100–200 mcg/g shows mild to moderate dysfunction. A PE1 of less than 100 mcg/g reflects moderate to severe pancreatic hypofunction. Chymotrypsin is another marker for testing pancreatic function. While it is affected by enzyme supplementation, it may be a good guide to follow the adequacy of enzyme supplementation.[89] Both chymotrypsin and fecal elastase-1 can be determined by a single random stool collection.[90]

Microbiology Testing

The merits of optimal GI microflora are discussed in the next part of this chapter. Of the nearly 400 species of bacteria that inhabit the gastrointestinal system, most of them are anaerobic. Bifidobacteriua account for approximately ¼ of the total flora. Other species found in large amounts include acidophilus and *E. coli*. Although it is well known that overgrowth of a pathogen can cause problems, it is less well understood that the presence of *beneficial* bacteria, or the substances that favor the growth of beneficial bacteria, can reduce the risk of conditions associated with inflammation.[91,92,93,94]

Stool culture has been used for years to assess the relative balance of beneficial vs. harmful microbes. Aerobic culture is common and readily available. It may be used to assess for beneficial and pathogenic bacteria, as well as for imbalance.[95,96,97]

Measurements of Inflammation in the Gut

Eosinophil protein X (EPX): EPX is a measure of eosinophil activity within the intestinal mucosa that can be evaluated by a non-invasive test on a stool sample. EPX is elevated in inflammatory bowel disease and can be useful for evaluating disease activity and predicting relapse.[98,99,100] Levels can also be elevated in a number of other common conditions (e.g., intestinal parasitic disease,[101] atopic dermatitis,[102] and eosinophilic gastroenteritis[103]), however, so its specificity is not very high.

Calprotectin: Calprotectin is a marker of leukocyte activity. It is well correlated with 111 indium labeled lymphocyte excretion testing and endoscopic biopsy assessment of leukocyte activity that is evaluated via a simple stool sample. Elevated calprotectin can help distinguish irritable bowel syndrome from inflammatory bowel disease[104,105] and is also seen in bowel cancer and polyp disease. Elevated calprotectin levels can also predict relapses of inflammatory bowel disease.[106]

Intestinal Permeability Testing

Mannitol-lactulose test: Mannitol is a small, non-metabolized sugar that is readily absorbed and excreted in urine unchanged. Lactulose is a large, non-metabolized sugar that is generally not absorbed and is excreted in stool. Lactulose can be absorbed paracellularly if the tight junctions between cells are "leaky." This test uses a known mixed dose of mannitol and lactulose. The recovery of each in urine is related to cellular absorption (mannitol) and paracellular leakiness (lactulose). The degree to which each is recovered is related to the degree of impaired barrier function of the GI mucosa; this relationship has been demonstrated in a variety of conditions.[107,108,109,110,111]

Food Allergy Testing

Another way of assessing leaky gut is via food allergy testing. If a patient is allergic to a large number of foods tested, leaky gut may be implicated. When intestinal permeability is increased, abnormal interactions between the gut luminal content and the immune system are more common.[112] If these interactions involve partially-digested food constituents, food allergy may develop. In cases of multiple food allergies, one should have a high degree of suspicion about leaky gut. Likewise, if a patient is placed on an elimination diet and initially improves, only to regress in one to six months, leaky gut should be suspected. The patient may have improved due to a lower overall immune load and then relapsed when the unresolved leaky gut resulted in more interactions with the new or resumed foods, resulting in allergy/intolerance of these new substances. A fully referenced discussion of leaky gut is presented in Chapter 31.

Visualization

Esophagogastroduodenoscopy (EGD).[113] This is a fiber optic test that allows visualization of the mucosa of the esophagus, stomach, and duodenum, and also biopsy evaluation. Biopsies may help with finding abnormalities that are not readily apparent to the naked eye. At times, the mucosa will appear normal, but a biopsy will show microscopic inflammatory changes or infiltrates with lymphocytes, eosinophils, or other leukocytes. In the case of eosinophils, it is suggestive of allergic or parasitic phenomenon. A number of chemical tests may also be performed on the biopsy, the most common of which is the urease test for detecting *H. pylori*. The gold standard for diagnosing celiac disease is a biopsy of the duodenum.

Colonoscopy.[114] This test allows fiber optic visualization of the colon. The same observations made about EGD apply. Biopsies can show inflammation and can differentiate inflammatory from non-inflammatory changes. The character of the infiltrate can also be helpful. As an example, an infiltrate of predominantly eosinophils may suggest an allergic or parasitic process, and cryptitis is typically seen in inflammatory bowel disease.

Summary

Based on the above discussion, we can identify some general guidelines for optimizing digestion and absorption, although it's important to remember that treatment in the functional medicine paradigm must be adapted to each patient's antecedents, triggers, mediators, and genetic predispositions.

1. An oligoantigenic elimination diet is an important first step, and can have significant clinical impact. Patients should follow the protocol shown in the Appendix for at least four weeks to clear the GI environment of antigens and toxic materials. Then, a careful and paced reintroduction of foods should be undertaken. This reintroduction is a vital part of the treatment intervention. The more careful the reintroduction of food types, the more specific the information gained from the challenge process.
2. The reduction of inflammation is extremely important. Use balanced anti-inflammatory strategies that do not increase leakiness of the gut. Many anti-inflammatory herbs and food have been identified. A complex and multi-targeted approach seems most likely to be successful.
3. The reduction of gut permeability should help to reduce dysfunctional immune/gut lumen interactions. This may reduce autoimmune activity by reducing molecular mimicry, and may balance Th1 vs. Th2 skewing. It will also reduce inflammatory immune complex formation. Several herbs and nutrients are known to reduce gut permeability, and the use of the elimination diet alone has been shown to reduce gut permeability.
4. Optimization of digestive constituents helps to break down food components, reduce the antigenicity of food constituents, and optimize the chyme for absorption. Enzymes typically have a fairly narrow pH range in which they operate efficiently. It is important to keep this in mind as you attempt to replete a patient with enzyme deficiency. Repletion will improve sterilization of the food bolus and help with unfolding of proteins for further enzymatic digestion. Bile is important for the saponification of fats. With the prevalence of gall bladder disease, relative bile salt deficiency is common. While the liver may be making bile salts normally, they are trickled into the duodenum rather than pumped in as a bolus at the appropriate time during fat ingestion.
5. Optimization of absorption by insuring adequate enzymatic and energy cofactors will improve repair and regeneration at all levels. The primary motive force for energy-dependent absorption is via the Na/K-ATPase pump. Steps should be taken to optimize the efficiency of this system.
6. Balancing immune interactions will have local and systemic effects on health. Leaky gut and abnormal immune interaction with the gut lumen contents are sources of autoimmunity that can be influenced through the use of herbal and food-based strategies designed to stabilize immune components. In addition, enzymes may be capable of cleaving immune complexes and reducing their inflammatory activity.
7. Stress management. While many of the so called "functional GI disorders" have now been found to have organic causes, the mind is still an active participant in the process. "Stress and emotions may trigger neuroimmune and neuroendocrine reactions via the brain-gut axis."[115] Helping patients achieve a sense of control over their illness can be powerful. Hypnosis, meditation, and other stress-management techniques may have a positive impact on GI health.

Balance of Flora, GALT, and Mucosal Integrity

Patrick Hanaway, MD

Introduction

The gastrointestinal tract, the tube within a tube, connects us to our environment through a dynamic interface that is larger than a doubles' tennis court. Over the course of our lifetimes, we will ingest many tons of macronutrients, micronutrients, chemicals, and toxins. (Experts vary on the tonnage, but figures range from 30 to 60 tons of food consumed in the lifetime of the average well-nourished adult.[116]) These materials provide the building blocks for everything human. Imbalances in our functional ability to make the most of these nutrients have ramifications for every aspect of our being. Imbalance in the gastrointestinal system has implications that extend far beyond gastrointestinal symptoms; thus, the clinician must be vigilant to gastrointestinal dysfunction in nearly every clinical interaction.

Classically, the functions of digestion and absorption are considered the principal roles of the gastrointestinal epithelium. The quality of discernment that Traditional Chinese Medicine (TCM) attributes to the "Small Intestine Official" is manifested through its ability to separate the wheat from the chaff,[117] but also in the embedded relationship of the innate and adaptive immune system within the gastrointestinal system. The impact of diet and nutrients on the balance of commensal flora is considerable. Digestion and absorption provide proper macronutrients and micronutrients, while responses such as appropriate physiologic inflammation, the development of oral tolerance, the production of neurochemicals by the "second brain" (Michael Gershon's term for the enteric nervous system[118]), and the appropriate excretion of waste must all function effectively and in balance with each other in order to foster health and well-being.

Dysfunction within the gastrointestinal system manifests in typical digestive diseases such as gastroesophageal reflux disease (GERD), irritable bowel syndrome (IBS), inflammatory bowel disease (IBD),[119] non-alcoholic steatohepatitis (NASH),[120] and even colorectal cancer (CRC).[121] Gastrointestinal dysfunction can also manifest as imbalanced immunologic function, thus creating and/or contributing to both atopic illness[122] (including allergy and asthma) and autoimmune dysfunction[123] (including rheumatoid arthritis, type 1 diabetes, and Hashimoto's thyroiditis). Other diseases of immune dysregulation and gastrointestinal dysfunction now include the autism spectrum disorders.[124] The evolution of these diseases begins long before the presentation of symptoms and thus the opportunity for prevention and early intervention can have tremendous impact on the burden of suffering and disease.

Dietary approaches provide the most effective means of restoring balance within the gastrointestinal system and there are many opportunities to bring these tools to patients. However, the profound dietary changes experienced by humans over the past 10,000 years—and greatly accelerated over the past 100 years—conflict with the nutritional input that our genetic structure evolved to maximize.[125] This discordance creates a much more complex array of clinical needs that require support for the whole being to regain balance and optimal function.

Functional medicine allows us to intervene along a continuum from illness to wellness, where the approach is of value at each level—addressing treatment of disease, relief of symptomatic imbalance even before pathologic disease has manifested, prevention, and optimal wellness. The determination of appropriate therapeutic approaches is contingent upon the degree of imbalance that is present. Observation of history, signs, and symptoms (including noting the patient's own antecedents, triggers, and mediators) helps with initial understanding. Diagnostic testing helps to further illuminate and clarify the degree of dysfunction.

Diagnostic considerations include, first and foremost, an extensive health history to gain an understanding of dietary inputs, utilization of antibiotics, laxatives, fiber, herbs, etc. In addition, one must elicit the current pattern of bowel movements, including frequency, history, abdominal pain, gas, bloating, relationship to meals, and duration. It is amazing how many patients consider their altered bowel movements to be normal. Western medicine does not have a defined norm of bowel movement frequency, while other forms of healing such as Ayurveda and Traditional Chinese Medicine view the regular functioning of the gastrointestinal tract to be a critical barometer of health and well-being, with one well-formed bowel movement per day as the norm.[126] Other diagnostic considerations include the evaluation of stool to gather information on parameters of digestion, absorption, inflammation, infection, and altered gut flora (known as dysbiosis).

Let us look more closely at the specific imbalances faced by clinicians as we examine how they manifest in pathophysiology and how they can be balanced to optimize health.

Gut Flora

Cordain[127] describes the dietary patterns most common today, and compares them with the characteristics of ancestral diets. He notes alterations in glycemic load, fiber content, essential fatty acid composition, pH balance, and macronutrient/micronutrient composition, all of which have tremendous effects on the balance of the commensal flora within the gastrointestinal tract.

The critical functions of the commensal flora are:

- Metabolic processes:
  - fermentation,
  - vitamin synthesis,
  - energy production;
- Trophic stimulation:
  - epithelial cell differentiation,
  - immunomodulation;
- Pathogen protection:
  - competing for nutrients, space, adherence;
  - producing bacteriocidins.

New evidence is evolving that the persistent interactions between host and bacteria that take place in the gut may constantly reshape the immune system.[128] Clinicians see the profound effects of altered commensal flora in the nearly 15% of the population who are affected by the functional GI disorder, IBS.[129] It is also becoming clear that the immune dysregulation of IBD is profoundly influenced by the role of gut flora.[130] Symptomatic evaluation of patients who have alterations in bowel patterns defined by the Rome II Criteria (see Table 28.1) meet the definition of IBS.[131]

Table 28.1 **IBS—Rome II Criteria**

12 or more weeks of continuous or recurrent abdominal pain or discomfort,

plus at least two of the following:
1. Relieved by defecation

and/or

2. Associated with change in frequency of stool

and/or

3. Associated with a change in form (appearance) of stool

and an absence of alarm symptoms:

- Anemia
- Fever
- Heme-positive stools
- New or recent onset if > 50 years old
- Nocturnal symptoms
- Palpable abdominal or rectal mass
- Persistent diarrhea or severe constipation
- Recent antibiotic use
- Weight loss

Studies have demonstrated the alteration in commensal flora present in IBS in both colonic biopsy samples[132] and stool analysis.[133] There is considerable research on optimal methodology for evaluating gut flora. Dysbiosis can be measured by stool analysis and culture, but 99% of colonic flora are facultative anaerobes and only ~50% will be picked up by culture methods. Alterations in the distribution of metabolic byproducts of bacterial fermentation, including n-butyrate, proprionate, and acetate, can provide a proxy for the distribution of colonic flora. Decrease or absence of normal *Lactobacillus*, *Bifidobacter*, and *E. coli* species in stool culture is an indication of imbalance.[134]

Recent studies on the pathogenesis of IBS have evaluated the common association with small bowel bacterial overgrowth (SBBO), also known as bacterial overgrowth of the small intestine (BOSI) and small intestinal bacterial overgrowth (SIBO). SBBO is noted when the coliform and anaerobic bacteria from the large intestine produce deleterious effects within the delicate environment of the small intestine. A simple breath test is performed by measuring hydrogen and methane gas produced after oral administration of lactulose. As gut bacteria ferment the lactulose, the gas production increases. Typically, the gas production will increase when the fermentable substrate has passed into the large intestine, but patients with SBBO have this increase in gas production much earlier. Intestinal dysbiosis has been noted to be present in 78% of IBS patients who tested positive for SBBO. When treated with antibiotic therapy, 48% of patients no longer met the Rome Criteria for IBS.[135] Studies have recently begun to evaluate probiotic therapy to improve the rate of SBBO, but results are not yet available.

It is well recognized that several other chronic diseases have a high degree of overlap with IBS, including fibromyalgia, interstitial cystitis, and chronic fatigue syndrome.[136] Studies in patients with fibromyalgia have shown that 100%[137] and 77%[138] of patients also have SBBO. It has been postulated that the immune response to bacterial antigens present in the small intestine provides a framework for understanding the hypersensitivity present in both IBS and fibromyalgia.[139] Thus, we begin to see that alteration in the distribution of gut flora is associated with clinical syndromes outside of the gastrointestinal tract. It is useful and important to modulate the gut flora for improved health by supplementing the diet with prebiotics and probiotics. Assessment of the overall microbiota community with stool culture allows for initial evaluation and the opportunity for evaluating treatment efficacy.

The word *probiotic* (derived from the Greek and meaning "for life") was first used in 1965 to describe a function that is opposite to that of antibiotics. It has subsequently been defined as "a preparation of or a product containing viable, defined microorganisms in sufficient numbers, which alter the microflora (by implantation or colonization) in a compartment of the host and by that exert beneficial health effects on the host."[140] A probiotic must be of human origin, be non-pathogenic in nature, be resistant to destruction by gastric acid and bile, adhere to intestinal epithelial tissue, and be able to colonize the gastrointestinal tract (if only for a short period).[141] Other common desirable properties include being able to produce antimicrobial substances, modulate immune responses, and influence human metabolic activities.

A prebiotic has been defined as "a non-digestible food ingredient which beneficially affects the host by selectively stimulating the growth of and/or activating the metabolism of one (or more) health-promoting bacteria in the intestinal tract, thus improving the host's intestinal balance."[142] Prebiotics induce antimicrobial effects via their selective stimulation of commensal strains that modulate immune function and compete with pathogens for receptors. Specific prebiotics are now being developed to help promote the growth of beneficial bacteria and selected probiotics.[143] Combinations of prebiotics and probiotics are collectively known as synbiotics.

The most common probiotic bacteria are:

- *Bifidobacterium*—25% of adult colonic bacteria and 95% of a breastfed newborn;
- *Lactobacillus*—several beneficial strains (GG, NCFM, acidophilus) have been identified;
- *Saccharomyces boulardii*—a patented yeast product that inhibits growth of pathogens.

Probiotic supplementation has been shown to be beneficial in antibiotic-associated diarrhea, necrotizing enterocolitis (NEC),[144] cancer prevention,[145] health promotion,[146] and *H. pylori* prevention.[147] Recently, researchers have also demonstrated the beneficial effect of probiotics for improving symptoms in IBS,[148] and for normalizing imbalances with inflammatory cytokine ratios.[149] Probiotics are moving into the mainstream of treatment options for IBS, as well as IBD.[150] Disease-specific activity and modulation of the immune system are bacterial species- and subspecies-dependent processes. Thus, the overall community of bacterial flora becomes a critical determining factor for promoting health and preventing/treating disease.

As the human host is highly adaptive to the presence of commensal bacteria, there is a dynamic learning opportunity that continues to unfold as probiotics and prebiotics are utilized therapeutically and preventively. What is the optimal endpoint for treatment? New quantitative molecular techniques with 16S ribosomal RNA probes are now being developed to characterize and quantify the 400+ bacterial families present within the colonic environment.[151] Questions abound regarding what constitutes optimal flora. This is an important limitation for treatment planning and health-promotion efforts. In the future, nutritional interventions may target probiotic strains based upon their specific characteristics to activate an inhibitory mucosal response. Until that time, phenotypic markers of digestion, absorption, inflammation, and dysbiosis will help clarify the patient's progress.

In addition to the benefit of probiotic therapies in IBS and IBD, additional studies have successfully used probiotics as a preventive strategy for infants at risk for atopic illness. Based upon the immunologic imbalance of T-helper cells offered in the hygiene hypothesis, researchers in Finland gave probiotics to infants with a family history of atopic illness and demonstrated a 50% reduction in incidence.[152] A follow-up study at four years confirmed these findings.[153] Isolauri and her colleagues showed that the anti-allergenic and anti-inflammatory activity of supplemental probiotics was mediated, at least in part, by a decrease in intestinal permeability.[154] These findings have been confirmed in children with moderate to severe atopic dermatitis, with the improvement in intestinal permeability correlating with improvements in the severity of eczema.[155]

Hygiene Hypothesis Reconsidered

Recent analyses have questioned the primacy of Th1/Th2 imbalance in the presence of both allergic (Th2) and autoimmune (Th1) diseases. Mammalian evolution has kept us in close contact with relatively harmless microorganisms over a very long period of time. In fact, it is clear that our innate immune system has evolved to recognize these old friends as harmless. However, in affluent countries, we may not have the necessary "friends" present to consistently stimulate the maturation of regulatory T cells (T_{reg})—the heart of the hygiene hypothesis. Thus, immunoregulation as determined by the $T_{effector}$ /T_{reg} balance may be a more crucial factor than Th1/Th2 balance.[156]

The innate immune system discriminates between potential pathogens and commensal bacteria by using a number of pattern-recognition receptors (PRRs). Mammalian cells express a series of toll-like receptors (TLRs) that recognize bacterial and microbial structures, including DNA.[157] When infection or pathogens are present, the inflammatory response can increase intestinal permeability. This allows for increased sampling of gut flora by the immune system—a physiologic process of checks and balances. In the presence of an alteration of the gut flora, immune dysregulation, or a genetic predisposition, there is a sustained chronic inflammation and release of calprotectin from neutrophils.[158] Conversely, the presence of healthy commensal flora and/or probiotics has been shown to have an anti-inflammatory effect on the gastrointestinal epithelium.[159]

Mucosal Integrity

Significant permeability changes in the gut mucosa can have profound effects on anatomic and immunologic barriers to disease.[160] Intestinal hyperpermeability, also known as leaky gut, can lead to increased inflammatory cytokine production and a propagation of inflammation within the intestine.[161] There is a great deal of evidence linking increased intestinal permeability with multiorgan system failure, systemic disease, and immune dysfunction.[162] Animal models also demonstrate that stress significantly increases intestinal permeability.[163] Studies have focused on animal models and the results are now being brought to bear on cases of trauma and sepsis.[164] Studies on ischemia and reperfusion injury have confirmed a disturbed intestinal barrier[165] and increases in intestinal permeability correlate with multiple organ failure.[166]

The assessment of intestinal permeability is performed with a standardized double sugar test. The client drinks a mixture of lactulose and mannitol. The larger lactulose molecule is only minimally absorbed (in the healthy patient) and the smaller mannitol molecule is absorbed through the microvilli of the duodenum and jejunum. Absorbed sugars are then excreted through the urine and measured individually. The relative ratio of urinary lactulose/mannitol is used as the determinant of increased permeability. Decreased levels of mannitol are indicative of poor absorption and may be an indication of microvilli damage.

While some have questioned the more simplistic model of leaky gut, the gastroenterology literature has validated the value of the double sugar test in studies using histology and electron microscopy.[167] Studies have demonstrated that the bacterial translocation across the gastrointestinal epithelium induces antibodies to bacterial components with antigenic cross-reactivity to HLA antigens.[168] *Klebsiella* has been associated with ankylosing spondylitis when cross-reactivity occurs with the HLA-B27 antigen.[169] Similarly, *Proteus mirabilis* has been associated with reactive arthritis and is known to cross-react with the HLA-DR4 antigen.[170] There is currently anecdotal evidence that the modification of gastrointestinal flora with antibiotics can have an effect on these arthritidies, although formal studies to confirm or deny this relationship are not currently available.

It has also been observed that a number of inflammatory conditions, such as asthma, eczema, psoriasis, and Crohn's disease, all affect the epithelial surfaces. Alterations in barrier defense and epithelial permeability are present in each of these diseases.[171] Further clinical studies have demonstrated that there is an increase in intestinal permeability in asthma, suggesting that the entire mucosal immune system is affected.[172] Intervention trials have not been reported, but anecdotal data from researchers and naturopathic physicians have suggested that there is a sub-set of asthmatic and atopic patients (~10–20%) who improve with treatments to decrease intestinal permeability.

The first approach to decreasing intestinal permeability is to effectively remove any inflammatory stimuli from the mucosal surface of the intestine. This entails an understanding of tools to assess digestive function, as well as the diagnostic tools that can be utilized to identify/quantify the degree of intestinal permeability. Sources of inflammation and increased intestinal permeability include infections and pathogens (including Candida), altered commensal flora (i.e., dysbiosis), celiac disease, lactose intolerance, and food allergies. Once the implicated agent has been effectively removed, clinical symptoms often begin to improve within 3–5 days, the turnover time of the intestinal epithelium.

Therapeutic agents include probiotics—to utilize their anti-inflammatory nature—along with the cultivation of appropriate metabolic substrates to assist in the differentiation of the epithelial lining. After removing the source of initial injury and inflammation, glutamine is one of the most powerful agents used to supply energy to enterocytes and colonocytes.[173] L-glutamine is a very useful clinical tool, but it is also a substrate for lymphocytes and macrophages, in addition to being a precursor of nitric oxide. Thus, it is necessary to ensure that inflammation is resolved before treating with this powerful trophic factor. Glutamine has also been noted to be a substrate for Candida synthesis, so this should be evaluated before initiating therapy.

Mucosal Immune System

As has been noted, the intestine is the primary immune organ in the body, containing nearly 70% of the immune cells—more than 10^6 lymphocytes/g of tissue.[174] The gut-associated lymphoid tissue (GALT) represents the largest mass of immunocompetent cells within the human body. The regulatory function occurs in several areas—e.g., the more organized Peyer's patches and the diffusely distributed intra-epithelial lymphocytes (IELs). These critical components of the innate immune system sample the luminal contents of the gastrointestinal tract, coordinate host responses, and synthesize inflammatory mediators as they differentiate between potential pathogens and commensal bacteria. Much of this process is mediated by the recently discovered toll-like receptors (TLRs), a sub-set of pattern recognition receptors that recognize different bacterial components and quickly respond with differential stimulation of the adaptive immune response.

The dialogue between host and bacteria at the mucosal interface plays an important part in the development of a competent immune system. Microbial colonization of the gastrointestinal tract affects the composition of the GALT. Many diverse interactions between microbes, epithelium, and gut-associated lymphoid tissue are involved in creating the memory of the immune system. For instance, commensal flora are intimately involved in the development of oral tolerance, part of the body's acceptance of something as self.[175] The ability to recognize food particles and commensal bacteria is critical for educating the adaptive immune system properly.

Immunologic Cross-Talk

Inflammatory bowel disease (IBD) is an important example we can use to understand how to evaluate imbalance within the mucosal immune system. Three factors are required for abnormal physiology to evolve into inflammatory bowel disease: altered intestinal permeability, access of gut contents to immunologic cells within the GALT and the MALT (mucosa-associated lymphoid tissue), and an abnormal immune response. Alterations in mucosal integrity that do not include an abnormal immune response will also tend to cause dysfunction within the system, though in a much more subtle manner. Luminal contents that can have a stimulatory effect on the immune system include bacteria, bacterial antigens, food antigens, and toxins. Translocation of bacteria can stimulate a physiologically normal inflammatory response when function is healthy and balanced.[176] When a significant number of pathogenic bacteria translocate across the epithelial lining, there is an overt inflammatory response from the gut-associated lymphoid tissue. The upregulation of inflammatory cytokines provides the body with a rapid response to invasion (see Chapter 23). Multiple mechanisms of cross-talk between the bacteria and epithelia that differentiate between the process of recognition and oral tolerance vs. effectively responding to pathogenic bacteria have been described.[177]

Oral Tolerance

Oral tolerance has been defined as the immunologic hypo-responsiveness to an antigen encountered through the enteric route, usually through oral administration.[178] The mucosal immune system is able to tolerate an abundance of dietary antigens and commensal bacteria, while still effectively repelling pathogens. Desensitization methods have been used to deal with allergic reactions, including food allergies, since the 1960s. Studies have been done in humans that apply the principles of oral tolerance to autoimmune and allergic diseases. In at least one such study, ~80% of patients with food allergies were desensitized to increasing doses over time;[179] however, treatments for autoimmune diseases such as IDDM, multiple sclerosis, and Reiter's syndrome have been less effective. Several trials with rheumatoid arthritis were effective, with therapeutic responses to oral collagen challenge.[180] The reason for this therapeutic effect is not clear, though it has been postulated that the source of initial antigen exposure may also be oral. Animal studies also seem to indicate that the relationship of maternal fatty acid ingestion during pregnancy may influence the induction of neonatal immunological tolerance. This means that mothers who had increased n-6/n-3 fatty acid ratios while pregnant had offspring with an increased prevalence of allergy.[181]

Different bacteria induce different immunologic responses. Nonpathogenic bacteria also elicit different cytokine responses from epithelial cells, inducing differential effects on the GALT and the adaptive immune system.[182] We can see from this dynamic interplay between the gut flora and the GALT that the immunologic response system can be modified, based upon dietary changes (in the form of prebiotics) and beneficial bacteria (in the form of probiotics).

One of the factors noted in the degree of immune response is the adhesion capacity of antigens to epithelial cells.[183] Strong adhesion of antigens to the epithelial cells is seen with increased immune response. Now it is seen that IBD patients are not tolerant of their own gut flora[184] but, interestingly, the administration of fecal flora derived from healthy controls has been shown to be effective.[185] A continuum of symptoms from IBS to IBD has been proposed[186] that includes alterations in gut flora, immune dysregulation and inflammation, altered mucosal permeability, and stress-induced symptoms. Epidemiologic evidence seems to bear out that some of the rapid increase in IBD may be due to large numbers of IBS patients, and the continuously increased risk of IBD detection in IBS patients favors a true association between the two.[187]

Food Allergies

These data indicate that commensal flora may play a paradoxical role in immune regulation, depending upon the antigen, intestinal permeability, degree of inflammation, and maturation of the GALT. This phenomenon is particularly important in early infancy. The intestinal barrier is more permeable with a physiologic inflammation present, as noted by elevated fecal calprotectin levels over the first six to 12 months of life. The cytokine profile is polarized toward humoral immunity (antibody production) and away from cell-mediated immunity.

This immunologic imbalance sets up the situation in which the immature gut is much more sensitive to oral antigens and food allergy. It is clear that allergic reactions to food are much more common in the first few years of life.[188] It has been postulated that the increased prevalence of formula feeding and subsequent loss of the critical immunologic factors present in breast milk have contributed to the increase in the incidence of immune-based disorders, such as allergy and asthma.[189] The studies by Isolauri et al. discussed earlier strongly support this hypothesis, as the prebiotic effect of breast milk encourages the growth of bifidobacteria and leads to significant differences in gastrointestinal flora at six months of age.[190]

The environmental setting of low-grade inflammation and increased mucosal permeability induces changes in antigen handling that lead to sensitization. This implies that allergic response to dietary antigens is caused by a failure of the GALT to maintain oral tolerance to these antigens.[191] It would follow that the role of probiotics in the treatment of food allergies in adults would be of benefit.[192] In general, the clinical approach to working with food allergies is to evaluate the client with an elimination/challenge diet (described briefly in the first part of this chapter and more extensively in Chapter 35). The removal of an antigen that is recognized as foreign for 21 to 28 days should improve symptoms, but it is necessary that all offending antigens be removed. Thus, a modified elimination diet may not have the requisite restrictions to be effective.

After removal of potentially offending food antigens for three to four weeks (the time period may be increased up to several months if needed), the patient carefully adds back a new food once every few days; frequency recommendations vary, but 2–4 days between foods is a common range for the reintroduction process. This time frame allows for recognition of delayed hypersensitivity responses. This methodical process is usually limited to the most common food allergens, including cow's milk, wheat, egg, corn, soy, and tree nuts; however, it can be adapted to eliminate and challenge any suspicious foods. This elimination/challenge process is the gold standard of allergy testing. No commercially available allergy tests, regardless of methodology, are as accurate. Patients are strongly encouraged to follow through with the elimination/challenge diet, but it is imperative that the clinician help the patient to embrace the process with adequate preparation and a positive attitude.

Considering the diversity of immunologic pathways, it is clear that using a single entity (such as serum IgG levels) to measure food allergies would be incomplete.[193] Functional assays to measure lymphocyte stimulation have not demonstrated good reproducibility. A recent study did demonstrate clinical utility in the utilization of IgG levels as a diagnostic tool to determine a modified elimination diet in patients with IBS. In comparison with a group receiving a sham diet, the patients whose diet was based upon eliminating foods with IgG reactivity were 30% improved.[194] In her commentary on this study, Isolauri notes the profound impact of low-grade inflammation and altered mucosal integrity on antigen transfer and the development of allergies: "A healthy gut microbiota is thus an indispensable component of gut barrier function."[195]

Once again, probiotics may have a therapeutic role in the case of food allergies. Bacteria produce a number of enzymes and products to assist with the metabolism of food. For example, *Lactobacillus rhamnosus* GG was able to hydrolyze casein and reduce the production of IL-4 in atopic infants with cow's milk allergy.[196] Probiotics modify the structure of potentially harmful antigens and lower their potential for harm. Current studies are now underway to evaluate the feasibility of creating a group of probiotic bacteria with the capacity to break down gluten in such a manner that people diagnosed with celiac disease will still be able to eat wheat products.[197]

Commensal bacteria have effects that extend across a range of immunologic imbalance. We have discussed the importance of commensal flora on stabilizing gut flora, promoting the integrity of the intestinal barrier, supporting host resistance to pathogenic bacteria, and modulating immune response. All of these qualities extend to the therapeutic use of probiotics. The anti-inflammatory and immunomodulatory effects of probiotics provide the basis for therapeutic intervention. Beneficial effects have been demonstrated in IBD,[198] IBS,[199] atopic illness,[200] and food allergies.[201]

Stool Analysis

Evaluating the effectiveness of probiotics in normalizing the gut flora may not be as simple as measuring the change in bacterial counts in stool culture at the species level, although these are the best clinical tools that we have right now. Microbial analysis of stool samples provides clinical insight into the flora population of the distal colon. Quantitative growth on the agar plate reflects the levels of bacteria in the distal colon. Results obtained from fecal samples demonstrate that 50–80% of total microscopic composition is recovered by fecal culture. There is good agreement on the degree of biodiversity when fecal culture is compared with 16S rDNA sequence analysis.[202]

The predominant beneficial bacteria in the large intestine are Bifidobacteria, strict anaerobes that constitute as much as 25% of the overall colonic flora in healthy adults. In the colon, obligate anaerobes such as Bifidobacteria predominate over facultative anaerobes such as Lactobacilli by 1000:1. Recovery of these organisms in stool culture should therefore ideally be in the 3+ or 4+ ranges. Lactobacilli, facultative anaerobes, have culture growth at 1+ or 2+ in healthy adults. Non-pathogenic *E. coli* populate the distal colon, although they are usually found in reduced quantities, comparable to levels of Lactobacilli. A growth of non-pathogenic *E. coli* from 1+ to 2+ is therefore considered normal.[203]

To date, it has been assumed (though not confirmed) that probiotics adhere to the gastrointestinal mucosa.[204] Only *in vitro* studies have been able to detect the presence of adhesive substances from probiotics and demonstrate adherence to tissue cells.[205] It is clear that probiotics exert a number of beneficial effects; however, effects from supplementation may occur from transient passage through the GI tract rather than actual colonization. Studies have shown that 3–14 days after exogenous supplementation ceases probiotics are no longer recovered from the stool.[206] It is therefore doubtful in the absence of supplementation that beneficial bacteria will be recovered unless they are of indigenous origin.[207] One can assess levels of beneficial bacteria when taking probiotics to ensure that they are delivered to the colon and thus are able to exert their beneficial effects on the host. Alternatively, one can re-evaluate the stool microbiology on a patient who has been treated for dysbiosis to ensure that the imbalance in stool flora has been corrected.

Probiotic Treatment

Probiotic dosage will vary based upon the indication for treatment (and/or prevention) and the age of the patient. Strain-specific effects are just beginning to be published and efficacy data on one sub-species or strain may not be applicable to another, even within the same species. Current data suggest that the intestinal flora in IBD is not normal, even as we strive to better understand the exact nature of the term "normal flora."[208] Epidemiologic data support the idea that insufficient protective commensal flora may impair immune system homeostasis.[209] Intervention studies are beginning to prove this therapeutic approach. Studies have demonstrated efficacy for maintenance treatment of pouchitis using 450 billion colony-forming units (cfu) per day.[210] Much higher doses are currently being studied for treatment of IBD.[211] Additional trials have demonstrated efficacy as adjunctive[212] and primary therapy[213] for ulcerative colitis, using doses of 10–75 billion cfu/day.

Treatment of IBS with probiotics has also been shown to be efficacious in six of eight trials, with response depending upon dosage and strain of probiotic used.[214] Several studies of IBS treatment with probiotics have utilized doses of 25–75 billion cfu/day of lactobacillus and bifidobacter, demonstrating decrease in flatus and improvement in quality-of-life symptom scores.[215,216,217] Post-antibiotic therapies have been recommended at 20–25 billion cfu/day to help normalize commensal flora.[218] Treatment is usually for 3–4 weeks and can begin during antibiotic treatment, as long as it is not taken concomitantly. Benefit in reducing antibiotic-associated diarrhea has also been demonstrated.[219]

In addition to studies on strain-specific effects, studies are needed to evaluate the appropriate dosages for various conditions. It has been assumed empirically that higher dosages may be effective for treatment of disease, and lower dosages are useful for health promotion and disease prevention. A meta-analysis of the utility of Lactobacillus in childhood diarrhea demonstrated its efficacy in reducing diarrhea an average of 0.7 days, with a reduction of bowel movements by 1.6/day on Day 2. A further evaluation of dose response was performed, demonstrating that the reduction in diarrheal days was directly correlated with dosages above 10 billion (10^{10}) cfu and up to 150 billion (10^{11}) cfu per day.[220] Synbiotics (the combination of prebiotics and probiotics) seem to be effective at lower dosages.[221]

A recent review summarizes the evidence that the immunostimulatory effect of probiotics extends far beyond the gastrointestinal tract to distant mucosal surfaces, including the respiratory and genito-urinary systems.[222] Further research has shown that probiotics enhance cell-mediated immunity in elderly patients, particularly in people whose immune systems showed poor response before treatment.[223]

Probiotics are extremely safe, even at high doses.[224] No pathogenic or virulence properties have been identified for Lactobacilli or Bifidobacteria.[225] To date, there are no documented cases of septicemia associated with Bifidobacteria. While Lactobacillus has been associated with bacteremia, it has only been documented in severely immunocompromised patients, with prolonged hospitalization and after surgery.[226] Data from Finland do not demonstrate any increase in bacteremia over the past 10 years of rapidly increasing probiotic consumption.[227]

Prebiotic Treatment

Fructooligosaccharides (FOS) may act as a fermentative substrate. Because they particularly favor the Bifidobacteria population in the gut, regular ingestion can help these organisms become predominant. A dose of 4 g/day appears sufficient to have this effect *in vivo*.[228] Even at a dose five times higher (i.e., 20 g/d), there is a negligible amount of intact FOS found in the stool, indicating that FOS have been nearly completely fermented in the colon.[229]

Summary

It is clear that there is a dynamic relationship involving the gastrointestinal flora, environmental inputs (food and other nutrients), and the health of the immune system. Recent research has taught us a great deal about the role of diet and commensal bacteria in promoting health. It appears that Nobel-laureate Eli Metchnikov may have been correct in his assertion that live bacterial cultures are "the elixir of life." We are unlocking a number of secrets about immune system functioning, but we keep coming back to a simple intervention that has an ever-expanding opus of research to support it, and an extremely low toxicity ratio.

Future studies will help us to clarify the best strains and the best dosages for individual patients and specific conditions. Assessment of commensal flora and a genomic scan for markers of immunologic dysregulation will be more accurate and more widely available. It appears, however, that the diagnostic and therapeutic tools we have to work with today can make a tremendous difference in reducing the burden of suffering for our patients. If "form follows function," as Buckminster

Fuller was fond of saying, then the form of our immune system may be following the precise functions that our commensal flora is dictating.

We have the opportunity to encourage breastfeeding, decrease unnecessary antibiotic and antimicrobial usage (especially in the first two years of life), improve oral tolerance with a healthy n-6/n-3 fatty acid ratio, and support the development of a healthy commensal flora. These actions on behalf of our immune systems will pay dividends for years to come.

The Enteric Nervous System

Michael D. Gershon, MD[i]

The Enteric Nervous System is Independent

The behavior of scientists and lemmings can sometimes have more in common than the scientists would like to admit. The actions of isolated lemmings are rarely exceptional; however, when they form a herd, lemmings have been known to stampede and follow the mass of their colleagues off a cliff. The actions of isolated scientists are also unexceptional and dictated by the scientific method, but like lemmings, scientists can abandon rational thought and follow their colleagues into the mass acceptance of a mistake. The history of the enteric nervous system (ENS) is a good example of the lemming approach to scientific thought. The idea that the gut contains an intrinsic nervous system (the ENS) that can, when it is called upon to do so, control the behavior of the bowel is old enough to have celebrated the beginnings of two new centuries.[230,231,232] The concept of intrinsic enteric neuronal control of gastrointestinal activity dates from the formulation of the "law of the intestine" by Bayliss and Starling as the 19th century came to a close. This "law" holds that increases in intraluminal pressure result in oral contraction and anal relaxation of the gut that persists in the face of ablation of the entire extrinsic innervation of the bowel. Bayliss and Starling attributed the "law of the intestine" to the "local nervous mechanism" (the ENS) of the gut, which had previously been shown by Auerbach (the myenteric plexus)[233,234] and Meissner (the submucosal plexus)[235] to be very large.

The "law of the intestine" is now called the peristaltic reflex and does not require the presence of the brain, spinal cord, dorsal root, or cranial nerve ganglia for its manifestation. Trendelenburg clearly demonstrated, while World War I raged in Europe, that the peristaltic reflex can be evoked in loops of guinea pig small intestine isolated *in vitro*.[236] In 1921, Langley established the ENS as a separate but equal division of the autonomic nervous system, which he defined.[237] Parasympathetic nerves were classified as those with cranial and sacral preganglionic connections to the central nervous system (CNS), while sympathetic nerves were those with thoracic and lumbar connections. Because Langley believed that the CNS did not directly innervate most enteric neurons, these neurons were grouped into their own autonomic division, called the ENS. After Langley, the lemming effect eclipsed the ENS, and it was almost universally dismissed as a collection of parasympathetic relay ganglia in the wall of the bowel. This eclipse has now blessedly ended and research on the ENS has effectively resumed, to the great practical benefit of clinical medicine.[238,239,240,241]

The ENS is Structurally and Chemically Similar to the CNS

The ENS has many unique organizational features. It lacks internal collagen, and enteric neurons are supported, not by Schwann cells, as in the remainder of the peripheral nervous system, but by enteric glia.[242,243,244,245,246] The small intestine contains at least as many neurons ($>10^8$ in humans) as the spinal cord,[247,248] and these neurons exhibit a phenotypic diversity that is unparalleled in other peripheral ganglia. By now, every class of CNS neurotransmitter has also been found in the ENS.[249,250] The ENS thus resembles the brain, and is, like the brain, too complex to be easily understood. Much of this complexity is manifested in microcircuits that are notoriously difficult to define.[251] Progress, however, has been made, and its rate has recently been accelerating.

[i]Article reprinted by permission from: Gershon MD. Nerves, reflexes and the enteric nervous system: Pathogenesis of the irritable bowel syndrome. J Clin Gastroenterol. 2005;39(4; Supp 3):S184-93. ©2005 Lippincott Williams & Wilkins.

Neuronal Detection of Intraluminal Conditions is Transepithelial

In order for the ENS to regulate the behaviors of the bowel, it is obviously necessary for it to be apprised of conditions (pressure, pH, nutrient concentrations, etc.) prevailing in the enteric lumen; nevertheless, nerve fibers do not enter the gastrointestinal lumen or even its epithelial lining. Sensation must therefore be accomplished transepithelially.[252,253,254] The ability of enteroendocrine cells to act as sensory transducers helps to make this possible. Enterochromaffin (EC) cells are the best characterized of these transducer cells.[255,256,257] Prodigious quantities of serotonin (5-hydroytryptamine; 5-HT) are stored in EC cells. The bowel contains about 95% of the body's serotonin and EC cells contain most of that 5-HT. What 5-HT is present in the gut that is not in EC cells is in the ENS, the myenteric plexus of which contains descending serotonergic interneurons.[258,259] Two isoforms of tryptophan hydroxylase (TpH1 and TpH2) have been identified.[260] Because of the presence of EC cells, the mucosa contains TpH1 and enteric neurons, like their counterparts in the CNS, contain TpH2.[261,262] The 5-HT storage granules of EC cells are distinctly basolateral in their intracellular distribution.[263] This distribution means that serotonin is primarily secreted from the basolateral surface of EC cells into the lamina propria (Figure 28.2). Here, the secreted 5-HT has access to nerve fibers.[264,265,266] The constitutive and stimulated secretion of 5-HT into the gut wall by EC cells has recently been confirmed in real time by means of electrochemical detection with small carbon electrodes.[267] EC cells constitutively secrete a great deal of 5-HT and even more in response to stimulation. 5-HT thus overflows into the portal circulation and intestinal lumen and this overflow increases postprandially.[268,269,270,271,272,273,274,275] The copious amounts of 5-HT that EC cells secrete may be necessitated by the large and variable distance that separates EC cells from the nerves that respond to them.[276] The enteric epithelium is constantly in the process of replacement; stem cells in intestinal crypts and gastric glands generate new cells, while old cells slough into the lumen. Nerves are not specialized to synapse with moving targets, and epithelial cells move from stem cell to sloughing zones. A paracrine method of 5-HT secretion thus has to suffice, in which specificity is determined by the ligand-receptor relationship, rather than by the anatomy. The large quantity of secreted 5-HT assures that a sufficient concentration reaches neural receptors. The mechanism is analogous to Niagara Falls. Because a great deal of water flows over Niagara, all boats in the vicinity of the Falls get wet. This type of signaling requires an efficient mechanism to remove 5-HT from the extracellular space. Signaling has to be terminated and 5-HT must be removed from contact with receptors, lest they desensitize. 5-HT is also toxic;[277] therefore, its overflow must be kept within tolerable limits.

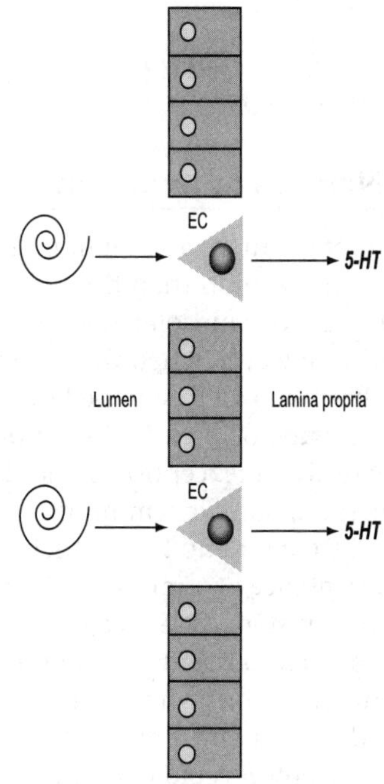

Figure 28.2 **Release of 5-HT from EC cells**

Pressure or other stimuli release 5-HT from EC cells. The primary direction of 5-HT secretion (arrows) is into the lamina propria.

SERT-Mediated Uptake Terminates Responses to 5-HT

In contrast to acetylcholine (ACh), which is catabolized by extracellular acetylcholinesterase, there are no extracellular enzymes that catabolize 5-HT. Reuptake is therefore required to terminate responses to 5-HT.[278,279] Diffusion of 5-HT away from its sites of action is too slow to prevent excessive potentiation of responses and eventual receptor desensitization. 5-HT, moreover, carries a charge at physiologic pH and thus will not cross the lipid bilayer of a plasma membrane. A specific serotonin reuptake transporter (SERT) is present in the plasma membranes of serotonergic neurons,[280,281,282] which mediates the transmembrane transport of 5-HT. The enteric mucosa, however, lacks a serotonergic innervation. Instead of nerves, therefore, other cells of the gastrointestinal mucosa must undertake the uptake of 5-HT (Figure 28.3). These cells appear to be enterocytes, which in mice, rats, guinea pigs, and humans have all been found to express SERT.[283,284,285,286] Mucosal and neuronal SERT are identical. Enterocytes probably catabolize the 5-HT after they take it up, not only by oxidative deamination catalyzed by monoamine oxidase, as in the brain, but also by O-glucuronidation.[287,288]

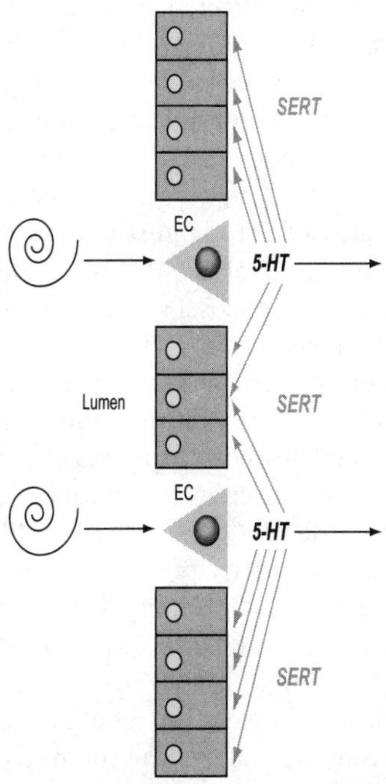

Figure 28.3 **5-HT is taken up by enterocytes**

Following its action in the lamina propria, 5-HT is taken up by enterocytes (gray arrows). This uptake terminates serotonergic signaling and thus prevents excessive stimulation of receptors and receptor desensitization.

Tricyclic antidepressants, serotonin selective reuptake inhibitors, and cocaine inhibit SERT.[289] These compounds all exert gastrointestinal effects,[290,291,292] but these actions are prevented from being catastrophic by the enteric expression of other transporters that can substitute for SERT; these molecules catalyze the uptake of 5-HT with a lower affinity than that of SERT, but they have a high capacity.[293] Backup transporters include organic cation transporters, the distributions of which resemble that of SERT, and the dopamine transporter, which is located in enteric dopaminergic neurons.[294] The basic serotonergic signaling unit of the mucosa thus consists of EC cells as the sensory transducers, 5-HT as the first messenger of sensory transduction, 5-HT receptor-expressing processes of intrinsic and extrinsic primary afferent nerves in the lamina propria as the receptive elements, and SERT-expressing enterocytes as the signal terminators.

Intrinsic Primary Afferent Neurons Enable the ENS to Mediate Reflexes Independently of CNS Input

The brain requires peripheral sensors to regulate behavior. Information from these sensors, of course, is transmitted to the CNS by means of dorsal root and cranial nerve ganglion cells. An analogous system operates in the gut. Independence from the CNS requires that the ENS be able to respond to sensors that detect luminal stimuli, and this ability, in turn, depends on the presence of intrinsic primary afferent neurons (IPANs), which are to the bowel what dorsal root and cranial nerve ganglion neurons are to the CNS. IPANs transmit information from sensors, such as EC cells, to the processing neurons of the ganglionated enteric plexuses (Figure 28.4). Both submucosal and myenteric IPANs have been described.[295,296,297,298] Mucosally-driven peristaltic and secretory reflexes appear to critically depend on submucosal IPANs.[299,300,301] Stretch-driven reflexes[302,303] and giant migrating contractions, which are ultrapropulsive,[304] may be mediated by myenteric IPANs. Both submucosal and myenteric IPANs are cholinergic in rodents[305,306,307] and humans.[308] Interestingly, myenteric IPANs display a characteristic bursting pattern of activity (about four action potentials per burst) when stimulated via the mucosa.[309] The significance of this bursting activity, in terms of the types of motility dependent on myenteric IPANs, has yet to be determined. Submucosal IPANs evidently secrete calcitonin gene-related peptide (CGRP) together with ACh.[310,311,312] Fast excitatory neurotransmission is cholinergic, while CGRP mediates slow excitatory neurotransmission,[313] which increases the excitability of submucosal ganglia. Inhibition of CGRP-mediated slow excitation thus interferes with the circumferential spread of excitation. In the guinea pig bowel, most myenteric IPANs exhibit a Dogiel Type II morphology and contain the calcium-binding protein, calbindin.[314,315,316] Calbindin, however, does not mark myenteric IPANs in all species.[317] In humans, myenteric IPANs have been reported to contain somatostatin, substance P, and another calcium binding protein, calretinin.[318] Certain differentiation antigens are commonly expressed by IPANs, dorsal root, and cranial nerve sensory ganglion cells;[319] nevertheless, submucosal and myenteric IPANs differ from dorsal root and cranial nerve sensory ganglion neurons in that IPANs are innervated, while dorsal root and cranial nerve sensory ganglion neurons are not; IPANs may thus be dual function cells, able to act as interneurons as well as initiators of enteric reflexes.[320,321,322,323,324]

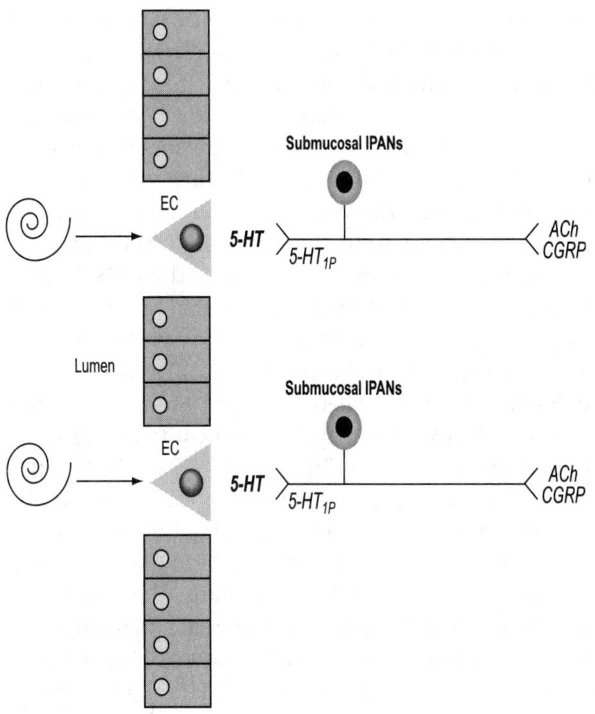

Figure 28.4 **5-HT secreted by EC cells activates IPANS**

5-HT secreted by EC cells activates intrinsic primary afferent neurons (IPANs) of the submucosal plexus. These cells, which are analogous in function to sensory neurons of dorsal root and cranial nerve ganglia, initiate peristaltic and secretory reflexes. The receptor activity that mediates stimulation of these cells by 5-HT is called 5-HT_{1P}. Neither 5-HT_3 nor 5-HT_4 receptors activate submucosal IPANs; thus, neither of these receptors, by themselves, initiates peristaltic or secretory reflexes.

5-HT_{1P} Receptor Activity Stimulates Submucosal IPANs

The submucosal IPANs that initiate peristaltic and secretory reflexes are activated in the mucosa by a uniquely enteric receptor activity, called 5-HT_{1P}[325,326,327,328] (Figure 28.4). Because a distinct 5-HT_{1P} receptor has not yet been cloned, it is defined operationally and by its transduction mechanism; the 5-HT_{1P} site is thus referred to here as a "receptor activity." 5-HT_{1P} receptor activity has not been described in the CNS, although it has been reported to be present in skin and lymphoid tissue as well as the gut.[329] 5-HT_{1P} receptor activity is activated by indoles with an unsubstituted hydroxyl moiety at the 5 or 6 position and is not affected by most conventional 5-HT antagonists. Hydroxylated indalpines have also been reported to be relatively selective 5-HT_{1P} agonists, while a dipeptide, N-acetyl-5-hydroxytryptophyl-5-hydroxytryptophan amide (5-HTP-DP) and renzapride have been reported to be 5-HT_{1P} antagonists.[330,331] Renzapride, which is also a 5-HT_4 agonist[332] and a 5-HT_3 antagonist,[333] is, of course, not at all selective. Submucosal IPANs are activated by mucosal stimulation and 5-HTP-DP blocks this activation.[334] 5-HTP-DP also inhibits the initiation of peristaltic and secretory reflexes.[335,336,337,338] In addition to its role in activating submucosal IPANs, 5-HT_{1P} activity mediates slow responses of enteric neurons to 5-HT and slow excitatory serotonergic neurotransmission in the ENS.[339,340,341] It seems likely that drugs that affect 5-HT_{1P} activity would not be good for the regulation of intestinal motility. Because 5-HT_{1P} activity initiates reflexes and activates submucosal IPANs, a 5-HT_{1P} antagonist might induce paralytic ileus by blocking peristaltic and secretory reflexes. Similarly, a 5-HT_{1P} agonist might, by activating submucosal IPANs, lead to severe diarrhea. 5-Hydroxyindalpine, for example, is a 5-HT_{1P} agonist and has been identified as the metabolite of indalpine in a clinical trial that induced unacceptable diarrhea.[342] Although drugs that activate IPANs are likely to be prokinetic and compounds that prevent their activation are likely to inhibit motility, neither would probably be useful in therapy. Agents that exhibit either of these effects would be expected to be difficult to control, leading respectively to unacceptable constipation or diarrhea. In contrast, the distal terminals of IPANs are a more attractive site to which to target a therapeutic agent because drugs that act at this site would strengthen or weaken neurotransmission in enteric microcircuits but would rely on natural stimuli to initiate reflexes.

5-HT$_4$ Receptors are Presynaptic and Strengthen Neurotransmission in Prokinetic Pathways

The secretion of ACh and CGRP from stimulated submucosal IPANs is increased by 5-HT.[343,344,345] 5-HT thus potentiates the effects of both of these transmitters and enhances neurotransmission from submucosal IPANs to second order neurons (Figure 28.5). The spread of excitation within the bowel from a point of application of a mucosal stimulus is thus made greater and propulsive peristaltic and secretory reflexes are enhanced. 5-HT$_4$ receptors mediate the 5-HT-induced increase in ACh and CGRP release from submucosal IPANs. Similarly, 5-HT$_4$ receptors also increase the secretion of ACh at nerve-nerve synapses in the myenteric plexus,[346,347] as well as at motor nerve-smooth muscle junctions.[348] All of these effects of 5-HT$_4$ receptor stimulation are prokinetic. Electrophysiologic recordings reveal that 5-HT$_4$ receptor agonists, such as tegaserod, renzapride, and cisapride, increase the amplitude of fast excitatory postsynaptic potentials (EPSP) or, in patch-clamp recordings, fast excitatory postsynaptic currents in myenteric neurons in response to presynaptic stimulation.[349,350,351] 5-HT$_4$ antagonists, such as GR113808, do not affect the EPSPs or ESPCs, which are mediated ACh acting at nicotinic receptors; however, 5-HT$_4$ antagonists prevent the enhancement of EPSPs or ESPCs elicited by 5-HT or 5-HT$_4$ agonists. 5-HT$_4$ agonists do not evoke postsynaptic responses and thus exert no direct effects on enteric neurons. Postsynaptic responses to 5-HT are all mediated by other subtypes of 5-HT receptors. The 5-HT-induced fast depolarization (or fast inward current in patch-clamp recordings) is 5-HT$_3$ mediated.[352,353] The 5-HT-evoked slow depolarization (or slow inward current in patch-clamp recordings) is 5-HT$_{1P}$ mediated.[354,355,356,357] The postsynaptic locations of the 5-HT$_3$[358,359] and 5-HT$_{1P}$ receptors,[360] determined by immunocytochemistry, are consistent with their pharmacological actions.

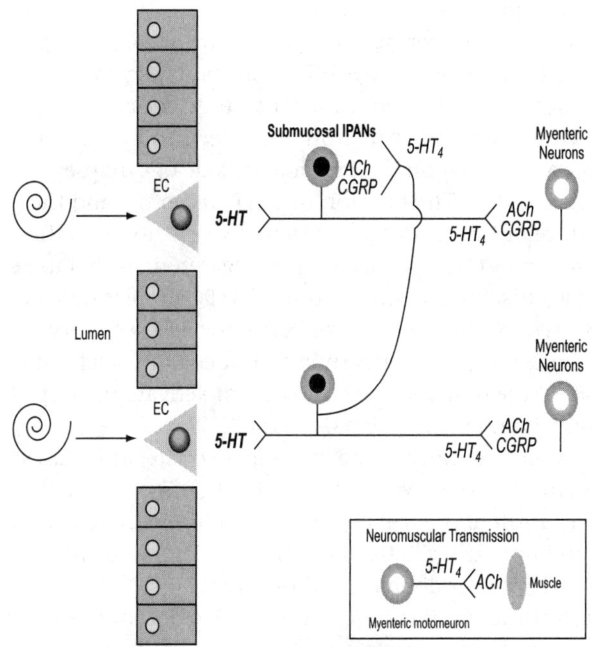

Figure 28.5 **5HT$_4$ receptors are presynaptic**

5-HT$_4$ receptors are presynaptic and are found at the terminals of submucosal IPANs, at synapses within the myenteric plexus, and at the neuromuscular junction. 5-HT$_4$ stimulation enhances the secretion of ACh and CGRP from stimulated nerve endings. The effect of activating 5-HT$_4$ receptors is to strengthen the neurotransmission in prokinetic pathways.

In contrast to 5-HT$_3$ and 5-HT$_{1P}$ receptors, enteric plasmalemmal 5-HT$_4$ receptors are exclusively presynaptic.[361] Neurons that express 5-HT$_4$ receptors have been identified by *in situ* hybridization, and the receptor protein has been located with selective antibodies. Rabbit antibodies react with the 5-HT$_{4a}$ isoform,[362,363] while chicken antibodies appear to recognize all isoforms of the 5-HT$_4$ receptor (personal observations). Subsets of both submucosal and myenteric neurons express 5-HT$_4$ as do some of the smooth muscle cells of the muscularis externa. 5-HT$_4$ immunoreactivity is especially dense in the neuropil at the light microscopic level. At the electron microscopic level, the 5-HT$_4$-immunoreactive receptor sites are found in the rough endoplasmic reticulum of neurons, the plasma membranes, internal vesicles of neurites (presumably axons), and on the presynaptic membranes of synapses. In contrast to the presynaptic membranes, the postsynaptic elements are not labeled by antibodies to 5-HT_4 receptors. The location of 5-HT_4 receptors, therefore, corresponds to the responses that have been observed to 5-HT_4 agonists. These compounds promote neurotransmission by enhancing release of excitatory neurotransmitters, and the receptors are located on the presynaptic side of synapses (Figure 28.5). The location of 5-HT_4 receptors and the nature of 5-HT_4 effects undoubtedly contribute to the safety of 5-HT_4 agonists, such as tegaserod, as therapeutic agents. To enhance motility, 5-HT_4 agonists depend on natural stimuli to evoke peristaltic and secretory reflexes. 5-HT_4 agonists thus do not constitutively activate these reflexes. They also do not activate nociceptors to send distress signals to the CNS.

When motility of the gut is inadequate, as in cases of chronic constipation or the constipation-predominant form of the irritable bowel syndrome (IBS-C), tegaserod provides relief and consistently outperforms a placebo in fair double-blind matches.[364,365,366,367,368,369,370] Unfortunately, if enteric neurons have degenerated, tegaserod cannot restore their function. When a drug acts presynaptically, it can only be of use if the presynaptic elements are present and contain transmitters to be released. Diabetic gastroparesis, therefore, is not likely to be susceptible to treatment with tegaserod. Obviously, when motility is normal or excessive, the presynaptic enhancement of neurotransmitter, release by tegaserod or a similar agent would be counterproductive. Tegaserod, or another 5-HT_4 agonist, would thus be contraindicated if motility or secretion is already excessive, as in the diarrhea-predominant form of irritable bowel syndrome (IBS-D). Tegaserod's use in IBS is thus restricted to the constipation-predominant form (IBS-C) of the condition.

5-HT_3 Receptors are Involved in Gut-to-Brain Signaling

IBS patients, who tend to focus on their visible symptoms of diarrhea or constipation, often overlook sensation from the bowel and attribute their discomfort to what they see. That leads these individuals to seek symptomatic treatment that fails to provide adequate relief. Overlooked or not, however, sensory reception from the bowel is an important component of IBS. Pain or discomfort is an integral component of IBS.[371] Visceral hypersensitivity, indeed, may be the most distressing component of IBS.[372,373,374] That should not be surprising, since more than 90% of vagal fibers are not centripetal but centrifugal, carrying information from the gut to the brain.[375,376,377] These sensory fibers, moreover, are supplemented by spinal nerves that transmit nociceptive data. Some of the information sent by the bowel to the brain, however, may not be perceived. Depression and epilepsy can be treated by stimulating the vagi, which also can improve learning and memory.[378,379,380,381] Natural stimulation of the vagus nerves in the bowel may thus influence the brain and affect mood, improving it when normal and disturbing it when abnormal.

Although the gut can, as noted earlier, function in the absence of CNS input, it does not normally do so. The ENS and the CNS can be thought of as two operators of an alimentary unit that have to work together. For the CNS to make informed decisions and worthwhile contributions to alimentation, it must, like the ENS, be informed about what is happening in the bowel and especially in the enteric lumen. Again, what the brain senses has to be the result of a transepithelial phenomenon because no nerves enter the lumen of the gut, but extrinsic visceral afferent neurons in cranial nerve and dorsal root ganglia, rather than IPANs, signal to the CNS. Instead of the 5-HT_{1P} receptor, which stimulates submucosal IPANs, the 5-HT_3 receptor is responsible for the activation of extrinsic primary neurons[382,383,384,385] (Figure 28.6). 5-HT_3 receptor immunoreactivity, therefore, is abundant on the enteric processes of extrinsic nerves.[386,387,388] 5-HT_3 antagonists can thus be used to prevent the activation by 5-HT of visceral afferent nerves in the gut. This action is therapeutically useful, and 5-HT_3 antagonists, such as ondansetron and granisetron, are used to alleviate the nausea and vomiting associated with cancer chemotherapy.[389,390] Alosetron and cilansetron are effective in counteracting the visceral hypersensitivity associated with IBS-D.[391,392,393]

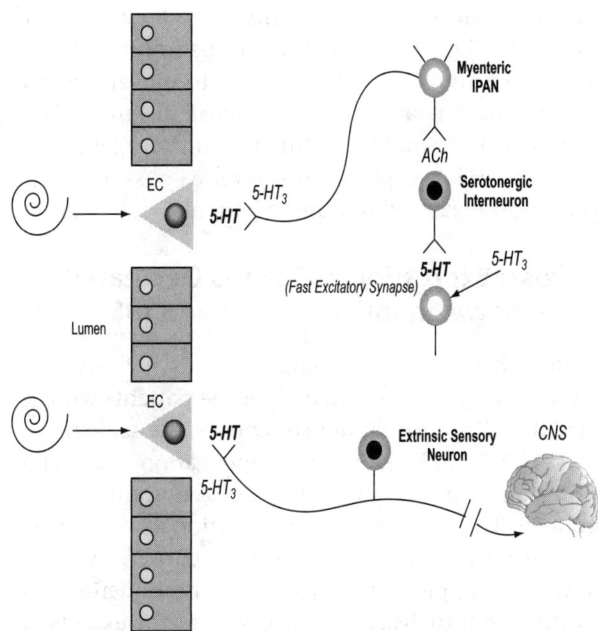

Figure 28.6 **5-HT$_3$ receptors are postsynaptic**

5HT$_3$ receptors are postsynaptic and are a ligand-gated ion channel. They are found on the terminals in the bowel of extrinsic sensory neurons and transmit noxious signals to the CNS. 5-HT$_3$ receptors are also located on neurons in the myenteric plexus, where they mediate fast excitatory neurotransmission from serotonergic interneurons and on the mucosal terminals of myenteric IPANs. Antagonism of 5-HT$_3$ receptors interferes with visceral hypersensitivity, but because of the location of 5-HT$_3$ receptors in the ENS and on myenteric IPANS, 5-HT$_3$ antagonists may also be constipating.

Importantly, it is the segregation in the gut of 5-HT receptor subtypes, 5-HT$_{1P}$ (Figure 28.4) and 5-HT$_4$ receptors to the submucosal IPANs (Figure 28.5) that initiate peristaltic and secretory reflexes, and 5-HT$_3$ to extrinsic visceral afferent nerve endings (Figure 28.6), that makes possible the pharmacologic manipulation of enteric serotonergic signaling. 5-HT$_3$ antagonists can be given to treat nausea or IBS-D without simultaneously blocking peristaltic or secretory reflexes. 5-HT$_4$ agonists can be used to enhance motility without simultaneously causing discomfort by stimulating the extrinsic visceral afferent nerve fibers that transmit nociceptive data to the CNS. Myenteric IPANs resemble extrinsic visceral afferent nerve fibers in that their responses to mucosal 5-HT are mediated by 5-HT$_3$ receptors[394,395] (Figure 28.6). The failure of 5-HT$_3$ antagonists to block peristaltic and secretory reflexes thus indicates that it is the submucosal IPANs, which lack 5-HT$_3$ receptors and are stimulated only via 5-HT$_{1P}$ receptor activity,[396] and not myenteric IPANs that initiate peristaltic and secretory reflexes.

Motility Can Be Slowed by Antagonizing 5-HT$_3$ Receptors Within the ENS

Extrinsic sensory nerves are not the only neural entities in the gut that express 5-HT$_3$ receptors (Figure 28.6). Enteric 5-HT$_3$ receptors are also found on myenteric neurons,[397,398,399] where they are responsible for serotonergic fast excitatory neurotransmission.[400,401,402,403] There is evidence that serotonergic interneurons and 5-HT$_3$ receptors participate in descending excitatory neural pathways.[404] 5-HT$_3$ receptors also activate the mucosal terminals of myenteric IPANs.[405,406] From a therapeutic point of view, the wide distribution of 5-HT$_3$ receptors is unfortunate. Not only do 5-HT$_3$ antagonists inhibit the transmission of sensory signals to the CNS by acting on the receptors expressed by extrinsic sensory nerves, they also interfere with serotonergic neurotransmission within the ENS and with the initiation of reflexes by myenteric IPANs. 5-HT$_3$ antagonism does not prevent the manifestation of peristaltic and secretory reflexes because these reflexes, which are triggered by submucosal IPANs, are activated by other 5-HT$_{1P}$ receptors and strengthened by 5-HT$_4$ receptors.[407,408,409] 5-HT$_3$ antagonists thus do not cause ileus; nevertheless, 5-HT$_3$ antagonists are constipating.[410,411,412] Constipation is an annoying "side effect" of the use of granisetron and ondansetron to alleviate the nausea and vomiting of cancer chemotherapy. It can also be a serious iatrogenic consequence of the misuse of alosetron or cilansetron in IBS. 5-HT$_3$ antagonists are thus useful in IBS only when the disease is associated with diarrhea. 5-HT$_3$ antagonists are contraindicated when constipation is a significant element of the condition. When alosetron was the only drug available to treat IBS, it was sometimes misused by physicians who did not understand its limitations and administered it to patients who were already constipated. This led to severe constipation and even rare instances of fecal impaction requiring surgical intervention. Now, however, tegaserod is available to treat IBS-C; tegaserod appears to provide adequate relief, not only from constipation but also from the consequences of visceral hypersensitivity.[413,414] The introduction of tegaserod should have made alosetron and cilansetron much safer in practice because the availability of another effective compound specifically for treating constipation should remove the temptation to mistakenly employ alosetron or cilansetron to treat IBS-C. It is not entirely clear how tegaserod relieves discomfort and bloating, because there is no evidence for the expression of 5-HT_4 receptors on extrinsic sensory nerves; conceivably, sensory disturbances from the gut disappear when intestinal motility, compliance, and tone are normalized by tegaserod treatment.

Colonic Motility Is Slowed by the Knockout of 5-HT_4 Receptors

Transgenic mice that lack 5-HT_4 receptors have been generated.[415] These mice show behavioral abnormalities, but they survive to adulthood. As might be expected from the prokinetic action of the 5-HT_4 receptor, colonic motility is abnormally slow in 5-$HT_4^{-/-}$ mice. This observation confirms that the 5-HT_4 receptor not only enhances motility when stimulated pharmacologically, but is also physiologically required for the maintenance of normal colonic motility. Surprisingly, the wall of the colon in some 5-HT_4 knockout mice is thinner than normal. The difference in wall thickness between knockout and normal mice is primarily in the muscularis externa; the thickness of the mucosa is similar in wild-type and 5-$HT_4^{-/-}$ mice. The numbers of neurons in both plexuses are also significantly reduced in older 5-HT_4 knockout animals, although the difference in neuronal numbers is not significant at birth. It is possible that a chronic or prolonged absence of 5-HT_4 receptor stimulation causes neurons and smooth muscle to atrophy in the colon. Alternatively, the poor motility of the colon in 5-$HT_4^{-/-}$ mice might impair the bowel's defense against pathogens, which in turn might exert toxic effects on neurons and muscle. Certainly, an abundance of bacteria can be observed in intestinal crypts in the colon and small intestine in the 5-$HT_4^{-/-}$ mice that is not evident in their wild-type littermates. The data from mice are compatible with the idea that long-standing failure to stimulate 5-HT_4 receptors and/or chronic constipation leads, in at least some animals, to deleterious changes in colonic nerve and muscle. If this is true, then by analogy to the mice, one wonders whether similar changes occur in human patients with chronic constipation or IBS-C. If so, then it might be important to intervene early with a 5-HT_4 agonist to prevent neuromuscular degeneration in the human intestine. It is impossible to restore 5-HT_4 function in transgenic mice that lack 5-HT_4 receptors; however, it is possible to administer tegaserod to human patients.

Mucosal Expression of SERT Is Decreased in the Bowel in Inflammation and IBS

IBS is defined as a symptom complex.[416,417] As a result, it is highly likely that all of the patients who carry that diagnosis do not suffer from the same disease.[418,419,420] The lack of general application of the same definition by physicians who treat IBS amplifies this problem. The fact that three international conferences have been called in Rome to arrive at consensus definitions of IBS implies that the condition is ill defined. To say this is not to disparage the efforts of the experts or the venue of the conferences, but to acknowledge that the absence of a tissue diagnosis impedes understanding the pathogenesis of IBS. This impediment has caused considerable grief to patients who have IBS. There is an underlying assumption among many lay people and some physicians that IBS is a mental illness and/or a character flaw. Unfortunately, there is no evidence that anyone with IBS can mentally will themselves to "get over it" and stop complaining. This anti-IBS prejudice may be, at least partially, behind the pronounced gender difference seen in referral practices in the incidence and prevalence of IBS;[421,422] females may predominate, in part, because men are too "macho" and ashamed to admit to being bothered by IBS. Certainly, anxiety can change bowel function; anxiety-associated diarrhea is common and well recognized. That phenomenon, however, is not IBS. On the contrary, IBS is itself depressing and may cause anxiety. No one who experiences the cramping abdominal pain, urgency, bloating, diarrhea, and/or constipation of IBS is likely to be happy about it. As discussed above, signals relayed from the bowel by way of the vagi might also alter mood without coming to consciousness. The public and medical questioning of the legitimacy of IBS as a disease, however, may soon change, because a molecular defect (mucosal SERT expression) has recently been found to be present in the colons of patients with IBS.

Mucosal enterocytes, as described earlier, express SERT in both rodents and humans.[423,424,425,426,427] Enterocyte SERT is required to terminate the action of 5-HT in the gastrointestinal mucosa, which lacks serotonergic nerves. Loss of SERT is not lethal because the gut expresses backup transporters, such as organic cation transporters 1 and 3 and the dopamine transporter, but motility cannot be controlled stably in the absence of mucosal SERT.[428] Mice that lack SERT exhibit diarrhea, constipation, or both in alternation. Patients with IBS also fail to stably regulate colonic motility, and they too may exhibit diarrhea, constipation, or both in alternation. The observation that drugs that affect mucosal serotonergic signaling exert beneficial effects in IBS suggested that mice that lack SERT and patients with IBS might possibly share a defect in SERT expression. Indeed, they do. The expression of SERT is reduced in mucosal biopsies of patients with IBS-C and in those with IBS-D.[429] A reduction in mucosal mRNA encoding SERT was documented by means of real-time reverse transcriptase polymerase chain reaction and found by immunocytochemistry to lead to decreased expression of SERT protein in colonic enterocytes. A loss of SERT would be expected to potentiate the action of 5-HT and lead to feedback inhibition of its biosynthesis. Feedback inhibition of 5-HT biosynthesis also occurs in the human colon in IBS. The expression of transcripts encoding TpH1, the isoform of TpH characteristic of EC cells, is decreased in the same colonic mucosal biopsies found to be deficient in SERT. Mucosal SERT expression decreases dramatically in guinea pig colon in which inflammation has been induced by administration of 2,4,6-trinitrobenzene sulfonic acid,[430] and in the human colon in ulcerative colitis.[431] That a reduction in SERT expression should be common to experimental colitis, ulcerative colitis, IBS-C, and IBS-D raises the possibility that inflammation is a common link in all of these entities. A linkage of IBS to inflammation has been suggested in the past, but not definitively established.[432,433,434,435,436,437,438] Certainly, the symptoms of discomfort, diarrhea, and constipation that are common to ulcerative colitis and IBS may all stem from a shared lesion in mucosal SERT and TpH1. Excessive accumulation of free and active 5-HT, with a resultant potentiation of serotonergic signaling, is the first effect to be anticipated to result from a decline in the function of SERT (Figure 28.3). Potentiation of the action of 5-HT at 5-HT_3 receptors would be expected to lead to discomfort, while a potentiation of the action of 5-HT at 5-HT_{1P}, 5-HT_4, and 5-HT_3 receptors would all lead to diarrhea. Constipation might be the result of receptor desensitization, and alternation between constipation and diarrhea could result from intermittent receptor desensitization. Indeed, a molecular change in 5-HT_3 receptors has been detected in transgenic mice that lack SERT; the receptors become less sensitive to 5-HT and more likely to desensitize.[439] A defect in mucosal SERT expression, whatever its cause, could thus explain the full extent of symptoms in IBS.

In summary, the ENS is an independent nervous system; as a result, the bowel, can uniquely exhibit reflexes even in the absence of input from the CNS. The ENS monitors luminal conditions, but has to do so transepithelially because no nerves enter the gastrointestinal lumen. Sensory transducer cells in the epithelium respond to mucosal stimuli and secrete transmitters that activate the mucosal processes of both intrinsic (IPANs) and extrinsic primary afferent (sensory) neurons. The best characterized of these cellular transducers is the EC cell, which acts through the secretion of 5-HT. Both the submucosal and myenteric plexuses contain IPANs. Submucosal IPANs initiate peristaltic and secretory reflexes; these cells are stimulated by a receptor activity called 5-HT_{1P}. The release of acetylcholine and CGRP at the terminals of submucosal IPANs and those of other enteric neurons is enhanced by 5-HT_4 receptors. These receptors are presynaptic and, by promoting transmitter release, 5-HT_4 receptors strengthen neurotransmission in prokinetic reflex pathways. 5-HT_3 receptors mediate serotonergic signaling to the CNS; however, they also activate myenteric IPANs and are responsible for fast serotonergic neurotransmission in the ENS. Because of the differential distribution of 5-HT receptor subtypes in the bowel, 5-HT_3 antagonists can be used to treat the nausea associated with cancer chemotherapy without blocking peristaltic and secretory reflexes. 5-HT_3 antagonists are also effective in treating the hypersensitivity of IBS and IBS-associated diarrhea. 5-HT_3 antagonists, however, can be constipating because of their effects on serotonergic neurotransmission within the ENS, and perhaps also because they stimulate myenteric IPANs. The use of 5-HT_3 antagonists in the treatment of IBS is therefore restricted to IBS-D. 5-HT_4 agonists can be used as prokinetic agents to relieve the discomfort as well as the constipation of IBS-C, and also to treat chronic constipation. The safety of 5-HT_4 agonists is enhanced because they do not initiate peristaltic and secretory reflexes but instead strengthen pathways that are activated by natural means. 5-HT_4 agonists also do not activate nociceptors and thus do not transmit noxious signals to the CNS. Serotonergic signaling in the mucosa and in the ENS is terminated by the action of a plasmalemmal serotonin transporter (SERT), which mediates the transmembrane uptake of 5-HT. Expression of SERT is decreased in the mucosa of patients with IBS-C, IBS-D, and ulcerative colitis. Transcripts encoding tryptophan hydroxylase-1 are also decreased, probably secondary to the potentiation of 5-HT that results from the diminished expression of SERT. SERT expression is also reduced in an experimentally inflamed mucosa. Potentiation of the effects of 5-HT due to the decrease in mucosal SERT expression, which may be followed by desensitization of overly stimulated 5-HT receptors, could account for the common symptoms seen in IBS and ulcerative colitis. Potentiation of 5-HT would be expected to cause discomfort and diarrhea, while desensitization of receptors would lead to constipation. Similar symptoms are seen in patients with IBS and transgenic mice that lack SERT. This commonality of symptoms in patients and animals that share a molecular defect in SERT expression supports the idea that the loss of mucosal SERT contributes to the pathogenesis of IBS.

The "4R" Program

Dan Lukaczer, ND

Introduction

To review briefly what has been covered so far in this chapter, gastrointestinal (GI) complaints are among the leading reasons patients seek out healthcare practitioners. In the United States, more than 70 million patients suffer some form of GI disorder, which can range from mild discomfort to life-threatening disease. Frequently diagnosed GI-related conditions include gastroesophageal reflux disease, gastritis, peptic ulcer, cholecystitis, diverticulitis, and inflammatory bowel disease. Even more common is the so-called "functional" disorder of irritable bowel syndrome.[440,441] Many of the most common GI disorders are found with greater frequency in people over 60 years of age and, therefore, are on the rise due to the aging of our population.[442]

While conditions localized to the GI tract make for an extensive list, GI dysfunction has also been linked to a number of other non-localized systemic conditions. This connection is likely related to a breach in the intestinal barrier, and is often referred to as "leaky gut." Increased intestinal permeability can lead to many systemic inflammatory and immune-related symptoms. It has been implicated in such unrelated conditions as rheumatoid arthritis, ankylosing spondylitis, eczema, non-alcoholic fatty liver disease, and chronic urticaria.[443,444,445,446,447,448,449,450] Thus, the normal integrity of the GI tract may be compromised, resulting in distant systemic complaints, even in the absence of overt GI symptomatology.

The ability of the body to maintain healthy GI function, and to heal the GI barrier when its integrity is breached, is integral to protection from many diseases and disorders. However, maintenance of healthy GI function is not a simple task, and understanding how to evaluate and therapeutically support GI function can be a difficult undertaking in a busy practice. For that reason, we will close this chapter with an in-depth discussion of a well-established functional medicine approach to treating GI dysfunction. This method for identifying clinical assessments and interventions that focus on normalizing and optimizing gastrointestinal function has been referred to as the "4R" program, in reference to its four basic clinical steps: remove, replace, reinoculate, and repair. It is designed to provide a focus for evaluation of the status of GI function, with interventions targeted to appropriate nutritional, digestive, probiotic/prebiotic, and antimicrobial therapy. The specific application of the program depends on the nature and course of the patient's condition, and should be individualized for maximum effectiveness.

The 4R Model

Often in conventional medicine, the clinician asks only how to suppress a particular symptom in a patient. The 4R model asks four primary questions in a patient with GI-related complaints, or complaints whose origins may stem from a breach of GI mucosal integrity:

1. What may need to be *removed* to support healthy GI function? The clinician may need to assess the presence/activity of pathogenic or potentially pathogenic yeast, bacteria, or protozoa in the intestinal

tract, or foods and additives that result in allergic or intolerant responses.

2. What may need to be *replaced* to support healthy GI function? Digestive enzymes, bile salts or stomach acid secretions should be considered.
3. What may be needed to support and/or reestablish a healthy balance of microflora? This step may include *reinoculation* with probiotic and/or prebiotics.
4. What may be needed to support regeneration and *repair* of a healthy mucosal layer? A variety of specific nutrients and phytonutrients are available for this purpose.

Remove

The "remove" aspect of this model focuses on eliminating pathogenic bacteria, viruses, fungi, parasites, and other environmentally-derived toxic substances from the gastrointestinal tract. Foods themselves may be the most important offending agents. Over the course of a lifetime, the gastrointestinal tract processes many tons of food, representing the largest antigenic load confronting the human immune system.[451] (Experts vary on the tonnage, but figures range from 30 to 60 tons of food consumed in the lifetime of the average well-nourished adult.[452]) During digestion, proteins and large peptides are broken down into amino acids or small peptides within the intestinal lumen, which removes or decreases their antigenic potential. In a healthy intestinal tract, more than 98% of ingested food antigens are blocked from entering circulation by a host of gastrointestinal barrier functions (described earlier in this chapter). In a compromised environment with increased intestinal permeability, significantly more antigens may penetrate to the systemic circulation. These protein fragments, recognized as foreign molecules, stimulate an immune response. In genetically susceptible individuals, autoimmune reactions may therefore result from this increased antigenic load.

Not every adverse response to food qualifies as an immunologically-mediated food allergy. By definition, an immune response only occurs when an antigen/antibody reaction has taken place. Therefore, if a person does not have antibodies against a specific food antigen, he or she cannot have an allergic reaction to that food. However, patients do respond in non-immunological ways. A simple example is a lactase insufficiency, which underlies lactose intolerance, and would not be considered an allergic reaction. Many food reactions fall into this category.

Some controversy exists with respect to the actual definition of food allergy. Some definitions describe a true food allergy as only an IgE-mediated response, which is also called a type 1 hypersensitivity, whereas a substance that elicits antibodies of any other class is termed antigenic. However, it is becoming clear that not all symptoms of allergic responses can be ascribed to IgE-mediated mechanisms.[453] Many allergic responses appear to involve some form of prolonged or delayed reaction to allergens.[454] IgG antibodies have been implicated as a possible etiological factor in conditions such as atopic dermatitis, asthma, and IBS.[455,456,457] Therefore, there appears to be some evidence for a role of both IgE and IgG antibodies in the provocation of both immediate and delayed reactions to food allergens.

Food allergies have been suggested as the cause of a variety of symptoms. Clinical studies suggest that 8% of U.S. children younger than six years have evidence of food intolerance, and 2 to 4% of those experience reproducible allergic reactions to foods, most often eggs, milk, peanuts, soy, fish, and wheat.[458,459] Surveys suggest that 1 to 2% of adult Americans are sensitive to foods, most commonly nuts, peanuts, fish, and shellfish.[460,461,462] Because delayed food reactions are often difficult to diagnose, these figures likely under-represent the extent of food allergy in the population. Table 28.2 lists some common symptoms and diseases that have been associated with food allergies.

The underlying mechanisms that elicit food-intolerant or allergic responses are complex and controversial, and a variety of assessment techniques for food allergy have been developed. Unfortunately, none are completely adequate, and it appears that the most cost-effective and accurate avenue to determine food allergy is the elimination or oligoantigenic diet, containing only those foods known to pose little risk of an allergic or intolerant reaction. Several studies have shown an association between food allergy and a variety of diseases and symptoms, with avoidance of the suspected foods leading to substantial improvement in clinical symptoms. Therefore, oligoantigenic diets are typically part of a "remove" protocol.[463,464] If a clinician or patient wants to confirm food sensitivity, the potentially offending food can be reintroduced and symptoms monitored.

Table 28.2 **Symptoms and Diseases that may be Associated with Food Allergy**

System	Symptoms/Disease
Gastrointestinal	Canker sores, celiac disease, chronic diarrhea, stomach ulcers, duodenal ulcers, recurrent mouth ulcers, indigestion, nausea, vomiting, diarrhea, constipation, gas, gastritis, irritable bowel syndrome, malabsorption, ulcerative colitis, Crohn's disease, colic (babies)
Genitourinary	Bed wetting, chronic bladder infections, nephrotic syndrome, frequent urination
HEENT	Serous otitis media, migraine headaches
Mental/Emotional	Attention deficit disorder, depression, anxiety, memory loss, epileptic seizures, schizophrenia
Musculoskeletal	Joint pain, myalgias, rheumatoid arthritis
Respiratory	Asthma, chronic or allergic sinusitis, constant runny or congested nose, nasal polyps
Cardiovascular	Irregular heart rhythm, vasculitis, inflammation of the veins producing purpura, spontaneous bruising, urticaria, edema
Skin	Eczema, psoriasis, urticaria, red itchy eyes, itchy skin

Equally important in assessment of antigenic stimuli is the myriad array of organisms that reside in or invade the gastrointestinal system. All too often, gut flora assessment is overlooked as a significant source of information concerning systemic or even local health problems. Recognition that intestinal flora could have a major impact on health and disease was first popularized by the Russian scientist Eli Metchnikoff at the turn of the 20th century. Metchnikoff put forth the idea of "dysbiosis," which he defined as a state of living with intestinal flora that may have harmful or detrimental effects. That idea is now receiving significant scientific validation. The indigenous flora was once thought to be relatively benign. It seems clear that the subject is far more complicated than previously believed.

The number of bacteria in the large bowel alone is greater than 100 billion, which is more than the total number of cells in the human body. These bacteria constitute a powerful chemical factory and can have important effects on human physiology, depending upon their activities. Intestinal bacteria produce toxins and antitoxins, alter chemical composition of foods and drugs, produce and degrade vitamins, produce short-chain fatty acids from fiber, degrade dietary toxins, and inhibit the growth of certain pathogens. Bacterial byproducts can inactivate brush border and pancreatic enzymes, deconjugate bile salts, and hydrolyze bile acids. Problems from a dysbiotic condition often relate to the prolific activity of an altered intestinal microflora. Additionally, through the process of microbial translocation, defined as the passage of both viable and nonviable microbes and microbial products (endotoxins) across an anatomically intact intestinal barrier, gut-derived products may play a role in increasing the systemic immune inflammatory response.[465] There is evidence that microflora share antigenic determinants with normal tissue and produce cross-reactive antibodies.[466,467] Bacterial lipopolysaccharides found in the cell walls of gram-negative bacteria have been shown to initiate immune responses and elevate proinflammatory cytokines.[468] For example, inflammatory diseases of the bowel such as Crohn's and ulcerative colitis, rheumatoid arthritis, and other spondyloarthropathies have been linked to indigenous flora of the gut.[469,470,471,472,473]

Yeast is another example of indigenous flora that may have detrimental consequences. There is evidence that, in certain individuals, intestinal yeast may result in diverse symptomatology.[474,475] Although still controversial, the "yeast syndrome" further supports the hypothesis that intestinal organisms can cause or exacerbate systemic or local disease.

The distinction between what is and what is not a pathogen becomes increasingly muddled when one looks at organisms that are clearly not indigenous. Certain parasites, yeasts, and bacteria are traditionally associated with local and systemic consequences. Examples are pathogenic strains of salmonella, giardia, shigella, and campylobacter. However, it does not appear that what has been traditionally described as a pathogen always elicits the same response. Diverse pathogens have been termed weak or strong, and pathogenicity may be determined in part by host immunological competence.[476] An example is the protozoa *Blastocystis hominis*. Experts disagree sharply on its pathogenicity. In certain studies, it has been associated with colitis, diarrhea, and other gastrointestinal complaints.[477,478,479,480] Other studies show it to be equally present in asymptomatic and symptomatic individuals, suggesting that it may not always be pathogenic.[481] Weak pathogens may cause disease in some people some of the time. Host resistance and virulence factors are important. Weakly pathogenic strains of salmonella, giardia, and yeast may be other examples of this theme.[482]

Pathogens can take up colonization anywhere in the GI mucosa, and cell wall components of bacteria, yeasts, and protozoa can be absorbed, which may cause systemic symptoms that are difficult to pinpoint to the pathogen directly. Laboratory tests evaluating microbiology, parasites, and presence of serum antibodies to pathogens are often useful to verify unwanted microbial organisms in the GI tract and monitor response to treatment.

Thus, bacteria, yeasts, and parasites may cause symptoms locally as well as systemically. Food proteins, gut bacterial breakdown products, and environmental toxins can and do reach the systemic circulation. Therefore, removal of offending antigens becomes key to a gastrointestinal restoration program.

Replace

The second clinical step in the 4R program, "replace," replenishes enzymes and other digestive factors which may be lacking or limited. Enzymes that may at times need to be replaced include proteases, lipases, cellulases, and saccharidases, which are normally secreted by cells lining the intestine or directly by the pancreas. Other digestive factors that may require replenishment include hydrochloric acid, pepsin, and intrinsic factor, normally secreted by cells in the stomach wall, and bile, synthesized by hepatocytes.

A key ingredient in replacement therapies is hydrochloric acid. Low stomach acidity can result in a variety of symptoms and digestive problems. It is particularly common among individuals older than 60. Reduced hydrochloric acid may impair the absorption of nutrients such as B6, folic acid, calcium, and iron and may also predispose an individual to increased intestinal infections. As hydrochloric acid production depends on zinc, decreased levels may indicate a zinc deficiency as well.[483]

The small intestine acts as the principal site of digestion and absorption. As mentioned, intact proteins and other large molecules can cross the intestinal lining, even in healthy individuals, to a certain extent.[484,485] Therapies that involve digestive enzyme supplementation enhance the breakdown of these particles and therefore help to exclude them from crossing that barrier intact. A variety of health conditions, including eczema and steatorrhea, may be ameliorated by enzyme therapy. For example, studies have shown that the digestive enzyme lipase, critical in fat digestion, can be supplemented to relieve problems of fat malabsorption.[486,487,488] Similarly, many people suffer from undiagnosed lactose intolerance. The digestive enzyme, lactase, has also been used successfully in individuals with the inability to digest lactose.[489]

Food allergies are another area where digestive enzymes may be helpful. Food allergies can be caused by several factors, including the increased supply of intact, poorly digested protein fragments that leak across the gut wall into the systemic circulation. By increasing digestion of dietary protein, protease enzymes decrease the supply of intact proteins available to leak into the bloodstream. Digestive protease enzymes taken orally may also help to digest dietary proteins that are encountered in the bloodstream. Table 28.3 provides some general information on the indications and approaches to the use of HCl and digestive enzymes. Laboratory tests such as gastric analyses, fat absorption tests, and stool analyses may be useful tools to verify the need to replace enzymes and other digestive factors.

Table 28.3 **Using Digestive Enzymes and Hydrochloric Acid**

Possible Symptoms of Low Stomach Acid	Taking HCl Supplements	Using Digestive Enzymes
• Bloating, belching, burning and flatulence immediately after meals • Dilated blood vessels in the nose or cheeks (Rosacea) • Excess gas in the upper intestine • Indigestion, diarrhea or constipation • Iron deficiency • Multiple food allergies • Nausea after taking supplements • Peeling or cracking fingernails • Rectal itching • Sense of "fullness" after eating • Undigested food in the stool	• Find supplements with at least 600 mg of betaine HCl per tablet or capsule. • Start with one right at the beginning of a meal or immediately after beginning to eat. • At every meal after that, use one more pill. • Continue until 5 tablets/capsules are consumed with each meal, or until warmth occurs in the stomach, whichever occurs first. • The warm feeling indicates too many were consumed, so cut back by one pill at the next meal. • Smaller meals need fewer pills, larger meals more. • Those who need 5 or so capsules should spread them throughout the meal. • After a while, and after repairing the digestive system, patients may produce their own HCl and need fewer capsules. The "warmth" will be present with fewer capsules. Just cut down the dose at that point.	Effective enzymes are available from both animal and plant sources; some are also available by prescription. Use 2–3 just before or at the beginning of a meal. They are generally well tolerated and without side effects. Look for a formula containing at least: • Protease 100,000 USP units • Lipase 20,000 USP units • Amylase 100,000 USP units Vegetarians can take a mixed plant-based form of digestive enzymes. Use 2–3 just before or at the beginning of a meal. Some of these are grown from Aspergillus fungus, so be careful if the patient has mold or yeast sensitivities. Others are derived from pineapple (bromelain) and papaya. Look for a formula with about 500 mg of enzymes per tablet or capsule and containing: • Amylase 100,000 USP units • Protease 100,000 USP units • Lipase 10,000 USP units • Lactase 1600 Lace Digestive bitters may also be tried. Swedish bitters or other aperitifs stimulate digestive function. Herbal bitters including gentian (most common) and artichoke, cardamom, fennel, ginger, and dandelion are also available in more concentrated forms that can be added to water.

Reinoculate

"Reinoculate" is the third step in the 4R gastrointestinal support program. Reinoculate refers to the reintroduction of desirable bacteria, or "probiotics," into the intestine to reestablish microfloral balance. Bacterial balance in the intestine is critical for proper intestinal permeability. Over 400 different species of microorganisms reside in the human GI tract, and the overall balance of these organisms can profoundly influence gut ecology and health.

Probiotics serve a variety of functions in the gastrointestinal tract. Perhaps the most important function of probiotics is antagonistic activity toward pathogens, which they perform in a variety of complementary ways. First, probiotics assist in colonization resistance—the ability of normal flora to protect against the unwanted establishment of pathogens. Second, probiotics may produce various antimicrobial substances. For instance, *Lactobacillus casei* GG has been shown to produce substances inhibitory toward a broad spectrum of gram-positive and gram-negative pathogens.[490] Competition for nutrients is a third mechanism. By competing for available nutrient substrate, beneficial bacteria can inhibit the growth of other less favorable flora. Competitive inhibition for bacterial adhesion sites is a fourth mechanism of probiotics. For instance, *Lactobacillus acidophilus* inhibits the adhesion of several enteric pathogens to human intestinal cells.[491] A final mechanism involves systemic host response. For instance, *L. casei* GG, administered orally to subjects with Crohn's disease, promoted a sIgA response.[492] These varied actions may decrease the likelihood that pathogens will develop resistance against probiotic agents. Thus, probiotics may be viewed as a vehicle to neutralize or inhibit pathogen activities, or increase or stimulate host immune stimulant activities to the intestinal tract, or both.[493]

A variety of supplemental sources may be considered helpful in reinoculation. These include cultured and fermented foods containing live bacteria, refrigerated liquid supplements containing live bacteria, or freeze-dried bacteria packaged in powder, tablet, or capsule form. Frequently supplemented species include *Lactobacillus acidophilus, Lactobacillus bulgaricus, Lactobacillus thermophilus, Lactobacillus sporogenes, Lactobacillus casei GG, Lactobacillus NCFM, Saccharomyces boulardii, Bifidobacterium bifidus, Bifidobacterium longum*, and *Bifidobacterium breve*.

In addition to directly reintroducing bacteria, the reinoculate step may also involve indirectly bolstering the healthy microflora with prebiotics, which selectively promote beneficial synergistic flora without simultaneously supporting pathogenic bacterial growth. When prebiotics are included in the diet, increased levels of fecal fermentation and intraluminal concentrations of short-chain fatty acids (SCFAs), such as propionate, acetate, and butyrate, are produced from fermentation of the fibers by the colonic microflora. SCFAs are thought to supply up to 70% of the energy used by colonic epithelial cells; therefore, prebiotics support improved intestinal integrity and promote intestinal mucosal cell regeneration.[494] Prebiotics include fructans, inulin and fructooligosaccharides, arabinogalactans, and some soy fibers.[495,496,497,498] The incorporation of soluble fiber, another important nutrient substrate for probiotics, may also help in the reinoculation process.

Repair

The fourth and final step in a 4R approach is "repair." Repair refers to providing nutritional support for regeneration and healing of the gastrointestinal mucosa. Part of the support for healing comes from removing insults that continually re-injure or irritate the mucosa, and from promoting healthy microflora. The repair phase of GI restoration benefits from all of the clinical approaches discussed so far.

The GI mucosal cells represent the largest mass (in normal individuals) of rapidly proliferating cells. Repair is necessary whenever there has been a loss of integrity of the GI mucosal structure, function, or both. This loss may be the result of chronic nutritional insufficiency, food allergen and xenobiotic exposure, dysbiosis, pathological intestinal infection, chronic inflammation as in ulcerative colitis, or other less common GI diseases. Assessment of individual need may include a dietary history, nutritional analysis, and any other investigative techniques that reveal the presence of dysfunction, disease, or nutritional insufficiencies.

Once the need for repair has been determined, remediation of any process that resulted in intestinal damage must be done first; second, direct nutritional support of the intestinal cells should be provided through foods or supplements critical to intestinal wall structure and function. Nutrients that play pivotal roles in GI mucosal cell differentiation, growth, functioning, and repair include glutamine, essential fatty acids, zinc, and pantothenic acid. For instance, dietary deficiency of glutamine is associated with atrophy and degenerative changes in the small intestine following intestinal injury, infection, stress, surgery, and radiation.[499,500,501] Fish oils, which contain eicosapentaenoic acid and docosahexaenoic acid, have also been shown to ameliorate mucosal injury and attenuate inflammatory conditions of the gut in animal studies.[502,503,504,505] Research has shown that supplementation with pantothenic acid is important to support the normal healing process.[506] It has also been found that pantothenic acid is concentrated in gut mucosa and may be important for stimulating the regeneration of the gastrointestinal mucosa in individuals who have chronic ulcerative or granulomatous colitis.[507] Many individuals with inflammatory bowel disease have zinc deficiencies.[508,509,510,511]

Summary

The Remove, Replace, Reinoculate, Repair clinical approach is a conceptual program, meant to outline the points to consider when clinically evaluating and applying therapies to a patient with underlying GI dysfunction. While this overall concept describes a basic approach, its use is individualized to the needs of each patient, based on his or her unique clinical condition and nutrient needs. The different steps in this gut restoration program can be applied together, in a unified therapy, or sequentially, beginning with *Remove*. When considered together, the steps of the 4R gastrointestinal support program may address a variety of clinical conditions. Proper assessment of gastrointestinal function and intervention in areas of dysfunction, imbalance, or impairment may have profound effects at the local as well as systemic level.

References

1. Lacy B, Lee R. Irritable bowel syndrome: a syndrome in evolution. J Clin Gastroenterology. 2005;39(5) Supplement 3:S230-42.
2. Mulak A, Bonza B. Irritable bowel syndrome: a model of the brain-gut interactions. Med Sci Monit. 2004;10(4):RA55-62.
3. De Giorgio R, Guerrini S, Barbara G, et al. Inflammatory neuropathies of the enteric nervous system. Gastroenterology. 2004;126(7):1872-73.
4. Gershon M. The Second Brain. Harper Collins, 1998.
5. Stipanuk MH. Biochemical and Physiological Aspects of Human Nutrition. WB Saunders Co: Philadelphia, 2000.
6. De Giorgio R, Guerrini S, Barbara G, et al. New insights into human enteric neuropathies. Neurogastroenterol Motil. 2004;16(Suppl 1):143-47.
7. Levin RJ. Digestion and absorption of carbohydrates—from molecules and membranes to humans. Am J Clin Nutr. 1994;59(3 Suppl):690S-98S.
8. Raul F. Lacroix B, Aprahamian M. Longitudinal distribution of brush border hydrolases and morphological maturation in the intestine of the preterm infant. Early Hum Dev. 1986;13(2):225-34.
9. Lester R, Smallwood RA, Little JM, et al. Fetal bile salt metabolism. The intestinal absorption of bile salt. J Clin Invest. 1977;59(6):1009-16.
10. Galluser M, Raul F, Canguilhem B. Adaptation of intestinal enzymes to seasonal and dietary changes in a hibernator: The European hamster (Cricetus cricetus). J Comp Physiol [B]. 1988;158(2):143-49.
11. Raul F, Goda T, Gosse F, Koldovsky O. Short-term effect of a high-protein/low-carbohydrate diet on aminopeptidase in adult rat jejunoileum. Site of aminopeptidase response. Biochem J. 1987;247(2):401-5.
12. Raul F, Gosse F, Doffoel M, et al. Age related increase of brush border enzyme activities along the small intestine. Gut. 1988;29(11):1557-63.
13. Acheson DW, Luccioli S. Microbial-gut interactions in health and disease. Mucosal immune responses. Best Pract Res Clin Gastroenterol. 2004;18(2):387-404.
14. Madara JL, Nash S, Parkos C. Neutrophil-epithelial cell interactions in the intestine. Adv Exp Med Biol. 1991;314:329-34.
15. Constant SL, Bottomly K. Induction of Th1 and Th2 CD4+ T cell responses: the alternative approaches. Annu Rev Immunol. 2997;15:297-322.
16. Hurwitz A, et al. Gastric acidity in older adults. JAMA. 1997;278 (8):659-62.
17. Kagan RS. Food allergy: an overview. Environ Health Perspect. 2003;111(2):223-25.
18. Hunter JO. Food allergy—or enterometabolic disorder? Lancet. 1991;338:495-96.
19. Federico MJ, Liu AH. Overcoming childhood asthma disparities of the inner-city poor. Pedatr Clin North Am. 2003;50(3):655-75, vii.
20. Nakamura Y, Hoshino M. TH2 cytokines and associated transcription factors as therapeutic targets in asthma. Curr Drug Targets Inflamm Allergy. 2005:4(2):267-70.
21. Isolauri E, Huurre A, Salminen S, Impivaara O. The allergy epidemic extends beyond the past few decades. Clin Exp Allergy. 2004;34(7):1007-10.
22. Maziak W. The asthma epidemic and our artificial habitats. BMC Pulmonary Medicine. 2005;5:5.
23. Halken S. What causes allergy and asthma? The role of dietary factors. Pediatr Pulmonol Suppl. 2004;26:223-24.
24. Roberts G, Lack G. Food allergy and asthma—what is the link? Paediatr Respir Rev. 2003;4(3):205-12.
25. Chen R, Hu Z, Seaton A. Eating more vegetables might explain reduced asthma symptoms. BMJ. 2004;328:1380.
26. Oddy WH, de Klerk NH, Kendall GE, et al. Ratio of omega-6 to omega-3 fatty acids and childhood asthma. J Asthma. 2004;41(3):319-26.
27. Peat JK, Mihrshahi S, Kemp AS, et al. Three-year outcomes of dietary fatty acid modification and house dust mite reduction in the Childhood Asthma Prevention Study. J Allergy Clin Immunology. 2004;114(4):807-13.
28. Surette ME, Koumenis IL, Edens MB, et al. Inhibition of leukotriene biosynthesis by a novel dietary fatty acid formulation in patients with atopic asthma: a randomized, placebo-controlled, parallel-group, prospective trial. Clin Ther. 2003;25(3):972-79.

29. Businco L, Meglio P, Amato G, et al. Evaluation of the efficacy of oral cromolyn sodium or an oligoantigenic diet in children with atopic dermatitis: a multicenter study of 1085 patients. J Investig Allergol Clin Immunol. 1996;6(2):103-9.
30. Fiocchi A, Bouygue GR, Martelli A, et al. Dietary treatment of childhood atopic eczema/dermatitis syndrome (AEDS). Allergy. 2004;59 Suppl 78:78-85.
31. Johnston GA, Bilbao RM, Graham-Brown RA. The use of dietary manipulation by parents of children with atopic dermatitis. Br J Dermatol. 2004;150(6):1186-89.
32. Niggemann B. Role of oral food challenges in the diagnostic work-up of food allergy in atopic eczema dermatitis syndrome. Allergy. 2004;59 (Suppl 78):32-34.
33. Saevik BK, Bergvall K, Holm BR, et al. A randomized, controlled study to evaluate the steroid sparing effect of essential fatty acid supplementation in the treatment of canine atopic dermatitis. Vet Dermatol. 2004;15(3):137-45.
34. Van Gool CJ, Zeegers MP, Thijs C. Oral essential fatty acid supplementation in atopic dermatitis—a meta-analysis of placebo-controlled trials. Br J Dermatol. 2004;150(4):728-40.
35. Egger J, Carter CM, Wilson J, et al. Is migraine food allergy? A double-blind controlled trial of oligoantigenic diet treatment. Lancet. 1983;2:865-69.
36. Carter CM, Egger J, Soothill JF. A dietary management of severe childhood migraine. Hum Nutr Appl Nutr. 1985;39(4):294-303.
37. Egger J, Carter CM, Soothill JF, Wilson J. Oligoantigenic diet treatment of children with epilepsy and migraine. J Pediatr. 1989;114(1):51-58.
38. Egger J, Carter CH, Soothill JF, Wilson J. Effect of diet treatment on enuresis in children with migraine or hyperkinetic behavior. Clin Pediatr (Phila). 1992;31(5):302-7.
39. Hadjivassiliou M, Davies-Jones GAB, Sanders DS, Grunewald RA. Dietary treatment of gluten ataxia. J Neurol Neurosurg Psychiatry. 2003;74:1221-24.
40. Hadjivassiliou M, Grunewald R, Sharrack B, et al. Gluten ataxia in perspective: epidemiology, genetic susceptibility and clinical characteristics. Brain. 2003;126:685-91.
41. Hadjivassiliou M, Williamson CA, Woodroofe N. The immunology of gluten sensitivity: beyond the gut. Trends Immunol. 2004;25(11):578-82.
42. Hadjivassiliou M, Sanders DS, Grunewald RA. Multiple sclerosis and occult gluten sensitivity. Neurology. 2005;64(5):933-34.
43. Hadjivassiliou M, Grunewald RA, Lawden M, et al. Headache and CNS white matter abnormalities associated with gluten sensitivity. Neurology. 2001;56(3):385-88.
44. Hadjivassiliou M, Williamson CA, Woodroofe N. The immunology of gluten sensitivity: beyond the gut. Trends Immunol. 2004;25(11):578-82.
45. Hadjivassiliou M, Sanders DS, Grunewald RA, Akil M. Gluten sensitivity masquerading as systemic lupus erythematosus. Ann Rheum Dis. 2004;63(11):1501-3.
46. Morinville V, Bernard C, Forget S. Foveolar hyperplasia secondary to cow's milk protein hypersensitivity presenting with clinical features of pyloric stenosis. J Pediatr Surg. 2004;39(1):E29-31.
47. Motrich RD, Gottero C, Rezzonico C, et al. Cow's milk stimulated lymphocyte proliferation and TNF-alpha secretion in hypersensitivity to cow's milk protein. Clin Immunol. 2003;109(2):203-11.
48. Pohjavuori E, Viljanen M, Korpela R. Lactobacillus GG effect in increasing IFN-gamma production in infants with cow's milk allergy. J Allergy Clin Immunol. 2004;114(1):131-36.
49. De Giorgio R, Guerrini S, Barbara G, et al. Inflammatory neuropathies of the enteric nervous system. Gastroenterology. 2004;126(7):1872-73.
50. McGonagle D, Gibbon W, Emery P. Classification of inflammatory arthritis by enthesitis. Lancet. 1998;352:1137-40.
51. Hadjivassiliou M, Williamson CA, Woodroofe N. The immunology of gluten sensitivity: beyond the gut. Trends Immunol. 2004;25(11):578-82.
52. Plotkin MJ. Tales of a Shaman's Apprentice. 1st Ed. Penguin Group: New York, 1993.
53. Gaspani L, Limiroli E, Ferrario P, Bianchi M. *In vivo* and *in vitro* effects of bromelain on PGE(2) and SP concentrations in the inflammatory exudates in rats. Pharmacology. 2002;65(2):83-86.
54. Hale LP, Greer PK, Sempowski GD. Bromelain treatment alters leukocyte expression of cell surface molecules involved in cellular adhesion and activation. Clin Immunol. 2002;104(2):183-90.
55. Monograph: Bromelain. Altern Med Rev. 1998;3(4):302-05.
56. Ishimaru K, Mitsuoka H, Unno N, et al. Pancreatic proteases and inflammatory mediators in peritoneal fluid during splanchnic arterial occlusion and reperfusion. Shock. 2004;22(5):467-71.
57. de la Mano AM, Sevillano S, Manso MA, et al. Cholecystokinin blockade alters the systemic immune response in rats with acute pancreatitis. Int J Exp Pathol. 2004;85(2):75-84.
58. Zhang F, Altorki NK, Mestre JR, et al. Curcumin inhibits cyclooxygenase-2 transcription in bile acid- and phorbol ester-treated human gastrointestinal epithelial cells. Carcinogenesis. 1999;20(3):445-51.
59. Yin X, Zhou J, Jie C, et al. Anticancer activity and mechanism of Scutellaria barbata extract on human lung cancer cell line A549. Life Sci. 2004;75(18):2233-44.
60. Chen X, Yang L, Zhang N, et al. Shikonin, a component of Chinese herbal medicine, inhibits chemokine receptor function and suppresses human immunodeficiency virus type 1. Antimicrob Agents Chemother. 2003;47(9):2810-16.
61. Shimizu T, Sano C, Akaki T, et al. [Effects of the Chinese traditional medicines "mao-bushi-saishin-to" and "yokuinin" on the antimycobacterial activity of murine macrophages against Mycobacterium avium complex infection.] Kekkaku. 1999;74(9):661-66.
62. Sandoval-Chacon M, Thompson JH, Zhang XJ, et al. Antiinflammatory actions of cat's claw: the role of NF-kappaB. Aliment Pharmacol Ther. 1998;12(12):1279-89.
63. Wallace JM. Nutritional and botanical modulation of the inflammatory cascade—eicosanoids, cyclooxygenases, and lipoxygenases—as an adjunct in cancer therapy. Integr Cancer Ther. 2002;1(1):7-37.
64. Aktas O, Prozorovski T, Smorodchenko A, et al. Green tea epigallocatechin-3-gallate mediates T cellular NF-kappa B inhibition and exerts neuroprotection in autoimmune encephalomyelitis. J Immunol. 2004;173(9):5794-800.
65. Hussain T, Gupta S, Adhami VM, Mukhtar H. Green tea constituent epigallocatechin-3-gallate selectively inhibits COX-2 without affecting COX-1 expression in human prostate carcinoma cells. Int J Cancer. 2005;113(4):660-69.
66. Ichikawa D, Matsui A, Imai M, et al. Effect of various catechins on the IL-12p40 production by murine peritoneal macrophages and a macrophage cell line, J774.1. Biol Pharm Bull. 2004;27(9):1353-58.
67. Kim DJ, Shin DH, Ahn B, et al. Chemoprevention of colon cancer by Korean food plant components. Mutat Res. 2003;523-524:99-107.
68. Greenwald P, Kelloff GJ, Boone CW, McDonald SS. Genetic and cellular changes in colorectal cancer: proposed targets of chemopreventive agents. Cancer Epidemiol Biomarkers Prev. 1995;4(7):691-702.
69. Constant SL, Bottomly K. Induction of Th1 and Th2 CD4+ T cell responses: the alternative approaches. Annu Rev Immunol. 1997;15:297-322.

70. Deters AM, Schroder KR, Hensel A. Kiwi fruit (Actinidia chinensis L.) polysaccharides exert stimulating effects on cell proliferation via enhanced growth factor receptors, energy production, and collagen synthesis of human keratinocytes, fibroblasts, and skin equivalents. J Cell Physiol. 2005;202(3):717-22.
71. Robinson R, Causey J, Slavin JL. Nutritional benefits of larch arabinogalactan. In: Advanced Dietary Fibre Technology, Eds. McCleary BV, Proskey L. Blackwell Science Ltd: 2001.
72. McGinnis WR. Oxidative stress in autism. Alt Ther. 2004;10(6):22-36.
73. Davidovic M, Trailov D, Milosevic D, et al. Magnesium, aging, and the elderly patient. Scientific World Journal. 2004;4:544-50.
74. Stipanuk MH. Biochemical and Physiological Aspects of Human Nutrition. WB Saunders Co: Philadelphia, 2000.
75. Dorup I, Skajaa K, Clausen T, Kjeldsen K. Reduced concentrations of potassium, magnesium, and sodium-potassium pumps in human skeletal muscle during treatment with diuretics. Br Med J (Clin Res Ed). 1988;296:455-58.
76. Clausen T. Clinical and therapeutic significance of the Na+, K+ pump*. Clin Sci (Lond). 1998;95(1):3-17.
77. Ibid.
78. De Giorgio R, Guerrini S, Barbara G, et al. Inflammatory neuropathies of the enteric nervous system. Gastroenterology. 2004;126(7):1872-73.
79. Saavedra JM, Tschernia A. Human studies with probiotics and prebiotics: clinical implications. Br J Nutr. 2002;87(Suppl 2):S241-46.
80. Brandtzaeg PE. Current understanding of gastrointestinal immunoregulation and its relation to food allergy. Ann N Y Acad Sci. 2002;964:13-45.
81. Constant SL, Bottomly K. Induction of Th1 and Th2 CD4+ T cell responses: the alternative approaches. Annu Rev Immunol. 1997;15:297-322.
82. McGonagle D, Gibbon W, Emery P. Classification of inflammatory arthritis by enthesitis. Lancet. 1998;352:1137-40.
83. Stavney LS, Hamilton T, Sircus W. Evaluation of the pH-sensitive telemetry capsule in the estimation of gastric secretory capacity. Am J Dig Dis. 1966;11:10.
84. Hardt PD, Hauenschild A, Jaeger C, et al. High prevalence of steatorrhea in 101 diabetic patients likely to suffer from exocrine pancreatic insufficiency according to low fecal elastase 1 concentrations: a prospective multicenter study. Dig Dis Sci. 2003;48(9):1688-92.
85. Cahill M. Handbook of Diagnostic Tests. Springhouse PA, Springhouse Corp 1995.
86. Pagaua KD. Mosby's Manual of Diagnostic and Laboratory Tests, St. Louis: Mosby Inc. 1998.
87. Hardt PD, Krauss A, Bretz L, et al. Pancreatic exocrine function in patients with type 1 and type 2 diabetes mellitus. Acta Diabetol. 2000;37(3):105-10.
88. Dominguez-Munoz JE, Hieronymus C, Sauerbruch T, Malfertheiner P. Fecal elastase test: evaluation of a new noninvasive pancreatic function test. Am J Gastroenterol. 1995;90(10):1834-37.
89. Richter ML, Wagner T. [Pancreatic exocrine insufficiency in patients with diabetes mellitus. Current state of our knowledge and practical consequences.] Fortschr Med Orig. 2001;119(Suppl 2):77-79.
90. Molinari I, Souare K, Lamireau T, et al. Fecal chymotrypsin and elastase-1 determination on one single stool collected at random: diagnostic value for exocrine pancreatic status. Clin Biochem. 2004;37(9):758-63.
91. Chin J. Prospects for beneficial health outcomes from intestinal microflora. Asia Pac J Clin Nutr. 2005;14(Suppl):S64-65.
92. Guarner F. Inulin and oligofructose: impact on intestinal disease and disorders. Br J Nutr. 2005;93(Suppl 1):S61-65.
93. Probiotics and prebiotics: A brief overview. J Ren Nutr. 2002;12(2):76-86.
94. von Wright A, Salminen S. Probiotics: established effects and open questions. Eur J Gastroenterol Heptaol. 1999;11(11):1195-98.
95. Chow J. Probiotics and prebiotics: A brief overview. J Ren Nutr. 2002;12(2):76-86.
96. Rastall RA, Maitin V. Prebiotics and synbiotics: towards the next generation. Curr Opinion Biotechnol. 2002;13(5):490-96.
97. Lund B, Adamsson I, Edlund C. Gastrointestinal transit survival of an Enterococcus faecium probiotic strain administered with or without vancomycin. Int J Food Microbiol. 2002;77(1-2):109-15.
98. Peterson CG, Eklund E, Taha Y, et al. A new method for the quantification of neutrophil and eosinophil cationic proteins in feces: establishment of normal levels and clinical application in patients with inflammatory bowel disease. Am J Gastroenterol. 2002;97(7):1755-62.
99. Saitoh O, Kojima K, Sugi K, et al. Fecal eosinophil granule-derived proteins reflect disease activity in inflammatory bowel disease. Am J Gastroenterology. 1999;94(12):13-20.
100. Bischoff SC, Grabowsky J, Manus MP. Quantification of inflammatory mediators in stool samples of patients with inflammatory bowel disorders and controls. Dig Dis Sci. 1997;42(2):394-403.
101. Del Pozo V, Arrieta I, Tunon T, et al. Immunopathogenesis of human gastrointestinal infection by Anisakis simplex. J Allergy Clin Immunol. 1999;104(3 Pt 1):637-43.
102. Pucci N, Novembre E, Cammarata MG, et al. Scoring atopic dermatitis in infants and young children: distinctive features of the SCORAD index. Allergy. 2005;60(1):113-16.
103. Bischoff SC, Mayer J, Nguyen QT, et al. Immunohistological assessment of intestinal eosinophil activation in patients with eosinophilic gastroenteritis and inflammatory bowel disease. Am J Gastroenterol. 1999;94(12):3521-29.
104. Silberer H, Kuppers B, Mickisch O, et al. Fecal leukocyte proteins in inflammatory bowel disease and irritable bowel syndrome. Clin Lab. 2005;51(3-4):117-26.
105. Tibble J, Teahon K, Thjodleifsson B, et al. A simple method for assessing intestinal inflammation in Crohn's disease. Gut. 2000;47(4):506-13.
106. Tibble JA, Sigthorsson G, Bridger S, et al. Surrogate markers of intestinal inflammation are predictive of relapse in patients with inflammatory bowel disease. Gastroenterology. 2000;119(1):15-22.
107. Tepper RE, Simon D, Brandt LJ, et al. Intestinal permeability in patients infected with the human immunodeficiency virus. Am J Gastroenterol. 1994;89(6):878-82.
108. Mack, Flick JA, Durie PR, et al. Correlation of intestinal lactulose permeability with exocrine pancreatic dysfunction. J Pediatr. 1992;120(95):696-701.
109. Lahesmaa-Rantala R, Magnusson KE, Granfors K, et al. Intestinal permeability in patients with yersinia triggered reactive arthritis. Ann Rheum Dis. 1991;50(2):91-94.
110. Jenkins AP, Trew DR, Crump BJ, et al. Do non-steroidal anti-inflammatory drugs increase colonic permeability? Gut. 1991;32(1):66-69.
111. Lunn PG, Northrop-Clewes CA, Downes RM. Intestinal permeability, mucosal injury, and growth faltering in Gambian infants. Lancet. 1991;338(8772):907-10.
112. Buhner S, Reese I, Kuehl F, et al. Pseudoallergic reactions in chronic urticaria are associated with altered gastroduodenal permeability. Allergy. 2004;59(10):1118-23.
113. eMedicine Esophagogastroduodenoscopy. http://www.emedicine.com/med/topic2965.htm
114. eMedicine Colonoscopy. http://www.emedicine.com/med/topic2966.htm
115. Mulak A, Bonza B. Irritable bowel syndrome: a model of the brain-gut interactions. Med Sci Monit. 2004;10(4):RA55-62.

116. Brandtzaeg P. Current understanding of gastrointestinal immunoregulation and its relation to food allergy. Ann N Y Acad Sci. 2002;964:13-45.
117. Jarrett LS. Nourishing Destiny: The Inner Tradition of Chinese Medicine. Spirit Path Press. 1999. p 327.
118. Gershon MD. The Second Brain: A Groundbreaking New Understanding of Nervous Disorders of the Stomach and Intestine. Harper Collins, NY, 1998.
119. Sansonetti PJ. War and peace at the mucosal surface. Nat Rev Immunol. 2004;4:953-64.
120. Angulo P. Nonalcoholic fatty liver disease. N Engl J Med. 2002;346:1221-31.
121. McGarr SE, Ridlon JM, Hylemon PB. Diet, anaerobic bacterial metabolism, and colon cancer: a review of the literature. J Clin Gastroenterol. 2005;39:98-109.
122. Brandtzaeg P. Current understanding of gastrointestinal immunoregulation and its relation to food allergy. Ann N Y Acad Sci. 2002;964:13-45.
123. Rook GAW, Adams G, Hunt J, et al. Mycobacteria and other environmental organisms as immunomodulators for immunoregulatory disorders. Springer Semin Immunol 2004. 25:237-55.
124. Ashwood P, Anthony A, Pellicer AA, et al. Intestinal lymphocyte populations in children with regressive autism: evidence for extensive mucosal immunopathology. J Clin Immunol. 2003;23:504-17.
125. Cordain L, Eaton SB, Sebastian A, et al. Origins and evolution of the Western diet: health implications for the 21st century. Am J Clin Nutr. 2005;81:341-54.
126. Svoboda R, Lade A. *Tao and Dharma*. Lotus Press. Twin Lakes, WI. 1988. p.75.
127. Cordain L, Eaton SB, Sebastian A, et al. Origins and evolution of the Western diet: health implications for the 21st century. Am J Clin Nutr. 2005;81:341-54.
128. Guarner F, Magdelena JR. Gut flora in health and disease. Lancet. 2003;361:512-19.
129. Drossman DA, Camilleri M, Whitehead WE. American Gastroenterological Association technical review on irritable bowel syndrome. Gastroenterology. 1997;112:2137-2149.
130. Shanahan F. Host-Flora interactions in inflammatory bowel disease. Inflamm Bowel Dis. 2004; 10(1):S16-S24.
131. Thompson WG, Longstreth GF, Drossman DA, et al. Functional bowel disorders and functional abdominal pain. Gut. 2000;45(Suppl 2):43-47.
132. Swidsinski A, Ladhoff A, Pernthaler A, et al. Mucosal flora in inflammatory bowel disease. Gastroenterology. 2002;122:44-54.
133. Nobaek S, Johansson ML, Molin G, et al. Alteration of intestinal microflora is associated with reduction in abdominal bloating and pain in patients with irritable bowel syndrome. Am J Gastroenterol. 2000;95:1231-38.
134. Fooks LJ, Gibson GR. Probiotics as modulators of the gut flora. Br J Nutr. 2002;88(Suppl 1):S39-S49.
135. Pimentel M, Chow EJ, Lin HC. Eradication of small intestinal bacterial overgrowth reduces symptoms of irritable bowel syndrome. Am J Gastro. 2000; 95:3503-6.
136. Aaron LA, Burke MM, Buchwald D. Overlapping conditions among patients with chronic fatigue syndrome, fibromyalgia, and temporomandibular disorder. Arch Intern Med. 2000;160:221-27.
137. Pimental M, Mayer AG, Park S, et al. Methane production during lactulose breath test is associated with gastrointestinal disease presentation. Dig Dis Sci. 2003;48:86-92.
138. Pimentel M, Chow EJ, Hallegua D, et al. Small intestinal bacterial overgrowth: A possible association with fibromyalgia. J Musculoskelet Pain. 2001;9:107-13.
139. Lin HC. Small intestinal bacterial overgrowth: a framework for understanding irritable bowel syndrome. JAMA. 2004;292:852-58.
140. Schrezenemeir J, deVrese M. Prebiotics, probiotics, and synbiotics—approaching a definition. Am J Clin Nutr. 2001;73:361S-64S.
141. Isolauri E, Sutas Y, Kankaanpaa, et al. Probiotics: effects on immunity. Am J Clin Nutr. 2001;73:444S-50S.
142. Gibson GR, Roberfroid MB. Dietary modulation of the human colonic microbiota: introducing the concept of prebiotics. J Nutr. 1995;125:1401-12.
143. Rastall RA, Maitlin V. Prebiotics and synbiotics: towards the next generation. Curr Opin Biotechnol. 2002;13:490-98.
144. Hoyos AB. Reduced incidence of necrotizing enterocolitis associated with enteral administration of *Lactobacillus acidophilus* and *Bifidobacterium infantis* to neonates in an intensive care unit. Int J Infect Dis. 1999;3:197-202.
145. McGarr SE, Ridlon JM, Hylemon PB. Diet, anaerobic bacterial metabolism, and colon cancer: a review of the literature. J Clin Gastroenterol. 2005;39:98-109.
146. Teitelbaum JE, Walker WA. Nutritional impact of pre-and probiotics as protective gastrointestinal organisms. Annu Rev Nutr. 2002;22:107-38.
147. Teitelbaum JE, Walker WA. Nutritional impact of pre-and probiotics as protective gastrointestinal organisms. Annu Rev Nutr. 2002;22:107-38.
148. Spiller R. Probiotics: an ideal anti-inflammatory treatment for IBS? Gastroenterology. 2005;128:783-85.
149. O'Mahony L, McCarthy J, Kelly P, et al. Lactobacillus and bifidobacterium in irritable bowel syndrome: symptom responses and relationship to cytokine profiles. Gastroenterology. 2005;128:541-51.
150. Sartor RB. Probiotic therapy for intestinal inflammation and infection. Curr Op Gastroenterol. 2005;21:44-50.
151. Macpherson AJ, Harris NL. Interactions between commensal intestinal bacteria and the immune system. Nat Rev Immunol. 2004;4:478-85.
152. Kalliomaki M, Salminen S, Avrilommi H, et al. Probiotics in primary prevention of atopic disease: a randomized placebo-controlled trial. Lancet. 2001;357:1076-79.
153. Kalliomaki M, Salminen S, Poussa T, et al. Probiotics and prevention of atopic disease: 4-year follow-up of a randomised placebo-controlled trial. Lancet. 2003;361:1869-71.
154. Isolauri E, Kirjavainen PV, Salminen S. Probiotics: a role in the treatment of intestinal infection and inflammation? Gut. 2002;50(S3):III54-59.
155. Rosenfeldt V, Benfeldt E, Valerius NH, et al. Effect of probiotics on gastrointestinal symptoms and small intestinal permeability in children with atopic dermatitis. J Pediatr. 2004;145:612-16.
156. Rook GAW, Brunet LR. Microbes, immuonregulation, and the gut. Gut. 2005;54:317-20.
157. Aderem A, Ulevitch RJ. Toll-like receptors in the induction of the innate immune response. Nature. 2000;406:782-787.
158. Mahida YR. Epithelial cell responses. Best Pract Res Clin Gastro. 2004;18:241-53.
159. Pessi T, Sutas Y, Saxelin M, et al. Antiproliferative effects of homogenates derived from five strains of candidate probiotic bacteria. Appl Environ Microbiol. 1999;65:475-78.
160. Baumgart DC, Dignass AU. Intestinal barrier function. Curr Opin Clin Nutr Metab Care. 2002;5:685-94.
161. Clayburgh DR, Shen L, Turner JR. A porous defense: the leaky epithelial barrier in intestinal disease. Lab Investig. 2004;84:282-91.
162. DeMeo MT, Mutlu EA, Keshavarzian A, Tobin MC. Intestinal permeation and gastrointestinal disease. J Clin Gastroenterol. 2002;34:385-96.
163. Baumgart DC, Dignass AU. Intestinal barrier function. Curr Op Clin Nutr Metab Care. 2002;5:685-694.
164. Wells CL, Hess DJ, Erlandsen SL. Impact of the indigenous flora in animal models of shock and sepsis. Shock. 2004;22:562-68.

165. Khanna A, Rossman JE, Fung HL, Caty MG. Intestinal and hemodynamic impairment following mesenteric ischemia/reperfusion. J Surg Res. 2001;99:114-19.
166. Fink MP. Intestinal epithelial hyperpermeability: update on the pathogenesis of gut mucosal barrier dysfunction in critical illness. Curr Opin Crit Care. 2003;9:143-51.
167. Bjarnason I, Peters TJ, Levi AJ. Intestinal permeability: clinical correlates. Dig Dis. 1986;4:83-92.
168. Wilson C, Rashid T, Tiwana H, et al. Cytotoxicity responses to peptide antigens in rheumatoid arthritis and ankylosing spondylitis. J Rheumatol. 2003;30:972-78.
169. Sahly H, Podschun R, Sass R, et al. Serum antibodies to Klebsiella capsular polysaccharides in ankylosing spondylitis. Arthritis Rheum. 1994;37:754-59.
170. Ebringer A, Khalafpour S, Wilson C. Rheumatoid arthritis and Proteus: a possible aetiological association. Rheumatol Int. 1989;9:223-28.
171. Cookson W. The immunogenetics of asthma and eczema: a new focus on the epithelium. Nat Rev Immunol. 2004;4:978-88.
172. Hijazi Z, Molla AM, Muawad WMRA, et al. Intestinal permeability is increased in bronchial asthma. Arch Dis Child. 2004;89:227-29.
173. Israeli E, Berenshtein E, Wengrower D, et al. Glutamine enhances the capability of rat colon to resist inflammatory damage. Dig Dis Sci. 2004;49:1705-12.
174. Salminen S, Bouley C, Boutron-Ruault MC, et al. Functional food science and gastrointestinal physiology and function. Br J Nutr. 1998;80:S147-S71.
175. Mayer L, Shao L. Therapeutic potential of oral tolerance. Nat Rev Immunol. 2004;4:407-19.
176. Fiocchi C. Inflammatory bowel disease: new insights into mechanisms of inflammation and increasingly customized approaches to diagnosis and therapy. Curr Opin Gastroenterol. 2004;20:309-10.
177. Lu L, Walker WA. Pathologic and physiologic interactions of bacteria with the gastrointestinal epithelium. Am J Clin Nutr. 2001;73:1124S-30S.
178. Strobel S, Mowat AM. Immune responses to dietary antigens: oral tolerance. Immunol Today. 1998;19:173-81.
179. Patriarcha G. Oral desensitization treatment in food allergy: clinical and immunological results. Aliment Pharmacol Ther. 2003;17:459-65.
180. McKown KM. Induction of immune tolerance to human type 1 collagen in patients with systemic sclerosis by oral administration of bovine type 1 collagen. Arthritis Rheum. 2000;43:1054-61.
181. Korotkova M, Telemo E, Yamashiro Y, et al. The ratio of n-6 to n-3 fatty acids in maternal diet influences the inducton of neonatal immunological tolerance to ovalbumin. Clin Exp Immunol. 2004;137:237-44.
182. Borruel N, Carol M, Casellas F, et al. Increased mucosal tumour necrosis factor alpha production in Crohn's disease can be downregulated ex vivo by probiotic bacteria. Gut. 2002;51:659-64.
183. Strober W, Kelsall B, Marth T. Oral tolerance. J Clin Immuno. 1998;18:1-30.
184. Shanahan F. Host-flora interactions in inflammatory bowel disease. Inflamm Bowel Dis. 2004;10(1):S16-S24.
185. Borody TJ, Warren EF, Leis S, et al. Treatment of ulcerative colitis using fecal bacteriotherapy. J Clin Gastroenterol. 2003;37:42-47.
186. Bradesi S, McRoberts JA, Anton PA, Mayer, EA. Inflammatory bowel disease and irritable bowel syndrome: separate or unified? Curr Opin Gastroenterol. 2003;9:336-42.
187. Rodriguez LAG, Ruigomez A, Wallander MA, et al. Detection of colorectal tumor and inflammatory bowel disease during follow-up of patients with initial diagnosis of irritable bowel syndrome. Scand J Gastroenterol. 2000;35:306-31.
188. Zeiger RS. Dietary aspects of food allergy prevention in infants and children. J Ped Gastro Nutr. 2000;30:S77-S86.
189. Kelly D, Coutts AGP. Early nutrition and the development of immune function in the neonate. Proc Nutr Soc. 2000;59:177-85.
190. Salminen S, Bouley C, Boutron-Ruault MC, et al. Functional food science and gastrointestinal physiology and function. Br J Nutr. 1998;80:S147-71.
191. Isolauri E, Sutas Y, Kankaanpaa P, et al. Probiotics: effects on immunity. Am J Clin Nutr. 2001;73:444S-50S.
192. Isolauri E, Rautava S, Kalliomaki M, et al. Role of probiotics in food hypersensitivity. Curr Op Aller Clin Immuno. 2002;2:263-71.
193. Brandtzaeg P. Current understanding of gastrointestinal immunoregulation and its relation to food allergy. Ann N Y Acad Sci. 2002;964:13-45.
194. Atkinson W, Sheldon TA, Shaath N, Whorwell PJ. Food elimination based upon IgG antibodies in irritable bowel syndrome: a randomized controlled trial. Gut. 2004;53:1459-64.
195. Isolauri E, Rautava S, Kalliomaki M. Food allergy in irritable bowel syndrome: new facts and old fallacies. Gut. 2004;53:1391-93.
196. Sutas Y, Hurme M, Isolauri E. Downregulation of antiCD3 antibody-induced IL-4 production by bovine caseins hydrolysed with Lactobacillus GG-derived enzymes. Scand J Immunol. 1996;43:687-89.
197. C DeSimone. Personal communication. March 12, 2005.
198. Gionchietti P, Rizello F, Helwig U, et al. Prophylaxis of pouchitis onset with probiotic therapy: a double blind placebo controlled trial. Gastroenterology. 2003;124:1202-9.
199. O'Mahony L, McCarthy J, Kelly P, et al. Lactobacillus and bifidobacterium in irritable bowel syndrome: symptom responses and relationship to cytokine profiles. Gastroenterology. 2005;128:541-51.
200. Kalliomaki M, Salminen S, Poussa T, et al. Probiotics and prevention of atopic disease: 4-year follow-up of a randomised placebo-controlled trial. Lancet. 2003;361:1869-71.
201. Sutas Y, Hurme M, Isolauri E. Downregulation of antiCD3 antibody-induced IL-4 production by bovine caseins hydrolysed with Lactobacillus GG-derived enzymes. Scand J Immunol. 1996;43:687-89.
202. Tannock GW. Molecular assessment of intestinal microflora. Am J Clin Nutr. 2001;73:410S-14S.
203. Tannock GW. The normal microflora: new concepts in health promotion. Microbiol Sci. 1988;5:4-8.
204. Bezkorovainy A. Probiotics: determinants of survival and growth in the gut. Am J Clin Nutr. 2001;73:399S-405S.
205. He F, Ouwehand AC, Isolauri E, et al. Differences in composition and mucosal adhesion of bifidobacteria isolated from healthy adults and healthy seniors. Curr Microbiol. 2001;43:351-54.
206. Isolauri E, Salminen S, Ouwehand AC. Probiotics. Best Prac Res Clin Gastro. 2004;18:299-313.
207. Reuter G. The Lactobacillus and Bifidobacterium microflora of the human intestine: composition and succession. Curr Issues Intest Microbiol. 2001;2:43-53.
208. Guarner F. The intestinal flora in inflammatory bowel disease: normal or abnormal? Curr Opin Gastroenterol. 2005;21:414-18.
209. Kleessen B, Kroesen AJ, Buhr HJ, Blauf M. Mucosal and invading bacteria in patients with inflammatory bowel disease compared with controls. Scand J Gastroenterol. 2002;37:1034-41.
210. Gionchetti P, Rizzello F, Venturi A, et al. Oral bacteriotherapy as maintenance treatment in patients with chronic pouchitis: a double-blind, placebo-controlled trial. Gastroenterol. 2000;119:305-309.
211. Mimura T, Rizzello F, Helwig U, et al. Once daily high dose probiotic therapy (VSL#3) for maintaining remission in recurrent or refractory pouchitis. Gut. 2004;53:108-14.

212. Kato K, Mizuno S, Umesaki Y, et al. Randomized placebo-controlled trial assessing the effect of bifidobacteria-fermented milk on active uncreative colitis. Aliment Pharmacol Ther. 2004;20:1133-41.
213. Kruis W, Frec P, Pokrotneiks J, et al. Maintaining remission of ulcerative colitis with the probiotic Escherichia coli Nissle 1917 is as effective as with standard mesalazine. Gut. 2004;53:1617-23.
214. Floch M. Use of diet and probiotic therapy in the irritable bowel syndrome: analysis of the literature. J Clin Gastro. 2005;39:S242-S46.
215. Niedzielin K, Kordecki H, Birkenfeld B. A controlled, double-blind, randomized study on the efficacy of Lactobacillus plantarum 299V in patients with irritable bowel syndrome. Eur J Gastroenterol Hepatol. 2001;13:1143-47.
216. Saggioro A. Probiotics in the treatment of irritable bowel syndrome. J Clin Gastroenterol. 2004;38:S104-S106.
217. Kim HJ, Camilleri M, McKinzie S, et al. A randomized controlled trial of probiotic. VLS#3, on gut transit and symptoms in diarrhoae-predominant irritable bowel syndrome. Aliment Pharmacol Ther. 2003;17:895-904.
218. Hatakka K, Savilahti E, Ponka A, et al. Effect of long term consumption of probiotic milk on infections in children attending day care centres: double blind, randomised trial. Br Med J. 2001;322:1327-29.
219. Vanderhoof JA, Whitney DB, Antonson DL, et al. Lactobacillus GG in the prevention of antibiotic-associated diarrhea in children. J Pediatr. 1999;135:564-68.
220. Van Niel CW, Feudtner C, Garrison MM, Christakis DA. Lactobacillus therapy for acute infectious diarrhea in children: a meta-analysis. Pediatrics. 2002;109:678-84.
221. Hatakka K, Savilahti E, Ponka A, et al. Effect of long term consumption of probiotic milk on infections in children attending day care centres: double blind, randomised trial. Br Med J. 2001;322:1327-29.
222. Cross HL. Immune-signalling by orally-delivered probiotic bacteria: effects on common mucosal immunoresponses and protection at distal mucosal sites. Int J Immunopathol Pharmacol. 2004;17:127-34.
223. Gill HS, Rutherfurd KJ, Cross ML, Gopal PK. Enhancement of immunity in the elderly by dietary supplementation with the probiotic *Bifidobacterium lactis* HN019. Am J Clin Nutr. 2001;74:833-39.
224. Cummings JH, Antoine JM, Azpiroz F, et al. PASSCLAIM—Gut health and immunity. Eur J Nutr. 2004;43(S2):118-73.
225. Aguirre M, Collins MD. Lactic acid bacteria and human clinical infection. J Appl Bacteriol. 1993;75:95-107.
226. Salminen MK, Rautelin H, Tynkkynen S, et al. Lactobacillus bacteremia, clinical significance, and patient outcome, with special focus on probiotic L. rhamnosus GG. Clin Infect Dis. 2004;38:62-69.
227. Salminen MK, Tynkkynen S, Rautelin H, et al. Lactobacillus bacteremia during a rapid increase in probiotic use of Lactobacillus rhamnosus GG in Finland. Clin Inf Dis. 2002;35:1155-60.
228. Gibson GR. Dietary modulation of the human gut microflora using prebiotics. Br J Nutr. 1998;80:S209-12.
229. Molis C, Flourie B, Ouarme F, et al. Digestion, excretion, and energy value of fructooligosaccharides in healthy humans. Am J Clin Nutr. 1996;64:324-28.
230. Bayliss WM, Starling EH. The movements and innervation of the small intestine. J Physiol. 1899;24:99-143.
231. Bayliss WM, Starling EH. The movements and innervation of the small intestine. J Physiol. 1900;26:125-38.
232. Bayliss WM, Starling EH. The movements and innervation of the large intestine. J Physiol. 1900;26:107-18.
233. Auerbach L. Über einen Plexus myentericus, einen bisher unbekannten ganglio-nervö sen Apparat im Darmkanal der Wirbeltiere. Vorlä ufige Mitteilung. E. Morgenstern, 1862.
234. Auerbach L. Fernere vorlaufige Mittielung über den Nervenapparat des Darmes. Arch Pathol Anat Physiol. 1864;30:457-60.
235. Meissner G. Über die Nerven der Darmwand. Z Ration Med. 1857;8.
236. Trendelenburg P. Physiologische und pharmakologische Versuche über die Dünndarm Peristaltick. Naunyn Schmiedebergs Arch Exp Pathol Pharmakol. 1917;81:55-129.
237. Langley JN. The Autonomic Nervous System, Part 1. Heffer, Cambridge, UK: W. Heffer, 1921.
238. Furness JB, Sanger GJ. Gastrointestinal neuropharmacology: identification of therapeutic targets. Curr Opin Pharmacol. 2002;2:609-11.
239. Gershon MD. Review article: serotonin receptors and transporters: roles in normal and abnormal gastrointestinal motility. Aliment Pharmacol Ther. 2004;20(suppl 7):3-14.
240. Gershon MD. Serotonin and its implication for the management of irritable bowel syndrome. Rev Gastroenterol Disord. 2003;3(suppl 2):25-34.
241. Gershon MD. Plasticity in serotonin control mechanisms in the gut. Curr Opin Pharmacol. 2003;3:600-7.
242. Gershon MD, Kirchgessner AL, Wade PR. Functional anatomy of the enteric nervous system. In: Johnson LR, Alpers DH, Jacobson ED., et al, eds. Physiology of the Gastrointestinal Tract, 3rd ed., vol. 1. New York: Raven Press, 1994:381-422.
243. Gershon MD, Rothman TP. Enteric glia. Glia. 1991;4:195-204.
244. Hanani M, Zamir O, Baluk P. Glial cells in the guinea pig myenteric plexus are dye coupled. Brain Res. 1989;497:245-49.
245. Gabella G. On the ultrastructure of the enteric nerve ganglia. Scand J Gastroenterol Suppl. 1982;71:15-25.
246. Bannerman PG, Mirsky R, Jessen KR. Analysis of enteric neurons, glia and their interactions using explant cultures of the myenteric plexus. Dev Neurosci. 1987;9:201-27.
247. Gershon MD, Kirchgessner AL, Wade PR. Functional anatomy of the enteric nervous system. In: Johnson LR, Alpers DH, Jacobson ED., et al, eds. Physiology of the Gastrointestinal Tract, 3rd ed., vol. 1. New York: Raven Press, 1994:381-422.
248. Furness JB, Costa M. The Enteric Nervous System. New York: Churchill Livingstone, 1987.
249. Furness JB, Sanger GJ. Gastrointestinal neuropharmacology: identification of therapeutic targets. Curr Opin Pharmacol. 2002;2:609-11.
250. Furness JB. Types of neurons in the enteric nervous system. J Auton Nerv Syst. 2000;81:87-96.
251. Thomas EA, Sjovall H, Bornstein JC. Computational model of the migrating motor complex of the small intestine. Am J Physiol Gastrointest Liver Physiol. 2004;286:G564-72.
252. Gershon MD. Review article: serotonin receptors and transporters: roles in normal and abnormal gastrointestinal motility. Aliment Pharmacol Ther. 2004;20(suppl 7):3-14.
253. Gershon MD. Serotonin and its implication for the management of irritable bowel syndrome. Rev Gastroenterol Disord. 2003;3(suppl 2):25-34.
254. Gershon MD. Plasticity in serotonin control mechanisms in the gut. Curr Opin Pharmacol. 2003;3:600-7.
255. Erspamer V. Über den 5-Hydroytryptamin-(Enteramin)Gehalt des Magen-Darmtraktes bei den Wirbelten. Naturwissenschaften. 1953;40:318-19.
256. Vialli M. Histology of the enterochromaffin cell system. In: Erspamer V, ed. Handbook of Experimental Pharmacology: 5-Hydroxytryptamine and Related Indolealkylamines, vol. 19. New York: Springer-Verlag, 1966:1-65.
257. Erspamer V. Occurrence of indolealkylamines in nature. In: Erspamer V, ed. Handbook of Experimental Pharmacology: 5-Hydroxytryptamine and Related Indolealkylamines, vol. 19. New York: Springer-Verlag, 1966:132-81.
258. Gershon MD. 5-HT (Serotonin) physiology and related drugs. Curr Opin Gastroenterol. 2000;16:113-20.

259. Wade PR, Tamir H, Kirchgessner AL, et al. Analysis of the role of 5-HT in the enteric nervous system using anti-idiotypic antibodies to 5-HT receptors. Am J Physiol. 1994;266:G403-16.
260. Walther DJ, Peter JU, Bashammakh S, et al. Synthesis of serotonin by a second tryptophan hydroxylase isoform. Science. 2003;299:76.
261. Ibid.
262. Coates MD, Mahoney CR, Linden DR, et al. Molecular defects in mucosal serotonin content and decreased serotonin reuptake transporter in ulcerative colitis and IBS. Gastroenterology. 2004;126:1657-64.
263. Wade PR, Westfall JA. Ultrastructure of enterochromaffin cells and associated neural and vascular elements in the mouse duodenum. Cell Tissue Res. 1985;241:557-63.
264. Gershon MD. Review article: serotonin receptors and transporters: roles in normal and abnormal gastrointestinal motility. Aliment Pharmacol Ther. 2004;20(suppl 7):3-14.
265. Gershon MD. Serotonin and its implication for the management of irritable bowel syndrome. Rev Gastroenterol Disord. 2003;3(suppl2):25-34.
266. Gershon MD. Plasticity in serotonin control mechanisms in the gut. Curr Opin Pharmacol. 2003;3:600-7.
267. Bertrand PP. Real-time detection of serotonin release from enterochromaffin cells of the guinea-pig ileum. Neurogastroenterol Motil. 2004;16:511-14.
268. Bearcroft CP, Perrett D, Farthing MJ. Postprandial plasma 5-hydroxytryptamine in diarrhoea predominant irritable bowel syndrome: a pilot study. Gut. 1998;42:42-46.
269. Grønstad KO, DeMagistris L, Dahlstrom A, et al. The effects of vagal nerve stimulation on endoluminal release of serotonin and substance P into the feline small intestine. Scand J Gastroenterol. 1985;20:163-69.
270. Fujimaya M, Okumiya K, Kuwahara A. Immunoelectron microscopic study of the luminal release of serotonin from rat enterochromaffin cells induced by high intraluminal pressure. Histochem Cell Biol. 1997;108:105-13.
271. Forsberg EJ, Miller RJ. Regulation of serotonin release from rabbit intestinal enterochromaffin cells. J Pharmacol Exp Ther. 1983;227:755-66.
272. Nilsson O, Ericson LE, Dahlstrom A, et al. Subcellular localization of serotonin immunoreactivity in rat enterochromaffin cells. Histochemistry. 1985;82:351-61.
273. Nilsson O, Ahlman H, Geffard M, et al. Bipolarity of duodenal enterochromaffin cells in the rat. Cell Tissue Res. 1987;248:49-54.
274. Racke K, Reimann A, Schworer H, et al. Regulation of 5-HT release from enterochromaffin cells. Behav Brain Res. 1996;73:83-87.
275. Feldberg W, Toh CC. Distribution of 5-hydroxytryptamine (serotonin, enteramine) in the wall of the digestive tract. J Physiol. 1953;119:352-62.
276. Wade PR, Westfall JA. Ultrastructure of enterochromaffin cells and associated neural and vascular elements in the mouse duodenum. Cell Tissue Res. 1985;241:557-63.
277. Gershon MD, Ross LL. Studies on the relationship of 5-hydroxytryptamine and the enterochromaffin cell to anaphylatic shock in mice. J Exp Med. 1962;115:367-82.
278. Iversen L. Neurotransmitter transporters: fruitful targets for CNS drug discovery. Mol Psychiatry. 2000;5:357-62.
279. Fuller RW, Wong DT. Serotonin uptake and serotonin uptake inhibition. Ann N Y Acad Sci. 1990;600:68-80.
280. Blakely RD, Berson HE, Fremeau RT, et al. Cloning and expression of a functional serotonin transporter from ratbrain. Nature. 1991;354:66-70.
281. Ramamoothy S, Bauman AL, Moore KR, et al. Antidepressant- and cocaine-sensitive human serotonin transporter: molecular cloning, expression, and chromosomal localization. Proc Natl Acad Sci U S A. 1993;90:2542-46.
282. Hoffman B, Mezey E, Brownstein M. Cloning of a serotonin transporter affected by antidepressants. Science. 1991;254:579-80.
283. Coates MD, Mahoney CR, Linden DR, et al. Molecular defects in mucosal serotonin content and decreased serotonin reuptake transporter in ulcerative colitis and IBS. Gastroenterology. 2004;126:1657-64.
284. Wade PR, Chen J, Jaffe B, et al. Localization and function of a 5-HT transporter in crypt epithelia of the gastrointestinal tract. J Neurosci. 1996;16:2352-64.
285. Chen J-X, Pan H, Rothman TP, et al. Guinea pig 5-HT transporter: cloning, expression, distribution and function in intestinal sensory reception. Am J Physiol. 1998;275:G433-48.
286. Chen JJ, Zhishan L, Pan H, et al. Maintenance of serotonin in the intestinal mucosa and ganglia of mice that lack the high affinity serotonin transporter (SERT): abnormal intestinal motility and the expression of cation transporters. J Neurosci. 2001;21:6348-61.
287. Gershon MD, Ross LL. Radioisotopic studies of the binding, exchange, and distribution of 5-hydroxytryptamine synthesized from its radioactive precursor. J Physiol. 1966;186:451-76.
288. Gershon MD, Sherman DL, Pintar JE. Type-specific localization of monoamine oxidase in the enteric nervous system: relationship to 5-hydroxytryptamine, neuropeptides, and sympathetic nerves. J Comp Neurol. 1990;301:191-213.
289. Fuller RW, Wong DT. Serotonin uptake and serotonin uptake inhibition. Ann N Y Acad Sci. 1990;600:68-80.
290. Wade PR, Chen J, Jaffe B, et al. Localization and function of a 5-HT transporter in crypt epithelia of the gastrointestinal tract. J Neurosci. 1996;16:2352-64.
291. Chen J-X, Pan H, Rothman TP, et al. Guinea pig 5-HT transporter: cloning, expression, distribution and function in intestinal sensory reception. Am J Physiol. 1998;275:G433-48.
292. Gorard DA, Libby GW, Farthing MJ. Effect of a tricyclic antidepressant on small intestinal motility in health and diarrhea-predominant irritable bowel syndrome. Dig Dis Sci. 1995;40:86-95.
293. Chen JJ, Zhishan L, Pan H, et al. Maintenance of serotonin in the intestinal mucosa and ganglia of mice that lack the high affinity serotonin transporter (SERT): abnormal intestinal motility and the expression of cation transporters. J Neurosci. 2001;21:6348-61.
294. Li ZS, Pham TD, Tamir H, et al. Enteric dopaminergic neurons: definition, developmental lineage, and effects of extrinsic denervation. J Neurosci. 2004;24:1330-39.
295. Pan H, Gershon MD. Activation of intrinsic afferent pathways in submucosal ganglia of the guinea pig small intestine. J Neurosci. 2000; 20:3295-309.
296. Kirchgessner AL, Tamir H, Gershon MD. Identification and stimulation by serotonin of intrinsic sensory neurons of the submucosal plexus of the guinea pig gut: activity-induced expression of Fos immunoreactivity. J Neurosci. 1992;12:235-49.
297. Furness JB, Kunze WA, Bertrand PP, et al. Intrinsic primary afferent neurons of the intestine. Prog Neurobiol. 1998;54:1-18.
298. Bertrand PP, Kunze WAA, Furness JB, et al. The terminals of myenteric intrinsic primary afferent neurons of the guinea pig ileum are excited by 5-HT acting at 5-HT_3 receptors. Neuroscience. 2000;101:459-69.
299. Pan H, Gershon MD. Activation of intrinsic afferent pathways in submucosal ganglia of the guinea pig small intestine. J Neurosci. 2000; 20:3295-309.
300. Sidhu M, Cooke HJ. Role for 5-HT and ACh in submucosal reflexes mediating colonic secretion. Am J Physiol Gastointest Liver Physiol. 1995;269:G346-51.

301. Cooke HJ, Sidhu M, Wang Y-Z. 5-HT activates neural reflexes regulating secretion in the guinea-pig colon. Neurogastroenterol Motil. 1997;9:181-86.
302. Kunze WAA, Furness JB, Bertrand PP, et al. Intracellular recording from myenteric neurons of the guinea-pig ileum that respond to stretch. J Physiol. 1998;506:827-42.
303. Grider JR, Jin J-G. Distinct populations of sensory neurons mediate the peristaltic reflex elicited by muscle stretch and mucosal stimulation. J Neurosci. 1994;14:2854-60.
304. Sethi AK, Sarna SK. Contractile mechanisms of canine colonic propulsion. Am J Physiol. 1995;268:G530-38.
305. Pan H, Gershon MD. Activation of intrinsic afferent pathways in submucosal ganglia of the guinea pig small intestine. J Neurosci. 2000;20:3295-309.
306. Li ZS, Furness JB. Immunohistochemical localisation of cholinergic markers in putative intrinsic primary afferent neurons of the guinea pig small intestine. Cell Tissue Res. 1998;294:35-43.
307. Bian XC, Heffer LF, Gwynne RM, et al. Synaptic transmission in simple motility reflex pathways excited by distension in guinea pig distal colon. Am J Physiol Gastrointest Liver Physiol. 2004;287:G1017-27.
308. Brehmer A, Croner R, Dimmler A, et al. Immunohistochemical characterization of putative primary afferent (sensory) myenteric neurons in human small intestine. Auton Neurosci. 2004;112:49-59.
309. Bertrand PP. Bursts of recurrent excitation in the activation of intrinsic sensory neurons of the intestine. Neuroscience. 2004;128:51-63.
310. Pan H, Gershon MD. Activation of intrinsic afferent pathways in submucosal ganglia of the guinea pig small intestine. J Neurosci. 2000;20:3295-309.
311. Grider JR. CGRP as a transmitter in the sensory pathway mediating peristaltic reflex. Am J Physiol. 1994;266:G1139-45.
312. Grider JR. Neurotransmitters mediating the intestinal peristaltic reflex in the mouse. J Pharmacol Exp Ther. 2003;307:460-67.
313. Pan H, Gershon MD. Activation of intrinsic afferent pathways in submucosal ganglia of the guinea pig small intestine. J Neurosci. 2000;20:3295-309.
314. Furness JB, Kunze WA, Bertrand PP, et al. Intrinsic primary afferent neurons of the intestine. Prog Neurobiol. 1998;54:1-18.
315. Song Z-M, Brookes SJH, Costa M. All calbindin-immunoreactive myenteric neurons project to the mucosa of the guinea pig small intestine. Neurosci Lett. 1994;180:219-22.
316. Li ZS, Furness JB. Inputs from intrinsic primary afferent neurons to nitric oxide synthase-immunoreactive neurons in the myenteric plexus of guinea pig ileum. Cel Tissue Res. 2000;299:1-8.
317. Furness JB. Types of neurons in the enteric nervous system. J Auton Nerv Syst. 2000;81:87-96.
318. Brehmer A, Croner R, Dimmler A, et al. Immunohistochemical characterization of putative primary afferent (sensory) myenteric neurons in human small intestine. Auton Neurosci. 2004;112:49-59.
319. Kirchgessner AL, Dodd J, Gershon MD. Markers shared between dorsal root and enteric ganglia. J Comp Neurol. 1988;276:607-21.
320. Bian XC, Heffer LF, Gwynne RM, et al. Synaptic transmission in simple motility reflex pathways excited by distension in guinea pig distal colon. Am J Physiol Gastrointest Liver Physiol. 2004;287:G1017-27.
321. Kunze WA, Furness JB, Bornstein JC. Simultaneous intracellular recordings from enteric neurons reveal that myenteric AH neurons transmit via slow excitatory postsynaptic potentials. Neuroscience. 1993;55:685-694.
322. Erde SM, Sherman D, Gershon MD. Morphology and serotonergic innervation of physiologically identified cells of the guinea pig's myenteric plexus. J Neurosci. 1985;5:617-33.
323. Linden DR, Sharkey KA. Enhanced excitability of myenteric AH neurones in the inflamed guinea-pig distal colon. J Physiol. 2003;547:589-601.
324. Linden DR, Sharkey KA, Ho W. Cyclooxygenase-2 contributes to dysmotility and enhanced excitability of myenteric AH neurones in the inflamed guinea pig distal colon. J Physiol. 2004;557:191-205.
325. Branchek T, Mawe G, Gershon MD. Characterization and localization of a peripheral neural 5-hydroxytryptamine receptor subtype with a selective agonist, ^{3}H-5-hydroxyindalpine. J Neurosci. 1988;8:2582-95.
326. Mawe GM, Branchek T, Gershon MD. Peripheral neural serotonin receptors: identification and characterization with specific agonists and antagonists. Proc Natl Acad Sci U S A. 1986;83:9799-803.
327. Mawe GM, Branchek T, Gershon MD. Blockade of 5-HT-mediated enteric slow EPSPs by BRL 24924: gastrokinetic effects. Am J Physiol Gastrointest Liver Physiol. 1989;257:G386-96.
328. Wade P, Branchek TA, Mawe GM, et al. Use of stereoisomers of zacopride to analyze actions of 5-hydroxytryptamine on enteric neurons. Am J Physiol. 1991;260:G80-90.
329. Branchek T, Mawe G, Gershon MD. Characterization and localization of a peripheral neural 5-hydroxytryptamine receptor subtype with a selective agonist, ^{3}H-5-hydroxyindalpine. J Neurosci. 1988;8:2582-95.
330. Mawe GM, Branchek T, Gershon MD. Blockade of 5-HT-mediated enteric slow EPSPs by BRL 24924: gastrokinetic effects. Am J Physiol Gastrointest Liver Physiol. 1989;257:G386-96.
331. Takaki M, Branchek T, Tamir H, et al. Specific antagonism of enteric neural serotonin receptors by dipeptides of 5-hydroxytryptophan: evidence that serotonin is a mediatory of slow synaptic excitation in the myenteric plexus. J Neurosci. 1985;5:1769-80.
332. Galligan JJ, Pan H, Messori E. Signalling mechanism coupled to 5-hydroxytryptamine4 receptor-mediated facilitation of fast synaptic transmission in the guinea-pig ileum myenteric plexus. Neurogastroenterol Motil. 2003;15:523-29.
333. Nagakura Y, Naitoh Y, Kamato T, et al. Compounds possessing 5-HT_3 receptor antagonistic activity inhibit intestinal propulsion in mice. Eur J Pharmacol. 1996;311:67-72.
334. Pan H, Gershon MD. Activation of intrinsic afferent pathways in submucosal ganglia of the guinea pig small intestine. J Neurosci. 2000;20:3295-309.
335. Wade PR, Tamir H, Kirchgessner AL, et al. Analysis of the role of 5-HT in the enteric nervous system using anti-idiotypic antibodies to 5-HT receptors. Am J Physiol. 1994;266:G403-16.
336. Sidhu M, Cooke HJ. Role for 5-HT and ACh in submucosal reflexes mediating colonic secretion. Am J Physiol Gastointest Liver Physiol. 1995;269:G346-51.
337. Cooke HJ, Sidhu M, Wang Y-Z. 5-HT activates neural reflexes regulating secretion in the guinea-pig colon. Neurogastroenterol Motil. 1997;9:181-86.
338. Frieling T, Cooke HJ, Wood JD. Serotonin receptors on submucous neurons in guinea pig colon. Am J Physiol. 1991;261:G1017-23.
339. Wade PR, Tamir H, Kirchgessner AL, et al. Analysis of the role of 5-HT in the enteric nervous system using anti-idiotypic antibodies to 5-HT receptors. Am J Physiol. 1994;266:G403-16.
340. Mawe GM, Branchek T, Gershon MD. Blockade of 5-HT-mediated enteric slow EPSPs by BRL 24924: gastrokinetic effects. Am J Physiol Gastrointest Liver Physiol. 1989;257:G386-96.
341. Takaki M, Branchek T, Tamir H, et al. Specific antagonism of enteric neural serotonin receptors by dipeptides of 5-hydroxytryptophan: evidence that serotonin is a mediatory of slow synaptic excitation in the myenteric plexus. J Neurosci. 1985;5:1769-80.

342. Branchek T, Mawe G, Gershon MD. Characterization and localization of a peripheral neural 5-hydroxytryptamine receptor subtype with a selective agonist, ^{3}H-5-hydroxyindalpine. J Neurosci. 1988;8:2582-95.
343. Pan H, Gershon MD. Activation of intrinsic afferent pathways in submucosal ganglia of the guinea pig small intestine. J Neurosci. 2000; 20:3295-309.
344. Grider JR. CGRP as a transmitter in the sensory pathway mediating peristaltic reflex. Am J Physiol. 1994;266:G1139-45.
345. Grider JR. Neurotransmitters mediating the intestinal peristaltic reflex in the mouse. J Pharmacol Exp Ther. 2003;307:460-67.
346. Galligan JJ, Pan H, Messori E. Signalling mechanism coupled to 5-hydroxytryptamine4 receptor-mediated facilitation of fast synaptic transmission in the guinea-pig ileum myenteric plexus. Neurogastroenterol Motil. 2003;15:523-29.
347. Pan H, Galligan JJ. 5-HT1A and 5-HT_4 receptors mediate inhibition and facilitation of fast synaptic transmission in enteric neurons. Am J Physiol. 1994;266:G230-38.
348. Craig DA, Clarke DE. Pharmacological characterization of a neuronal receptor for 5-hydroxytryptamine in guinea pig ileum with properties similar to the 5-hydroxytryptamine4 receptor. J Pharmacol Exp Ther. 1990;252:1378-86.
349. Galligan JJ, Pan H, Messori E. Signalling mechanism coupled to 5-hydroxytryptamine4 receptor-mediated facilitation of fast synaptic transmission in the guinea-pig ileum myenteric plexus. Neurogastroenterol Motil. 2003;15:523-29.
350. Pan H, Galligan JJ. 5-HT1A and 5-HT_4 receptors mediate inhibition and facilitation of fast synaptic transmission in enteric neurons. Am J Physiol. 1994;266:G230-38.
351. Liu M-T, Fiorica-Howells E, Gershon MD. Alternative splicing of enteric 5-HT_4 receptors and a patch-clamp analysis of function. Gastroenterology. 2003;124:A342.
352. Liu MT, Rayport S, Jiang Y, et al. Expression and function of 5-HT_3 receptors in the enteric neurons of mice lacking the serotonin transporter. Am J Physiol Gastrointest Liver Physiol. 2002;283:G1398-G1411.
353. Derkach V, Surprenant A, North RA. 5-HT_3 receptors are membrane ion channels. Nature. 1989;339:706-9.
354. Mawe GM, Branchek T, Gershon MD. Peripheral neural serotonin receptors: identification and characterization with specific agonists and antagonists. Proc Natl Acad Sci U S A. 1986;83:9799-803.
355. Mawe GM, Branchek T, Gershon MD. Blockade of 5-HT-mediated enteric slow EPSPs by BRL 24924: gastrokinetic effects. Am J Physiol Gastrointest Liver Physiol. 1989;257:G386-96.
356. Wade P, Branchek TA, Mawe GM, et al. Use of stereoisomers of zacopride to analyze actions of 5-hydroxytryptamine on enteric neurons. Am J Physiol. 1991;260:G80-90.
357. Takaki M, Branchek T, Tamir H, et al. Specific antagonism of enteric neural serotonin receptors by dipeptides of 5-hydroxytryptophan: evidence that serotonin is a mediatory of slow synaptic excitation in the myenteric plexus. J Neurosci. 1985;5:1769-80.
358. Glatzle J, Sternini C, Robin C, et al. Expression of 5-HT_3 receptors in the rat gastrointestinal tract. Gastroenterology. 2002;123:217-26.
359. Mazzia C, Hicks GA, Clerc N. Neuronal location of 5-hydroxytryptamine3 receptor-like immunoreactivity in the rat colon. Neuroscience. 2003;116:1033-41.
360. Wade PR, Tamir H, Kirchgessner AL, et al. Analysis of the role of 5-HT in the enteric nervous system using anti-idiotypic antibodies to 5-HT receptors. Am J Physiol. 1994;266:G403-16.
361. Fiorica-Howells E, Liu M-T, Ponimaskin EG, et al. Distribution of 5-HT_4 receptors in wild-type mice and analysis of intestinal molity in 5-HT_4 knockout mice. Gastroenterology. 2003;124:A342.
362. Ibid.
363. Ponimaskin EG, Heine M, Joubert L, et al. The 5-hydroxytryptamine(4a) receptor is palmitoylated at two different sites, and acylation is critically involved in regulation of receptor constitutive activity. J Biol Chem. 2002;277:2534-46.
364. Norman P. Tegaserod (Novartis). IDrugs. 2002;5(2):171-79.
365. Scott LJ, Perry CM. Tegaserod. Drugs. 1999;58(3):491-96.
366. Camilleri M. Review article: tegaserod. Aliment Pharmacol Ther. 2001;15:277-89.
367. Muller-Lissner SA, Fumagalli I, Bardhan KD, et al. Tegaserod, a 5-HT_4 receptor partial agonist, relieves symptoms in irritable bowel syndrome patients with abdominal pain, bloating and constipation. Aliment Pharmacol Ther. 2001;15:1655-66.
368. Prather CM, Camilleri M, Zinsmeister AR, et al. Tegaserod accelerates orocecal transit in patients with constipation-predominant irritable bowel syndrome. Gastroenterology. 2000;118:463-68.
369. Camilleri M, Talley NJ. Pathophysiology as a basis for understanding symptom complexes and therapeutic targets. Neurogastroenterol Motil. 2004;16:135-42.
370. Nyhlin H, Bang C, Elsborg L, et al. A double-blind, placebo-controlled., randomized study to evaluate the efficacy, safety and tolerability of tegaserod in patients with irritable bowel syndrome. Scand J Gastroenterol. 2004;39:119-26.
371. Camilleri M. What's in a name? Roll on Rome II. [editorial]. Gastroenterology. 1998;114:23-27.
372. Al-Chaer ED., Kawasaki M, Pasricha PJ. A new model of chronic visceral hypersensitivity in adult rats induced by colon irritation during postnatal development. Gastroenterology. 2000;119:1276-85.
373. Mayer EA, Collins SM. Evolving pathophysiologic models of functional gastrointestinal disorders. Gastroenterology. 2002;122:2032-48.
374. Drossman DA. Review article: an integrated approach to the irritable bowel syndrome. Aliment Pharmacol Ther. 1999;13(suppl2):3-14.
375. Smith GP, Jerome C, Norgren R. Afferent axons in abdominal vagus mediate satiety effect of cholecystokinin in rats. Am J Physiol. 1985;249:R638-41.
376. Hoffman HH, Schnitzlein HN. The number of vagus nerves in man. Anat Rec. 1961;139:429-35.
377. Sengupta JN, Gebhart GF. Gastrointestinal afferent fibers and sensation. In: Johnson LR, Alpers DH, Jacobson ED., et al, eds. Physiology of the Gastrointestinal Tract, 3rd ed., vol. 1. New York: Raven Press,1994:483-520.
378. Clark KB, Naritoku DK, Smith DC, et al. Enhanced recognition memory following vagus nerve stimulation in human subjects. Nat Neurosci. 1999;2:94-98.
379. George MS, Sackeim HA, Rush AJ, et al. Vagus nerve stimulation: a new tool for brain research and therapy [see comments]. Biol Psychiatry. 2000;47:287-95.
380. Van Laere K, Vonck K, Boon P, et al. Vagus nerve stimulation in refractory epilepsy: SPECT activation study. J Nucl Med. 2000;41:1145-54.
381. Rosenbaum JF, Heninger G. Vagus nerve stimulation for treatment-resistant depression [editorial; comment]. Biol Psychiatry. 2000;47:273-75.
382. Hillsley K, Grundy D. Sensitivity to 5-hydroxytryptamine in different afferent subpopulations within mesenteric nerves supplying the rat jejunum. J Physiol. 1998;509:717-27.
383. Blackshaw LA, Grundy D. Effects of 5-hydroxytryptamine on discharge of vagal mucosal afferent fibres from the upper gastrointestinal tract of the ferret. J Auton Nerv Syst. 1993;45:41-50.
384. Hillsley K, Kirkup AJ, Grundy D. Direct and indirect actions of 5-hydroxytryptamine on the discharge of mesenteric afferent fibers innervating the rat jejunum. J Physiol. 1998;506:551-61.

385. Camilleri M, Mayer EA, Drossman DA, et al. Improvement in pain and bowel function in female irritable bowel patients with alosetron, a 5-HT_3 receptor antagonist. Aliment Pharmacol Ther. 1999;13:1149-59.
386. Glatzle J, Sternini C, Robin C, et al. Expression of 5-HT_3 receptors in the rat gastrointestinal tract. Gastroenterology. 2002;123:217-26.
387. Mazzia C, Hicks GA, Clerc N. Neuronal location of 5-hydroxytryptamine3 receptor-like immunoreactivity in the rat colon. Neuroscience. 2003;116:1033-41.
388. Raybould HE, Glatzle J, Robin C, et al. Expression of 5-HT_3 receptors by extrinsic duodenal afferents contribute to intestinal inhibition of gastric emptying. Am J Physiol Gastrointest Liver Physiol. 2003;284:G367-72.
389. Gregory RE, Ettinger DS. 5-HT_3 receptor antagonists for the prevention of chemotherapy-induced nausea and vomiting: a comparison of their pharmacology and clinical efficacy. Drugs. 1998;55:173-89.
390. Rudd JA, Naylor RJ. Effects of 5-HT_3 receptor antagonists on models of acute and delayed emesis induced by cisplatin in the ferret. Neuropharmacology. 1994;33:1607-8.
391. Mangel AW, Northcutt AR. Review article: the safety and efficacy of alosetron, a 5-HT_3 receptor antagonist, in female irritable bowel syndrome patients. Aliment Pharmacol Ther. 1999;13(suppl 2):77-82.
392. Humphrey PP, Bountra C, Clayton N, et al. Review article: the therapeutic potential of 5-HT_3 receptor antagonists in the treatment of irritable bowel syndrome. Aliment Pharmacol Ther. 1999;13(suppl 2):31-38.
393. Coremans G, Clouse RG, Carter F, et al. Cilansetron, a novel 5-HT_3 antagonist, demonstrated efficacy in males with irritable bowel syndrome with diarrhea predominance (IBS-D). Gastroenterology. 2004;126(Suppl 2):105454.
394. Bertrand PP, Kunze WAA, Furness JB, et al. The terminals of myenteric intrinsic primary afferent neurons of the guinea pig ileum are excited by 5-HT acting at 5-HT_3 receptors. Neuroscience. 2000;101:459-69.
395. Bertrand PP, Furness JB, Bornstein JC. 5-HT and ATP stimulate the mucosal terminals of some myenteric sensory neurons and cause increases in excitability in a population of sensory neurons, In: Falk Symposium No. 112. Neurogastroenterology: From the Basics to the Clinics. Freiburg, Germany, 1999.
396. Pan H, Gershon MD. Activation of intrinsic afferent pathways in submucosal ganglia of the guinea pig small intestine. J Neurosci. 2000; 20:3295-309.
397. Glatzle J, Sternini C, Robin C, et al. Expression of 5-HT_3 receptors in the rat gastrointestinal tract. Gastroenterology. 2002;123:217-26.
398. Mazzia C, Hicks GA, Clerc N. Neuronal location of 5-hydroxytryptamine3 receptor-like immunoreactivity in the rat colon. Neuroscience. 2003;116:1033-41.
399. Raybould HE, Glatzle J, Robin C, et al. Expression of 5-HT_3 receptors by extrinsic duodenal afferents contribute to intestinal inhibition of gastric emptying. Am J Physiol Gastrointest Liver Physiol. 2003;284:G367-72.
400. Galligan JJ. Electrophyiological studies of 5-hydroxytryptamine receptors on enteric neurons. Behav Brain Res. 1996;73:199-201.
401. Galligan JJ. Mechanisms of excitatory synaptic transmission in the enteric nervous system. Tokai J Exp Clin Med. 1998;23:129-36.
402. Galligan JJ, LePard KJ, Schneider DA, et al. Multiple mechanisms of fast excitatory synaptic transmission in the enteric nervous system. J Auton Nerv Syst. 2000;81:97-103.
403. Galligan JJ. Pharmacology of synaptic transmission in the enteric nervous system. Curr Opin Pharmacol. 2002;2:623-29.
404. Monro RL, Bertrand PP, Bornstein JC. ATP and 5-HT are the principal neurotransmitters in the descending excitatory reflex pathway of the guinea-pig ileum. Neurogastroenterol Motil. 2002;14:255-64.
405. Bertrand PP, Kunze WAA, Furness JB, et al. The terminals of myenteric intrinsic primary afferent neurons of the guinea pig ileum are excited by 5-HT acting at 5-HT_3 receptors. Neuroscience. 2000;101:459-69.
406. Bertrand PP, Furness JB, Bornstein JC. 5-HT and ATP stimulate the mucosal terminals of some myenteric sensory neurons and cause increases in excitability in a population of sensory neurons, In: Falk Symposium No. 112. Neurogastroenterology: From the Basics to the Clinics. Freiburg, Germany, 1999.
407. Monro RL, Bertrand PP, Bornstein JC. ATP and 5-HT are the principal neurotransmitters in the descending excitatory reflex pathway of the guinea-pig ileum. Neurogastroenterol Motil. 2002;14:255-64.
408. Kadowaki M, Wade PR, Gershon MD. Participation of 5-HT_3, 5-HT_4, and nicotinic receptors in the peristaltic reflex of the guinea pig distal colon. Am J Physiol. 1996;271:G849-57.
409. Nagakura Y, Kontoh A, Tokita K, et al. Combined blockade of 5-HT_3-and 5-HT_4-serotonin receptors inhibits colonic functions in conscious rats and mice. J Pharmacol Exp Ther. 1997;281:284-90.
410. Mangel AW, Northcutt AR. Review article: the safety and efficacy of alosetron, a 5-HT_3 receptor antagonist, in female irritable bowel syndrome patients. Aliment Pharmacol Ther. 1999;13(suppl 2):77-82.
411. Beck IT. Possible mechanisms for ischemic colitis during alosetron therapy. Gastroenterology. 2001;121:231-32.
412. Friedel D, Thomas R, Fisher RS. Ischemic colitis during treatment with alosetron. Gastroenterology. 2001;120:557-60.
413. Muller-Lissner SA, Fumagalli I, Bardhan KD, et al. Tegaserod, a 5-HT_4 receptor partial agonist, relieves symptoms in irritable bowel syndrome patients with abdominal pain, bloating and constipation. Aliment Pharmacol Ther. 2001;15:1655-66.
414. Coffin B, Farmachidi JP, Rueegg P, et al. Tegaserod, a 5-HT_4 receptor partial agonist, decreases sensitivity to rectal distension in healthy subjects. Aliment Pharmacol Ther. 2003;17:577-85.
415. Gazzara RA, Compan V, Mullan D, et al. Behavioral characterization of 5-HT_4 receptor knockout mice. In: Society for Neuroscience. Orlando, FL, 2002.
416. Talley NJ. Irritable bowel syndrome: disease definition and symptom description. Eur J Surg Suppl. 1998;583:24-28.
417. Kay L, Jorgensen T, Lanng C. Irritable bowel syndrome: which definitions are consistent? J Intern Med. 1998;244:489-94.
418. Camilleri M. What's in a name? Roll on Rome II. [editorial]. Gastroenterology. 1998;114:23-27.
419. Talley NJ. Irritable bowel syndrome: disease definition and symptom description. Eur J Surg Suppl. 1998;583:24-28.
420. Kay L, Jorgensen T, Lanng C. Irritable bowel syndrome: which definitions are consistent? J Intern Med. 1998;244:489-94.
421. Talley NJ. Scope of the problem of functional digestive disorders. Eur J Surg Suppl. 1998;582:35-41.
422. Locke G, Yawn B, Wollan P, et al. Incidence of a clinical diagnosis of the irritable bowel syndrome in a United States population. Aliment Pharmacol Ther. 2004;19:1025-31.
423. Gershon MD. Plasticity in serotonin control mechanisms in the gut. Curr Opin Pharmacol. 2003;3:600-7.
424. Coates MD, Mahoney CR, Linden DR, et al. Molecular defects in mucosal serotonin content and decreased serotonin reuptake transporter in ulcerative colitis and IBS. Gastroenterology. 2004;126:1657-64.
425. Wade PR, Chen J, Jaffe B, et al. Localization and function of a 5-HT transporter in crypt epithelia of the gastrointestinal tract. J Neurosci. 1996;16:2352-64.
426. Chen J-X, Pan H, Rothman TP, et al. Guinea pig 5-HT transporter: cloning, expression, distribution and function in intestinal sensory reception. Am J Physiol. 1998;275:G433-48.

427. Chen JJ, Zhishan L, Pan H, et al. Maintenance of serotonin in the intestinal mucosa and ganglia of mice that lack the high affinity serotonin transporter (SERT): abnormal intestinal motility and the expression of cation transporters. J Neurosci. 2001;21:6348-61.
428. Ibid.
429. Coates MD, Mahoney CR, Linden DR, et al. Molecular defects in mucosal serotonin content and decreased serotonin reuptake transporter in ulcerative colitis and IBS. Gastroenterology. 2004;126:1657-64.
430. Linden DR, Chen JX, Gershon MD, et al. Serotonin availability is increased in mucosa of guinea pigs with TNBS-induced colitis. Am J Physiol Gastrointest Liver Physiol. 2003;285:G207-16.
431. Coates MD, Mahoney CR, Linden DR, et al. Molecular defects in mucosal serotonin content and decreased serotonin reuptake transporter in ulcerative colitis and IBS. Gastroenterology. 2004;126:1657-64.
432. Mayer EA, Collins SM. Evolving pathophysiologic models of functional gastrointestinal disorders. Gastroenterology. 2002;122:2032-48.
433. Bueno L, Fioramonti J. Effects of inflammatory mediators on gut sensitivity. Can J Gastroenterol. 1999;13(suppl A):42-46.
434. Spiller RC, Jenkins D, Thornley JP, et al. Increased rectal mucosal enteroendocrine cells, T lymphocytes, and increased gut permeability following acute Campylobacter enteritis and in post-dysenteric irritable bowel syndrome. Gut. 2000;47:804-11.
435. Verdu EF, Collins SM. Microbial-gut interactions in health and disease: irritable bowel syndrome. Best Pract Res Clin Gastroenterol. 2004;18:315-21.
436. Bercik P, Wang L, Verdu EF, et al. Visceral hyperalgesia and intestinal dysmotility in a mouse model of postinfective gut dysfunction. Gastroenterology. 2004;127:179-87.
437. Collins SM, Piche T, Rampal P. The putative role of inflammation in the irritable bowel syndrome. Gut. 2001;49:743-45.
438. Spiller RC. Inflammation as a basis for functional GI disorders. Best Pract Res Clin Gastroenterol. 2004;18:641-61.
439. Liu MT, Rayport S, Jiang Y, et al. Expression and function of 5-HT_3 receptors in the enteric neurons of mice lacking the serotonin transporter. Am J Physiol Gastrointest Liver Physiol. 2002;283:G1398-G1411.
440. Horwitz BJ, Fisher RS. The irritable bowel syndrome. N Engl J Med. 2001;344(24):1846-50.
441. Mayer EA. Emerging disease model for functional gastrointestinal disorders. Am J Med. 1999;107(5A):12S-19S.
442. Camilleri M, Lee JS, Viramontes B, et al. Insights into the pathophysiology and mechanisms of constipation, irritable bowel syndrome, and diverticulosis in older people. J Am Geriatr Soc. 2000;48(9):1142-50.
443. Mielants H, De Vos M, Goemaere S, et al. Intestinal mucosal permeability in inflammatory rheumatic diseases. J Rheumatol. 1991;18(3):394-400.
444. Andre C, Andre F, Colin L. Effect of allergen ingestion challenge with and without cromoglycate cover on intestinal permeability in atopic dermatitis, urticaria and other symptoms of food allergy. Allergy. 1989;44 (Suppl 9):47-51.
445. Smith MD, Gibson RA, Brooks PM. Abnormal bowel permeability in ankylosing spondylitis and rheumatoid arthritis. J Rheumatol. 1985;12(2):299-305.
446. Isolauri E, Juntunen M, Wiren S, et al. Intestinal permeability changes in acute gastroenteritis: effects of clinical factors and nutritional management. J Pediatr Gastroenterol Nutr. 1989;8(4):466-73.
447. Munkholm P, Langholz E, Hollander D, et al. Intestinal permeability in patients with Crohn's disease and ulcerative colitis and their first degree relatives. Gut. 1994;35(1):68-72.
448. Olaison G, Sjodahl R, Tagesson D. Abnormal intestinal permeability in Crohn's disease. A possible pathogenic factor. Scand J Gastroenterol. 1990;25(4):321-28.
449. Hollander D. Intestinal permeability, leaky gut, and intestinal disorders. Curr Gastroenterol Rep. 1999;1(5):410-16.
450. DeMeo MT, Mutlu EA, Keshavarzian A, Tobin MC. Intestinal permeation and gastrointestinal disease. J Clin Gastroenterol. 2002;34(4):385-96.
451. Sampson HA, Anderson JA. Summary and recommendations: Classification of gastrointestinal manifestations due to immunologic reactions to foods in infants and young children. J Pediatr Gastroenterol Nutr. 2000;30 (Suppl):S87-94.
452. Brandtzaeg PE. Current understanding of gastrointestinal immunoregulation and its relation to food allergy. Ann N Y Acad Sci. 2002;964:13-45.
453. Carini C, Brostoff J, Wraith DG. IgE complexes in food allergy. Ann Allergy. 1987;59(2):110-17.
454. Halpern GM, Scott JR. Non-IgE antibody mediated mechanisms in food allergy. Ann Allergy. 1987;58(1):14-27.
455. el Rafei A, Peters SM, Harris N, Bellanti JA. Diagnostic value of IgG4 measurements in patients with food allergy. Ann Allergy. 1989;62(2):94-99.
456. Atkinson W, Sheldon TA, Shaath N, Whorwell PJ. Food elimination based on IgG antibodies in irritable bowel syndrome: a randomised controlled trial. Gut. 2004;53(10):1459-64.
457. Zar S, Kumar D, Benson MJ. Food hypersensitivity and irritable bowel syndrome. Aliment Pharmacol Ther. 2001;15(4):439-49.
458. Sampson HA. Clinical manifestations of adverse food reactions. Pediatr Allergy Immunol. 1995;6(Suppl 8):29-37.
459. Burks A, Sampson HA. Diagnostic approaches to the patient with suspected food allergies. J Pediatr. 1992;121(5 Pt 2):S64-71.
460. Carini C, Brostoff J, Wraith DG. IgE complexes in food allergy. Ann Allergy. 1987;59(2):110-17.
461. Halpern GM, Scott JR. Non-IgE antibody mediated mechanisms in food allergy. Ann Allergy. 1987;58(1):14-27.
462. Sampson HA. Clinical manifestations of adverse food reactions. Pediatr Allergy Immunol. 1995;6(Suppl 8):29-37.
463. Sicherer SH. Manifestations of food allergy: evaluation and management. Am Fam Physician. 1999;59(2):415-24, 429-30.
464. Sicherer SH, Sampson HA. Food hypersensitivity and atopic dermatitis: pathophysiology, epidemiology, diagnosis, and management. J Allergy Clin Immunol. 1999;104(3 Pt 2):S114-22.
465. Alexander JW, Boyce ST, Babcock GF, et al. The process of microbial translocation. Ann Surg. 1990;212(4):496-510.
466. Ebringer A, Khalafpour S, Wilson C. Rheumatoid arthritis and Proteus: a possible aetiological association. Rheumatol Int. 1989;9(3-5):223-28.
467. Rashid T, Leirisalo-Repo M, Tani Y, et al. Antibacterial and antipeptide antibodies in Japanese and Finnish patients with rheumatoid arthritis. Clin Rheumatol. 2004;23(2):134-41.
468. Pledger JV, Pearson AD, Craft AW, et al. Intestinal permeability during chemotherapy for childhood tumours. Eur J Pediatr. 1988;147(2):123-27.
469. Pirzer U, Schonhaar A, Fleischer B, et al. Reactivity of infiltrating T lymphocytes with microbial antigens in Crohn's disease. Lancet. 1991; 338(8777):1238-39.
470. Falgarone G, Jaen O, Boissier MC. Role for innate immunity in rheumatoid arthritis. Joint Bone Spine. 2005;72(1):17-25.
471. Mills JA. Do bacteria cause chronic polyarthritis? N Engl J Med. 1989;320(4):245-46.
472. Rashid T, Leirisalo-Repo M, Tani Y, et al. Antibacterial and antipeptide antibodies in Japanese and Finnish patients with rheumatoid arthritis. Clin Rheumatol. 2004;23(2):134-41.

473. Gautam V, Sehgal R, Paramjeet SG, Arora DR. Detection of anti-Proteus antibodies in sera of patients with rheumatoid arthritis. Indian J Pathol Microbiol. 2003;46(1):137-41.
474. Kane JG, Chretien JH, Garagusi VF. Diarrhoea caused by Candida. Lancet. 1976;1(7955):335-36.
475. Bolivar RBG. Candidiasis of the gastrointestinal tract, in Candidiasis, F.V. Bodey GP, Editor. 1985, Raven Press: New York.181-201.
476. Lee M. Parasites, yeasts and bacteria in health and disease. J Adv Med. 1995;8(8):121-29.
477. Tungtrongchitr A, Manatsathit S, Kositchaiwat C, et al. Blastocystic hominis infection in irritable bowel syndrome patients. Southeast Asian J Trop Med Public Health. 2004;35(3):705-10.
478. Carrascosa M, Martinez J, Perez-Castrillon JL. Hemorrhagic proctosigmoiditis and Blastocystis hominis infection. Ann Int Med. 1996:124(2):278-79.
479. Yarze JC. Hemorrhagic proctosigmoiditis and Blastocystis hominis. Ann Int Med. 2996;125(10):860-61.
480. Yakoob J, Jafri W, Jafri N, et al. Irritable bowel syndrome: in search of an etiology: role of Blastocystis hominis. Am J Trop Med Hyg. 2004;70(4):383-85.
481. Udkow MP, Markell EK. Blastocystis hominis: prevalence in asymptomatic versus symptomatic hosts. J Infect Dis. 1993;168(1):242-44.
482. Lee M. Parasites, yeasts and bacteria in health and disease. J Adv Med. 1995;8(8):121-29.
483. Cho CH. Zinc: absorption and role in gastrointestinal metabolism and disorders. Dig Dis. 1991;9(1):49-60.
484. Salamat-Miller N, Johnston TP. Current strategies used to enhance the paracellular transport of therapeutic polypeptides across the intestinal epithelium. Int J Pharm. 2005;294(1-2):201-16.
485. Gardner ML. Gastrointestinal absorption of intact proteins. Annu Rev Nutr. 1988;8:329-50.
486. Lu C-L, Chen C-Y, Luo J-C, et al. Impaired gastric myoelectricity in patients with chronic pancreatitis: role of maldigestion. World J Gastroenterol. 2005;11(3):372-76.
487. Griffin SM, Alderson D, Farndon JR. Acid resistant lipase as replacement therapy in chronic pancreatic exocrine insufficiency: a study in dogs. Gut. 1989;30(7):1012-15.
488. Schneider MU, Knoll-Ruzicka ML, Domschke S, et al. Pancreatic enzyme replacement therapy: comparative effects of conventional and enteric-coated microspheric pancreatin and acid-stable fungal enzyme preparations on steatorrhoea in chronic pancreatitis. Hepatogastroenterology. 1985;32(2):97-102.
489. Barillas C, Solomons NW. Effective reduction of lactose maldigestion in preschool children by direct addition of beta-galactosidases to milk at mealtime. Pediatrics. 1987;79(5):766-72.
490. Silva M, Jacobus NV, Deneke C, Gorbach SL. Antimicrobial substance from a human Lactobacillus strain. Antimicrob Agents Chemother. 1987;31(8):1231-33.
491. Bernet MF, Brassart D, Neeser JR, Servin AL. Lactobacillus acidophilus LA 1 binds to cultured human intestinal cell lines and inhibits cell attachment and cell invasion by enterovirulent bacteria. Gut. 1994;35(4):483-89.
492. Malin M, Suomalainen H, Saxelin M, Isolauri E. Promotion of IgA immune response in patients with Crohn's disease by oral bacteriotherapy with Lactobacillus GG. Ann Nutr Metab. 1996;40(3):137-45.
493. Elmer GW, Surawicz CM, McFarland LV. Biotherapeutic agents. A neglected modality for the treatment and prevention of selected intestinal and vaginal infections. JAMA. 1996;275(11):870-76.
494. Gibson GR, Roberfroid MB. Dietary modulation of the human colonic microbiota: introducing the concept of prebiotics. J Nutr. 1995;125(6):1401-12.
495. Ibid.
496. Roberfroid MB. Chicory fructooligosaccharides and the gastrointestinal tract. Nutrition. 2000;16(7-8):677-79.
497. Robinson RR, Feirtag J, Slavin JL. Effects of dietary arabinogalactan on gastrointestinal and blood parameters in healthy human subjects. J Am Coll Nutr. 2001;20(4):279-85.
498. Buddington RK, Williams CH, Chen SC, Witherly SA. Dietary supplement of neosugar alters the fecal flora and decreases activities of some reductive enzymes in human subjects. Am J Clin Nutr. 1996;63(5):709-16.
499. Klimberg VS, Salloum RM, Kasper M, et al. Oral glutamine accelerates healing of the small intestine and improves outcome after whole abdominal radiation. Arch Surg. 1990;125(8):1040-45.
500. Souba WW, Klimberg VS, Plumley DA, et al. The role of glutamine in maintaining a healthy gut and supporting the metabolic response to injury and infection. J Surg Res. 1990;48(4):383-91.
501. Soeters PB, van de Poll MC, van Gemert WG, Dejong CH. Amino acid adequacy in pathophysiological states. J Nutr. 2004;134(6 Suppl):1575S-82S.
502. Belluzzi A, Brignola C, Campieri M, et al. Effects of new fish oil derivative on fatty acid phospholipid-membrane pattern in a group of Crohn's disease patients. Dig Dis Sci. 1994;39(12):2589-94.
503. Bjorkkjaer T, Brunborg LA, Arslan G, et al. Reduced joint pain after short-term duodenal administration of seal oil in patients with inflammatory bowel disease: comparison with soy oil. Scand J Gastroenterol. 2004;39(11):1088-94.
504. Gil A. Polyunsaturated fatty acids and inflammatory diseases. Biomed Pharmacother. 2002;56(8):288-96.
505. Inui K, Fukuta Y, Ikeda A, et al. The nutritional effect of a-linolenic acid-rich emulsion with total parenteral nutrition in a rat model with inflammatory bowel disease. Ann Nutr Metab. 1996;40(4):227-33.
506. Lacroix B, Didier E, Grenier JF. Role of pantothenic and ascorbic acid in wound healing processes: *in vitro* study on fibroblasts. Int J Vitam Nutr Res. 1988;58(4):407-13.
507. Ellestad-Sayed JJ, Nelson RA, Adson MA, et al. Pantothenic acid, coenzyme A, and human chronic ulcerative and granulomatous colitis. Am J Clin Nutr. 1976;29(12):1333-38.
508. Ojuawo A, Keith L. The serum concentrations of zinc, copper and selenium in children with inflammatory bowel disease. Cent Afr J Med. 2002;49(9-10):116-19.
509. Geerling BJ, Badart-Smook A, Stockbrugger RW, Brummer RJ. Comprehensive nutritional status in recently diagnosed patients with inflammatory bowel disease compared with population controls. Eur J Clin Nutr. 2000;54(6):514-21.
510. Fleming CR, Huizenga KA, McCall JT, et al. Zinc nutrition in Crohn's disease. Dig Dis Sci. 1981;26(10):865-70.
511. Hendricks KM, Walker WA. Zinc deficiency in inflammatory bowel disease. Nutr Rev. 1988;46(12):401-8.

Chapter 29
Clinical Approaches to Structural Imbalance

- ***Physical Fitness and Exercise***
- ***Manipulative Therapy and Functional Medicine: Clinical Interactions between Structure and Function***

Physical Fitness and Exercise

David Musnick, MD

Introduction

It is important for the functional medicine practitioner to understand the physiological and health benefits of exercise and to be able to prescribe, and help patients achieve compliance with, exercise recommendations. In Chapter 13, the extensive evidence base documenting the many significant health effects of regular exercise was reviewed. In this chapter, we examine the clinical applications of the evidence—how clinicians can build into their practices the prescribing of exercise as a therapeutic and for prevention-oriented intervention. Many health improvement goals are difficult or impossible to achieve without specific "doses" of exercise. This is especially true for people with conditions such as obesity, metabolic syndrome, type 2 diabetes, hypertension, and for cardiovascular prevention. Aerobic exercise is essential for maximum cardiovascular risk reduction, stress management, and mood stabilization. Strength training is essential for injury prevention, slowing of sarcopenia, improvement of lean body mass, and for increasing resting metabolic rate for weight loss. Balance training can decrease injuries and reduce the risk of falling for people with neurodegenerative diseases, as well as for elderly patients and those with osteoporosis.

Overview

The most important elements for integrating exercise prescriptions into clinical care are:

- Include an exercise history as an integral part of the patient's health history.
- Pay special attention during the physical examination to any cardiac, pulmonary, or orthopedic findings that may restrict the patient's exercise choices.
- Ask the patient to identify symptoms and key health goals that can be benefited by exercise.
- Educate and motivate the patient about the benefits of exercise.
- Design an exercise program that includes elements of aerobic exercise, strength training, and balance training.
- Ensure that the program you design accommodates the patient's level of abilities, personal preferences, any orthopedic or medical conditions, and financial resources.

The Exercise History

The following questions can be added to a written patient health history form, or they may be asked in person (in which case, the answers need to be noted in the chart).

Aerobic Exercise

- Do you do any regular cardio/aerobic exercise? If yes, what do you do and how many minutes per day do you do it?
- How many exercise sessions in the average week do you do?
- Do you monitor your pulse rate or perceived level of exertion and, if so, what is your average pulse rate or level of exertion during your exercise?
- Do you have any pain or other uncomfortable symptoms from your aerobic exercise?

Strength Training

- Do you do any strength training/weight lifting?
- What exercises do you do and how many sets, reps, and how much weight do you use?
- What are your goals for your strength training?

Balance Training

- Do you do any lunges or balance exercises?
- Do you tend to fall or feel that you have any difficulties with your balance?
- Do you do any tai chi or other exercise that works on balance?

Personal Issues

- Are you happy with your weight? If not, what do you think is a reasonable weight for you?
- How would you like to look?
- Are you satisfied with your exercise program? If not, why not?
- Are you able to schedule exercise and follow through with your schedule? If not, what is your internal dialog about that?
- What are your controllable and uncontrollable roadblocks to doing your exercise?

Exercise Goals

- What are your goals for exercise? Are you meeting them?
- Do you have any activity goals such as running a race, skiing, etc.? If yes, are you doing any special training for these goals?
- Are you aware of the health benefits that regular exercise can provide in terms of preventing strokes, cancer, and heart attacks?

Health Issues Affecting Exercise

- Do you have any cardiac, lung, neurological, hormonal, or orthopedic problems that might influence your ability to do aerobic or strength-training exercise?

Exercise: Risks and Risk Assessment

Aerobic exercise done at a moderate intensity has some cardiovascular, pulmonary, and musculoskeletal risks, although benefits of exercise strongly outweigh risks.[1] Patients should be adequately screened and given precise exercise prescriptions and education to help them receive the benefits and avoid the risks. Strength training, for example, can lead to strains, back injuries, and tendonitis.

General Health Screening

Before prescribing an exercise program, patients should be screened for a history of angina, MI, arrhythmias, hypertension, valvular heart problems (especially aortic stenosis), peripheral vascular disease, and vascular and neurogenic claudication. Screening is also advised for endocrine disorders, including adrenal dysfunction, diabetes, and the metabolic syndrome. It is very important to screen for pulmonary problems, including asthma and COPD. Remember that precipitation of asthma or exercise oxygen desaturation and hypoxia can occur in patients with compromised pulmonary status. Finally, screen for a history of unresolved musculoskeletal injuries, including bursitis, tendonitis, sacroiliac and spine injuries, meniscus and ligament injuries.

Screening for Cardiovascular Risks

Cardiovascular risk factors that should be considered before prescribing exercise include:

- diabetes (fasting glucose and HbA1C)
- high homocysteine levels
- smoking
- positive family history of CAD
- lipid risk factors (high Lip(a), high total and LDL cholesterol, high triglycerides, and trig/HDL ratio >3)
- elevation of cardioselective CRP and fibrinogen

Order an EKG and consider a stress test in a man over 40 or a woman over 50 if a moderate intensity aerobic program (70–85% of max heart rate) is planned or if the individual has significant risk factors for symptomatic coronary artery disease.

Screening for Pulmonary Risks

Assess for pulmonary risks and functional limitations, including exercise-induced asthma. Consider evaluating the patient with COPD pre and post mild exercise (such as walking). If the O2 saturation drops below 91, the patient will be a candidate for oxygen during exercise. If the patient is already on oxygen, consider increasing the flow rate during exercise.

Screening for Musculoskeletal Conditions

The following tests can be included in the physical exam if the clinician is trained in and comfortable with basic orthopedic testing. Results will help determine which types of exercise and aerobic equipment are correct for the patient.

- Screen for range of motion, muscle weakness and imbalances, and balance deficits that might increase the risk of injury or degenerative joint disease (DJD) from exercise.
- Do quick scanning exams of the feet, ankles, knees, hips, shoulders, elbows, wrist, and hands.
- Evaluate for adequate range of motion (ROM) and pain with joint motion to assess whether your patient can do the movement patterns of indoor aerobic equipment and classes and outdoor aerobic activities (hiking, skating, running, rowing, etc.).
- Check ankle dorsiflexion (DF)—10 degrees of ankle DF would be preferred for treadmill, stairmaster, and EFX elliptical trainer.
- Check great toe dorsiflexion to see if there is at least 45 degrees for walking, hiking, and treadmill.
- Check for hallux valgus and pes planus to evaluate for orthotic needs during exercise to prevent tendonitis of the foot or knee and excessive stress on the hip and low back. If significant foot flattening (pronation) exists, prescribe orthotics (generic or custom) and more stable shoes.
- Check for knee extension and flexing abilities to evaluate for walking stride and bike seat height.
- Check for tightness in the quads, hamstrings, and IT bands, and prescribe flexibility exercises if tight.
- Check for crepitus in the kneecap joint and pain with squats or lunges. If kneecap pain is present, avoid exercises that require excessive knee flexing (such as bikes or stairmasters), and avoid step aerobics classes.
- Check hip extension. If there is less than 10 degrees, which would be consistent with DJD, limit walking, running, and cross country skiing until extension improves; prescribe cycling and swimming instead.
- Check the strength of the ankle dorsiflexors, knee flexors, and extensors.
- Check gluteal muscle strength in supine and prone positions.
- Do a neurological exam and straight-leg raise to evaluate for lumbosacral sensory or motor radiculopathies.

Characteristics and Benefits of Aerobic Exercise

Aerobic exercise is the repetitive use of muscle in an indoor or outdoor activity that is demanding enough to lead to a demand for increased blood flow to the muscles and a rise in heart rate. Oxygen is used in the electron transport chain and leads to an increase in ATP production compared to anaerobic metabolism. Aerobic metabolism produces 18 times the ATP of anaerobic metabolism. Anaerobic exercise (such as interval high intensity training) generates only 2 ATP, builds up lactic acid, and has higher risks for the heart and musculoskeletal system.

The Benefits of Aerobic Exercise

The health benefits of aerobic exercise have been extensively studied. Researchers have examined different exercise dose-response effects from varying the duration, intensity, and frequency of exercise. Many studies have used a "minimum program," which is 30 minutes of aerobic exercise in the target heart rate zone, 5–6 days per week. Other studies have reported benefit from two separate 15-minute exercise sessions. The benefits of aerobic exercise do vary depending on the dose of the exercise.[2,3] It is important to understand these benefits, to educate your patients about them, and to help patients connect their own personal health goals with what can be achieved through proper exercise.

Cardiovascular Benefits of Aerobic Exercise

- Can decrease the risk of all-cause mortality by as much as 30%.[4,5,6]
- Can decrease the risk of coronary mortality and the risk of fatal myocardial infarction by 40%.
- Can reduce the risk of stroke by up to 25%.[7]
- Can decrease blood pressure.[8] Systolic and diastolic blood pressures can be reduced by 5–10 mm Hg if the patient is hypertensive. The maximum systolic pressure reduction from exercise alone is estimated to be 10–15 points. If there is weight loss, the drop in BP may be even greater. If a patient is normotensive, exercise can help to maintain a normal blood pressure over time.
- Can increase the ejection fraction and decrease the resting heart rate, both of which may prolong heart function.[9,10]
- Improves the heart rate reserve.[11]
- Decreases platelet aggregation.

Cardio CRP. Aerobic exercise can lower an elevated CRP[12] and decrease the risk of elevated normal CRP over time. (Note that if the cardio CRP is elevated, there is a 2–5 times increased risk of MI and other coronary events, and an increased risk for developing type 2 diabetes; in fact, if CRP >2.9, there is a RR increase of 2.7 of developing type 2 DM.) Increased CRP is seen in infections, smoking, type 2 DM, and obesity, all of which are risk factors themselves for developing vascular disease. The most significant drop in CRP is when sedentary adults change to a regular, low-to-moderate intensity exercise program. As exercise intensity, frequency, and duration increase, the CRP continues to drop. Of note is that anaerobic high-intensity training (interval training) can lead to an acute phase reaction and elevate CRP temporarily, so patients should be cautious with interval training.

Cholesterol. Not exercising is as harmful as a high cholesterol. Exercise can decrease the total cholesterol, LDL, and triglycerides.[13,14] A 1% decrease in total cholesterol is associated with a 2–3% risk reduction of coronary disease. The total cholesterol drop is variable, but appears to be 10–25 points. It is higher when combined with other interventions in obese patients with the metabolic syndrome. Exercise can also help increase the HDL; this is most noticeable in syndrome X patients and others who are overweight and have higher triglycerides. Endurance exercise leads to increased lipoprotein lipase, more breakdown of triglycerides, and more transfer to HDL.

Endocrine Benefits of Aerobic Exercise

- Improves insulin sensitivity[15] and decreases the likelihood of developing NIDDM.
- Decreases the need for medication for hypertension, hyperlipidemia, and dysglycemia if syndrome X or NIDDM is present.
- Decreases the need for insulin use if insulin-dependent diabetic.
- Facilitates weight loss.[16,17]
- Reduces total body fat.

Other Aerobic Exercise Benefits

- Improves immune function and resistance to infection.[18]
- Reduces stress.
- May decrease constipation (improved motility).
- Improves sleep (sleep onset can be disturbed if exercise starts after 8 pm).
- Decrease the risk of developing depression or reduces the severity of depression.[19,20]
- Improves symptoms of seasonal affective disorder (SAD) from lack of light.
- Facilitates detoxification.
- Reduces the risk of several common cancers: colon, breast, prostate.[21,22,23]

The Aerobic Exercise Prescription

It is very important to design a specific exercise program for each patient and to write it down. A sample Patient Exercise Calendar is provided in Figure 29.1. For aerobic exercise, the prescription should address the following issues:

Frequency: The number of exercise sessions per day and per week. To achieve basic health goals, patients should do 5–6 aerobic exercise sessions a week. (Patients can do two sessions per day of shorter duration if this is the only way that they can get the exercise in.)

Duration (Length): You would like your patients to do the minimum program of 30 minutes in their target heart rate zone each day. If they are just starting out, they can begin at 15 minutes and add a minute each session until they reach that 30-minute goal. For weight loss, 45–50 minutes a day of aerobic exercise is advised, in either one session or split sessions. Patients can work up to this target gradually. It is reasonable to walk for this long, but most patients should try two different modes of exercise for 20–25 minute sessions each (per day). An example would be 25 minutes on a bike and 20 minutes on a treadmill.

Patient Exercise Calendar

Name ______________________ Date ____________

Circle below all the benefits that you want to experience.

I want to:

- Reduce my risk for fatal heart attacks by as much as 50%.
- Reduce my risk of strokes by as much as 40%.
- Improve my cholesterol.
- Have better blood sugar for diabetes control or prevention.
- Decrease my blood pressure.
- Reduce my risk of injuries.
- Decrease my risk of colon cancer.
- Build muscle.
- Improve my immune system.
- Improve my tone and look better.
- Unload daily stress.
- Decrease my risk of falling.
- Improve my sleep.
- Slow down my aging process.
- Improve my mood.
- Improve my performance in a sport.
- Improve my endurance.
- Improve my flexibility.
- Lose weight.
- Improve strength.

Your maximum heart rate is calculated in this way:

220 - _____ (your age) = _____ (your maximum heart rate).

Your **heart rate training zones** are a pulse rate per minute of ______ -_______.

Your Exercise Prescription

Aerobic Exercise:

The suggested **length** of your aerobic sessions in your training heart rate zone is ____ minutes.

The suggested **frequency** of your exercise sessions is _____ times per week.

Your suggested **progress** schedule is: ______________________

Your **exercise options** are: ______________________

Strength Training Exercises:

Lunges ______________ Chest Press ______________
Squats ______________ Lat Pull Down ______________
Biceps curls ______________ Push ups (against the wall) ______________
Triceps ______________ Basic row ______________

Balance Training: ______________________

____

Stretching:

Achilles ______________ Quads ______________
Hamstrings ______________ Other: ______________

Figure 29.1 **Patient exercise calendar**

Intensity: The intensity of the aerobic workout should be in the heart rate zone you have recommended, or via a rating of perceived exertion.

Heart rate (pulse) zones are appropriate if a patient is not on a beta blocker or calcium channel blocker that could increase vagal tone and slow the heart rate. These zones are figured as a percentage of the patient's maximum calculated heart rate, which is 220 minus the patient's age. (This may be an underestimate in very fit people.) Multiply the calculated maximum heart rate by 60%, 70%, or 80% to determine the heart rate zone for the patient. Most patients should be in the 70–80% zone, which has been most studied for health benefits. Obese patients or those with a cardiac or pulmonary condition should start in the 60–70% zone and move up when they feel that this zone is too easy (and if there are no symptoms created by the exercising).

For patients with whom heart rate zones are not applicable, a perceived exertion scale can be used. Patients are asked to exercise at an intensity that represents 5–6 on a scale of 10; they should perceive that they are working somewhat hard, but not too hard.

Remind all patients that they should not be excessively winded and should be able to talk during their exercise.

Mode: Select the two or three most appropriate exercise options, taking into account the patient's medical conditions, life patterns and work demands, and health goals. Also consider any findings from the orthopedic exam, as well as what the patient finds enjoyable and can do pain free. It's a good idea for any clinician who is physically able to go to a gym and try out the different aerobic machines with a trainer, acquiring a good feel for the demands these machines make on the body. That will help with individualizing recommendations for your patients. See below for "Exercise Prescriptions for Special Conditions."

Progression: It's important that patients understand how and when to make the initial program more rigorous. For sedentary patients, it is advisable to underdose the duration initially; start at 15 minutes and add a minute for each subsequent exercise session until the desired duration is reached. Sedentary patients can normally begin at 60% of their maximum heart rate, raising it to 70% or the 70–80% zone within a few weeks. Patients who are already exercising, but not to the recommended dose (frequency, duration, or intensity) can start at 70% of the calculated maximum heart rate.

Evaluation: Follow up is essential. Check patient compliance with the aerobic prescription by using a Patient Exercise Record (sample provided in Figure 29.2) and scheduling return visits to discuss results and problems.

Characteristics and Benefits of Strength Training

Strength training can:

- Build more lean body mass (muscle).[24]
- Improve resting metabolic rate and aid in weight loss.
- Slow sarcopenia (loss of muscle with aging).[25]
- Build strength[26] to decrease the likelihood of injuries and falls.
- Improve function in activities of daily living.
- Stimulate growth hormone release.[27]
- Improve self confidence.
- Create a positive proactive attitude for other healthy life changes.

Strength Training Prescriptions

In order to write an individualized, specific strength training prescription, the concepts of sets, reps, and resistance must be understood, as well as how body regions work together and what precautions or restrictions to give, depending on the patient's musculoskeletal problems.

The exercise calendar (Figure 29.1) provides space to identify the specific strength training exercises for each patient. Individual recommendations should include those least likely to cause any pain or exacerbation of a current musculoskeletal problem. Instruct patients to do 2–3 sets of 10 repetitions per set; remind them that sets should be pain free. Arm and upper body exercises can be done with free weights or on machines at a gym. Recommend some training before beginning strength training—by reading about the approach, the risks, and how to ensure safe practices, or by enrolling for an in-person training session (or course) with a qualified instructor. For patients with medical or orthopedic problems, an experienced personal trainer who understands how to work with clients of varying abilities and for general health goals is probably an excellent idea.

Patient Exercise Record

Write the dates of each day in the month below. Record in each box the exercise activity you engaged in, the amount of time you spent doing it, and your heart rate (for aerobic exercise). If you did nothing that day, write a note to explain why you did not exercise. Bring this page with you to every clinic visit.

Month: ______________

Sunday	Monday	Tuesday	Wednesday	Thursday	Friday	Saturday
☐	☐	☐	☐	☐	☐	☐
☐	☐	☐	☐	☐	☐	☐
☐	☐	☐	☐	☐	☐	☐
☐	☐	☐	☐	☐	☐	☐
☐	☐	☐	☐	☐	☐	☐
☐	☐	☐	☐	☐	☐	☐

Record any problems associated with exercise:

Date	Type of Exercise	Description of Problem

Figure 29.2 **Patient exercise record**

Location of Strength Training

A complete strength training program is best done at a gym because of the variety of the equipment available and the multiple options for each type of exercise. If a patient exercises only at home, biceps curls, lunges, and squats will be their primary exercises. With a bench, patients can add a basic row, chest press, and triceps exercise. For the average patient, it is easier to use machines at a gym for most exercises, and to use free weights primarily for biceps curls and lunges.

A Basic Strength Training Program

Prescribe the following exercises to help your patient achieve most of the goals above:

- Biceps curls (with free weights)
- Triceps extensions
- Latissimus pulldowns
- Chest press
- Basic row
- Squats
- Lunges

It is recommended that the healthcare provider learn each of these exercises so as to understand the movement patterns and the muscles used.

Recommending Resistance Levels

Most patients should choose the amount of free weight or the amount on a machine or pulley system that will allow them to do two sets of 10–12 repetitions. In each set, they should experience fatigue in the last 1–2 repetitions. In general, patients should choose a weight that allows performance of the exercise without pain and with normal motion. A fitness trainer can usually choose an appropriate amount of weight for each exercise.

Patients for whom stimulating growth hormone is advisable will need to add squats[28] with a bar, use higher resistance, and do three sets of 10 repetitions of each exercise. The last two reps in each set should be very difficult but still safe.

Choosing Strength and Aerobic Exercise Based on Orthopedic Conditions

Wrist sprain or DJD: Strength training—avoid heavy weight lifting (biceps curls), pull-ups, and other forces that lead to wrist distraction. Avoid end-range dorsiflexion in push-ups. Aerobic—avoid boxing and tae bo classes. Avoid rowing and cross-country skiing, and hold on to the stationary bar while using an elliptical machine.

Elbow pain: Strength training—avoid excessive resistance and repetitive wrist extensions with significant loads. Limit rows, biceps curls, and latissimus (lat) pull downs. Aerobic—avoid rowing and cross-country skiing, caution with kickboxing.

Shoulder AC sprains and rotator cuff tendonitis: Strength training—avoid abduction and flexion above 90 degrees; avoid overhead press, pull-ups and lat pull-downs. Aerobic—avoid cross-country ski machines, rowing machines, tae bo classes and swimming.

Cervical sprain and DJD: Strength training—avoid quick rapid motions such as military press; avoid heavy squats with the neck loaded; avoid lat pull-downs to the posterior neck, overhead press and abdominal crunches with hands on the head, pulling the neck into flexion. Aerobic—avoid running, step aerobics, blading, downhill skiing, snow boarding, tae bo, kick boxing. Caution with bicycling on a road bike. A comfort bike with upright bars and a high stem is better.

Lumbosacral sprain, disc problems: Strength training—avoid lumbar extensions, military press, heavy squats, rapid knee extensions; avoid standing toe touches. Aerobic—avoid diving, snow boarding, downhill skiing, blading, tae bo, and soccer.

Sacroiliac conditions: Avoid exercises that will posteriorly rotate the pelvis in the position of dysfunction. Avoid excessive hamstring stretching. Minimize adductor (groin) exercises. Avoid exercises that involve lumbar flexion and rotation at the same time. Aerobic—avoid running, step aerobics, tae bo and boxing classes.

Hip DJD: Strength training—avoid high resistance and deep squats; avoid walking lunges. Be careful with hip exercises. Aerobic—avoid cross-country ski machines and skiing, Avoid fast swimming, blading, and soccer.

Patellofemoral (kneecap) conditions and IT band syndrome (similar precautions for severe DJD of the knee): Strength training—avoid deep squats, limit depth of lunges. Aerobic—caution with running, step aerobics, steep or fast downhill hiking, bicycling, and stairmaster. With patella tendonitis, all of the above recommendations stand, except bicycling is OK and volleyball, basketball, and all jumping should be avoided.

Ankle sprains: Avoid high-impact aerobic activities initially; avoid basketball, kick boxing, tae bo classes, and other jumping activities.

Balance Exercises for Older Patients and Those with Neurodegenerative Disorders

It is essential to test balance in any patient with a neurodegenerative disorder and in patients over age 60. Preventing falls in your patients is extremely important. Patients who fall can break their hips and wrists or injure their spine. A broken hip is a high risk factor for a deep vein thrombosis. Studies have indicated that physical training can improve balance in the elderly,[29] and in people with neurodegenerative diseases like Parkinson's.[30,31] It is the author's clinical experience of 10 years that balance training can be effective in improving gait, decreasing falls, and decreasing the pain of lower extremity musculoskeletal syndromes.

Testing Balance

There are three planes of balance: the sagittal plane, which is in front and back of the patient; the frontal plane, which is to the left and right; and the transverse plane, which is a rotational plane. Patients can have dysfunction in any or all of these planes. Dysfunction in the sagittal plane and frontal plane are the most common, are the easiest to test, and improve with basic exercises. If the patient shows signs of dysfunction when using a specific balance test, use the test itself as the exercise. Signs of balance dysfunction are wobbling and quick motions of the arms, legs or torso. In general, most static balance exercises can be done in sets of 8–10 and practiced for 5 seconds each, working up to 10 seconds. Patients should work toward equal balance on both legs.

Sagittal Plane Static Balance Tests

Start with these tests if a patient is frail or has questionable balance. The patient stands with both knees bent slightly to engage the quadriceps, and raises one foot slightly off the floor. Measure the time that balance can be maintained on one foot without touching the floor with the raised foot, and without abruptly moving the arms; perform on the other foot, and compare results. At least 5–10 seconds on each foot is desirable. If performing this exercise is too difficult, have the patient stand with hands holding onto a chair back or the exam table. One foot is raised with toes touching the floor, and then the amount of pressure needed for holding onto the chair is gradually lessened. The challenge can be intensified by lifting the raised foot completely off the ground while still holding on. When balance improves with this approach, the exercise can progress to raising the foot, toe touching the ground, but the hands no longer holding onto the chair. These exercises should be done 5 times on each foot, every other day. Patients should be trained on how to progress to the next level of difficulty, and the instructions should be written down. When patients can do at least 5 seconds on each leg with the foot completely off the floor and without holding on, they can progress to the next set of tests and exercises.

With knees slightly bent and one foot raised completely (or with toe touching the floor), add the following movements: <u>Level 1</u>—Arm swinging, both arms together, forwards and backwards in short ranges of motion, up to 45 degrees in front of them. <u>Level 2</u>—Arm swinging that reaches an angle of 90 degrees with the floor. <u>Level 3</u>—Swing the arms to 90 degrees and increase speed to intensify the challenge in the sagittal plane. Patients should begin with the level that is difficult but possible, and work their way up to the third level. These exercises should be done 5 times on each foot for 5–10 seconds at a time.

Patients with poor sitting balance can do the following exercises while seated on a chair or a physioball. Perform the arm swings as described above, with both feet firmly on the floor (<u>Level 1</u>); only the heels touching the ground (<u>Level 2</u>); one foot firmly on the floor and the other foot off the floor (<u>Level 3</u>).

Sagittal Plane Dynamic Balance Tests

Sagittal plane lunge. The lunge exercise is one of the most functional exercises patients can do for lower body strength and balance. It is useful for virtually anyone who is trying to improve balance and build lower extremity strength. The beginning exercise is 5 lunges on each foot, done at a level in which the patient is slightly unsteady.

For a forward lunge, the patient starts in a standing position with feet parallel to one another and 1–2 shoe widths apart. One foot is moved about 1½ to 2 feet forward of the other, allowing the front knee to bend. The excursion of the lunge is the length from where the toe begins in the start position to where the heel makes first contact with the surface after the lunge. Patients shorter than 5'5" may wish to start with a one-foot excursion and progress the lunge excursion gradually. Most lunges should be performed within a 1½ to 2-foot excursion, although some may exceed this range if there is an activity that requires longer lunge movements. Before progressing to longer lunges, however, these guidelines should be followed:

1. The movement should be pain-free.
2. Wobbling or swaying of the knees or torso should be minimal.
3. The low back should be in a neutral position, with minimal forward or side-to-side motion of the back with the lunge.
4. Before increasing the excursion of the lunge past 2 feet, try increasing the speed of the lunges while maintaining good control of motion.

Control the speed of knee flexion and stop at about 55–60 degrees. Eventually, patients may go into a deeper lunge. Allow the back knee to bend and the back foot to lift up at the heel. Try to align the forward knee over the first and second toes. Return to the start position by pushing off the front foot. Initially do the lunge with one foot going forward and back.

Same side lunges. Lunge on the right foot for a set of 5–6 repetitions, and then do another set on the left foot.

Alternating lunges. When the form is steady and the patient is not wobbling, the exercise can be done by alternating the feet on each lunge, working up to a set that includes 5–10 lunges on each side.

In most workout routines, patients should do two sets of whichever lunge variation has been chosen.

Tips and precautions. If the forward lunge is painful, try decreasing the depth of knee flexion and add lunges in different directions, especially to the sides. If a lunge is still painful, try unloading it with the arms, as described below. In any lunge, make sure the knee is in line with the foot.

The unloaded lunge, or "no-knee-pain lunge." Patients may unload a lunge to decrease kneecap pain or if this is the only way they can do a lunge. Ski poles, dowels, or 2 chair backs are used to support part of the body weight through the arms as the knee is bent in the basic lunge. Enough weight should be supported by the arms so that the knees do not hurt and the patient does not wobble.

Static Frontal Plane Balance Tests

Some patients with neurodegenerative disorders and some elderly patients will demonstrate balance dysfunction in the frontal plane, and will benefit from exercises done in this plane.

Frontal plane balance test with arm swing. Have the patient balance on one foot with the knee slightly bent and the opposite foot raised (or toe touching the floor beside the balance foot). Test for balance and time the position can be maintained; as balance improves, progress to a level where balancing is a challenge and work there. Exercises should be practiced five times on each foot. Level 1—Swing the arms together across the front of the body, side to side in short ranges of motions, at first initially up to 45 degrees. Level 2—Do Level 1, but swing the arms faster to increase the momentum and challenge in the frontal plane.

Dynamic Frontal Plane Balance Tests

Frontal plane lunge. This test is performed by having the patient lunge 90 degrees to the right with the right foot, keeping the lunge foot parallel to the non-lunge foot (fixed foot) while bending the ankles, knees, and hips and keeping the back upright. Then the patient pushes off the lunge foot to return to the start position. Patient should do three consecutive lunges to the right and three to the left. Compare their stability, form, and ability to keep the torso steady and the back in good alignment. If there are differences between the sides, or difficulties on both sides, assign this as an exercise with five lunges each to the right and left in a set, and two sets every other day.

Exercise Prescription for Special Conditions

Osteoporosis Prevention Program

Patients with osteopenia or osteoporosis (and perimenopausal females) need exercise as an important element in maintaining bone mass.[32] Physical activity provides mechanical stress to bone, which stimulates bone formation. It is important to impact-load both the forearms every other day and the legs on most days. Strength training with the arms can help prevent significant declines in arm bone density, which can lead to a Colles fracture of the radius. Instruct the patient to do a squat with an arm assist by holding onto the backs of two chairs with the feet firmly on the ground. Once they reach a partial squat position, they simultaneously straighten their knees and elbows. Have them do two sets of these along with two sets of 10 biceps curls.

Aerobic exercise that involves moderate-impact loading through the feet and legs can help slow bone loss in the hips and spine. Walking, treadmill, aerobics classes, hiking, elliptical trainer, stairmaster, or jogging are all viable options. Note that the elliptical machine and stairmaster are less impact-loading and should be used with the other more impact-loaded aerobic workouts.

Exercise for CFIDS, Multiple Chemical Sensitivities (MCS), and Fibromyalgia Patients

Patients with fibromyalgia, MCS or CFIDS can benefit from an exercise program,[33] but be very cautious with aerobic exercise, as they may have prolonged fatigue after an aerobic exercise session. Evaluate the level of fatigue they experience with activities of daily living and with aerobic exercise. If significant fatigue is experienced, start with a strength and balance program. Use a functional medicine approach and consider supplements to improve energy.

When the patient reports that enough energy is available to do daily living tasks, consider a low-intensity (50% of max HR) and short-duration (10 minutes) aerobic program two times/week. If the patient tolerates this program, add 1 minute duration every two sessions until the patient has reached 30 minutes per session. Increase the intensity cautiously by 2–5% per week until the patient has reached 60–70% max HR (or the perceived level of effort that is manageable). Decrease the intensity and duration if significant post-exercise fatigue returns.

Supplements may improve a patient's ability to do aerobic exercise. Trying a supplement program for patients with fatigue in daily life activities or for those who can't tolerate brisk walking is a reasonable step. Consider supplementation with CoQ10, 200–300 mg/day and L-carnitine, 1000 mg 3x/day.

Patients with fibromyalgia should be started on a careful strength training program, using only a few upper body exercises at a time (such as biceps curls and triceps exercises). Add one new exercise per week, and use a lower amount of resistance, as these patients are prone to strains and cervical injury. Initiate a walking program, or exercise in a gym, at lowered intensity for 15 minutes, adding one minute every other workout until a duration of 30 minutes, at 60–70% intensity, is reached. Progress to the next intensity level as the patient is able.

Obesity

As noted in the aerobic exercise discussion above, obese patients benefit from longer duration aerobic sessions so they can burn more fat for fuel and more calories. Follow the aerobics guidelines under duration above and progress to 45–50 minute workouts. Incorporate strength training, but let the patient know that this will slow weight loss initially and then will enhance it by helping to increase muscle mass. Most overweight individuals can do stationary bike and the elliptical machines, as well as water aerobics.

The Metabolic Syndrome

Aerobic exercise done as in the paragraph above will increase a patient's sensitivity to insulin and will benefit all aspects of the metabolic syndrome. Patients should experience an improvement in blood pressure and blood sugars within the first two weeks. With only 10–20 pounds lost, significant improvements can be achieved in energy levels, blood sugar, and blood pressure. HDL can be raised and triglycerides lowered. If patients are on numerous insulin-sensitizing supplements and on drug therapy, it is important to monitor their progress closely. After three weeks of regular daily exercise, it is important to monitor the blood pressure and blood sugar to watch out for hypoglycemia. If blood sugars are coming down, medications such as metformin and other drugs may need to be reduced. Blood pressure medication may also be decreased over time, especially if the patient loses weight (10–20 pounds). For overweight patients, ½–1 pound lost per week is a reasonable outcome. If a moderate-intensity exercise program is desired, it is a good idea to obtain a treadmill stress test first to rule out significant ischemia with exercise, as there are many vascular risk factors with diabetes and metabolic syndrome.

Gaining Compliance with an Exercise Calendar

Achieving compliance with the exercise prescription is very important. Emphasize to patients that the exercise calendar and patient record (see Figures 29.1 and 29.2) can be very helpful—particularly when the health benefits have been circled on the top of the page to remind patients daily of their goals. Write in the aerobic exercise prescription with all the details about how you would like them to start and progress.

Circle the strength training exercises at the bottom and write in the balance exercises you are recommending. A normal program would be to recommend aerobic exercise five to six times per week, three strength training sessions per week, and balance exercises every other day. Provide handouts explaining the balance exercises in detail; providing pictures is helpful, as is demonstrating the exercises in the office until the patient can reproduce them accurately.

Other suggestions for improving patient compliance include the following:

- Ask patients to bring their calendar and patient record with them to every clinic visit, so that their program can be evaluated and updated if needed.
- Explain that it's important to record when exercise is not done, and the reason, so that if there are continuing obstacles to performing the complete program, they can be identified and resolved.
- Ask patients to note any symptoms or problems with their exercise, so they can be evaluated and addressed.

When patients bring in their records and calendars, review them, make sure the information is being recorded completely, address any problems, and answer any questions. If you change the prescription, fill out another calendar (and remind patients to circle their goals as well).

If a patient is missing many exercise sessions, gently address the issue by asking questions to elicit the reasons:

1. What do you think is in the way of fitting in all your exercise sessions?
2. Are you having any worrisome symptoms or scheduling problems?
3. If you were to advise me, as if I were your patient, on how to schedule all the recommended exercise, what would be your suggestions?

The most common reasons for poor compliance are:

1. Scheduling difficulties. (Patients may say, "I do not have enough time. I am working too much.")
2. Pain on exercising (usually knee, hip, or back pain).
3. It is too hard.

Whatever the patient's excuse, it is important to address the problem, avoiding criticism or judgment. Any pain problems should be immediately evaluated and addressed—changing the program may be the answer. If the program level is too difficult, move it down a step or two. Help with planning and time management can be offered, as well as scheduling suggestions (see below). Remind patients of their health goals and the role that exercise plays in achieving them. Validate <u>any</u> exercise that they do. As discussed in Chapter 36, it's rare that a person will immediately adopt new health behaviors and never relapse. Most of us cycle through our process of change several times, and we all need support.

Scheduling Exercise

There are issues to consider in scheduling exercise. Most people will exercise when they have the most energy or when they want to relieve stress; they look for times when there are no other more important demands to be met. It is best to write the schedule down on a daily calendar so that it is not left to memory or chance. In general, patients are more likely to exercise first thing in the morning or at lunch time. If they are going to exercise at lunch time and will be doing moderate intensity exercise, they will likely need at least an hour in their schedule to fit in the 30 minute basic exercise session along with changing and showering. Most people are tired at the end of the day and will not exercise then unless they are very committed to their program. Patients can also schedule and do their exercise in two short periods, such as a 10–15 minute walk at their break times or during their lunch period.

Ask patients when they can schedule exercise sessions and, if they miss the planned time, whether there is a backup time they could use. Note that, for patients with sleep problems, exercise after 8 pm is not a good idea.

Charging and Billing for the Exercise-focused Visit

Visits focusing on exercise should be encouraged. Practitioners can bill for an office visit using the standard time-based procedure codes. If you demonstrate balance or strength exercises, you can add codes such as Kinetic Activities (1–2 units, 15 or 30 minute sessions). You can combine the visit focusing on exercise with reviewing labs or another billable concern or activity.

Summary

Prescribing exercise is a skill that can take a while to develop. Your prescription should be individualized to each patient. It is important to encourage and monitor your patients' compliance to see that goals are being met. For more information on aerobic machines and balance and strength exercise options, there are numerous references including *Conditioning for Outdoor Fitness: Functional Exercise and Nutrition for Every Body*.[34] Your patients will notice improved health and wellness outcomes as they achieve their exercise goals.

Manipulative Therapy and Functional Medicine: Clinical Interactions between Structure and Function

David Wickes, DC

Introduction

Changes in structure can affect the function of any component within the body, from the cell to major organ systems. At the simplest level, it is relatively easy to attribute local symptoms and visible asymmetry to structural imbalances. Most practitioners have encountered patients with an antalgic posture secondary to lumbar disc herniation, swelling and ecchymosis from an acute ankle sprain, and the distorted chest wall and unleveled shoulders seen in severe kyphoscoliosis. Cause-and-effect relationships in these presentations are often easily determined, and a therapeutic management plan can be logically derived. Often unrecognized and unappreciated, however, are the more subtle structural imbalances involving macro- and micro-systems. The rest of this chapter will explore how these structural imbalances may result in local and remote system malfunctions and resulting signs and symptoms.

Structural integrity is essential to optimal function. In biology, as is the case with architecture and engineering, structure influences function. In genomics, amino acid type and sequence determine genetic structure, which in turn affects protein synthesis. Cell and organelle membrane structure affect many local functions, including hormone receptor activity, energy production, permeability, transportation, and storage. In turn, altered cell function affects organ function. Attention is devoted in functional medicine to structural imbalances at all levels in the organism, as well as to the concept that disturbed function can, in turn, lead to changes in structure. Thus, instead of a unidirectional, linear pathway, a more appropriate view is of a complex interactive relationship.

Structural Changes at the Micro Level

The changes that occur in cell membranes incorporating abnormal lipid moieties serve to illustrate the relationship between structure and function at the cellular and tissue level. Cell membranes are composed of a complex double layer of phospholipids, intermixed with cholesterol and glycoproteins. The protein component includes receptors, transport mechanisms, and enzymes. Rather than a static structure, the cell membrane is constantly in a state of flux, reshaping its dynamic structure as function requires.[35] During the course of cell and organelle membrane formation or repair, phospholipids and free fatty acids are incorporated into the structure. The free fatty acids are primarily present in the *cis* configuration, although small amounts of *trans* configured fatty acids may also be present normally. Although *trans* fatty acids can be found in dairy products and can also be synthesized by colonic bacteria, most *trans* fatty acids entering the body come from fried or mass-produced foods. If abnormal amounts of *trans* fatty acids are in the bloodstream and interstitial fluids, they may be taken up by the cell and incorporated into the membranes in place of the *cis* fatty acids normally used. Similarly, changes in the relative concentration and availability of normal essential fatty acids may result in alterations of membrane composition. It is now recognized that the changes effected by fatty acids extend beyond the simple concept of membrane lipid replacement to include binding of fatty acids to nuclear receptors and subsequent alteration of gene transcription.[36] As these fatty acid abnormalities occur, the cell may develop different membrane characteristics.[37] Replacement of membrane lipids with *trans* fatty acids or saturated fats reduces cell membrane fluidity.[38] Cell receptors may become inhibited or defective, leading to neurotransmitter or hormonal blockade.[39] Prostaglandin synthesis may become disturbed, either due to changes in the type and availability of fatty acids, or to changes in the function of formational enzymes. High levels of *trans* fatty acids may lead to deficiency of essential fatty acids. Membrane permeability and carrier-mediated transport can become disturbed, resulting in intracellular nutrient deficiencies and a reduction in protein formation and secretion. These structural changes at the molecular level have widespread implications in health and disease, including alteration of insulin receptor function and the potential evolution of the metabolic syndrome and type 2 diabetes, alterations in the immune response to infectious agents and mutagenic stimuli, response to inflammatory disease, and the development of cardiac disease.

Structural Changes at the Macro Level

At the other end of the structural spectrum, the practitioner must consider the possibility that organ functional abnormalities might be the result of, or aggravated by, osseous, connective tissue, and muscle structural lesions. The chiropractic and osteopathic professions were founded after observation and theorization that neuromusculoskeletal abnormalities could lead to organ system dysfunction and frank pathology. In the 1890s, these professions were based upon hypotheses that vertebral malpositioning ("subluxation" or joint "lesion") could cause spinal nerve or vascular impingement and lead to both local symptoms as well as remote pathophysiology. This evolved over the subsequent decade into a monocausal theory in which the subluxation was felt to be the sole or primary cause of disease. The monocausal philosophy crumbled under scientific scrutiny and was gradually replaced by the current conceptual model, in which the subluxation is considered as one of many possible contributory factors to illness. The subluxation itself has been redefined as an articular dysfunction (joint fixation), with a wide spectrum of theoretical neurobiologic local and remote effects. This current model fits the functional medicine concept in which the clinician must look for the presence of core clinical imbalances, one of which is structural, and any of which may disturb or influence the web-like communication pathways of the body.

Structural imbalances may develop in any part of the neuromusculoskeletal system and may have a primary influence on organ function (i.e., they may cause pathophysiology); or, they may be secondary to either organ system dysfunction or other structural problems. In the functional medicine context, the respective terms somatovisceral and viscerosomatic are too limiting unless conceptually these terms are expanded to include more than just the organ or tissue (see Figure 29.3).

Structural imbalances can be due to congenital or developmental deficits, or they can be acquired. The ability of the organism to adapt to these deficits will determine both short- and long-term effects. Examples of congenital/developmental deficits include anatomical short legs, joint deformities, hemivertebrae, cervical ribs, absent muscles, and foot deformities. Acquired deficits can result from poor posture, trauma, stress, psychological factors, irritation (e.g., inflammation, toxins), and hormonal alterations (e.g., myalgias and myopathy in hypothyroidism).

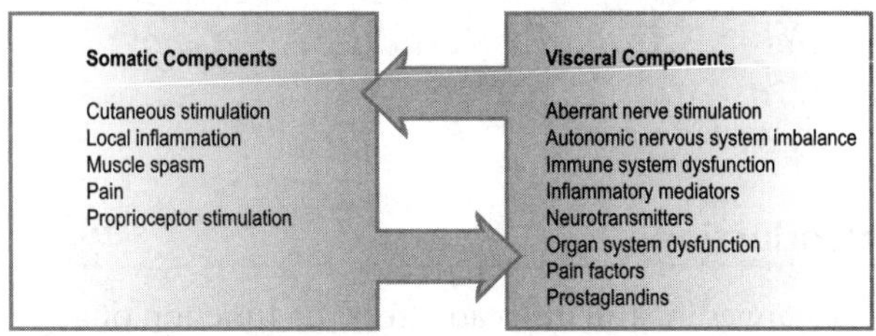

Figure 29.3 **Somatovisceral interrelationships**

The mechanisms by which structural abnormalities at the macro-level result in pathophysiology are diverse (see Table 29.1). Some of these, such as sciatic nerve irritation in vertebral disc disorders, are relatively easy to determine clinically; however, other presentations are subtler. Cervical spine facet injuries and asymmetric facet motion may result in errant proprioceptive signals, initiating dizziness, vertigo, nausea, and possible ocular dysfunction. Aberrant stimulation of afferent and efferent nerves by altered joint motion or local inflammatory mediators may cause both local as well as remote effects. Local changes might consist of pain and muscle spasm. Remote changes include possible referred pain syndromes, facilitation or blockade of spinal cord reflex pathways, and irritation of the reticular activating system. These changes, in turn, may lead to fatigue, disruption of sleep patterns, changes in circulating adrenal hormones, other hormonal fluctuations, and changes in autonomic tone.

Table 29.1 **Pathophysiologic Mechanisms in Structural Abnormalities**

Aberrant nerve stimulation
Arterial compression (e.g., vascular outlet syndromes)
Autonomic nervous system regulatory abnormalities
Compromised respiration and thoracic cage movement
Focal hypoxia
Mechanical pressure (e.g., herniated intervertebral disc)
Proprioceptive disturbances
Secondary inflammatory changes
Venous and lymphatic congestion

Conditions Associated with Structural Imbalances

Fibromyalgia

Isolated trigger or tender points may be responsible for both local and referred pain patterns. Fibromyalgia is an example of a clinical disorder primarily presenting with somatic complaints, which may become complicated by other organ system dysfunctions if not appropriately managed. When tender points occur in multiple locations, then fibromyalgia or chronic myofascial pain syndrome should be considered. A thorough somatic assessment should include assessment of the 18 classic locations of fibromyalgia tender (trigger) points, with appreciation that the diagnostic criteria for that disorder include finding tender points at 11 or more of these sites.[40] Fibromyalgia patients may develop dyspepsia, abdominal pain, and other symptoms of the irritable bowel syndrome, and these patients tend to be more sensitive to somatic pain stimuli.[41] Animal studies have demonstrated that noxious somatic afferent stimulation promotes visceral hyperalgesia via spinal cord interactions, establishing a means for the production of intestinal symptoms.[42,43] It therefore seems reasonable to assess irritable bowel syndrome patients for signs and symptoms of fibromyalgia, and to institute treatment of the somatic component in the hopes of amelioration of visceral symptoms. Fibromyalgia, chronic fatigue syndrome, irritable bowel disease, and other chronic functional disorders often co-exist, so the presence of one of these should prompt a physical assessment for fibromyalgic tender points.

Vascular Changes

Stagnation and congestion of interstitial, lymphatic, and venous fluids is another pathophysiologic state with a somatic component. Although peripheral edema is often dismissed as simply a fluid imbalance, the clinician must keep in mind that these fluids are rich in cellular and humeral components. Accumulation of these fluids in the interstitial compartment may lead to decreased cell nutrition, impaired tissue repair, and compromised immune function. Appropriate exercise, support garments, limb positioning, and lymphatic massage therapy can help reduce edema.

Various outlet disorders can compromise peripheral nerve, arterial, and venous function. Most outlet disorders, including the common thoracic outlet and carpal tunnel syndromes, have predominantly a neurological presentation because the nerves are more vulnerable to compression than the vascular components. Assessment for these conditions typically involves attempts to reproduce symptoms by functional maneuvers and sustained limb positions. What is often underappreciated is the potential for these outlet syndromes to develop in patients with abnormal spinal function associated with nerve root compression proximal to the additional compression at the outlet (i.e., a "double-crush" injury). Other subtle disorders, including vitamin B12 deficiency, mild hypothyroidism, and inflammatory joint disorders may further predispose the nerve to dysfunction. These conditions, in turn, may also explain why some patients do not respond to manual therapy alone.

Inflexibility and Contractions

A gradual loss of flexibility often goes unnoticed by the patient. Chronic contractions and shortening of ligaments and tendons lead to abnormal compensatory positions and motions, contributing to overall physical stress and a tendency for patients to avoid physical exercise. Sit-and-reach testing assesses for decreased low-back, hip, hamstring, and calf flexibility. Routine evaluation should also include range of motion testing of the neck, trunk, shoulders, and ankles. Abnormalities of peripheral musculoskeletal structures may result in secondary abnormalities of the axial musculoskeletal system..

Vertigo

Another example of the structure-function relationship is benign positional vertigo. This syndrome is characterized by episodic vertigo triggered by certain head positions. The pathophysiologic explanation for this disorder is that calcium carbonate debris suspended in the inner ear fluid becomes lodged or displaced and abnormally stimulates vestibular reflexes. Pharmacologic therapy is generally ineffective; however, a physical maneuver (canalith repositioning procedure, "Epley maneuver") that places the patient's head in a particular sequence of positions designed to promote the movement of the debris back into the utricle has shown to be very effective.[44] Unfortunately, many patients with benign positional vertigo are ineffectively treated because the physician has neglected to perform the simple functional head positioning tests needed to diagnose the disorder.

The Functional Assessment

Changes in spinal motion can lead to irritation of other spinal structures and possible secondary neurobiological phenomena. Unless accompanied by pain, the patient may be unaware of the restricted motion. Gross screening procedures such as toe touching and assessment of head flexion and extension may fail to detect subtle restrictions. The functional medicine assessment for structural deviations from optimal health should include postural and morphological observations, evaluation for signs of lymphatic or venous congestion, palpation for abnormal muscle tone and fibromyalgia tender points, evaluation of flexibility and joint motion, assessment of respiratory chest motion, and dynamic palpation of the spine (see Table 29.2). Careful postural evaluation can reveal changes in muscle symmetry, scoliosis, and antalgic positioning, but may miss more subtle intersegmental motion abnormalities. Because of this, it is recommended that the functional assessment minimally include direct posterior-to-anterior dynamic palpation using the thumb and index finger or the palm of the hand to test for blocks of restricted intersegmental motion. Respiratory excursion should also be assessed. Unfortunately, the musculoskeletal examination is an oft-neglected component in medical education, and many non-orthopedist clinicians lack competence in the diagnosis and management of musculoskeletal disorders.[45] Should the functional screening demonstrate abnormalities, or if the practitioner is unfamiliar with the assessment procedures, the patient can be referred to a chiropractic or osteopathic physician for more comprehensive evaluation.

Treatment Approaches

Manipulation in Musculoskeletal Disorders

Back pain. There is substantial evidence that manipulative therapy is effective in the management of many musculoskeletal disorders. Most of this type of therapy is in the form of high-velocity, low-amplitude directional thrusts. Other forms of manipulative therapy, including lower-velocity procedures, localized distraction, general joint mobilization, soft-tissue manipulation, and instrument-assisted procedures may be useful in specific situations. The most common musculoskeletal complaints seen by chiropractic physicians are low-back pain, neck pain, and cervicogenic headache. Numerous randomized clinical trials have assessed the efficacy of manipulative therapy in acute low-back pain. A meta-analysis in 1992 concluded that spinal manipulation is often of short-term benefit in uncomplicated, acute low-back pain.[46] A large study in 1995 demonstrated that patients with low-back pain showed rapid improvement with chiropractic manipulation.[47] A 2004 multicenter randomized clinical trial demonstrated that manipulation improves back function, and that the improvement could be increased by the addition of an exercise program.[48] Both U.S. and British national clinical practice guidelines for the management of low-back pain recommended the inclusion of manipulation, although the former was not updated in the decade following issuance and is now considered obsolete.[49,50] A systematic review of 17 clinical guidelines for acute low-back pain found that one of the consistent recommendations was spinal manipulation for pain relief.[51]

Table 29.2 Screening Assessment for Structural Dysfunction

Gait
Posture
- Asymmetry
- Abnormal curves
- Deformity
- Shoulder and iliac crest heights
- Patellar and ankle relationships

Body habitus
Shoe (sole and heel) wear pattern
Compression marks from clothing
Edema
Venous distension and skin discoloration
Fibromyalgia tender point survey
Flexibility assessment
Spinal and large joint ranges of motion
Spinal passive motion
Paraspinal muscle palpation
Respiratory thoracic cage excursion

Neck pain and headache. The application of manipulation in the management of neck pain has also been studied, although not as extensively. A 2004 review assessed the efficacy of manipulation in neck pain and low-back pain and found that the evidence was inconclusive regarding its value in acute neck pain, but for acute and chronic low-back pain and chronic neck pain, manipulation was a viable treatment option.[52] A Cochrane review concluded that manipulation, when done in conjunction with exercise, is beneficial for chronic mechanical neck disorders.[53] Cervicogenic headache, i.e., headache caused by cervical spine dysfunction, is commonly treated with manipulation and other physical modalities. These headaches are often associated with autonomic nervous system symptoms, such as nausea and photophobia, and may be confused with migraine headache. A study comparing the effects of high-velocity, low-amplitude manipulation to soft-tissue therapy showed manipulation to be superior, to result in decreased medication reliance, and to decrease the duration and frequency of headaches.[54]

Manipulation and Non-musculoskeletal Disorders

Although the treatment of musculoskeletal disorders with manipulation and other forms of physical medicine is well established, the evidence for the integration of this therapy into the management of non-musculoskeletal conditions is less supported by the literature. Historical perspectives and numerous published anecdotal or small studies suggest that manipulation has a role to play, but rigorous scientific study has lagged well behind the theoretical explanations of mechanism and efficacy.

Structural asymmetry or gait abnormalities may place an additional burden upon the organ systems. In patients with cardiac failure, chronic obstructive lung disease, or other cardiopulmonary disorders, it is easy for the clinician to neglect the musculoskeletal system as a possible contributory factor. Patients with symptomatic knee or hip arthritis have diminished walking speed and a resultant energy cost.[55] Leg length inequality, either congenital or acquired, may result in compensatory postural adaptations, including pelvic tilt and changes in pelvic and lumbar muscle activity and resultant increased energy demands.

There are complex and overlapping interactions between structure and function at the tissue and organ level. Stimulation of spinal afferent nerves from local spinal and paraspinal tissues or distant organs or somatic structures can result in reflex stimulation of autonomic efferent nerves (i.e., "somatovisceral" reflex) as well as referred pain. These normal reflex pathways can become sustained or exaggerated, leading to dysfunction of the effector organs. The autonomic nervous system has complex interactions with other organ systems, and changes in the activity or tone of the parasympathetic or sympathetic components can trigger a cascade of pathophysiologic events that extend beyond the directly innervated structure. Table 29.3 lists some of the disorders (excluding those classic conditions associated with total autonomic failure) linked to changes in autonomic nervous system balance or regulation.

Table 29.3 **Pathophysiology Linked to Autonomic Nervous System Dysfunction**

Anxiety
Asthma
Cardiac arrhythmias
Chronic fatigue syndrome
Depression
Fibromyalgia
Gastroesophageal reflux disease
Hypertension
Idiopathic carpal tunnel syndrome
Infertility
Irritable bowel syndrome
Menstrual disorders
Metabolic syndrome
Migraine
Neuropathic pain syndromes
Orthostatic hypotension
Peptic ulcer
Raynaud's phenomenon

As an example of the effects of altered structure upon the autonomic nervous system, movement of inflamed peripheral joints can result in increased blood pressure and heart rate.[56] Patients with chronic myofascial pain or inflammatory arthritis have heightened sympathetic nervous system activity coupled with diminished cardiac parasympathetic activity.[57] In fibromyalgia, patients frequently have fatigue, anxiety, headache, weakness, and irritable bowel symptoms. The primary fibromyalgia pain, as well as these accompanying symptoms, may be attributed to a sympathetic hyperdynamic state.[58] Fibromyalgia patients appear to respond favorably to manipulative care, and such care may further enhance the positive effects of medications.[59]

Some genitourinary disorders have been shown to have a structural basis. The pelvic floor fascia and musculature provide mechanical support to the lower urinary tract and interact with the somatic and autonomic nervous systems to coordinate sphincter and bladder activity. It has long been appreciated that pelvic floor exercises can be useful in controlling minor stress incontinence. It has now become apparent that interstitial cystitis and the urethral syndrome may also respond to myofascial therapy aimed at the pelvic floor. In a study of 52 patients with some form of interstitial cystitis or the urgency-frequency syndrome, more than 70% had moderate or marked improvement after treatment with manual trigger point therapy to the pelvic floor muscles.[60] Another study showed that a transvaginal application of a massage technique first described in the 1930s as an intrarectal therapy for coccydynia was effective in relieving symptoms of interstitial cystitis and restoring proper pelvic floor tone.[61]

Even in the absence of specific causal relationships between spinal dysfunction and organ dysfunction, the presence of somatovisceral and viscerosomatic reflexes can obscure the clinical presentation. A study of back pain and abdominal pain revealed that the vast majority of patients with abdominal pain experienced concomitant back pain and the vast majority of patients with back pain also had abdominal abnormalities on physical examination.[62] Whether induced by pain or lifestyle, decreased physical activity and increased caloric intake further complicate these disorders by isturbing diurnal rhythms and shifting the balance between the sympathetic and parasympathetic nervous systems.[63]

A Common Pathway of Pathophysiology Initiated by Structural Change

Regardless of the initial etiology of the patient's disorder, in many patients there is an associated common pathway of pathophysiology characterized by aberrant activity or noxious stimulation of the nervous system or other feedback mechanisms. This irritation may simply result in localized discomfort or other regional symptoms, or may result in widespread changes in cardiovascular, neurological, humeral, or immune dysfunction. Conversely, primary disorders in those systems may result in secondary dysfunction of the neuromusculoskeletal system. From a functional medicine perspective, clinical improvement may result from introducing a change in one or more of the many interconnected pathophysiologic pathways. The nature and number of these interventions is determined by the patient's anatomical, biochemical, functional, environmental, and psychological individuality. For example, a patient with low-back pain due to a facet disorder may respond well to manipulation aimed at restoring joint motion, to botanical or pharmacologic agents aimed at neutralizing inflammatory mediators, to massage or biofeedback aimed at relaxing spastic muscles, to acupuncture to restore balance of energy pathways, or to some combination of those modalities. A patient with a non-musculoskeletal disorder resistant to initial therapy should be assessed for possible contributory structural faults, the correction of which might be sufficient to shift the balance towards recovery. Figure 29.4 shows some of the complex interrelationships between structural and functional factors in disease. From this diagram, one can see how different therapeutic approaches may produce the same outcome, and how a management plan that fails to appreciate the web-like connectivity of the body may fail to break a disorder's vicious cycle.

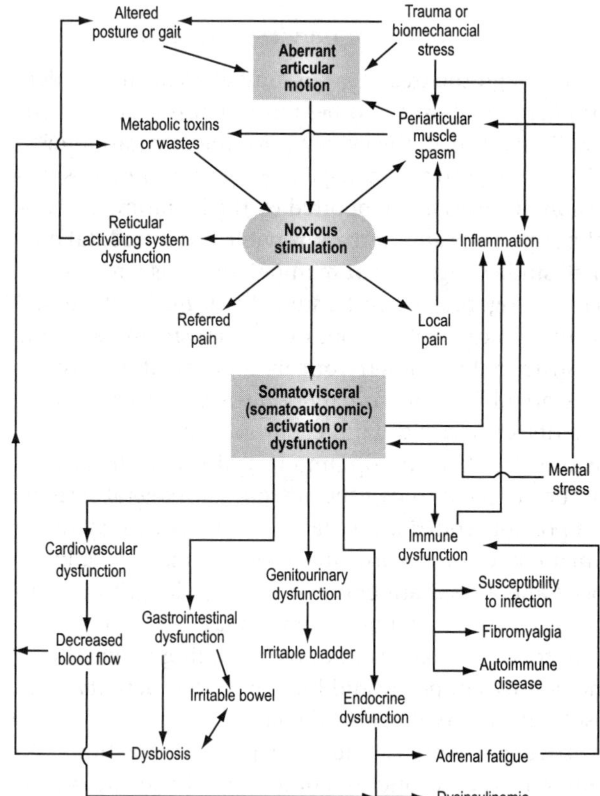

Figure 29.4 **Pathophysiology in structural imbalance and autonomic nervous system dysfunction**

Summary

Structure is a major determinant of function and this axiom applies to all levels of the body, from the genes to the axial skeleton and body organs. Structural change at the cellular level can result in altered cell metabolism, changes in receptor activity, defective enzyme and protein synthesis, abnormal repair and reproduction, abnormal membrane permeability, and defective signaling. At the other end of the structure spectrum, changes in the neuromusculoskeletal system can result in pathophysiology ranging from pain syndromes to increased energy consumption, somatoautonomic reflex activation, and organ reserve depletion. Because of the complex interactions of the musculoskeletal, humeral, immune, autonomic, and central nervous systems, the clinician should look for imbalances in any of those systems that might contribute to dysfunction in the others. A structural survey should be included in the assessment of any patient with chronic illness.

References

1. Melzer K, Kayser B, Pichard C. Physical activity: the health benefits outweigh the risks. Curr Opin Clin Nutr Metab Care. 2004;7(6):641-47.
2. Oja P. Dose response between total volume of physical activity and health and fitness. Med Sci Sports Exerc. 2001;33(6 Suppl):S428-37.
3. Kohl HW 3rd. Physical activity and cardiovascular disease: evidence for a dose response. Med Sci Sports Exerc. 2001;33(6 Suppl):S472-83.
4. Hu G, Tuomilehto J, Silventoinen K, et al. The effects of physical activity and body mass index on cardiovascular, cancer and all-cause mortality among 47,212 middle-aged Finnish men and women. Int J Obes Relat Metab Disord. 2005;Feb 22:Epub ahead of print.
5. Barengo NC, Hu G, Lakka TA, et al. Low physical activity as a predictor for total and cardiovascular disease mortality in middle-aged men and women in Finland. Eur Heart J. 2004;25(24):2204-11.
6. Lee IM, Skerrett PJ. Physical activity and all-cause mortality: what is the dose-response relation? Med Sci Sports Exerc. 2001;33(6 Suppl):S459-71.
7. Lee CD, Folsom AR, Blair SN. Physical activity and stroke risk: a meta-analysis. Stroke. 2003;34:2475-82.
8. Pescatello LS, Franklin BA, Fagard R, et al. American College of Sports Medicine position stand. Exercise and hypertension. Med Sci Sports Exerc. 2004;36(3):533-53.
9. Ueshima K, Suzuki T, Nasu M, et al. Effects of exercise training on left ventricular function evaluated by the Tei index in patients with myocardial infarction. Circ J. 2005;69(5):564-66.
10. Blumenthal JA, Sherwood A, Babyak MA, et al. Effects of exercise and stress management training on markers of cardiovascular risk in patients with ischemic heart disease: a randomized controlled trial. JAMA. 2005;293(13):1626-34.
11. Cheng YJ, Macera CA, Church TS, Blair SN. Heart rate reserve as a predictor of cardiovascular and all-cause mortality in men. Med Sci Sports Exerc. 2002;34(12):1873-78.
12. Goldhammer E, Tanchilevitch A, Maor I, et al. Exercise training modulates cytokines activity in coronary heart disease patients. Int J Cardiol. 2005;100(1):93-99.
13. Kelley GA, Kelley KS, Tran ZV. Walking and non-HDL-C in adults: a meta-analysis of randomized controlled trials. Prev Cardiol. 2005;8(2):102-7.
14. Carroll S, Dudfield M. What is the relationship between exercise and metabolic abnormalities? A review of the metabolic syndrome. Sports Med. 2004;34(6):371-418.
15. Hayashi Y, Nagasaka S, Takahashi N, et al. A single bout of exercise at higher intensity enhances glucose effectiveness in sedentary men. J Clin Endocrinol Metab. 2005;Apr 19:Epub ahead of print.
16. Bond Brill J, Perry AC, Parker L, et al. Dose-response effect of walking exercise on weight loss. How much is enough? Int J Obes Relat Metab Disord. 2002;26(11):1484-93.
17. Dubnov G, Brzezinski A, Berry EM. Weight control and the management of obesity after menopause: the role of physical activity. Maturitas. 2003;44(2):89-101.
18. Venjatraman JT, Fernandes G. Exercise, immunity and aging. Aging (Milano). 1997;9(1-2):42-56.
19. Manger TA, Motta RW. The impact of an exercise program on posttraumatic stress disorder, anxiety, and depression. Int J Emerg Ment Health. 2005;7(1):49-57.
20. Kirby S. The positive effect of exercise as a therapy for clinical depression. Nurs Times. 2005;101(13):28-9.
21. Samad AK, Taylor RS, Marshall T, Chapman MA. A meta-analysis of the association of physical activity with reduced risk of colorectal cancer. Colorectal Dis. 2005;7(3):204-13.
22. Barnard RJ. Prevention of cancer through lifestyle changes. eCAM. 2004;1(3):233-39.
23. Torti DC, Matheson GO. Exercise and prostate cancer. Sports Med. 2004;34(6):363-69.
24. Evans WJ. Protein nutrition, exercise and aging. J Am Coll Nutr. 2004;23(6 Suppl):601S-9S.
25. Ibid.
26. Schlicht J, Camaione DN, Osen SV. Effect of intense strength training on standing balance, walking speed, and sit-to-stand performance in older adults. J Gerontol A Biol Sci Med Sci. 2001;56(5):M281-86.
27. Hakkinen K, Pakarinen A, Hannonen P, et al. Effects of strength training on muscle strength, cross-sectional area, maximal electromyographic activity, and serum hormones in premenopausal women with fibromyalgia. J Rheumatol. 2002;29(6):1287-95.
28. Kraemer WJ, Hakkinen K, Newton RU, et al. Effects of heavy-resistance training on hormonal response patterns in younger vs. older men. J Appl Physiol. 1999;87(3):982-92.
29. Gauchard GC, Jeandel C, Tessier A, Perrin PP. Beneficial effect of proprioceptive physical activities on balance control in elderly human subjects. Neurosci Lett. 1999;273(2):81-84.
30. Hirsch MA, Toole T, Maitland CG, Rider RA. The effects of balance training and high-intensity resistance training on persons with idiopathic Parkinson's disease. Arch Phys Med Rehabil. 2003;84(8):1109-17.
31. Toole T, Hirsch MA, Forkink A, et al. The effects of a balance and strength training program on equilibrium in Parkinsonism: A preliminary study. NeuroRehabilitation. 2000;14(3):165-74.
32. Ott C, Fulton MK. Osteoporosis risk and interest in strength training in men receiving androgen ablation therapy for locally advanced prostate cancer. J Am Acad Nurse Pract. 2005;17(3):113-22.
33. Karper WB, Stasik SC. A successful, long-term exercise program for women with fibromyalgia syndrome and chronic fatigue and immune dysfunction syndrome. Clin Nurse Spec. 2003;17(5):243-48.

34. Musnick D. Conditioning for Outdoor Fitness: Functional Exercise and Nutrition for Every Body. Mountaineers Books, 2004.
35. Vereb G, Szollosi J, Matko J, et al. Dynamic, yet structured: the cell membrane three decades after the Singe-Nicolson model. Proc Natl Acad Sci U S A. 2003;100(14):8053-58.
36. Sampath H, Ntambi J. Polyunsaturated fatty acid regulation of gene expression. Nutr Rev. 2004;62:333-39.
37. Valenzuela A, Morgado N. Trans fatty acid isomers in human health and in the food industry. Biol Res. 1999;32:273-87.
38. Roach C, Feller SE, Ward JA, et al. Comparison of cis and trans fatty acid containing phosphatidylcholines on membrane properties. Biochemistry. 2004;43:6344-51.
39. Murphy MG. Dietary fatty acids and membrane protein function. Nutr Biochem. 1990;1:68-79.
40. Wolfe F, Smythe HA, Yunus MB, et al., The American College of Rheumatology 1990 criteria for the classification of fibromyalgia: Report of the Multicenter Criteria Committee. Arth Rheum. 1990; 33:160-72.
41. Chang L, Mayer EA, Johnson T, et al. Differences in somatic perception in female patients with irritable bowel syndrome with and without fibromyalgia. Pain. 2000;84(2-3):297-307.
42. Miranda A, Peles S, Rudolph C, et al. Altered visceral sensation in response to somatic pain in the rat. Gastroenterology. 2004;126:1082-89.
43. Coffin B, Bouhassira D, Sabate JM, et al. Alteration of the spinal modulation of nociceptive processing in patients with irritable bowel syndrome. Gut. 2004;53:1465-70.
44. Woodworth BA, Gillespie MB, Lambert PR. The canalith repositioning procedure for benign positional vertigo: a meta-analysis. Laryngoscope. 2004;114:1143-46.
45. Freedman KB, Bernstein J. Educational deficiencies in musculoskeletal medicine. J Bone Joint Surg. 2002;84:604-8.
46. Anderson R, Meeker WC, Wirick BE, et al. A meta-analysis of clinical trials of spinal manipulation. J Manipulative Physiol Ther. 1992;15(3):181-94.
47. Meade T, Dyer S, Browne W, Frank A. Randomised comparison of chiropractic and hospital outpatient management for low back pain: results from extended follow up. BMJ. 1995;311:349-51.
48. UK BEAM Trial Team. United Kingdom back pain exercise and manipulation (UK BEAM) randomised trial: effectiveness of physical treatments for back pain in primary care. BMJ. 2004 329(7479):1377.
49. U.S. Agency for Health Care Policy and Research. Acute low back pain problems in adults: assessment and treatment. Quick Reference Guide for Clinicians. Clinical Practice Guideline #14, 1994.
50. Waddell G, McIntosh A, Hutchinson A, et al. Clinical guidelines for the management of acute low back pain. London: Royal College of General Practitioners, 1999.
51. van Tulder MW, Tuut M, Pennick V, et al. Quality of primary care guidelines for acute low back pain. Spine. 2004;29:E357-62.
52. Bronfort G, Haas M, Evans RL, Bouter LM. Efficacy of spinal manipulation and mobilization for low back pain and neck pain: a systematic review and best evidence synthesis. Spine J. 2004;4:335-56.
53. Gross AR, Hoving JL, Haines TA, et al. Cervical overview group. A Cochrane review of manipulation and mobilization for mechanical neck disorders. Spine. 2004; 29(14):1541-48.
54. Nilsson N, Christensen HW, Hartvigsen J. The effect of spinal manipulation in the treatment of cervicogenic headache. J Manipulative Physiol Ther. 1997;20:326-30.
55. Waters RL, Conaty PJ, Lunsford B, O'Meara P. The energy cost of walking with arthritis of the hip and knee. Clin Orthop. 1987;214:278-84.
56. Sato A, Sato Y, Schmidt R. Changes in blood pressure and heart rate induced by movements of normal and inflamed knee joints. Neurosci Lett. 1984;52(1-2):55-60.
57. Perry F, Heller PH, Kamiya J, Levine JD. Altered autonomic function in patients with arthritis or with chronic myofascial pain. Pain. 1989;39:77-84.
58. Martinez-Lavin M, Vidal M, Barbosa RE, et al. Norepinephrine-evoked pain in fibromyalgia. A randomized pilot study [ISRCTN70707830]. BMC Musculoskelet Disord. 2002;3(1):2.
59. Gamber RG, Shores JH, Russo DP, et al. Osteopathic manipulative treatment in conjunction with medication relieves pain associated with fibromyalgia syndrome: results of a randomized clinical pilot project. J Am Osteopath Assoc. 2002;102:321-25.
60. Weiss JM. Pelvic floor myofascial trigger points: manual therapy for interstitial cystitis and the urgency-frequency syndrome. J Urol. 2001;166:2226-31.
61. Oyama IA, Rejba A, Lukban JC, et al. Modified Thiele massage as therapeutic intervention for female patients with interstitial cystitis and high-tone pelvic floor dysfunction. Urology. 2004;64:862-65.
62. Jorgensen LS, Fossgreen J. Back pain and spinal pathology in patients with functional upper abdominal pain. Scand J Gastroenterol. 1990;25:1235-41.
63. Kreier F, Yilmaz A, Kalsbeek A, et al. Hypothesis: shifting the equilibrium from activity to food leads to autonomic unbalance and the metabolic syndrome. Diabetes. 2003;52:2652-56.

Chapter 30
Clinical Approaches to Energy Production and Oxidative Stress

- *Bioenergetics, Mitochondrial Function and Oxidative Stress in Functional Medicine*
- *Oxidative Stress and Autism*
- *Oxidative Stress and Glycemic Control*

Bioenergetics, Mitochondrial Function and Oxidative Stress in Functional Medicine

Jeffrey S. Bland, PhD

Introduction

This chapter will develop the concept of oxidative stress from the functional medicine perspective, which represents a mosaic of basic chemistry, biochemistry, cellular physiology, molecular biology, and clinical medicine. There are still gaps in our understanding of this emerging area of basic and clinical science. In order to make clinical connections, the trajectory of the current scientific understanding of oxidative stress will be formulated into a functional model. This model reflects an integration of the principles of energy metabolism and oxidative stress and their relationship to coronary heart disease (CHD), neurodegenerative diseases, autism, diabetes, cancer, arthritis, and syndromes such as fibromyalgia, chronic fatigue syndrome (CFS), and multiple chemical sensitivity.

Knowledge of oxidative stress has significant clinical payoffs. It provides the clinician a lens through which to filter observations that result in new clinical options for both prevention and treatment. The clinical implications of oxidative stress apply to a wide variety of conditions, such as environmental toxicity and the chronic inflammatory disorders of various organs and systems, including the GI system, the liver, heart, brain, joints, and vascular endothelium. Patients with clinical presentations in these areas would be candidates on whom to focus the lens of oxidative stress.

The topic also relates to the controversy surrounding antioxidants. The word "antioxidant" is a non-specific term that can lead to as much confusion as clarity. In this chapter, a more functional understanding of what is meant by antioxidant will be provided, allowing the clinician to better evaluate new information, such as the discussion concerning vitamin E in cancer and heart disease prevention, and what the data really mean.

We will focus mainly on five learning objectives for this chapter:

- This organelle, the mitochondrion, is the so-called energy powerhouse of the cell and has a significant relationship to oxidative stress. We will examine this energy-producing function in some detail.
- We will explore the role of altered bioenergetics in the diathesis of chronic disease. Energy is defined as the ability to do work. What does that really mean in terms of health and disease?
- We want to understand the role of antioxidants in cellular redox control. Redox is a chemical term describing reduction/oxidation reactions, or the transfer of electrons that occurs in oxidative chemistry and cellular physiology.

- We will analyze how various nutrients play a role in establishing proper bioenergetics. Nutrition not only provides the body's fuel (macronutrients), but also facilitates (through micronutrients) proper energy utilization.
- Finally, we will review how all these concepts are related to some common clinical conditions.

Many articles in the literature touch upon these topics. One such article is "New Targets for Heart Failure Therapy: Endothelin, Inflammatory Cytokines and Oxidative Stress."[1] These cardiac disease issues are not cholesterol-related phenomena; they are related to oxidative stress, inflammation, and altered bioenergetics. New observations suggest there may be other factors beyond the traditional risk factors associated with cardiovascular disease (CVD) that contribute to myocardial remodeling. Among the growing list of possibilities are endothelin, inflammatory cytokines, and nitric oxide (NO). NO, along with citrulline, is produced in the vascular endothelium from the amino acid arginine by the enzyme endothelial NO synthase. This process is tightly controlled in order to regulate blood pressure and vascular tone. Other reactive oxygen species (ROS), including superoxide, hydroxyl, peroxynitrite, peroxyl radicals, hydroxyl radicals, and singlet oxygen, must also be rigorously controlled. These generally reactive molecules react with cellular components that alter biochemical and/or genetic potential. Most ROS originate internally, due to inefficiencies within the mitochondria, and are part of the price we pay for living in an oxygen-enriched atmosphere. The judicious use of both micro- and macronutrients can minimize their impact on chronic inflammation.

Mitochondria and Energy Production

The mitochondria are our ultimate energy producers. However, they don't release energy in one big burst, but rather as metabolic bumps along the road, analogous to a metabolic Pachinko game. (Pachinko is a Japanese pinball game.) The person playing the game tries to get as much energy out of his or her pinball investment as possible. If the player is good at the game (efficient), the ball can be kept in play for a long time, getting a lot more fun for the money. That's what good metabolism does. It tries to get a lot more activity for the energy by taking many steps along the way in the redox/oxidative pathway. That's why there are so many metabolic control points in bioenergetic transformation. You don't want to light a fire in your metabolic fireplace and have all the energy lost in one large flame before important metabolic work is completed. People who have lost their metabolic degrees of freedom experience loss of energy efficiency.

The mitochondrion not only generates the bulk of the energy currency of the cell, it is responsible for distributing it. It is the center of bioenergetics. The cells that have the greatest mitochondrial activity are those that do the most aerobic work, such as the cells of the heart and nervous system. Cardiac tissue is an excellent example, in that it is doing the work of muscle contraction 24 hours a day. Seventy-five percent of the heart cell volume, the cardiocyte, is occupied by mitochondria, very tightly packed. In cells that are engaged in a lot of aerobic work and consuming a lot of oxygen (resulting in high energy production), the mitochondria are plentiful and very active. In a sense, the mitochondrion is an organelle that transduces the potential energy in macronutrients into high-energy molecules through the process of oxidation. The mitochondrion takes the chemical potential energy available in food—fatty acids, glucose, and amino acids—and, through the process of redox, converts potential energy into high-energy biomolecules (e.g., ATP, NADH, and FADH2) that are used by the cell to accomplish its varied tasks. When the mitochondrion is working effectively, it is a clean-burning, oxygen-utilizing, metabolic engine.

The control of this process is closely tied to mitochondrial electron transport through the balance of catabolism (i.e., breaking down large molecules to small ones) and anabolism (i.e., building up large molecules from small ones). Efficient metabolism is controlled by many factors, including hormones, trophic factors, cytokines, neurotransmitters, cofactors, and coenzymes.

The cell membrane is ultimately responsible for the import of nutrients and export of waste products. Macronutrients are broken down to lower molecular weight molecules that can enter the mitochondrion for their terminal oxidation. The mitochondrion is a cellular organelle bounded by a double membrane. The inner membrane is highly folded, creating what are referred to as cristae. Attached to the surface of the cristae are the proteins and enzymes that actually perform the work.

(The cristae of the mitochondrion make one think of a battery wherein energy is stored through an electrical-chemical process of metabolism. No one really knows how these electrons in oxidative metabolism travel through this system. We think we have the answer through our knowledge of the electron transport chain in the mitochondrion, but we don't really know exactly how it occurs. The electron transport chain involves abstracting energy from food, ultimately generating ATP. This is an amazing process that occurs on the surface of the electron-transporting cytochromes, iron-containing proteins present in the mitochondria. Therefore, the mitochondrion is paramagnetic because there are iron atoms present; it can be polarized in a magnetic or electric field. Studies have been done placing animals in a very high magnetic field strength and noting changes in their mitochondrial bioenergetics.[2] This raises interesting questions about the influence of electromagnetic energy on mitochondrial bioenergetics. [3])

As the molecules move across the outer mitochondrial membrane through the inner membrane, they gain access to the enzymes of the Krebs cycle and electron transport chain that are bound to the surface of the inner membrane. As electrons are removed from the di- and tricarboxylic acids of the Krebs cycle, they are captured by proteins of the electron transport chain and transferred in an orderly manner to molecular oxygen. By accepting these electrons, oxygen is reduced to water. Whenever there is oxidation, there must be a concomitant reduction. Electrons are neither lost nor gained; energy and matter are conserved. The electrons exchanged in this process travel down a wire, just as they would from a hydroelectric power generator to an electrical outlet. In this case, the "wire" is the electron transport chain that has various cofactors that assist in the proper regulation of electron flow. Without the integrity of the electron transport chain, the electrons could fly off the wire, as they might in the case of a short circuit on the cord of a lamp. Just as a short circuit can destroy a house, electrons leaking from the electron transport chain can destroy a cell.

It is important to recognize that oxygen, which constitutes 21% of the air we breathe, is a corrosive gas to carbon-based life. Therefore, we have a "love-hate" relationship with oxygen. Using it in the mitochondria as an oxidizing agent (for energy production) provides an energy advantage over the anaerobic organisms that cannot use oxygen. The flip side is that the use of oxygen increases the risk of oxidative injury. This is why complex antioxidant defense systems evolved over millennia to protect against oxidative injury.

On average, about 1% of the oxygen we breathe is converted into high-energy, corrosive oxygen materials, such as superoxide, hydrogen peroxide, and hydroxyl radical. The mitochondria, which are very vulnerable because they are rich in membrane-associated unsaturated fatty acids, have evolved an effective system for protection against oxidation. The protective agents, analogous to the insulation on a wire, are antioxidants present at high levels within the mitochondrion. A high level of antioxidants, consisting of both small molecules and enzymes such as superoxide dismutase and glutathione peroxidase/reductase, can be found in the mitochondria. The small-molecule antioxidants that contribute to the system include lipoic acid, coenzyme Q10, and carnitine (which transports fatty acids across the outer mitochondrial membrane). Together, the components of the system protect the mitochondrion and cell against oxidative stress/injury. In a sense, these agents may be considered "redox buffering agents" that help resist oxidative stress.

If mitochondrial oxidative phosphorylation is blocked or inhibited, then energy production is taken up through metabolic activities occurring in the cytosol. This cytosolic capability results in the reduction of pyruvate to lactate (anaerobic glycolysis). The lactate fermentation is not as energy efficient as oxidative phosphorylation. The process of pyruvate/lactate metabolism is a back-up energy production system. It is a legacy from our anaerobic evolutionary history. When a tissue becomes oxygen deprived, it is shifted to this metabolic state. For example, what happens if you're in a marathon and you run to the 20th mile and "hit the wall"? Biochemically, you have just exceeded your mitochondrial bioenergetic, aerobic, high-efficiency capacity and you are now starting to shift to lactate fermentation, or anaerobic metabolism, as the backup-up system. Lactate is accumulating in your tissues, which lowers cellular pH. As a consequence, you may feel fatigue and pain, as well as changes in mood.

The question therefore arises whether fibromyalgia syndrome could be considered lactic acidosis due, in part, to mitochondrial inhibition occurring at certain trigger points in the muscle body. There are a number of chronic pain syndromes associated with poor muscle performance related to altered mitochondrial bioenergetics. One also wonders about statin drugs and the various kinds of rhabdomyolyses[i] that are associated with muscle pain from these medications. Are these consequences of the statins altering oxidative chemistry at the mitochondria? One of the important factors for the electron transport pathway is coenzyme Q10 (CoQ10). Statins have been found to decrease CoQ10, which results in interruption of electron transport, thereby blunting mitochondrial oxidative phosphorylation, and possibly inducing a transition to anaerobic metabolism that produces lactic acid. The whole reduction/oxidation balance of the tissue has changed. It's like a 12-volt storage battery that tries to run on eight volts. It doesn't power the system nearly as well at the reduced voltage.

Mitochondrial DNA

For nearly 100 years, it was felt that the source of DNA in cells was restricted to the nucleus and packaged in structures called chromosomes. Isolation of DNA from cells implied the extraction solely of nuclear DNA. We now recognize that while the majority of the DNA in cells is indeed found in the nucleus, a small amount is found in the mitochondria. The mitochondrial DNA, though small in magnitude relative to genomic DNA, serves an important function. The mitochondrial DNA encodes proteins and RNA molecules that are essential for mitochondrial activity. Mutations in mitochondrial DNA can occur in the absence of mutations that occur in the chromosomes within the nucleus. Despite the fact that several mitochondrial enzymes are encoded on the mitochondrial genome, most are encoded within the nucleus.

The mitochondrion appears to be a very primitive organelle. In fact, molecular paleontologists have dated its origin back 1.6 billion years, so it predates anything we're familiar with in terms of our species. Dr. Lynn Margulis has postulated that long ago a bacterium infected a nucleated cell and so was born the mitochondrion.[4] If we look at the anatomy of the mitochondria, it would be like taking a facial tissue and packing it into a balloon. That is what the inner mitochondrial membranes are like. On the surface of the inner membrane are bound many enzymes that are like little molecular machines engaged in the process of energy production. All the bioenergetics reactions are occurring on the surface of those inner mitochondrial membranes. Given the similarity of the mitochondrial DNA to that of bacterial DNA, a number of well-respected medical researchers have discussed the possible origin of the mitochondria in eukaryotic biology.[5,6] Bacteria lived inside the nucleated cell as symbiotes, providing a competitive edge for the "infected" cell by allowing it to use oxygen more effectively in metabolism.

This provides an explanation for a number of clinical observations—for instance, the example of chloramphenicol-induced hemolytic anemia. Hemolytic anemia is a problem associated with many third-generation antibiotics. If the mitochondrion has the "personality" of a bacteria-like genome, then, when exposed to a hard-hitting antibiotic, it is possible that it can become damaged, resulting in an energy-deficit disorder that leads to conditions such as anemia. Chloramphenicol-induced hemolytic anemia seems to be associated with the sensitivity of the mitochondrion to this antibiotic; it has been found to be sex linked to the maternal genome. The mitochondrial DNA is inherited predominantly from the mother.[7,8,9] Sperm have mitochondria (necessary to make energy in order to swim), but they are mostly contained in a section near the tail (the midpiece, a cytologically distinct region between the head and tail) that falls off after fertilization; thus, rarely do mitochondria from sperm enter the ovum. The ovum, on the other hand, is large and has a tremendous number of mitochondria. Therefore, mitochondrial function and mitochondria-associated diseases are largely a maternally-inherited characteristic.

Mitochondrial DNA is far more susceptible to oxidative injury than nuclear DNA. In the nucleus, the DNA is bound up and tightly coated for protection by histone and non-histone proteins. These protective proteins wrap the DNA in a beautiful helical configuration so that it will not be exposed to agents that might damage it. Through this mechanism, the body has developed protection against nuclear injury to the genome. The genome, when it needs to be read, has mechanisms to selectively unwrap the coat on the DNA so that the reader enzymes can come in. These selective reactions occur by deacetylation and demethylation of the genome that results in reading the specific message on the DNA. In contrast, the mitochondrial DNA is not well protected against injury.[10] It is laid bare, almost like

[i] The destruction or degeneration of skeletal muscle tissue (as from traumatic injury, excessive exertion, or stroke) that is accompanied by the release of muscle cell contents (as myoglobin and potassium) into the bloodstream resulting in hypovolemia, hyperkalemia, and sometimes acute renal failure. (Source: Medline Medical Dictionary.)

the circular chromosome of the bacterium, contrasted to the nucleosome structure of the nuclear DNA.

Mitochondria and Oxidative Stress

Oxidative stress is associated with reactive oxygen species (ROS) that have high reactivity with unsaturated lipids in membranes, proteins, and nucleic acids, thereby changing cellular function. Certain steps in the electron transport chain are facilitated by the reduced form of Q10 and its relationship to the oxidized form of Q10. CoQ10 might then be perceived as an "insulator" on the wire of the electron transport chain. Lipoic acid is also part of this "insulation" through the dihydrolipoic and lipoic acid couple. The enzymes glutathione peroxidase and glutathione reductase help control the concentration of reduced and oxidized forms of glutathione, which is also part of the mitochondrial protection system. Vitamin E also plays a role to shuttle electrons and provide insulation on the wire. If electrons are lost along the electron transport chain, they can do cellular damage. Those electrons are very promiscuous oxidizing agents. Electrons don't want to be alone. They're going to find something to react with. The process by which this occurs is called oxidative stress.

The oxidants released as a result of mitochondrial oxidative stress include superoxide, hydrogen peroxide, singlet oxygen, and hydroxyl radical. These oxidants, in turn, generate lipid peroxides, nitrogen, and sulfur oxide free radical species. Hydroxyl radical is oxidant material produced in cells. In 1975, research I was involved in at the Functional Medicine Research Center (HealthComm International) indicated that hydroxyl radical was produced by cellular systems in humans. (Chemically, hydroxyl radical is the product of the Fenton reaction by which, in the presence of iron, hydrogen peroxide generates a molecule each of hydroxy radical and hydroxide ion.) This hypothesis was criticized by a number of scientists at the time who asserted that there was no way hydroxyl radical could ever be formed in physiological systems because it's only found in high atmosphere particle physics and only occurs in the ionosphere due to high-energy, cosmic radiation exposure. The thought was that we would never get hydroxyl at normal oxygen tension and physiological temperature in the human. Today, however, it is well recognized that hydroxyl radical is generated in human processes and contributes to oxidative stress, along with other organic molecules in the body, by producing a whole family of other peroxyl radicals that also initiate oxidative stress.

This process is more prevalent when a person has a high level of free, available iron, such as seen in hemochromatosis. In such cases, pulmonary and cardiac disease is common because of iron-induced hydroxyl radical pathology. (The only effective treatment is phlebotomy to reduce iron levels.) In tissues that have experienced a hemorrhage, there is a release of free iron from hemoglobin that initiates oxidative stress at the site of the hemorrhage. If you can either decrease the bleeding or increase the antioxidant protection at that site, there will be lowered scarring and tissue injury post-trauma. The antioxidant defense is provided by cellular enzymes such as glutathione peroxidase, glutathione reductase, catalase, and superoxide dismutase.

Normal metabolic processes all produce enough oxidants to rancidify the body each day. Fortunately, our antioxidant enzyme systems defend us from most oxidant damage. The body is working all the time through these enzyme processes and other antioxidants to defend against superoxide, hydrogen peroxide, and hydroxyl radical.

One of the most paradoxical concepts is that the time of greatest oxidative stress is when tissues have the lowest oxygen levels. This sounds counterintuitive, but it's a very important concept clinically. Any time there are low levels of oxygen in a tissue, there are high levels of oxygen radicals. Conditions such as ischemia, hypoxia, anemia, or anything that causes poor delivery of oxygen to tissues (e.g., vascular bed defect, vasoconstriction, trauma to the vessels, infection, edema) create reduced blood flow and oxygen delivery to the tissues. The tissue downstream from the blockade of oxygen is then under high oxidative stress. This is what happens in reperfusion ischemia as a result of coronary artery bypass surgery or a stroke. When a patient is on the pump, it changes the oxygen tension, and when the waiting blood is reoxygenated, it delivers a large shock of oxidants and free radicals.

Every tradition in medicine has had a way of delivering oxygen to tissues to reduce problems of oxidative stress. Today, there is intubation, but before that, there was yoga, deep breathing, respiratory exercises, and physical manipulation, all of which help to deliver oxygen to tissues. If tissues are not being oxygenated, the person is under oxidative stress. Sleep apnea is a good clinical example of a pro-oxidant situation. Cardiac damage occurs with sleep apnea as a result of oxidative stress-induced phenomena.

Oxidative stress is a cumulative effect of all the factors that increase oxidant production and mitochondrial dysfunction, and decrease antioxidant defense. Let's look at a simplistic example of a vacation in a sunny environment. Before going on vacation, the person has been sedentary. While on vacation, he or she drinks excessive alcohol and exercises very heavily. The person also eats a lot of fried foods and sugar, and is allergic to something during the whole vacation. Finally, the person gets sunburned. All of these factors contribute to oxidative stress; incurring them all at once may overload the body's defense systems. Increased oxidative stress is generally a consequence of a number of factors perpetuating free radical injury to cells.

Mitochondrial Dysfunction and Age-Related Illness

There are several hundred (up to 3,000) mitochondria per cell. The total number of mitochondria in the body obviously greatly exceeds the total number of cells. Over a lifetime, these mitochondria can sustain injury from any number of sources. For example, the mitochondria "remember" many of the toxic exposures that occur over a lifetime, resulting in a decline in their function, including a decline in the synthesis of useful compounds, detoxification capacity, and a loss of control over apoptosis, or cellular suicide. Premature neuronal apoptosis leads to dementia. We want to protect neurons against premature apoptosis unless we really need to get rid of them. If we accelerate apoptosis, we are creating excessive cellular suicide in post-mitotic tissues. The brain is a post-mitotic tissue. Once it's developed, its cells don't get replaced very rapidly. The heart and the muscles are also post-mitotic tissues. We know we can regenerate a liver cell, but it's not so easy for the brain, the heart, or the muscles. That's why these cells are more vulnerable, with age, to cumulative injury. Mitochondrial bioenergetic dysfunctions result in accelerated apoptosis in these tissues.

Think about patients who have been exposed to occupational toxins or xenobiotics, those who are under chronic high stress, those who are heavy smokers or alcoholics and may not be eating properly, those who are taking certain drugs like the nucleoside analog drugs used for HIV treatment, or even those who have been on repetitive, long-term antibiotics. These are all factors that are injurious to mitochondrial bioenergetics. The lipodystrophy of HIV/AIDS is caused by drugs that injure the mitochondria and alter fat metabolism and the way fat is stored, resulting in diabetes or cardiopathy.

A highly visible example of age-related (i.e., cumulative) oxidative stress was seen on a 2001 cover of *Science News*, showing a photograph of two men of the same age. One is a Navajo chief, looking very old; the other is a Buddhist monk, looking much younger. The principal difference between them was their exposure to the sun. Sun exposure generates free radical oxidative injury to the collagen in subcutaneous tissues, causing them to crosslink and form little puckers in the connective fascia that affect the outer surface of the skin. That's the origin of a sun-induced wrinkle—an example of free radical injury. Another visible example of sun-induced free radical damage is the greater wrinkling on the left versus the right cheek of a truck driver. He is his own "control" because one cheek sustains constant sun exposure over the course of his career, while the other does not. The greater wrinkling on his left cheek is due to radiation-induced free radical injury that is not occurring on his right cheek. These highly visible examples of what cumulative free radical oxidative injury can do to aging tissues help us to understand the similar processes—invisible to the naked eye—that are taking place in our bodies every day.

Mitochondria and Cell Death

There are people who spend their lives trying to figure out the complex processes by which bioenergetics influences all the set points, trigger points, and control points in metabolism. These control points are closely tied to the process of cell suicide, or apoptosis. It seems reasonable that the body would have a built-in way of getting rid of damaged cells to prevent future problems. Over the course of a life, each person will sustain damage to many cells. They can be sloughed off or they can undergo necrosis, but the most common way that damaged cells are removed is through apoptosis. There are cellular signaling pathways that have recently been identified for the control of apoptosis.[11] Some of these pathways involve the mitochondria.[12,13] The mitochondria may receive signals to uncouple their oxidative processes and produce an excess of free radicals, triggering apoptosis.

There are many protective mechanisms that prevent cells from undergoing apoptosis prematurely. Proper regulation of mitochondrial redox is an important part of the protective mechanism against apoptosis. Therefore, the mitochondria have multiple purposes. If cells are damaged or altered, it is important that those cells die before replicating the injury in a daughter cell. However, we don't want our normal, healthy cells receiving a message that unleashes apoptosis and oxidative injury. (We're talking about the release of unpaired electron species that are oxidants, like peroxyl or nitroxyl radicals, where there is an oxygen with a single electron on it, and it's hunting for a partner.) In neurology, the word excitotoxicity has to do with processes like the excessive stimulation of the NMDA receptor site in neuronal cells that can activate apoptosis, resulting in premature death. This has been suggested as one possible mechanism resulting in neurodegenerative disorders such as Parkinson's disease.[14,15,16]

Assessing Oxidative Stress and Oxidative Damage

Free radical oxidative stress can be assessed, not only by analyzing lipid peroxides, but also by measuring levels of isoprostanes in biological samples. These prostaglandin-like molecules are produced in the body by way of oxidative injury to arachidonic acid. Hydroxynonenal can also be measured as an indication of oxidative stress. Another way of assessing is the evaluation of blood levels of another byproduct of oxidation called 8-hydroxy-deoxyguanosine (8OHdG). 8OHdG is produced as a consequence of oxidation of guanosine residues in DNA. It has a close correlation with neuronal oxidative stress, in that about 50% of 8OHdG comes from the central nervous system.

Glutathione status can also be measured as an indication of oxidative stress. Glutathione is an important mitochondrial protector against the production of oxidants. Cellular levels of reduced glutathione are elevated by improving redox and increasing protection of the cell against oxidative injury. The use of N-acetylcysteine supplementation results in a shift of the reduction/oxidation level of the cell more toward a reduced state. This results in a higher glutathione-to-glutathione disulfide ratio in cells. It is important to increase the reduced glutathione levels to increase the total cellular redox capability. During clinical situations demanding increased glutathione reserves, it is important to supplement with N-acetylcysteine, but it is also very important to focus on the reduction of triggers to oxidative stress, along with increasing cellular antioxidant status and mitochondrial function. Clinicians should make sure the patient is getting adequate sulfur-rich proteins in the diet (i.e., methionine and cysteine), in that these are the building blocks for glutathione.

Oxidative damage can be analyzed by measuring substances in the plasma, such as serum lipid peroxides, which are an indirect measurement for the amount of oxidative injury that is occurring to unsaturated lipids, particularly the membrane lipids. If you measure serum peroxide levels by the thiobarbituric acid (TBA) test, you're indirectly measuring the "cinders" that result from the oxidative injuries that have occurred to membrane lipids.

Nutrients and Mitochondrial Function

Vitamins and Antioxidants

ATP is the ultimate product of the energy-production process and it is generated by oxidative phosphorylation utilizing electrons that are generated in the oxidation of the organic acids of the Krebs cycle. In order to function properly, the Krebs cycle utilizes a number of coenzymes and cofactors that are derived from vitamins and minerals. Cofactors include thiamine pyrophosphate from thiamin (vitamin B1), riboflavin (vitamin B2) that occurs as flavin-adenine-dinucleotide (FAD), niacin (vitamin B3) that occurs as nicotinamide dinucleotide (NAD), and pyridoxine (vitamin B6) that occurs as pyridoxal phosphate. All of these play a role in serving as facilitators of specific biochemical reactions that occur within the Krebs cycle and, subsequently, in energy production within the mitochondria.

NAD is derived from vitamin B3. It is coupled with its reduced relative, NADH, to store the energy of metabolism. The oxidized form of NAD^+ is chemically reduced to the higher energy NADH that, in turn, can serve as a reducing agent in specific metabolic reactions. The specific vitamin B3-derived cofactor NAD is, therefore, of critical importance in controlling energy processes in every cell. The symptoms of vitamin B3 deficiency—diarrhea, dermatitis, and dementia—demonstrate its important role in maintaining the energy processes in these target tissues. The same explanation holds true for the other B vitamins, and minerals such as iron and magnesium that regulate enzyme function.

As oxidative stress occurs, the high-energy intermediates (the reduced intermediates) are lower, and the oxidized intermediates are higher, resulting in a decrease in the capacity to produce energy. It's like losing the voltage in the battery of a car. It may still be able to crank, but not on a cold morning. It has lost its energy reserve. People who have lost their energy reserve have higher susceptibility to infection, stress, or trauma. Under conditions of oxidative stress, the ratio of reduced to oxidized intermediates is lower. One of the most important of these ratios is the oxidized-to-reduced-glutathione ratio. When glutathione is oxidized, it yields glutathione disulfide. Under oxidative stress, the ratio of reduced glutathione to glutathione disulfide is reduced from the normal level of 100:1.

It is similar with flavin adenine dinucleotide (FAD), derived from riboflavin. When this coenzyme is reduced by metabolic processes in the mitochondria, it produces the reduced derivative FADHz. The reduced flavin, as does the oxidized flavin, absorbs visible light in the blue, so it has a yellow color. When you consume B vitamins and have color in your urine, what you are really doing is indirectly measuring the riboflavin in the urine as it gets excreted.

Does taking vitamins just produce "expensive urine"? Why would you take nutrient supplements if they are "wasted" by excretion? First of all, if you didn't excrete any vitamins over the course of your life, you would accumulate a lot of vitamins in your body that could build up to a toxic level. They have to be excreted. The question becomes, what happens as they pass through the body? Just because they're eventually excreted doesn't mean they didn't achieve an important health effect on the way through. Vitamins spilled in the urine are neither useless nor detrimental. What we need to know is what happened while they were present in the body. Because they control and influence many bioenergetic reactions, including glycolysis, aminolysis, and lipolysis, vitamins are critically important for functions beyond prevention of deficiency symptoms. Individual vitamin and mineral needs can vary greatly. As Bruce Ames, PhD has described, there is considerable genetic variation from person to person in how specific nutrients influence their cellular function.[17] Robert Heaney, MD, PhD recently termed the health problems that result from nutrient intake below the level of individual genetic need as "long-latency diseases."[18] Heart disease, diabetes, osteoporosis, and cancer are all long-latency diseases.

Dietary antioxidants such as vitamin E play an important role. We are all aware that the vitamin E story is still emerging and is more complex than was thought in the 1980s. Clinical trials have suggested that vitamin E supplementation does not have favorable effects in CVD[19] and certain cancers[20,21] (although studies of other types of cancer have had more positive outcomes[22]). Vitamin E appears to play a complex role in modulating oxidative stress through its direct and indirect influence on signaling processes associated with oxidative stress. Indirectly, vitamin E appears to influence inflammatory pathways that, in turn, influence oxidative stress. Vitamin E also has direct effects on cellular mitochondrial redox, altering the signaling pathways so that redox signaling is modified. In some sense, vitamin E might be seen as a cell-signaling messenger. It's not just trapping oxidants. It has a specific cellular effect on regulation of the redox signal to the nucleus. Vitamin E works in combination with many other factors to control redox signaling. In studies that have used vitamin E by itself, the outcome on cellular function is different than when a complex array of antioxidant nutrients is provided, as is found in whole phytonutrient-rich foods.[23] The intervention studies with vitamin E alone may, therefore, not be evaluating the actual contribution of vitamin E, as found in the complex diet, to redox control. This might help explain why results of the Nurses' Study demonstrated a significant reduction in heart disease in women who consumed a diet high in vitamin E,[24] but the intervention trials with vitamin E alone have not demonstrated this protective effect.[25]

What about beta-carotene? In the Finnish smokers' study, the supplemental beta-carotene in the smoking group generated a small but statistically significant increase in lung cancer, a result which disappeared during post-intervention follow-up, confirming the effect.[26] The participants in this study were 2- to 3-pack-per-day smokers who were known to consume high levels of alcohol. Smoking and drinking large amounts of alcohol are activities that increase hepatic oxidative stress. It has been demonstrated that oxidative injury to beta-carotene produces harmful oxidation products that can subsequently damage tissue.[27,28] This suggests that supplementation with high doses of beta-carotene while smoking and consuming excess alcohol loads the dice in favor of potential carcinogenesis.

Charles Lieber, MD, who is at the Bronx VA Hospital and an expert in studying the effects of alcoholism in animals, showed that if you gave beta-carotene supplements to baboons that had been forced to drink alcohol, they had a high incidence of hepatoxicity.[29] A subsequent study in human smokers confirmed this tendency.[30] The oxidation products of beta-carotene created the higher risk. Once again, the question that emerges is whether antioxidants, as part of a complex diet, may have a different physiological effect than taking supplemental pharmacological doses of antioxidants.

As was previously mentioned, regulation of redox is tightly tied to control of the glutathione cycle, which is an important part of cellular defense. Glutathione participates in cellular protection in two ways—as an antioxidant through its role in regenerating glutathione from glutathione disulfide, and as a direct conjugate for detoxification. Glutathione conjugation is a fundamental process in the detoxification of drugs and xenobiotics. If a patient has an upregulated detoxification process requiring glutathione, he or she is going to deplete hepatic glutathione, resulting in less available glutathione for the antioxidant function. The result is that the liver is under oxidative stress. The patient develops a functional glutathione insufficiency that alters cellular redox, because the most important single antioxidant in liver cells is the glutathione-to-glutathione disulfide couple.

Fatty Acids

The mitochondrial membrane is a lipid bilayer, made up of phospholipids such as phosphatidylserine, phosphatidylinositol, and phosphatidylethanolamine. These phospholipids are highly unsaturated fatty acid derivatives. Much of the mitochondrial membrane is made up of omega-3 fatty acids. Just as we don't want to cook on the stove with omega-3 fatty acids because they are easily oxidized and become rancid, we also don't want to expose the mitochondrial membrane to excessive free radical oxidants that would cause injury and oxidative damage. Protecting the lipid bilayers of the mitochondrial membrane appears to be one important role of antioxidants.

Fatty acids don't diffuse across the mitochondrial membrane. They're first conjugated to carnitine, which is outside the mitochondria, and then the enzyme carnitine palmitoyl transferase 1 (CPT1) transports the conjugated fatty acid across the mitochondrial membrane. Once within the mitochondrial matrix, the fatty acid is deconjugated with a second enzyme, CPT2, an isozyme of CPT1. A carnitine deficiency in the cell would affect its ability to burn fats because, without adequate carnitine, fats can't be transported into the mitochondria where they can be metabolized; clinically, this would raise triglyceride levels. There are examples in the literature of the treatment of hypertriglyceridemia by the administration of therapeutic doses of L-carnitine to both humans[31] and animals.[32] (Carnitine is not an essential nutrient. It's called a "conditionally essential nutrient," meaning that a person's need for carnitine at times may exceed his or her own body's ability to manufacture it. There are some nutrients that are essential to everybody, and there are also conditionally essential nutrients that may be, under certain conditions, essential because the body can't make enough of them. CoQ10, lipoic acid, and gammalinolenic acid, or dihomogammalinolenic acid would be examples of conditionally essential nutrients.

It has also been shown that omega-3 fatty acids, which make up the mitochondrial membrane, are potentially important therapeutic agents to regenerate healthy mitochondrial membranes. Cell membrane fluidity and the role of the membrane in regulation and transport depend on unsaturated fatty acids such as docosahexaenoic acid, or DHA. Brain, mitochondria, and spermatozoa membranes have very high levels of DHA in their composition.[33,34,35]

The mitochondria have a close relationship with other organelles, like the peroxisomes. The peroxisomes are very important organelles for maintaining energy dynamics. They have the responsibility for breaking down the long-chain fatty acids into smaller, bite-sized pieces that can be transported across the mitochondrial membrane. The mitochondria don't transport long-chain fatty acids. They like shorter fatty-acid chains. The peroxisome is controlled, in part, through regulating factors called orphan nuclear receptors, such as peroxisome proliferator activated receptors (PPARs). The glitazone drugs have been found to work as PPAR gamma (PPARγ) agonists and the fibrates are PPAR alpha (PPARα) agonists. Both these families of drugs influence fatty acid metabolism and its relationship to diabetes and heart disease. (There is a new family of drugs that is probably going to be approved soon that are mixed agonists of PPARα and γ, so that they will better manage the conversation between fats, the mitochondria, and insulin.)

There is a connection between insulin, diabetes, and mitochondrial dysfunction. In diabetes, fatty acid metabolism is altered, resulting in fat infiltration of the liver. Diabetes is not just a sugar problem; it's also a fat problem. When we talk about oxidative chemistry, we are also talking about proper regulation of fatty acid metabolism through control of peroxisome function, and the interface with the nuclear orphan receptor family that signals to the peroxisomes to break down the fats so they can enter the mitochondria for proper energy regulation. That process can be activated by sending a signal to the nuclear orphan receptors to come up to speed and activate fat and sugar metabolism.

Foods

It has been discovered that there are foods in our normal diets that are mixed PPARα and γ agonists.[36] If you eat a phytonutrient-rich diet, you are already getting molecules that speak to your nuclear orphan receptors and cause signaling to occur. More and more foods that contain these PPARα and γ agonists are being identified. Cinnamon, for instance, contains compounds that influence insulin signaling. Momordica, or bitter melon, has been identified to have PPARα and γ activity. Licorice[37] and ginseng[38] also have PPARα and γ agonist capability. Gymnema also contains phytochemicals that modulate PPAR activity. Conjugated linolenic acid (CLA)[39] is a PPAR agonist. Historically, we have been eating foods that have a nutrigenomic influence on these energy control processes. Unfortunately, we've taken a lot of these nutrients out of our food through processing. Certain diseases that have their origin in altered cellular bioenergetics might be caused, at least in part, by the loss of nutrients in our diet that are associated with the control of these important energy-signaling processes.

Clinical Conditions Associated with Altered Mitochondrial Function

What are the clinical conditions that have been associated with altered bioenergetics and mitochondrial dysfunction? The list is long and growing. Oxidative stress, inflammatory cytokines, and changes in endothelial dynamics all appear to be related to heart failure. Strategies designed to modify their pathological effects represent new therapeutic potentials. These often involve improvements in mitochondrial function and redox control. The conditions and diagnoses associated with mitochondrial defects cut across most sub-specialties in medicine. The list includes skeletal muscle weakness, fatigue, myopathy, including conditions like fibromyalgia syndrome and other myopathic syndromes.

In cardiac disease, it is recognized that Wolff-Parkinson-White syndrome is a mitochondria-associated disorder.[40] A cardiac mitochondrial defect can lead to a sudden conduction velocity disorder and cardiac failure. Even in fit people, these mitochondrial myopathies can have serious, adverse effects. Leber's optic neuropathy[41] is an inborn error of metabolism relative to mitochondria; certain hepatopathies, specific kidney dysfunctions, and certain endocrine pancreatic dysfunctions, including diabetes, are all associated with mitochondrial problems. Also included in this list are certain colonic obstructive disorders and certain types of sensory deafness and hearing impairment in older-age individuals that occur as a consequence of mitochondrial dysfunction (for which acetyl-L-carnitine has been shown to improve auditory thresholds[42]). Conditions associated with mitochondrial dysfunction cut across multiple organs, but they cluster in tissues that have the greatest degree of oxygen-processing and bioenergetic activity.

Fatigue-Related Syndromes and Mitochondrial Injury

Greg LeMond is a previous world-class bicyclist and Tour de France winner who retired at the peak of his career with what his physician defined as "acquired mitochondrial myopathy." There is some evidence from the sports world, particularly in endurance events, that elite performance capacity can be lost as a result of overtraining.[43] Studies have been published showing mutations in mitochondrial DNA in muscle biopsies from athletes with sustained fatigue.[44] Their symptoms mimic those of chronic fatigue syndrome, or CFS.[45]

These findings raise the question of whether CFS could be, in part, a clinical syndrome associated with lowered bioenergetic capability due to chronic mitochondrial dysfunction, or mitochondrial injury. Paul Cheney, MD, PhD, a member of IFM in its founding years, was a world expert and one of the original researchers on CFS.[46] He did some work with us in the early 1990s showing that his most severe CFS patients had very marked oxidative injury to their mitochondria, resulting in the accumulation of 8-hydroxy-deoxyguanosine (8OHdG), which is a measurement of damaged DNA from oxidative stress. When a certain level of mitochondrial injury was reached (the point at which around 70% of the mitochondrial genome was damaged, according to Dr. Cheney), he found that it was not possible to bring these patients back to health. They died of many different diagnoses, including cardiopathies.

The mitochondria, in some philosophical sense, has the role of generating the energy necessary to maintain cellular organization, from which the body maintains its structure and function against the natural disordering tendency in the universe, which is called entropy. The reason people eventually die is that the ordering and stabilizing energy systems of the body are exceeded by the natural disordering tendency of the universe. The mitochondrion is constantly supplying the energy to keep order—regeneration, healing, inflammatory response, and rebuilding. If mitochondrial energy production is lost in a certain organ or tissue, that organ or tissue starts shifting its function into a degenerative mode, because it no longer has enough ordering energy.

Maintenance of mitochondrial function in tissues that are high-oxygen consumers is a critical part of a molecular preventive medicine program. The clinician needs to be aware of how to protect the mitochondria against injury, particularly in the post-mitotic tissues (brain, heart, and muscle). These tissues do not regenerate very rapidly. If they are injured, their mitochondria may have a chance to replicate, but if they have mutational injuries, they will replicate the mutation. The problem can then be perpetuated, and a downward cycle can begin.

This situation can be characteristic of patients who present with CFS, fibromyalgia, multiple chemical sensitivities, or anything related to a chronic, mitochondrial, bioenergetic dysfunction. These patients appear worn out; they are dragging around, ragged, and tired. They have lymphadenopathy, fatigue of unknown origin, intolerance to previously well-tolerated exercise, and sleep disturbances. The reasonable assumption that there is an underlying bioenergetic deficit begs the question, why would patients with something like a post-viral fatigue syndrome stay fatigued for years? Why don't they just get over it, like any other kind of limiting infection?

The association with bioenergetics can be understood by taking a look at the general pattern:

- Upregulation and activation of the immune system increase inflammatory mediators and enhance mitochondrial oxidative stress.
- The oxidative injuries are clustered in the gut, liver, muscles, and brain.
- The inflammatory mediators work at the mitochondrial level to alter cell signaling, which causes a reduction of ATP in the mitochondria.
- A reduction in ATP causes the cell membrane binding and transport processes to be modified.
- The membrane pumps are altered and extracellular calcium goes into cells. Cytosolic calcium goes up and, as it does, activation of mitochondrial oxidative stress occurs.

To break the cycle, clinicians and patients must work together to remove the precipitating factors (triggers and mediators) that are activating the immune system. As discussed extensively in other chapters of this book, important steps in such a process may include a detoxification diet, elimination of toxic exposures, removal from the diet of antigens to which the patient is sensitive, and support of intestinal immune function through the 4R program. Then, a metabolic program to regenerate mitochondrial function to the greatest extent possible should be initiated. Depending upon the individual patient's history and condition, a variety of therapeutic agents for mitochondrial resuscitation have been investigated (although significantly more research is needed): CoQ10,[47,48] lipoic acid,[49] N-acetylcarnitine,[50] N-acetylcysteine,[51] vitamin E,[52,53,54] flavonoids,[55,56] and omega-3 fatty acids[57] have all demonstrated beneficial (although often different) effects on mitochondrial function. Finally, basic lifestyle changes to support the treatment program on an ongoing basis should be implemented—as you would expect, these changes include a healthy diet, rich in phytonutrients; moderate exercise suited to the patient's physical condition; decreased stress and improved stress management; and adequate rest. All of these interventions help to break the oxidative stress cycle.

Summary

Clinicians are just starting to learn how important maintaining mitochondrial function is from the functional medicine perspective. Because symptoms indicative of oxidative stress can present with so many different complaints, conditions, and diseases, it is vital to understand the common underlying mechanisms in order to develop clinical strategies that can affect multiple organs and systems through the improvement of mitochondrial function. Although the evidence base is far from complete, there are strong indications of approaches that can be used effectively. These approaches are highly consistent with therapeutic interventions presented throughout this book for multiple conditions and diseases, providing confirmation of the functional medicine principles upon which they are based.

Oxidative Stress and Autism

Woody R. McGinnis, MD[ii]

Introduction

Both indirect and direct markers suggest increased oxidative stress in autism. Indirect markers include lower antioxidant enzymes and glutathione, lower antioxidant nutrients, higher toxin levels, impaired energetics, impaired cholinergic function, greater excitotoxicity, and greater free-radical production.

Direct markers for oxidative injury to biomolecules are abnormal in autism: higher red-cell lipid peroxides; higher urinary isoprostanes, and accelerated lipofuscin deposition in autistic cortex. Brain and gut, pathological in autism, are inherently sensitive to oxidative injury. Double-blind, placebo-controlled trials of potent antioxidants—vitamin C or carnosine—have significantly improved autistic behavior. Benefits of these and other nutritional interventions may be due to reduction of oxidative stress. Understanding the role of oxidative stress should help illuminate the pathophysiology of autism, its environmental and genetic influences, new treatments, and prevention.

Oxidative Stress in Autism

As described earlier in this chapter, when oxidants exceed the antioxidant defense, biological systems suffer oxidative stress, with damage to biomolecules and functional impairment. Autism is a behavioral disorder, with hallmark communication and social deficits. It has been suggested that oxidative stress may play a role in the pathophysiology that underlies the behaviors that define autism.[58] Another serious behavioral disorder, schizophrenia, features high oxidative biomarkers[59] and clinical response to vitamin C.[60] Many neuroleptic medications used in the treatment of schizophrenia are, in fact, potent antioxidants.[61]

Oxidized Biomolecules in Autism

Lipids, proteins, glycoproteins, and nucleic acids are subject to oxidative injury, and a number of analytical methods exist for measurement of oxidative by-products in urine, blood, breath, and organ tissue samples. Oxidized lipids and their protein adducts are commonly used as oxidative biomarkers. Lipids, which comprise biological membranes, are easily oxidized, particularly if highly unsaturated. Direct markers for lipoxidation are higher in autism. In a published study that carefully eliminated dietary and medicinal confounders, levels of red-cell thiobarbituric reactive substance (TBARS, a measure of lipoxidation) in autistic children were twice as high as those in age-matched controls.[62] Other, preliminary studies found serum lipid peroxides[63] and urinary isoprostanes[64] significantly higher in the autistic group.

Indirect markers are consistent with greater lipoxidation in autism. Low concentrations of highly unsaturated lipids in autistic subjects' red-cell membrane[65] suggest oxidative depletion. Higher phospholipase A_2[66] and loss of membrane lipoprotein asymmetry[67] in autism comport with oxidative effects.

Lipofuscin is a non-degradable matrix of oxidized lipid and cross-linked protein that forms in tissues as a result of oxidative injury. Co-localization of lipofuscin with specific subcellular components or injurious agents may provide clues to neuropathogenesis. In Alzheimer's disease, lipofuscin is associated with oxidized mitochondrial DNA.[68] Examination of lipofuscin itself can be informative: a documented case of human mercury poisoning with psycho-organic symptoms measured elevated brain mercury, which localized in lipofuscin 17 years after exposure.[69]

Lipofuscin is experimentally induced by strong prooxidants such as iron[70] or kainic acid.[71] In animal experiments, lipofuscin forms initially in the hippocampus, later in the cortical brain.[72] Also in animals, lipofuscin deposition is retarded by supplementation with vitamins C and E[73] or carnitine.[74] Measurable brain activity is inversely correlated with lipofuscin content.[75]

[ii] Adapted, with permission, from McGinnis WR. Oxidative stress in autism. Altern Ther Health Med. 2004;10(6):22-36.

Edith Lopez-Hurtado and Jorge Prieto found greater lipofuscin in areas of the autistic cortical brain concerned with language and communication, deficits of which are integral to the diagnosis of autism. After age seven, in comparison to controls, greater lipofuscin was measured in autistics in Broadmann area 22 (Wernicke's, speech recognition), area 39 (reading), and area 44 (Broca's, language production).[76] (See Figure 30.1.)

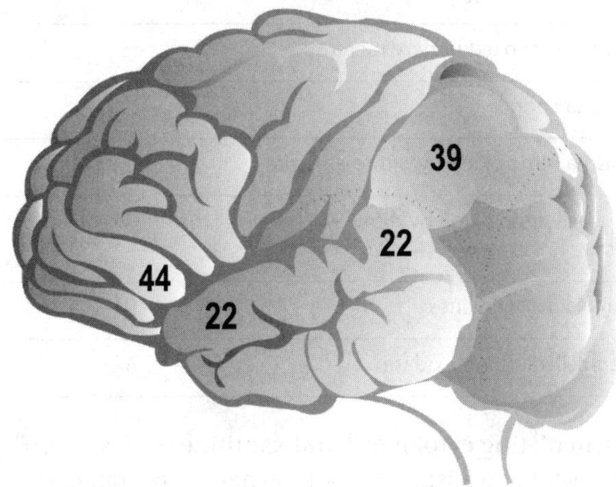

Figure 30.1 **Areas of greater lipofuscin in autistic brain**

In both autistic and control subjects, lipofuscin was always more prominent in Brodmann area 44 at all ages. Analysis by cortical layers showed that the number of cells (both pyramidal and non-pyramidal neurons) containing lipofuscin was larger in layers II and IV. A significant decrease in neuronal cell numbers was found in layers II and IV.[77] Greater lipofuscin also has been reported in Rett syndrome,[78] on the autistic spectrum.

The retina, a virtual extension of the brain, is very sensitive to oxidative stress. Greater oxidative stress is associated with flattened electroretinograms and increased retinal lipid peroxides in animal experiments.[79] In autism, abnormal retinograms with flattened b-waves[80,81] suggest oxidative retinal injury. Data implying greater oxidation of biomolecules in autism are summarized in Table 30.1.

Table 30.1 **Oxidized Biomolecules in Groups of Autistic Children vs. Controls**

Elevation/Abnormality	Reference
Red-cell lipid peroxides by TBARS	62
Serum lipid peroxides	63
Urinary isoprostanes	64
Lipofuscin in cortical brain	75
Abnormal retinograms	80, 81

Indirect Markers are Consistent with Greater Oxidative Stress

Indirect markers for greater oxidative stress in autism include lower endogenous antioxidant enzymes and glutathione, lower antioxidant nutrients, higher organic toxins and heavy metals, higher xanthine oxidase and cytokines, and higher production of nitric oxide ($NO^{\bullet}$), a toxic free radical.

Lower levels of antioxidant enzymes and glutathione in autism (Table 30.2) may stem from lesser production or greater consumption, and impose greater vulnerability to oxidants. Lower antioxidant nutrients (Table 30.3) may be attributed to lower intake or absorption, and/or greater depletion by oxidants. A substantial literature documents increased oxidation of biomolecules and cell injury in relevant nutrient-deficient states.[82] Nutrient levels affect the status of glutathione and antioxidant enzymes. The glutathione-boosting effect of vitamin C and vitamin E supplementation is well known. Marginal deficiency of vitamin B6 is associated with lower glutathione peroxidase (GPx) and glutathione reductase.[83] All forms of GPx contain selenium, and strong correlations exist between low and low-normal blood selenium levels and GPx activity.[84]

Table 30.2 **Antioxidant Enzymes and Glutathione in Groups of Autistic Children and Controls**

Lower in Autism	Reference
Red-cell GSHPx	337, 338
Plasma GSHPx	93, 343
Red-cell SOD	337
Platelet SOD	338
Red-cell catalase	62
Total plasma glutathione	374
Plasma GSH/GSSG	374

Table 30.3 **Antioxidant Nutrients in Groups of Autistic Children vs. Controls**

Lower in Autism	Reference
Plasma vitamins C, E and A	211
Red-cell activated B6 (P5P)	160
Red-cell B6 activity by EGOT	211
Red-cell magnesium	211
Red-cell selenium	211
Plasma zinc	244
Red-cell zinc	211

Organic toxins[85,86] and heavy metals[87] are strongly pro-oxidant. Impaired detoxification in autism[88] undoubtedly contributes to higher toxin levels (see Table 30.4). Toxins incite the production of oxidative species by various mechanisms. The volatile organic compounds and insecticides stimulate nitric oxide synthase (NOS).[89] Copper catalyzes the production of potent hydroxyl radical (OH•), especially when catalase is insufficient.[90] Mercury is known to increase oxidative stress by blocking mitochondrial energy production and depleting glutathione.

Table 30.4 **Higher Pro-oxidants in Groups of Autistic Children vs. Controls**

Higher in Autism	Reference
Plasma perchloroethylene, hexane, pentane	211
Red-cell mercury, lead and arsenic	211
Higher provoked urinary mercury	436
Plasma copper	299
Plasma nitric oxide by *nitrite* + *nitrate*	94, 95
Red-cell nitric oxide by *nitrite* + *nitrate*	96
Circulating cytokines	91
Red-cell xanthine oxidase	62

Circulating cytokines[91] and xanthine oxidase (XO)[92] are greater in autism, and both generate free radicals. XO actually results from oxidative alteration of xanthine dehydrogenase. Cytokines and XO can be both cause and effect of greater oxidative stress.

Higher Free-Radical Production in Autism

NO•, which is short-lived, is measured indirectly as total *nitrite* + *nitrate*, stable derivatives of NO•. In autism, red-cell[93] and plasma[94,95] total *nitrite* + *nitrate* are elevated, and plasma *nitrite* + *nitrate* levels correlate positively with TBARS.[96] Excess NO• production is suspected to play a role in other neurobehavioral disorders, including schizophrenia,[97] Alzheimer's disease, Down syndrome,[98] and multiple sclerosis.[99] It is undetermined whether production of excess NO• in autism localizes to specific organs or tissues. Cytokine-producing cells anywhere can stimulate NO•. Inflammation in the autistic gut and/or brain might contribute significantly to overall NO• production. Excess NO• in the brain would be a serious matter, as it increases apoptosis,[100] leaky blood-brain barrier (BBB),[101] and demyelination,[102] any of which might influence neurodevelopment in autism.

Decreased activity of oxidant-sensitive receptors is found in the autistic brain, and this may relate to greater concentrations of NO• specifically, or greater oxidative stress generally. Cholinergic receptor activity is decreased in the autistic cortex,[103] and cholinergic receptors are sensitive to NO• toxicity.[104] Gamma-aminobutyric acid (GABA) receptors, generically sensitive to oxidative stress,[105] are reduced in the autistic hippocampus.[106] It is conceivable that a GABA polymorphism associated with autism may lead to an increase in the sensitivity of this receptor to oxidative stress.[107]

In the existing literature, lesser cerebellar Purkinje cell numbers and smaller neurons in the entorhinal cortex and medial amygdala are consistent findings in autism,[108] with marked Purkinje cell loss described as the most consistent finding.[109] "Stunted" pyramidal neurons and decreased complexity and extent of dendritic spines are found in the hippocampus.[110] These findings are unexplained. Current technology would allow quantification and localization of specific oxidative (and nitrosative) biomarkers and any corresponding microscopic pathology in autistic brain.

Gross and microscopic gut inflammation is very common in autism (see Table 30.5). Corresponding symptoms—pain, constipation or diarrhea, gastroesophageal reflux,[111] and increased intestinal permeability[112]—are also frequent. Inflammation of the distal ileum with adenopathy can be particularly prominent.[113,114] The inflamed autistic gut probably contributes substantially to greater NO• production in autism, as inflammation of the gut is associated with greater NO• production in other clinical conditions. Plasma *nitrite + nitrate* is elevated in childhood colitis.[115] In chronic diarrhea, urinary *nitrite + nitrate* excretion correlates with leaky gut.[116]

NO• is potently antimicrobial.[117] Certain viruses and bacteria provoke massive local production of NO• in the gut[118] and brain.[119] Unfortunately, massive NO• also oxidizes host tissue.[120,121] Thus, in the gut, excess NO• is known to increase inflammation and permeability.[122] The young gut is uniquely sensitive to damage by NO•, especially the ileum.[123,124] Too much NO• can deplete the antioxidant defense, depressing levels of reduced glutathione (GSH).[125,126] Low GSH, in turn, increases NO•.[127] Nitrite is known to bind GSH.[128] In essence, a mutually amplifying positive-feedback loop exists between gut inflammation and NO•.

Table 30.5 **Gut Abnormalities in Subgroups of Autistic Children**

Abnormality		Autistic Sub-group	Reference
High intestinal permeability	42%	Asymptomatic	112
Reflux esophagitis	69%	Abdominal symptoms	178
Chronic gastritis	42%	Abdominal symptoms	178
Chronic duodenitis	67%	Abdominal symptoms	178
Ileal lymphonodular hyperplasia	89%	Regressed, gut symptoms	113
Colitis	88%	Regressed, gut symptoms	113

A particularly ominous result of excess NO• is increased formation of peroxynitrite ($ONOO^-$), which savages biomolecules. $ONOO^-$ is formed by reaction of NO• with superoxide ($O^{-\bullet}$); it is much more reactive than its parent radicals. Known targets of $ONOO^-$ attack with possible relevance to autistic pathophysiology include: tyrosine groups (as in glutamine synthetase and glutathione reductase inhibition), sulfhydryl (-SH) groups, superoxide dismutase (SOD), neurofilaments, ceruloplasmin (releasing pro-oxidant copper), membrane receptors, ion channels, G-proteins, and methionine. $ONOO^-$ aggressively depletes antioxidants, peroxidizes lipids, and breaks DNA.[129,130]

NO• is too ephemeral for distant transport. Hypothetically, however, excess NO• originating in one site could cause damage in more distant tissue via higher circulating nitrite and nitrate. Experimentally, intravenous nitrite injures the BBB.[131] Conceivably, higher levels of circulating nitrite from the inflamed autistic gut may be injurious to the brain.

It is thought that excess NO• production outside the gut, by raising levels of circulating stable products of NO• (nitrite, nitrate, and S-nitrosohemoglobin), may lead to greater production of NO• in the gut, with resultant gut inflammation.[132,133] Nitrite and nitrate are selectively removed from the circulation by the gut.[134,135] Various bowel flora convert nitrite and nitrate to NO• by enzymatic reduction,[136,137] which is catalytically favored by low oxygen tension,[138] as found in the gut. In the case of S-nitrosohemoglobin, NO• release is facilitated by low oxygen tension and the presence of sulfides produced by certain bacteria.[139]

As modulated by gastrointestinal flora, excess production of NO• from any site in the body—including brain or non-localized immune activation—might serve to inflame the autistic gut. Alternatively, a primary inflammatory process in the gut—whether infectious, toxic, or autoimmune—could account for greater total NO• production in autism.

Brain and BBB Sensitivity to Oxidative Stress

The brain is inherently sensitive to oxidative stress due to its higher energy requirements, higher amounts of lipids, iron and auto-oxidizable catecholamines, and lower levels of certain endogenous antioxidant molecules.[140,141] The protective BBB is relatively sensitive to oxidative damage.[142] Clinical and laboratory findings suggest a leaky BBB in autism. (See Table 30.6.)

Table 30.6 **Leaky Blood-Brain Barrier in Autism?**

Clues and Predisposing Factors	Reference
High antibodies to brain proteins	150, 151, 152, 153
Sleep disturbance in autism	146, 178
Perivascular lymphocytic cuffing	95
Higher NO/nitrite	94, 95, 96
Lower zinc	211, 244
Higher circulating cytokines	91
Higher heavy metals	211, 436

Clinicians report immediate behavioral improvement in some autistic children at the time of infusion with GSH.[143] In healthy animals, transit of GSH across the intact BBB is practically nonexistent, so this clinical response in autistic children may be consistent with leaky BBB in autism.

Also in animals, experimental oxidative injury to the BBB preferentially injures the reticular formation.[144,145] In autism, widely reported difficulties with falling asleep or staying asleep[146] suggest the possibility of reticular formation dysfunction. Further, the specific nature of rapid eye movement (REM) abnormalities found in autistic sleep disturbance is more typically associated with neurodegenerative disorders in which oxidative stress has been documented.[147] Other than melatonin, which has proved effective in autistic sleep disorders,[148] the effect of antioxidants on autistic sleep disturbance has not been investigated.

Laboratory observations also suggest leaky BBB in autism. Perivascular lymphocytic cuffs reported in three of seven autistic brains[149] are sentinel, though nonspecific. High autoimmune titers to central nervous system proteins in autism[150,151,152,153] suggest abnormal exposure of the immune system to brain antigens via leaky BBB.

The autoimmune response to brain antigen may be promoted by generation of neoepitopes, which can result from oxidative alteration of host proteins.[154] If they co-exist, autoimmune and oxidative mechanisms in the autistic brain may be mutually reinforcing, as NO• production is increased significantly in autoimmune disease of the central nervous system.[155]

Conditions that have been documented in autism are associated with a porous BBB in animals. Higher levels of circulating cytokines,[156] heavy metals,[157] NO•,[158] and nitrite[159] produce leaky BBB in animals. Lower zinc status in autism[160,161] may be relevant to BBB status. Zinc at physiological concentrations protects the BBB from injury,[162] while zinc deficiency increases BBB permeability, particularly in conjunction with oxidative stress.[163]

Intriguingly, preliminary data suggest overgrowth of gram-negative aerobes in autistic throat and rectal cultures.[164] These organisms produce endotoxin, renowned for permeabilization of the BBB.

Investigation of the autistic BBB is warranted. Enhanced magnetic resonance imaging technology can demonstrate BBB leaks,[165,166] and scanning electron microscopy can visualize BBB injury, including luminal protrusion, endothelial craters, vacuolation, inclusion bodies, and necrosis, though such visible lesions may be sparse.[167]

Greater Oxidative Stress and the Gut

Ischemia/reperfusion studies demonstrate that the gut is very sensitive to oxidative injury.[168,169] Ingested toxins such as peroxidized fats, electrophilic food contaminants, allergens, and microbial metabolites present a large oxidative burden to the intestinal epithelium.[170] Sufficient quantities of GPx (to reduce peroxides), GST (to reduce electrophiles), and GSH (to facilitate both GPx and GST), are required to protect the gut from oxidation.

As indicated earlier, ileal inflammation and adenopathy are conspicuous in autistic children with gastrointestinal symptoms. Ileum appears more vulnerable to oxidative injury. In animals, GST is 36-fold lower in the distal ileum than in the proximal intestine.[171] Double knock-out genes for gastrointestinal GPx result in mucosal inflammation of the ileum, but not other parts of the intestine.[172] In human inflammatory bowel disease, NOS expression is most prominent in the ileum, and the ileum is most sensitive to NO•-dependent oxidative injury.[173]

Excess NO• is a plausible mediator for common autistic gastrointestinal abnormalities. (See Table 30.7.) NO• degrades mucin, which protects the gut from a wide variety of irritants.[174] Excess NO• increases intestinal permeability,[175] prevalent in autism.[176] In excess, NO• relaxes the esophageal sphincter,[177] and two-thirds of autistic children with gastrointestinal symptoms have reflux esophagitis.[178]

Table 30.7 Autistic Gut Abnormalities Possibly Mediated by Excess NO•

Abnormality in Autism	Reference
Inflammation	108, 111, 113, 114
Increased intestinal permeability	112
Low esophageal sphincter tone	177
Poor gall-bladder contraction	352
Slow-transit constipation	113

Excess NO• inhibits gall bladder contraction,[179] perhaps accounting for lighter-colored stools observed in many autistic children by parents and clinicians. Poor bile flow impairs nutrition and limits delivery of protective GSH to the gut mucosa.

Excess NO• mediates slow-transit constipation.[180] Many autistic children are constipated, some with very large caliber stools. It is possible that malabsorption and floral overgrowths offset clinical constipation in even larger numbers of autistic children.

Oxidative Stress, Low Energy Production, and Excitotoxicity

Oxidative stress, impaired energy production, and excitotoxicity are dynamically related. For instance, energy-producing mitochondria are sensitive to oxidative injury,[181,182,183,184,185,186,187] and injured mitochondria leak more oxidants into the cellular environment.[188,189,190] Impaired energy production predisposes to activation of excitatory receptors, decreased intracellular calcium buffering, and increased oxidizing species—as well as apoptosis.[191,192]

Overstimulation of excitatory receptors results in oxidative neuronal injury,[193,194] and greater oxidative stress increases release of glutamate and subsequent stimulation of excitatory receptors.[195,196] Subcellular anatomy correlates with this functional relationship: excitatory glutamate receptors and NOS in the brain and gut[197] are co-localized.

As a general rule, oxidative biochemistry adheres to the following construct, which is both consistent and useful:

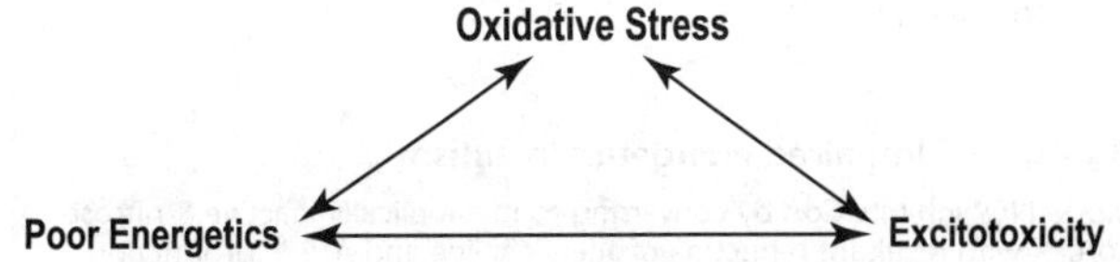

Accordingly, greater oxidative stress in autism implies associated problems in energy production and excitotoxicity.

Impaired Energetics in Autism

Magnetic resonance imaging has demonstrated decreased ATP levels in the autistic brain.[198] In blood, higher lactate,[199,200] higher pyruvate,[201] higher ammonia, and lower carnitine[202] have been documented in groups of autistic children. Collectively, these differences suggest impaired mitochondrial function in autism and, in fact, mitochondrial abnormalities are reported in autistic case studies.[203,204]

Excess NO• in autism may impair energy production, directly or via $ONOO^-$. Excess NO• reduces oxidative phosphorylation, lowering ATP and increasing lactate.[205] NO• directly inhibits complex IV, causing leakage of superoxide and inhibition of GPx.[206] $ONOO^-$ selectively damages complexes I and III.[207] NO• inactivates coenzyme A (CoA), depriving mitochondria of this precious "energy currency."[208] (See Figure 30.2.)

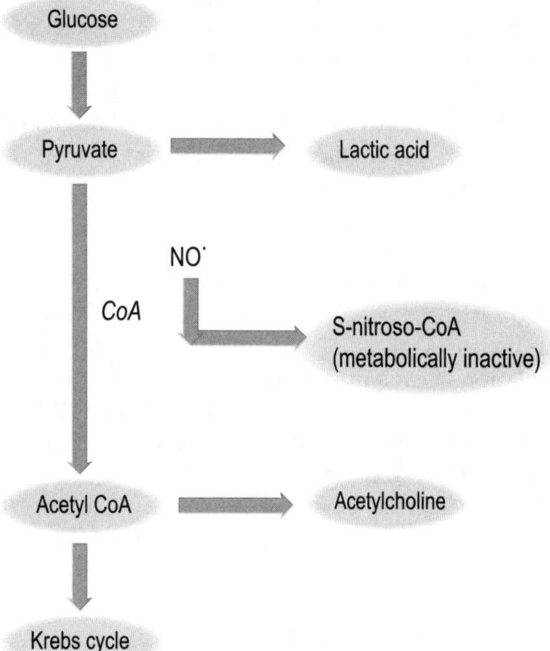

Figure 30.2 **Impaired energetics in autism**

Excess NO• inhibits CoA by conversion to metabolically inactive S-nitroso-CoA,[132] with resultant reduction of acetylcholine and ATP[198] production. Lower ATP,[198] higher lactate[199,200] and higher pyruvate[201] are found in autism.

Excitotoxic Markers in Autism

Higher extracellular glutamate in the brain is associated with excitotoxicity, especially if energy metabolism is compromised.[209] Glutamic acid decarboxylase (GAD) converts glutamate to GABA, and GABA lessens excitotoxicity. A decrement in brain GAD favors excitotoxicity by increasing glutamate and decreasing GABA.

There is ample suggestion that GAD is depressed in autism. The quantity of GAD in the post-mortem autistic brain is decreased by half.[210] Peripheral measurements are consistent. Red-cell GAD binding affinity is lower,[211] plasma glutamate higher,[212,213] and plasma glutamine lower[214] in autism. GAD,[215] glutamine synthetase,[216] the glutamate transporter,[217] and inhibitory GABA receptors[218] are sensitive to oxidative stress.[219] (See Figure 30.3.)

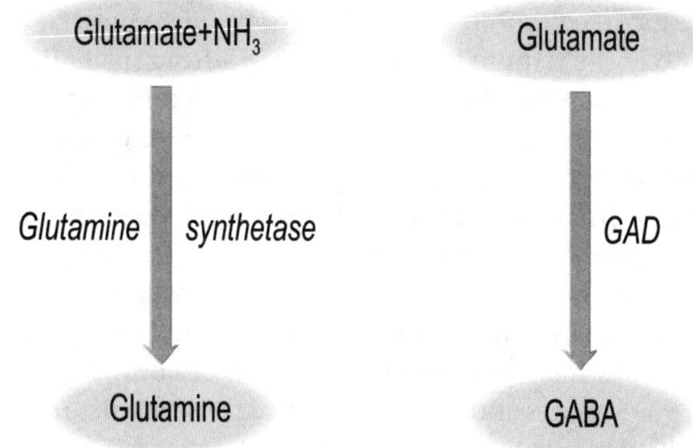

Figure 30.3 **Excitotoxicity in autism**

Higher extra-cellular glutamate and lower GABA increase excitotoxicity. GAD quantity and activity are lower in autism. GAD, glutamine synthetase, and glutamate transporter are sensitive to oxidative stress.

Whether cause or effect of greater oxidative stress in autism, greater excitotoxicity is a reasonable hypothetical and clinical concern. Excitotoxicity can be aggravated by oral ingestion of excitotoxic compounds,[220] and the author joins many other clinicians in advising autistic patients to avoid flavor enhancers such as monosodium glutamate (MSG) and aspartame in food and drink.

Impaired Cholinergics in Autism

Laboratory and clinical observations suggest a significant cholinergic deficit in autism, and this also is consistent with greater oxidative stress. Cholinergic receptor activity is lower in the autistic cerebral cortex.[221] Treatment with cholinergic agonists[222,223] or a precursor (deanol) for acetylcholine[224] is associated with improved behavior in autism.

Response to bethanecol, a specific agonist for the muscarinic subtype of cholinergic receptors, is suggestive. Oral bethanecol (2.5–12.5 mg bid) normalizes dilated pupils, increases bowel motility, and improves sleep pattern and behavior in many autistic children. Occasionally, sudden behavioral improvement is reported immediately after a single dose of bethanecol,[225] and the author confirms this observation.

Neuroimaging reveals cerebral hypoperfusion in autism,[226,227] worsening with age,[228] and vasodilatation of cerebral microvessels is the province of muscarinic receptors.[229,230] A possible explanation for the rapid bethanecol response is sudden improvement in cerebral perfusion. Bethanecol may stimulate readily accessible muscarinic receptors in the small blood vessels that perfuse the brain.

Muscarinic impairment in autism may potentiate greater oxidative stress. Experimentally, muscarinic signals are neuroprotective, shielding cells from oxidative stress and apoptosis.[231] Muscarinic receptor numbers are decreased by oxidative stress.[232] They are sensitive to NO• toxicity[233] and, relative to other receptor subtypes, preferentially sensitive to inhibition by $ONOO^-$[234] and other oxidants.[235]

As discussed earlier, excess NO• in autism may depress CoA, which is important in energy production and a necessary precursor for the cholinergic neurotransmitter, acetylcholine. (See Figure 30.2.) Insufficient CoA renders cholinergic neurons more vulnerable to a variety of toxic insults, including the effects of excess NO•.[236] CoA function has not been studied in autism, but does appear to play an important role in encephalopathies.[237]

Antioxidant Nutrients in the Treatment of Autism

A double-blind, placebo-controlled university trial utilized 8 grams per 70 kg body weight per day of oral vitamin C in two or three divided doses in institutionalized autistic children.[238] Some of the cohort had been on doses of up to 4 grams of vitamin C prior to the trial. The cross-over design, comprised of three 10-week periods, included treatment of all subjects with vitamin C for the first 10 weeks. In the second and third phases of the trial, half the children received placebo and then vitamin C. The other half received vitamin C and then placebo.

Psychometric testing was performed after each 10-week phase of the study, but not prior. Total scores on the Ritvo-Freeman (RF) scale, which rates 47 social, affective, sensory, and language behaviors, demonstrated improvement in the group going from placebo to vitamin C, and worsening in the group going from vitamin C to placebo ($p=0.02$). Pacing, flapping, rocking, and whirling behaviors, in particular, corresponded to vitamin C manipulation, and a group of "strong responders" was described as "obvious" to the investigators. No serious side effects were reported in this study, but clinicians report that excessive stool softening sometimes limits vitamin C dosing in autistic children.

Vitamin C is strongly antioxidant. This suggests—but does not prove—an antioxidant mechanism for its therapeutic effect in these autistic subjects. Antioxidant effects of vitamin C do seem to match known abnormalities in autism. Vitamin C provides good protection against excess NO• and $ONOO^-$.[239] Vitamin C is known to protect neurons from glutamate neurotoxicity,[240] as glutamate re-uptake involves exchange for vitamin C.[241] Vitamin C blocks the inhibition of glutamate transport by NO•,[242] an effect seen particularly in the presence of copper,[243] higher in autistic blood.[244]

Carnosine

Carnosine, a naturally-occurring amino acid found in high concentrations in the brain, is a strong antioxidant and neuroprotectant.[245,246] A double-blind, placebo-controlled 8-week trial of carnosine (400 mg by mouth twice daily) produced significant improvement in autistic children compared with placebo. Psychometric testing demonstrated improvements in vocabulary ($p=0.01$), socialization ($p=0.01$), communication ($p=0.03$), and behavior ($p=0.04$).[247] Side effects were inconsequential: sporadic hyperactivity responded to lowering the dose of carnosine, and no child had to discontinue the study due to side effects.

Possible physiological mechanisms for the carnosine effect in autism include its prevention of NO• toxicity,[248] binding of free radicals and reactive hydroperoxides, and the ability to complex with metals such as copper.[249] The copper:carnosine complex demonstrates antioxidant, SOD-like activity *in vitro*.[250]

Vitamin B6

Any mechanistic hypothesis for autism should accommodate the successful application of high-dose vitamin B6 pioneered by Bernard Rimland. Multiple controlled trials demonstrate that, in combination with magnesium, B6 improves behavior in many autistic children.[251,252,253] While serum B6 levels usually are normal, B6 activity, as reflected by erythrocyte glutamic oxaloacetic transaminase (EGOT) assay, is lower in autistic children.[254]

There is some evidence that pyridoxal kinase, which converts B6 to its active form, pyridoxal-5-phosphate (P5P), is impaired in autism. A preliminary study found poor binding affinity of pyridoxal kinase in autistic red cells, as reflected by high K_m (Michaelis constant).[255] P5P activity in blood is below normal in over 40% of autistic subjects.[256] Pyridoxal kinase has many modulators. Lower zinc[257,258] and energy status in autism may be operant in this context, as pyridoxal kinase requires ATP-facilitated release of zinc from metallothionein for activation.[259] The potential role of inhibiting agents should be considered. The strongest pyridoxal kinase inhibitors are the carbonyl agents, which are exogenous compounds such as hydrazine, from jet fuel.[260] Endogenous carbonyls result from oxidative alteration of lipids, proteins, and sugars, and are broadly elevated in clinical conditions associated with excess NO•.[261] It is not established whether endogenous carbonyls inhibit pyridoxal kinase.

While the cause of poor B6 function in autism is not fully articulated, we can be sure that B6 impairment favors greater oxidative stress. As discussed earlier, even marginal B6 deficiency is associated with lower GPx and glutathione reductase activity, lower reduced-to-oxidized glutathione ratios, and higher lipid peroxide levels.[262]

B6 deficiency results in mitochondrial decay and, consequently, oxidative stress.[263,264] P5P is required for the synthesis of key mitochondrial components: iron-sulfur crystals (for complexes I, II and III), heme (for complex IV),[265] and coenzyme Q10.[266] Experimentally, P5P protects neurons from oxidative stress, apparently by increasing ATP production and stemming extracellular glutamate.[267]

Lagging B6 function lowers the excitotoxic threshold. P5P is a necessary cofactor for GAD, impairment of which can increase glutamate receptor activation, NO•, and oxidative stress.[268] P5P protects GAD, sensitive to oxidative impairment,[269] from inactivation.[270] (Likewise, P5P protects gastrointestinal GPx by complex formation.[271]) Predictably, P5P administration to animals increases brain GAD activity.[272]

High doses of B6 may benefit autistic patients by increasing energy production, lessening excitotoxicity, increasing GABA, and reducing oxidative stress. Treatment with B6 also may relieve a state of functional B6 deficiency caused by excess oxidants. The B6 vitamers are highly vulnerable to damage by oxidative species such as hydroxyl (OH•) and singlet oxygen ($^1O_2$).[273,274,275] Oxidative impairment of B6 potentially impairs myriad enzymes and neurotransmitters in autism.

Magnesium

In animal experiments, magnesium deficiency increases NO•,[276] increases lipid peroxides,[277] and lowers plasma antioxidants.[278] Magnesium supplementation lowers oxidative stress experimentally in animals with higher oxidative stress.[279] So, low magnesium favors oxidation.

As a group, autistic children have lower magnesium, as measured sensitively in red cells.[280] Double-blind trials demonstrate behavioral improvement and normalization of evoked potential recordings in autistic children receiving combined high-dose B6 and magnesium, but no significant improvement with high-dose B6 or magnesium alone.[281] The synergism may be a cofactor function. For instance, B6-dependent kinase, which affects diverse muscarinic and GABA-nergic functions, requires both B6 and magnesium.[282]

Magnesium also protects against oxidative stress via functions unrelated to B6. Production of NADPH requires magnesium for reduction of glutathione. ATP synthase, which catalyzes energy production by oxidative phosphorylation, is magnesium sensitive.[283] In the brain, magnesium normally blocks overactivity of excitatory receptors by modulating calcium channels.[284]

Zinc

Lower zinc status in autism has been well documented. Red-cell zinc, a sensitive indicator of zinc sufficiency, is significantly lower in the autistic group[285] and, in individual cases, may be half the lower limit for age-matched controls.[286] Plasma zinc is sub-normal in 40% of autistic children.[287]

Low zinc potentiates oxidative stress. In animals, zinc-deficient diets decrease total glutathione, vitamin E, GST, GPx, and SOD levels, while increasing lipid peroxides and free radicals in tissue, mitochondria, and cell membranes.[288,289,290,291] In elderly adults, zinc supplementation decreases lipid peroxides.[292] In diabetics with retinopathy, zinc supplementation increases GPx and decreases lipid peroxides.[293]

Zinc status affects the intestine. Zinc deficiency in animals increases gastrointestinal NOS and susceptibility to gastrointestinal infection.[294] Conversely, supplemental zinc decreases intestinal lipoxidation[295] and lessens intestinal permeability.[296]

Clinicians increasingly appreciate zinc as a mainstay in the treatment of autism. William Walsh, who organized zinc and copper data on over 3,500 autistic children at the Pfeiffer Treatment Center, finds that high doses of zinc (2–3 mg per kg body weight per day, of highly absorbable zinc picolinate) are often needed to achieve optimal behavioral response.[297]

Periodic measurement of plasma zinc is used to assure that zinc is not pushed above the normal laboratory range. Zinc is withheld on the day of testing to avoid artifacts. Zinc supplementation lowers copper, and this is usually desirable. Serum copper monitoring is used to avoid subnormal levels.[298]

Copper excess is evident in autism. Higher total serum copper,[299] lower ceruloplasmin,[300] and higher unbound copper in serum[301] are reported in autistic children. Copper, especially unbound, is highly pro-oxidant. Supplemental copper is rarely needed in autism, and even small doses of copper in supplements have been observed to produce negative behavioral effects.[302] Higher serum copper-to-plasma zinc ratios (in autism, mean 1.63 vs. 1.15 in controls, $p<0.0001$),[303] are correlated significantly with systemic oxidative stress in neurodegenerative disease.[304] Sufficient zinc supplementation normalizes copper/zinc ratios.[305]

High zinc dosing can suppress manganese. A balancing dose of manganese, administered separately from zinc at dosages of approximately 5 mg manganese to 30 mg of zinc, is often beneficial, and serum manganese levels can be monitored to avoid excess.[306]

The antioxidant functions of zinc are prodigious. There are several important mechanisms:

- **Zinc protects SH (sulfhydryl) groups against oxidation**, as, for example, in the protection of the key antioxidant enzyme, GPx.[307] The initial event in experimental zinc deficiency is loss of membrane SH groups, with consequent membrane fragility.[308]
- **Zinc competes with pro-oxidant metals such as copper and iron** for binding sites, preventing metal-catalyzed free-radical formation.[309] Copper-containing enzymes are inherently prone to auto-oxidation, which is prevented by zinc.[310] Copper-induced membrane oxidation is prevented by zinc.[311]
- **Zinc is an essential constituent of copper-zinc SOD**, a key antioxidant enzyme. Even marginal zinc deficiency in humans decreases SOD activity.[312] Zinc-deficient SOD becomes pro-oxidant, catalyzing biomolecular attack by $ONOO^-$.[313] Zinc-less SOD is neurotoxic.[314]
- **Zinc induces the synthesis of metallothionein (MT)**,[315] an effective scavenger of free radicals (including $ONOO^-$)[316] and sequestrant for copper and other heavy metals.[317,318] In animals, high-dose zinc induces measurably higher gastrointestinal MT levels.[319] Moderate zinc deficiency in animals, in which overt negative health effects are not manifest, is associated with significant reduction of retinal MT.[320] MT normally increases as a protective response to oxidative stress, but actually decreases in response to oxidants when zinc is deficient.[321] MT also blocks copper toxicity, but this protective effect is lost in the presence of excess $NO^•$, which releases copper from MT, causing lipid peroxidation and apoptosis.[322] In the brain, MT_{III}, a neuronal growth inhibiting factor, is particularly sensitive to copper displacement by oxidants.[323] This suggests a mechanism for reported greater gross brain size in younger autistic children.[324]
- **Zinc provides a physiological glutamate receptor blockade**,[325] lessening excitotoxicity.
- **Diverse biomolecules are protected from oxidation by zinc.** By complexing with phospholipids,[326] zinc blocks oxidation of fatty membranes.[327] Zinc blocks peroxidation of polyunsaturated fat unbound to membrane.[328] Zinc generally inhibits the oxidation of enzymes and other proteins,[329] including those with functional SH groups vulnerable to mild oxidative conditions: Na,K-ATPase, Ca-ATPase, aquaporin, the voltage-gated calcium channel, and the NMDA-calcium channel.[330]

Future studies may establish that oxidative stress decreases clinical zinc retention. At a molecular level, oxidants (including $NO^•$) displace zinc from proteins, including MT.[331,332,333,334] This phenomenon may extrapolate to lesser whole-body zinc retention under greater oxidative stress. Schizophrenics have diminished urinary zinc loss in response to high doses of B6,[335] possibly associated with antioxidant effects of B6.

Selenium

Mean red-cell selenium levels are lower in autistic children,[336] and this may contribute to reported lower GPx in autism.[337,338] As stated previously, GPx activity correlates with low-normal and borderline selenium levels.[339] Clinicians frequently include oral selenium,

50–300 mcg/d, in nutritional supplementation for children with autism.

GPx is irreplaceable in the antioxidant defense, especially for protection of mitochondria, which do not contain catalase for protection from peroxide.[340] In addition, GPx confers sole protection from organic hydroperoxides, which sustain the devastating lipoxidation chain reaction.[341,342]

Lower GPx activity in frank selenium deficiency is associated with peroxidative damage and mitochondrial dysfunction.[343] The physiological effects of selenium deficiency can be compensated partially by administration of vitamin E.[344] GPx is sensitive to inactivation by copper[345] and mercury.[346] Human mercury exposure is associated with decreased GPx activity and increased lipid peroxides.[347] In animals, GPx is protected by P5P[348] and zinc supplementation.[349]

Lower GPx in autism favors greater membrane lipid peroxidation, which is known to impair receptor and enzyme functions, presumably due to conformational changes and altered binding.[350] Lipid peroxidation has been shown to inhibit muscarinic, adrenergic, serotonergic, and insulin receptors, as well as Na,K-ATPase, and glutamine synthase.[351]

Reduced Glutathione

In an open-label trial, daily intravenous GSH improved patients with early Parkinson's disease.[352] Likewise, intravenous GSH improves behavior in many autistic children, including very rapid extinction of perseverative behaviors such as hand-flapping. Rarely, apparent histamine-mediated reactions (sneezing, coughing, pruritic eyes) are noted.[353]

Oral GSH, up to 30 mg per kg body weight per day, has been beneficial in some children with cystic fibrosis, a high-oxidant state.[354] The author finds similar doses of oral GSH helpful in some autistic children. Reversible adverse behavioral reactions to oral GSH have been reported in children with low plasma zinc levels. It is thought such GSH intolerance may result from rapid induction of metallothionein, which may deleteriously affect circulating zinc.[355]

Oral GSH is relatively well-absorbed. In animals, plasma GSH doubles within two hours of a large oral dose, mostly from absorption of intact GSH.[356] Increased animal organ levels of GSH are attributed to absorption of intact GSH.[357] In healthy humans, a 15 mg per kg oral dose of GSH increases plasma GSH levels by two- to five-fold.[358]

High intestinal mucosal demand for GSH can exceed synthesizing capacity,[359] as would be expected in inflamed autistic gut. The intestinal mucosa imports intact GSH from both the intestinal lumen[360,361] and the plasma[362] to combat oxidation. In normal physiology, biliary excretion of GSH represents a significant portion of total hepatic GSH production, and bile regularly bathes the intestinal mucosa with GSH.

Severe degeneration of the epithelium of the small intestine and colon, with mitochondrial swelling and degeneration, results from experimental GSH deficiency; these changes are prevented by the administration of oral GSH, which is associated with increased mucosal GSH levels.[363] In animals, mucosal GSH levels increase rapidly and significantly after oral GSH, but less in the ileum than elsewhere.[364] Oral GSH may lower oxidative stress in the autistic gut.

Strong *in vitro* antiviral properties of GSH are noted,[365] and chronic viral infection in autism has not been ruled out.

An Oxidative Perspective on Newer Treatments for Autism

Subcutaneous vitamin B12 injections, as preservative-free methylcobalamin, 1250–7500 mcg weekly to daily, reportedly improve behavior in autistic children.[366] One B12 intermediate, cob(I)alamin, is exquisitely sensitive to oxidative inactivation,[367] so functional B12 deficiency may result from greater oxidative stress in autism.

NO• and nitrite elevations in autism should sound the "B12 alarm." An intermediate form of B12 reacts specifically with NO•,[368,369,370] and nitrite inactivates methylcobalamin.[371] NO• binds B12 to impair enzyme function, as with *in vivo* inhibition of methionine synthase by NO• at physiological concentrations.[372] Large parenteral doses of B12 are thought to scavenge and reverse the physiological effects of excess NO•.[373]

Oral folinic acid supplementation improves glutathione levels and GSH-to-GSSG ratios in autistic children.[374] Tetrahydrofolate is very sensitive to oxidation,[375,376] and degradation may be significant under conditions of greater oxidative stress.[377] Folate deficiency (which may be aggravated by B12 impairment) is known to decrease ATP levels and increase reactive oxygen species and excitotoxicity.[378]

Amino acid supplementation may be useful in autism. Plasma cysteine levels were much lower in a series of 286 supplement-naïve autistic children.[379] Cysteine is produced endogenously from methionine, and provides a full third of the substituent molecules in glutathione and metallothionein.

Oral N-acetylcysteine (NAC), as a source of cysteine, is generally well-tolerated in autistic children, while direct supplementation with cysteine is not. Intravenous NAC (150–600 mg NAC + 1000–2000mg vitamin C + 1 ml sodium bicarbonate) treatments were reported to improve behavior in autistic children.[380]

The Pfeiffer Treatment Center follows generous zinc loading with a proprietary oral supplement[381] containing the amino acid constituents of MT. Initial data suggest that this formula increases levels of MT.[382] Some parents report improvement in autistic behavior coincident with greater exposure to natural sunlight. Ultraviolet radiation rapidly induces metallothionein,[383] so sunlight may be of benefit if zinc is sufficient.

Thiamine tetrahydrofurfuryl disulfide (TTFD) via rectal suppository improved behavior and increased heavy metals clearance in autistic children.[384] TTFD provides high cellular levels of thiamine, which boosts three mitochondrial enzymes known to be especially sensitive to oxidative stress.[385,386] One of these, α-ketoglutarate dehydrogenase complex, is a rate limiter in energy metabolism and is inactivated by NO•, both directly and via $ONOO^-$.[387]

Casein- and gluten-free diets improved behavior in autistic children, possibly by reducing excess central opioid effects.[388] Higher peripheral opioid peptides from casein and gluten are demonstrable in the urine of autistic patients,[389] possibly due to oxidative inhibition of the enzyme needed to complete digestion of dietary casein and gluten.[390] In addition, a shift towards oxidation in the redox environment is known to strengthen opioid binding, and GSH to weaken it.[391]

Fatty acid supplementation has been found beneficial in autism.[392] Lower concentrations of highly-unsaturated fatty acids in plasma[393] and red-cell membranes[394,395] may be due to oxidative depletion of these key membrane building blocks and prostaglandin precursors. Depletion of omega-3 and omega-6 polyunsaturated fatty acids also is seen in schizophrenia, and these changes are associated with increased lipid peroxide levels.[396]

Eicosapentaenoic acid (EPA, an omega-3) was lower in the red-cell membranes of autistic children generally; arachidonic acid (AA, omega-6) was lower in the regressed subgroup.[397] Fish oil, high in EPA, suppresses production of NO• and other free radicals[398,399] and increases expression of GST and mitochondrial SOD.[400] Brain levels of NO• and lipid peroxides are less in animals on diets supplemented with fish oil.[401]

Administration of fish oil to even marginally B6-deficient animals can result in increased tissue lipid peroxide levels.[402] Prior administration of vitamin B6 and other antioxidants is suggested in autism, to avoid generation of toxic lipid peroxides.

Ongoing administration of fish oil to autistic children is associated with significant lowering of red-cell membrane dihomogamma-linolenic acid (DGLA).[403] DGLA is an essential omega-6 precursor for prostaglandin-1, which tightens leaky gut and boosts immunity. Accordingly, autistic children receiving fish oil may benefit from a balancing dose of evening primrose oil, which provides gamma linolenic acid (GLA), a DGLA precursor.

Clinical and laboratory assessment helps titrate fatty acid dosing. After antioxidant loading, many autistic children do well on an initial dose of 3 grams fish oil and 1 gram evening primrose oil.[404] Optimal doses vary individually, and over time.

Laboratory Assessment of Oxidative Stress

The use of oxidative biomarkers in the clinical management of autism is nascent. Various blood, urine, stool, and breath assays[405] are potentially useful in determining optimal doses and combinations of nutrients and other interventions.

Some available assays include lipid peroxides, 4-hydroxynonenal (4-HNE), malondialdehyde (MDA), isoprostanes, levuglandin adducts, nitrotyrosine, oxidized nucleic acids, protein carbonyls, advanced glycation end-products, cellular apoptosis, nutrient and antioxidant enzyme concentrations, total *nitrite + nitrate*, enzyme-binding affinities, and luminal NO• by rectal catheter. Ten-fold higher levels of neopterin,[406] a marker for upregulation of NO• synthesis,[407] suggest possible clinical utility of this measurement in autism.

In research, autistic brain and gut tissues certainly should be examined for specialized oxidative and nitrosative markers. Conventional pathologic assessment of autistic brain tissue may not detect neuronal loss due to apoptosis, a marker for oxidative stress[408] that can be obscured by rapid removal of apoptotic cells.[409]

Testing for Oxidative Biomarkers

Jointly, formal research and case-by-case testing by clinicians will determine the utility of oxidative biomarkers in the management of oxidative stress in autism. Potential assays vary in specificity, sensitivity, sample stability, and cost. Fundamentally, the most useful biomarkers will be those which best correlate with clinical improvement. Utility may vary among individual patients.

It is established that various blood fractions for GSH, GPx, and catalase are quite low in autism, and it is known that these parameters are affected by antioxidant treatments in other illnesses. Besides their more general usefulness, tissue concentrations of antioxidant nutrients (vitamins C, E, A; Zn, Mg, Se, fatty acids) or pro-oxidants (Cu, Fe, heavy metals) imply an oxidative diathesis. Cellular markers such as natural killer cytotoxicity or apoptosis may prove useful.

Non-invasive biomarkers are appealing. Breath-testing for ethane and pentane are limited presently to research. DNA-adducts in urine are available commercially, but have not been measured systematically in autism. Pre-publication data from two studies indicate that urinary isoprostanes are much higher in autism; these are more stable than lipid peroxides, and less prone to artifact from fats ingested prior to collection.

By survey, we identified a commercial American laboratory—BioHealth Diagnostics—that offers urinary isoprostane testing. Simultaneous measurement of urinary creatinine improves accuracy of urinary isoprostane assay. A number of progressive commercial laboratories (Great Smokies, Great Plains, Immunosciences, Metametrix, Vitamin Diagnostics) measure the various oxidative biomarkers, including indirect assessment of hydroxyl radical production and energy profiling by urinary organic acid analysis.

Future Directions

Leading thinkers are now giving serious consideration to the potential significance of greater oxidative stress in autism. If oxidative stress proves important in autism, there are many implications. For instance, nutritional management of autism[410] to modulate oxidative stress would presumably gain importance.

We may need to reconsider ingrained living habits. Consumption of free radicals via foods fried in polyunsaturated oils[411] may need to be curbed. Ingestion of excitotoxic flavor enhancers, chlorine, nitrite, nitrate, and copper in water may need reassessment. Pro-oxidant[412,413,414] and antioxidant[415,416,417,418] drug profiles may become more pertinent.

We may need to consider how oxidative influences during pregnancy can affect neurodevelopment, including post-partum development. Gestational zinc deficiency, for instance, produces oxidative DNA damage in newborn primates.[419] The ubiquitous flavor enhancer and excitotoxin MSG traverses the placenta and causes fetal neurotoxicity in rodents.[420]

Higher $NO^{\bullet}$ is now a well-established fact of autism that may provide clues to specific etiologies, aggravants, and treatments. Viral infections can greatly increase $NO^{\bullet}$ production in brain and other tissues, so high $NO^{\bullet}$ in autism should increase the demand for a systematic examination of autistic tissues for viral antigen.

Higher $NO^{\bullet}$ in autism might focus useful attention on treatment with antioxidants with specificity for $NO^{\bullet}$. Vitamin C is a good $NO^{\bullet}$ quencher,[421] and so are melatonin and uric acid. Melatonin effectively scavenges both $NO^{\bullet}$ and $ONOO^{-}$.[422] Melatonin has excellent potential for relief of oxidative stress in both brain and gut,[423,424] increases expression of GPx,[425] and has proved effective in autistic sleep disorders.[426]

Uric acid normally represents up to 60% of total plasma antioxidant capacity.[427] It effectively binds transition metals and reactive species, and is especially effective at quenching $NO^{\bullet}$[428] and $ONOO^{-}$.[429] Careful upward titration of uric acid levels with oral inosine, a uric acid precursor, may be of benefit in high-$NO^{\bullet}$ states such as multiple sclerosis[430] and autism.

Testing and treating mitochondrial function to improve energy production probably merits a higher priority in autism. Acetyl-L-carnitine (ALC) and α-lipoic acid (ALA) enhance mitochondrial function and reduce oxidative stress in senescent animals.[431] Oral administration of the mitochondrial metabolite L-carnitine has improved behavior in children with Rett syndrome,[432] and initial trials of high carnitine doses in autism are underway.

A leading university clinic often treats patients referred for suspected mitochondrial disease with a combination of CoQ10, vitamin E, and balanced B vitamins.[433] CoQ10, in combination or alone, is an attractive potential intervention in autism. It facilitates ATP production by carrying electrons and protons in the electron transport chain, and also acts in its reduced form to protect mitochondria by quenching oxidants.[434] Vitamin B3 is crucial to mitochondrial energy production and effective in the high-oxidative state of schizophrenia,[435] but has received little attention in autism.

Many key biochemical functions are sensitive to oxidative impairment (Table 30.8). We need to examine systematically the functions of the enzymes, receptors, G-proteins, and vitamin cofactors in autism, and integrate findings into clinical management. Glucose-6-phosphate dehydrogenase (G-6-PD) activity, given its central role in the reduction of GSH, is but one of many oxidant-sensitive functions that deserve scrutiny. We should not be surprised to encounter a very broad enzymopathy in autism.

Table 30.8 **Sensitive to Oxidative or Nitrosative Impairment**

Enzyme or Cofactor	Reference
Glutamic acid decarboxylase	215
Glutamate transporter	217
Glutamine synthetase	216, 351
GABA channels	105
B6 vitamers	273, 274, 275
Pyridoxal kinase by carbonyl inhibition	261
B6-dependent enzymes by carbonyl inhibition	437
Tetrahydrofolate	371, 376
Methionine synthase	438
B12 vitamers	367, 368, 369, 370, 371
Glucose-6-phosphate dehydrogenase	439
CoenzymeA	208
α-KGDHC	239, 386, 388
Na,K-ATPase, Ca^{++} Channels, Aquaporin	308, 351
Catalase	440
Glutathione peroxidase	271

Summary

The evidence strongly supports the presence of greater oxidative stress in autism. The clinical response to antioxidant nutrients also suggests that increased oxidative stress does affect the expression of autistic symptoms. The important issues surrounding this topic are (a) how oxidative stress creates these effects, and (b) what are the most effective therapeutic interventions.

Antioxidant therapeutic trials measuring oxidative biomarkers could help elucidate the mechanisms. While such research is progressing, clinicians and parents are advised to implement safe nutritional interventions—sooner, rather than later. It is also time to start applying laboratory biomarkers for oxidative stress to optimize doses and combinations of nutrients.

The preliminary lipofuscin data are potentially very important, and replicative and expansive studies are indicated. It is conceivable that lipofuscin analysis might identify specific toxic or infectious etiologies. Greater lipofuscin in the autistic brain is a concrete suggestion that neurodevelopment in autism is altered by oxidative influences.

By analogy, chronic neonatal vitamin E deficiency may help us understand how excess oxidative stress in early life can indeed affect neurodevelopment. Vitamin E deficiency is a neurological disease that clearly results from low antioxidant protection from birth.[436,437] Lipofuscin deposition is prominent. Neurological symptoms—gait disturbance, abnormal ocular movements—present at 18–24 months,[438] are a common chronology in autistic regression.

Beyond analogy, we simply might consider the clinical potential of vitamin E in autism, or in ostensibly healthy children prior to regression. Besides enteropathy, autistic children demonstrate an immune profile very similar to common variable immune deficiency (CVID).[439] Neurological complications of vitamin E deficiency are seen in patients with CVID and enteropathy, and vitamin E screening has been recommended for patients with these conditions.[440] Preliminary data suggest lower plasma vitamin E levels in autistic children,[441] and functional testing by red-cell hemolysis may be even more sensitive.

Optimistically, we note that oxidative damage to biomolecules is not always permanent. Oxidative inactivation of enzymes, for instance, is reversed when sufficient antioxidant is provided.[442] Even structural elements such as cytoskeleton can undergo restoration by GSH.[443]

If we learn that oxidative stress is an important mechanism in autism, then our search for genetic and environmental causes gains focus. A spatial or chronological map of oxidative changes in the autistic brain may conform to the effects of one or more toxins. Lipofuscin may contain an etiologic agent. Perhaps an efficient approach to genetic research should prioritize the examination of genes affecting autism that may also be relevant to oxidative stress. From the oxidative wounds, science may more rapidly deduce the causes, treatments, and prevention of autism.

Oxidative Stress and Glycemic Control

Dan Lukaczer, ND

Introduction

Type 2 diabetes (T2D) is a chronic, progressive disease that is becoming increasingly common throughout much of the world, with the incidence rising most rapidly among younger people. With the epidemic explosion of T2D in the United States, glycemic control has become an increasingly important clinical issue. Hyperglycemia, an inevitable consequence of T2D, is the source of most of the deleterious effects usually associated with this disease. Hyperglycemia leads to generation of free radicals or reactive oxygen species (ROS), a state known as oxidative stress. There is strong evidence that this oxidative stress is at least partly responsible for the development or exacerbation of insulin resistance during diabetes,[444] and for the complications, morbidity, and mortality associated with diabetes.[445] The body's defenses against oxidative stress (discussed in detail earlier in this chapter) are accomplished by an interconnecting system of endogenous antioxidant micronutrients, phytonutrients, and enzymes.[446] T2D is associated not only with increased ROS, but in many instances with a reduction in these antioxidant defenses as well.

We review in Chapters 19 and 34, respectively, glucose dysregulation and its many manifestations, and a practical clinical approach to the diagnosis and treatment of insulin resistance. Here we will focus specifically on an approach to controlling the oxidative stress that can often accompany this dysregulation. While clearly overlapping, it is important to understand T2D from this standpoint as well.

It is well established that tight glycemic control is the most effective way of preventing or decreasing diabetic complications. However, supplementation with antioxidant micronutrients has been proposed as an important adjunctive therapy. In a comprehensive review of oxidative stress and the use of antioxidants in diabetes in 2005, Johansen et al.[447] point out some of the problems with the evidence base on this topic: most of the studies have been done on animals, each one examining only a small part of the underlying mechanisms involved in the overall process; very few antioxidants have been studied in depth (primarily studied have been vitamins C and E and alpha-lipoic acid); the majority of clinical trials were not designed to study diabetic patients specifically; and "none of the studies to date effectively assessed the baseline oxidative stress of the enrolled patients using any of the commonly accepted markers of inflammation." Given all of these caveats, we nonetheless feel that the high level of oxidative stress present in diabetics warrants a review of the current evidence, and a judicious application of that evidence by clinicians.

The Link between Oxidative Stress and Glycemic Control

T2D is characterized by an increased risk for the development of macrovascular disease (coronary heart disease, cerebrovascular disease, and peripheral vascular disease) and microvascular complications (diabetic retinopathy, nephropathy, and peripheral neuropathy). Cardiovascular (CV) complications are the leading cause of mortality and morbidity in T2D.[448] Additionally, there is a strong relationship between poor glycemic control and the progression of diabetic complications such as retinopathy and polyneuropathy.[449]

Clearly, frank diabetes carries the most risk; however, the development of CV complications does not end precisely at the boundary of defined hyperglycemia. Even mild increases in blood sugar (referred to as impaired glucose tolerance) can contribute to microvascular injury, atherosclerotic changes, and cardiovascular disease.[450] It is clear that the progressive relationship between glucose levels and cardiovascular risk extends well below the diabetic threshold.[451]

While the mechanisms by which hyperglycemia produces these complications are complex and not completely understood, much evidence points to the association between hyperglycemia and increased oxidative stress.[452] Blood glucose control and vascular complications affect both free radical indices and antioxidant status in T2D patients.[453] In addition, many endothelial functions can be affected by ROS and oxidative stress (and may be ameliorated by exogenous antioxidants).[454]

Two primary mechanisms by which hyperglycemia promotes the generation of ROS are activation of the polyol pathway and increased glucose auto-oxidation. Reactive oxygen species affect vascular smooth muscle cell growth, migration, and endothelial function.[455] Elevated levels of ROS can also cause general damage to proteins through cross-linking, fragmentation, and lipid oxidation. Radical-generating reactions cause formation of advanced glycation end products (AGEs) due to elevated nonenzymatic glycation of proteins, lipids, and nucleic acids. Once formed, AGEs can influence cellular function by attaching to various binding sites. Binding of AGEs can result in generation of intracellular oxidative stress and subsequent activation of NFκB.[456] Additionally, there is specific evidence that in chronic hyperglycemia, apoptosis induced by oxidative stress causes reduction of beta-cell mass.[457] Overall, there is sufficient human and animal research to support the hypothesis that hyperglycemia results in increased oxidative stress and increased formation of advanced glycation end products.[458] There is also evidence that hyperinsulinemia, in the face of normal to near-normal glucose levels, may enhance free radical generation and thus contribute to oxidative stress as well.[459] Elevated insulin itself may inhibit proper metabolism of fatty acids, promoting the proinflammatory arachidonic acid cascade and resulting in increased free radical generation and oxidative stress.[460]

Hyperglycemia and Antioxidants

The body possesses defense mechanisms that, in the healthy individual, adequately control ROS concentrations under most conditions. In T2D, however, increased ROS generation results in increased oxidative stress, which in turn can lead to many of the hallmark complications of the disease. Reduction of oxidative stress is therefore an important goal for management of this condition. As discussed earlier in this chapter, antioxidant nutrients may help to reduce oxidative stress. In various studies of humans and animals, dietary supplementation with antioxidants is associated with decreased risk of T2D and induces changes that can be beneficial in reducing insulin resistance and protecting various tissues from injury.[461] Below is a review of certain antioxidants that may be of particular importance.

Lipoic Acid

Some of the most convincing evidence for a beneficial effect of antioxidant therapy in diabetes has been done on lipoic acid,[462,463,464] which is a potent lipophilic free radical scavenger. Since oxidative stress appears to play an important role in the pathogenesis of diabetic neuropathy, it is important to consider the benefits of lipoic acid in this condition. Several clinical studies reveal that lipoic acid is generally safe and effective in reducing symptoms of diabetic peripheral neuropathy. Doses of 600–1200 mg/d of ALA may improve microcirculation and diabetic polyneuropathy.[465,466] Oral treatment for 4–7 months tended to reduce neuropathic deficits and improve cardiac autonomic neuropathy.[467] Oral treatment also decreased urinary albumin excretion after 18 months, suggesting that the antioxidative effects of alpha-lipoic acid may play a promising role in the pathogenesis of diabetic nephropathy as well.[468] In a 2004 double-blind study, 600 mg of intravenous ALA rapidly and significantly improved neuropathic sensory symptoms.[469]

Vitamins

Studies of vitamin E have produced conflicting results. In an animal model, vitamin E supplementation significantly improved glycemic control, possibly by minimizing free radical damage to the pancreatic β-cells.[470] In humans, a low plasma vitamin E concentration was associated with a 3.9-fold increased risk of incident diabetes.[471] Vitamin E may reduce LDL-cholesterol oxidation and therefore may decrease cardiovascular risk in T2D.[472] However, not all human studies have been positive. For instance, the Heart Outcomes Prevention Study, using a dose of 400 IU/day of d-alpha tocopherol, did not show improvement in microvascular or cardiovascular damage.[473] Overall, human studies with vitamin E have been mixed.[474]

Similarly, studies of vitamin C have shown positive effects, negative effects, and no effects, depending on the parameters (and subjects) being studied. When administered alone or in combination with vitamin E, vitamin C has been shown to lower oxidative stress parameters in diabetic animals.[475,476] Supplementation with vitamin C and/or E in animal models has been shown to modulate late pathological changes in the retina and peripheral nerves.[477,478,479] Two grams/day of vitamin C demonstrated a beneficial effect on both glycemic control and blood lipids in T2D subjects.[480] In another 1995 study, the percent increase in plasma vitamin C levels was correlated with the percent decline in plasma free radicals.[481] A 2002 study demonstrated that 1.25 g of vitamin C and 680 IU of vitamin E significantly lowered urinary albumin excretion rate, a marker of progression to end-stage renal disease.[482] One gram of vitamin C alone lowered the urinary albumin excretion in diabetic subjects,[483] but the same dose in a study of effects on microcirculation in T2D patients found no effect on microvascular reactivity, and no effect on inflammatory cytokines or ox-LDL.[484] Doses of 100 or 600 mg/d of vitamin C reduced sorbitol accumulation and therefore may be useful in preventing diabetic retinopathy complications.[485] On the other hand, a 2004 study[486] concluded that "high vitamin C intake from supplements is associated with an increased risk of cardiovascular disease mortality in postmenopausal women with diabetes." Interestingly, increased vitamin C from dietary changes did not show a similar pattern.

Riboflavin is an antioxidant that regenerates glutathione, which plays a major role in the detoxification of ROS. Riboflavin deficiency has been noted in T2D, but little interventional work has been done with this nutrient.

Minerals

Zinc and selenium have been shown to improve certain aspects of the oxidative stress of T2D. Selenium acts as a coenzyme in glutathione peroxidase (GPx) activity. It has been suggested that selenium, through its effect on GPx, may decrease NFκB activity, which has been associated with hyperglycemia and oxidative stress.[487] Selenium supplementation to diabetic rats prevents not only oxidative stress but renal structural injury as well, suggesting that selenium plays a role in reducing the oxidative stress associated with diabetes.[488,489] Human studies have also shown positive results in oxidative stress markers following selenium supplementation.[490]

Zinc is bound to insulin and stabilizes the molecule; decreased zinc uptake may be one of the features of diabetic patients.[491] Zinc supplementation has been shown to increase glucose disposal,[492] and a study of skeletal muscle cells indicated a positive effect on insulin signaling leading to glucose uptake.[493] Zinc depletion appeared to increase the susceptibility of insulin to free radicals, and it has been suggested that zinc is protective against free radical injury.[494,495] Supplementation with zinc may decrease antioxidant damage.[496]

Vanadium appears to exhibit antioxidant properties.[497] However, vanadium can become toxic and even a pro-oxidant at high levels.[498,499] Copper and manganese are both cofactors in superoxide dismutase. This suggests a physiological role for these nutrients as antioxidants in T2D. However, little work has been done with these nutrients to validate their usefulness.

Taurine, CoQ10, and Other Accessory Nutrients

Taurine and coenzyme Q10 are endogenous antioxidants that, while not essential nutrients, may be beneficial in T2D at higher levels. In rats with diabetes induced by chemical destruction of β-cells, taurine supplementation reduced renal oxidant injury by decreasing lipid peroxidation and inhibiting the accumulation of advanced glycation end products within the kidney.[500] The effects of oral treatment with coenzyme Q10 (60 mg twice daily) were examined in a randomized, double-blind trial of 30 patients with coronary heart disease. After eight weeks, the treatment group receiving coenzyme Q10 had reduced plasma levels of insulin (fasting and 2-hr), glucose, and lipid peroxides as compared to the control group.[501] In another trial, 200 mg of CoQ10 daily improved HA1C and blood pressure in T2D patients, but there did not appear to be a specific antioxidant effect that could be measured by the plasma levels of isoprostanes (markers of oxidative stress).[502] Results overall with CoQ10 are inconsistent,[503] but a 2004 review did conclude that CoQ10 might "improve endothelial dysfunction by 'recoupling' eNOS and mitochondrial oxidative phosphorylation."[504]

Other antioxidant phytonutrients have been reported to be beneficial. Dietary flavonoids such as catechins and quercetin may protect against oxidative stress in T2D.[505] *In vitro* and animal studies have shown that catechins in particular may help as antioxidants in protection of pancreatic beta cells.[506,507,508]

Summary

While there is still controversy over the role of antioxidants and oxidative stress in T2D, there appears to be sufficient evidence to show that oxidative stress in the diabetic patient is greater than normal antioxidant defenses can withstand; and this increased oxidative stress is associated with the onset and progression of diabetic complications. Overall, but by no means unanimously, results indicate that dietary supplementation with micronutrients may be a complement to conventional therapies for preventing and treating diabetes and its complications.[509] It seems likely that oxidative stress is only one factor contributing to diabetic complications; thus, antioxidant treatment would most likely be more effective if it were coupled with other treatments. While supplementation is expected to be more effective when a deficiency in these micronutrients exists, studies have reported beneficial effects in individuals without deficiencies. Some of these positive studies were short term and had small sample sizes, but there are other, placebo-controlled, multicenter trials that have shown significant improvements in diabetic complications by addressing the oxidative stress component of diabetes. Treatment with antioxidants has been demonstrated to preserve beta-cell function, protect the vascular endothelium, and ameliorate polyneuropathy, retinopathy, and nephropathy. Results of these reviewed studies, and others, indicate that dietary supplementation with antioxidant nutrients may be a safe and simple complement to conventional therapies for preventing and treating diabetic complications. (Practitioners should also remember that dietary interventions to increase consumption of antioxidants have few safety problems, may produce an improvement in redox status parameters,[510] and undoubtedly produce significant other benefits as well, as discussed in many other chapters of this book.)

References

1. Givertz MM, Colucci WS. New targets for heart failure therapy: endothelin, inflammatory cytokines and oxidative stress. Lancet. 1998;352(suppl):34-38.
2. Schmitz C, Keller E, Freuding T, et al. 50-Hz magnetic field exposure influences DNA repair and mitochondrial DNA synthesis of distinct cell types in brain and kidney of adult mice. Acta Neuropathol (Berl). 2004;107(3):257-64.
3. Kurup RK, Kurup PA. Hypothalamic digoxin, geomagnetic fields and human disease—a hypothesis. Med Hypotheses. 2003;60(2):237-42.
4. Margulis L, Dolan MF, Guerrero R. The chimeric eukaryote: Origin of the nucleus from the karyomastigont in amitochondriate protests. Proc Natl Acad Sci U S A. 2000;97(13):6954-59.
5. Gray MW, Lang BF, Burger G. Mitochondria of protests. Annu Rev Genet. 2004;38:477-524.
6. Andersson SG, Karlberg O, Canback B, Kurland CG. On the origin of mitochondria: a genomics perspective. Philos Trans R Soc Lond B Biol Sci. 2003;358(1429):165-77.
7. Chan KM, Levin SA. Leaky prezygotic isolation and porous genomes: rapid introgression of maternally inherited DNA. Evolution Int J Org Evolution. 2005;59(4):720-29.
8. Bandelt HJ, Kong QP, Parson W, Salas A. More evidence for non-maternal inheritance of mitochondrial DNA? J Med Genet. 2005;May 27:Epub ahead of print.
9. Pakendorf B, Stoneking M. Mitochondrial DNA and human evolution. Annu Rev Genomics Hum Genet. 2005;Feb 15;Epub ahead of print.
10. Fosslien E. Mitochondrial medicine—molecular pathology of defective oxidative phosphorylation. Ann Clin Lab Sci. 2001;31(1):25-67.
11. Modrowski D, Orosco A, Thevenard J, et al. Syndecan-2 overexpression induces osteosarcoma cell apoptosis: Implication of syndecan-2 cytoplasmic domain and JNK signaling. Bone. 2005;June 2;Epub ahead of print.
12. Groenendyk J, Michalak M. Endoplasmic reticulum quality control and apoptosis. Acta Biochim Pol. 2005;June 1;Epub ahead of print.
13. Park JB, Lee JK, Park SJ, et al. Mitochondrial involvement in fas-mediated apoptosis of human lumbar disc cells. J Bone Joint Surg Am. 2005;87(6):1338-42.
14. Przedborski S. Pathogenesis of nigral cell death in Parkinson's disease. Parkinsonism Relat Disord. 2005;11(Suppl 1):S3-7.
15. Dawson VL, Dawson TM. Deadly conversations: nuclear-mitochondrial cross-talk. J Bioenerg Biomembr. 2004;36(4):287-94.
16. Berg D, Youdim MB, Riederer P. Redox imbalance. Cell Tissue Res. 2004;318(1):201-13.
17. Ames BN. The metabolic tune-up: Metabolic harmony and disease prevention. J Nutr. 2003;133:1544S-48S.
18. Heaney RP. Long-latency deficiency disease: insights from calcium and vitamin D. Am J Clin Nutr. 2003;78:912-19.
19. Duvall WL. Endothelial dysfunction and antioxidants. Mt Sinai J Med. 2005;72(2):71-80.
20. Lonn E, Bosch J, Yusuf S, et al. Effects of long-term vitamin E supplementation on cardiovascular events and cancer: a randomized controlled trial. JAMA. 2005;293(11):1338-47.
21. Bairati I, Meyer F, Gelinas M, et al. A randomized trial of antioxidant vitamins to prevent second primary cancers in head and neck cancer patients. J Natl Cancer Inst. 2005;97(7):481-88.
22. Meyer F, Galan P, Doubille P, et al. Antioxidant vitamin and mineral supplementation and prostate cancer prevention in the SU.VI.MAX trial. Int J Cancer. 2005;116(2):182-86.
23. Ito Y, Kurata M, Hioki R, et al. Cancer mortality and serum levels of carotenoids, retinol, and tocopherol: a population-based follow-up study of inhabitants of a rural area of Japan. Asian Pac J Cancer Prev. 2005;6(1):10-15.
24. Emmert DH, Kirchner JT. The role of vitamin E in the prevention of heart disease. Arch Fam Med. 1999;8(6):537-42.
25. Alkhenizan AH, Al-Omran MA. The role of vitamin E in the prevention of coronary events and stroke. Meta-analysis of randomized controlled trials. Saudi Med J. 2004;25(12):1808-14.
26. Virtamo J, Pietinen P, Huttunen JK, et al. Incidence of cancer and mortality following alpha-tocopherol and beta-carotene supplementation: a postintervention follow-up. JAMA. 2003;290(4):476-85.

27. Sommerburg O, Langhans CD, Arnhold J, et al. Beta-carotene cleavage products after oxidation mediated by hypochlorous acid—a model for neutrophil-derived degradation. Free Radic Biol Med. 2003;35(11):1480-90.
28. Yeh SL, Hu ML. Induction of oxidative DNA damage in human foreskin fibroblast Hs68 cells by oxidized beta-carotene and lycopene. Free Radic Res. 2001;35(2):203-13.
29. Leo MA, Kim C, Lowe N, Lieber CS. Interaction of ethanol with beta-carotene: delayed blood clearance and enhanced hepatotoxicity. Hepatology. 1992;15(5):883-91.
30. Leo MA, Lieber CS. Alcohol, vitamin A, and beta-carotene: adverse interactions, including hepatotoxicity and carcinogenicity. Am J Clin Nutr. 1999;69(6):1071-85.
31. Elisaf M, Bairaktari E, Katopodis K, et al. Effect of L-carnitine supplementation on lipid parameters in hemodialysis patients. Am J Nephrol. 1998;18(5):416-21.
32. Kim E, Park H, Cha YS. Exercise training and supplementation with carnitine and antioxidants increases carnitine stores, triglyceride utilization, and endurance in exercising rats. J Nutr Sci Vitaminol (Tokyo). 2004;50(5):335-43.
33. Bazan NG. Neuroprotectin D1 (NPD1): a DHA-derived mediator that protects brain and retina against cell injury-induced oxidative stress. Brain Pathol. 2005;15(2):159-66.
34. Chapkin RS, Hong MY, Fan YY, et al. Dietary n-3 PUFA alter colonocyte mitochondrial membrane composition and function. Lipids. 2002;37(2):193-99.
35. Lenzi A, Gandini L, Maresca V, et al. Fatty acid composition of spermatozoa and immature germ cells. Molec Hum Reprod. 2000:6(3):226-31.
36. McCarty MF. Nutraceutical resources for diabetes prevention—an update. Med Hypotheses. 2005;64(1):151-58.
37. Mae T, Kishida H, Nishiyama T, et al. A licorice ethanolic extract within peroxisome proliferators-activated receptor-gamma ligand-binding activity affects diabetes in KK-Ay mice, abdominal obesity in diet-induced obese C57BL mice and hypertension in spontaneously hypertensive rates. J Nutr. 2003;133(11):3369-77.
38. Yoon M, Lee H, Jeong S, et al. Peroxisome proliferator-activated receptor alpha is involved in the regulation of lipid metabolism by ginseng. Br J Pharmacol. 2003;138(7):1295-302.
39. Lampen A, Leifheit M, Voss J, Nau H. Molecular and cellular effects of cis-9, trans-11-conjugated linoleic acid in enterocytes: effects on proliferation, differentiation, and gene expression. Biochim Biophys Acta. 2005;Feb 16;Epub ahead of print.
40. Silva-Oropeza E, Reyes EG, Hernandez LR, Palencia LB. Mitochondrial hypertrophic cardiomyopathy associated with Wolff-Parkinson-White syndrome. Arq Bras Cardiol. 2004;82(5):490-92.
41. Qian Y, Zhou X, Hu Y, et al. Clinical evaluation and mitochondrial DNA sequence analysis in three Chinese families with Leber's hereditary optic neuropathy. Biochem Biophys Res Commun. 2005;332(2):614-21.
42. Seidman MD, Khan MJ, Bai U, et al. Biologic activity of mitochondrial metabolites on aging and age-related hearing loss. Am J Otol. 2000;21(2):161-67.
43. Angeli A, Minetto M, Dovio A, Paccotti P. The overtraining syndrome in athletes: a stress-induced disorder. J Endocrinol Invest. 2004;27(6):603-12.
44. Collins M, Renault V, Grobler LA, et al. Athletes with exercise-associated fatigue have abnormally short muscle DNA telomeres. Med Sci Sports Exerc. 2003;35(9):1524-28.
45. Derman W, Schwellnus MP, Lambert MI, et al. The 'worn-out athlete': a clinical approach to chronic fatigue in athletes. J Sports Sci. 1997;15(3):341-51.
46. Lapp, CW, Cheney PR, Rest J, et al. The chronic fatigue syndrome. Ann Int Med. 1995:123(1):74-76.
47. Rosenfeldt F, Marasco S, Lyon W, et al. Coenzyme Q10 therapy before cardiac surgery improves mitochondrial function and *in vitro* contractility of myocardial tissue. J Thorac Cardiovasc Surg. 2005;129(1):25-32.
48. Groneberg DA, Kindermann B, Althammer M, et al. Coenzyme Q10 affects expression of genes involved in cell signaling metabolism and transport in human CaCo-2 cells. Int J Biochem Cell Biol. 2005;37(6):1208-18.
49. Savitha S, Sivarajan K, Haripriya D, et al. Efficacy of levo carnitine and alpha lipoic acid in ameliorating the decline in mitochondrial enzymes during aging. Clin Nutr. 2005;May23;Epub ahead of print.
50. Ames BN, Liu J. Delaying the mitochondrial decay of aging with acetylcarnitine. Ann N Y Acad Sci. 2004;1033:108-16.
51. Cocco T, Sgobbo P, Clemente M, Tissue-specific changes of mitochondrial functions in aged rats: effect of a long-term dietary treatment with N-acetylcysteine. Free Radic Biol Med. 2005;38(6):796-805.
52. Valko M, Morris H, Cronin MT. Metals, toxicity and oxidative stress. Curr Med Chem. 2005;12(10):1161-208.
53. Fariss MW, Chan CB, Patel M, et al. Role of mitochondria in toxic oxidative stress. Mol Interv. 2005;5(2):94-111.
54. Hart PE, Lodi R, Rajagopalan B, et al. Antioxidant treatment of patients with Friedreich ataxia: four-year follow-up. Arch Neurol. 2005;62(4):621-26.
55. Wenzel U, Schoberl K, Lohner K, Daniel H. Activation of mitochondrial lactate uptake by flavone induces apoptosis in human colon cancer cells. J Cell Physiol. 2005;202(2):379-90.
56. Montero M, Lobaton CD, Hernandez-Sanmiguel E, et al. Direct activation of the mitochondrial calcium uniporter by natural plant flavonoids. Biochem J. 2004;384(Pt 1):19-24.
57. Rosenfeldt F, Miller F, Nagley P, et al. Response of the senescent heart to stress: clinical therapeutic strategies and quest for mitochondrial predictors of biological age. Ann N Y Acad Sci. 2004;1019:78-84.
58. Ross MA. Could oxidative stress be a factor in neurodevelopmental disorders? Prostaglandins Leukot Essent Fatty Acids. 2000;63:61-63.
59. Prabakaran S, Swatton JE, Ryan MM, et al. Mitochondrial dysfunction in schizophrenia: evidence for compromised brain metabolism and oxidative stress. Mol Psychiatry. 2004;9:684-697.
60. Sandyk R, Kanofsky JD. Vitamin C in the treatment of schizophrenia. Int J Neurosci. 1993;68:67-71.
61. Jeding I, Evans PJ, Akanmu D, et al. Characterization of the potential antioxidant and pro-oxidant actions of some neuroleptic drugs. Biochem Pharmacol. 1995;49:359-65.
62. Zoroglu SS, Armutcu F, Ozen S, et al. Increased oxidative stress and altered activities of erythrocyte free radical scavenging enzymes in autism. Eur Arch Psychiatry Clin Neurosci. 2004;254:143-47.
63. Chauhan A, Chauhan VP, Brown WT, et al. Oxidative stress in autism: Increased lipid peroxidation and reduced serum levels of ceruloplasmin and transferrin–the antioxidant proteins. Life Sci. 2004;75:2539-49.
64. Ming X, Stein TP, Brimacombe M, et al. Increased lipid peroxidation in children with autism. International Meeting for Autism Research. Sacramento, California: May 7-8, 2004. p. 85.
65. Bell JG, MacKinlay EE, Dick JR, et al. Essential fatty acids and phospholipase A2 in autistic spectrum disorders. Prostaglandins Leukot Essent Fatty Acids. 2004;71:201-4.
66. Ibid.
67. Chauhan V, Chauhan A, Cohen IL, et al. Alteration in amino-glycerophospholipids levels in the plasma of children with autism: a potential biochemical diagnostic marker. Life Sci. 2004;74:1635-43.
68. Hirai K, Aliev G, Nunomura A, et al. Mitochondrial abnormalities in Alzheimer's disease. J Neurosci. 2001;21:3017-23.

69. Opitz H, Schweinsberg F, Grossmann T, et al. Demonstration of mercury in the human brain and other organs 17 years after metallic mercury exposure. Clin Neuropathol. 1996;15:139-44.
70. Zs-Nagy I, Steiber J, Jeney F. Induction of age pigment accumulation in the brain cells of young male rats through iron-injection into the cerebrospinal fluid. Gerontology. 1995;41(Suppl 2):145-58.
71. Kim HC, Bing G, Jhoo WK, et al. Oxidative damage causes formation of lipofuscin-like substances in the hippocampus of the senescence-accelerated mouse after kainate treatment. Behav Brain Res. 2002;131:211-20.
72. Nakano M, Oenzil F, Mizuno T, et al. Age-related changes in the lipofuscin accumulation of brain and heart. Gerontology. 1995;41(Suppl 2):69-79.
73. O'Donnell E, Lynch MA. Dietary antioxidant supplementation reverses age-related neuronal changes. Neurobiol Aging. 1998;19:461-67.
74. Arockia Rani PJ, Panneerselvam C. Carnitine as a free radical scavenger in aging. Exp Gerontol. 2001;36:1713-26.
75. Sharma D, Singh R. Age-related decline in multiple unit action potential of cerebral cortex correlates with the number of lipofuscin-containing neurons. Indian J Exp Biol. 1996;34:776-81.
76. Lopez-Hurtado E, Prieto JJ. Immunocytochemical analysis of interneurons in the cerebral cortex of autistic patients. International Meeting for Autism Research. Sacramento, California. May 7-8, 2004. p. 153.
77. Jellinger K, Armstrong D, Zoghbi HY, et al. Neuropathology of Rett syndrome. Acta Neuropathol (Berl). 1988;76:142-58.
78. Ibid.
79. Qingfen T, Xirang G, Weijing Y, et al. An experimental study on damage of retina function due to toxicity of carbon disulfide and lipid peroxidation. Acta Opthalmol Scand. 1999;77:298-301.
80. Ritvo ER, Creel D, Realmuto G, et al. Electroretinograms in autism: a pilot study of b-wave amplitudes. Am J Psychiatry. 1988;145:229-32.
81. Realmuto G, Purple R, Knobloch W, et al. Electroretinograms (ERGs) in four autistic probands and six first-degree relatives. Can J Psychiatry. 1989;34:435-39.
82. Fang YZ, Yang S, Wu G. Free radicals, antioxidants and nutrition. Nutrition. 2002;18:872-79.
83. Cabrini L, Bergami R, Fiorentini D, et al. Vitamin B6 deficiency affects antioxidant defences in rat liver and heart. Biochem Mol Biol Int. 1998;46:689-97.
84. Halliwell B, Gutteridge JM. Free Radicals in Biology and Medicine. 3rd ed. New York: Oxford University Press; 1999.
85. Bondy SC, LeBell CP. Oxygen radical generation as an index of neurotoxic damage. Biomed Environ Sci. 1991;4:217-23.
86. Thomas CE, Aust SD. Free radicals and environmental toxins. Ann Emerg Med. 1986;15:1075-83.
87. Stohs SJ, Bagchi D. Oxidative mechanisms in the toxicity of metal ions. Free Radic Biol Med. 1995;18:321-36.
88. Edelson SB, Cantor DS. Autism: xenobiotic influences. Toxicol Ind Health. 1998;14:553-63.
89. Pall ML. NMDA sensitization and stimulation by peroxynitrite, nitric oxide, and organic solvents as the mechanism of chemical sensitivity in multiple chemical sensitivity. FASEB J. 2002;16:1407-17.
90. Bondy SC, LeBell CP. Oxygen radical generation as an index of neurotoxic damage. Biomed Environ Sci. 1991;4:217-23.
91. Croonenberghs J, Bosmans E, Deboutte D, et al. Activation of the inflammatory response system in autism. Neuropsychobiology. 2002;45:1-6.
92. Zoroglu SS, Armutcu F, Ozen S, et al. Increased oxidative stress and altered activities of erythrocyte free radical scavenging enzymes in autism. Eur Arch Psychiatry Clin Neurosci. 2004;254:143-47.
93. Sogut S, Zoroglu SS, Ozyurt H, et al. Changes in nitric oxide levels and antioxidant enzyme activities may have a role in the pathophysiological mechanisms involved in autism. Clin Chim Acta. 2003;331:111-17.
94. Zoroglu SS, Yurekli M, Meram I, et al. Pathophysiological role of nitric oxide and adrenomedullin in autism. Cell Biochem Funct. 2003;21:55-60.
95. Sweeten TL, Posey DJ, Shankar S, et al. High nitric oxide production in autistic disorder: a possible role for interferon-gamma. Biol Psychiatry. 2004;55:434-37.
96. Sogut S, Zoroglu SS, Ozyurt H, et al. Changes in nitric oxide levels and antioxidant enzyme activities may have a role in the pathophysiological mechanisms involved in autism. Clin Chim Acta. 2003;331:111-17.
97. Shinkai T, Ohmori O, Hori H, et al. Allelic association of the neuronal nitric oxide synthase (NOS1) gene with schizophrenia. Mol Psychiatry. 2002;7:560-563.
98. de la Monte SM, Bloch KD. Aberrant expression of the constitutive endothelial nitric oxide synthase gene in Alzheimer disease. Mol Chem Neuropathol. 1997;30:139-59.
99. Scott GS, Spitsin SV, Kean RB, et al. Therapeutic intervention in experimental allergic encephalomyelitis by administration of uric acid precursors. Proc Natl Acad Sci U S A. 2002;99:16303-308.
100. Liu S, Kawai K, Tyurin VA, et al. Nitric oxide-dependent pro-oxidant and pro-apoptotic effect of metallothioneins in HL-60 cells challenged with cupric nitrilotriacetate. Biochem J. 2001;354(Pt 2):397-406.
101. Giovannoni G, Miller RF, Heales SJ, et al. Elevated cerebrospinal fluid and serum nitrate and nitrite levels in patients with central nervous system complications of HIV-l infection: a correlation with blood-brain-barrier dysfunction. J Neurol Sci. 1998;156:53-58.
102. Acar G, Idiman F, Idiman E, et al. Nitric oxide as an activity marker in multiple sclerosis. J Neurol. 2003;250:588-92.
103. Perry EK, Lee ML, Martin-Ruiz CM, et al. Cholinergic activity in autism: abnormalities in the cerebral cortex and basal forebrain. Am J Psychiatry. 2001;158:1058-66.
104. Szutowicz A, Tomaszewicz M, Jankowska A, et al. Acetyl-CoA metabolism in cholinergic neurons and the susceptibility to neurotoxic inputs. Metab Brain Dis. 2000;15:29-44.
105. Sah R., Galeffi F, Ahrens R, et al. Modulation of the GABA(A)-gated chloride channels by reactive oxygen species. J Neurochem. 2002;80:383-91.
106. Blatt GJ, Fitzgerald CM, Guptill JT, et al. Density and distribution of hippocampal neurotransmitter receptors in autism: an autoradiographic study. J Autism Dev Disord. 2001;31:537-43.
107. Buxbaum JD, Silverman JM, Smith CJ, et al. Association between a GABRB3 polymorphism and autism. Mol Psychiatry. 2002;7:311-16.
108. Bauman ML, Kemper TL. The neuropathology of the autism spectrum disorders: what have we learned? Novartis Found Symp. 2003;251:112-22.
109. Kern JK. Purkinje cell vulnerability and autism: a possible etiological connection. Brain Dev. 2003;25:377-82.
110. Raymond GV, Bauman ML, Kemper TL. Hippocampus in autism: a Golgi analysis. Acta Neuropathol. 1996;91:117-19.
111. Horvath K, Perman JA. Autistic disorder and gastrointestinal disease. Curr Opin Pediatr. 2002;14:583-87.
112. D'Eufemia P, Celli M, Finocchiaro R, et al. Abnormal intestinal permeability in children with autism. Acta Paediatr. 1996:85:1076-79.
113. Wakefield AJ, Anthony M, Murch SH, et al. Enterocolitis in children with developmental disorders. Am J Gastroenterol. 2000;95:2285-95.
114. Torrente F, Ashwood P, Day R., et al. Small intestinal enteropathy with epithelial IgG and complement deposition in children with regressive autism. Mol Psychiatry. 2002;7:375-82.

115. Levine JJ, Pettei MJ, Valderrama E, et al. Nitric oxide and inflammatory bowel disease: evidence of local intestinal production in children with active colonic disease. J Pediatr Gastroenterol Nutr. 1998;26:34-38.
116. Charmandari E, Meadows N, Patel M, et al. Plasma nitrate concentrations in children with infectious and noninfectious diarrhea. J Pediatr Gastroenterol Nutr. 2001;32:418-20 (comment), 423-27.
117. Kukuruzovic R, Brewster DR, Gray E, et al. Increased nitric oxide production in acute diarrhoea is associated with abnormal gut permeability, hypokalaemia and malnutrition in tropic Australian aboriginal children. Trans R Soc Trop Med Hyg. 2003;97:115-20.
118. Kukuruzovic R, Robins-Browne RM, Anstey NM, et al. Enteric pathogens, intestinal permeability and nitric oxide production in acute gastroenteritis. Pediatr Infect Dis J. 2002;21:730-39.
119. Hooper DC, Ohnishi ST, Kean R, et al. Local nitric oxide production in viral and autoimmune diseases of the central nervous system. Proc Natl Acad Sci U S A. 1995;92:5312-16.
120. Kukuruzovic R, Robins-Browne RM, Anstey NM, et al. Enteric pathogens, intestinal permeability and nitric oxide production in acute gastroenteritis. Pediatr Infect Dis J. 2002;21:730-39.
121. Wallace JL, Miller MJ. Nitric oxide in mucosal defense: a little goes a long way. Gastroenterology. 2000;119:512-20.
122. Banan A, Fields JZ, Zhang Y, et al. iNOS upregulation mediates oxidant-induced disruption of F-actin and barrier of intestinal monolayers. Am J Physiol Gastrointest Liver Physiol. 2001;280:G1234-46.
123. Salzman AL. Nitric oxide in the gut. New Horiz. 1995;3:33-45.
124. Morin MJ, Karr SM, Faris RA, et al. Developmental variability in expression and regulation of inducible nitric oxide synthase in rat intestine. Am J Physiol Gastrointest Liver Physiol. 2001;281:G552-59.
125. Menconi MJ, Unno N, Smith M, et al. Nitric oxide donor-induced hyperpermeability of cultured intestinal epithelial monolayers: role of superoxide radical, hydroxyl radical, and peroxynitrite. Biochim Biophys Acta. 1998;1425:189-203.
126. Chen Y, Vartiainen NE, Ying W, et al. Astrocytes protect neurons from nitric oxide toxicity by glutathione-dependent mechanism. J Neurochem. 2001;77:1601-10.
127. Heales SJ, Bolanos JP, Clark JB. Glutathione depletion is accompanied by increased neuronal nitric oxide synthase activity. Neurochem Res. 1996;21:35-39.
128. Kuo WN, Kocis JM, Nibbs J. Nitrosation of cysteine and reduced glutathione by nitrite at physiological pH. Front Biosci. 2003;8:a62-69.
129. Halliwell B, Gutteridge JM. Free Radicals in Biology and Medicine. 3rd ed. New York: Oxford University Press; 1999.
130. Pall ML. Common etiology of posttraumatic stress disorder, fibromyalgia, chronic fatigue syndrome and multiple chemical sensitivity via elevated nitric oxide/peroxynitrite. Med Hypotheses. 2001;57:139-45.
131. Weyerbrock A, Walbridge S, Pluta RM, et al. Selective opening of the blood-tumor barrier by a nitric oxide donor and long-term survival in rats with C6 gliomas. J Neurosurg. 2003;99:728-37.
132. Roediger WE. Nitric oxide damage to colonocytes in colitis-by-association: remote transfer of nitric oxide to the colon. Digestion. 2002;65:191-95.
133. Roediger WE, Babidge WJ. Nitric oxide effect on colonocyte metabolism: co-action of sulfides and peroxide. Mol Cell Biochem. 2000;206:159-67.
134. Thayer JR, Chasko JH, Swartz LA, et al. Gut reactions of radioactive nitrite after intratracheal administration in mice. Science. 1982;217:151-53.
135. Schultz DS, Deen WM, Karel SF, et al. Pharmacokinetics of nitrate in humans: role of gastrointestinal absorption and metabolism. Carcinogenesis. 1985;6:847-52.
136. Cutruzzola F, Rinaldo S, Centola F, et al. NO production by Pseudomonas aeruginosa cd1 nitrite reductase. IUBMB Life. 2003;55(10-11):617-21.
137. van Niel EW, Braber KJ, Robertson LA, et al. Heterotrophic nitrification and aerobic denitrification in Alcaligenes faecalis strain TUD. Antonie Van Leeuwenhoek. 1992;62:231-37.
138. Robertson LA, Kuenen JG. Aerobic denitrification—old wine in new bottles? Antonie Van Leeuwenhoek. 1984;50:525-44.
139. Roediger WE. Nitric oxide damage to colonocytes in colitis-by-association: remote transfer of nitric oxide to the colon. Digestion. 2002;65:191-95.
140. Juurlink BH, Paterson PG. Review of oxidative stress in brain and spinal cord injury: suggestions for pharmacological and nutritional management strategies. J Spinal Cord Med. 1998;21:309-34.
141. Coyle JT, Puttfarcken P. Oxidative stress, glutamate, and neurodegenerative disorders. Science. 1993;262:689-95.
142. Noseworthy MD, Bray TM. Effect of oxidative stress on brain damage detected by MRI and *in vivo* 31P-NMR. Free Radic Biol Med. 1998;24:942-51.
143. Jeff Bradstreet, personal communication.
144. Belova I, Jonsson G. Blood-brain barrier permeability and immobilization stress. Acta Physiol Scand. 1982;116:21-29.
145. Belova TI. [Immobilization stress-induced lesions of structures of the midbrain reticular formation]. Biull Eksp Biol Med. 1989;108:101-5.
146. Richdale AL. Sleep problems in autism: prevalence, cause, and intervention. Dev Med Child Neurol. 1999;41:60-66.
147. Thirumalai SS, Shubin RA, Robinson R. Rapid eye movement sleep behavior disorder in children with autism. J Child Neurol. 2002;17:173-178.
148. Ishizaki A, Sugama M, Takeuchi N. [Usefulness of melatonin for developmental sleep and emotion/behavioral disorders—studies of melatonin trials on 50 patients with developmental disorders]. No To Hattatsu. 1999;31:428-37.
149. Sweeten TL, Posey DJ, Shankar S, et al. High nitric oxide production in autistic disorder: a possible role for interferon-gamma. Biol Psychiatry. 2004;55:434-37.
150. Singh VK, Warren RP, Odell JD, et al. Antibodies to myelin basic protein in children with autistic behavior. Brain Behav Immun. 1993;7:97-103.
151. Singh VK, Warren R, Averett R, et al. Circulating autoantibodies to neuronal and glial filament proteins in autism. Pediatr Neurol. 1997;17:88-90.
152. Connolly AM, Chez MG, Pestronk A, et al. Serum autoantibodies to brain in Landau-Kleffner variant, autism, and other neurological disorders. J Pediatr. 1999;134:607-613.
153. Vojdani A, Campbell AW, Anyanwu E, et al. Antibodies to neuron-specific antigens in children with autism: possible cross-reaction with encephalitogenic proteins from milk, Chlamydia pneumoniae and Streptococcus group A. J Neuroimmunol. 2002;129:168-77.
154. Palinski W, Witztum JL. Immune responses to oxidative neoepitopes on LDL and phospholipids modulate the development of atherosclerosis. J Intern Med. 2000;247:371-80.
155. Hooper DC, Ohnishi ST, Kean R, et al. Local nitric oxide production in viral and autoimmune diseases of the central nervous system. Proc Natl Acad Sci U S A. 1995;92:5312-16.
156. Blamire AM, Anthony DC, Rajagopalan B, et al. Interleukin-1beta - induced changes in blood-brain barrier permeability, apparent diffusion coefficient, and cerebral blood volume in the rat brain: a magnetic resonance study. J Neurosci. 2000;20:8153-59.
157. Romero IA, Abbott NJ, Bradbury MW. The blood-brain barrier in normal CNS and in metal-induced neurotoxicity. In Toxicology of Metals. Chang LW, ed. Boca Raton, New York, London and Tokyo: CRC Lewis Publishers;1996. p. 561-85.

158. McClain C, Morris P, Hennig B. Zinc and endothelial function. Nutrition. 1995;11(1 Suppl):117-20.
159. Weyerbrock A, Walbridge S, Pluta RM, et al. Selective opening of the blood-tumor barrier by a nitric oxide donor and long-term survival in rats with C6 gliomas. J Neurosurg. 2003;99:728-37.
160. Raiten DJ, Massaro TF, Zuckerman C. Vitamin and trace element assessment of autistic and learning disabled children. Nutr Behav. 1984;2:9-17.
161. Fang YZ, Yang S, Wu G. Free radicals, antioxidants and nutrition. Nutrition. 2002;18:872-79.
162. McClain C, Morris P, Hennig B. Zinc and endothelial function. Nutrition. 1995;11(1 Suppl):117-20.
163. Noseworthy MD, Bray TM. Zinc deficiency exacerbates loss in blood-brain barrier integrity induced by hyperoxia measured by dynamic MRI. Proc Soc Exp Biol Med. 2000;223:175-82.
164. Rosseneau S. Aerobic throat and gut flora in children with regressive autism and gastrointestinal signs. Defeat Autism Now (DAN) Conference. Washington, D.C. April 16-19, 2004 Defeat Autism Now Conference. p. 101-105.
165. Gilgun-Sherki Y, Melamed E, Offen D. Oxidative stress induced-neurodegenerative diseases: the need for antioxidants that penetrate the blood brain barrier. Neuropharmacology. 2001;40:959-79.
166. Harris NG, Gauden V, Fraser PA, et al. MRI measurement of blood-brain barrier permeability following spontaneous reperfusion in the starch microsphere model of ischemia. Magn Reson Imaging. 2002;20:221-30.
167. Romero IA, Abbott NJ, Bradbury MW. The blood-brain barrier in normal CNS and in metal-induced neurotoxicity. In Toxicology of Metals. Chang LW, ed. Boca Raton, New York, London and Tokyo: CRC Lewis Publishers;1996. p. 561-85.
168. Halliwell B, Gutteridge JM. Free Radicals in Biology and Medicine. 3rd ed. New York: Oxford University Press; 1999.
169. Kruidenier L, Kuiper I, Lamers CB, et al. Intestinal oxidative damage in inflammatory bowel disease: semi-quantification, localization and association with mucosal antioxidants. J Pathol. 2003;201:28-36.
170. Von Ritter C, Lamont JT, Smith BF, et al. Effects of oxygen-derived free radicals on gastric mucin. In: Free Radicals in Digestive Disease. Tsuchiya M, Kawai K, Kondo M, et al, eds. Amsterdam, New York, Oxford: Excerpta Medica; 1988:73-80.
171. Ogasawara T, Hoensch H, Ohnhaus EE. Distribution of glutathione and its related enzymes in small intestinal mucosa of rats. Arch Toxicol Suppl. 1985;8:110-13.
172. Esworthy RS, Aranda R, Martin MG, et al. Mice with combined disruption of Gpx1 and Gpx2 genes have colitis. Am J Physiol Gastrointest Liver Physiol. 2001;281:G848-55.
173. Morin MJ, Karr SM, Faris RA, et al. Developmental variability in expression and regulation of inducible nitric oxide synthase in rat intestine. Am J Physiol Gastrointest Liver Physiol. 2001;281:G552-59.
174. Von Ritter C, Lamont JT, Smith BF, et al. Effects of oxygen-derived free radicals on gastric mucin. In: Free Radicals in Digestive Disease. Tsuchiya M, Kawai K, Kondo M, et al, eds. Amsterdam, New York, Oxford: Excerpta Medica; 1988:73-80.
175. Xu DZ, Lu Q, Deitch EA. Nitric oxide directly impairs intestinal barrier function. Shock. 2002;17:139-45.
176. D'Eufemia P, Celli M, Finocchiaro R, et al. Abnormal intestinal permeability in children with autism. Acta Paediatr. 1996:85:1076-79.
177. Hornby PJ, Abrahams TP. Central control of lower esophageal sphincter relaxation. Am J Med. 2000;108(Suppl 4a):90S-98S.
178. Horvath K, Papadimitriou JC, Rabsztyn A, et al. Gastrointestinal abnormalities in children with autistic disorder. J Pediatr. 1999;135:559-63.
179. Konturek JW, Konturek SJ, Pawlik T, et al. Physiological role of nitric oxide in gallbladder emptying in men. Digestion. 1997;58:373-78.
180. Salzman AL. Nitric oxide in the gut. New Horiz. 1995;3:33-45.
181. Coyle JT, Puttfarcken P. Oxidative stress, glutamate, and neurodegenerative disorders. Science. 1993;262:689-95.
182. Packer, L. Ed. Oxygen Radicals in Biological Systems. Methods in Enzymology. Vol 105. New York: Academic Press; 1984.
183. Kowaltowski AJ, Vercesi AE. Mitochondrial damage induced by conditions of oxidative stress. Free Radic Biol Med. 1999;26:463-71.
184. Kirkinezos IG, Moraes CT. Reactive oxygen species and mitochondrial diseases. Semin Cell Dev Biol. 2001;12:449-57.
185. Lenaz G. Role of mitochondria in oxidative stress and ageing. Biochim Biophys Acta. 1998;1366:53-67.
186. Hagen TM, Liu J, Lykkesfeldt J, et al. Feeding acetyl-L-carnitine and lipoic acid to old rats significantly improves metabolic function while decreasing oxidative stress. Proc Natl Acad Sci U S A. 2002;99:1870-75.
187. Gibson GE, Zhang H. Interactions of oxidative stress with thiamine homeostasis promote neurodegeneration. Neurochem Int. 2002;40:493-504.
188. Wei YH, Lu CY, Lee HC, et al. Oxidative damage and mutation to mitochondrial DNA and age-dependent decline of mitochondrial respiratory function. Ann N Y Acad Sci. 1998;854:155-70.
189. Lenaz G. The mitochondrial production of reactive oxygen species: mechanisms and implications in human pathology. IUBMB Life. 2001;52:159-64.
190. Chen Q, Vazquez EJ, Moghaddas S, et al. Production of reactive oxygen species by mitochondria: central role of complex III. J Biol Chem. 2003;278:36027-31.
191. Coyle JT, Puttfarcken P. Oxidative stress, glutamate, and neurodegenerative disorders. Science. 1993;262:689-95.
192. Simonian NA, Coyle JT. Oxidative stress in neurodegenerative disease. Annu Rev Pharmacol Toxicol. 1996;36:83-106.
193. Farooqui AA, Horrocks LA. Excitotoxicity and neurological disorders: involvement of membrane phospholipids. Int Rev Neurobiol. 1994;36:267-323.
194. Bishop C. GSH augmentation therapy in CF: an initial protocol for interested physicians. http://members.tripod.com/uvicf/gsh/gshaugment.htm.
195. Bondy SC. The relation of oxidative stress and hyperexcitation to neurological disease. Proc Soc Exp Biol Med. 1995;208:337-45.
196. Milusheva E, Sperlagh B, Shikova L, et al. Non-synaptic release of[3H] noradrenaline in response to oxidative stress combined with mitochondrial dysfunction in rat hippocampal slices. Neuroscience. 2003;120:771-81.
197. Talman WT, Dragon DN, Ohta H, et al. Nitroxidergic influences on cardiovascular control by NTS: a link with glutamate. Ann N Y Acad Sci. 2001;940:169-78.
198. Minshew NJ, Goldstein G, Dombrowski SM. A preliminary 31P MRS study of autism: evidence for undersynthesis and increased degradation of brain membranes. Biol Psychiatry. 1993;33:762-73.
199. Coleman M, Blass JP. Autism and lactic acidosis. J Autism Dev Disord. 1985;15:1-8.
200. Chugani DC, Sundram BS, Behen M, et al. Evidence of altered energy metabolism in autistic children. Prog Neuropsychopharmacol Biol Psychiatry. 1999;23:635-41.
201. Moreno H, Borjas L, Arrieta A, et al. [Clinical heterogeneity of the autistic syndrome: a study of 60 families] [article in Spanish]. Invest Clin. 1992;33:13-31.
202. Filipek PA, Juranek J, Nguyen MT, et al. Relative carnitine deficiency in autism. J Autism Dev Disord. 2004;34:615-23.

203. Graf WD, Marin-Garcia J, Gao HG, et al. Autism associated with the mitochondrial DNA G8363A transfer RNA(Lys) mutation. J Child Neurol. 2000;15:357-61.
204. Filipek PA, Juranek J, Smith M, et al. Mitochondrial dysfunction in autistic patients with 15q inverted duplication. Ann Neurol. 2003;53:801-4.
205. Maletic SD, Dragicevic LM, Zikic RV, et al. Effects of nitric oxide donor, isosorbide dinitrate, on energy metabolism of rat reticulocytes. Physiol Res. 1999;48:417-27.
206. Halliwell B, Gutteridge JM. Free Radicals in Biology and Medicine. 3rd ed. New York: Oxford University Press; 1999.
207. Pearce LL, Epperly MW, Greenberger JS, et al. Identification of respiratory complexes I and III as mitochondrial sites of damage following exposure to ionizing radiation and nitric oxide. Nitric Oxide. 2001;5:128-36.
208. Roediger WE. Nitric oxide damage to colonocytes in colitis-by-association: remote transfer of nitric oxide to the colon. Digestion. 2002;65:191-95.
209. Siegel GJ, Agranoff BW, Albers RW, et al, Eds. Basic Neurochemistry: Molecular, Cellular and Medical Aspects. 6th ed. Philadelphia: Lippincott Williams and Wilkins; 1998.
210. Fatemi SH, Halt AR, Stary JM, et al. Glutamic acid decarboxylase 65 and 67 kDa proteins are reduced in autistic parietal and cerebellar cortices. Biol Psychiatry. 2002;52:805-10.
211. Audhya T, McGinnis WR. Nutrient, toxin and enzyme profile of autistic children. International Meeting for Autism Research. Sacramento CA, May 7-8, 2004. p. 74.
212. Moreno H, Borjas L, Arrieta A, et al. [Clinical heterogeneity of the autistic syndrome: a study of 60 families] [article in Spanish]. Invest Clin. 1992;33:13-31.
213. Aldred S, Moore KM, Fitzgerald M, et al. Plasma amino acid levels in children with autism and their families. J Autism Dev Disord. 2003;33:93-97.
214. Ibid.
215. Davis K, Foos T, Wu JY, et al. Oxygen-induced seizures and inhibition of human glutamate decarboxylase and porcine cysteine sulfinic acid decarboxylase by oxygen and nitric oxide. J Biomed Sci. 2001;8:359-64.
216. Bondy SC, Guo SX. Effect of ethanol treatment on indices of cumulative oxidative stress. Eur J Pharmacol. 1994;270:349-55.
217. Trotti D, Danbolt NC, Volterra A. Glutamate transporters are oxidant-vulnerable: a molecular link between oxidative and excitotoxic neurodegeneration? Trends Pharmacol Sci. 1998;19:328-34.
218. Chauhan V, Chauhan A, Cohen IL, et al. Alteration in amino-glycerophospholipids levels in the plasma of children with autism: a potential biochemical diagnostic marker. Life Sci. 2004;74:1635-43.
219. Sah R., Galeffi F, Ahrens R, et al. Modulation of the GABA(A)-gated chloride channels by reactive oxygen species. J Neurochem. 2002;80:383-91.
220. Olney JW. Excitotoxic food additives—relevance of animal studies to human safety. Neurobehav Toxicol Teratol. 1984;6:455-62.
221. Perry EK, Lee ML, Martin-Ruiz CM, et al. Cholinergic activity in autism: abnormalities in the cerebral cortex and basal forebrain. Am J Psychiatry. 2001;158:1058-66.
222. Mary Megson, personal communication.
223. Hardan AY, Handen BL. A retrospective open trial of adjunctive donepezil in children and adolescents with autistic disorder. J Child Adolesc Psychopharmacol. 2002;12:237-41.
224. Ames BN, Elson-Schwab I, Silver EA. High-dose vitamin therapy stimulates variant enzymes with decreased coenzyme binding affinity (increased K(m)): relevance to genetic disease and polymorphisms. Am J Clin Nutr. 2002;75:616-58.
225. Mary Megson, personal communication.
226. Boddaert N, Zilbovicius M. Functional neuroimaging and childhood autism. Pediatr Radiol. 2002;32:1-7.
227. Boddaert N, Chabane N, Barthelemy C, et al. [Bitemporal lobe dysfunction in infantile autism: positron emission tomography study] [article in French]. J Radiol. 2002;83(12 Pt 1):1829-33.
228. Wilcox J, Tsuang MT, Ledger E, et al. Brain perfusion in autism varies with age. Neuropsychobiology. 2002;46:13-16.
229. Elhusseiny A, Hamel E. Muscarinic—but not nicotinic—acetylcholine receptors mediate a nitric oxide-dependent dilation in brain cortex arterioles: a possible role for the M5 receptor subtype. J Cereb Blood Flow Metab. 2000;20:298-305.
230. Fukuyama H, Ouchi Y, Matsuzaki S, et al. Focal cortical blood flow activation is regulated by intrinsic cortical cholinergic neurons. Neuroimage. 1996;3(3 Pt 1):195-201.
231. De Sarno P, Shestopal SA, King TD, et al. Muscarinic receptor activation protects cells from apoptotic effects of DNA damage, oxidative stress, and mitochondrial inhibition. J Biol Chem. 2003;278:11086-93.
232. Gajewski M, Laskowska-Bozek H, Orlewski P, et al. Influence of lipid peroxidation and hydrogen peroxide on muscarinic cholinergic receptors and ATP level in rat myocytes and lymphocytes. Int J Tiss Reac. 1988:5:281-90.
233. Fass U, Panickar K, Personett D, et al. Differential vulnerability of primary cultured cholinergic neurons to nitric oxide excess. Neuroreport. 2000;11:931-36.
234. De Sarno P, Jope RS. Phosphoinositide hydrolysis activated by muscarinic or glutamatergic, but not adrenergic, receptors is impaired in ApoE-deficient mice and by hydrogen peroxide and peroxynitrite. Exp Neurol. 1998;152:123-28.
235. Joseph JA, Denisova NA, Bielinski D, et al. Oxidative stress protection and vulnerability in aging: putative nutritional implications for intervention. Mech Ageing Dev. 2000;116:141-53.
236. Szutowicz A, Tomaszewicz M, Jankowska A, et al. Acetyl-CoA metabolism in cholinergic neurons and the susceptibility to neurotoxic inputs. Metab Brain Dis. 2000;15:29-44.
237. Buxbaum JD, Silverman JM, Smith CJ, et al. Association between a GABRB3 polymorphism and autism. Mol Psychiatry. 2002;7:311-16.
238. Dolske MC, Spollen J, McKay S, et al. A preliminary trial of ascorbic acid as supplemental therapy for autism. Prog Neuropsychopharmacol Biol Psychiatry. 1993;17:765-74.
239. Halliwell B, Gutteridge JM. Free Radicals in Biology and Medicine. 3rd ed. New York: Oxford University Press; 1999.
240. MacGregor DG, Higgins MJ, Jones PA, et al. Ascorbate attenuates the systemic kainate-induced neurotoxicity in the rat hippocampus. Brain Res. 1996;727:133-44.
241. Rebec GV, Pierce RC. A vitamin as neuromodulator: ascorbate release into the extracellular fluid of the brain regulates dopaminergic and glutamatergic transmission. Prog Neurobiol. 1994;43:537-65.
242. Korcok J, Wu F, Tyml K, et al. Sepsis inhibits reduction of dehydroascorbic acid and accumulation of ascorbate in astroglial cultures: intracellular ascorbate depletion increases nitric oxide synthase induction and glutamate uptake inhibition. J Neurochem. 2002;81:185-93.
243. Sorg O, Horn TF, Yu N, et al. Inhibition of astrocyte glutamate uptake by reactive oxygen species: role of antioxidant enzymes. Mol Med. 1997;3:431-40.
244. Isaacson HR, Moran MM, Hall A. Autism: a retrospective outcome study of nutrient therapy. J Appl Nutr. 1996;48:110-18.
245. Horning MS, Blakemore LJ, Trombley PQ. Endogenous mechanisms of neuroprotection: role of zinc, copper and carnosine. Brain Res. 2000;852:56-61.

246. Wang AM, Ma C, Xie ZH, et al. Use of carnosine as a natural anti-senescence drug for human beings. Biochemistry (Mosc). 2000;65:869-71.
247. Chez MG, Buchanan CP, Aimonovitch MC, et al. Double-blind, placebo-controlled study of L-carnosine supplementation in children with autistic spectrum disorders. J Child Neurol. 2002;17:833-37.
248. Fontana M, Pinnen F, Lucente G, et al. Prevention of peroxynitrite-dependent carnosine and related sulphonamido pseudodipeptides. Cell Mol Life Sci. 2002;59:546-551.
249. Kohen R, Yamamoto Y, Cundy KC, et al. Antioxidant activity of carnosine, homocarnosine, and anserine present in muscle and brain. Proc Natl Acad Sci U S A. 1988;85:3175-79.
250. Kohen R, Misgav R, Ginsburg I. The SOD like activity of copper:carnosine, copper:anserine and copper:homocarnosine complexes. Free Radic Res Commun. 1991;12-13 Pt 1:179-85.
251. Ames BN, Elson-Schwab I, Silver EA. High-dose vitamin therapy stimulates variant enzymes with decreased coenzyme binding affinity (increased K(m)): relevance to genetic disease and polymorphisms. Am J Clin Nutr. 2002;75:616-58.
252. Rimland B, Callaway E, Dreyfus P. The effect of high doses of vitamin B6 on autistic children: a double-blind crossover study. Am J Psychiatry. 1978;135:472-75.
253. Kleijnen J, Knipschild P. Niacin and vitamin B6 in mental functioning: a review of controlled trials in humans. Biol Psychiatry. 1991;29:931-41.
254. Audhya T, McGinnis WR. Nutrient, toxin and enzyme profile of autistic children. International Meeting for Autism Research. Sacramento CA, May 7-8, 2004. p. 74.
255. Ibid.
256. Raiten DJ, Massaro TF, Zuckerman C. Vitamin and trace element assessment of autistic and learning disabled children. Nutr Behav. 1984;2:9-17.
257. Audhya T, McGinnis WR. Nutrient, toxin and enzyme profile of autistic children. International Meeting for Autism Research. Sacramento CA, May 7-8, 2004. p. 74.
258. Isaacson HR, Moran MM, Hall A. Autism: a retrospective outcome study of nutrient therapy. J Appl Nutr. 1996;48:110-18.
259. Realmuto G, Purple R, Knobloch W, et al. Electroretinograms (ERGs) in four autistic probands and six first-degree relatives. Can J Psychiatry. 1989;34:435-39.
260. Churchich JE, Scholz G, Kwok F. Activation of pyridoxal kinase by metallothionein. Biochim Biophys Acta. 1989;996:181-86.
261. Webb JL. Enzyme and Metabolic Inhibitors. Vol II. New York and London: Academic Press; 1966.
262. Cabrini L, Bergami R, Fiorentini D, et al. Vitamin B6 deficiency affects antioxidant defences in rat liver and heart. Biochem Mol Biol Int. 1998;46:689-97.
263. Park LC, Zhang H, Sheu KF, et al. Metabolic impairment induces oxidative stress, compromises inflammatory responses, and inactivates key mitochondrial enzyme in microglia. J Neurochem. 1999;72:1948-58.
264. Atamna H, Walter PB, Ames BN. The role of heme and iron-sulfur clusters in mitochondrial biogenesis, maintenance, and decay with age. Arch Biochem Biophys. 2002;397:345-53.
265. Benderitter M, Hadj-Saad F, Lhuissier M, et al. Effects of exhaustive exercise and vitamin B6 deficiency on free radical oxidative process in male trained rats. Free Radic Biol Med. 1996;21:541-49.
266. Willis R, Anthony M, Sun L, et al. Clinical implications of the correlations between coenzyme Q10 and vitamin B6 status. Biofactors. 1999;9:359-63.
267. Yamashima T, Zhao L, Wang XD, et al. Neuroprotective effects of pyridoxal phosphate and pyridoxal against ischemia in monkeys. Nutr Neurosci. 2001;4:389-97.
268. Weber GF. Final common pathways in neurodegenerative diseases: regulatory role of the glutathione cycle. Neurosci Biobehav Rev. 1999;23:1079-86.
269. Davis K, Foos T, Wu JY, et al. Oxygen-induced seizures and inhibition of human glutamate decarboxylase and porcine cysteine sulfinic acid decarboxylase by oxygen and nitric oxide. J Biomed Sci. 2001;8:359-64.
270. Porter TG, Martin DL. Rapid inactivation of brain glutamate decarboxylase by aspartate. J Neurochem. 1987;48:67-72.
271. Das D, Bandyopadhyay D, Banerjee RK. Oxidative inactivation of gastric peroxidase by site-specific generation of hydroxyl radical and its role in stress-induced gastric ulceration. Free Radic Biol Med. 1998;24:460-69.
272. Villela GG, Calcagnotto AM. Effect of vitamin B6 on L-glutamate dehydrogenase activity in mice brain. J Nutr Sci Vitaminol (Tokyo). 1977;23:19-22.
273. Moorthy PN, Hayon E. One-electron redox reactions of water-soluble vitamins. III. Pyridoxine and pyridoxal phosphate (vitamin B6). J Am Chem Soc. 1975;97:2048-52.
274. Bilski P, Li MY, Ehrenshaft M, et al. Vitamin B6 (pyridoxine) and its derivatives are efficient singlet oxygen quenchers and potential fungal antioxidants. Photochem Photobiol. 2000;71:129-34.
275. Devasagayam TP, Kamat JP. Biological significance of singlet oxygen. Indian J Exp Biol. 2002;40:680-92.
276. Rock E, Astier C, Lab C, et al. Magnesium deficiency in rats induces a rise in plasma nitric oxide. Magnes Res. 1995;8:237-42.
277. Rayssiguier Y, Gueux E, Bussiere L, et al. Dietary magnesium affects susceptibility of lipoproteins and tissues to peroxidation in rats. J Am Coll Nutr. 1993;12:133-37.
278. Hans CP, Chaudhary DP, Bansal DD. Magnesium deficiency increases oxidative stress in rats. Indian J Exp Biol. 2002;40:1275-79.
279. Hans CP, Chaudhary DP, Bansal DD. Effect of magnesium supplementation on oxidative stress in alloxanic diabetic rats. Magnes Res. 2003;16:13-19.
280. Audhya T, McGinnis WR. Nutrient, toxin and enzyme profile of autistic children. International Meeting for Autism Research. Sacramento CA, May 7-8, 2004. p. 74.
281. Martineau J, Barthelemy C, Garreau B, et al. Vitamin B6, magnesium, and combined B6-Mg: therapeutic effects in childhood autism. Biol Psychiatry. 1985;20:467-78.
282. Siegel GJ, Agranoff BW, Albers RW, et al, Eds. Basic Neurochemistry: Molecular, Cellular and Medical Aspects. 6th ed. Philadelphia: Lippincott Williams and Wilkins; 1998.
283. Rodriguez-Zavala JS, Moreno-Sanchez R. Modulation of oxidative phosphorylation by Mg2+ in rat heart mitochondria. J Biol Chem. 1998;273:7850-55.
284. Danysz W, Parsons CG. The NMDA receptor antagonist memantine as a symptomatological and neuroprotective treatment for Alzheimer's disease: preclinical evidence. Int J Geriatr Psychiatry. 2003:18(Suppl 1):S23-32.
285. Audhya T, McGinnis WR. Nutrient, toxin and enzyme profile of autistic children. International Meeting for Autism Research. Sacramento CA, May 7-8, 2004. p. 74.
286. Joan Jory, personal communication.
287. Isaacson HR, Moran MM, Hall A. Autism: a retrospective outcome study of nutrient therapy. J Appl Nutr. 1996;48:110-18.
288. Bray TM, Bettger WJ. The physiological role of zinc as an antioxidant. Free Radic Biol Med. 1990;8:281-91.
289. Ames BN. A role for supplements in optimizing health: the metabolic tune-up. Arch Biochem Biophys. 2004;423:227-34.
290. Maret W. Metallothionein/disulfide interactions, oxidative stress, and the mobilization of cellular zinc. Neurochem Int. 1995;27:111-17.

291. Powell SR. The antioxidant properties of zinc. J Nutr. 2000;130(5S Suppl):1447S-54S.
292. Maret W. Metallothionein/disulfide interactions, oxidative stress, and the mobilization of cellular zinc. Neurochem Int. 1995;27:111-117.
293. Faure P, Benhamou PY, Perard A, et al. Lipid peroxidation in insulin-dependent diabetic patients with early retina degenerative lesions: effects of an oral zinc supplementation. Eur J Clin Nutr. 1995;49:282-88.
294. Wapnir RA. Zinc deficiency, malnutrition and the gastrointestinal tract. J Nutr. 2000;130(5S Suppl):1388S-92S.
295. Joseph RM, Varela V, Kanji VK, et al. Protective effects of zinc in indomethacin-induced gastric mucosal injury: evidence for a dual mechanism involving lipid peroxidation and nitric oxide. Aliment Pharmacol Ther. 1999;13:203-8.
296. Lambert JC, Zhou Z, Wang L, et al. Prevention of alterations in intestinal permeability is involved in zinc inhibition of acute ethanol-induced liver damage in mice. J Pharmacol Exp Ther. 2003;305:880-86.
297. Walsh WJ, Usman A, Tarpey J, et al. Metallothionein and Autism, 2nd edition, Monograph. Health Research Institute. Naperville, Illinois. 2002.
298. William Walsh, personal communication.
299. Walsh W. Metallothionein deficiency in autism spectrum disorders. National Conference of the Autism Society of America. Seattle, Washington. July 7-10,2004. p. 342-349.
300. Chauhan A, Chauhan VP, Brown WT, et al. Oxidative stress in autism: Increased lipid peroxidation and reduced serum levels of ceruloplasmin and transferrin–the antioxidant proteins. Life Sci. 2004;75:2539-49.
301. William Walsh, personal communication.
302. Ibid.
303. Walsh W. Walsh W. Metallothionein deficiency in autism spectrum disorders. National Conference of the Autism Society of America. Seattle, Washington. July 7-10,2004. p. 342-349.
304. Sayre LM, Perry G, Smith MA. Redox metals and neurodegenerative disease. Curr Opin Chem Biol. 1999;3:220-25.
305. William Walsh, personal communication.
306. Ibid.
307. Bray TM, Bettger WJ. The physiological role of zinc as an antioxidant. Free Radic Biol Med. 1990;8:281-91.
308. Xia J, Browning JD, O'Dell BL. Decreased plasma membrane thiol concentration is associated with increased osmotic fragility of erythrocytes in zinc-deficient rats. J Nutr. 1999;129:814-19.
309. Faure P, Benhamou PY, Perard A, et al. Lipid peroxidation in insulin-dependent diabetic patients with early retina degenerative lesions: effects of an oral zinc supplementation. Eur J Clin Nutr. 1995;49:282-88.
310. Powell SR. The antioxidant properties of zinc. J Nutr. 2000;130(5S Suppl):1447S-54S.
311. Chvapil M, Elias SL, Ryan JN, et al. Pathophysiology of zinc. Int Rev Neurobiol. 1972;1:104-24.
312. Ruz M, Cavan KR, Bettger WJ, et al. Indices of iron and copper status during experimentally induced, marginal zinc deficiency in humans. Biol Trace Elem Res. 1992;34:197-212.
313. Ames BN, Elson-Schwab I, Silver EA. High-dose vitamin therapy stimulates variant enzymes with decreased coenzyme binding affinity (increased K(m)): relevance to genetic disease and polymorphisms. Am J Clin Nutr. 2002;75:616-58.
314. Estevez AG, Crow JP, Sampson JB, et al. Induction of nitric oxide-dependent apoptosis in motor neurons in zinc-deficient superoxide dismutase. Science. 1999;286:2498-500.
315. Haq F, Mahoney M, Koropatnick J. Signaling events for metallothionein induction. Mutat Res. 2003;533:211-26.
316. Li X, Chen H, Epstein PN. Metallothionein protects islets from hypoxia and extends islet graft survival by scavenging most kinds of reactive oxygen species. J Biol Chem. 2004;279:765-71.
317. Miceli MV, Tate DJ, Alcock NW, et al. Zinc deficiency and oxidative stress in the retina of pigmented rats. Invest Opthalmol Vis Sci. 1999;40:1238-44.
318. Tate DJ, Miceli MV, Newsome DA. Zinc protects against oxidative damage in cultured human retinal pigment epithelial cells. Free Radic Biol Med. 1999;26:704-13.
319. Mulder TP, Van Der Sluys Veer A, Verspaget HW, et al. Effect of oral zinc supplementation on metallothionein and superoxide dismutase concentrations in patients with inflammatory bowel disease. J Gastroenterol Hepatol. 1994;9:472-77.
320. Miceli MV, Tate DJ, Alcock NW, et al. Zinc deficiency and oxidative stress in the retina of pigmented rats. Invest Opthalmol Vis Sci. 1999;40:1238-44.
321. Tate DJ, Miceli MV, Newsome DA. Zinc protects against oxidative damage in cultured human retinal pigment epithelial cells. Free Radic Biol Med. 1999;26:704-13.
322. Liu S, Kawai K, Tyurin VA, et al. Nitric oxide-dependent pro-oxidant and pro-apoptotic effect of metallothioneins in HL-60 cells challenged with cupric nitrilotriacetate. Biochem J. 2001;354(Pt 2):397-406.
323. Maret W. Cellular zinc and redox states converge in the metallothionein/thionein pair. J Nutr. 2003;133(5 Suppl 1):1460S-62.
324. Walsh WJ, Usman A, Tarpey J, et al. Metallothionein and Autism, 2nd edition, Monograph. Health Research Institute. Naperville, Illinois. 2002.
325. Siegel GJ, Agranoff BW, Albers RW, et al, Eds. Basic Neurochemistry: Molecular, Cellular and Medical Aspects. 6th ed. Philadelphia: Lippincott Williams and Wilkins; 1998.
326. Cunnane SC. Role of zinc in lipid and fatty acid metabolism and in membranes. Prog Food Nutr Sci. 1988;12:151-88.
327. Ruz M, Cavan KR, Bettger WJ, et al. Indices of iron and copper status during experimentally induced, marginal zinc deficiency in humans. Biol Trace Elem Res. 1992;34:197-212.
328. Peterson DA, Gerrard JM, Peller J, et al. Interactions of zinc and arachidonic acid. Prostaglandins Med. 1981;6:91-99.
329. Powell SR. The antioxidant properties of zinc. J Nutr. 2000;130(5S Suppl):1447S-54S.
330. Xia J, Browning JD, O'Dell BL. Decreased plasma membrane thiol concentration is associated with increased osmotic fragility of erythrocytes in zinc-deficient rats. J Nutr. 1999;129:814-19.
331. Maret W. Metallothionein/disulfide interactions, oxidative stress, and the mobilization of cellular zinc. Neurochem Int. 1995;27:111-17.
332. Maret W. Cellular zinc and redox states converge in the metallothionein/thionein pair. J Nutr. 2003;133(5 Suppl 1):1460S-62S.
333. Lapenna D, De Gioia S, Ciofani G, et al. Hypochlorous acid-induced zinc release from thiolate bonds: a potential protective mechanism towards biomolecules oxidant damage during inflammation. Free Radic Res. 1994;20:165-70.
334. Fliss H, Menard M. Oxidant-induced mobilization of zinc from metallothionein. Arch Biochim Biophys. 1992;293:195-199.
335. Pfeiffer CC. Mental and Elemental Nutrients. New Canaan, Connecticut: Keats Publishing; 1975.
336. Audhya T, McGinnis WR. Nutrient, toxin and enzyme profile of autistic children. International Meeting for Autism Research. Sacramento CA, May 7-8, 2004. p. 74.
337. Golse B, Debray-Ritzen P, Durosay P, et al. [Alterations in two enzymes: superoxide dismutase and glutathione peroxidase in developmental infantile psychosis (infantile autism) (author's transl)]. Rev Neurol (Paris). 1978;134:699-705.

338. Yorbik O, Sayal A, Akay C, et al. Investigation of antioxidant enzymes in children with autistic disorder. Prostaglandins Leukot Essent Fatty Acids 2002;67:341-43.
339. Halliwell B, Gutteridge JM. Free Radicals in Biology and Medicine. 3rd ed. New York: Oxford University Press; 1999.
340. Rokutan K, Hosokawa T, Aoike A, et al. Hydroperoxide-induced mitochondrial damage: inactivation of 2-oxoglutarate dehydrogenase in liver mitochondria by its substrate and t-butyl hydroperoxide. In: Free radicals in digestive diseases. Tsuchiya M. et al, eds. Amsterdam, New York, Oxford: Excerpta Medica; 1988:131-45.
341. Juurlink BH, Paterson PG. Review of oxidative stress in brain and spinal cord injury: suggestions for pharmacological and nutritional management strategies. J Spinal Cord Med. 1998;21:309-34.
342. Rokutan K, Hosokawa T, Aoike A, et al. Hydroperoxide-induced mitochondrial damage: inactivation of 2-oxoglutarate dehydrogenase in liver mitochondria by its substrate and t-butyl hydroperoxide. In: Free radicals in digestive diseases. Tsuchiya M. et al, eds. Amsterdam, New York, Oxford: Excerpta Medica; 1988:131-45.
343. Fang YZ, Yang S, Wu G. Free radicals, antioxidants and nutrition. Nutrition. 2002;18:872-79.
344. Halliwell B, Gutteridge JM. Free Radicals in Biology and Medicine. 3rd ed. New York: Oxford University Press; 1999.
345. Das D, Bandyopadhyay D, Banerjee RK. Oxidative inactivation of gastric peroxidase by site-specific generation of hydroxyl radical and its role in stress-induced gastric ulceration. Free Radic Biol Med. 1998;24:460-69.
346. Bem EM, Mailer K, Elson CM. Influence of mercury (II), cadmium (II), methylmercury and phenylmercury on the kinetic properties of rat liver glutathione peroxidase. Can J Biochem Cell Biol. 1985;63:1212-16.
347. Bulat P, Dujic I, Potkonjak B, et al. Activity of glutathione peroxidase and superoxide dismutase in workers occupationally exposed to mercury. Int Arch Occup Environ Health. 1998;71:S37-39.
348. Bem EM, Mailer K, Elson CM. Influence of mercury (II), cadmium (II), methylmercury and phenylmercury on the kinetic properties of rat liver glutathione peroxidase. Can J Biochem Cell Biol. 1985;63:1212-16.
349. Santon A, Irato P, Medici V, et al. Effect and possible role of Zn treatment in LEC rats, an animal model of Wilson's disease. Biochim Biophys Acta. 2003;1637:91-97.
350. Abe K, Kogure K, Arai H, et al. Ascorbate induced lipid peroxidation results in loss of receptor binding in tris, but not in phosphate, buffer. Implications for the involvement of metal ions. Biochem Int. 1985;11:341-48.
351. Farooqui AA, Horrocks LA. Lipid peroxides in the free radical pathophysiology of brain diseases. Cell Mol Neurobiol. 1998;18:599-608.
352. Gilgun-Sherki Y, Melamed E, Offen D. Oxidative stress induced-neurodegenerative diseases: the need for antioxidants that penetrate the blood brain barrier. Neuropharmacology. 2001;40:959-79.
353. Jeff Bradstreet, personal communication.
354. Bishop C. GSH augmentation therapy in CF: an initial protocol for interested physicians. http://members.tripod.com/uvicf/gsh/gshaugment.htm.
355. Walsh WJ, Usman A, Tarpey J. Disordered metal metabolism in a large autism population. Abstract NR-823. Amer Psychiatr Assn. New Orleans, Louisiana. 2001.
356. Hagen TM, Wierzbicka GT, Sillau AH, et al. Bioavailability of dietary glutathione: effect on plasma concentration. Am J Physiol. 1990;259(4 Pt 1):G524-29.
357. Favilli F, Marraccini P, Iantomasi T, et al. Effect of orally administered glutathione on glutathione level in some organs of rats: role of specific transporter. Br J Nutr. 1997;78:293-300.
358. Hagen TM, Wierzbicka GT, Sillau AH, et al. Bioavailability of dietary glutathione: effect on plasma concentration. Am J Physiol. 1990;259(4 Pt 1):G524-29.
359. Ibid.
360. Lash LH, Hagen TM, Jones DP. Exogenous glutathione protects intestinal epithelial cells from oxidative injury. Proc Nat Acad Sci U S A. 1986;83:4641-45.
361. Hagen TM, Jones DP. Transepithelial transport of glutathione in vascularly perfused small intestine or rat. Am J Physiol. 1987;252:G607-13.
362. Lash LH, Hagen TM, Jones DP. Exogenous glutathione protects intestinal epithelial cells from oxidative injury. Proc Nat Acad Sci U S A. 1986;83:4641-45.
363. Martensson J, Jain A, Meister A. Glutathione is required for intestinal function. Proc Nat Acad Sci U S A. 1990;87:1715-19.
364. Palamara AT, Perno CF, Ciriolo MR, et al. Evidence for antiviral activity of glutathione: *in vitro* inhibition of herpes simplex virus type 1 replication. Antiviral Res. 1995;27:237-53.
365. Hagen TM, Wierzbicka GT, Bowman BB, et al. Fate of dietary glutathione: disposition in the gastrointestinal tract. Am J Physiol. 1990;259:G530-35.
366. Jerry Kartzinel, personal communication.
367. Yamada K, Yamada S, Tobimatsu T, et al. Heterologous high level expression, purification, and enzymological properties of recombinant rat cobalamin-dependent methionine synthase. J Biol Chem. 1999;274:35571-76.
368. Pall ML. Cobalamin used in Chronic Fatigue Syndrome therapy is a nitric oxide scavenger. J Chronic Fatigue Syndr. 2001;8:39-44.
369. Wolak M, Zahl A, Schneppensieper T, et al. Kinetics and mechanism of the reversible binding of nitric oxide to reduced cobalamin B(12)(Cob(II)alamin). J Am Chem Soc. 2001;123:9780-91.
370. Kruszyna H, Magyar JS, Rochelle LG, et al. Spectroscopic studies of nitric oxide (NO) interactions with cobalamins: reaction of NO with superoxocobalamin(III) likely accounts for cobalamin reversal of the biological effects of NO. J Pharmacol Exp Ther. 1998;285:665-71.
371. Abu Khaled M, Watkins CL, Krumdieck CL. Inactivation of B12 and folate coenzymes by butyl nitrite as observed by NMR: implication on one carbon transfer metabolism. Biochem Biophys Res Commun. 1986;135:201-7.
372. Zheng D, Yan L, Birke RL. Electrochemical and spectral studies of the reactions of aquocobalamin with nitric oxide and nitrite ion. Inorganic Chem. 2002;41:2548-55.
373. Bem EM, Mailer K, Elson CM. Influence of mercury (II), cadmium (II), methylmercury and phenylmercury on the kinetic properties of rat liver glutathione peroxidase. Can J Biochem Cell Biol. 1985;63:1212-16.
374. James SJ, Cutler P, Melnyk S, et al. Metabolic biomarkers of increased oxidative stress and impaired methylation capacity in children with autism. Am J Clin Nutr. 2004; 80:1611-17.
375. Abu Khaled M, Watkins CL, Krumdieck CL. Inactivation of B12 and folate coenzymes by butyl nitrite as observed by NMR: implication on one carbon transfer metabolism. Biochem Biophys Res Commun. 1986;135:201-7.
376. Widner B, Enzinger C, Laich A. Hyperhomocysteinemia, pteridines and oxidative stress. Curr Drug Metab. 2002;3:225-32.
377. Bondy SC. Reactive oxygen species: relation to aging and neurotoxic damage. Neurotoxicology. 1992;13:87-100.
378. Mattson MP, Shea TB. Folate and homocysteine metabolism in neural plasticity and neurodegenerative disorders. Trends Neurosci. 2003;26:137-46.
379. Jerry Kartzinel, personal communication.
380. Maret W. Cellular zinc and redox states converge in the metallothionein/thionein pair. J Nutr. 2003;133(5 Suppl 1):1460S-62.

381. Walsh W, Usman A. Nutrient Supplements and Methods for Treating Autism and for Preventing the Onset of Autism. U.S. Patent Application 09/998,342. November, 2001.
382. Zoroglu SS, Yurekli M, Meram I, et al. Pathophysiological role of nitric oxide and adrenomedullin in autism. Cell Biochem Funct. 2003;21:55-60.
383. Janssen YM, Van Houten B, Borm PJ, et al. Cell and tissue responses to oxidative damage. Lab Invest. 1993;69:261-74.
384. Lonsdale D, Shamberger RJ, Audhya T. Treatment of autism spectrum children with thiamine tetrahydrofurfuryl disulfide: a pilot study. Neuro Endrocrinol Lett. 2002;23:303-8.
385. Gibson GE, Zhang H. Interactions of oxidative stress with thiamine homeostasis promote neurodegeneration. Neurochem Int. 2002;40:493-504.
386. Gibson GE, Zhang H, Xu H, et al. Oxidative stress increases internal calcium stores and reduces a key mitochondrial enzyme. Biochim Biophys Acta. 2002;1586:177-89.
387. Gibson GE, Zhang H. Interactions of oxidative stress with thiamine homeostasis promote neurodegeneration. Neurochem Int. 2002;40:493-504.
388. Knivsberg AM, Reichelt KL, Hoien T, et al. A randomised, controlled study of dietary intervention in autistic syndromes. Nutr Neurosci. 2002;5:251-61.
389. Reichelt KL, Knivsberg AM. Can the pathophysiology of autism be explained by the nature of the discovered urine peptides? Nutr Neurosci. 2003;6:19-28.
390. Karl Reichelt, personal communication.
391. Liu YF, Quirion R. Modulatory role of glutathione on μ-opioid, substance P/neurokinin-1, and kainic acid receptor binding sites. J Neurochem. 1992;59:1024-32.
392. Johnson SM, Hollander E. Evidence that eicosapentaenoic acid is effective in treating autism. J Clin Psychiatry 2003;64:848-49.
393. Vancassel S, Durand G, Bathelemy C, et al. Plasma fatty acid levels in autistic children. Prostaglandins Leukot Essent Fatty Acids. 2001;65:1-7.
394. Bell JG, MacKinlay EE, Dick JR, et al. Essential fatty acids and phospholipase A2 in autistic spectrum disorders. Prostaglandins Leukot Essent Fatty Acids. 2004;71:201-4.
395. Bell JG, Sargent JR, Tocher DR, et al. Red blood cell fatty acid composition in a patient with autistic spectrum disorder: a characteristic abnormality in neurodevelopmental disorders? Prostaglandins Leukot Essent Fatty Acids. 2000;63:21-25.
396. Evans DR, Parikh VV, Khan MM, et al. Red blood cell membrane essential fatty acid metabolites in early psychotic patients following antipsychotic drug treatment. Prostaglandins Leukot Essent Fatty Acids. 2003;69:393-99.
397. Bell JG, MacKinlay EE, Dick JR, et al. Essential fatty acids and phospholipase A2 in autistic spectrum disorders. Prostaglandins Leukot Essent Fatty Acids. 2004;71:201-4.
398. Cabrini L, Bergami R, Fiorentini D, et al. Vitamin B6 deficiency affects antioxidant defences in rat liver and heart. Biochem Mol Biol Int. 1998;46:689-97.
399. Takahashi M, Tsuboyama-Kasaoko N, Nakatani T, et al. Fish oil feeding alters liver gene expression to defend against PPAR-a activation and ROS production. Am J Physiol Gastrointest Liver Physiol. 2002;282:G338-48.
400. Ibid.
401. Sarsilmaz M, Songur A, Ozyurt H, et al. Potential role of dietary α-3 essential fatty acids on some oxidant/antioxidant parameters in rats' corpus striatum. Prostaglandins Leukot Essent Fatty Acids. 2003;69:252-59.
402. Cabrini L, Bergami R, Maranesi M, et al. Effects of short-term dietary administration of marginal levels of vitamin B6 and fish oil on lipid composition and antioxidant defences in rat tissues. Prostaglandins Leukot Essent Fatty Acids. 2001;64:265-71.
403. Bell JG, MacKinlay EE, Dick JR, et al. Essential fatty acids and phospholipase A2 in autistic spectrum disorders. Prostaglandins Leukot Essent Fatty Acids. 2004;71:201-4.
404. Gordon Bell, personal communication.
405. Frei B, McCall MR. Antioxidant vitamins: evidence from biomarkers in humans. In: Hornig WP, Moser U, eds. Functions of Vitamins beyond Recommended Dietary Allowances. Basel, Karger: Bibl Nutr Dieta 2001;51:46-67.
406. Messahel S, Pheasant AE, Pall H, et al. Urinary levels of neopterin and biopterin in autism. Neurosci Lett. 1998;241:17-20.
407. Kuo WN, Kocis JM, Nibbs J. Nitrosation of cysteine and reduced glutathione by nitrite at physiological pH. Front Biosci. 2003;8:a62-69.
408. Jones DP, Brown LA, Sternberg P. Variability in glutathione-dependent detoxication *in vivo* and its relevance to detoxication of chemical mixtures. Toxicology. 1995;105:267-74.
409. Corcoran GB, Fix L, Jones DP, et al. Apoptosis: molecular control point in toxicity. Toxicol Appl Pharmacol. 1994;128:169-81.
410. Kidd PM. Autism, an extreme challenge to integrative medicine. Part 2: Medical management. Alt Med Rev. 2002;7:472-99.
411. Donnelly JK, Robinson DS. Free radicals in foods. Free Radic Res. 1995;22:147-76.
412. Parikh V, Khan MM, Mahadik SP. Differential effects of antipsychotics on expression of antioxidant enzymes and membrane lipid peroxidation in rat brain. J Psychiatr Res. 2003;37:43-51.
413. Banerjee RK. Nonsteroidal anti-inflammatory drugs inhibits gastric peroxidase activity. Biochim Biophys Acta. 1990;1034:275-80.
414. Loeb AL, Raj NR, Longnecker DE. Cerebellar nitric oxide is increased during isoflurane anesthesia compared to halothane anesthesia: a microdialysis study in rats. Anesthesiology. 1998;89:723-30.
415. Biswas K, Bandyopadhyay U, Chattopadhyay I, et al. A novel antioxidant and antiapoptotic role of omeprazole to block gastric ulcer through scavenging of hydroxyl radical. J Biol Chem. 2003;278:10993-11001.
416. Li XM, Chlan-Fourney J, Juorio AV, et al Differential effects of olanzapine on the gene expression of superoxide dismutase and the low affinity nerve growth factor receptor. J Neurosci Res. 1999;56:72-75.
417. Braughler JM. Lipid peroxidation-induced inhibition of gamma-aminobutyric acid uptake in rat brain synaptosomes: protection by glucocorticoids. J Neurochem. 1985;44:1282-88.
418. Bagchi D, Carryl OR, Tran MX, et al. Protection against chemically-induced oxidative gastrointestinal tissue injury in rats by bismuth salts. Dig Dis Sci. 1997;42:1890-1900.
419. Olin KL, Shigenaga MK, Ames BN, et al. Maternal dietary zinc influences DNA strand break and 8-hydroxy-2'-deoxyguanosine levels in infant rhesus monkey liver. Proc Soc Exp Biol Med. 1993;203:461-66.
420. Gao J, Wu J, Zhao XN, et al. [Transplacental neurotoxic effects of monosodium glutamate on structures and functions of specific brain areas of filial mice]. Sheng Li Xue Bao. 1994;46:44-51.
421. Whiteman M, Halliwell B. Protection against peroxynitrite-dependent nitration and a-1-antiproteinase inactivation by ascorbic acid. A comparison with other biological antioxidants. Free Radic Res. 1996;25:275-83.
422. Reiter RJ, Tan DX, Burkhardt S. Reactive oxygen and nitrogen species and cellular and organismal decline: amelioration with melatonin. Mech Ageing Dev. 2002;123:1007-19.

423. Bubenik GA, Blask DE, Brown GM, et al. Prospects of the clinical utilization of melatonin. Biol Signals Recept. 1998;7:195-219.
424. Bandyopadhyay D, Biswas K, Bhattacharyya M, et al. Involvement of reactive oxygen species in gastric ulceration: protection by melatonin. Indian J Exp Biol. 2002;40:693-705.
425. Kotler M, Rodriguez C, Sainz RM, et al. Melatonin increases gene expression for antioxidant enzymes in rat brain cortex. J Pineal Res. 1998;24:83-89.
426. Ishizaki A, Sugama M, Takeuchi N. [Usefulness of melatonin for developmental sleep and emotion/behavioral disorders—studies of melatonin trials on 50 patients with developmental disorders]. No To Hattatsu. 1999;31:428-37.
427. Gilgun-Sherki Y, Rosenbaum Z, Melamed E, et al. Antioxidant therapy in acute central nervous system injury: current state. Pharmacol Rev. 2002;54:271-84.
428. Halliwell B, Gutteridge JM. Free Radicals in Biology and Medicine. 3rd ed. New York: Oxford University Press; 1999.
429. Regoli F, Winston GW. Quantification of total oxidant scavenging capacity of antioxidants for peroxynitrite, peroxyl radicals, and hydroxyl radicals. Toxicol Appl Pharmacol. 1999;156:96-105.
430. Scott GS, Spitsin SV, Kean RB, et al. Therapeutic intervention in experimental allergic encephalomyelitis by administration of uric acid precursors. Proc Natl Acad Sci U S A. 2002;99:16303-308.
431. Hagen TM, Liu J, Lykkesfeldt J, et al. Feeding acetyl-L-carnitine and lipoic acid to old rats significantly improves metabolic function while decreasing oxidative stress. Proc Natl Acad Sci U S A. 2002;99:1870-75.
432. Ellaway CJ, Peat J, Williams K, et al. Medium-term open label trial of L-carnitine in Rett syndrome. Brain Dev 2001;23(Suppl 1):S85-89.
433. Naviaux RK. The spectrum of mitochondrial disease. Mitochondrial and Metabolic Disorders—a Primary Physician's Guide. Special supplement to Exceptional Parent Magazine. Pp. 3-10. http://biochemgen.ucsd.edu/mmdc/ep-toc.htm
434. Albano CB, Muralikrishnan D, Ebadi M. Distribution of coenzyme Q homologues in brain. Neurochem Res. 2002;27:359-68.
435. Abram Hoffer, personal communication.
436. Brody T. Nutritional Biochemistry. 2nd ed. San Diego and London: Academic Press; 1999. p 631-33.
437. Fryer MJ. The possible role of nitric oxide and impaired mitochondrial function in ataxia due to severe vitamin deficiency. Med Hypotheses 1998;50:353-44.
438. Brody T. Nutritional Biochemistry. 2nd ed. San Diego and London: Academic Press; 1999. p 631-33.
439. Rimland B, McGinnis W. Vaccines and autism. Lab Med. 2002;9:708-17.
440. Larnaout A, Belal S, Zouari M, et al. Friedreich's ataxia with isolated vitamin E deficiency: neuropathological study of a Tunisian patient. Acta Neuropathol (Berl). 1997;93:633-37.
441. Audhya T, McGinnis WR. Nutrient, toxin and enzyme profile of autistic children. International Meeting for Autism Research. Sacramento CA, May 7-8, 2004. p. 74.
442. Webb JL. Enzyme and Metabolic Inhibitors. Vol II. New York and London: Academic Press; 1966.
443. Stohs SJ. The role of free radicals in toxicity and disease. J Basic Clin Physiol Pharmacol. 1995;6:205-28.
444. Bitar MS, Al-Saleh E, Al-Mulla F. Oxidative stress-mediated alterations in glucose dynamics in a genetic animal model of type II diabetes. Life Sci. 2005;June3; Epub ahead of print.
445. Johansen JS, Harris AK, Rychly DJ, Ergul A. Oxidative stress and the use of antioxidants in diabetes: Linking basic science to clinical practice. Cardiovasc Diabetol. 2005;4:5-15.
446. Opara EC. Oxidative stress, micronutrients, diabetes mellitus and its complications. J R Soc Health. 2002;122(1):28-34.
447. Johansen JS, Harris AK, Rychly DJ, Ergul A. Oxidative stress and the use of antioxidants in diabetes: Linking basic science to clinical practice. Cardiovasc Diabetol. 2005;4:5-15.
448. Ibid.
449. Fedele D, Giugliano D. Peripheral diabetic neuropathy. Current recommendations and future prospects for its prevention and management. Drugs. 1997;54(3):414-21.
450. Kawamori R. Asymptomatic hyperglycaemia and early atherosclerotic changes. Diabetes Res Clin Pract. 1998;40 Suppl:S35-S42.
451. Coutinho M, Gerstein HC, Wang Y, Yusuf S. The relationship between glucose and incident cardiovascular events. A metaregression analysis of published data from 20 studies of 95,783 individuals followed for 12.4 years. Diabetes Care. 1999;22(2):233-40.
452. Duckworth WC. Hyperglycemia and cardiovascular disease. Curr Atheroscler Rep. 2001;3(5):383-91.
453. Komosinska-Vassev K, Olczyk K, Olczyk P, Winsz-Szczotka K. Effects of metabolic control and vascular complications on indices of oxidative stress in type 2 diabetic patients. Diabetes Res Clin Pract. 2005;68(3):207-16.
454. Pratico D. Antioxidants and endothelium protection. Atherosclerosis. 2005;May 11;Epub ahead of print.
455. Son SM, Whalin MK, Harrison DG, et al. Oxidative stress and diabetic vascular complications. Curr Diab Rep. 2004;4(4):247-52.
456. Mohamed AK, Bierhaus A, Schiekofer S, et al. The role of oxidative stress and NF-KB activation in late diabetic complications. Biofactors. 1999;10(2-3):157-67.
457. Kaneto H, Kajimoto Y, Miyagawa J, et al. Beneficial effects of antioxidants in diabetes: possible protection of pancreatic beta-cells against glucose toxicity. Diabetes. 1999;48(12):2398-406.
458. Watts GF, Playford DA. Dyslipoproteinaemia and hyperoxidative stress in the pathogenesis of endothelial dysfunction in non-insulin dependent diabetes mellitus: an hypothesis. Atherosclerosis. 1998;141(1):17-30.
459. Paolisso G, Esposito R, D'Alessio MA, Barbieri M. Primary and secondary prevention of atherosclerosis: is there a role for antioxidants? Diabetes Metab. 1999;25(4):298-306.
460. Brenner RR. Nutritional and hormonal factors influencing desaturation of essential fatty acids. Prog Lipid Res. 1981;20:41-47.
461. Bonnefont-Rousselot D. The role of antioxidant micronutrients in the prevention of diabetic complications. Treat Endocrinol. 2004;3(1):41-52.
462. Smith AR, Shenvi SV, Widlansky M, et al. Lipoic acid as a potential therapy for chronic diseases associated with oxidative stress. Curr Med Chem. 2004;11(9):1135-46.
463. Bernkop-Schnurch A, Reich-Rohrwig E, Marschutz M, et al. Development of a sustained release dosage form for alpha-lipoic acid. II. Evaluation in human volunteers. Drug Dev Ind Pharm. 2004;30(1):35-42.
464. Negrisanu G, Rosu M, Bolte B, et al. Effects of 3-month treatment with the antioxidant alpha-lipoic acid in diabetic peripheral neuropathy. Rom J Intern Med. 1999;37(3):297-306.
465. Ziegler D, Hanefeld M, Ruhnau KJ, et al. Treatment of symptomatic diabetic polyneuropathy with the antioxidant alpha-lipoic acid: a 7-month multicenter randomized controlled trial (ALADIN III Study). ALADIN III Study Group. Alpha-Lipoic Acid in Diabetic Neuropathy. Diabetes Care. 1999;22(8):1296-1301.
466. Haak E, Usadel KH, Kusterer K, et al. Effects of alpha-lipoic acid on microcirculation in patients with peripheral diabetic neuropathy. Exp Clin Endocrinol Diabetes. 2000;108(3):168-174.
467. Ziegler D, Reljanovic M, Mehnert H, Gries FA. Alpha-lipoic acid in the treatment of diabetic polyneuropathy in Germany: current evidence from clinical trials. Exp Clin Endocrinol Diabetes. 1999;107(7):421-30.

468. Morcos M, Borcea V, Isermann B, et al. Effect of alpha-lipoic acid on the progression of endothelial cell damage and albuminuria in patients with diabetes mellitus: an exploratory study. Diabetes Res Clin Pract. 2001;52(3):175-83.
469. Ametov AS, Barinov A, Dyck PJ, et al. The sensory symptoms of diabetic polyneuropathy are improved with alpha-lipoic acid: the SYDNEY trial. Diabetes Care. 2003;26(3):770-76.
470. Ihara Y, Toyokuni S, Uchida K, et al. Hyperglycemia causes oxidative stress in pancreatic beta-cells of GK rats, a model of type 2 diabetes. Diabetes. 1999;48(4):927-32.
471. Salonen JT, Nyyssonen K, Tuomainen TP, et al. Increased risk of non-insulin dependent diabetes mellitus at low plasma vitamin E concentrations: a four year follow up study in men. BMJ. 1995;311(7013):1124-27.
472. Upritchard JE, Sutherland WH, Mann JI. Effect of supplementation with tomato juice, vitamin E, and vitamin C on LDL oxidation and products of inflammatory activity in type 2 diabetes. Diabetes Care. 2000;23(6):733-38.
473. Gerstein HC, Bosch J, Pogue J, et al. Rationale and design of a large study to evaluate the renal and cardiovascular effects of an ACE inhibitor and vitamin E in high-risk patients with diabetes. The MICRO-HOPE Study. Microalbuminuria, cardiovascular, and renal outcomes. Heart Outcomes Prevention Evaluation. Diabetes Care. 1996;19(11):1225-28.
474. Scott JA, King GL. Oxidative stress and antioxidant treatment in diabetes. Ann N Y Acad Sci. 2004;1031:204-13.
475. Gaede P, Poulsen HE, Parving HH, Pedersen O. Double-blind, randomised study of the effect of combined treatment with vitamin C and E on albuminuria in Type 2 diabetic patients. Diabet Med. 2001;18(9):756-60.
476. Cameron NE, Cotter MA. Effects of antioxidants on nerve and vascular dysfunction in experimental diabetes. Diabetes Res Clin Pract. 1999;45(2-3):137-46.
477. Kowluru RA, Kennedy A. Therapeutic potential of anti-oxidants and diabetic retinopathy. Expert Opin Investig Drugs. 2001;10(9):1665-76.
478. Koya D, Haneda M, Kikkawa R, King GL. d-alpha-tocopherol treatment prevents glomerular dysfunctions in diabetic rats through inhibition of protein kinase C-diacylglycerol pathway. Biofactors. 1998;7(1-2):69-76.
479. Koya D, Lee IK, Ishii H, et al. Prevention of glomerular dysfunction in diabetic rats by treatment with d-alpha-tocopherol. J Am Soc Nephrol. 1997;8(3):426-35.
480. Eriksson J, Kohvakka A. Magnesium and ascorbic acid supplementation in diabetes mellitus. Ann Nutr Metab. 1995;39(4):217-23.
481. Paolisso G, Balbi V, Volpe C, et al. Metabolic benefits deriving from chronic vitamin C supplementation in aged non-insulin dependent diabetics. J Am Coll Nutr. 1995;14(4):387-92.
482. Gaede P, Poulsen HE, Parving HH, Pedersen O. Double-blind, randomised study of the effect of combined treatment with vitamin C and E on albuminuria in Type 2 diabetic patients. Diabet Med. 2001;18(9):756-60.
483. McAuliffe AV, Brooks BA, Fisher EJ, et al. Administration of ascorbic acid and an aldose reductase inhibitor (tolrestat) in diabetes: effect on urinary albumin excretion. Nephron. 1998;80(3):277-84.
484. Lu Q, Bjorkhem I, Wretlind , et al. Effect of ascorbic acid on microcirculation ini patients with Type II diabetes: a randomized placebo-controlled cross-over study. Clin Sci (Lond). 2005;108(6):507-13.
485. Cunningham JJ, Mearkle PL, Brown RG. Vitamin C: an aldose reductase inhibitor that normalizes erythrocyte sorbitol in insulin-dependent diabetes mellitus. J Am Coll Nutr. 1994;13(4):344-50.
486. Lee DH, Folsom AR, Harnack L, et al. Does supplemental vitamin C increase cardiovascular disease risk in women with diabetes? Am J Clin Nutr. 2004;80(5):1194-200.
487. Faure P. Protective effects of antioxidant micronutrients (vitamin E, zinc and selenium) in type 2 diabetes mellitus. Clin Chem Lab Med. 2003;41(8):995-98.
488. Reddi AS, Bollineni JS. Selenium-deficient diet induces renal oxidative stress and injury via TGF-beta1 in normal and diabetic rats. Kidney Int. 2001;59(4):1342-53.
489. Mukherjee B, Anbazhagan S, Roy A, et al. Novel implications of the potential role of selenium on antioxidant status in streptozotocin-induced diabetic mice. Biomed Pharmacother. 1998;52(2):89-95.
490. Skripchenko ND, Sharafetdinov K, Plotnikova OA, et al. [Effect of selenium enriched diet on lipid peroxidation in patients with diabetes mellitus type 2]. Vopr Pitan. 2003;72(1):14-17.
491. Agte VV, Nagmote RV, Tarwadi KV. Comparative *in vitro* uptake of zinc by erythrocytes of normal vs Type 2 diabetic individuals and the associated factors. Diabetes Nutr Metab. 2004;17(6):343-49.
492. Grungreiff K, Reinhold D. Liver cirrhosis and "liver" diabetes mellitus are linked by zinc deficiency. Med Hypotheses. 2005;64(2):316-17.
493. Miranda ER, Dey CS. Effect of chromium and zinc on insulin signaling in skeletal muscle cells. Biol Trace Elem Res. 2004;101(1):19-36.
494. Faure P, Lafond JL, Coudray C, et al. Zinc prevents the structural and functional properties of free radical treated-insulin. Biochim Biophys Acta. 1994;1209(2):260-64.
495. Bray TM, Bettger WJ. The physiological role of zinc as an antioxidant. Free Radic Biol Med. 1990;8(3):281-91.
496. Anderson RA, Roussel AM, Zouari N, et al. Potential antioxidant effects of zinc and chromium supplementation in people with type 2 diabetes mellitus. J Am Coll Nutr. 2001;20(3):212-18.
497. Thompson KH, McNeill JH. Effect of vanadyl sulfate feeding on susceptibility to peroxidative change in diabetic rats. Res Commun Chem Pathol Pharmacol. 1993;80(2):187-200.
498. Oster MH, Llobet JM, Domingo JL, et al. Vanadium treatment of diabetic Sprague-Dawley rats results in tissue vanadium accumulation and pro-oxidant effects. Toxicology. 1993;83(1-3):115-30.
499. Lapenna D, Ciofani G, Bruno C, et al. Vanadyl as a catalyst of human lipoprotein oxidation. Biochem Pharmacol. 2002;63(3):375-80.
500. Trachtman H, Futterweit S, Maesaka J, et al. Taurine ameliorates chronic streptozocin-induced diabetic nephropathy in rats. Am J Physiol. 1995;269(3 Pt 2):F429-38.
501. Singh RB, Niaz MA, Rastogi SS, et al. Effect of hydrosoluble coenzyme Q10 on blood pressures and insulin resistance in hypertensive patients with coronary artery disease. J Hum Hypertens. 1999;13(3):203-8.
502. Hodgson JM, Watts GF, Playford DA, et al. Coenzyme Q(10) improves blood pressure and glycaemic control: a controlled trial in subjects with type 2 diabetes. Eur J Clin Nutr. 2002;56(11):1137-42.
503. Watts GF, Playford DA, Croft KD, et al. Coenzyme Q(10) improves endothelial dysfunction of the brachial artery in Type II diabetes mellitus. Diabetologia. 2002;45(3):420-26.
504. Chew GT, Watts GF. Coenzyme Q10 and diabetic endotheliopathy: oxidative stress and the 'recoupling hypothesis'. AJM. 2004;97(8);537-48.
505. Lean ME, Noroozi M, Kelly I, et al. Dietary flavonols protect diabetic human lymphocytes against oxidative damage to DNA. Diabetes. 1999;48(1):176-181.
506. Mori M, Hasegawa N. Superoxide dismutase activity enhanced by green tea inhibits lipid accumulation in 3T3-L1 cells. Phytother Res. 2003;17(5):566-67.
507. Kim MJ, Ryu GR, Chung JS, et al. Protective effects of epicatechin against the toxic effects of streptozotocin on rat pancreatic islets: *in vivo* and *in vitro*. Pancreas. 2003;26(3):292-99.

508. Han MK. Epigallocatechin gallate, a constituent of green tea, suppresses cytokine-induced pancreatic beta-cell damage. Exp Mol Med. 2003;35(2):136-39.
509. Bonnefont-Rousselot D. The role of antioxidant micronutrients in the prevention of diabetic complications. Treat Endocrinol. 2004;3(1):41-52.
510. Giammarioli S, Filesi C, Vitale B, et al. Int J Vitam Nutr Res. 2004;74(5):313-20.

Section VI

A Practical Clinical Approach

Chapter 31
Clinical Approaches to Detoxification and Biotransformation

- ***Genetic and Environmental Influences on Detoxification***
- ***Systemic In-office Detoxification***
- ***Home-based Detoxification***
- ***The Gut-Liver Axis***

Genetic and Environmental Influences on Detoxification

Michael Lyon, MD, Jeffrey Bland, PhD, and David S. Jones, MD

In Chapter 22, the basic mechanisms and potential dysfunctions of detoxification and biotransformation were presented in detail. In this chapter, we will review some of those elements from a more clinical perspective. This initial part of the chapter provides a comprehensive overview of detoxification/biotransformation issues, followed by two examples of specific clinical protocols for detoxification—one for in-office use under the clinician's supervision, and the other for in-home use by patients—and ending with an in-depth discussion of the gut-liver connections (and the clinical implications of those relationships for this topic).

Introduction

Throughout evolution, we have developed complex protection systems against endogenous and exogenous substances. Scientists working in the early 1970s discovered the first enzyme of the detoxification family. This enzyme contained iron and emitted absorbed ultraviolet radiation of 450 nanometers, so it was called a cytochrome P450. A high level of this cytochrome P450 enzyme was found to be localized in the liver, and researchers soon discovered it was responsible for converting lipophilic (fat-loving) toxins into bio-transformed intermediates that were more water-soluble (*phase I detoxification*).

Later research revealed that most of these biotransformed intermediates undergo further biotransformation in the liver by a second series of enzymes called conjugases. They called this *phase II detoxification*. The conjugases were enzymes that attached molecules to the biotransformed intermediate, such as glucuronic acid, sulfate, glutathione, glycine, taurine, or methyl groups. Hormones and other signaling molecules are detoxified (biotransformed) and eliminated through specific phase I and phase II processes. The most common phase II pathways include sulfation, glucuronidation, and methylation. Drugs and xenobiotics, along with hormones and other endogenous metabolites, compete for these same detoxification pathways and specific phase I enzymes. As research continued into the 1980s and 1990s, investigators discovered a tremendous number of phase I cytochrome P450s and phase II conjugases. We now know that phase I cytochrome P450s are members of a "super-family" of enzymes,[1] for which more than 58 different genes exist in humans.

Genetic Variability in Detoxification Function

The complexity of detoxification and biotransformation is intensified by the widespread genetic polymorphisms for the expression of cytochrome P450 enzymes within the human species. Researchers have discovered that great variability exists among humans in not only the structure and function of the phase I cytochrome P450s but the phase II conjugases as well.[2] Recent molecular genetic analysis has identified hundreds of single nucleotide polymorphisms (SNPs) that modify the structure and function of the various detoxification enzymes. As a consequence of this inter-individual variation in detoxification enzyme function, very significant differences exist from person to person in the way we metabolize specific substances. (This material was covered in detail in Chapter 22.)

The full extent and significance of this phenomenon have not been completely ascertained, and there is no strong consensus in the literature about specific relationships, but a number of studies have suggested a correlation between genetic deficiency of certain cytochrome P450 enzymes and susceptibility to environmentally mediated disorders.[3,4,5,6,7] Early cancer indications, for example, have not always been reproducible, particularly lung cancer and prostate cancer.[8] In a 2003 review, Guengerich[9] observed that "Difficulties in studying the association of cancers with toxic chemicals in the environment are made more complex by the usually very limited numbers of patients available, the need to identify individual chemicals and levels of exposure, and the long latency period (up to 20 years) from exposure to onset of cancer."

These differences in the metabolism of drugs are not only genetic; they also relate to environmental and nutritional influences that modify gene expression and proteomic activity of the cytochrome P450 and conjugase family of enzymes. We are now aware that dietary factors can play a significant role in modifying first-pass detoxification or biotransformation in an individual by inducing or inhibiting transport and metabolism.[10]

The majority of the research in this area presents epidemiological, animal-based, basic science, small human clinical trials, or case-based information. As a consequence, it is difficult to recommend with certainty specific patient intervention techniques from the literature. Given, however, that patients and practitioners alike have increasing concerns about environmentally-related illnesses, we believe it is important to explore the role that diet and lifestyle may play in prevention, risk reduction, and therapeutics. The concepts described in this chapter frame an important component of the functional medicine model.

Genetics of Detoxification and the Diet

Heritable polymorphisms are also known for several conjugating enzymes (phase II detoxification) that are extensively involved in the metabolism of exogenous chemicals,[11] a significant factor conferring susceptibility to environmental toxins. An example of this genetic variation is the activation of glutathione S-transferase (GST), an important phase II detoxification enzyme involved in glutathione conjugation.[12] There are a number of polymorphisms of GST, including those within the *mu* and *theta* classes (GSTM and GSTT).

Certain foods may contain constituents that activate the expression of a specific detoxification process, while other foods may contain substances that inhibit its activity. For example, in humans, consumption of Brussels sprouts leads to the induction of one isoform of glutathione-S-transferase only, and the administration of the terpene eugenol from thyme oil inhibits the activity of two different isoforms of glutathione-S-transferase at the same time.[13] Studies of the induction of individual isozymes of glutathione transferase in humans have shown that Brussels sprouts and garlic induce these activities in similar ways.

The findings that food/drug interactions are associated with alterations in the detoxification of hormones have important clinical implications. Foods may interact with hormones during key metabolic processes:

1. before and during gastrointestinal absorption,
2. during distribution,
3. during metabolism, and
4. during elimination.[14]

Specific macro- and micronutrients in foods may influence the biotransformation process of both phase I and phase II enzyme systems, and thus have an impact on all four of these fundamental physiological processes. For example, nondigestible carbohydrate (fiber) that is not digested in the intestinal tract may be quite bioactive toward the detoxification enzyme systems. The most important effects of food on biotransformation and its relationship to detoxification are observed through the influence on metabolism and elimination of various substances.

Influencing Detoxification

Phytochemicals

Dr. Paul Talalay and his colleagues from the Johns Hopkins University School of Medicine have been working for the past 40 years to elucidate the mechanisms by which various phytochemicals in plant foods modify the activity of phase I and phase II enzyme systems.[15,16] Animal studies reveal that a surprising number of phytochemicals protect rodents against neoplastic, mutagenic, and other toxic effects when the animals are exposed to various types of carcinogens. Dr. Talalay points out that these chemoprotective agents often belong to totally unrelated chemical classes, such as substituted phenols, coumarins, sulfur compounds such as isothiocyanates, flavones, indoles, retinoids, tocopherols, and selenium compounds.[17]

Specific chemical substances in various foods have specific effects on the expression and activity of the biotransformational detoxification system. For many years, we have known, in general, that certain foods seemed to promote improved detoxification. As a consequence of the work of Talalay and others, however, we now know that certain phytochemicals have specific influences on the various isoforms of cytochrome P450 and the variety of conjugases involved with phase II activity.[18]

The discovery that specific phytochemicals influence the activity of different components of the phase I and phase II biotransformational detoxification system poses a challenge to the clinician concerning what specific foods or phytonutrients to recommend to improve the unique detoxification systems of individual patients. Upregulation of the activity of phase I cytochrome P450, without proper balance with phase II detoxification capability, can result in a more harmful outcome by producing higher levels of highly reactive biotransformed intermediates. The clinical focus should not be solely on inducing increased detoxification activity, but rather on trying to establish balance in the patient between phase I and phase II detoxification systems.

Mono- and Multifunctional Modulators of Detoxification

The challenge of finding the appropriate clinical support program to balance phase I and phase II detoxification systems was simplified by Talalay's discovery of specific phytochemicals that are bifunctional modulators of detoxification effects. These phytochemicals have an influence on modulating specific phase I cytochrome P450s and phase II conjugases simultaneously, thereby leading, potentially, to balanced detoxification.[19] Some agents act in a monofunctional manner. They have only single effects on either cytochrome P450 isoforms or phase II conjugases.

The impact of any factor upon detoxification status is the sum of all effects upon phase I and phase II enzyme systems. For example, moderately high-protein diets bring about upregulation of P450s in a pattern that may either increase or decrease susceptibility to pesticides and other xenobiotics, depending upon whether the protein is of animal or vegetable origin, while diets that are deficient in protein may increase pesticide toxicity because of P450 downregulation. On the other hand, cigarette smoking brings about a monofunctional induction of P450, biotransforming certain xenobiotics into potent carcinogens while simultaneously increasing oxidative stress.[20]

Numerous phytochemicals are known to exert potent effects upon both phase I and phase II enzyme activities. With few exceptions (such as grapefruit slowing drug metabolism, or St. John's wort accelerating drug metabolism), plant foods common to the human diet have been shown to have important effects upon detoxification systems. Onions and garlic, cruciferous vegetables, chlorophyll, terpenoids (e.g., citrus, *Ginkgo biloba*, menthol, camphor), bioflavonoids (e.g., citrus, pine bark, grape seed, green tea) and others all act in a complex, highly beneficial manner to improve balanced detoxification capability.[21]

In a landmark article titled "Dietary Carcinogens and Anti-carcinogens," Ames explained that although some foods are known to contain substances that may be potential carcinogens, whole foods, particularly those in the vegetable family, contain phytochemicals that modulate the potential carcinogenic activity of other substances through their ability to modify detoxification.[22] Further evidence indicates this bifunctional aspect of various phytochemicals is important in establishing a higher degree of tolerance and safety in their influence on hepatic bifunctional detoxification systems.

A diet rich in bifunctional modulators, as well as monofunctional phase II regulators, influences the detoxification and elimination of neuroendocrine modulators. According to research by Lanai et al., "Compounds acting as inducers of anti-carcinogenic enzymes are divided into two classes: (1) bifunctional inducers, which induce those phase I xenobiotic-metabolizing enzymes ... and subsequently generate intermediates which transcriptionally activate genes encoding phase II enzymes including QR (quinone reductase); and (2) mono-functional inducers, which induce phase II enzymes directly without inducing the phase I enzymes."[23]

Talalay pointed out that protection against endogenous and exogenous toxins is achieved through the proper balance between monofunctional inducers of the selective phase II enzymes and appropriate bifunctional inducers that help regulate both phase I and phase II activities, resulting in "balanced detoxification."[24]

Monofunctional and Bifunctional Inducers and Cancer Risk

Dr. Johanna Lampe and her colleagues at the Fred Hutchinson Cancer Research Center in Seattle, Washington, have been actively involved in clinical evaluation of these concepts in studies of human patients. In one paper, Dr. Lampe discusses the effects of genetic polymorphisms on detoxification systems and the role of specific diets rich in phase II monofunctional and bifunctional inducers in reducing carcinogenic risk.[25] According to Dr. Lampe, a diet/gene interaction that works through the detoxification mechanisms is likely to contribute significantly to the observed inter-individual variations in cancer risk in response to exposures to various carcinogens. Her work once again emphasizes the importance of supporting balanced detoxification through proper activity of both phase I cytochrome P450s and phase II conjugases.

Phase II enzymes, such as glutathione-S-transferase, N-acetyltransferase, sulfotransferase, UDP-glucuronosyltransferase, and catechol-methyl transferase, are extra-ordinarily important in providing balanced detoxification. Upregulation of phase I cytochrome P450 without a concomitant balance with phase II enzymes can result in significant increase in reactive intermediary metabolites, which may increase the risk of cellular injury. The scheme that relates to the balance between phase I and phase II detoxification enzymes is shown in Figure 31.1. (Another version can be seen in Figure 22.1, in Chapter 22.)

Glucuronidation

Dr. Lampe has focused on the role of specific nutrients in the regulation of phase II glucuronidation. Glucuronidation is a major detoxification process catalyzed by UDP glucuronysyltransferases that convert a vast variety of endogenous compounds, including bilirubin, steroid and thyroid hormones, and retinoids or bile acids, as well as a remarkable number of lipophilic xenobiotics, into more hydrophilic and therefore excretable metabolites.

UDP glucuronosyltransferase enzymes are members of a super-family of enzymes with considerable genetic polymorphisms. Individuals who have specific polymorphisms in specific UDP glucuronosyltransferases are more susceptible than others to Gilbert's syndrome. Reduced glucuronidation ability of specific substances in these individuals may make them more susceptible to the effects of endo- and exotoxins. [26] Glucuronidation is under dual regulatory control. The first control, carried out on the genetic expression level of the isoenzymes, determines the amount of a different isoform available. The second control is modulation of the activity of individual isoforms to their "functional state" by specific substances, including certain nutrients. [27]

Individual differences in glucuronidation ability. Lampe et al. discovered that UDP glucuronosyltransferase polymorphisms result in significant differences in glucuronidation ability from person to person, and that dietary factors may significantly influence the activity of the phase II biotransformation function.[28] Interestingly, Dr. Lampe has found considerable differences in the activity of UDP glucuronosyltransferase isoforms between Caucasians and individuals of Asian ethnicity, suggesting the origin of possible differences in certain disease incidence upon exposure to various toxins.[29]

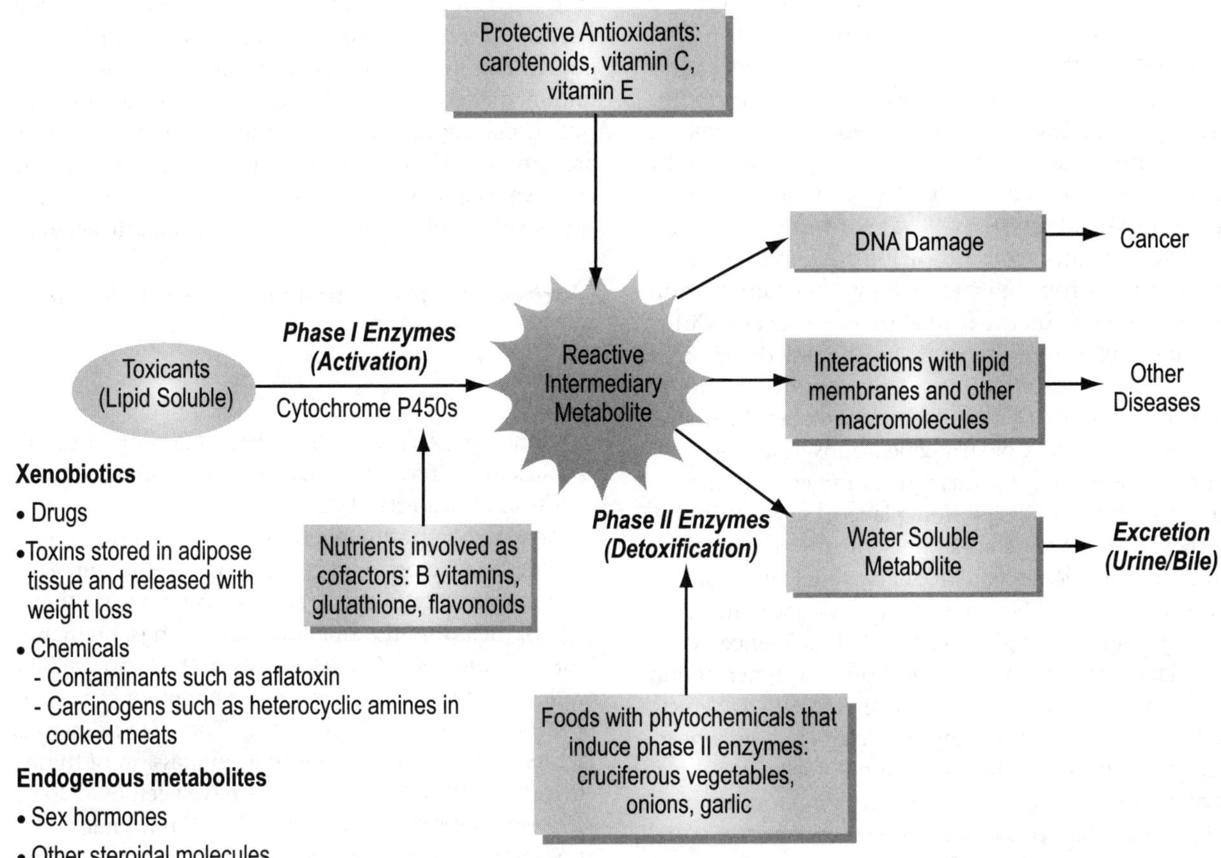

Figure 31.1 **Interrelationships among the biotransformation enzyme systems**

In a pilot study, Lampe found the consumption of different vegetables, including members of the allium (garlic and onion), apiaceae (carrot), and cruciferous (broccoli and Brussels sprouts) families had different influences on phase II GST enzyme activity.[30] In another study, researchers found that garden cress, a relative of the cruciferous vegetables, contains specific glucosinolates that increase glucuronidation activity. According to the authors of this study, "Our findings suggest that the chemoprotective effect of GC (garden cress) is mediated through enhancement of detoxification of IQ (2-amino-3-methyl-imidazo [4,5-1) quinoline by UDPGT."[31]

Once again, these studies demonstrate the important concept that clinical response in biotransformation is a result of genomically determined factors and environmental influences on gene and protein expression. The clinical application of this emerging information is to find dietary programs containing the right balance of monofunctional inducers of phase II enzymes and bifunctional inducers of the appropriate isoforms of phase I and phase II enzymes to provide balanced detoxification in the majority of genotypes represented in a genomically heterogeneous population such as that in the United States.

Factors that induce glucuronidation. With specific reference to UDP glucuronosyltransferase induction, researchers have demonstrated that a number of flavonoids have the ability to induce specific glucuronidases, which will increase glucuronidation. Luteolin is one example of a flavonoid that can induce glucuronidation; another is chrysin, which induces UGT1A1.[32]

Thyroid hormone T_3 is also involved in the expression of UGT1A1 and UGT1A6. UGTIA1 is responsible for the glucuronidation of bilirubin, while UGT1A6 is responsible for the glucuronidation of potentially xenobiotic phenolic compounds. The influence of T_3 on UGT expression was also found to depend on vitamin A retinol status. A deficiency of vitamin A resulted in inhibition of the expression of UGT1A1 and 1A6, even in the absence of administered T_3. The investigators conclude, "Our results demonstrate for the first time the existence of a strong interaction between vitamin A and thyroid hormone on the regulation of genes encoding cellular detoxification enzymes, in this case the UGT." [33]

The role of dietary fiber in glucuronidation. It has also been found that certain sources of dietary fiber will influence the activity of UDP-glucuronosyltransferase. A comparative study of various forms of fiber in animals found that intestinal microflora played a key role in the effects of fiber on xenobiotic-metabolizing enzyme systems, not just as a consequence of bacterial fermentation of various types of fiber. In examining wheat bran, carrot, cocoa, and oat bran fibers and their influence as potential modulators of detoxification, researchers found that cocoa fiber seemed to influence phase II UDP glucuronosyltransferase activity more than fibers from wheat or carrot.[34] This result suggests that colonic bacteria may play an important role in modulating glucuronidation, and that diet-derived substrates for colonic bacteria can influence detoxification. (Clinically, the important application of this concept is to focus on gastrointestinal restoration and recolonization of the colon with symbiotic bacteria and prebiotics, while also providing a nutritional support program for hepatic detoxification phase I and phase II balance.)

Silymarin and glucuronidation. Milk thistle concentrate containing silymarin is another botanical medicine that influences cytochrome P450 and UDP glucuronosyltransferase activity. In a human cell culture study, researchers reported that silymarin significantly reduced cytochrome P450-3A4 enzyme activities, as well as those of glucuronosyltransferase 1A6 and 1A9. [35] This result may have potential clinical importance because these are hepatic drug-metabolizing enzyme systems that are important for first-pass detoxification of a variety of pharmaceuticals. Although this was a cell culture study, it does call into question the potential effects of milk thistle concentrate, when administered with specific pharmaceuticals, on their detoxification.

One can learn from this study to be aware that specific substances in botanical medicines may have influence on specific aspects of either phase I or phase II detoxification systems and alter the metabolism of certain medications. One should always ask patients what nutritional supplements and botanical medicines they are currently taking and assess potential interaction of these various substances with their detoxification processes before administering other therapeutic agents.

Biochemical Individuality and Toxic Response

Modifying Susceptibility to Environmental Toxicants: Diet, Lifestyle, Environment

Although genetic predisposition may confer certain absolute risks in the response of an individual to toxic agents, most aspects of detoxification and resistance involve highly modifiable nutritional, environmental, and lifestyle factors. The cytochrome P450 enzymes are located primarily in the liver. However, several other organs, including the small intestine, lungs, brain and kidneys, contribute in a lesser way to the P450-mediated oxidation of both xenobiotics and endobiotics such as hormones and neurotransmitters. There are numerous factors that influence phenotypic expression of these critical enzymes. Although there have been over 30 different P450s characterized in detail in humans, it appears that the majority of P450 activity is carried out by about six different isoforms.[36] The impact of various physical, chemical, and microbiological agents upon P450 activity is highly complex and may involve upregulation, downregulation, inhibition, or stimulation of enzyme activity.

Fasting. One significant consideration for the natural medicine clinician is the impact of fasting upon detoxifying enzyme function. For the most part, P450 enzymes are relatively resistant to depletion during fasting, and may even be significantly induced by products of starvation such as ketones and xenobiotics released from stored fat. On the other hand, the conjugating enzymes are highly dependent upon dietary provision of adequate amounts of substrate and are consumed rapidly under states of high xenobiotic load or oxidative stress.[37] Complete fasting, juice fasts, or other nutritionally marginal fasting regimens may exacerbate systemic toxicity,[38] particularly if the fluid intake is low and there is reduced fecal elimination. This may result in a marked rise in highly toxic bioactive intermediates and free radicals, with a concomitant decrease in phase II detoxification activity, because those regimens don't provide adequate substrate for phase II detoxification. For example, sulfation is particularly susceptible to inhibition due to compromised cofactor status, and the serum sulfate level is decreased in individuals who are fasting. Humans excrete approximately 20 to 25 millimoles of sulfate in 24 hours; therefore, sulfate reserves must be maintained through dietary intake of sulfur-containing amino acids or inorganic sulfate, both of which have been shown to support increased serum sulfate levels.[39]

As discussed in Chapter 22, imbalanced detoxification can result in marked oxidative stress and may be particularly deleterious to chronically ill patients whose antioxidant reserves are already exhausted or significantly weakened. Perhaps in the past, when tissue burdens of xenobiotics and heavy metals were low, complete fasting regimens were of significant benefit. However, the modern human is probably ill advised to follow such traditional detoxification methods for lengthy periods of time.

Amino acid needs in phase II detoxification. Phase II detoxification systems are particularly dependent upon and responsive to adequacy of substrates to carry out the conjugation of oxidized intermediates. Adequate amounts of protein, with special attention to glycine, L-glutamine, methionine, L-cysteine, and N-acetylcysteine, along with inorganic sulfate, selenium and additional taurine, are all very important in the support of phase II activity.[40,41,42,43] Lipoic acid supplementation markedly enhances the level of intracellular glutathione in states of adequate sulfur amino acid intake.[44] Undenatured whey protein, rich in glutathione precursors, has been shown in several studies to increase cellular and plasma glutathione.[45] Cruciferous vegetables significantly upregulate phase II enzyme activity.[46] Antioxidants also provide a highly supportive role in liver detoxification by reducing oxidative stress resulting from phase I activity and by preventing glutathione consumption by reactive oxygen species. Milk thistle, curcumin, and green tea extracts are particularly useful antioxidants for the liver;[47,48,49] silymarin (milk thistle) is mediated through the upregulation of phase II enzymes such as glutathione-S-transferase.

Other dietary factors. Other nutritional factors impact detoxification. High carbohydrate diets bring about downregulation of P450s in a pattern that results in an undesirable reduction in the metabolism of several drugs and hormones. Intestinal dysbiosis may inhibit specific P450 activity through altered enzyme activity. On the other hand, supplementation with probiotic bacteria can markedly reduce the adverse effects of bacterial endotoxin upon the liver, as well as decreasing gut permeability.[50] Inhibition of nitric oxide synthesis may improve detoxification in inflammatory liver conditions.[51] Certain types of dietary fiber markedly enhance the activity of both phase I and phase II detoxification systems in the liver.[52] Fiber also decreases stool transit time, acts to sequester conjugated xenobiotics and endobiotics located in the bile, and reduces the level of bacterial deconjugating enzymes in the stool. All of these effects reduce the recycling of xenobiotics and endobiotics through the enterohepatic circulation.[53,54]

Exercise. Exercise, if accompanied by adequate calories and protein, has been shown to result in liver hypertrophy and a multifunctional induction of detoxification enzyme systems, as well as a marked increase in antioxidant enzymes and reduced glutathione in several organs.[55,56,57] Additionally, exercise results in a mobilization of extracellular fluid and lymph where xenobiotics often temporarily reside after being released from cells by exocytosis or other mechanisms. Sweating augments the liver's detoxification mechanisms as it is an important route of elimination for both organic [58,59] and metallic [60,61] toxicants.

Nutritional and Environmental Regulation of Toxic Metals

Nutritional adequacy has a marked influence upon the absorption, retention, toxicity, and excretion of toxic metals. For example, the effect of lead on cognitive and behavioral development is increased with iron deficiency, which also leads to increased gastrointestinal absorption of cadmium. Cadmium competes with zinc for binding sites on metallothionein.[62] Iron deficiency also increases the uptake of aluminum.[63] The absorption of several other toxic metals may be enhanced by increased intestinal permeability. Inadequacy of certain minerals can lead to enhanced retention of toxic metals. Through increased absorption, calcium deficiency increases both lead and cadmium body burden, and selenium deficiency increases mercury retention.

Toxic metals compete with nutritional minerals, leading to displacement of nutrient minerals from protein binding sites, as well as excessive loss of minerals from the body.[64] Because of this, the requirement for several nutrient minerals may rise significantly above the RDA in the metal-toxic patient. The clinician must also be aware that certain nutritionally necessary metals (e.g., iron, copper) can become conditionally toxic, and perhaps should only be supplemented if a deficiency is determined. The best example of this is excessive iron stores in patients who are homozygous or heterozygous for a hemochromatosis mutation, the most common genetic disorder. Although homozygotes are relatively uncommon, heterozygotes for this disorder may be as high as one in five in certain populations, and these individuals may be at risk for manifestations of iron toxicity, particularly if iron supplementation is administered.[65] Other nutrient metals (e.g., manganese) may be nontoxic unless control of absorption is bypassed through inhalation or injection.[66]

The excretion of toxic metals is governed by a complex chain of interwoven activities. If any link in this chain is broken, proper elimination of the toxic metal may not take place. Toxic metals must be released from the cell, moved from the extracellular fluid into the blood, transported from the blood to the liver or kidneys, and then transported from the kidneys to the urine or from the liver into the bile. Once the metal is in the bile, it must then be transported out of the body in the stool before it can be reabsorbed back into the circulation.

For example, the first step in mercury excretion involves binding of the mercury to metallothionein (MT) or glutathione within the cell. Metallothionein production, in turn, is highly inducible through exercise and nutritional adequacy of zinc (zinc deficiency results in MT depletion). Metallothionein production is also induced by supplementary L-cysteine or by brief periods of oxidative stress (as with aerobic exercise).[67] MT works in cooperation with glutathione in the initial mobilization of mercury from cells and it also shares intracellular antioxidant activity with glutathione.[68] Selenium may also play a role in binding to mercury within the cell and forming a transportable complex. Therefore, selenium supplementation has been recommended in the treatment of mercury toxicity.[69]

Once mercury is mobilized by MT or glutathione, it is transported through the cell membrane (probably by exocytosis). Mercury must then be carried away from the cell to limit toxicity upon the cell membrane and to transport mercury to the liver. Exercise is probably helpful in accelerating the movement of mercury from the extracellular fluid through the lymph and into the blood. Hyperthermic therapy (e.g., sauna) may be helpful in mobilizing mercury directly from the extracellular fluid.[70] Once the mercury reaches the liver, it usually undergoes conjugation with glutathione and is transformed into a mercapturate. The mercury mercapturate is then released into bile.[71]

Both the liver and the kidneys are highly sensitive to glutathione depletion by mercury. Hepatic and renal glutathione production can be enhanced by supplementing the diet with L-cysteine, N-acetylcysteine, glutathione, cruciferous vegetables, dietary fiber, undenatured whey protein, lipoic acid, onions, and garlic. Lipoic acid may also assist in this process by directly binding inorganic mercury in the liver and accelerating its excretion into the bile, while simultaneously inducing the formation of glutathione.[72]

Once mercury has entered the intestine through the release of bile, it must leave the body via the stool. Optimal gastrointestinal function is very important to prevent recycling of mercury through the enterohepatic circulation. Fiber has been shown to have a significant effect in lowering total body burden of mercury through sequestration of intestinal mercury and reduction in stool transit time.[73] Other factors, including increased gut permeability and intestinal dysbiosis resulting in deconjugating bacterial enzymes, help determine how efficiently mercury can leave the body once it has passed from the liver into the small intestine. Since 90% of excreted mercury leaves the body through the enteric route, colonic elimination is a vital component in maintaining an unbroken and efficient chain of excretion from the cell to the outside of the body for mercury as well as a host of other toxicants.

Assessing the Toxicologically Impaired Patient

Patient History

A carefully gathered toxic exposure history is a vital part of the clinical evaluation. The mnemonic **C(H2) OP(D4)** will aid in remembering important elements of the toxic exposure history.

- Community .... City and neighborhood air quality, noise, electromagnetic fields
- Home .... Home heating and ventilation, cleaning chemicals, pesticides, paints, carpets, building materials, molds, allergens, water
- Hobbies .... Toxic chemicals, paints, solvents, metal fumes
- Occupation .... Workplace air quality, toxic chemicals
- Personal habits .. Smoking, drinking, drug use, sun exposure, exercise, stress management
- Diet .... Overall quality of diet, over- or undereating, meat eater or vegetarian, fast foods, snack foods, deep fried foods, fish and seafood, organic or non-organic foods, food allergies or intolerances, leaky gut syndrome, abnormal microbial ecology of the digestive tract
- Drugs .... Prescription and nonprescription
- Dental .... Amalgams placed and removed, extractions, root canals
- Development ..... Mother's pregnancy history (e.g., smoking, drugs, drinking, toxic exposures, dental work), childhood exposures (e.g., leaded paints, pesticides, secondhand smoke)

Patients may not be aware of important sources of toxic exposure. They may also have genetic, nutritional, or lifestyle factors that place them at elevated risk for toxicologically-mediated health problems.

Laboratory Assessment

The field of toxicogenomics is in its infancy, but several labs have begun to offer toxicogenomic assays to help in evaluating a patient's genetic risk of toxin-mediated illness. Evaluations of SNPs to assess cytochrome P450 variability, DNA or RNA amplification techniques (primarily polymerase chain reaction—PCR) to assess adequacy of metallothionein or glutathione S-transferase activity are examples of toxicogenomic tests that are (or are becoming) commercially available to the clinician.

Some laboratories have developed panels that include evaluation of several factors relative to a particular toxicologic system. For example, an available metallothionein profile measures serum zinc, serum copper, serum ceruloplasmin, serum ceruloplasmin copper, non-ceruloplasmin ("free") copper, whole blood reduced glutathione, whole blood metallothioneins, copper/zinc ratio, reduced glutathione/metallothionein ratio, zinc/metallothionein ratio. Other examples include the functional liver detoxification profiles offered through several commercial laboratories. In these tests, patients are given drugs (often acetaminophen, aspirin, and caffeine) as a single oral dose. Urine is gathered following the ingestion of the test substance, and levels of metabolites processed through phase I and phase II detoxification are measured. Although no profile currently exists which assays the function of more than a few out of the several dozen possible detoxification enzymes, these tests often do provide useful information for the clinician.

Organic toxicants. In some cases, an occupational history will provide clues about specific toxicants to be searched for. Some toxicology laboratories offer extensive panels to quantify the level of organic toxins in blood, urine, or adipose tissue. Available panels include such things as PCBs, organochlorine pesticides, PBDE fire retardants, furans, and dioxins. Body burdens for these agents are accurately assessed by providing a small sample of adipose tissue (often taken through a small incision under the umbilicus). For example, an electric utility worker with chronic fatigue syndrome was shown to have a high body burden of PCBs, as measured in a provided fat biopsy. In this case, PCB tissue levels can be monitored in a serial fashion following detoxification efforts. Such assessment may also help a patient to support a disability or worker's compensation claim.

However, unless a specific chemical or family of chemicals can be suggested by an exposure history, the range of possible organic toxicants is far too vast to be determined practically and financially in most cases. It is generally more realistic to assume that all functionally impaired patients carry a wide range of synergistically active organic toxicants at various levels, and focus instead upon engaging the patient in a comprehensive detoxification program using outcome-based measures and functional testing to gauge success.

Metal toxicants. On the other hand, the definitive assessment of a patient's heavy metal burden is relatively simple and probably should be performed early in the assessment of most patients with poly-symptomatic, chronic illness. Metal-toxic patients present a unique clinical challenge and, if a significant toxic metal burden is present, the outcome of clinical intervention may be disappointing unless the metal burden is effectively diminished. Once metal burdens are diminished, patients often respond far more effectively to other clinical interventions.

There is a limited number of toxic metals commonly found in the human and most labs provide panels that include most of these metals. Hair analysis is a simple and inexpensive screening test for levels of a few metals such as lead or methylmercury (from seafood). However, there are confounding factors that can make it difficult to use for individual patient diagnosis—for example, some anecdotal reports indicate that low levels of hair mercury in autistic children may indicate poor excretion rather than normality, whereas high levels of hair mercury may indicate normal mercury excretion patterns. Furthermore, the precision of this methodology in determining long-standing body burdens of most other metals is probably too low to base confident clinical decisions upon, and some toxicology authorities suggest that hair analysis be limited to population screening.[74]

Conventional toxicologists generally rely upon other methodologies of assessing metal burden to gauge clinical decision making. "Acceptable" blood levels of lead in children and adults, as well as blood and urine levels of several other metals in industrial settings, have been widely suggested in published literature. However, the limitation of blood or urine tests is that they largely reflect only the level of ongoing exposure to the metal and may bear little relationship to tissue levels. Since tissue biopsy for heavy metal levels is impractical, post-provocative urine testing is probably the most reliable means to assess body burden of metals acquired through long-standing, low-level exposure, especially in the assessment of low-level inorganic mercurialism.[75]

The Detoxification Lifestyle

When working with chronically ill patients whose health is impacted by toxicological stresses, clinicians need to provide education to help these individuals develop habits of living that will reduce their exposure to toxicological factors and improve the efficiency of their detoxification mechanisms. The mnemonic **A NERD** will help the clinician to remember the important elements of a detoxification lifestyle. Patients who learn to follow these habits of living are creating a foundation for better long-term health, and their response to more extensive clinical interventions will be more successful.

Avoid exposure to all known sources of toxicity. Chemical dependencies, smoking, excessive alcohol, unnecessary prescription drugs, toxic work environments, homes with leaded paint, severe air pollution, polluted drinking water, and standard North American diets—particularly sugary drinks, junk foods, processed meats, fast foods, and deep fried foods—should be avoided. For some patients, removal of dental amalgam fillings might be indicated.

Nutrition must be optimized for efficient detoxification. The diet must be based upon whole foods (plenty of vegetables, fruits, and fiber) and should emphasize foods with a net alkalinizing impact with lower amounts of acid-forming foods. Generous portions of cruciferous vegetables should be eaten daily, along with modest amounts of olive oil, as well as onions, garlic, and modest amounts of lean, unprocessed protein. Supplements can include alkalinizing minerals (Ca, Mg, K, Zn), along with multivitamin/trace elements, essential fatty acids (DHA/EPA), N-acetylcysteine, lipoic acid, and antioxidant support (vitamins C and E, grape seed extract, green tea extract). Undenatured whey protein supports synthesis of glutathione. Detoxification medical food products are available with a base of undenatured whey, rice, or pea protein, along with a range of nutrients to support detoxification. These can be used as a supplement to, or in replacement of, one meal per day to simplify the daily detoxification supplement program.

Exercise accelerates lymphatic flow, induces sweating, and increases metabolism and detoxification efficiency. Exercise should be a daily part of the detoxification lifestyle.

Rest, including proper sleep, relaxation, and stress management, is an essential element in the detoxification lifestyle.

Detoxification as a specific therapeutic activity should be considered as a periodic means to improve vitality and reduce toxic body burdens. Traditions of fasting and purification have been incorporated into the way of life and healthcare systems of most traditional cultures, and variations on fasting are central to the practices of natural, integrative, and functional medicine. Taking a few days to rest and rejuvenate the gastrointestinal tract and bolster the excretion of xenobiotics is a lifestyle habit that can improve a patient's vitality.

Nutritionally-Controlled Detoxification

Rigden has described the "enterohepatic resuscitation program for chronic fatigue syndrome" and reported significant improvement in the majority of patients studied.[76] In this uncontrolled study, subjects consumed a limited, low-calorie diet supplemented by a medical food product designed to provide nutritional support of hepatic detoxification phase I (antioxidants) and phase II (conjugation substrates).

Bland, in another uncontrolled study, utilized a similar program with a high degree of success in 106 patients with a variety of chronic illnesses.[77] Using a much different approach, clinicians prescribing exercise and saunas combined with supplementary niacin, calcium, magnesium, and polyunsaturated oil report a significant reduction in tissue PCBs and other fat-soluble xenobiotics in toxic patients.[78,79,80] Europeans have successfully utilized sauna treatment to decrease mercury levels in exposed workers.[81] None of these approaches have been validated with controlled clinical trials.

Many clinicians have successfully prescribed a nutritionally-controlled detoxification program that follows this general approach:

- Mild to moderate caloric restriction to promote fat loss
- No fast foods, junk foods, deep fried foods
- High quantities of fresh vegetables and often fresh vegetable juice
- Very simple, low processed, oligoantigenic (low allergy potential) foods—protein from chicken, fish, and legumes, and whole grains such as brown rice, millet, and quinoa
- Medical food product designed to support detoxification (1–3 times per day, depending upon quantities of other foods eaten)
- Light exercise daily
- Sauna 3–5 times per week

This program is continued for 5 to 21 days or more, depending upon the patient's condition and the clinician's experience.

Gastrointestinal Rehabilitation

Gastrointestinal rehabilitation is a concept familiar to practitioners of functional medicine. Many clinicians consider gastrointestinal rehabilitation an essential part of any detoxification program, and will often institute such a program before beginning any detoxification interventions. In this text, we refer to the process of GI rehabilitation as the 4R Program (Remove, Replace, Reinoculate, and Repair), and it is described fully in Chapter 28. An effective GI rehab program will reduce intestinal permeability, improve nutrient absorption, and increase immune response to gut pathogens while diminishing hypersensitivities.

Summary

The study of detoxification mechanisms, processes, and influences is a young field. The growing body of research is helping clinicians understand their patients better, particularly in three main areas:

- the role of genetic individuality in detoxification,
- influences of diet, nutrition, environment, and lifestyle on detoxification, and
- the importance of staying current with emerging data on food/drug and herb/drug interactions that affect detoxification.

Even without a mature evidence base, knowledge of basic mechanisms and processes can guide clinicians in assessing and improving detoxification and biotransformation in their patients. Specific nutrients play key roles in supporting both phase I and phase II detoxification, and a number of clinical approaches are available to those with the proper knowledge and training.

Detoxification Procedures—A Disclaimer

The following two subsections of this chapter will provide the reader a glimpse into clinical approaches that may help patients decrease their toxic burdens. We have presented in Chapters 13, 22, and elsewhere in this chapter a portion of the large and growing evidence base about the presence and persistence of exogenous toxic substances in humans, their effects upon our physiology and biochemistry, and some interventions that may help to strengthen and balance the body's own detoxification systems. Unfortunately, there is a dearth of evidence about how to actually detoxify patients whose illnesses are caused by, or exacerbated by, a toxic burden. As Dr. Crinnion explains below, even the differential diagnosis is difficult.

Healthcare practitioners are often faced with the challenge of when to act and what to do in the absence of compelling evidence. Historical uses and clinical experience do form a portion of the evidence that informs all clinical decisions. It seemed to us that, in the face of the significant and well-documented body burden of toxins we all carry, providing practitioners with some clinically-derived views on clinical detoxification procedures is important. We have, therefore, invited Dr. Walter Crinnion and Dr. Peter Bennett to share with you the approaches they have used with their patients for many years. It is our hope that by increasing awareness of such practices, we may help to stimulate interest in research on these and other approaches that may be of benefit to patients. That research is badly needed.

— The Editors

Systemic In-office Detoxification

Walter J. Crinnion, ND

Introduction

"Is this patient toxic?" The answer to this question is "Yes." Virtually all patients today have a body burden of toxins. According to one recent study, the average number of toxins found per person was 91.[82] The CDC has also picked up the challenging question of how many toxins are in us. They have already published two reports and will continue to publish their research.[83]

Instead of asking *whether* the client is toxic, the more clinically relevant questions are:

- Is this patient's toxic burden a causative factor in his or her illness?
- If so, is it an obstacle to cure?
- If yes, what can be done to help the patient?

Unfortunately, the answers to these questions can be hard to come by. The subject has not been adequately researched in even small clinical trials (see sidebar). Connecting the toxic burden directly to the patient's illness is very difficult and sometimes impossible. However, as a clinician who has worked in this field for more than 20 years, I strongly believe that many patients with chronic illness will benefit from the procedures I am about to describe. Where there is evidence to share, I will cite it. As always, each individual practitioner must decide what to recommend for his or her patients.

Absence of Good Research on Toxicity and Illness

Although the evidence base describing many mechanisms of toxic insult is well developed for a host of different environmental toxins and pharmaceuticals, there is a notable lack of evidence to help clinicians differentiate the clinical presentation of symptoms that may involve a toxic exposure from those that do not. Most of our clinical knowledge of toxic effects has been derived from acute exposures in amounts far in excess of what is likely to be found in the everyday environment of most patients (or from animal studies, which do not extrapolate fully to human patients). Researchers have not yet clearly described and quantified, in ways that lead to good differential diagnosis, detectable long-term clinical effects of low-level exposures to multiple toxic sources (many of which may be working through common pathways). So, the clinician's challenge is very difficult. Common complaints such as vomiting, diarrhea, nausea, and abdominal pain may stem from a vast array of causes; endocrine disruption and neurological symptoms likewise have multiple etiologies. Many of the subtle effects that we might expect to see in patients, based on bench science and animal research, would (for now) only be detected in large population-based studies over long periods of time; and those studies have, for the most part, not been performed. Factors that further complicate clinical assessment are the age of the patient and the role of individual susceptibility. Infants and young children have different (and often fewer) defenses than adults; elderly people may be more vulnerable to certain toxic agents than younger adults. And individual variability in response to toxic agents, both for environmental toxins and for pharmaceuticals, can be great—never has it been more true that "one man's meat is another man's poison." An excellent summary of what we still need to learn about endocrine disrupters (just one example of environmental toxins) can be found in a 2003 article by Daston et al.[84] The April 2004 issue of *Pediatrics* had a special focus on toxicity problems in infants and children; two reviews of GI toxins[85] and pesticides[86] are particularly recommended.

Assessing and Treating Toxic Burden

Determining whether the toxic burden of your patients must be dealt with in order for them to get better requires, in part, an understanding of what organs and systems are affected by the common toxins. In-depth discussion of those topics can be found in the earlier parts of this chapter and in Chapter 22. It also requires recognizing the common signs and symptoms of toxin buildup—a more difficult task, as described above. Recognition of these signposts greatly assists the clinician in designing the most efficacious treatment program. In addition to recognizing the telltale signs of toxicities in a good history and physical exam, clinicians should also be aware of laboratory markers that reflect toxin load, as these assessments can help to clarify the patient's condition. A limited number of tests are useful in establishing that patients could benefit from lowering their toxic burden. Measurements of chlorinated compounds and solvents can be done from both serum and adipose samples. Urinary measurements can be taken for heavy metals, organophosphate pesticide metabolites, and phthalates. Fecal measurement of toxic metals is also available and can be used for testing pediatric clients.

Finding the Source of Exposure

The documentation of xenobiotic presence in an individual's serum, adipose tissue, stool or urine can be important in formulating an effective therapeutic protocol. This initial testing provides a basis on which to initiate treatment, a baseline to refer back to in order to help judge your progress, clear motivation for the client to follow your recommendations (depending upon how well the practitioner presents this information), and an indication as to possible sources of toxin exposure. The importance of finding the source of toxin exposure in an individual cannot be overemphasized. For many persons, the identification and elimination of the source comprises the majority of necessary treatment. Other individuals will need more help to reduce the total toxic burden.

Finding the source of exposure typically includes taking a detailed environmental history (past and present) of the person, checking out towns she or he has resided in, and possibly doing some home air-quality testing. Finding exposure sources in various towns can be accomplished with the help of two websites: www.scorecard.org (just enter the zip code for a listing of local polluters and pollutants) and www.atsdr.cdc.gov/hazdat.html.

If the exposure is ongoing, it is imperative that the source be removed before beginning a detoxification program. Once the exposure has been identified and dealt with, the depuration program can be safely started. The program should be based on the type(s) of xenobiotics that appear to be the causative agents in the client's illness. Heavy metals will often be dealt with differently from lipophilic xenobiotics, as they can be easily and directly chelated, while the lipophilic chemicals cannot.

Heavy Metal Chelation

Measuring heavy metals in clients for whom toxicity is suspected as a factor in their illness is a useful step. When these compounds are found, a protocol can be initiated to mobilize the heavy metals, utilizing dimercaptosuccinic acid (DMSA). This compound is FDA approved, and is well researched for safety and efficacy in clearing mercury, lead, and other heavy metals from animals and humans.[87,88,89] DMSA is available from pharmacies under the names Chemet and Succimer, as well as from other sources.

DMSA is given in a body-weight dose of 30 mg/kg, and has been shown to be safe in that dose for children (including infants) who have been poisoned with both mercury and lead.[90,91] Using the published body-weight dose of DMSA, the two protocols that seem to be most commonly used are three days of DMSA followed by 11 days without, or five days of DMSA followed by nine days without. A repeat urinalysis at the beginning of every fifth round (at week 10, 20, 30, etc.) can be used to monitor the client's progress. Over the years, we found that most of our clients did 20 or 25 rounds before stopping. On the days they were not taking DMSA, they were supplemented with low levels of zinc, copper, molybdenum, and manganese to replete any possible micromineral loss from the DMSA.[92] Fairly high levels of magnesium were required, often accompanied by magnesium sulfate shots, to avoid magnesium depletion. While magnesium does not appear on the affinity list for DMSA, it appears to be mobilized from the body in this process.

Lipophilic Xenobiotics

While the clearance of heavy metals through chelation is fairly straightforward, the mobilization of lipophilic compounds is not. The body burden studies previously mentioned, along with numerous smaller studies worldwide, have alerted us to the presence of chlorinated pesticides and PCBs in everyone tested. The majority of the compounds found in everyone tested are lipophilic rather than water-soluble. Lipophilic substances have no efficient means of exit from the body, as the bowels are designed to retain fat-soluble substances. In order to help these compounds leave the body, saunas have been employed with documented success.[93,94,95,96] Sauna therapy allows the xenobiotics stored in the subcutaneous fat pads to be released through the skin, while those in deeper fat stores are released into the circulation. The compounds in the subcutaneous fat pads include both substances absorbed through the skin[97] and some compounds from the circulation (including medications). Numerous compounds have been documented to exit the body via the skin, including necessary minerals,[98,99] zinc, copper, iron and manganese; the heavy metals lead,[100,101] cadmium,[102] and mercury;[103] plus various medications.

Compounds that are moved out through the skin are often grossly detectable by smell and by their damaging effect on articles of clothing. Clinical experience with numerous patients undergoing thermal chamber depuration has provided many indisputable olfactory encounters with chemical compounds being released in the sweat. Two patients undergoing thermal chamber depuration experienced disintegration of clothing that was worn in the chambers. There are two published accounts of thermal chamber depuration being successfully used in the treatment of chemically sensitive persons,[104,105] including the reduction of serum hydrocarbon levels.

The fat-soluble compounds released into the circulation through sauna therapy do not exit the body easily. These compounds must again be processed by the same phase I and II detoxification pathways that were unable to successfully transform and excrete them before. Therefore, it is important to attempt to increase the excretion of fat-soluble items from the bowels when sauna depuration is used. Increased use of dietary fiber and chlorophyll,[106] and use of dietary substances that interrupt the enterohepatic circulation[107] may be useful. When proper nutrition and other physical therapy modalities are included with thermal chambers, good clinical results, such as those with chemically sensitive persons,[108,109] can be achieved.

Summary

Utilizing these approaches (chelation for heavy metals, sauna and enhanced fecal excretion for lipophilic toxins), the author has noted significant improvements in numerous chronic illness states. By reducing the body burden on the client (through avoidance of the source, chelation, and mobilization of lipophilic substances), the self-healing functions of the body can work unfettered.

Home-based Detoxification

Peter Bennett, ND

Introduction

Historically, detoxification therapies have been applied in clinical settings, in medical spas, and at home. Although early practitioners of this approach did not call it "detoxification therapy," their methods of hydrotherapy, fasting, regulated diet, and Nature Cure are similar to many modern detoxification methods.[110] By studying the work of Sebastian Kneipp,[111] John Harvey Kellogg,[112] O. G. Carroll, and John Bastyr,[113] one gets the impression that doctors and healers found that the best results happened in a setting where the patient could be closely watched. Just preceding this part of the current chapter, a doctor-supervised program was described. Unfortunately, time and cost prohibit this for many patients today, so a home-based program may be recommended to patients, within certain guidelines.

A complete detoxification program should focus on three targets:

1. Retrieve gut functioning (4R program—see Chapter 28);
2. Reduce heavy metals; and
3. Reduce organic chemicals stored in fat tissue.

A one-week home-based program may help patients detoxify key dysregulating influences that are obstacles to regaining stability and balance in their health. On a biochemical level, such a program can help to support cellular functioning, improve the filtration capacity of the liver, stimulate the excretion of toxins through the kidneys, bowel, and skin, support gut repair, and improve neuroendocrine balance in the hypothalamic-pituitary system.

Such claims may seem exaggerated in a world that relies heavily on expensive and high-risk interventions for patient complaints, and—unfortunately—these natural approaches to detoxification have rarely been researched. However, even a brief review of the literature detailing the powerful negative health effects of toxicity (see Chapters 13 and 22 and the first parts of the current chapter) demonstrates that it may be important to help certain patients relieve some of the body burden that modern living imposes.[114,115]

The home detoxification program described here has been used by thousands of patients with reportedly excellent results. It is fairly easy and effective but the clinician needs to be prepared to teach patients what to do, and to offer the appropriate cautions. Patient instructions must be provided and reviewed carefully, and the practitioner must be available to answer questions after patients have started the program. A patient handout such as the one shown in Figure 31.2 can be used to guide your patients.

Elements of the Detoxification Program

The essential steps of this home-based program are:

- Brief water fasting (two days),
- Oligoantigenic diet (five days) and slow reintroduction of omitted foods,
- Saunas and hydrotherapy (one month), and
- Nutritional supplements (one month).

In the author's experience, using all these elements together gives reliable results.

Fasting

Fasting on water for a short period can be a safe and powerful way to rejuvenate the mind and body. While water fasting may not be suitable for severely compromised patients (see recommendations earlier in this chapter), research has shown that calorie restriction and fasting help to alleviate hypertension,[116,117] diabetes,[118] epilepsy,[119,120] and rheumatoid arthritis.[121] Recent research has shown that calorie restriction may be the most powerful way known yet to extend lifespan.[122,123] Studies have shown that high glucose and insulin damage mitochondria, and calorie restriction (fasting) reduces the total amount of oxidative stress within the cellular mitochondria.[124,125]

Fasting may improve liver function. Fasting has traditionally been thought to enhance the liver's ability to clear out metabolic byproducts from the blood stream, and regenerate the liver's ability to function in a healthy way. There are indications from a few animal studies that dietary restriction may help to reduce the risk of age-related diseases associated with impaired lipid metabolism.[126,127] However, caution is indicated because long-term fasting or fasting in a polluted environment can deprive the body of nutrients that are critical to a patient's health. Fasting should be done for short periods of time in a pure environment and, in my practice, I recommend taking vitamin C during fasting in the range of one to four grams per day.

Fasting may benefit cognitive functioning. Several studies have shown that as severe liver toxicity progresses, the patient fails to break down valium-like compounds that create a toxic state.[128,129] One might hypothesize a continuum of such effects for patients who are not nearly so ill. Patients who fast often report a sense of renewal and clearer thinking. Fasting allows the liver to reduce the presence of recycled chemical messengers like adrenalin and other stress hormones, which often have a second chance to restimulate the nervous system when they are not biotransformed and excreted appropriately.

Caloric restriction improves immune function. Caloric restriction, which can be achieved by short-term fasting, appears to have measurable benefit for the immune system.[130,131] It rests the intestines and liver, both key sites of immune function. It is estimated that 60% of our immune system resides in our intestines. By resting this major site of immune function with fasting, the patient's immune function may be potentiated. A fast of 36 or 60 hours significantly increases the power of white blood cells to destroy pathogenic bacteria.[132] Conversely, eating can depress immune function and have a proinflammatory effect,[133,134] whereas energy restriction may restore the impaired immune response.[135] Studies have shown that a glucose challenge increases the generation of reactive oxygen species (ROS), while nutritional restriction can inhibit ROS generation by leucocytes.[136,137]

Patient Handout for Home Detoxification

Practitioner's Name
Address
Phone
Email (if you choose)

Seven Day Detoxification Plan

Please follow precisely all the instructions in this one-week home-based detoxification plan. It has been used with thousands of patients, many experiencing excellent results. This program of rest and renewal for your body can reduce aches and pains and symptoms of chronic disease; it can help you feel healthier and more energetic.

How Does It Work?

The body has its own self-healing mechanisms This seven-day program strengthens your body's healing forces in a short period of time. By stimulating your natural capacity to release and excrete toxins, you can remove some of the obstacles that are keeping you from being completely healthy. Detoxification is like an oil change for your car. It cleans and improves the filtering of your internal fluids in a way that prevents your body's engine from breaking down, and produces immediate benefits in fighting existing disease. It is a simple program using a special diet, supplements, heat, and contrast hydrotherapy.

Detoxification Program Summary

- Two day water fast with bed rest if necessary
- Five days of rice, fruit and vegetables
- Protein shakes 1-2x/day daily during days 3 to 7
- Supplements as recommended
- Shower hydrotherapy treatment at least once per day
- Daily saunas. Don't do the sauna on the fasting days
- Sleep at least 6-7 hours a night
- Avoid "enervation" at night (TV, theater, movies, parties)

Diet

The program begins with a two-day water fast followed by five days of rice, fruit, and vegetables. (Additional details on the fast and the diet are shown below.) While on this diet, you should supplement these foods twice a day with a whey or rice protein-based powder. Add 2 rounded scoops in juice, blended, 2-3 times a day for breakfast and snacks to improve protein status during detoxification.

Days 1 and 2

Consume water, lemon water, and herbal tea only. Be sure to drink a minimum of 8 glasses of these fluids per day. This fluid fast is extremely helpful in achieving optimal detoxification. Some people cannot tolerate this two-day fast, can't afford to lose any weight, or are in a debilitated condition. These people should add the rice or whey protein and fruit juice 2 to 3 times per day to the other fluids.

Days 3 to 7

Following the water fast, a typical day's menu should reflect the general choices shown below. (You may need to eat more or less depending on your appetite.)

Reintroduction of Omitted Foods

Following your seven-day program, you should reintroduce foods back into your diet slowly - one food at a time, every 1 to 2 days. This process may take up to a month. Focus first on protein sources from lean meat, fish, or eggs. Then add back beans and grains (other than wheat). Then introduce nuts. Finally, slowly reintroduce wheat, dairy, and soy. Each time a food is reintroduced, note any reactions - physical, mental, or emotional. Write them down and bring your notes to your next appointment.

Figure 31.2 **Sample patient handout for home detoxification**

Typical Menus

Upon arising . . . . 8 ounces of hot lemon water
Breakfast . . . . .A protein shake made with fresh fruit and fruit juice; rice cakes; fresh fruit; herbal tea
Snack . . . . .Fruit and/or a rice protein shake; herbal tea
Lunch . . . . Salad and soup, or rice and steamed vegetables, or yam and steamed vegetables (hot or cold)
Snack . . . . .Fruit and/or rice protein shake; rice crackers; herbal tea
Dinner . . . . Rice and mixed vegetables (steamed or lightly sautéed), or soup and salad, or salad and baked sweet potato
Note . . . . Drink plenty of water and lemon water in these days as well.

Foods to Use and Avoid

Carbohydrates

Use: Brown rice, basmati rice, jasmine rice, wild rice, rice cakes/crackers, rice bread, rice pasta, and rice pancake mix (read labels to avoid any wheat content). If variety is required, you can use quinoa, millet, and amaranth grains.

Avoid: Sugar, honey, molasses, jams, artificial sweeteners, corn, wheat, spelt, kamut, barley and any products with these in them.

Legumes

Use: Mung beans, red lentils

Avoid: All other beans

Vegetables and Fruits

Use: All varieties of fresh produce can be used. They can be steamed, baked, lightly sautéed in a small amount of extra virgin olive oil, eaten raw, or juiced. Vegetables can be used in any combination and quantity desired. Fruits are to be eaten one variety at a time and away from other foods.

Fats and Oils

Use: Extra virgin olive oil and unheated flaxseed oil.

Avoid: All other oils including butter and margarine.

Beverages

Use: Non-caffeinated herbal teas, purified water (spring or filtered), lemon water (organic lemons only). (Squeeze 1/2 lemon into 1 litre of water and then drop the squeezed lemon peel into the water; at least 1 litre of this lemon water to be drunk per day.) Diluted fruit and vegetable juices (ideally, made fresh from a juicer).

Avoid: Coffee, black tea, all alcohol, soda pop and caffeinated/decaffeinated herbal teas/coffees.

Condiments

Use: Vegetable salt, sea salt, apple cider/balsamic/rice vinegars, Bragg's amino acids, wheat-free tamari, all spices

Avoid: Ketchup, mayonnaise, Worcestershire sauce, barbecue sauce, relishes, mustards, salad dressings and any packaged oil/liquid-based seasonings (i.e., chutneys; Indian, Thai, Chinese seasonings, etc.)

General Categories of Foods to Avoid

During your seven day detox program, all of the following foods put too much burden on the liver's detoxification ability and often disrupt digestion. They must be avoided.

- meat
- fish
- poultry
- eggs
- dairy products
- chocolate
- nuts
- beans (other than mung and listed soybean products)
- grains (other than rice, quinoa, amaranth, millet)
- preservatives and food coloring
- all packaged/processed/ canned foods

Shower Hydrotherapy

This home therapy enhances circulation, detoxification, and metabolism. Ideally, it should be done every day. Take a hot shower for 3 minutes then switch to cold water for 30 seconds. Repeat the cycle 3 times, ending with the cold rinse. Make sure your entire body is showered this way. After you've finished three rounds, get out of the shower, dry off quickly, and go to bed or dress warmly till you refresh the body heat.

Sauna

Sauna therapy is extremely safe, and is a critical step in removing fat-stored toxins through the skin. As you sweat, many toxins that are stored in the fat and blood (PCBs, cadmium, lead, and industrial chemicals) are excreted through the skin. Do not sauna during the first two days of the program (the water fast).

Sauna Method

Use a low-temperature or infra red sauna, choosing a temperature from 150 to 170 degrees Fahrenheit. Drink 1 quart of warm water before entering and take water into the sauna with you, continuing to drink throughout the length of your sweat. Begin by staying in the sauna for fifteen minutes, then come out for a cold-water rinse.

Repeat this process for up to one hour. As you become more acclimated to the heat, you may increase your time a little each day until you reach two hours. The cold rinse is important because it stimulates circulation in the skin and removes waste material being excreted through it.

Dry Skin Brushing

The skin regulates body temperature, functions as an organ of elimination and has even been called the "third kidney." It averages 3,100 square inches of surface area, acting as a protective shield to the outside world. Dry skin brushing is an old natural healing method used to increase blood and lymphatic circulation. It removes dead skin cells, keeps the skin soft, improves blood and lymph circulation, and helps rid the body of toxins.

Skin Brushing Method

Brush your whole body once a day with a natural-bristle dry skin brush that you can find at health food stores. Start with your arms, front and back, moving from the fingertips up into the armpit, always brushing toward the heart. Then do each leg, front and back, starting at the feet and brushing upward. Follow each leg up through the pelvis, buttocks, abdomen, and lower back. Then do the chest and upper back, always brushing toward the heart.

If you wish, you can lightly do the face and head, using downward strokes. Keep the brush dry (never get it wet). Just as you wouldn't use someone else's toothbrush, be sure that only you use your skin brush. If skin brushing is painful, do it lightly and persevere-the discomfort will pass. The chest, abdomen, and inner thigh should be done gently and carefully.

Supplements

During this detox, the filtering mechanisms of the liver can become overloaded. Feelings of fatigue, headache, muscle pain, and nausea are common as toxins are mobilized and excreted. Taking certain supplements is a necessary step to support the liver, promote better detoxification, and prevent symptoms as much as possible. Follow the supplements listed on your treatment program by your doctor. Supplements are prescribed according to your personal needs, but here are some general guidelines that will be followed:

1. The supplement program is for enhancing detoxification and improving circulation. It will be reviewed after 4 weeks.
2. The recommended supplements work by feeding the internal mechanisms of cells involved in detoxification. Work inside of the cells is driven by mini power plants called mitochondria (my-toe-con-dria). Toxins interfere with their energy production and this upsets the functioning of the entire cell.
3. The supplement program will not interfere with other supplements or medications that you are taking. All prescription medications are to be maintained unless directed by your physician.
4. You will not be asked to take any supplement that you do not absolutely need.

Fasting benefits arthritis. It has been demonstrated in research settings that fasting benefits arthritis.[138] The best results in treating autoimmune arthritis are achieved when a short fast is combined with a change to a vegetarian diet, and foods to which the patient is sensitive or allergic are removed.[139,140] Fasting may be involved in changing the bacterial flora in a favorable way for patients with rheumatoid arthritis. Abnormal bacteria or microflora are present in the stool in patients with a variety of autoimmune problems such as Crohn's disease,[141] rheumatoid arthritis,[142] and ankylosing spondylitis.[143] Anaerobic bacterial species such as *Klebsiella* and *Proteus* have been implicated.[144] Fasting may play a role in changing bacterial flora, perhaps by enhancing competition and thereby giving dominance to probiotics. Changes in intestinal flora from a vegan diet have been documented.[145]

Fasting contraindications. A two-day water fast is safe for most patients. Certain exclusions are important, such as diabetics, hypoglycemics, and severely nutritionally deficient individuals. The biggest risks to most patients are hypoglycemia and orthostatic hypotension with vertigo, sometimes resulting in fainting. Although these reactions are generally harmless, they can cause a fall. Patients should be warned to take extra care in standing up—i.e., getting out of bed or a hot bath, or getting up from a chair. If faintness or vertigo does not resolve within a very few minutes, patients should contact their practitioner.

There is medical literature to suggest that fasting for a prolonged period of time can diminish the body's stores of glutathione, making it more susceptible to aging and disease. Low tissue antioxidant status is found under dietary restriction because fasting lowers glutathione detoxification in the liver.[146,147] People who are fasting should be very careful to avoid any chemical exposure, because lack of dietary protein makes the liver unable to process toxins optimally due to lack of adequate amino acid precursors that are important to the detoxification pathways. (As an aside, patients who are preparing to undergo surgery might have fewer complications to the anesthetic if they were put on a protein-dense regimen instead of clear fluids.[148,149])

Oligoantigenic Diet

After a two-day water fast, a simple diet of rice, fruit and vegetables is then followed for five days. This is similar to an oligoantigenic diet, used for allergic, behavioral, and digestive problems.[150] This simple diet provides enough caloric input to sustain the patient, but is very easy on the intestinal environment to allow optimum rest. The rationale for vegetarian fare is two-fold: vegetarian diets contain fewer potential food allergens that can cause activation of the gut-associated lymphoid tissue, and enhanced vegetable intake provides more soluble fiber, bioflavonoids, antioxidants, and complex carbohydrates. Some patients experience fatigue on this program; if it is not ameliorated with rice- or whey-based protein shakes, it will resolve upon resuming normal protein intake (unless, of course, the patient is allergic to the food being reintroduced). Chapters 28 and 35 provide detailed information on the use of oligoantigenic diets.

Sauna and Hydrotherapy

Sauna therapy (discussed earlier in this chapter) can support the removal of fat-soluble toxins from the body, and has been shown to provide relief of symptoms for patients with toxicity conditions.[151,152] Sauna programs need to be carefully tailored to the individual patient and supervised closely, particularly with more compromised patients. Hydrotherapy has been employed for hundreds of years because of its ability to stimulate circulation. Although medical studies on the effectiveness of hydrotherapy for detoxification have not been done, there is a modest research base documenting its usefulness in symptomatic relief of many conditions, including rheumatoid arthritis,[153] osteoarthritis,[154,155] chronic heart failure,[156] management of spasticity,[157] and other similar conditions. Although the mechanisms are not fully understood, many seasoned clinicians recommend its use.

Theoretically, application of alternating hot and cold water to the body stimulates regulation of sympathetic tone in the extracellular matrix, and generates a "pumping" action that stimulates circulation of blood and lymph. The extracellular matrix is now understood to influence cellular development, movement, reproduction, and shape, as well as biochemical function. Dr. Alfred Pischinger, professor of histology and embryology at the University of Vienna, saw the importance of the extracellular matrix. In 1991, he wrote that the extracellular matrix is the support system for the cell and the foundation substance in which all cells are embedded. The extracellular matrix is made up of collagens and polysaccharides that form proteoglycans. These two molecules form a water-filled, gel-like "ground substance" in which the connective tissue fibers are embedded. The condition of the space around a cell is as important to health as what occurs within the cell and in the membrane that encloses it.

Supplements

There is a complex set of variables involved in choosing the appropriate supplements for detox patients. Supplement programs should be adapted to the individual patient's need, using the following general strategies:

- Antioxidants for cellular protection
- Amino acids for phase II detoxification
- Cholagogues (bile stimulants)
- Bile binding
- Replacing probiotic bacteria
- Repairing intestinal permeability
- Vitamins, minerals, and nutritional cofactors
- Cathartics
- Antiparasitics

Additional tips:

- No supplements during the water fasting except for vitamin C.
- Structuring supplement recommendations for twice-a-day dosing improves compliance.
- Ensure that there is some sort of protein shake for the patient to use, if needed.

Post-Detox Recommendations

After the seven-day program, it is best to continue the hydrotherapy and/or saunas and the supplement strategies for at least a month. The patient should slowly reintroduce foods, starting with foods least likely to irritate the intestinal mucosa. Since the diet is relatively low in essential amino acids, the introduction of eggs, fish, or lean meat on a daily basis helps to restore proper protein balance. After several days of this regimen, begin adding foods that seem prudent for the individual patient; last, introduce known allergens like dairy products, wheat, and soy foods (one at a time and allowing a day or two between each new food to determine any reactions).

Patients may be surprised to discover how well they have adapted to the new diet. Some people experience fewer cravings for many of the foods they gave up during their detox week. The best advice is to support patients to do the best they can throughout this detox program, following the guidelines as closely as possible but being flexible when necessary. However, patients who are highly allergic to certain foods shouldn't eat them—ever. Eating the right diet is the first step, but digesting it properly is critical for long-term health.

Summary

A home-based detoxification program is within the capacity of many patients, and may generate a significant increase in well being for them. Resting the gut, relaxing the body, the use of heat to release toxic agents, an oligoantigenic diet, and supportive supplementation are all techniques that can be managed at home, provided the patient is given information, advice, and support.

The Gut-Liver Axis

Mary James, ND

Introduction

It is primarily through the gastrointestinal (GI) tract that we "taste" the external environment, including both good and bad. In a healthy system, nutrients critical to health are efficiently absorbed through the small bowel, whereas the bulk of potentially toxic molecules are barred entry. This dual role of the intestine necessitates that this barrier be an incomplete one, which poses a tremendous challenge to the rest of the system. The gut's long list of defense mechanisms, including mechanical, immunologic, and metabolic, speaks to the enormous potential of compounds entering the body to exert toxic effects.

Although enterocytes are separated by "tight junctions" that serve to minimize this potential, a certain amount of passive transfer of particles is normal, and even necessary (e.g., penetration of the intestinal epithelium by enteric antigens is a necessary step in the development of oral tolerance).[158] A variety of factors, however, including exogenous substances, intestinal imbalances, and systemic disease states, can abnormally increase intestinal permeability to the point that toxins and macromolecules overwhelm the body's defense mechanisms and gain entry into the body.[159] Associations between increased permeability ("leaky gut") and systemic disorders have been well documented for conditions such as inflammatory arthritides,[160] ankylosing spondylitis,[161] chronic dermatological conditions,[162] AIDS,[163] and alcoholism.[164]

The likelihood of an adverse outcome depends in part on intestinal factors (e.g., flora balance, mucosal integrity, the type and size of particles presented) and partly on hepatic health and response to these antigens. This is because the liver is the first organ that comes into contact with all enterically-derived molecules, thus playing a crucial role in the metabolism of endogenous and exogenous compounds, as well as the phagocytosis and elimination of immune complexes and other antigenic molecules.[165]

Here we see an extraordinary metabolic cooperation between the GI tract and the liver. Abnormal gut permeability (low or high) and/or compromised hepatic function, such as impairments in hepatic metabolism or excessive immunological responses in the liver, can quickly imbalance the gut-liver axis, resulting in systemic toxicity and/or inflammatory responses that contribute to illness.

This part of the chapter will review aspects of this intimate relationship between the gut and liver, briefly highlighting a few of the key clinical disorders resulting from imbalances in this system, specifically in the categories of impaired metabolism and upregulated inflammatory reactions. Finally, it will lay the groundwork for optimal preservation of a healthy gut-liver axis, for both intestine and liver.

The Gut-Liver Axis and Biotransformation

The Role of the Liver

Unlike other organs that receive 100% of their blood supply as arterial, 75% of the liver's blood supply is venous, delivered through the portal vein that travels directly from the intestine, pancreas, and other abdominal organs.[166] Upon arrival at the liver, this venous blood flows through capillary-like vessels called sinusoids to the hepatocytes, the primary functional cells of the liver.

In addition to their other myriad and complex functions, hepatocytes transform gut-derived compounds into safe by-products before excreting them through the bile or releasing them into the arterial circulation. The process of detoxification has been discussed both earlier in this chapter and in Chapter 22; here, we will review only what is necessary for the discussion that follows.

The detoxification/biotransformation process is mediated by two types of reactions that usually, although not always, occur sequentially.[167,168] Phase I metabolism serves to biotransform fat-soluble molecules (via oxidation, reduction or hydroxylation) by the cytochrome P450 mixed-function oxidase system. (Most water-soluble drugs and compounds are eliminated from the body through the kidneys). While phase I is a necessary preparatory step for most compounds requiring phase II, its activity concomitantly generates free radicals and renders these compounds into biologically more active forms that may cause damage to surrounding tissues, particularly the mitochondrial-rich hepatocyte that houses this system. In an efficient system, phase II reactions convert these reactive compounds into water-soluble and inactive forms by conjugating them with hydrophilic molecules such as glucuronic acid or glutathione.[169] All of these phase II enzyme reactions are highly dependent upon nutrients, especially sulfhydryl amino acids. Consequently, nutritional deficits, especially when accompanied by upregulated cytochrome P450 enzymes (all of which are inducible by various drugs or xenobiotics), can contribute to toxicity and the accumulation of reactive molecules in the body.

The Role of the GI Tract

The term "first pass" is often applied to the hepatic filtering of exogenous compounds, since the liver inspects all gut-derived substances before releasing them into the systemic circulation. Indeed, most biotransformation reactions in the body take place in the liver. However, given the extensive metabolism that occurs initially in the intestine, hepatic filtering may be more accurately classified as "second pass."

For example, almost all of the hepatic phase I and II reactions occur as well in the intestinal mucosa, serving to minimize the systemic uptake of xenobiotics.[170] The intestinal microflora is also a major player in biotransformation. Many substances that have taken a "second pass" through the liver are returned to the intestine through bile canaliculi for biliary excretion. Some of these compounds are, in turn, reactivated by bacterial enzymes such as beta-glucuronidase, and routed once again to the portal system through enterohepatic recirculation. This normal process serves to recycle essential compounds such as bile acids, estrogen, and vitamin

D.[171,172] It also ensures the bioavailability of certain sought-after compounds like medications (the eradication of gut microorganisms by antibiotics can reduce the enterohepatic drug recirculation by 8–22%).[173]

Conversely, microbial enzymes may augment toxicity in the body. For example, levels of beta-glucuronidase (elaborated by *Escheriacea coli*, *Bacteroides*, and *Clostridium*)[174,175] have been observed to be 12.1 times higher in colon cancer patients compared to healthy controls,[176] consistent with the increased reactivation of local carcinogens in the bowel. Animal studies have also demonstrated reductions in breast cancer risk by administering calcium D-glucarate, an inhibitor of beta-glucuronidase.[177] Bacterial azoreductases are able to reduce dietary additives, such as monoazo dyes, into aromatic amines, which can be further metabolized by gut microbes into carcinogens.[178]

It is reasonable to assume that enhanced gut permeability would serve to increase the concentration of potentially toxic compounds in the portal circulation, thus burdening the liver's detoxification system. This very premise, in fact, drives ongoing research on the use of the Zonula occluden toxin (produced by *Vibrio cholerae*) for the deliberate induction of leaky gut to enhance drug delivery to the rest of the system.[179]

Impaired Hepatic Metabolism and Illness

As mentioned above, reactive intermediates that are generated in phase I metabolism may contribute to illness if not neutralized by subsequent phase II conjugation reactions. The impact of liver disease on hepatocyte function and blood levels of potentially toxic substances can be profound. Inefficient filtering and removal of toxins and bacterial products results in increased delivery of these substances to the systemic circulation. Indeed, elevated levels of circulating gut-derived endotoxin (described below) are often demonstrated in individuals with chronic liver disease.[180]

Hepatic Encephalopathy and Neuropeptides

The intimate relationship between the GI tract and the liver is well demonstrated in hepatic encephalopathy (HE). With liver injury, the organ's ability to clear bacterial end products declines and greater amounts of toxic compounds enter the systemic circulation. Some of these compounds are able to pass directly into the brain and exert neurotoxic effects on the central nervous system.[181]

Features of hepatic encephalopathy range from confusion to coma. Minimal hepatic encephalopathy (MHE) in patients with liver cirrhosis is a milder form of the disorder that is defined by the presence of otherwise unexplained cognitive dysfunction (only detectable on neurophysiological testing), in the absence of overt hepatic encephalopathy.[182] The disorder is common and can seriously impair a patient's daily functioning.

Observations of developmental regression in some autistic children with intestinal pathology has led to speculation that analogous mechanisms may exist between HE in patients with liver failure and autistic patients who have similar symptoms.[183]

Partial digestion of dietary casein and gluten can lead to the release of "exorphins" (β-casomorphins and gliadomorphins, respectively) that cross the blood-brain barrier and exert opioid-like effects.[184] Here we have an example of a clinical reaction to food proteins that has nothing to do with allergy. Reactions to opiate peptides may also explain some cerebral effects (e.g., gluten-induced schizophrenic symptoms)[185] that cannot be understood from a classical allergy perspective.

Although these biochemical imbalances in autistic individuals are assumed to stem from a breach in the intestinal mucosa rather than from a diseased liver (the case in HE), the net result is the same: the flood of compounds from the gut exceeds the liver's ability to metabolize them, causing neuroactive peptides to escape into the systemic circulation. Consequently, some overlap in therapeutic approaches for autism and hepatic encephalopathy makes sense.

Initially, ammonia was thought to be the driving factor in the pathogenesis of HE and MHE, as it is often elevated in the plasma of patients with liver failure and impaired mental function and it readily diffuses into the brain.[186] Forty percent of ammonia is generated in the intestine from ingested nitrogenous substances and is primarily metabolized in the liver through its conversion to urea.[187]

Ammonia's contribution to HE pathogenesis, however, is debatable. First, the actions of ammonia are essentially neuroexcitatory, whereas HE is characterized by an increase in neuronal inhibition, not excitation. Furthermore, blood ammonia levels do not strongly correlate with HE, suggesting that other factors are likely involved.[188] Indeed, numerous gut flora-derived nitrogenous compounds, if allowed to enter the bloodstream, have been shown to produce adverse effects on brain function, including false neurotransmitter activity.

One such class of compounds is endogenously-produced benzodiazepine-like compounds, likely synthesized by intestinal bacteria from amino acids.[189] *In vitro* production of gamma-aminobutyric acid (GABA), the major inhibitory neurotransmitter in the mammalian brain, has been demonstrated by *E. coli* and *Bacteroides fragilis*.[190] Other studies have shown the ability of rifaximin (an oral, non-absorbable antibiotic) to lower endogenous benzodiazepine levels by 40%.[191]

Interestingly, ammonia enhances the activity of GABA receptors, as well as the actions of endogenous benzodiazepine receptor agonists like tetrahydroprogesterone and tetrahydrodeoxycorticosterone (neuroactive steroid derivatives of progesterone and deoxycorticosterone, respectively).[192]

Interventions for HE are usually aimed at reducing gut-derived toxins, especially ammonia. Common recommendations include a low-protein diet, antibiotics directed against colonic bacteria, and the use of non-digestible disaccharides, such as lactulose, which pass through the small bowel without being digested.[193] Lactulose is conventionally regarded as a treatment for constipation.[194] However, insoluble fibers such as lactulose offer the added advantage of lowering colonic pH through bacterial fermentation, thus creating an environment that discourages the growth of urease-producing microorganisms like *Klebsiella* and *Proteus*.[195]

Probiotics are helpful, in part, because the bacterial strains used in these formulations are non-urease-producing. In one study of cirrhotic patients with MHE, a 30-day course of two lactobacillus strains (with or without fiber) was shown to reverse the condition in 50% of patients (13% in placebo group).[196] Fiber, alone, was also of benefit.

The Gut-Liver Axis and Immunologic Responses

The Role of the Intestine

Given the fact that the GI tract encounters more antigen than any other part of the body and must be able to discriminate between invasive organisms and harmless antigens (e.g., commensal bacterial and food proteins), it is not surprising that the majority of the body's immune system is housed there.[197]

The gut-associated lymphoid tissue (GALT) is comprised of lymphocytes in the mucosal epithelium and lamina propria (the underlying connective tissue), mesenteric lymph nodes, and aggregates of lymphoid follicles called Peyer's patches. The intestinal lumen is separated from these lymphoid areas by a single layer of columnar epithelial cells, which is infiltrated by B cells, T cells, macrophages, dendritic cells, and M (microfold) cells. All of these cellular components work in concert to maintain a homeostatic balance between oral tolerance and active immunity.[198]

The immunologic fate of orally-administered antigen ultimately depends on where and how antigen is taken up and presented to T cells.[199] Invasive pathogens and other antigens are taken up by M cells, which then pass the intact antigen to antigen-presenting cells (APCs) such as dendritic cells. Alternatively, antigen may enter the lamina propria directly through the villus epithelium. APCs, in turn, present the antigen to T cells in either the Peyer's patch or mesenteric lymph nodes. In the case of pathogens, a microbe-induced inflammatory response leads to full maturation of dendritic cells and release of IL-12, with subsequent induction of T-helper-1 (Th1) cellular differentiation and the release of proinflammatory cytokines.

In the absence of inflammation (as is normally the case with dietary proteins and commensal bacteria), the release of prostaglandin E2, transforming growth factor-β, and IL-10 (an inhibitory cytokine) results in partial maturation of dendritic cells. In the mesenteric lymph node or Peyer's patch, antigen is presented to naïve CD4+ T cells, which differentiate into regulatory T cells. The immunologic consequences are local IgA production and systemic tolerance.[200,201]

Although the intestinal immune system is clearly capable of generating protective immune responses when necessary, oral tolerance appears to be the default response to antigen. A breakdown in this process, leading to inappropriate immune responses to foods or commensal bacteria, may underlie inflammatory conditions such as Crohn's disease and ulcerative colitis.[202]

The Role of the Liver

While hepatocytes assume the responsibility of metabolizing and excreting compounds such as xenobiotics and hormones, it is the monocyte-derived Kupffer cells in the liver that manage larger compounds such as immune complexes and bacterial products.[203] Kupffer cells represent 80–90% of the fixed macrophage population in the body. Because these cells are situated in the sinusoids of the liver, they are some of the first to come into contact with invading microorganisms and other gut-derived products.[204]

As macrophages, Kupffer cells act as phagocytes that clear the portal blood of circulating debris, including bacterial toxins. Lipopolysaccharide, a component of gram-negative bacterial cell wall (also referred to as LPS or endotoxin), is one of the most immunogenic toxins in this group.[205] Kupffer cells are activated in the process of removing LPS, stimulating in the process the production of inflammatory mediators, including eicosanoids, interleukin-1 (IL-1), IL-6, tumor necrosis factor-α (TNF-α), superoxide, and nitric oxide.[206]

LPS is not the only bacterial component known to stimulate cytokine synthesis. Components of both gram-negative and gram-positive bacteria, including proteins, glycoproteins, lipoproteins, carbohydrates, and lipids, are also capable of inducing inflammatory cytokines.[207]

Kupffer cell activation is a normal immunologic response, serving to limit the entry of endotoxins and other antigenic molecules into the systemic circulation. In fact, Kupffer cells are always in a low-grade state of activation due to the small quantities of bacterial toxins that continually penetrate the intestinal mucosa.[208] Typically, these endotoxins are not measurable beyond the liver. Only when the ability of the liver to sequester LPS is overwhelmed does endotoxemia occur. Either increased intestinal permeability (with translocation of LPS from the gut) or impaired hepatic clearance (as seen in liver damage) can disrupt this balance, resulting in an exaggerated immune/inflammatory response.

Intestinal permeability increases within hours of exposure to a bacterial toxin,[209] further increasing hepatic load. This may be a direct effect of endotoxin on enterocytes or an indirect effect mediated through inflammatory cytokines like TNF-α, blood levels of which are typically elevated following endotoxin administration.[210] The finding that metronidazole can prevent NSAID-induced hyperpermeability emphasizes the role of bacterial toxins in this process.[211]

Endotoxins are capable of producing multiple adverse effects within the liver, ranging from neutrophil accumulation and oxidant stress-induced mitochondrial dysfunction,[212] to enhanced coagulation,[213] reduced bile formation[214] (hence impaired excretion of waste), and downregulation of cytochrome P450 enzymes.[215] Although speculated to be a protective effect (upregulated phase I generates potentially toxic reactive intermediates), suppressed cytochrome P450 activity may contribute over time to impaired clearance of xenobiotics from the body.

Endotoxin-induced overactivation of Kupffer cells has been implicated in a number of disorders, including multiple organ dysfunction syndrome, alcoholic and non-alcoholic liver disease, spontaneous bacterial peritonitis, celiac disease, and inflammatory bowel disease. A few of these conditions are reviewed here.

Multiple Organ Dysfunction Syndrome (MODS)

Patients who experience severe trauma frequently develop a significant systemic inflammatory response. In some individuals, this response is followed by progressive deterioration and subsequent failure of various organ systems, a syndrome that has been referred to as "death in slow motion."[216] Multiple Organ Dysfunction Syndrome (MODS) is one of the major causes of morbidity and mortality in the Intensive Care Unit (ICU).[217] Although this inflammatory response and organ failure may develop from uncontrolled sepsis, it is frequently seen without any evidence of sepsis.[218]

Studies have increasingly implicated the gut as an important factor in the pathogenesis of MODS.[219,220] In fact, a study by Doig and colleagues demonstrated that the only variable statistically associated with the development of secondary MODS in the ICU was increased intestinal permeability on admission or during a patient's stay in the ICU.[221] Furthermore, the severity of organ failure correlated with the degree of gut permeability upon admission.

Bacterial translocation from the intestine following multiple trauma and hemorrhage has been documented in animal models, and endotoxemia has been observed during hemorrhagic shock in humans, suggesting that critical illness can directly impact intestinal permeability.[222] Doig's study of ICU patients did not assume a causal relationship between leaky gut and MODS. However, the observed correlation between baseline intestinal permeability and subsequent organ failure supports the premise that gastrointestinal dysfunction may be an important stimulus in the development of the syndrome.

Alcoholic Liver Disease

Increased intestinal permeability is a major factor in the pathogenesis of alcoholic liver disease.[223] In the intestine, ethanol and its derivatives, especially acetaldehyde, loosen tight junctions between enterocytes, independent of inflammation and nutritional state.[224,225] Alcohol also favors the growth of gram-negative bacteria, thereby increasing the concentration of endotoxin.[226] As gut permeability increases, endotoxin and other macromolecules activate Kupffer cells. Inflammatory cytokines are released, culminating in hypoxia, neutrophil activation, increased sinusoidal permeability in the liver, and the generation of free radicals.[227] Supporting a strong role for intestinal translocation of endotoxin in alcoholic liver disease, levels of endotoxin-specific IgA have been found to correlate closely with alcohol intake and with levels of SGOT and C-reactive protein (markers of inflammation).[228] Furthermore, ethanol-fed rats are protected from alcohol-induced liver injury when fed, together with ethanol, oral non-absorbable antibiotics, polymyxin (a binder of LPS), or lactobacilli.[229]

Hepatocytes contain two primary pathways for the metabolism of ethanol: cytosolic alcohol dehydrogenase and the mitochondrial phase I enzyme, CYP2E1. Alcohol dehydrogenase activity generates NADH, while CYP2E1 converts ethanol to acetaldehyde, producing reactive oxygen species (ROS) in the process.[230] Acetaldehyde can inhibit DNA repair and trap reduced glutathione (GSH), an important peptide for detoxification as well as the neutralization of ROS via GSH-peroxidase (GSH-Px).[231] An elevated level of NADH enhances ROS production by altering the intra-mitochondrial redox (reduction-oxidation) potential.[232] Mitochondria are a major source of ROS and contain no catalase (the alternative to GSH-Px for neutralizing peroxides). Therefore, mitochondrial GSH plays a critical role in preserving mitochondrial function. Depletion of GSH in the mitochondria has been shown to sensitize alcohol-exposed hepatocytes to the pro-oxidant effects of cytokines and free radicals generated during ethanol metabolism.[233]

One of the cardinal features of alcoholic liver disease is fatty liver, or steatosis.[234] Various mechanisms, including reduced oxidation of free fatty acids due to mitochondrial damage, have been proposed for the ethanol-induced accumulation of fats in the liver.[235] Fatty acids are highly reactive. Hepatic peroxidation of these lipids results in the generation of potentially toxic intermediates that further augment inflammatory responses in the liver.[236] Fibrosis is a common reaction to ongoing parenchymal inflammation and injury. If unchecked, cirrhosis can result, characterized by widespread fibrosis, disorganized liver architecture, nodule formation, and dramatic reductions in hepatocellular function.[237]

Non-alcoholic Steatohepatitis (NASH)

Non-alcoholic steatohepatitis (NASH) is part of a spectrum of non-alcoholic fatty liver disease (NAFLD) that ranges from simple steatosis (fatty liver) to cirrhosis.[238] NASH, the most common form of progressive liver disease in the United States,[239] is an intermediate state between the two. NAFLD is very common in diabetics and obese individuals,[240] including children.[241]

NASH is strongly associated with features of the metabolic syndrome, including insulin resistance, central (visceral) obesity, dysglycemia, hyperlipidemia, and cardiovascular disease.[242,243] Insulin resistance and obesity both play a role in increased intrahepatic production of free fatty acids from glucose that is not efficiently taken up by peripheral adipocytes.[244] High levels of insulin also inhibit mitochondrial fatty acid oxidation, further adding to fat accumulation.[245] As described, steatosis sets the stage for liver damage.

Despite the contrasting initial contributing factors (alcohol vs. obesity and insulin resistance), the histologic features of alcoholic- and non-alcoholic liver disease are identical. Hepatocellular injury in both disorders appears to be mediated by lipid peroxidation and oxidative stress.[246] Hepatic mitochondria are the main source of this oxidant stress, as beta-oxidation of fatty acids normally produces reactive oxygen species. A vicious cycle develops that involves continual generation of ROS, inflammatory cytokine release, Kupffer cell damage, and depletion of antioxidants.[247] Obesity is thought to exacerbate liver injury by sensitizing hepatocytes to TNF-α toxicity and reducing Kupffer cell phagocytosis of toxic debris.[248]

There are at least two mechanisms by which intestinal bacteria may contribute to liver injury. As mentioned earlier, LPS and other bacterial toxins stimulate Kupffer cells in the liver, resulting in a cascade of cytokines and other inflammatory mediators.[249] If chronic, the induced oxidative stress causes hepatic steatosis and fibrosis. Interestingly, bacterial overgrowth in the small intestine has been found in 50% of NASH patients, compared to 22% of healthy controls.[250]

A second mechanism involves microbe-mediated endogenous production of alcohol and its metabolites. The ability of yeast to ferment sugars into alcohol is well established. Endogenous ethanol production has been documented in various studies and, in some subjects with yeast infection, high ethanol concentrations have been reported following the ingestion of carbohydrate-rich foods.[251] Yeasts and various gut bacteria have alcohol dehydrogenase activity, thus are capable of oxidizing ethanol to acetaldehyde.[252] On the other hand, microbial activity of aldehyde dehydrogenase (converting acetaldehyde to acetate) is limited.[253] As a result, acetaldehyde may accumulate to toxic levels in the face of gut flora imbalances.

Acetaldehyde is a potent toxin capable of inducing leaky gut and systemic absorption of endotoxin.[254] As discussed earlier, endotoxin stimulates the release of TNF-α from Kupffer cells. TNF-α further promotes insulin resistance (and subsequent steatosis) in NASH by inhibiting insulin-initiated signal transduction.[255] Probiotics may help to reduce levels of acetaldehyde in the gut. Although lactobacilli and bifidobacteria are weak producers of acetaldehyde, they appear to be more efficient than other intestinal bacteria at removing acetaldehyde.[256]

Hepatic CYP2E1, which is normally induced upon exposure to fatty acids and ethanol, is overexpressed in both NASH and alcoholic liver disease.[257] Upregulated CYP2E1 is associated with free radical production[258] and the conversion of xenobiotics such as petrochemicals and organic solvents to toxic metabolites, which can contribute to inflammation and fibrosis in the liver.[259] Availability of antioxidants is critical for protection.

Celiac Disease

Celiac disease (CD) is a familiar disorder characterized by intolerance to gluten, small bowel mucosal atrophy, malabsorption and abdominal symptoms that are typically reversed by removing gluten from the diet.[260] Increased intestinal permeability has been documented in CD,[261] and has been hypothesized to predispose untreated celiac patients to some of the extra-intestinal symptoms sometimes seen in these patients.[262]

Hepatic dysfunction in patients with celiac disease is common. At the time of diagnosis of CD, a mild disturbance of liver function is reported in up to 42% of adults and 54% of children.[263] In most of these cases, elevated liver enzymes tend to normalize within 12 months of gluten removal from the diet. In mild cases where biopsy has been performed, histological changes in the liver are similar to those seen in NASH: Kupffer cell hyperplasia, mononuclear cell infiltration, steatosis, and mild fibrosis. In more severe cases, severe fibrosis, cirrhosis, and chronic hepatitis have been observed in both adults and children.[264]

Celiac disease is not always apparent in patients with associated liver disease. Elevated liver enzymes may, in fact, be the sole manifestation of CD.[265] In one study of adults being investigated for raised transaminases, but without gastrointestinal symptoms, the prevalence of CD was 9%.[266] Thirty NASH patients who also tested positive for anti-gliadin antibodies were placed on a gluten-free diet. After three months, both steatosis and serum transaminase levels were reduced. At one year from diagnosis, enzyme levels were normal, intestinal histology had improved, and there was no further evidence of steatosis on ultrasound.[267]

The exact mechanisms for these associations are unknown, although theories have been proposed. Because a high prevalence of autoantibodies exists in CD patients, the disturbed liver function in this disorder may be mediated by an autoimmune process.[268] In many of these individuals, antibodies become undetectable following a period of gluten exclusion. The malabsorption and leaky gut induced by celiac enteropathy have also been proposed to place undue stress on the liver. The fact that cow's milk allergy can induce liver dysfunction in some individuals suggests that it may not be the gluten as much as the mucosal damage that leads to the hepatic injury.[269] Other proposed mechanisms include viral triggers[270] (hepatitis C is the most common liver disease associated with CD[271]) and genetic predisposition.[272]

Because gluten exclusion so often helps to ameliorate hepatic inflammation, testing for celiac disease in patients with liver disorders, and hepatic evaluation in CD patients, would be prudent.

Promoting a Healthy Gut-Liver Axis

As discussed, optimal functioning of the gut-liver axis depends on an intact intestine, as well as a healthy liver that is balanced in both immunologic response to toxins and biotransformation of endogenous and exogenous compounds. A leaky gut places undue burden on the liver, whereas hepatocellular injury enhances the likelihood of toxic metabolites escaping into the systemic circulation. Consequently, a broad-spectrum approach is fundamental.

Intestinal Support

Gut mucosal integrity can be compromised by a host of factors, including malnutrition,[273] antibiotics,[274] small bowel bacterial overgrowth,[275] intestinal infections,[276,277] food allergies,[278] gluten intolerance,[279] enterotoxic agents such as NSAIDs[280] or alcohol,[281] immune dysregulation,[282] mucosal hypoxia,[283] dysmotility,[284] and various systemic disorders.[285] (For a comprehensive review of intestinal permeability, please see Chapter 28.) What follows is a brief summary of a few key areas that are pertinent to the current discussion.

Nutrition. Enterocytes have one of the highest turnover rates in the body.[286] As a result, they are particularly vulnerable to low levels of nutrients that are critical to epithelial cell renewal. One such nutrient is glutamine, the principal metabolic fuel used by cells of the small intestine. Patients given glutamine-free total parenteral nutrition develop atrophy of the intestinal mucosa, impaired immune activity, and leaky gut. Addition of L-glutamine reverses these changes.[287]

In the large intestine, short-chain fatty acids (SCFAs), specifically n-butyrate, provide energy for the colonocytes and exert a trophic effect on the intestinal lining.[288] Although the anaerobic bacterial fermentation of all non-absorbed dietary fibers generates SCFAs, the slower-to-ferment forms (e.g., resistant starch) are generally most effective at raising butyrate levels along the entire length of the bowel.[289]

Flora balance. Alterations in the complex microflora of the intestine can induce changes that adversely affect intestinal permeability. Those factors that reduce the concentration of beneficial organisms are particularly damaging, such as broad-spectrum (or frequent) antibiotic use. The resulting overgrowth of yeast and gram-negative coliforms may amplify the production of acetaldehyde and endotoxin. As mentioned, endotoxin increases gut permeability and sensitizes Kupffer cells in the liver.

Exposure to stress is associated with reduced levels of beneficial bacteria and decreased production of both secretory IgA[290] and protective mucins on the mucosal surface.[291] Stress stimulates catecholamine release. High concentrations of norepinephrine, in particular, appear to encourage the growth of possible pathogens in the intestine.[292]

Replenishing "friendly" strains of bacteria, such as lactobacilli and bifidobacteria, has been shown to support the gut-liver axis in multiple ways. Probiotics appear to be adaptogenic in the gut. That is, they can stimulate humoral immune responses to pathogens, but also downregulate proinflammatory cytokines when excessive.[293] In cases of bacterial sensitization (and associated gut inflammation), probiotics may help to restore oral tolerance.[294] Probiotics have also been shown to reduce levels of acetaldehyde[295] and ammonia[296] in the intestine, and to help process food antigens. Finally, these organisms have demonstrated a stimulating effect on gastric mucin production.[297] Regular ingestion of *Lactobacillus* GG, for example, has been shown to protect the integrity of the gastric mucosal barrier against indomethacin, although it showed no effect at the intestinal level. *Pre*biotics, such as fructooligosaccharides, can encourage a healthy balance via the selective feeding of bifidobacteria and other beneficial strains.[298]

Dietary influences. Diets high in meats and meat fat can stimulate the activity of bacterial enzymes such as azoreductase and beta-glucuronidase, high levels of which are capable of producing reactive metabolites in the bowel.[299] High amounts of simple sugars in the diet tend to slow bowel transit, thus increasing the exposure of the gut mucosa to potentially toxic compounds; they also promote the production of secondary bile acids in the colon.[300]

Some individuals are sensitive to large amounts of foods rich in sulfur compounds, principally sulfates and sulfites. These compounds may foster the growth of anaerobic sulfate-reducing bacteria, which reduce the sulfur compounds to hydrogen sulfide. This gas is thought to damage the intestinal mucosa by inhibiting butyrate oxidation, as well as to induce hyperpermeability by degrading mucin.[301]

Continued ingestion of gluten in gluten-sensitive individuals not only predisposes them to malabsorption through microvilli damage, but also to tight junction injury and gut hyperpermeability. Laboratory measurement of anti-gliadin, anti-endomysial, and anti-tissue transglutaminase antibodies can help to rule out the condition.[302] Hyperpermeability is also frequently aggravated by ingestion of allergenic foods. This increase is often prevented by the mast cell stabilizer, cromolyn, suggesting that the release of mediators like histamine and serotonin from mast cells is responsible for the increased permeability.[303] Quercetin, a flavonoid that also reduces gut permeability via mast-cell stabilization, may serve as a natural alternative to cromolyn.[304]

Small intestine bacterial overgrowth (SIBO). Far fewer bacteria normally inhabit the small intestine compared to the colon. However, factors such as chronic hypochlorhydria or stasis of gut contents can lead to overgrowth of organisms in the small bowel,[305] typically coliforms and strict anaerobes.[306] SIBO facilitates the translocation of endotoxin and other bacterial toxins from the gut lumen to the portal blood, thereby increasing the risk of liver injury. Interestingly, the prevalence of SIBO in patients with chronic liver disease may be as high as 75%.[307]

Laboratory Assessment of the GI Tract

Preventive or therapeutic regimens for the gut-liver axis are ideally based on an initial assessment of gastrointestinal function and balance, especially since GI imbalances frequently present without symptoms. Comprehensive digestive stool analysis provides information about several aspects of the gut environment, including flora balance and metabolism (e.g., beneficial bacteria, potential pathogens, yeast, and parasites), as well as digestion, absorption, and immunologic reactions in the gut.

Flora imbalances may also be assessed by measuring specific by-products of microbial activity in a morning urine specimen. The patterns of these organic acids may suggest anaerobic bacterial imbalances, the presence of specific pathogenic organisms, or intestinal malabsorption.

Intestinal permeability and absorption can be assessed by measuring the ability of two non-metabolized sugars—lactulose and mannitol—to permeate the intestinal mucosa.[308] Following the ingestion of a challenge drink containing these sugars, their clearance is measured in a urine collection. Mannitol is easily absorbed, thus serving as a marker for transcellular uptake (nutrient absorption). Lactulose is a much larger molecule that is only able to enter the system between enterocytes. Consequently, high amounts of lactulose in the urine, or an elevated lactulose/mannitol ratio, suggest increased intestinal permeability ("leaky gut"). Indirect measures of gut permeability are also available, which include titers of antibody directed against enteric microbial antigens.

Although SIBO is most directly diagnosed through culture of a small bowel aspirate,[309] breath testing for SIBO is a more comfortable and cost-effective alternative that still demonstrates good sensitivity. After a baseline breath collection and the ingestion of a lactulose challenge drink, several more breath specimens are collected over a two-hour period. In the laboratory, sequential levels of breath hydrogen and methane are measured and recorded, reflecting bacterial fermentation of the lactulose. An early gas peak (within the first 90 minutes) suggest SIBO. Treatment typically involves the administration of broad-spectrum, anti-microbial agents[310] and attention to underlying contributing factors such as hypochlorhydria or stasis of gut contents.[311]

Hepatic Support

The liver is the largest organ in the body and is extremely complex, with a vast array of metabolic and immunologic functions. The liver's role in neutralizing and excreting xenobiotics and other potentially toxic compounds is delicately balanced with its immunologic response to bacterial toxins and other macromolecules. As demonstrated, imbalances in either area can lead to toxicity or tissue injury, both local and systemic.

Nutrition. Maintaining adequate broad-spectrum nutritional reserves is of paramount importance for optimal liver function. Numerous amino acids are used in phase II conjugation reactions, and both phase I and phase II reactions utilize a wide array of vitamins and minerals.[312]

Glutathione, in the form of GSH-S-transferase, helps to process a large number of xenobiotics. GSH-peroxidase helps prevent oxidative stress by catalyzing the reduction of lipid peroxides and hydrogen peroxide.[313] Hepatic mitochondria represent a major source of ROS during ethanol metabolism and are also particularly vulnerable to oxidative damage.[314] Mitochondria do not contain catalase (an alternative means of neutralizing peroxides); therefore, GSH plays a critical role in this organelle. Animal models of NASH typically show reduced levels of GSH.[315] Availability of GSH depends on sufficient amounts of its constituent amino acids (cysteine, glycine, and glutamic acid), magnesium (an essential cofactor in GSH synthesis), B vitamins for methionine recycling, and reducing agents.[316]

S-adenosylmethionine (SAMe) is a major methyl donor and precursor of GSH.[317] The hepatic form of the enzyme that converts methionine to SAMe is highly vulnerable to oxidative stress.[318] Low SAMe levels have been documented in experimental liver injury, and administration of SAMe has been shown to attenuate alcohol-induced liver injury, at least in part by preventing mitochondrial GSH depletion.[319]

Low SAMe (hence impaired methylation) is commonly associated with elevated homocysteine.[320] It is interesting to note that increased levels of homocysteine are frequently observed in NASH patients.[321] Critical to methionine recycling are adequate levels of vitamins B2, B6, B12, folic acid, and serine.[322] Betaine serves as an alternative methyl donor, and has been shown to increase SAMe and also to reduce hepatic enzymes, steatosis, and fibrosis in NASH patients.[323]

Measures aimed at inhibiting the activity of inflammatory cytokines can help to "quiet" an overactive immune response and associated liver injury, such as that found in MODS, alcoholic liver disease, and NASH. Examples of inflammatory cytokine inhibitors include alpha-lipoic acid,[324] zinc,[325] curcumin,[326] and fish oils,[327] all of which act to inhibit NFκB, a transcription factor for inflammatory cytokines and other immune mediators of inflammation.

Fish oils (EPA/DHA), besides modifying prostaglandin-mediated inflammation, have been shown to blunt the systemic inflammatory response to endotoxin.[328] In contrast, corn oil (linoleic acid) appears to increase NFκB activity in activated rat Kupffer cells *in vitro*. When the rats were pretreated with glycine (an agent that inactivates Kupffer cells), this increase was almost completely prevented. The omega-6 fatty acid, arachidonic acid, has been shown to directly induce superoxide production by Kupffer cells.[329]

Medium-chain triglycerides (MCTs) appear to benefit the gut-liver axis. In addition to providing immediate energy by virtue of their ability to be absorbed intact across the gut wall and transported into the mitochondria independent of the carnitine shuttle,[330] MCTs are also anti-inflammatory. *In vitro* research has shown that MCTs blunt linoleic acid-induced increases in TNF-α production by ~45%. MCTs also appear to prevent endotoxemia-induced liver damage in mice.[331]

Lipotropic factors, such as L-carnitine, L-methionine, choline, and inositol, help prevent steatosis by facilitating the oxidation of fatty acids in the liver.[332] These nutrients (often used in combination with liver botanicals) also enhance the flow of bile from the liver and gall bladder, thereby assisting in the removal of toxins. Phosphatidylcholine (from lecithin) has been shown to protect against alcoholic cirrhosis, enhance collagenase activity, and prevent acetaldehyde-induced collagen accumulation *in vitro*.[333] Supplementation with pantethine (a derivative of pantothenic acid) may help to reduce the toxic effects of acetaldehyde by increasing the activity of aldehyde dehydrogenase.[334]

It is beyond the scope of this book to review the wide array of botanicals that effectively support the liver. The reader is encouraged to consult relevant texts for listings of choleretics, cholagogues, and antioxidant herbs.

Lifestyle. As mentioned, insulin resistance is a common feature of NASH. When glucose is not efficiently taken up by peripheral adipocytes and myocytes, the liver converts this glucose to free fatty acids. Over time, the increased fat deposition contributes to steatosis, the precursor to NASH. Obesity, irrespective of insulin resistance, predisposes to hepatic steatosis by increasing the amount of free fatty acids entering the hepatocyte.[335] CYP2E1 is upregulated by this process.[336] Increased CYP2E1 activity has been demonstrated in type 2 diabetes, insulin resistance, central obesity, and NASH.[337] It is also upregulated by a high-fat, low-carbohydrate diet.[338] Finally, obesity is associated with impaired phagocytic function by Kupffer cells.[339]

Dietary adjustments, customized nutritional supplementation, and attention to exercise, weight control, and stress management all impact insulin sensitivity. (Insulin resistance is discussed in Chapter 32, and glycemic control is discussed in Chapter 30.) Stress also directly impacts the development of fatty liver. Adrenal catecholamines directly activate hormone-sensitive lipase, which in turn promotes the release of free fatty acids from adipose tissue.[340] In the liver, these free fatty acids contribute to triglyceride accumulation within hepatocytes.[341]

Laboratory Assessment of Liver Function

The functional capacity of the liver to metabolize and clear xenobiotics from the blood can be evaluated by measuring the clearance of specific challenge substances in the saliva and urine. Caffeine is almost completely absorbed by the intestine and metabolized by cytochrome P450 enzymes.[342] Comparing its clearance in two sequential saliva specimens provides insight into up- or downregulated microsomal enzyme activity. Inborn tendencies for excessive or impaired enzyme activity in both phase I and phase II pathways and clinical correlations can be evaluated by examining a patient's blood for genetic polymorphisms. Some key phase II pathways that may be evaluated for polymorphisms include methylation,[343] glutathione conjugation, and acetylation.[344] The two step conversion of cysteine to inorganic sulfate (sulfoxidation) ensures availability of sulfate for the phase II sulfation pathway. Impaired sulfoxidation (a frequent occurrence in neurological disorders such as Parkinson's)[345] can be evaluated by measuring these compounds in the blood.

The body's redox balance can be evaluated by examining antioxidants as well as markers of oxidative stress. Fasting blood measurements of GSH and the endogenous antioxidant enzymes, GSH-peroxidase and superoxide dismutase, reflect varying degrees of protection against ROS, while markers such as urine lipid peroxides can reveal oxidative damage in the body.

Finally, variations in the genes that code for phase I and phase II enzymes are known to influence an individual's ability to neutralize toxic compounds. Polymorphisms in these genes have been associated with adverse drug reactions, as well as cancer and other clinical disorders.[346] Genomic testing can reveal susceptibility to imbalances in the detoxification system that may promote illness, and provide direction for more customized prevention and treatment of gut-liver axis disorders.

Summary

Functional medicine practitioners are generally appreciative of the concept of leaky gut and its potential impact on organ systems beyond the intestine. What is sometimes overlooked is the exceptionally tight interplay between gut and liver, and how dramatically imbalances in one organ can affect the performance of the other.

Imbalanced intestinal flora, dysregulated gut immune function, and compromised gut mucosal integrity can all lead to alterations in gut permeability. Malabsorption of critical nutrients impacts every organ system in the body, including hepatic metabolism of potentially toxic compounds. Leaky gut places an undue burden on hepatic detoxification and leads to overactivity of Kupffer cells and excessive release of free radicals and fibrosis-promoting cytokines. Conversely, compromised hepatic function can cause gut-derived compounds, including toxic metabolites and neuroactive peptides, to escape into the systemic circulation and have an impact on far-reaching organs such as the brain. As liver injury progresses, systemic toxicity increases as well. Analyses of disorders such as hepatic encephalopathy, MODS, and NASH have helped to illuminate this close partnership between gut and liver.

Awareness of the interconnectedness and frequency of asymptomatic functional imbalances should inspire healthcare practitioners to evaluate hepatic function in chronic GI disorders and vice versa. Maintenance of a healthy gut-liver axis is not only achievable through a variety of measures, but is critical to long-term health.

References

1. Coon MJ. Cytochrome P450: nature's most versatile biological catalyst. Annu Rev Pharmacol Toxicol. 2005;45:1-25.
2. Yu AM, et al. Potential role for human cytochrome P450 CYP3A4 in estradiol homeostasis. Endocrinology. 2005 Apr 7; [Epub ahead of print].
3. Ingelman-Sundberg M. Genetic susceptibility to adverse effects of drugs and environmental toxicants. The role of the CYP family of enzymes. Mut Res.2001;482:11-19.
4. McFadden SA. Phenotypic variation in xenobiotic metabolism and adverse environmental response: focus on sulfur-dependent detoxification pathways. Toxicology. 1996;111:43-65.
5. Gonzalez F, Gelboin H. Role of human cytochrome P450s in risk assessment and susceptibility to environmentally based disease. J Toxicol Environ Health. 1993;40:289-308.
6. Kurth M, Kurth J. Variant cytochrome P450 CYP2D6 allelic frequencies in Parkinson's disease. Am J Med Genet. 1993;48:166-8.
7. Kawajiri K, Nakachi K, Imai K, et al. Identification of genetically high risk individuals to lung cancer by DNA polymorphisms of the cytochrome P450IA1 gene. FEBS Lett. 1990;263:131-3.
8. Guengerich FP. Cytochromes P450, drugs, and diseases. Mol Interventions. 2003;3(4):194-204.
9. Ibid.
10. Ames BN, et al. High-dose vitamin therapy stimulates variant enzymes with decreased coenzyme binding affinity (increased Km): relevance to genetic disease and polymorphisms. Am J Clin Nutr. 2002;75:616-58.
11. Weber WW. Influence of heredity on human sensitivity to environmental chemicals. Environ Mol Mutagen. 1995;25 Suppl 26:102-14.
12. Hayes JD, Strange RC. Glutathione S-transferase polymorphisms and their biological consequences., Pharmacology. 2000;61:154-66.
13. Van Bladeren PJ. Influence of non-nutrient plant components on biotransformation enzymes. Biomed Pharmacother. 1997;151:324-327.
14. Singh BN. Effects of food on clinical pharmacokinetics. Clin Pharmacokinet. 1999;37(3):213-255.
15. Fahey JW, Stephenson KK, Dinkova-Kostova AT, et al. Chlorophyll, chlorophyllin and related tetrapyrroles are significant inducers of mammalian phase 2 cytoprotective genes. Carcinogenesis. 2005 Mar 17; [Epub ahead of print].
16. Shapiro TA, Fahey JW, Wade KL, et al. Chemoprotective glucosinolates and isothiocyanates of broccoli sprouts: metabolism and excretion in humans. Cancer Epidemiol Biomarkers Prev. 2001 May;10(5):501-8.

17. Prochaska HJ, De Long MJ, Talalay P. On the mechanisms of induction of cancer-protective enzymes: a unifying proposal. Proc Natl Acad Sci USA. 1985;82:8232-8236.
18. Talalay P, Prochaska HJ, Spencer SR. Regulation of enzymes that detoxify the electrophilic forms of chemical carcinogens. Princess Takamastsu Symp. 1990;21:177-187.
19. Prochaska HJ, Talalay P. Regulatory mechanisms of monofunctional and bifunctional anticarcinogenic enzyme inducers in murine liver. Cancer Res. 1988;48:4776-4782.
20. Mori Y, Iimura K, Furukawa F, et al. Effect of cigarette smoke on the mutagenic activation of various carcinogens in hamster. Mutat Res. 1995;346:1-8.
21. Kitts D. Bioactive substances in food: identification and potential uses. Can J Physiol Pharmacol. 1994;72:423-34.
22. Ames B. Dietary carcinogens and anticarcinogens. Oxygen radicals and degenerative diseases. Science. 1983;221:1256-1264.
23. Yannai S, Day AJ, Williamson G, Rhodes MJ. Characterization of flavonoids as monofunctional or bifunctional inducers of quinone reductase in murine hepatoma cell lines. Food Chemical Toxicol. 1998;36:623-630.
24. Talalay P. Chemoprotection against cancer by induction of phase 2 enzymes. BioFactors. 2000;12:5-II.
25. Rock CL, Lampe JW, Patterson RE. Nutrition, genetics, and risks of cancer. Ann Rev Public Health. 2000;21:47-64.
26. De Morais SM, Uetrecht JP, Wells, PG. Decreased glucuronidation and increased bioactivation of acetaminophen in Gilbert's syndrome. Gastroenterol. 1992;102:577-586.
27. Gueraud F, Paris A. Glucuronidation: a dual control. Gen Pharmac. 1998;131(5):683-688.
28. Lampe JW, Bigler J, Horner NK, Potter JD. UDP-glucuronosyltransferase (UGT1A1*28), and UGT1A6*2) polymorphisms in Caucasians and Asians: relationships to serum bilirubin concentrations. Pharmacogenetics. 1999;9:341-349.
29. Lampe JW, Bigler J, Bush AC, Potter JD. Prevalence of polymorphisms in the human UDP-glucuronosyltransferase 2B family: UGT2B4(D458E), UGT2B7(H268Y), and UGT2BI5(D85Y). Cancer Epidemiol Biomarkers Prev. 2000;9:329-333.
30. Lampe JW, King IB, Li S, et al. Brassica vegetables increase and apiaceous vegetables decrease cytochrome P450 IA2 activity in humans: changes in caffeine metabolite ratios in response to controlled vegetable diets. Carcinogenesis. 2000;21(6):II57-II62.
31. Kassie F, Rabot S, Uhl M, et al, Chemoprotective effects of garden cress (Lepidium sativum) and its constituents towards 2-amino-3-methyl-imidazol[4,5-flquinoline (IQ)-induced genotoxic effects and colonic preneoplastic lesions. Carcinogenesis. 2002;23(7):II55II61.
32. Walle UK, Walle T. Induction of human UDP-glucuronosyltransferase UGTIA1 by flavonoids-structural requirements. Drug Metab Disposition. 2002;30(5):564-569.
33. Haberkorn V, Heydel JM, Mounie J, et al. Influence of vitamin A status on the regulation of uridine (5'-)diphosphate-glucuronosyltransferase (UGT) 1AI and UGTIA6 expression by L-triiodothyronine. British J Nutr. 2001;85:289-297.
34. Nugon-Baudon L, Roland N, Flinois JP, Beaune P. Hepatic cytochrome P450 and UDP-glucuronosyl transferase are affected by five sources of dietary fiber in germ-free rats. J Nutr. 1996,126:403-409.
35. Venkataramanan R, Ramachandran V, Komoroski BJ, et al. Milk thistle, an herbal supplement, decreases the activity of CYP3A4 and uridine diphosphoglucuronosyl transferase in human hepatocyte cultures. Drug Metab Disposition. 2000;28(II):1270-1273.
36. Guengerich F. Influence of nutrients and other dietary materials on cytochrome P450 enzymes. Am J Clin Nutr. 1995;61:651S-658S.
37. Bray T, Taylor C. Tissue glutathione, nutrition, and oxidative stress. Can J Physiol Pharmacol. 1993;71:746-51.
38. Rubio-Gozalbo ME, Bakker JA, Waterham HR, Wanders RJ. Carnitine-acylcarnitine translocase deficiency, clinical, biochemical and genetic aspects. Mol Aspects Med. 2004;25(5-6):521-32.
39. Mulder GJ. Sulfate availability *in vivo*. In: Mulder GJ, ed. Sulfation of drugs and related compounds. Boca Raton, FL: CRC Press, Inc; pp. 31-52.
40. Birdsall T. Therapeutic applications of taurine. Altern Med Rev. 1998;3:128-36.
41. Kelly G. Clinical applications of N-acetylcysteine. Altern Med Rev. 1998;3:II4-27.
42. Gregus Z, Fekete T, Varga F, Klaassen C. Dependence of glycine conjugation on availability of glycine: role of the glycine cleavage system. Xenobiotica. 1993;23:141-53.
43. Hong R, Rounds J, Helton W, et al. Glutamine preserves liver glutathione after lethal hepatic injury. Ann Surg. 1992;215:II4-9.
44. Han D, Handelman G, Marcocci L, et al. Lipoic acid increases de novo synthesis of cellular glutathione by improving cystine utilization. Biofactors. 1997;6:321-38.
45. Micke P, Beeh KM, Buhl R. Effects of long-term supplementation with whey proteins on plasma glutathione levels of HIV-infected patients. Eur J Nutr. 2002;41:12-8.
46. Nho CW, Jeffery E. The synergistic upregulation of phase II detoxification enzymes by glucosinolate breakdown products in cruciferous vegetables. Toxicol Appl Pharmacol. 2001;174:146-52.
47. Zhao J, Agarwal R. Tissue distribution of silibinin, the major active constituent of silymarin, in mice and its association with enhancement of phase II enzymes: implications in cancer chemoprevention., Carcinogenesis. 1999;20:2101-8.
48. Rukkumani R, Aruna K, Varma PS, et al. Comparative effects of curcumin and an analog of curcumin on alcohol and PUFA induced oxidative stress. J Pharm Pharm Sci. 2004;7:274-83.
49. Cai YJ, Ma LP, Hou LF, et al, Antioxidant effects of green tea polyphenols on free radical initiated peroxidation of rat liver microsomes. Chem Phys Lipids. 2002;120: 109-17.
50. Nanji A, Khettry U, Sadrzadeh S. Lactobacillus feeding reduces endotoxemia and severity of experimental alcoholic liver (disease). Proc Soc Exp Biol Med. 1994;205:243-7.
51. Veihelmann A, Brill T, Blobner M, et al. Inhibition of nitric oxide synthesis improves detoxication in inflammatory liver dysfunction *in vivo*. Am J Physiol. 1997;273:G530-6.
52. Roland N, Nugon-Baudon L, Flinois JP, Beaune P. Hepatic and intestinal cytochrome P450, glutathione-S-transferase and UDP-glucuronosyl transferase are affected by six types of dietary fiber in rats inoculated with human whole fecal flora. J Nutr. 1994;124:1581-7.
53. Reddy B, Engle A, Simi B, Goldman M. Effect of dietary fiber on colonic bacterial enzymes and bile acids in relation to colon cancer. Gastroenterology. 1992;102:1475-82.
54. Story J, Furumoto E, Buhman K. Dietary fiber and bile acid metabolism—an update. Adv Exp Med Biol. 1997;427:259-66.
55. Leeuwenburgh C, Hollander J, Leichtweis S, et al. Adaptations of glutathione antioxidant system to endurance training are tissue and muscle fiber specific. Am J Physiol. 1997;272:R363-9.
56. Yiamouyiannis C, Sanders R, Watkins JD, Martin B. Chronic physical activity: hepatic hypertrophy and increased total biotransformation enzyme activity. Biochem Pharmacol. 1992;44:121-7.
57. Duncan K, Harris S, Ardies C. Running exercise may reduce risk for lung and liver cancer by inducing activity of antioxidant and phase II enzymes. Cancer Lett. 1997;II6:151-8.
58. Schnare D, Robinson P. Reduction of the human body burdens of hexachlorobenzene and polychlorinated biphenyls. IARC Sci Pub. 1986;77:596-603.
59. Schnare D, Denk G, Shields M, Brunton S. Evaluation of a detoxification regimen for fat stored xenobiotics. Med Hypotheses. 1982;9:265-82.

60. Lovejoy H, Bell ZJ, Vizena T. Mercury exposure evaluations and their correlation with urine mercury excretions. 4. Elimination of mercury by sweating. J Occup Med. 1973;15:590-1.
61. Fuzailov I. The role of the sweat glands in excreting antimony from the body in people living in the biogeochemical provinces of the Fergana Valley. Gig Tr Prof Zabol (RUSSIA) 1992;5:13-5
62. Goyer R. Nutrition and metal toxicity. Am J Clin Nutr. 1995;61:646S-650S.
63. Ittel T, Kinzel S, Ortmanns A, Sieberth H. Effect of iron status on the intestinal absorption of aluminum: a reappraisal. Kidney Int. 1996;50:1879-88.
64. Goyer R. Toxic and essential metal interactions. Annu Rev Nutr. 1997;17:37-50.
65. Sham R, Ou C, Cappuccio J, et al. Correlation between genotype and phenotype in hereditary hemochromatosis: analysis of 61 cases. Blood Cells Mol Dis. 1997;23:314-20.
66. Fell J, Reynolds A, Meadows N, et al. Manganese toxicity in children receiving long-term parenteral nutrition. Lancet. 1996;347:1218-21.
67. Dalton T, Li Q, Bittel D, et al. Oxidative stress activates metal-responsive transcription factor-1 binding activity. Occupancy *in vivo* of metal response elements in the metallothionein-I gene promoter. J Biol Chem. 1996;271:26233-41.
68. Miura T, Muraoka S, Ogiso T. Antioxidant activity of metallothionein compared with reduced glutathione. Life Sci. 1997;60:PL 301-9.
69. Cuvin-Aralar ML, Furness R. Mercury and selenium interaction: a review. Ecotoxicol Environ Saf. 1991;21:348-64.
70. Lovejoy H, Bell ZJ, Vizena T. Mercury exposure evaluations and their correlation with urine mercury excretions. 4. Elimination of mercury by sweating. J Occup Med. 1973;15:590-1.
71. Foulkes E. Metallothionein and glutathione as determinants of cellular retention and extrusion of cadmium and mercury. Life Sci. 1993;52:1617-20.
72. Gregus Z, Stein A, Varga F, Klaassen C. Effect of lipoic acid on biliary excretion of glutathione and metals. Toxicol Appl Pharmacol. 1992;II4:88-96.
73. Rowland I, Mallett A, Flynn J, Hargreaves R. The effect of various dietary fibres on tissue concentration and chemical form of mercury after methylmercury exposure in mice. Arch Toxicol 1986;59:94-8
74. Bencko V. Use of human hair as a biomarker in the assessment of exposure to pollutants in occupational and environmental settings. Toxicology. 1995;101:29-39.
75. Aposhian HV, Maiorino RM, Gonzalez-Ramirez D, et al. Mobilization of heavy metals by newer, therapeutically useful chelating agents. Toxicology. 1995;97:23-38.
76. Rigden S. Entero-hepatic resuscitation program for CFIDS. CFIDS Chronicle. Spring 1995.
77. Bland J, Barrager E, Reedy R, Bland K. A medical food-supplemented detoxification program in the management of chronic health problems. Altern Ther Health Med. 1995;1:67-71.
78. Kilburn K, Warsaw R, Shields M. Neurobehavioral dysfunction in firemen exposed to polychlorinated biphenyls (PCBs): possible improvement after detoxification [see comments]. Arch Environ Health. 1989;44:345-50.
79. Schnare D, Robinson P. Reduction of the human body burdens of hexachlorobenzene and polychlorinated biphenyls. IARC Sci Pub. 1986;77:596-603.
80. Schnare D, Denk G, Shields M, Brunton S. Evaluation of a detoxification regimen for fat stored xenobiotics. Med Hypotheses. 1982;9:265-82.
81. Lovejoy H, Bell ZJ, Vizena T. Mercury exposure evaluations and their correlation with urine mercury excretions. 4. Elimination of mercury by sweating. J Occup Med. 1973;15:590-1.
82. http://www.ewg.org/reports/bodyburden/es.php
83. http://www.cdc.gov/exposurereport/
84. Daston GP, Cook JC, Kavlock RJ. Uncertainties for endocrine disrupters: Our view on progress. Toxicological Sciences. 2003;74:245-52.
85. Sreedharan R, Mehta DI. Gastrointestinal tract. Pediatrics. 2004;113(4):1044-50.
86. Weiss B, Amler S, Amler RW. Pesticides. Pediatrics. 2004;113(4):1030-36.
87. Graziano, JH. Role of 2,3-dimercaptosuccinic acid in the treatment of heavy metal poisoning. Med Toxicol. 1986;1:155-62.
88. Aposhian HV. DMSA and DMPS—water soluble antidotes for heavy metal poisoning. Ann Rev. Pharmacol Toxicol. 1983;23:193-215.
89. Aposhian HV, Maiorino RM, Rivera M, et al. Human studies with the chelating agents DMPS and DMSA. Clin Toxicol. 1992;30(4):505-28.
90. Forman J, Moline J, Cernichiari E, et al. A cluster of pediatric metallic mercury exposure cases treated with meso-2,3-dimercaptosuccinic acid (DMSA). Environ Health Perspect. 2000;108(6):575-77.
91. Chisolm J. Safety and efficacy of meso-2,3-dimercaptosuccinic acid (DMSA) in children with elevated blood lead concentrations. Clin Toxicol. 2000;38(4):365-75.
92. Quig D. Personal communication
93. Schnare D, Ben M, Shields M. Body burden reductions of PCBs, PBBs and chlorinated pesticides in human subjects. Ambio. 1984;13(5-6):77-380.
94. Root D, Lionelli G. Excretion of a lipophilic toxicant through the sebaceous glands: a case report. J. Toxicol—Cut Ocular Toxicol. 1987;6(1):13-17.
95. Tretjak Z, Shields M, Beckmann S. PCB reduction and clinical improvement by detoxification: and unexploited approach. Hum Exp Toxicol. 1990;9:235-44.
96. Krop J. Chemical sensitivity after intoxication at work with solvents: response to sauna therapy. J Alt Comp Med. 1998;4(1):77-86.
97. Lilley SG, Florence TM, Stauber JL. The use of sweat to monitor lead absorption through the skin. Sci Total Environ. 1988;76(2-3):267-78.
98. Cohn JR, Emmett EA. The excretion of trace metals in human sweat. Ann Clin Lab Sci. 1978;8(4):270-75.
99. Omokhodion FO, Howard JM. Trace elements in the sweat of acclimatized persons. Clin Chim Acta. 1994; 231(1):23-28.
100. Lilley SG, Florence TM, Stauber JL. The use of sweat to monitor lead absorption through the skin. Sci Total Environ. 1988;76(2-3):267-78.
101. Omokhodion FO, Crockford GW. Lead in sweat and its relationship to salivary and urinary levels in normal healthy subjects. Sci Total Environ. 1991;103(2-3):113-22.
102. Stauber JL, Florence TM. A comparative study of copper, lead, cadmium and zinc in human sweat and blood. Sco Total Environ. 1988;74:235-47.
103. Sunderman FW. Clinical response to therapeutic agents in poisoning from mercury vapors. Ann Clin Lab Sci. 1978;8(4):259-69.
104. Krop J. Chemical sensitivity after intoxication at work with solvents: response to sauna therapy. J Altern Complement Med. 1998;4(1):77-86.
105. Rea WJ, Pan Y, Johnson AR, et al. Reduction of chemical sensitivity by means of heat depuration, physical therapy and nutritional supplementation in a controlled environment. J Nutr Environ Med. 1996;6:141-48.
106. Nagayama J, Takasuga T, Tsuji H, et al. Active elimination of causative PCDFs/DDs congeners of Yusho by one year intake of FBRA in Japanese people. Fukuoka Igaku Zasshi. 2003;94(5):118-25.
107. Jandacek RJ, Tso P. Factors affecting the storage and excretion of toxic lipophilic xenobiotics. Lipids. 2001;36(12):1289-305.

108. Krop J. Chemical sensitivity after intoxication at work with solvents: response to sauna therapy. J Altern Complement Med. 1998;4(1):77-86.
109. Rea WJ, Pan Y, Johnson AR, et al. Reduction of chemical sensitivity by means of heat depuration, physical therapy and nutritional supplementation in a controlled environment. J Nutr Environ Med. 1996;6:141-48.
110. Kilburn KH, Warsaw RH, Shields MG. Neurobehavioral dysfunction in firemen exposed to polychlorinated biphenyls (PCBs): possible improvement after detoxification. Arch Environ Health. 1991;46(4):254-55.
111. Watrous LM. Constitutional hydrotherapy: from nature cure to advanced naturopathic medicine. J Nat Med. 1997;7(2):72-79.
112. Jackson LS, Dudrick SJ, Sumpio BE. John Harvey Kellogg; surgeon, inventor, nutritionist (1852-1943). J Am Coll Surg. 2004;199(5):817-821.
113. On the cover: John Bastyr. J Naturopath Med. 1991;2(1):39.
114. Institute for Functional Medicine. Clinical Nutrition, 2nd Ed., Chapter 9: Environment and Toxicity. Gig Harbor, WA: Institute for Functional Medicine, 2004.
115. Krop J. Chemical sensitivity after intoxication at work with solvents: response to sauna therapy. J Altern Complement Med. 1998;4(1):77-86.
116. Michalsen A, Weidenhammer W, Melchart D, et al. [Short-term therapeutic fasting in the treatment of chronic pain and fatigue syndromes—well-being and side effects with and without mineral supplements.] Forsch Komplementarmed Klass Naturheilkd. 2002;9(4):221-27.
117. McCarty MF. A preliminary fast may potentiate response to a subsequent low-salt, low-fat vegan diet in the management of hypertension—fasting as a strategy for breaking metabolic vicious cycles. Med Hypotheses. 2003;60(5):624-633.
118. Kimura KD, Tissenbaum HA, Liu Y, Ruvkun G. Daf-2, an insulin receptor-like gene that regulates longevity and diapause in Caenorhabditis elegans. Science. 1997;277:942-46.
119. Greene AE, Todorova MT, Seyfried TN. Perspectives on the metabolic management of epilepsy through dietary reduction of glucose and elevation of ketone bodies. J Neurochem. 2003;86(3):529-37.
120. Mantis JG, Centeno NA, Todorova MT, et al. Management of multifactorial idiopathic epilepsy in EL mice with caloric restriction and the ketogenic diet: role of glucose and ketone bodies. Nutr Metab (Lond). 2004;1(1):11.
121. Iwashige K, Kouda K, Kouda J, et al. Calorie restricted diet and urinary pentosidine in patients with rheumatoid arthritis. J Physiol Anthropol Appl Human Sci. 2004;23(1):19-24.
122. Lee C-K L, Weindruch R. Calorie intake, gene expression and aging. In Functional Medicine Approaches to Endocrine Disturbances of Aging, 8th International Symposium on Functional Medicine, 2001. Gig Harbor, WA: Institute for Functional Medicine.
123. Guarente L, Kenyon C. Genetic pathways that regulate ageing in model organisms. Nature. 2000;408:255-62.
124. Merry BJ. Oxidative stress and mitochondrial function with aging—the effects of calorie restriction. Aging Cell. 2004;3(1):7-12.
125. Lambert AJ, Merry BJ. Effect of caloric restriction on mitochondrial reactive oxygen species production and bioenergetics: reversal by insulin. Am J Physiol Regul Integr Comp Physiol. 2004;286(1):R20-21.
126. Mulas MF, Demuro G, Mulas C, et al. Dietary restriction counteracts age-related changes in cholesterol metabolism in the rate. Mech Ageing Dev. 2005;126(6-7):648-54.
127. Araki S, Goto S. Dietary restriction in aged mice can partially restore impaired metabolism of apolipoprotein A-IV and C-III. Biogerontology. 2004;5(6):445-50.
128. Basile AS, Hughes RD, Harrison PM, et al. Elevated brain concentrations of 1.4-benzodiazepenes in fulminate hepatic failure. New Engl J Med. 1991;325(7):473-78.
129. Mullen KD. Benzodiazepine compounds and hepatic encephalopathy. New Engl J Med. 1991;325(7):509-11.
130. Sun D, Krishnan A, Su J, et al. Regulation of immune function by calorie restriction and cyclophosphamide treatment in lupus-prone NZB/NZW F1 mice. Cell Immunol. 2004;228(1):54-65.
131. Jolly CA, Muthukumar A, Avula CP, et al. Life span is prolonged in food-restricted autoimmune-prone (NZB x NZW)F(1) mice fed a diet enriched with (n-3) fatty acids. J Nutr. 2001;131(19):2753-60.
132. Sanchez A, Reeser JL, et al. Role of sugars in human neutrophilic phagocytosis. Am J Clin Nutr. 1973;26:1180-84.
133. Aljada A, Ghanim H, Mohanty P, et al. Glucose intake induces an increase in activator protein 1 and early growth response 1 binding activities, in the expression of tissue factor and matrix metalloproteinase in mononuclear cells, and in plasma tissue factor and matrix metalloproteinase concentrations. Am J Clin Nutr. 2004;80:51-7.
134. Aljada A, Mohanty P, Ghanim H, et al. Increase in intranuclear nuclear factor kB and decrease in inhibitor kB in mononuclear cells after a mixed meal: evidence for a proinflammatory effect. Am J Clin Nutr. 2004;79:682-90.
135. Lamas O, Martinez JA, Marti A. Energy restriction restores the impaired immune response in overweight (cafeteria) rats. J Nutr Biochem. 2004;15(7):418-25.
136. Mohanty P, Hamouda W, Garg R, et al. Glucose challenge stimulates reactive oxygen species (ROS) generation by leucocytes. J Clin Endocrinol Metab. 2000;85(8):2970-73.
137. Dandona P, Mohanty P, Hamouda W, et al. Inhibitory effect of a two day fast on reactive oxygen species (ROS) generation by leucocytes and plasma ortho-tyrosine and meta-tyrosine concentrations. J Clin Endocrinol Metab. 2001:86(6):2899-902.
138. Adam O. Anti-inflammatory diet and rheumatic diseases. Eur J Clin Nutr. 1995;49:703-17.
139. Kjeldsen-Kragh J. Rheumatoid arthritis treated with vegetarian diets. Am J Clin Nutr. 1999;70(Suppl.):594S-600S.
140. Gamlin L, Brostoff J. Food sensitivity and rheumatoid arthritis. EnviroTox Pharm. 1997;4:43-49.
141. Mylonaki M, Langmead L, Pantes A, et al. Enteric infection in relapse of inflammatory bowel disease: importance of microbiological examination of stool. Eur J Gastroenterol Hepatol. 2004;16(8):775-78.
142. Benno P, Alam M, Henriksson K, et al. Abnormal colonic microbial function in patients with rheumatoid arthritis. Scand J Rheumatol. 1994;23(6):311-15.
143. Stebbings S, Munro K, Simon MA, et al. Comparison of the faecal microflora of patients with ankylosing spondylitis and controls using molecular methods of analysis. Rheumatology (Oxford). 2002;41(12):1395-401.
144. Hunter J.O. Food allergy or enterometabolic disorder. Lancet. 1991;338:495-96.
145. Toivanen P, Eerola E. A vegan diet changes the intestinal flora. Rheumatology (Oxford). 2002;41:950-51.
146. Vogt BL, Richie JP Jr. Fasting-induced depletion of glutathione in the aging mouse. Biochem Pharmacol. 1993;46(2):257-63.
147. Godin DV, Wohaieb SA. Nutritional deficiency, starvation and tissue antioxidant status. Free Radical Biol Med. 1988;5:165-76.
148. Boyd EM, Taylor FL. The acute oral toxicity of chlordane in albino rats fed for 28 days from weaning on a protein-deficient diet. Input Med Surg. 1969;1:213-51.
149. Godin DV, Wohaieb SA. Nutritional deficiency, starvation and tissue antioxidant status. Free Radical Biol Med. 1988;5:165-76.

150. Paganelli R, Fagiolo U, Cancian M, et al. Intestinal permeability in irritable bowel syndrome. Effect of diet and sodium cromoglycate administration. Ann Allergy. April 1990;64:377-380.
151. Krop J. Chemical sensitivity after intoxication at work with solvents: response to sauna therapy. J Altern Complement Med. 1998;4(1):77-86.
152. Kilburn KH, Warsaw RH, Shields MG. Neurobehavioral dysfunction in firemen exposed to polychlorinated biphenyls (PCBs): possible improvement after detoxification. Arch Environ Health. 1989;44(6):345-50.
153. Kavuncu V, Evcik D. Physiotherapy in rheumatoid arthritis. Medscape General Medicine. 2004;6(2):http://www.medscape.com/viewarticle/474880_print.
154. Stener-Victorin E, Kruse-Smidje C, Jung K. Comparison between electro-acupuncture and hydrotherapy, both in combination with patient education and patient education alone, on the symptomatic treatment of osteoarthritis of the hip. Clin J Pain. 2004;20(3):179-85.
155. Foley A, Halbert J, Hewitt T, Crotty M. Does hydrotherapy improve strength and physical function in patients with osteoarthritis—a randomized controlled trial comparing a gym based and a hydrotherapy based strengthening programme. Ann Rheum Dis. 2003;62:1162-67.
156. Michalsen A, Ludtke R, Buhring M, et al. Thermal hydrotherapy improves quality of life and hemodynamic function in patients with chronic heart failure. Am Heart J. 2003;146(4):E11.
157. Kesiktas N, Paker N, Erdogan N, et al. The use of hydrotherapy for the management of spasticity. Neurorehabil Neural Repair. 2004;18(4):268-73.
158. Editorial. Lancet. 1978;9:715-17.
159. Miller A. The pathogenesis, clinical implications, and treatment of intestinal hyperpermeability. Alt Med Review. 1997;2(5):330-45.
160. Rooney PJ, Jenkins RT, Buchanan WW. A short review of the relationship between intestinal permeability and inflammatory joint disease. Clin Exp Rheumatol. 1990;8(1):75-83.
161. Smith MD, Gibson RA, Brooks PM. Abnormal bowel permeability in ankylosing spondylitis and rheumatoid arthritis. J Rheumatol. 1985;12(2):299-305.
162. Andre C, Andre F, et al. Effect of allergen ingestion challenge with and without cromoglycate cover on intestinal permeability in atopic dermatitis, urticaria and other symptoms of food allergy. Allergy. 1989;44(9):47-51.
163. Tepper RE, Simon D, et al. Intestinal permeability in patients infected with the human immunodeficiency virus. Am J Gastroenterol. 1994;89(6):878-82.
164. Bjarnason I, Peters TJ, et al. The leaky gut of alcoholism: possible route of entry for toxic compounds. Lancet. 1984;1(8370):179-82.
165. Zeuzem S. Gut-liver axis. Int J Colorectal Dis. 2000;15:59-82.
166. Berkow R, Bondy DC, Bondy PK, et al, editors. Hepatic and biliary disorders. In: The Merck Manual of Diagnosis and Therapy, 14th Edition. Rathway, NJ: Merck Sharp & Dohme Research Laboratories; 1982. p. 808.
167. Timbrell JA. Principles of biochemical toxicology. 2nd ed. London: Taylor & Francis; 1991.
168. Anders MW, Dekant W, editors. Conjugation-dependent carcinogenicity and toxicity of foreign compounds. New York: Academic Press, 1994.
169. Liska DJ. The detoxification enzyme systems. Altern Med Rev. 1998;3(3):187-98.
170. Zeuzem S. Gut-liver axis. Int J Colorectal Dis. 2000;15:59-82.
171. Adlercreutz H, Martin F, Pulkkinen M, et al. Intestinal metabolism of estrogens. J Clin Endocrin Metab. 1976;43(3):497-505.
172. Gorbach SL, Bengt E. Function of the normal human microflora. Scand J Infect Dis Suppl. 1986;49:17-30.
173. Parker RJ, Hirom PC, Millburn P. Enterohepatic recycling of phenolphthalein, morphine, lysergic acid diethylamide (LSD) and diphenylacetic acid in the rat. Hydrolysis of glucuronic acid conjugates in the gut lumen. Xenobiotica. 1980;10(9):689-703.
174. Benno Y, Mitsuoka T. Impact of Bifidobacterium longum on human fecal microflora. Microbiol Immunol. 1992;36(7):683-94.
175. Cole CB, Fuller R, Mallet AK, Rowland IR. The influence of the host on expression of intestinal microbial enzyme activities involved in metabolism of foreign compounds. J Appl Bacteriol. 1985;59(6):549-53.
176. Kim DH, Jin YH. Intestinal bacterial beta-glucuronidase activity of patients with colon cancer. Arch Pharm Res. 2001;24(6):564-67.
177. Walaszek Z, Hanausek-Walaszek M, Minton JP, Webb TE. Dietary glucarate as anti-promoter of 7,12-dimethylbenz[a]anthracene-induced mammary tumorigenesis. Carcinogenesis. 1986;7(9):1463-66.
178. Roland N, Nugon-Baudon L, Rabot S. Interactions between the intestinal flora and xenobiotic metabolizing enzymes and their health consequences. World Rev Nutr Diet. 1993;74:123-48.
179. Marinaro M, Fasano A, De Magistris MT. Zonula occludens toxin acts as an adjuvant through different mucosal routes and induces protective immune responses. Infect Immun. 2003;71(4):1897-902.
180. Zeuzem S. Gut-liver axis. Int J Colorectal Dis. 2000;15:59-82.
181. Zeneroli ML, Venturini I, Stefanelli S, et al. Antibacterial activity of rifaximin reduces the levels of benzodiazepine-like compounds in patients with liver cirrhosis. Pharmacol Res. 1997;35(6):557-60.
182. Liu Q, Duan ZP, Ha da K, et al. Synbiotic modulation of gut flora: effect on minimal hepatic encephalopathy in patients with cirrhosis. Hepatology. 2004;39(5):1441-49.
183. Wakefield AJ, Puleston JM, Montgomery SM, et al. Review article: the concept of entero-colonic encephalopathy, autism and opioid receptor ligands. Aliment Pharmacol Ther. 2002;16(4):663-74.
184. White JF. Intestinal pathophysiology in autism. Exp Biol Med (Maywood). 2003;228(6):639-49.
185. Dohan FC. Genetics and idiopathic schizophrenia. Am J Psychiatry. 1989;146(11):1522-23.
186. Abou-Assi S, Vlahcevic ZR. Hepatic encephalopathy. Metabolic consequence of cirrhosis often is reversible. Postgrad Med. 2001;109(2):52-54, 57-60.
187. Ibid.
188. Basile AS, Jones EA. Ammonia and GABA-ergic neurotransmission: interrelated factors in the pathogenesis of hepatic encephalopathy. Hepatology. 1997;25(6):1303-5.
189. Zeneroli ML, Venturini I, Stefanelli S, et al. Antibacterial activity of rifaximin reduces the levels of benzodiazepine-like compounds in patients with liver cirrhosis. Pharmacol Res. 1997;35(6):557-60.
190. Schafer DF, Jones EA. Hepatic encephalopathy and the gamma-aminobutyric-acid neurotransmitter system. Lancet. 1982;1(8262):18-20.
191. Zeneroli ML, Venturini I, Stefanelli S, et al. Antibacterial activity of rifaximin reduces the levels of benzodiazepine-like compounds in patients with liver cirrhosis. Pharmacol Res. 1997;35(6):557-60.
192. Basile AS, Jones EA. Ammonia and GABA-ergic neurotransmission: interrelated factors in the pathogenesis of hepatic encephalopathy. Hepatology. 1997;25(6):1303-5.
193. Abou-Assi S, Vlahcevic ZR. Hepatic encephalopathy. Metabolic consequence of cirrhosis often is reversible. Postgrad Med. 2001;109(2):52-4, 57-60.
194. Locke GR 3rd, Pemberton JH, Phillips SF. AGA technical review on constipation. American Gastroenterological Association. Gastroenterology. 2000;119(6):1766-78.
195. Riordan SM, Williams R. Treatment of hepatic encephalopathy. N Engl J Med. 1997;337(7):473-79.

196. Liu Q, Duan ZP, Ha da K, et al. Synbiotic modulation of gut flora: effect on minimal hepatic encephalopathy in patients with cirrhosis. Hepatology. 2004;39(5):1441-49.
197. Mowat AM. Anatomical basis of tolerance and immunity to intestinal antigens. Nat Rev Immunol. 2003;3(4):331-41.
198. Ibid.
199. Ibid.
200. Ibid.
201. Khoo UY, Proctor IE, Macpherson AJ. CD4+ T cell down-regulation in human intestinal mucosa: evidence for intestinal tolerance to luminal bacterial antigens. J Immunol. 1997;158(8):3626-34.
202. Bouma G, Strober W. The immunological and genetic basis of inflammatory bowel disease. Nat Rev Immunol. 2003;3:521-33.
203. Brown TA, Russell MW, Mestecky J. Elimination of intestinally absorbed antigen into the bile by IgA. J Immunol. 1984;132(2):780-82.
204. Kuiper J, Brouwer A, Knook DL, van Berkel TJC. Kupffer and sinusoidal endothelial cells. In: Arias IM, Boyer JL, Fausto N, et al, editors. The Liver: Biology and Pathobiology. New York: Raven Press; 1994. p 791-818.
205. O'Dwyer ST, Michie HR, Ziegler TR, et al. A single dose of endotoxin increases intestinal permeability in healthy humans. Arch Surg. 1988;123(12):1459-64.
206. Marubayashi S, Fukuma K, Okada K, et al. Effect of monoclonal antibodies to adhesion molecules, nitric oxide synthase inhibitors, methylprednisolone and lazaroid on endotoxin-induced liver cell injury. In: Yoshikawa T, editor. Oxidative Stress and Digestive Diseases. Kyoto, Japan: Karger Press; 2001. p 119-136.
207. Henderson B, Poole S, Wilson M. Bacterial modulins: a novel class of virulence factors which cause host tissue pathology by inducing cytokine synthesis. Microbiol Rev. 1996;60(2):316-41.
208. Callery MP, Mangino MJ, Flye MW. A biologic basis for limited Kupffer cell reactivity to portal-derived endotoxin. Surgery. 1991;110(2):221-30.
209. O'Dwyer ST, Michie HR, Ziegler TR, et al. A single dose of endotoxin increases intestinal permeability in healthy humans. Arch Surg. 1988;123(12):1459-64.
210. Ibid.
211. Davies GR, Wilkie ME, Rampton DS, Effects of metronidazole and misoprostol on indomethacin-induced changes in intestinal permeability. Dig Dis Sci. 1993;38(3):417-25.
212. Jaeschke H. Reactive oxygen and neutrophil-induced liver injury. In: Yoshikawa T, editor. Oxidative Stress and Digestive Diseases. Kyoto, Japan: Karger Press; 2001. p. 13-24.
213. Zeuzem S. Gut-liver axis. Int J Colorectal Dis. 2000;15:59-82.
214. Ibid.
215. Masubuchi Y, Horie T. Resistance to indomethacin-induced down-regulation of hepatic cytochrome P450 enzymes in the mice with non-functional Toll-like receptor 4. J Hepatol. 2003;39(3):349-56.
216. Doig CJ, Sutherland LR, Sandham JD, et al. Increased intestinal permeability is associated with the development of multiple organ dysfunction syndrome in critically ill ICU patients. Am J Respir Crit Care Med. 1998;158(2):444-51.
217. Ibid.
218. Faries PL, Simon RJ, Martella AT, et al. Intestinal permeability correlates with severity of injury in trauma patients. J Trauma. 1998;44(6):1031-5; discussion 1035-6.
219. Ibid.
220. Anup R, Aparna V, Pulimood A, Balasubramanian KA. Surgical stress and the small intestine: role of oxygen free radicals. Surgery. 1999;125(5):560-69.
221. Doig CJ, Sutherland LR, Sandham JD, et al. Increased intestinal permeability is associated with the development of multiple organ dysfunction syndrome in critically ill ICU patients. Am J Respir Crit Care Med. 1998;158(2):444-51.
222. Faries PL, Simon RJ, Martella AT, et al. Intestinal permeability correlates with severity of injury in trauma patients. J Trauma. 1998;44(6):1031-5; discussion 1035-6.
223. Thurman RG. II. Alcoholic liver injury involves activation of Kupffer cells by endotoxin. Am J Physiol. 1998;275(4 Pt 1):G605-11.
224. Parlesak A, Schafer C, Bode C. IgA against gut-derived endotoxins: does it contribute to suppression of hepatic inflammation in alcohol-induced liver disease? Dig Dis Sci. 2002;47(4):760-66.
225. Bjarnason I, Peters TJ, Wise RJ. The leaky gut of alcoholism: possible route of entry for toxic compounds. Lancet. 1984;1(8370):179-82.
226. Zeuzem S. Gut-liver axis. Int J Colorectal Dis. 2000;15:59-82.
227. Thurman RG. II. Alcoholic liver injury involves activation of Kupffer cells by endotoxin. Am J Physiol. 1998;275(4 Pt 1):G605-11.
228. Parlesak A, Schafer C, Bode C. IgA against gut-derived endotoxins: does it contribute to suppression of hepatic inflammation in alcohol-induced liver disease? Dig Dis Sci. 2002;47(4):760-66.
229. Solga SF, Diehl AM. Non-alcoholic fatty liver disease: lumen-liver interactions and possible role for probiotics. J Hepatol. 2003;38(5):681-87.
230. Song Z, Zhou Z, Chen T, et al. S-adenosylmethionine (SAMe) protects against acute alcohol induced hepatotoxicity in mice small star, filled. J Nutr Biochem. 2003;14(10):591-97.
231. Seitz HK, Poschl G, Simanowski UA. Alcohol and cancer. Recent Dev Alcohol. 1998;14:67-95.
232. Song Z, Zhou Z, Chen T, et al. S-adenosylmethionine (SAMe) protects against acute alcohol induced hepatotoxicity in mice small star, filled. J Nutr Biochem. 2003;14(10):591-97.
233. Ibid.
234. Berkow R, Bondy DC, Bondy PK, et al, editors. Liver disease due to alcohol. In: The Merck Manual of Diagnosis and Therapy, 14th Edition. Rathway, NJ: Merck Sharp & Dohme Research Laboratories; 1982. p. 846-49.
235. Baraona E, Lieber CS. Effects of ethanol on lipid metabolism. J Lipid Res. 1979;20(3):289-315.
236. Lieber CS. CYP2E1: from ASH to NASH. Hepatol Res. 2004;28(1):1-11.
237. Berkow R, Bondy DC, Bondy PK, et al, editors. Liver disease due to alcohol. In: The Merck Manual of Diagnosis and Therapy, 14th Edition. Rathway, NJ: Merck Sharp & Dohme Research Laboratories; 1982. p. 846-49.
238. Angulo P, Lindor KD. Insulin resistance and mitochondrial abnormalities in NASH: a cool look into a burning issue. Gastroenterology. 2001;120(5):1281-85.
239. Clark JM, Diehl AM. Defining nonalcoholic fatty liver disease: implications for epidemiologic studies. Gastroenterology. 2003;124(1):248-50.
240. Sheth SG, Gordon FD, Chopra S. Nonalcoholic steatohepatitis. Ann Intern Med. 1997;126(2):137-45.
241. Franzese A, Vajro P, Argenziano A, et al. Liver involvement in obese children. Ultrasonography and liver enzyme levels at diagnosis and during follow-up in an Italian population. Dig Dis Sci. 1997;42(7):1428-32.
242. Reid AE. Nonalcoholic steatohepatitis. Gastroenterology. 2001;121(3):710-23.
243. Patrick L. Nonalcoholic fatty liver disease: relationship to insulin sensitivity and oxidative stress. Treatment approaches using vitamin E, magnesium, and betaine. Altern Med Rev. 2002;7(4):276-91.
244. Pessayre D, Mansouri A, Fromenty B. Nonalcoholic steatosis and steatohepatitis. V. Mitochondrial dysfunction in steatohepatitis. Am J Physiol Gastrointest Liver Physiol. 2002;282(2):G193-99.

245. Reid AE. Nonalcoholic steatohepatitis. Gastroenterology. 2001;121(3):710-23.
246. Ibid.
247. Pessayre D, Mansouri A, Fromenty B. Nonalcoholic steatosis and steatohepatitis. V. Mitochondrial dysfunction in steatohepatitis. Am J Physiol Gastrointest Liver Physiol. 2002;282(2):G193-99.
248. Yang SQ, Lin HZ, Lane MD, et al. Obesity increases sensitivity to endotoxin liver injury: Implications for the pathogenesis of steatohepatitis. Proc Natl Acad Sci U S A. 1997;94:2557-62.
249. Marubayashi S, Fukuma K, Okada K, et al. Effect of monoclonal antibodies to adhesion molecules, nitric oxide synthase inhibitors, methylprednisolone and lazaroid on endotoxin-induced liver cell injury. In: Yoshikawa T, editor. Oxidative Stress and Digestive Diseases. Kyoto, Japan: Karger Press; 2001. p 119-136.
250. Lichtman SN, Keku J, Schwab JH, Sartor RB. Hepatic injury associated with small bowel bacterial overgrowth in rats is prevented by metronidazole and tetracycline. Gastroenterology. 1991;100(2):513-19.
251. Logan BK, Jones AW. Endogenous ethanol 'auto-brewery syndrome' as a drunk-driving defence challenge. Med Sci Law. 2000;40(3):206-15.
252. Nosova T, Jousimies-Somer H, Jokelainen K, et al. Acetaldehyde production and metabolism by human indigenous and probiotic Lactobacillus and Bifidobacterium strains. Alcohol Alcohol. 2000;35(6):561-68.
253. Ibid.
254. Ibid.
255. Cope K, Risby T, Diehl AM. Increased gastrointestinal ethanol production in obese mice: implications for fatty liver disease pathogenesis. Gastroenterology. 2000;119(5):1340-47.
256. Nosova T, Jousimies-Somer H, Jokelainen K, et al. Acetaldehyde production and metabolism by human indigenous and probiotic Lactobacillus and Bifidobacterium strains. Alcohol Alcohol. 2000;35(6):561-68.
257. Lieber CS. CYP2E1: from ASH to NASH. Hepatol Res. 2004;28(1):1-11.
258. Robertson G, Leclercq I, Farrell GC. Nonalcoholic steatosis and steatohepatitis. II. Cytochrome P-450 enzymes and oxidative stress. Am J Physiol Gastrointest Liver Physiol. 2001;281(5):G1135-39.
259. Cotrim HP, Andrade ZA, Parana R, et al. Nonalcoholic steatohepatitis: a toxic liver disease in industrial workers. Liver. 1999;19(4):299-304.
260. Berkow R, Bondy DC, Bondy PK, et al, editors. Celiac disease. In: The Merck Manual of Diagnosis and Therapy, 14th Edition. Rathway, NJ: Merck Sharp & Dohme Research Laboratories; 1982. p. 775-77.
261. Vogelsang H, Schwarzenhofer M, Steiner B, et al. *In vivo* and *in vitro* permeability in coeliac disease. Aliment Pharmacol Ther. 2001;15(9):1417-25.
262. Fasano A. Intestinal zonulin: open sesame! Gut. 2001;49(2):159-62.
263. Zeuzem S. Gut-liver axis. Int J Colorectal Dis. 2000;15:59-82.
264. Davison S. Coeliac disease and liver dysfunction. Arch Dis Child. 2002;87(4):293-96.
265. Vajro P, Fontanella A, Mayer M, et al. Elevated serum aminotransferase activity as an early manifestation of gluten-sensitive enteropathy. J Pediatr. 1993;122(3):416-19.
266. Volta U, De Franceschi L, Lari F, et al. Coeliac disease hidden by cryptogenic hypertransaminasaemia. Lancet. 1998;352(9121):26-29.
267. Grieco A, Miele L, Pignatoro G, et al. Is coeliac disease a confounding factor in the diagnosis of NASH? Gut. 2001;49(4):596.
268. Ventura A, Neri E, Ughi C, et al. Gluten-dependent diabetes-related and thyroid-related autoantibodies in patients with celiac disease. J Pediatr. 2000;137(2):263-65.
269. Lindberg T, Berg NO, Borulf S, Jakobsson I. Liver damage in coeliac disease or other food intolerance in childhood. Lancet. 1978;1(8060):390-91.
270. Fine KD, Ogunji F, Saloum Y, et al. Celiac sprue: another autoimmune syndrome associated with hepatitis C. Am J Gastroenterol. 2001;96(1):138-45.
271. Davison S. Coeliac disease and liver dysfunction. Arch Dis Child. 2002;87(4):293-96.
272. Sollid LM, Thorsby E. HLA susceptibility genes in celiac disease: genetic mapping and role in pathogenesis. Gastroenterology. 1993;105(3):910-22.
273. van der Hulst RR, von Meyenfeldt MF, van Kreel BK, et al. Gut permeability, intestinal morphology, and nutritional depletion. Nutrition. 1998;14(1):1-6.
274. Berg RD. Bacterial translocation from the gastrointestinal tract. J Med. 1992;23(3-4):217-44.
275. Wigg AJ, Roberts-Thomson IC, Dymock RB, et al. The role of small intestinal bacterial overgrowth, intestinal permeability, endotoxaemia, and tumour necrosis factor alpha in the pathogenesis of non-alcoholic steatohepatitis. Gut. 2001;48(2):206-11.
276. De Magistris L, Secondulfo M, Sapone A, et al. Infection with Giardia and intestinal permeability in humans. Gastroenterology. 2003;125(1):277-79.
277. Isolauri E, Juntunen M, Wiren S, et al. Intestinal permeability changes in acute gastroenteritis: effects of clinical factors and nutritional management. J Pediatr Gastroenterol Nutr. 1989;8(4):466-73.
278. Andre C, Andre F, et al. Effect of allergen ingestion challenge with and without cromoglycate cover on intestinal permeability in atopic dermatitis, urticaria and other symptoms of food allergy. Allergy. 1989;44(9): 47-51.
279. Pearson AD, Eastham EJ, et al. Intestinal permeability in children with Crohn's disease and coeliac disease. Br Med J. 1982;285(6334):20-21.
280. Bjarnason I, Williams P, et al. Effect of non-steroidal anti-inflammatory drugs and prostaglandins on the permeability of the human small intestine. Gut. 1986;27(11):1292-97.
281. Bjarnason I, Peters TJ, Wise RJ. The leaky gut of alcoholism: possible route of entry for toxic compounds. Lancet. 1984;1(8370):179-82.
282. Nagler-Anderson C. Man the barrier! Strategic defences in the intestinal mucosa. Nat Rev Immunol. 2001;1(1):59-67.
283. Faries PL, Simon RJ, Martella AT, et al. Intestinal permeability correlates with severity of injury in trauma patients. J Trauma. 1998;44(6):1031-5; discussion 1035-6.
284. Kirsch M. Bacterial overgrowth. Am J Gastroenterol. 1990;85(3):231-37.
285. Rose S, Young MA, Reynolds JC. Gastrointestinal manifestations of scleroderma. Gastroenterol Clin North Am. 1998;27(3):563-94.
286. Miller A. Therapeutic considerations of L-glutamine: a review of the literature. Altern Med Rev. 1999;4(4):239-48.
287. Li J, King BK, Janu PG, et al. Glycyl-L-glutamine-enriched total parenteral nutrition maintains small intestine gut-associated lymphoid tissue and upper respiratory tract immunity. JPEN J Parenter Enteral Nutr. 1998;22(1):31-36.
288. Royall D, Wolever TMS, Jeejeebhoy KN. Clinical significance of colonic fermentation. Am J Gastroenterol 1990;85(10):1307-12.
289. Phillips J, Muir JG, Birkett A, et al. Effect of resistant starch on fecal bulk and fermentation-dependent events in humans. Am J Clin Nutr. 1995;62:121-30.
290. Lizko NN. Stress and intestinal microflora. Nahrung. 1987;31(5-6):443-47.
291. Ibid.

292. Freestone PP, Haigh RD, Williams PH, Lyte M. Stimulation of bacterial growth by heat-stable, norepinephrine-induced autoinducers. FEMS Microbiol Lett. 1999;172(1):53-60.
293. Isolauri E, Sutas Y, Kankaanpaa P, et al. Probiotics: effects on immunity. Am J Clin Nutr. 2001;73(2 Suppl):444S-450S.
294. Ibid.
295. Nosova T, Jousimies-Somer H, Jokelainen K, et al. Acetaldehyde production and metabolism by human indigenous and probiotic Lactobacillus and Bifidobacterium strains. Alcohol Alcohol. 2000;35(6):561-68.
296. Liu Q, Duan ZP, Ha da K, et al. Synbiotic modulation of gut flora: effect on minimal hepatic encephalopathy in patients with cirrhosis. Hepatology. 2004;39(5):1441-49.
297. Gotteland M, Cruchet S, Verbeke S. Effect of Lactobacillus ingestion on the gastrointestinal mucosal barrier alterations induced by indomethacin in humans. Aliment Pharmacol Ther. 2001;15(1):11-17.
298. Bornet FR, Brouns F. Immune-stimulating and gut health-promoting properties of short-chain fructo-oligosaccharides. Nutr Rev. 2002;60(10 Pt 1):326-34.
299. Reddy BS, Weisburger JH, Wynder EL. Fecal bacterial beta-glucuronidase: control by diet. Science. 1974;183(123):416-17.
300. Kruis W, Forstmaier G, Scheurlen C, Stellaard F. Effect of diets low and high in refined sugars on gut transit, bile acid metabolism, and bacterial fermentation. Gut. 1991;32(4):367-71.
301. Hawrelak JA, Myers SP. The causes of intestinal dysbiosis: a review. Altern Med Rev. 2004;9(2):180-97.
302. Fasano A, Catassi C. Current approaches to diagnosis and treatment of celiac disease: an evolving spectrum. Gastroenterology. 2001;120(3):636-51.
303. Falth-Magnusson K, Kjellman N-IM et al. Gastrointestinal permeability in children with cow's milk allergy: effect of milk challenge and sodium cromoglycate as assessed with polyethyleneglycols (PEG 400 and PEG 1000). Clin Allergy. 1986;16(6):543-51.
304. Szabo A, Boros M, Kaszaki J, Nagy S. Mucosal permeability changes during intestinal reperfusion injury. The role of mast cells. Acta Chir Hung. 1997;36(1-4):334-36.
305. Kirsch M. Bacterial overgrowth. Am J Gastroenterol. 1990;85(3):231-37.
306. [No authors listed]: Small intestinal bacterial overgrowth syndrome. Gastroenterology. 1981;80:834-45.
307. Zeuzem S. Gut-liver axis. Int J Colorectal Dis. 2000;15:59-82.
308. Bjarnason I, Peters TJ, et al. Intestinal permeability: clinical correlates. Dig Dis. 1986;4(2):83-92.
309. Kirsch M: Bacterial overgrowth. Am J Gastroenterol. 1990;85:231-237.
310. Ibid.
311. [No authors listed]: Small intestinal bacterial overgrowth syndrome. Gastroenterology. 1981;80:834-45.
312. Liska DJ. The detoxification enzyme systems. Altern Med Rev. 1998;3(3):187-98.
313. Groff JL, Gropper SS, Hunt SM. The regulatory nutrients. In: Advanced Nutrition and Human Metabolism, 2nd Edition. St Paul, MN: West Publishing Co; 1995. p 382-83.
314. Song Z, Zhou Z, Chen T, et al. S-adenosylmethionine (SAMe) protects against acute alcohol induced hepatotoxicity in mice small star, filled. J Nutr Biochem. 2003;14(10):591-97.
315. Robertson G, Leclercq I, Farrell GC. Nonalcoholic steatosis and steatohepatitis. II. Cytochrome P-450 enzymes and oxidative stress. Am J Physiol Gastrointest Liver Physiol. 2001;281(5):G1135-39.
316. Kidd PM. Glutathione: Systemic protectant against oxidative and free radical damage. Alt Med Review. 1997;2(3):155-72.
317. Groff JL, Gropper SS, Hunt SM. Macronutrients and their metabolism. In: Advanced Nutrition and Human Metabolism, 2nd Ed. St Paul, MN: West Publishing Co; 1995. p 175.
318. Avila MA, Corrales FJ, Ruiz F, et al. Specific interaction of methionine adenosyltransferase with free radicals. Biofactors. 1998;8(1-2):27-32.
319. Song Z, Zhou Z, Chen T, et al. S-adenosylmethionine (SAMe) protects against acute alcohol induced hepatotoxicity in mice small star, filled. J Nutr Biochem. 2003;14(10):591-97.
320. Miller AL, Kelly GS. Homocysteine metabolism: Nutritional modulation and impact on health and disease. Alt Med Rev. 1997;2(4):234-54.
321. Saeian K, Curro K. Binion DG, et al. Plasma total homocysteine levels are higher in nonalcoholic steatohepatitis. Hepatology. 1999;30:436A.
322. Kidd PM. Glutathione: Systemic protectant against oxidative and free radical damage. Alt Med Review. 1997;2(3):155-72.
323. Abdelmalek MF, Angulo P, Jorgensen RA, et al. Betaine, a promising new agent for patients with nonalcoholic steatohepatitis: results of a pilot study. Am J Gastroenterol. 2001;96(9):2711-17.
324. Lee HA, Hughes DA. Alpha-lipoic acid modulates NF-kappaB activity in human monocytic cells by direct interaction with DNA. Exp Gerontol. 2002;37(2-3):401-10.
325. Ho E, Quan N, Tsai YH, et al. Dietary zinc supplementation inhibits NfkappaB activation and protects against chemically induced diabetes in CD1 mice. Exp Biol Med (Maywood). 2001;226(2):103-11.
326. Lukita-Atmadja W, Ito Y, Baker GL, McCuskey RS. Effect of curcuminoids as anti-inflammatory agents on the hepatic microvascular response to endotoxin. Shock. 2002;17(5):399-403.
327. Das UN. Beneficial effect(s) of n-3 fatty acids in cardiovascular diseases: but, why and how? Prostaglandins Leukot Essent Fatty Acids. 2000;63(6):351-62.
328. Zhao Y, Joshi-Barve S, Barve S, Chen LH. Eicosapentaenoic acid prevents LPS-induced TNF-alpha expression by preventing NF-kappaB activation. J Am Coll Nutr. 2004;23(1):71-78.
329. Rusyn I, Bradham CA, Cohn L, et al. Corn oil rapidly activates nuclear factor-kappaB in hepatic Kupffer cells by oxidant-dependent mechanisms. Carcinogenesis. 1999;20(11):2095-100.
330. Calabrese C, Myer S, Munson S, et al. A cross-over study of the effect of a single oral feeding of medium chain triglyceride oil vs. canola oil on post-ingestion plasma triglyceride levels in healthy men. Altern Med Rev. 1999;4(1):23-28.
331. Kono H, Fujii H, Asakawa M, et al. Protective effects of medium-chain triglycerides on the liver and gut in rats administered endotoxin. Ann Surg. 2003;237(2):246-55.
332. Patrick L. Nonalcoholic fatty liver disease: relationship to insulin sensitivity and oxidative stress. Treatment approaches using vitamin E, magnesium, and betaine. Altern Med Rev. 2002;7(4):276-91.
333. Li J, Kim CI, Leo MA, et al. Polyunsaturated lecithin prevents acetaldehyde-mediated hepatic collagen accumulation by stimulating collagenase activity in cultured lipocytes. Hepatology. 1992;15(3):373-81.
334. Watanabe A, Hobara N, Kobayashi M, et al. Lowering of blood acetaldehyde but not ethanol concentrations by pantethine following alcohol ingestion: different effects in flushing and nonflushing subjects. Alcohol Clin Exp Res. 1985;9(3):272-76.
335. Pessayre D, Mansouri A, Fromenty B. Nonalcoholic steatosis and steatohepatitis. V. Mitochondrial dysfunction in steatohepatitis. Am J Physiol Gastrointest Liver Physiol. 2002;282(2):G193-9.
336. Lieber CS. CYP2E1: from ASH to NASH. Hepatol Res. 2004;28(1):1-11.

337. Chitturi S, Farrell GC. Etiopathogenesis of nonalcoholic steatohepatitis. Semin Liver Dis. 2001;21(1):27-41.
338. Robertson G, Leclercq I, Farrell GC. Nonalcoholic steatosis and steatohepatitis. II. Cytochrome P-450 enzymes and oxidative stress. Am J Physiol Gastrointest Liver Physiol. 2001;281(5):G1135-39.
339. Yang SQ, Lin HZ, Lane MD, et al. Obesity increases sensitivity to endotoxin liver injury: Implications for the pathogenesis of steatohepatitis. Proc Natl Acad Sci U S A. 1997;94:2557-62.
340. Guyton AC. Hormonal regulation of fat utilization. In: Textbook of Medical Physiology, 8th Edition. Philadelphia, PA: W.B. Saunders Company; 1991. p. 759.
341. Patrick L. Nonalcoholic fatty liver disease: relationship to insulin sensitivity and oxidative stress. Treatment approaches using vitamin E, magnesium, and betaine. Altern Med Rev. 2002;7(4):276-91.
342. Jost G, Wahlländer A, von Mandach U, Preisig R. Overnight salivary caffeine clearance: a liver function test suitable for routine use. Hepatology 1987;7(2):338-44.
343. Manniso PT, Kaakkola S. Catechol-O-methyltransferase (COMT): biochemistry, molecular biology, pharmacology, and clinical efficacy of the new selective COMT inhibitors. Pharmacol Rev. 1999;51(4):593-628.
344. Norppa H. Genetic polymorphisms and chromosome damage. Int J Hyg Environ Health. 2001;204(1):31-38.
345. Heafield MT, Fearn S, Steveton GB, et al. Plasma cysteine and sulphate levels in patients with motor neurone, Parkinson's and Alzheimer's disease. Neurosci Lett. 1990;110:216-20.
346. Friedberg T. Cytochrome P450 polymorphisms as risk factors for steroid hormone-related cancers. Am J Pharmacogenomics. 2001;1(2):83-91.

Chapter 32
Clinical Approaches to Hormonal and Neuroendocrine Imbalances

Cellular Messaging, Part I

Jeffrey S. Bland, PhD and David S. Jones, MD

Introduction

Functional medicine provides the model for the new medical paradigm upon which medicine of the 21st century will be based. Core principles of the functional medicine model include the following:

- The predisposition for disease is related to the interplay of antecedents, triggers, and mediators that give rise to an individual's clinical signs and symptoms.
- Individuals are genetically, metabolically, and biochemically unique and their medical care must support a patient-centered, rather than a disease-centered approach.
- Health is a state of positive vitality related to maintenance of a homeodynamic physiology that reflects a balance both between and among internal and external factors.
- Disease in the adult is often the result of a progressive loss of physiological, cognitive, emotional, and physical function and flexibility (that is, loss of organ reserve).

The antecedents of disease in an individual are dictated in part by the unique set of genetic characteristics derived from the 23 pairs of chromosomes that the individual inherited from his or her parents. Many of these genetic characteristics demonstrate *pleiomorphism*, which means they can be expressed in different ways, depending upon external and internal triggers. The phenotype (health patterns) the individual expresses results from the interplay between the genetic antecedents and the environmental triggers. Triggers include infectious organisms, stress, toxic exposures, electromagnetic radiation, trauma, and—probably most important of all—poor nutrition and activity/exercise patterns. It is now recognized that specific environmental exposures can have an epigenetic influence on genetic expression in the offspring that can be passed on to subsequent generations.[1] This relationship ties genes and environment together in ways that go beyond simple Mendelian genetics.

The mediators released as a result of exposure to these triggers represent a broad array of intercellular communication agents. These can be large and protein-like in structure (e.g., insulin) or small (e.g., the sex hormones). Table 32.1 provides a list of representative intercellular communication mediators, their type, and their function.

Table 32.1 **Representative Classes of Intercellular Communication Agents**

Communication Agent	Type	Function
Prostaglandins	Small molecules derived from arachidonic acid	Cellular regulators
Leukotrienes and thromboxanes	Small molecules derived from arachidonic acid	Proinflammatory
Nitric oxide	Small molecule derived from arginine via nitric oxide synthase	Immune, neurological, vascular effects
Dopamine, serotonin, acetylcholine	Small molecules derived from tyrosine, tryptophan, and choline, respectively	Neurotransmitters
Cortisol, aldosterone	Small molecules derived from cholesterol	Stress hormones and electrolyte control
Estrogen, testosterone, DHEA	Small molecules derived from cholesterol	Sex hormones
Melatonin	Small molecule derived from tryptophan	Sleep regulation
N-methyl D-aspartate (NMDA), glutamate	Small molecules derived from aspartic and glutamic acids	Excitotoxins
Endorphins	Polypeptide	Pain and immune regulation
Insulin, glucagon, somatostatin	Polypeptide	Blood sugar control
Interleukins, tumor necrosis factor, interferon	Protein	Inflammation process and immune function
NFκB/IκB	Protein	Control of oxidant response
ICAM/VCAMs	Protein	Cellular and vascular adhesion
Leptin	Protein	Appetite control
Vasopressin, ACTH, TSH, oxytocin	Polypeptides	Pituitary hormones
Bombesin, vasoactive intestinal peptide	Peptide	Gut-brain transmitters
C-reactive protein (CRP), serum amyloid A (SAAO)	Protein and protein-carbohydrate complex, respectively	Inflammatory markers
Natriuretic peptides (atrial, brain, and C-type natriuretic peptide)	Peptide	Diuretic, vasorelaxant

In many cases, these intercellular communication agents are produced when a trigger modifies gene expression. Imbalances of these agents in response to a trigger result in various signs and symptoms of dysfunction or illness. These signs and symptoms frequently express across multiple organ systems, because the intercellular communication agents are produced in many types of cells that clinically impact myriad conventional medical specialty domains. A more technical discussion of these processes can be found in Chapter 15. Here, we will focus on understanding the cellular communication process from a more clinical perspective.

Research into intercellular communication and intracellular signal transduction is evolving rapidly. Intracellular signal transduction refers to the way cells modify their function when they are exposed to molecules of intercellular communication. These two related fields of investigation, which have emerged from our increased understanding of genetic structure and expression, have practical clinical applications. A notable facet of the emerging research—particularly to the functional medicine practitioner—is the recognition of the importance of lifestyle, nutrition, and environment in determining which intercellular communication agents are expressed at a particular time from a person's pluripotential "card catalogue" of genes. This rapidly accumulating knowledge base has made it possible in many clinical situations to develop a personalized approach to health care that reflects an individual's genetic uniqueness. Practitioners who evaluate the signs and symptoms associated with imbalanced intercellular communication agents (hormonal, neurotransmitter, and immune-modulating molecules) can develop a program to normalize those agents using specific and individually-tailored lifestyle, diet, nutritional, and environmental interventions.

The Impact of Environment on Cellular Messenging

Chronic Stress as a Trigger for Intercellular Communication Dysfunction

More than 25 years ago, Austrian physician Hans Selye, MD, borrowed the term stress from physics to describe an organism's physiological response to perceived stressful events in the environment.[2] Stress triggers the *fight or flight* response and the short-term release of glucocorticoids, such as cortisol, from the adrenal glands. The result is a temporary increase in energy production, at the expense of processes that are not required for immediate survival. An imbalance in intercellular communication agents, therefore, naturally results from this stress response.

A chronic stress response, extended over a long period of time, may produce a variety of age-related pathologies, including increased risk of dementia. In animals (as in human Alzheimer's disease), high cortisol levels correlate with increasing disease severity, which is associated, in turn, with degeneration of the substructure in the brain called the hippocampus.[3,4] Studies attempting to link high cortisol levels directly with reduced hippocampal volume and consequent loss of cognitive function have begun to emerge,[5] with the association being particularly strong in depression.[6] None of the research has yet described the precise pathway by which the effects occur.[7] In healthy subjects, the link between high cortisol and age-related cognitive decline may not actually be accompanied by brain atrophy.[8] Clearly, there is much we do not yet know, but there is also a growing body of knowledge that can help clinicians improve patient management.

In a 1998 study, researchers measured cortisol levels in 51 individuals over five to six years and determined whether each person's cortisol level was rising or falling over time. They were able to divide the subjects into three groups: those whose cortisol levels were high and increasing (the *high-stress group*); those whose cortisol levels were moderate but increasing (the *moderate-stress group*); and those with decreasing cortisol levels (the *low-stress group*). The researchers found that individuals in the high-stress group had greater memory impairment than those in the low-stress group.[9] Magnetic resonance imaging (MRI) and additional memory tests were performed on some of the individuals; the results showed that the six individuals in the high-stress group and the five in the moderate-stress group had 14% lower hippocampal volume than those in the low-stress group. They also had reduced hippocampal energy production. This study supports other investigations that indicate long-term, chronic stress may be damaging to the brain and may increase the risk of Alzheimer's and other neurodegenerative diseases.[10,11]

A 2005 study reported a "new personality construct," the type D, which is "characterized by the joint tendency to experience negative emotions and to inhibit these emotions while avoiding social contacts with others."[12]

The research revealed that both characteristics were associated with greater cortisol reactivity to stress; the author hypothesized, therefore, that "Elevated cortisol may be a mediating factor in the association between type D personality and the increased risk for coronary heart disease and, possibly, other medical disorders."

In 1995, Licinio, Gold, and Wong[13] proposed a molecular mechanism for stress-induced alterations in the susceptibility to disease. In this model, they evoked the concept of how stress influences gene expression to describe the origin of *stress-induced* diseases ranging from heart disease to arthritis to cancer. They found that the hypothalamic hormone, corticotropin-releasing hormone (CRH), had gene complementarity with proinflammatory molecules (as well as cancer oncogenes); they postulated that events elevating CRH levels could increase the risk of many age-related chronic diseases. This model is consistent with the older view of Axelrod and Reisine, who also stated that CRH regulates release of ACTH, which subsequently influences the adrenal catecholamines and glucocorticoids.[14]

Since that 1995 study, elevated CRH has been associated with anxiety and all common manifestations of stress, including fear, startle reflex, decreased food intake, and others.[15] Elevated CRH has also been associated with increased proinflammatory response as a result of secretion of TNF-α, IL-I, and IL-6.[16,17,18] The link with inflammation is being demonstrated through studies of many different conditions, including alterations in gut motility and mucosal function,[19] ulcerative colitis,[20] and endometriosis.[21]

Xenobiotics as a Trigger for Intercellular Communication Dysfunction

As mentioned earlier, stress is not the only environmental modifier of cellular communication agents. Environmental xenobiotics have also been identified as "endocrine disrupters" that can modify intercellular communication and cellular function.[22] For example, xenobiotic estrogens (environmental compounds with estrogenic activity), can modify the way a woman metabolizes estrogen. Estrogen is metabolized through three hydroxylation reactions—one at the carbon position 2, one at carbon 4, and the third at carbon 16 in the estrogen structure. Investigators have found that the hydroxylation of estrogen and its methylation at carbon 2 result in an estrogen metabolite that **does not** signal the genes of the mammary cells to engage in proliferation. The absence of a cell proliferation message reduces the risk of breast cancer. On the other hand, hydroxylation at carbon 4 or 16 results in production of a metabolite in the breast tissue that **does** create potential metaplastic changes associated with premalignancy.[23]

Environmental pollutants can modify the hydroxylation of estrogen, producing a higher ratio of the 4 and 16 hydroxylated estrogen derivatives that are potentially more genotoxic. Pesticides were found to significantly increase the ratio of 16-hydroxyestrone to 2-hydroxyestrone.[24] The investigators suggested that the ratio of 16-hydroxyestrone to 2-hydroxyestrone may provide a marker for analyzing breast cancer risk (prognostic indices) and for generating preventive nutritional strategies and interventions. Subsequent studies have often,[25] but not always,[26] supported the 2-to-16 ratio hypothesis, although the ability of xenobiotics to disrupt hormone function does not appear to be in doubt.[27,28]

Environmental xenobiotics may affect the detoxification of estrogen by modifying genetic expression and activity of the detoxification enzymes, which are members of the cytochrome P450 family. Some cytochrome P450 isoforms detoxify estrogen by hydroxylation at the 2 position, and others act at the 16 position. We can speculate that environmental chemicals may modify intercellular communication and shift the expression of genes toward the isoforms of cytochrome P450 that result in production of the potentially harmful metabolites produced by position 16 hydroxylation. This could explain why postmenopausal women with the highest circulating estradiol (E2) levels have the greatest frequency of breast cancer. (Earlier evidence from epidemiological and animal studies indicated a causal relationship between high estradiol levels and breast cancer risk in postmenopausal women.[29] However, subsequent research has revealed that these issues are more complex. Studies in women have reported that high testosterone levels may be more accurate than estradiol for predicting older women at risk for breast cancer,[30] that increased sex steroid levels do **not** translate into a measurable increased breast cancer risk in postmenopausal women with the CYP1 genotype,[31] and even that estradiol has either no effect or even a positive influence in breast cancer progression and mortality.[32,33])

Stress and environmental xenobiotics are just two of many external agents that can influence intercellular communication and either decrease or increase a person's risk of age-related diseases. Common constituents of the diet, including both macro- and micronutrients, can also influence cellular messenging and genetic expression.[34]

Chronic Infection as a Trigger for Intercellular Communication Dysfunction

Research clearly indicates that infectious organisms can modify intercellular communication and signal transduction, and shift the physiological state toward inflammation and risk of heart disease and cerebrovascular disorders. A few examples include the following:

- Chronic *Helicobacter pylori* infection is associated not only with peptic ulcers, but also with increased heart disease risk.[35] Possibly because it upregulates intercellular agents involved with chronic inflammation, chronic *H. pylori* infection represents an independent risk factor for cerebrovascular and ischemic heart disease.[36] Interestingly, however, one study compared *H. pylori* patients who had been treated with those who had not, and found that eradication treatment had "no effect on metabolic and inflammatory parameters."[37] Current knowledge does not yet rise to the level of demonstrating a causal relationship, nor does it definitely implicate the inflammatory pathways as the link between *H. pylori* infection and heart disease.[38]
- Infection with *Chlamydia pneumoniae* has also been associated with increased risk of heart disease and cell signals related to inflammation.[39,40]
- Individuals with certain genetic susceptibilities, such as the apo E4 allele, have increased risk of expressing dementia (including Alzheimer's dementia) as a consequence of chronic infection with the *Herpes simplex* virus.[41,42]

All of this information indicates that many substances and external agents can initiate altered cellular communication and signal transduction, which can shift a cell into an alarm state associated with altered function and later-stage disease risk.

The Influence of Nutrients on Gene Expression and Intercellular Communication

In the past, nutritionists and other healthcare professionals believed the only role of macronutrients (protein, carbohydrate, and fat) was to provide calories, with little or no effect on the regulatory cycles of the cell. This assumption is changing rapidly, and practitioners of all disciplines must be able to adapt their clinical practice to the new information. Research indicates that various amino acids in protein, fatty acids in dietary fat, and certain types of carbohydrate affect cell recognition, receptor site function, and genetic expression. Discovery of novel nuclear receptors is increasing and rapidly gaining biological and medical significance. These nuclear receptors are members of a family of supergenes used to control expression of important genes under different physiological circumstances. Four examples of dietary components that interact with receptors and activate their gene regulatory networks are: specific fatty acids,[43] antioxidants,[44] vitamin A,[45] and trace minerals.[46]

Fatty acids. Omega-3, omega-6, omega-9, medium-chain, and long-chain fatty acids are known to influence cellular membrane structure and function. As a consequence of altered structure and function of membranes, receptor affinity for intercellular mediators can also be altered, thereby affecting signal transduction. Beyond that, among the most important nutrients serving as intercellular communication agents and influencing the control of gene expression are fatty acids that interact with the peroxisome proliferator activated receptors (PPARs).[47,48] Different fatty acids, members of the omega-6 or omega-3 families, have different influences on the PPARs, as do their metabolic by-products, prostaglandins, and leukotrienes.[49] In animal studies, dietary n-3 and n-6 polyunsaturated fatty acids have been found to influence expression of the cyclooxygenase-1 and -2 genes that are involved in prostaglandin biosynthesis[50] and levels of P2I^{ras} protein. These studies demonstrate that dietary n-6 unsaturated fatty acids can upregulate expression of cyclooxygenase-2 and, to some extent, cyclooxygenase-1, which can increase inflammation. On the other hand, n-3 fatty acids did not increase cyclooxygenase-2 activity.[51,52]

Fatty acids have been shown to positively affect the postprandial lipoprotein cascade in diabetic patients,[53] a gene expression pattern that may hold promise for dietary and nutritional treatments that could affect the high rate of heart disease in diabetic patients.

Dietary fat also plays a role in this process via the absorption of fat-soluble vitamins. By its own composition, it can also modify the expression of nuclear receptors that, in turn, can influence, for example, thyroid hormone activity. Some important aspects of this complex pathway are depicted in Figure 32.1.

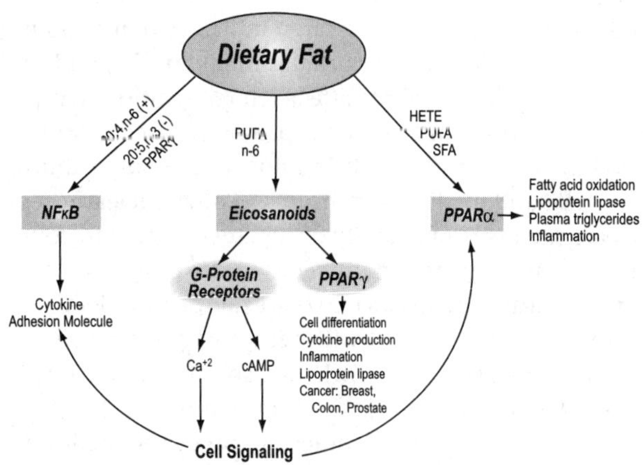

Figure 32.1 **Influence of dietary fat on cell signaling**

Studies indicate that DHA, a member of the omega-3 fatty acid family, increases TSH concentration in animals.[54] Substances that increase PPAR activity improve thyroid function, and this influence may occur as a consequence of the effects of T_3 on induction of enzymes involved with mitochondrial activity.[55] Some of the effects of T_3 on mitochondrial activity may occur as a consequence of activation of PPARs located in the mitochondrial matrix.[56]

In 1998, investigators of dietary prevention of cancer at the Division of Nutritional Carcinogenesis at the American Health Foundation found that omega-3 eicosapentaenoic acid (EPA, fish oil concentrate) inhibited the expression of farnesyl protein transferase, a critical step in oncogenesis.[57] EPA, therefore, helped prevent colon tumor development in animals. Subsequent studies by other researchers seemed to identify the effect of the fish oil as an ability to differentially modulate Ras activation, without affecting farnesyl protein transferase.[58,59] Although the precise mechanisms of action are not yet clear, this research opens the door for improved understanding of the potential role of specific macronutrients as cell-signaling substances in modifying gene expression.

Antioxidants. Control of cellular physiology and response to various external signals are both related to the expression of various substances that interact with the genes. A principal example is nuclear factor-kappaB (NFκB). NFκB regulates a number of genes that are necessary for normal immune responses and secretion of intercellular communication agents involved in the inflammatory process. Included among those agents are interleukin-2 (IL-2), interleukin-6 (IL-6), and tumor necrosis factor-α (TNF-α). Activation of T lymphocytes to engage in inflammatory response requires at least two signals: one that stimulates an increase in intercellular calcium and another that stimulates enzymatic processes, including kinases.

Similarly, evidence indicates that NFκB is activated by a number of intracellular signals. Hydrogen peroxide and other reactive oxygen species induce T cell signals, and modification of the reduction/oxidation (redox) potential within a cell modifies NFκB activation.[60] As the cellular environment shifts toward oxidative chemistry and away from a balance between oxidation and reduction, the presence of oxidized species in the cell (including glutathione disulfide and lipid peroxides) increases. Proteins become oxidatively damaged as well, with the production of such proteins as oxidized low-density lipoprotein. This oxidative shift in intercellular chemistry promotes the transcription from the genes of adhesion molecules that participate in the inflammatory process, including the intercellular adhesion molecules (ICAMs), endothelial leukocyte adhesion molecules, and vascular adhesion molecules, as well as cytokines.

Strong evidence suggests that the shift of intracellular redox toward an oxidative state is a principal process that signals the genes to shift their transcription and move into an "alarm state." Knowledge of the increased level of NFκB associated with oxidative stress and its subsequent association with the expression of cell adhesion molecules and interleukins forms an advancing understanding of how inflammation results from external signals of alarm, infection, or toxicity.

Oxidative signals are capable of inducing NFκB-binding activity. Glutathione is a principal intracellular redox buffering agent that helps protect against oxidative stress. As glutathione is consumed, and glutathione disulfide is produced as a consequence of oxidative exposure, NFκB is activated and gene expression signals are modified toward inflammation and alarm.

A number of antioxidant substances play an important role along with glutathione to maintain proper intracellular redox. One that is under current investigation is α-lipoic acid. R-α-lipoic acid occurs naturally as a prosthetic group in α-keto acid dehydrogenase complexes of the mitochondria. However, investigators have found that α-lipoic acid affects cellular metabolic processes *in vitro* and that it has the ability to alter the redox status of cells and interact with glutathione and other antioxidants to help maintain redox buffering.[61] Most of the clinical studies to date with lipoic acid have been done with intravenous administration, but the evidence indicates that agents that improve cellular redox, such as lipoic acid and N-acetylcysteine, can reduce inflammatory signaling.

In 1998, researchers conducted human clinical trials with intravenous α-lipoic acid supplementation in the treatment of various types of inflammatory conditions involving altered intercellular communication. Among the conditions studied are alcohol-induced liver damage, mushroom poisoning, metal intoxication, and carbon tetrachloride poisoning. Doses of 600 mg per day of lipoic acid have shown positive therapeutic value in the management of insulin-resistant individuals as well. Lipoic acid has a hypoglycemic effect, and it helps improve insulin sensitivity and lowers the risk of diabetic polyneuropathy in type 2 diabetics.[62]

Because these processes are associated with NFκB activation and oxidative stress reactions, the expression of ICAM-1 and VCAM-1, which is induced by TNF-α, is inhibited by increasing activity of glutathione peroxidase and production of reduced glutathione.[63] In part, this may explain why glutathione-related antioxidant defense mechanisms help prevent human atherosclerotic plaques.[64] The influence of antioxidants in preventing atherosclerosis and other diseases of aging may not be as simple as a free radical antioxidant effect. It may, instead, be mediated through a complex interaction of cellular communication agents like NFκB, their relationship to genetic expression of interleukins and adhesion molecules, and their subsequent relationship to white cell attachment to mucosal surfaces and the origin of disease.

In support of this model, it has been reported that vitamin E inhibits the production of cell adhesion molecules and, therefore, also inhibits the attachment of monocytes to cultured human endothelial cells.[65] In 1994, researchers found that the cardiac drug probucol (which is known to act as an antioxidant) and N-acetylcysteine also inhibited the elaboration of adhesion molecules and the attachment of monocytes to human endothelial cells.

These studies may provide a mechanistic explanation for the clinical observation that antioxidant supplements help block the loss of endothelial function in healthy subjects with normal cholesterol who have consumed a high-fat meal. In a 1997 randomized clinical trial,[66] 20 individuals with normal cholesterol, who were presumed to be healthy, were administered one of three breakfasts. They received either a high-fat meal, a low-fat meal, or a high-fat meal following pretreatment with oral administration of 1000 mg of vitamin C and 800 IU of vitamin E. A subgroup of 10 subjects also ate the low-fat meal following the same vitamin pretreatment. High-resolution ultrasound assessed flow-mediated (endothelium-dependent) brachial artery vasodilation, measured as percent diameter change before the meal and hourly for six hours following each meal. In this study, flow-mediated vasodilation fell significantly in the high-fat breakfast group. In the low-fat meal group or the high-fat meal group with antioxidant vitamin supplements, there was no such drop. The same researchers published a similar study in 2003,[67] demonstrating that dietary interventions (e.g., a fruit and vegetable concentrate)—with or without supplemented phytonutrients—could "reverse the immediate adverse impact of high-fat meals on flow-mediated vasoactivity ... ."

The authors conclude that a single high-fat meal transiently reduces endothelial function for up to four hours in healthy subjects with normal cholesterol, probably through the accumulation of triglyceride-rich lipoproteins and the subsequent effects on the elaboration of adhesion molecules. This decrease was blocked both by dietary intervention and by pretreatment with antioxidant supplements (vitamin C and vitamin E, in the study described above), and, in another study, postprandial supplementation with vitamin C,[68] suggesting an oxidant/antioxidant mechanism and the potential interrelationship with NFκB/IκB modulation of cellular communication agents such as ICAMs and VCAMs. Reduced superoxide dismutase and glutathione peroxidase activities have also been associated with increased risk of endothelial injury.[69] This is potentially related to their role in quenching the cellular oxidant superoxide, thereby reducing the contribution of oxidative stress to inflammatory signaling. (This topic is addressed further in Chapter 30.)

Vitamin A. Similarly, vitamin A is required for regulation of various receptors. Investigators at the University of Alabama reported in 1998 that vitamin A strongly interacts with the proinflammatory molecules interleukin-4 and interferon-γ to regulate the expression of an immunoglobulin receptor.[70] Their data suggest vitamin A may be required, therefore, for the regulation of secretory IgA transport in response to mucosal infections.

Vitamin A has also demonstrated both an ability to inhibit expression of TNF-α and iNOS in animals,[71] and a regulatory effect on human intercellular adhesion molecule-1 (ICAM-1).[72,73]

Although the mechanisms responsible for the anti-inflammatory effect of retinoic acid are still uncertain, researchers are looking for the underlying explanation.[74]

Trace elements. The trace element zinc also plays a very important role in modifying gene expression through its ability to serve as an intercellular messenger. In animals, zinc deficiency increases the output of hypothalamic neuropeptide Y and may explain why appetite is suppressed in zinc deficiency and why anorexia results.[75,76]

The trace element selenium is also a powerful signaling agent. In a prospective study in 1998,[77] investigators at the Harvard School of Public Health and at Harvard Medical School used the level of selenium in human toenails as an indicator of selenium status. (The use of toenail and plasma levels as biomarkers of selenium exposure has been validated in further studies.[78]) In this study, low selenium level was associated with increased risk of advanced prostate cancer in males. This study supports a previous report from the cancer study group at the Arizona Cancer Center in 1963, in which oral selenium supplementation at 200 mg per day significantly reduced the incidence of and mortality from carcinomas of several sites, including prostate.[79] The importance of selenium in cancer prevention has been validated by numerous additional studies in the intervening years.[80,81,82]

Selenium is an essential nutrient. One of its major roles is as a component of the antioxidant enzyme glutathione peroxidase, which is involved with the recycling of glutathione disulfide to reduced glutathione. In healthy individuals, glutathione is recycled very rapidly and exists principally in the reduced state. As an individual ages or becomes ill, his/her reduced glutathione level decreases, and the amount of oxidized glutathione disulfide increases. This change in status may indicate an increase in oxidative stress that cannot be accommodated by the existing antioxidant systems.[83]

Insufficient selenium could be one contributor to reduced antioxidant protection. Although selenium does not participate in this process as an intercellular communication agent, it indirectly relates to the influence of an enzyme engaged in establishing proper cellular reduction/oxidation potential. Redox potential, in turn, has been found to be an important determinant of intercellular communication. Selenium has also been found to be the central mineral atom in the deiodinase enzyme that converts thyroid hormone T_4 to T_3. As such, its deficiency may play a role in secondary hypothyroidism.

As reported in a 2005 review, "selenium is capable of exerting multiple actions on endocrine systems by modifying the expression of at least 30 selenoproteins. ... Selenoenzymes are capable of modifying cell function by acting as antioxidants and modifying redox status and thyroid hormone metabolism."[84] The authors point out that the most important factor in selenoprotein expression is selenium supply—a fact that is critically important in thyroid function.

Altered Cellular Communication and the Risk of Various Diseases

The 1998 Nobel Prize in Medicine was awarded to three researchers who discovered the role of nitric oxide in physiology. One of the recipients was Ferid Murad, MD, PhD. At the Fourth International Symposium on Functional Medicine in 1997, Dr. Murad presented information showing that many chronic illnesses are associated with imbalances in nitric oxide production in their early stages.

Nitric oxide (NO) is associated with apparently contradictory actions—both proinflammatory effects and protective influences have been identified.[85,86] NO, an example of a second-signal messenger, alters levels or types of cellular messengers and can play a key role in triggering effects that are associated with a variety of diseases (cutting across numerous ICD-9 diagnostic codes). According to Dr. Murad in 1996, "NO can be recognized as an intracellular second messenger, a local substance for regulation of neighboring cells, a neurotransmitter in central and peripheral neurons, and perhaps a hormone that can act at distant sites and has been shown to have beneficial or deleterious biological effects, depending on its concentration, the system, and the cellular environment."[87] In particular, diseases associated with altered nitric oxide elaboration and physiology (both adverse and beneficial) include atherosclerosis,[88] AIDS,[89,90] cancer,[91] schizophrenia,[92] and certain inflammatory conditions.[93,94]

Nitric oxide has several dichotomous effects within the stages of cancer. Chronic inflammation can lead to production of chemical intermediates, including nitric oxide, as part of the inflammatory cascade. This process, in turn, can mediate damage to DNA. Nitric oxide also appears to be involved with both tumor-promoting and tumoricidal activities.[95,96] Understanding the balance and activity of nitric oxide within the context of other cellular communication agents associated with the immune and the inflammatory process may help clinicians develop therapies that focus on ameliorating the cause of the disease.

Grouping dysfunctions on the basis of altered cellular communication may be much more useful for understanding the predisposition to disease than is the categorization of disease from a taxonomic perspective. By understanding the triggers that influence elaboration of intercellular mediators and how these mediators influence signs and symptoms, the clinician may be better able to identify and treat the causes of disease, rather than just the symptoms. Once the nature of the imbalance of the cellular communication agent has been identified and evaluated for activity levels, its function may be improved by modification of lifestyle, environment, nutritional pharmacology, or specific medications. For example, supplemental use of L-arginine and other nitric oxide stimulators or inhibitors appears to modify nitric oxide production under some conditions.[97,98,99]

Administration of the nitric oxide donor S-nitroso-N-acetylpenicillamine reduced the severity of myocardial injury in animals with experimental atherosclerosis that were fed a high-cholesterol, high-fat diet.[100] Nitric oxide protects against the attachment of leukocytes and monocytes to the vascular endothelium, and it helps prevent the early stages of atherogenesis associated with hypercholesterolemia.[101] In an animal model using pigs, L-arginine supplementation as a stimulator of nitric oxide production reduced endothelial inflammation and the elaboration of inflammatory messengers during ischemic episodes.[102]

In a human clinical trial in 1998, 26 patients without significant coronary artery disease, as measured by coronary angiography and intravascular ultrasound, were blindly randomized to either oral L-arginine, 3 g tid, or a placebo. Endothelium-dependent coronary blood flow reserve to acetylcholine administration was assessed at baseline and after six months of therapy. After six months, the coronary blood flow in response to acetylcholine in subjects who were taking L-arginine increased compared with the placebo group. The results reached statistical significance ($p<.05$) and were associated with a decrease in the plasma level of vascular adhesion molecules and an improvement in patients' symptom scores in the L-arginine treatment group, compared to the placebo group.[103]

Many other diseases associated with aging also exhibit altered nitric oxide dynamics. They include the metastatic events of cancer, inflammatory destruction of the joints in arthritis,[104,105] glial cell activation and dementia,[106] and vascular and secondary side effects associated with type 2 diabetes.[107] Evaluating altered intercellular communication by looking at nitric oxide alone, therefore, may provide insight into a disease process that cuts across many conditions. That insight can be lost if one examines only the end-stage disease.

Neurotransmitters as Intercellular Communication Agents

The first and second signal messengers of inflammation and cellular adhesion are not the only substances with a relationship to oxidative stress mechanisms and mitochondrial function. An array of biologically active peptides with molecular weights between 1 and 5 Kd also has neurotransmission and neuroregulatory effects and communicates with the immune system. These peptides are predominantly distributed in the nervous system and gut of most animals. The significance of these patterns of distribution is still uncertain, but one possibility is that these molecules represent the interface between the external environment and the internal physiological process. Therefore, they are information molecules that translate external events to the internal environment.[108]

Within the brain, the anatomic localization of peptides is most notably associated with those regions concerned with neuroendocrine and autonomic regulation. These neuropeptides cross the blood/brain barrier and, therefore, can influence the activity of both glia and neurons. Before these discoveries, almost no one believed that intact peptides could cross the blood/brain barrier. This erroneous belief was based on unsupported opinions rather than on substantiated data.[109] In the evolution of our understanding of peptides, we now recognize that these small molecular weight, protein-like molecules can be transported intact across both the gastrointestinal mucosa and the blood/brain barrier. Therefore, food-derived, peptide-like molecules may, in fact, influence neurotransmission and immune function through mechanisms not directly related to allergy or traditional immunoglobulin-mediated processes.[110,111,112]

It is also now recognized that certain food proteins—including gluten from grains and casein from dairy products—can be partially digested to yield bioactive peptides such as gliadorphin and casomorphin that have opioid-like activities in the central nervous system.[113,114]

In the 1970s, while she was working at the National Institutes of Health, Dr. Candace Pert discovered peptide binding sites for endorphin substances on the surface of white blood cells. This discovery pointed to a connection between brain chemistry and immune function. From this discovery came a strong impetus for the further development of mind/body medicine, in which the distinction between external and internal influences on physiological, cognitive/emotional, and physical functioning is not as important as the interplay among all these elements.[115,116]

The field of psychoneuroimmunology developed from this exciting series of discoveries in basic neurophysiology and immunology. The mechanisms by which stress, toxins, thoughts, attitudes, and beliefs influence physiological function and later disease are beginning to find a mechanistic explanation. Figure 32.2 describes the increasing understanding of how cellular communication agents interconnect external phenomenology, as taken in through the senses, with internal physiological function.[117]

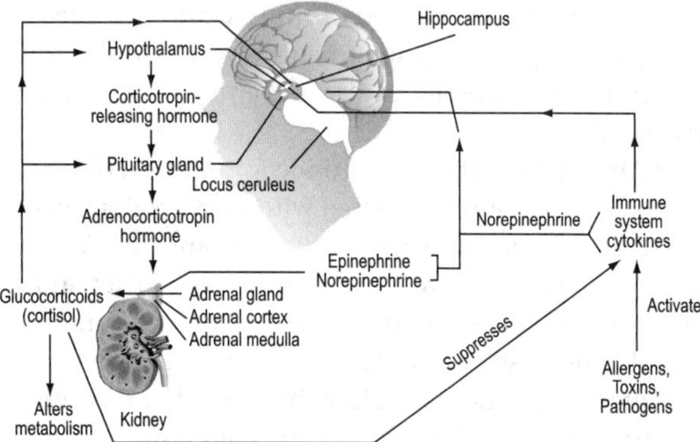

Figure 32.2 **Interactions between the nervous and immune systems**

Summary

As shown in Table 32.1, there are many representative classes of intercellular communication agents (hormonal, neurotransmitter, and immune-modulating molecules). They are released as a well-orchestrated response to both internal and external factors and stressors, with the clear intent to maintain total organism stability and adaptability. This maintenance of stability is an active process for which the term homeodynamics has been coined from the original model of homeostasis. The responses can be either negative or positive. It has become increasingly apparent that many chronic diseases result from failures in these regulatory processes. As stated by Dr. Gary Darland in Chapter 15: "Evolution has resulted in the elaboration of sophisticated mechanisms to maintain cells (and whole organisms) in an optimal state. The systems are not foolproof. If balance is significantly disturbed, it can be difficult to return to a state of grace."

Cellular Messaging, Part II—Tissue Sensitivity and Intracellular Response

Jeffrey S. Bland, PhD and David S. Jones, MD

Introduction

A full exploration of the interface of neurochemical and endocrine function (the neuroendocrine system) would require another book. Because this area is so broad, we will focus on a few topics that are particularly relevant to clinical care and that exemplify the complex actions and interactions characteristic of the neuroendocrine system as a whole. In this chapter, we will primarily address thyroid signaling hormones, stress, adrenal function and the HPA axis, growth hormone and insulin-like growth factor-1, and melatonin in the context of the menopausal female neuroendocrine system.

Establishing a healthy balance of hormonal and neurotransmitter signaling function should include consideration of a number of critical activities and mechanisms: production of the messenger substance; transport of the messenger substance; tissue sensitivity to the message; intracellular response to the message; and detoxification and excretion of the messenger substance. In the previous discussion, we focused on internal and external triggers promoting the production of the messenger substances. Here, the focus is on transport, tissue sensitivity, and intracellular response to the messenger substance and to some specifics of detoxification and excretion of messenger molecules.

We have chosen our topics very deliberately; thyroid signaling hormones, stress, adrenal function, and the HPA axis illustrate the dynamic interplay among the functional factors that create balance or imbalance within endocrine system signaling. Clinicians too often consider only one or two of these factors in developing a patient-management strategy. A clinician who measures the level of a specific messenger substance in a biological fluid and finds it to be low, often makes the assumption that this substance should be replaced with exogenous hormone or neurotransmitter repletion, either natural or synthetic. However, the low level of a substance may, in fact, reflect a series of disordered feedback steps related to transport, tissue sensitivity, and metabolism. Supplementing the substance without inspecting these other factors may aggravate the imbalance, producing even more dramatic signs and/or symptoms. The converse is also true. When a substance is present in an elevated level in a biological fluid, one might assume too much is being produced and an antagonist is needed to block its secretion or function. This assumption might also be inappropriate. Excess production of the substance may be a consequence of reduced tissue sensitivity, as in the case of the hyperinsulinemia/insulin resistance syndrome.

Assessing and Balancing Neuroendocrine Mediators

We will explore ways of assessing the symphony of various neuroendocrine mediators. Developing various approaches to normalizing their balance might involve the use of secretagogues, hormone precursors, hormones themselves, tissue-sensitizing substances, agents that improve bioavailability and/or transport of the substance, or substances that initiate improved metabolism and excretion. As noted in the previous essay, healthy neuroendocrine balance is a very complex issue.

In an ideal world, we would base our understanding of neuroendocrine function on the results of large prospective studies in which a comprehensive panel of neuroendocrine mediators had been measured sequentially throughout the course of a large cohort of representative individuals' lives, recording as well the changes in health patterns during the study. We would have measurements of thyroid congeners, cortisol, dehydroepiandrosterone, progesterone, estrogen, testosterone, estrogen and testosterone metabolites, melatonin, growth hormone, insulin-like growth factor-1, noradrenaline, serotonin, dopamine, leptin, and tumor necrosis factor-α (TNF-α), over decades of living and a variety of circumstances. Using this information, we could understand the relationship of neuroendocrine modulators to central questions of healthy or unhealthy aging. Unfortunately, in this less-than-ideal world, these studies have not been done. Therefore, our assessment will necessarily depend on a variety of inferential and incomplete data that we must weave together to guide us in making decisions to support healthy aging, vis-à-vis hormonal, neurotransmitter, and immuno-modulating messaging molecules.

A Changing View of Neuroendocrine Signaling and Hormone Balance

Indeed, data from the hypothetical prospective studies described above may never be available. Even if they were, the conclusions that could be drawn *for a specific individual* would likely be equivocal because of the unique variations in his/her polymorphisms and resultant physiology and biochemistry. From midlife on, individuals, in consultation with their healthcare provider(s), make decisions about managing their health concerns based on less-than-complete information. These therapeutic plans are often based on the assumption that aging is a disease process and can be managed like illness (single disease with a focused pharmacological intervention). However, according to the model presented in this book, to assess neuroendocrine function, we must take into account the web-like interaction of multiple messaging processes that cut across discrete organ systems and function through complex feedback control systems.

Using this model, we should, for example, view estrogen and progesterone not solely as reproductive hormones in the female, but rather as signaling substances that also affect function in the central and peripheral nervous system,[118] the musculoskeletal system,[119,120] adipocyte physiology, and immunological response.[121] Receptor sites for steroid hormones have been identified on the surface of virtually every type of cell in the body.[122] It would, therefore, be safe to say that steroid hormones represent a component of the body's overall cell signaling processes and influence the way tissues, organs, and organ systems respond to their environment.[123,124]

Our perception of neuroendocrine function is rapidly changing. Within the past decade, many nuclear receptors have been identified, along with a series of agonist and antagonist substances—hormone transporters whose important physiological function had previously not been recognized.[125,126,127] For example, we have moved beyond the belief that the steroid-based endocrine system is principally the sex steroid hormone-modulated pathways.[128,129] We now understand the importance of an array of collateral activities of substances, including dehydroepiandrosterone, omega-3 fatty acids, and lipoic acid. This improved understanding of neuroendocrine mediators will help clinicians design programs to balance function and promote healthy aging. Function of the endocrine system plays a central role in defining many aspects of the natural, biological aging process.

Also, woven into this complex interchange is the oxidative/reductive balance of the system. The process of free radical production can damage mitochondrial DNA, which is approximately 10 times more susceptible to oxidative damage than nuclear DNA, and the majority of oxidants are produced in the mitochondria. As mitochondrial DNA (mtDNA) undergoes injury, the daughter mitochondria become less able to provide energy production for the cell, and redox imbalances result. These imbalances can be seen as altered cell messages that may affect both neuroendocrine and immune functions. These alterations can act as feed-forward mechanisms leading to unhealthy aging, with changes in neuroendocrine function resulting in altered cellular energy production. This, in turn, produces more free radicals, further damaging mtDNA, and thus continuing the "aging" of the neuroendocrine system.

The contribution of neuroendocrine imbalance to aging may be, in part, a manifestation of a fundamental process of altered reduction/oxidation potential within the mitochondrion, creating cellular messages that alter the expression of the genome. As cellular physiology changes, different messages are expressed from the genome, cellular debris accumulates, and the immune system may become sensitive to the body itself. The result can be autoimmunity disorders. Autoimmune diseases like rheumatoid arthritis, systemic lupus erythematosus, and myasthenia gravis are immune dysfunctions associated with alteration in neuroendocrine function that increase in prevalence with age and are associated with unhealthy aging.

In the early 1990s, a study from the University of Pisa in Italy reported that healthy centenarians had serum plasma titers of thyroid autoantibodies similar to controls aged less than 50.[130] This observation, and other supportive research, suggests that one principle of healthy aging is to avoid becoming "allergic to yourself" by lowering the load of antigenic substances that generate immune vigilance and cross-reactivity with products of the endocrine glands.

No single explanation to adequately address all aspects of biological aging has been developed.[131] The recognition is emerging that accelerated biological aging occurs in concert with a variety of physiological changes in the immune, endocrine, musculoskeletal, neurological, and cardiovascular systems. All these changes may interrelate with fundamental processes at the cellular level, altered gene expression, modification of intracellular reduction/oxidation balance, and alterations in neuroendocrine messenging.

Neuroendocrine System as Indicator of Cellular Changes in Aging

The neuroendocrine system may be a barometer for changes occurring at the cellular level that reflect aspects of the aging processes. Changes in neuroendocrine function may reflect underlying alterations in cellular physiology associated with unhealthy aging, rather than these changes themselves being the primary cause of aging. The inclusion of these interactions brings us full circle in the development of a more complete model of neuroendocrine and immune system interchanges. Often, it is not possible to establish cause/effect relationships; but it is clear that changes in neuroendocrine function throughout life are associated with significant changes in physiology and vitality.

Therefore, in this chapter we will address the neuroendocrine system, not as the primary seat of aging, but as a reflective component of the overall process of the body and its various rhythms associated with functional status. We should not assume a neuroendocrine system that will promote healthy aging in a 50-year-old is the same as that required for health in a 15-, 25-, or 35-year-old. Changes in endocrine function occur throughout life and are orchestrated by the temporal characteristics of gene expression. These functional changes may have specific advantages at specific times. For example, aggression is often associated with youthful males whose androgenic hormone levels are typically much higher than in older-age males for whom reason, judgment, and control of passion become dominant survival features. Characteristics advantageous in youth for reproduction and protecting the young may become disadvantageous in older age when reproduction is not vital and maintaining function becomes more important. Thus, it is important to evaluate neuroendocrine system function with the objective of achieving healthy balance for individuals of a specific age.

The neuroendocrine system translates sensory input from the environment into physiochemical actions that modify the phenotype. Complex interactions take place among all the organs involved in neuroendocrine function. One should be cautious in evaluating neuroendocrine function based on simple, single-point analysis of one component of this web. There is a certain rhythmic pattern to neuroendocrine function, with cycles that are daily, monthly, yearly, and even longer. These cycles may be tied to environmental events such as the full moon, solar spots, and perhaps even low-level electromagnetic fields. All these complexities make evaluation of neuroendocrine function challenging. Taking a single blood or saliva sample of two or three hormones and trying to understand the rhythmic nature of endocrine balance in the individual may be overly simplistic and can lead to inappropriate clinical decisions.

Evaluating Thyroid Function

A common clinical presentation of patients with age-related functional changes of the neuroendocrine/immune system is *altered thyroid function*, although a number of studies have demonstrated that in the elderly the clinical picture is often atypical and misattributed to aging or disease.[132,133] We have chosen this system to more fully illustrate the model of a functional neuroendocrinological investigation. Typical symptoms of low thyroid function include low energy, cold hands and feet, fatigue, hypercholesterolemia, muscle pain, depression, and cognitive deficits, although in the elderly these complaints can also be related to cardiovascular, gastrointestinal, and neuropsychiatric disorders.[134] The conditions of either hypo- or hyperthyroidism[135] are often related to altered thyroid hormone sensitivity and cellular response.

As mentioned earlier, maintaining thyroid hormone function throughout the aging process may be an important hallmark of healthy aging.[136,137] In 1992, a group of investigators from the National Research Council in Italy performed a series of studies to examine the thyroid's importance during aging. They compared parameters of thyroid function in 34 healthy centenarians, ranging in age from 100 to 108 years, to that of 40 younger subjects, aged 70 to 85. They found a significantly lower level of thyroid antibodies in the sera of healthy centenarians than in the sera of 75- to 80-year-olds who had varying degrees of chronic illness. This observation led the authors to suggest that the absence of circulating thyroid autoantibodies in healthy centenarians is not mere coincidence.[138] Since unhealthy aging is associated with a progressively increasing prevalence of organ-specific and non-organ-specific autoantibodies,[139,140] the absence of these antibodies may represent a reduced risk in older age for cardiovascular disease and other chronic age-related disorders,[141] and therefore could be a hallmark of age-related healthy neuroendocrine-immune signaling.

Subclinical Hypothyroidism: A Case Report

Subclinical hypothyroidism represents, for many individuals, the first signs of thyroid hormone dysfunction. A case report in *The New England Journal of Medicine* in 2001 described a 59-year-old woman in whom routine screening revealed serum thyrotropin (TSH) of 7 mU per liter. (Normal reference range for this case study was reported as 1-5 mU per liter.) Her symptoms, although mild, had been present for more than 10 years.

The results of the physical examination were normal, except that her thyroid was small and firm, with a slightly irregular surface. Her serum cholesterol level was 220 mg per deciliter; her low-density lipoprotein cholesterol was 140 mg per deciliter; and a test for antibodies against thyroperoxidase (TPO) was positive. She had difficulty losing weight. The author of this clinical case presentation, David S. Cooper, MD, asked if treatment with thyroxin replacement therapy should be initiated in this patient.[142] The answer to this was a conditional "yes."

From a functional medicine perspective, that answer begs the question of how to more fully assess a patient with a diagnosis of borderline subclinical thyroid dysfunction before asking the downstream question about hormone replacement therapy (HRT). This patient may be at risk for age-related chronic diseases as a consequence of imbalances in the hypothalamus/pituitary/thyroid axis; the antecedents and triggers to her elevated TSH require further elucidation. Recent evidence suggests that jumping into thyroid hormone replacement therapy before thoroughly evaluating thyroid hormone metabolism may be inappropriate.[143,144] Additionally, a placebo-controlled trial of the administration of 100 mg of L-thyroxine to patients who expressed symptoms of borderline hypothyroidism (*cf.* this 59-year-old woman) found thyroxine HRT to be no more effective than placebo in improving cognitive function, mood, or well being.[145]

Low serum TSH level in conjunction with normal concentrations of circulating thyroid hormones is associated with increased mortality from all causes in people 60 years or older.[146] This does not necessarily mean that the increased mortality is related to a primary hypothyroidism requiring thyroid hormone replacement. The increased mortality may reflect altered hypothalamic or pituitary function or alteration in metabolism or cell signaling of thyroid hormones at the peripheral tissue. The diagnosis of low serum TSH is simply a first step in the much more complex evaluation of function within this system.

Laboratory Thyroid Screening

Laboratory blood testing has often been used as the *sine qua non* in determining hypo- or hyperthyroidism in a patient. The TSH test (aka: thyroid-stimulating hormone or thyrotropin hormone test), free T_4, free T_3, and thyroid peroxidase activity (TPO) tests have become a routine part of a panel for evaluating primary and secondary thyroid hormone dysfunction.[147]

Considerable controversy exists regarding whether the laboratory in and of itself can define borderline thyroid dysfunctions[148,149] and, if so, what is the most sensitive analyte(s) to evaluate. A study in 2001 evaluated TSH concentrations as a potential first-line test of thyroid function. Using a combination of TSH and thyroxine (free T_4) assays, investigators analyzed 56,000 tests for a population of 471,000 people over a period of 12 months. The study identified 17 patients with secondary hypothyroidism whose thyrotropin concentrations were within the normal reference range (0.17-3.20 mU/L). In most cases, TSH proved useful for evaluating pituitary function regulation of thyroid hormone secretion from the thyroid gland. But in this study, it did not pick up secondary hypothyroidism and related disorders, such as thyroid hormone resistance.[150]

Baisier and colleagues suggest the 24-hour urinary excretion of free T_3 may also prove beneficial in defining patients with functional borderline hypothyroidism.[151] However, these authors agree that the evidence indicates TSH measurement, free T_4, and serum free T_3 all have clinical limitations in their ability to identify all cases of thyroid hormone dysfunction.

Cardiac laboratory thyroid screening. In subclinical hypothyroidism (SH), impaired diastolic function has been documented at rest and on effort, while systolic dysfunction has only been assessed on effort. A study was performed to further assess systolic function at rest in SH and to ascertain whether cardiac dysfunction could precede TSH increase in euthyroid patients with a high risk of developing SH. All subjects underwent pulsed wave tissue Doppler imaging (PWTDI) to accurately quantify the global and regional left ventricular function. PWTDI proved to be a sensitive technique that allowed detection of both diastolic and systolic abnormalities, not only in patients with SH, but also in euthyroid subjects with a high risk of developing thyroid failure. Futhermore, the significant correlations of several PWTDI indices with serum free T_3 and TSH concentrations strongly supported the concept of a continuum of slight thyroid failure in autoimmune thyroiditis extending to subjects with serum TSH still within the normal range.[152] Other studies in the cardiac laboratory have substantiated the importance of these cardiac lab modalities in the evaluation of SH.[153]

Alternatives to laboratory testing. According to Damien Downing, MD, an important clinical adjunctive is to approach functional thyroid problems from careful evaluation of the patient, not simply treating the laboratory test. The combination of good clinical acumen and a functional assessment based on patient-centered review, combined with laboratory information, provides a much more robust and reliable review of dysfunctions of the hypothalamic-pituitary-thyroid (HPT) axis.[154]

Additional criteria for evaluating thyroid dysfunction. The following nine symptoms appear to be among the most reliable indicators of dysfunction in the HPT axis:

1. Fatigue, usually persistent, especially on waking; less toward the evening, with slow recovery
2. Depression; psychological melancholia with a tendency toward depression

3. Coldness, deep as well as peripheral
4. Elevated cholesterol, generally seen as LDL cholesterol increases
5. Muscle cramps and pain in the calves, thighs, and upper arms
6. Constipation: hard bowel movements and decreased frequency (at most, every two days)
7. Arthritis; rheumatoid-like pain in the joints, muscle swelling, and muscle pain
8. Neurological symptoms, such as prolonged Achilles tendon reflex time
9. Easy bruising and/or evidence of clotting defects[155,156,157]

Using this extended list of clinical signs and symptoms associated with dysfunction of the HPT axis,[158,159] it is possible to hypothesize that subclinical hypothyroidism may be more common in a population of patients with early signs of age-related diseases than most practitioners realize. For example, elevated TSH concentrations have reportedly been found in nearly 10% of women older than 60 years.[160]

Prevalence of Subclinical Thyroid Dysfunction

It is apparent from this discussion that subclinical thyroid dysfunction is common in individuals with symptoms of unhealthy aging. It may be seen across a number of organ systems, including peripheral nerve dysfunction, depression, increased seasonal affective disorder (SAD), memory deficits, elevated LDL levels and risk of atherosclerosis,[161,162] skeletal muscle problems including pain, sarcopenia, and fibromyalgia, and exacerbation of allergic disorders and sleep problems.

Thyroid dysfunctions are related not only to the primary thyroid gland, but also to a range of secondary metabolic challenges associated with unhealthy aging and poor nutritional status, all of which reduce the efficiency of the HPT axis and control of intermediary metabolism and cellular physiology by thyroid hormones.[163] Furthermore, high levels of cortisol, along with high levels of inflammatory cytokines, have been associated with depressed levels of the active thyroid hormone T_3 in fibromyalgia patients, suggesting they may down-regulate the activity of the HPT axis.[164] Increased urinary cortisol metabolites have been associated with reduction in peripheral thyroid hormone metabolism and symptoms of functional hypothyroidism as well.[165]

Stress increases the levels of glucagon, lowers levels of T_3, and elevates levels of rT_3, producing the outcome of secondary borderline hypothyroidism.[166] Reports have indicated that thyroxine replacement therapy in patients with neuromuscular symptoms and subclinical hypothyroidism can result in improved function.[167] Therefore, psychological, chemical, and physical stresses have a significant impact on the HPT axis and may account for the high prevalence of functional thyroid problems in aging individuals.

Effects of Maternal Thyroid Dysfunction

Abnormalities in TSH, T_4, and T_3 are often related to depressive illnesses and melancholia.[168] Thyroid hormones play an important role in the development of the nervous system in the fetus, as well as in neonates and children. Hypothyroidism in the pregnant woman or low thyroid function in the neonate can have a long-term impact on the child's behavior, locomotor ability, speech, hearing, and cognitive function.[169] T_3 reportedly stimulates gene expression of myelin basic protein in oligodendrocytes.[170] Therefore, data suggest that in the developing central nervous system, thyroid hormones regulate processes of terminal brain differentiation, such as dendritic and axonal growth, synaptogenesis, and myelination.

Iodination of Thyroxine and Related Biochemical Processes

Thyroglobulin is a precursor of all thyroid hormone and contains approximately 110 tyrosine residues. These residues are iodinated by a peroxidase enzyme that ultimately forms the thyroid hormones. The iodination of thyroxine by the peroxidase enzyme depends on the availability of adequate dietary iodine, as well as active thyroperoxidase (TPO). Iodide is actively transported from the extracellular fluid into the thyroid follicular cell.

Substances such as thiocyanate and sulfhydryl compounds (e.g., 5-vinyloxalidine-2-thione) inhibit thyroid hormone by blocking the iodination of thyroglobulin. A number of dietary sulfhydryl compounds may, when an individual consumes them at high levels, have similar adverse impact on the iodination of thyroglobulin. These compounds include members of the Brassica family of vegetables: cabbage, Brussels sprouts, broccoli, and cauliflower.[171,172,173,174]

It is important to point out, however, that the level of intake that renders these phytochemicals "goitrogenic" is higher than individuals would get in their normal diet. Most studies have been performed in animals with high intake levels and using uncooked vegetables. Although there are some anecdotal reports of women developing goiters after consuming large amounts of cabbage juice, human studies provide no clear evidence that normal intake of the Brassica family of vegetables induces thyroid abnormalities.

Once iodinated tyrosine residues in thyroglobulin have been formed, there is a coupling of these molecules to produce the principal thyroid hormone thyroxine (T_4). Secretion of T_4 and, to a smaller extent, T_3 from the thyroid gland, depends on TSH stimulation from the pituitary gland, which takes its message from stimulation by thyrotropin-releasing hormone (TRH), secreted by the hypothalamus. Stressors that influence the function of the hypothalamus and pituitary system, therefore, influence not only the secretion of catecholamines and glucocorticoids from the adrenal gland, but also thyroid hormone and its metabolism.

Thyroxine (T_4) represents the majority of the thyroid hormone secreted by the thyroid gland. T_3, which is the more active thyroid hormone, is produced principally by deiodination reactions at the peripheral tissues through the activity of the 5′-deiodinase enzyme. The iodine atom can be removed from T_4 in one of two ways: producing that result via the type 1 and type 2 deiodinases results in active T_3; the deiodinase type 3 pathway results in an inactive rT_3. Deiodination of T_4 to T_3 through type 1 deiodinase requires an adequate level of selenium nutrition, because this enzyme is a selenoenzyme.

On a relative scale of biological activities, T_3 is three to eight times more active than T_4 in influencing physiological function, and rT_3 has less than 1% of the activity of T_4. T_3, therefore, is considered a "step up" hormonal message, whereas rT_3 is considered a "step-down" hormonal message. Psychosocial, chemical, and physical stressors increase the production of rT_3 through the activity of deiodinase type 3, at the expense of lowering the physiologically active levels of T_3.[175]

To be active, T_3 must both bind to one of its receptors in the cell, and the receptor-T_3 complex must then bind and activate specific DNA sequences in the cell's nucleus, which are present on T_3 target genes.[176] The activation of the T_3-nuclear receptor-transcription depends on heterodimerization of T_3 receptors with retinoic acid-specific receptors, and therefore may be dependent on vitamin A nutriture and metabolism.

Molecular Biology of Thyroid Hormone Action

Our understanding of the molecular biology of thyroid hormone action is improving. We know it is mediated by multiple thyroid hormone receptor isoforms derived from two distinct genes. The thyroid hormone receptors belong to a nuclear receptor super-family that includes receptors for other small hormones such as vitamin A-derived retinoic acid and vitamin D-derived 1,25-dihydroxy vitamin D.[177]

The appropriate conversion of T_4 to T_3, transport of T_3 to specific cells, the binding of T_3 to receptors within these cells, and the binding and activation of unique regions of the genome are important in establishing proper thyroid hormone-mediated function. This is another example of the important role of modulator substances on genomics and proteomics. It once again emphasizes the importance of nutrition and environment in modifying gene expression and cellular physiology. Nutrition and the environment can play multiple roles in modifying thyroid hormone metabolism, activity of the HPT axis, sensitivity of the hormone at the receptor site, and its ultimate effect on cellular transcription.

The peripheral metabolism of T_4 to T_3 occurs principally in the liver. Low levels of circulating T_3 with high or adequate levels of T_4 have been associated with such conditions as the "euthyroid sick syndrome," or the "low T_3 syndrome."[178] We might consider T_4 a "prohormone" that must be converted to T_3 to have its full physiological functional impact on cellular physiology.[179] Because of their important role in deiodinating T_4 to T_3, the thyroid hormone deiodinases have been called the "gatekeepers" of thyroid hormone action.[180] Selenium deficiency may reduce the function of this enzyme and result in lowered T_3 production.

Effects of Soy Consumption on Thyroid Function

Isoflavones from soy have been found to be iodinated by TPO and it was therefore hypothesized that they might compete with thyroglobulin as sites for iodination. Further studies have shown conflicting results. A high level of soybean intake in animals has been implicated in diet-induced goiter in a number of studies. *In vitro* incubation of soy isoflavones with TPO shows that the isoflavones can compete with thyroglobulin.[181] Genistein, the principal isoflavone found in soybeans, is known to inactivate TPO *in vitro*, but in animal studies it did not induce an apparent hypothyroid effect. In contrast, rats that consumed a diet supplemented with genistein at up to 500 parts per million showed no difference in levels of T_3, T_4, and TSH compared to rats on a non-soy diet.[182]

In one clinical observation study, when a group of adult humans had a high daily intake of soybeans (30 g per day), half of those on the three-month program experienced such hypometabolic symptoms as malaise, constipation, sleepiness, and goiters. No differences were seen in thyroid hormone levels, and the symptoms were shown to disappear within one month after soybeans were removed from the diet. In a subgroup of these subjects, dietary iodide levels were lower during the administration of soybeans, and TSH levels were increased.[183]

Information from both animal and human studies seems to suggest that as soy isoflavones are increased in the diet, a reasonable precaution is to also increase iodide in the diet. Iodide is available either in organic sources, such as seaweed, or in inorganic form. Soy isoflavones and thyroid function may be of clinical concern in the use of soy formulas in the first years of life. Increased intake of isoflavones may be contraindicated for infants who already have hypothyroid symptoms.[184] Reports indicate that increasing soy consumption can reduce the absorption of exogenous thyroid hormone administered to infants who have thyroid dysfunction.[185] This is not a consequence of the adverse effect of soy isoflavones on thyroid metabolism; it is a consequence of soy's impact on the absorption of exogenous thyroid that has been orally administered as a medication. Many individuals have expressed strong concern that infants with hypothyroidism who received soy formula may have exacerbation of their thyroid symptoms and that the use of soy-based formula should be approached cautiously.[186]

This information suggests that normal levels of intake of soy isoflavones such as genistein are not "goitrogenic," but adequate dietary levels of iodide and selenium should be maintained while one consumes these isoflavones to support proper hormone production and metabolism. One study in 2003 demonstrated that soy isoflavones did not adversely affect thyroid function in iodine-replete subjects.[187] And, for individuals on exogenous thyroid supplements, thyroid hormone should be monitored when a person changes to a high soy protein-supplemented diet.

Other Thyroid Hormone Antagonists

More important than the soy isoflavones in terms of thyroid metabolism are specific bioflavonoids, which, if given at high levels on a continued basis, have been shown *in vitro* and in animal studies to demonstrate antagonistic effects on both TPO and the iodinase enzymes, thereby lowering thyroid hormone activity.[188,189,190] It has come to light that certain types of flavonoids derived from plant foods may participate as inhibitors of T_4 production. Studies indicate a "prohormone" variety of flavonoids, including fisetin, kaempferol, naringenin, and quercetin, have the ability to inhibit TPO.[191] As noted above, TPO is involved in the iodination of thyroglobulin, after which T_4 is produced from the iodinated thyroglobulin.

One other recently identified antagonist of thyroid hormone metabolism is L-carnitine. One study demonstrated that supplementation with L-carnitine at the level of 2 to 4 g/day provided successful treatment of patients with hyperthyroidism.[192] L-carnitine lowered thyroid hormone entry into the nucleus of hepatocytes, neurons, and fibroblasts. This clinical study follows from previous work suggesting that carnitine is a naturally occurring inhibitor of thyroid hormone nuclear uptake.[193] Therefore, high levels of carnitine in a hypothyroid patient could result in exacerbation of symptoms.

Resistance to Thyroid Hormone

Beyond the production of T_4 and its conversion to T_3 is the transport of the hormone and its ultimate activity as a transcription activator at the nuclear receptor site.[194] Resistance to this process at the subsequent steps can result in what has been called "thyroid resistance." A number of genetic polymorphisms are associated with thyroid resistance. Therapy for thyroid resistance can be compared to therapy for insulin resistance, which is often treated clinically by administering high doses of insulin to overcome the resistance. Similarly, high levels of thyroid hormone replacement have been used clinically to overcome thyroid receptor hormone insensitivity.[195]

Animals with mutations in the thyroid hormone receptor genes exhibit impaired growth and resistance to thyroid hormone activity.[196] This resistance could be seen as "euthyroid sick syndrome," in which the individual has reasonably normal levels of T_4, T_3, and TSH but exhibits symptoms associated with thyroid dysfunction.[197] Recognizing the existence of multiple forms of thyroid hormone receptors that can produce multiple phenotypes based upon the environment of the individual has improved the understanding of ways to manage some forms of thyroid dysfunction. Variations may exist in all areas of thyroid metabolism, including polymorphisms in the deiodinase enzymes as well as the alterations of T_3 activities.[198,199]

Heterodimerization

Thyroid hormone receptors are part of the nuclear steroid hormone family of receptors, which also includes peroxisome proliferated activated receptors (PPARs) and the retinoic acid receptors. One recent development in this field is the recognition that thyroid hormones must properly bind to the nuclear hormone receptor to be active at the genomic level, and this binding may depend upon what is called "heterodimerization" with other receptors.[200] Alterations in the genotype of these receptor proteins can result in significantly different DNA binding activities in different individuals.[201] A number of studies have attempted to identify how the thyroid receptor interacts with other receptors to induce specific effects on gene expression.[202,203,204,205,206,207]

Effect of Vitamin A on Thyroid Function

As discussed in the previous essay, a number of environmental and nutritional agents (triggers) can modify orphan nuclear receptors. These modifications have the potential to alter the effect of T_3 at the gene transcription level.[208,209] One such modifiable factor is vitamin A intake and its effect on retinoic acid synthesis and activation of the retinoic acid receptor.[210,211] (Another that we won't explore here is insulin sensitivity and its relationship to the activity of the PPAR receptor.[212]) Studies have found PPAR agonists have thyromimetic effects,[213] suggesting that substances like omega-3 fatty acids, including EPA and DHA as well as conjugated linoleic acid (CLA), may play roles in thyroid function.

Chronic illnesses associated with aging may adversely influence thyroid function. In addition, it has been shown in animals that gene expression changes with aging result in decreased abundance of the retinoic acid and T_3 nuclear receptors.[214] The binding of T_3 to its nuclear receptor is retinoic acid-dependent, suggesting that factors that lower retinoic acid levels may result in lower thyroid hormone effect at the nuclear receptor.

Factors that either produce vitamin A (retinol) insufficiency or prevent the conversion of vitamin A to retinoic acid may result in reduced thyroid nuclear signaling.[215,216,217] One source of vitamin A is through conversion of beta-carotene to an active form of vitamin A in the intestinal mucosa.[218] Homocysteine elevation has also been shown to inhibit the conversion of retinol to retinoic acid in cell cultures.[219] Excess alcohol consumption may also reduce the production of retinoic acid.[220]

The increasing understanding that specific nutrients influence hormone receptor gene interactions that then influence disease expression is a remarkable new chapter in understanding the etiology of chronic disease.[221] Vitamins A and D have been identified as important "prohormones" that help regulate these gene expression pathways shared with T_3.

It seems remarkable that specific dietary fats and vitamin A could have such dramatic impact on thyroid hormone activity but, as this story of nuclear receptor regulatory factors emerges, it appears clear that these relationships do exist.[222] This is an extraordinarily complex story because multiple polymorphisms are related to multiple steps in this process. We cannot simply say, therefore, that all people with thyroid hormone resistance are suffering from vitamin A insufficiencies.

The Mitochondrial Connection to Thyroid Hormone Activity

Increasing evidence in the literature indicates that T_3 has a direct impact on mitochondrial function. It is interesting to note that diiodo-L-thyronine (T_2) seems to have binding sites in the mitochondria.[223] T_2 is generated from T_3 and rT_3. Recent data suggest T_2 can stimulate mitochondrial respiration and, therefore, thyroid hormone status can influence mitochondrial function.[224,225]

In essence, we are beginning to recognize that thyroid hormones play a role, through receptor activities, in mitochondrial function. Conditions that either prevent the proper formation of T_3, or increase the formation of rT_3, or inhibit the appropriate binding of T_3 to its nuclear receptor, may result in symptoms of thyroid insufficiency. Increased levels of rT_3 are also associated with increased autoantibodies in the thyroid gland. A patient may start developing a general autoimmunity to his or her endocrine function, associated with increased senescence and a range of age-related chronic illnesses.[226,227] Proper metabolism of T_4 to T_3 and, subsequently, T_3 to T_2 is critical in controlling the communication to the mitochondria and their subsequent energy reduction.[228,229] Through this process, thyroid hormones can exert both a genomic expression effect on cellular physiology and a rapid response effect that does not require protein synthesis on mitochondrial energy production.[230] Deficiencies in the regulation of this thyroid-modulated mitochondrial pathway can also have adverse impact on growth hormone synthesis and regulation of other anabolic functions.

In essence, this two-step process associated with metabolic regulation by thyroid hormones may account for many of the features associated with healthy or unhealthy aging. Thyroid hormones, particularly T_3, have a profound effect on cellular respiration and mitochondrial function, both indirectly through activity of the nuclear receptor family on gene transcription, and directly on the impact of T_3 on the mitochondrial respiratory enzymes.[231,232,233,234]

Clinical Effects of Thyroid Imbalance

The clinical effects of thyroid imbalance or dysfunction may be observed as poor thermogenic responsiveness and a tendency to gain weight associated with insulin resistance, hypercortisolemia, and under-conversion hypothyroidism. This clinical picture is further characterized by elevated postprandial insulin, decreased level of T_3 with increased rT_3, low axillary body temperature on waking, elevated triglycerides with a reduced HDL level, and a tendency to gain weight as visceral adipose tissue with an increase in waist-to-hip ratio.

T_3 is important for activating thermogenesis in adipocyte cells.[235] It appears to accomplish this thermogenic effect by activating what are called uncoupling proteins (UCPs) in various tissues.[236,237] The proper ratio of T_3 to rT_3 is critically important in expressing mitochondrial UCPs. Patients with energy production problems, poor thermogenesis, and symptoms of functional hypothyroidism may be suffering from either underproduction of T_3 or overproduction of rT_3, both of which are often found in states of overactivation of the HPT axis.

Once again, this calls for the application of the functional medicine model that ties together the activity of the adrenal axis with that of the thyroid axis. If a patient is suffering from hyperactivity of adrenocortical function, this needs to be stabilized while also focusing on appropriate T_3 production and sensitivity.

Thyroid Autoantibodies

One contributor to lack of proper T_3 production is higher titers of antithyroidal antibodies that impair proper thyroid hormone metabolism and sensitivity. In the extreme case, one might think of Hashimoto's disease as the diagnosis of autoimmune thyroiditis. Well before that disease sets in, however, there are states of functional impairment of thyroid activity[238] that result from marginally elevated antithyroid antibodies against many of the thyroid proteins.[239,240]

Down syndrome and thyroid abnormalities. One clinical condition in which elevated levels of antithyroid antibodies are quite common is in Down syndrome. Children with Down syndrome are often found to have thyroid abnormalities.[241] One study has found an association between low serum levels of selenium and thyroid hypofunction in Down's patients.[242] Down syndrome children appear to develop thyroid autoantibodies as they age past eight years.[243,244] The literature suggests that thyroid autoimmunity and resulting thyroid dysfunction in children with Down syndrome may be one of the principal determinants of some of the functional problems they encounter as they grow older. Researchers have recently observed an association between the presence of thyroid autoantibodies and gastrointestinal abnormalities in Down syndrome infants with congenital hypothyroidism.[245]

Gut-associated lymphoid tissue (GALT) and thyroid function. It may at first seem incongruous to suggest that the gut is somehow connected to the thyroid gland, but we have recently learned that the gut-associated lymphoid tissue (GALT) plays a role in priming the rest of the body's immune system. Therefore, when the gut encounters antigens for which antibodies are produced, an impact may occur on inflammatory mediators elsewhere in the body. An association between autoimmune thyroid disease and celiac disease has been noted in a study that reports the presence of anti-endomysium antibodies was ten-fold higher than expected in patients with celiac disease who had autoimmune thyroid disorders, suggesting the two share common immunopathogenic mechanisms.[246]

Managing thyroid autoantibodies with gluten-free diet. A case report in 1999 described a 23-year-old woman with a diagnosis of hypothyroidism due to Hashimoto's thyroiditis and autoimmune Addison's disease, who was found to have elevated anti-endomysium antibodies. Over a three-month period on a gluten-free diet, this woman showed remarkable clinical improvement in both her gastrointestinal-related symptoms and, more importantly, in her thyroid function. She required progressively less thyroid and adrenal replacement therapy. After six months, her endomysium antibodies became negative, her antithyroidal antibody titer decreased significantly, and thyroid medication was discontinued.[247] This case points out the potential impact of a hypoallergenic diet on thyroid function in the reduction of antithyroidal antibodies. Gluten sensitivity is being reported with increasing frequency in numerous conditions (discussed further in Chapter 31); a 2002 review of diagnostic tests in IBS concluded, for example, that the only screening test likely to be useful in that patient population was the routine performance of serological testing for celiac disease.[248]

The same theme is mirrored in a number of other studies. An article in the *American Journal of Gastroenterology* described the importance of gluten in the induction of endocrine autoantibodies and organ system dysfunction in adolescent celiac patients.[249] Another study evaluated 48 patients with celiac disease and thyroid dysfunction. It found that those individuals who carried the DQ131*0502 genotype had a strong risk of thyroid autoantibodies as a consequence of gluten sensitivity.[250] A *Journal of Pediatrics* article reported that gluten-dependent diabetes and thyroid-related autoantibodies found in patients with celiac disease were abolished after a gluten-free diet was followed.[251] And a study published in the *Canadian Journal of Gastroenterology* described a 66-year-old woman with dermatitis herpetiformis and biopsy-defined celiac disease who developed a thyroid mass that later proved to be a T cell lymphoma.[252]

The congenital gastrointestinal abnormalities in Down syndrome suggest a potential connection between gluten sensitivity and autoantibodies to the thyroid gland. According to a 2001 study describing the immune-endocrine status in celiac disease in children with Down syndrome, "Dietary antigens may represent a continuous stimulus for the immune system in this syndrome and interfere with normal immune responses. Altered intestinal absorption of nutrients may in turn affect endocrine functions, brain development, and cognitive performances."[253]

Similarly, a study in the *American Journal of Gastroenterology* (also in 2001) reported that there is a high prevalence of thyroid disorders in untreated adult celiac disease patients and that gluten withdrawal through dietary avoidance may single-handedly reverse this abnormality.[254]

It is obvious from this discussion that a low-antigen dietary approach is desirable in patients with thyroid autoantibodies and altered thyroid function. Gluten is an important dietary variable that can modify thyroid hormone activity. Since rice has low antigenicity and is gluten-free, a rice-based diet may be desirable in these patients.

Inflammatory cytokines and thyroid function. Psychosocial, chemical, and physical stressors can also increase the level of inflammatory mediators (the cytokines) that alter thyroid hormone function and activity. One study, which looked at military cadets involved in special forces training, found the extensive stress of this training resulted in elevated cortisol, reduced testosterone, and increased TSH, but significant reductions in T_3.[255] This study also found evidence of elevated inflammatory cytokines and increased gastrointestinal permeability as a consequence of these inflammatory factors.

Treating patients with proinflammatory cytokines such as interleukin-2, may lead to hypothyroidism as a consequence of the production of antithyroidal antibodies in cancer patients.[256] A study evaluating the cytokine levels in hypothyroid patients contrasted to age-matched, sex-matched euthyroid controls, found a significant elevation in IL-2 in the hypothyroid patients, once again potentially linking activation of the inflammatory system with the production of autoantibodies to the thyroid.[257]

A study in 2000 indicated that hypothyroid patients with autoimmune thyroiditis have a disruption in the normal balance between the Th1 and Th2 cytokines.[258] Patients with subclinical hypothyroidism (SH), irrespective of gender, have higher serum hs-CRP, insulin, total and LDL cholesterol levels than healthy subjects. The conclusion drawn from this study was that an elevated hs-CRP level (and therefore low-grade inflammation) may be associated with fasting hyperinsulinemia before insulin resistance becomes evident in patients with SH.[259] Reduction in inflammatory cytokines can be achieved through a variety of dietary, lifestyle, and environmental factors, including lowering physical and emotional stressors, reducing antigens and toxin exposure and improving nutritional factors associated with the support of balanced immune function.

Vitamin D. One nutrient that is critically important for establishing immune balance and preventing the production of autoantibodies is vitamin D. Vitamin D suppresses the development of autoimmune diseases, such as arthritis and multiple sclerosis, in experimental animal models.[260] Vitamin D insufficiency increases the severity of experimental autoimmune encephalitis. It is interesting to speculate that the role of vitamin D in the immune system may have a downstream effect on thyroid hormone activity.

Vitamin D is considered a prohormone that is converted by activity at the liver and kidney into 1,25-dihydroxy vitamin D3, a hormone with immunomodulatory properties. 1,25-dihydroxy D3 has antiproliferative, differentiating, and immunosuppressive activities.[261] Animals fed vitamin D-insufficient diets had profound increases in serum levels of interleukin-2,[262] which, as noted above, may be associated with thyroid autoantibodies. Vitamin D appears to work with other nutritional factors to help regulate immune sensitivity and to protect against development of autoantibodies.

Zinc. Another nutrient that is beneficial in establishing hormone balance is zinc. Plasma zinc levels are often compromised in Down syndrome children, and zinc therapy can reduce thyroidal antibodies and improve thyroid function.[263] Research suggests that zinc supplementation affects the metabolism of thyroid hormones and reduces antithyroidal antibodies in Down syndrome children.[264] Supplementation with zinc sulfate improves thyroid function in Down syndrome children, and reduces the incidence of subclinical hypothyroidism.[265]

In a clinical trial with disabled patients who displayed compromised thyroid parameters, supplementation with 4 to 10 mg of zinc sulfate per kg body weight (50–100 mg of elemental zinc) resulted in increased levels of serum free T_3, reduced levels of rT_3 and normalized TSH levels.[266] A study of older-aged individuals found that the low T_3-to-T_4 ratio was related to impaired zinc and/or selenium status.[267] This follows closely the previous discussions of the role of both selenium and zinc in promoting proper thyroid function, selenium through its deiodination, the activity of thyroid hormones, and zinc by its role as a cofactor for the thyroid receptor.

Xenobiotics and their Relationship to Thyroid Function

Other environmental factors are known to influence antithyroidal antibodies and thyroid hormone metabolism. The developing brain of the fetus has significant vulnerability to thyroid abnormalities caused by environmental insults *in utero*.[268] In both fetal and neonatal stages, the nervous system is vulnerable to the adverse effects of toxic substances on thyroid gland function or activities.

Porterfield pointed out that a number of the environmental toxins to which we are now exposed, such as dioxins and PCBs, have abnormal effects on thyroid function that can result in neurological impairment. These compounds appear to act as agonists or antagonists for receptors of the thyroid steroid retinoic acid super-family of nuclear receptors.[269] The resulting "twisted molecules" serve as endocrine disruptors that have an adverse influence on the function of the thyroid axis. Organochlorine compounds interact with thyroid-binding globulin and disrupt thyroid hormone metabolism.[270]

Citizens of a small town in Colombia had a significant prevalence of autoimmune thyroiditis, which was traced back to the contamination of drinking water with phenolic chemicals. Those chemicals adversely influenced the immune system, resulting in production of antithyroidal antibodies.[271,272] When the water supply was purified, the prevalence of autoimmune thyroiditis was significantly reduced in the community.

A number of mechanisms of chemical injury to the thyroid gland have been identified. They include inhibition of the iodine-trapping mechanism, blockage of organic binding of iodine, coupling of iodothyronines to thyroxine, and inhibition of thyroid hormone activity, as well as the production of thyroid antibodies.[273] Clinically, this may be seen as resistance to thyroid hormones, and the person may experience refractory response to hormone replacement therapy.[274] The suggestion has been made that exposure to even modest levels of PCBs in the food supply might result in the production of mild hypothyroidism.[275] Sensitivity to these chemicals may be most profound in the thyroid function of infants and children; however, it could have impact on thyroid function in adults as well.[276]

Approaches to Managing HPT Axis Imbalances

Our understanding of thyroid function, its relationship to hypothalamic and pituitary function, and the interrelationship with aspects of adrenal and immune function, is developing at the clinical, cellular, and molecular biological levels. In a paper in *The New England Journal of Medicine*,[277] Klein and Ojamaa describe the relationship of thyroid hormones to the cardiovascular system, and the pleiotropic effects of thyroid hormone across a wide range of functions. All of these effects are triggered through the binding of T_3 to the thyroid hormone response elements in the genome and the inducing of transcription and translation of proteins that alter the phenotype, such as that of the cardiac myocyte. This is just one of a number of papers describing the role of the hypothalamus/pituitary/thyroid axis across a wide range of organs and organ systems, and clarifying how these functional attributes relate to chronic disease in aging individuals.

Taking into account many aspects of this extended essay on cellular messenging as it relates to thyroid function, one can develop a checklist of criteria for clinicians in evaluating patients with imbalances in the function of their hypothalamus/pituitary/thyroid axis:

1. *Provide adequate precursors for the formation of thyroxine (T_4).* Iodide is a limiting nutrient in many individuals for the production of thyroxine. Adequate levels of organic iodide, which can come from seaweed, are important in thyroxine production.[278,279] Supplementation with tyrosine does not appear to have a beneficial effect on elevating thyroid hormones. However, adequate dietary protein intake is important in establishing proper protein-calorie nutrition.
2. *Reduce antithyroidal antibodies.* A variety of food antigens can induce antibodies that cross-react with the thyroid gland. The relationship between celiac disease and autoimmune hypothyroidism has been discussed. A food elimination diet utilizing gluten-free grains and possible elimination of dairy proteins that contain casein, the predominant milk protein, may be desirable in patients with hypothyroidism of unexplained origin. It has also been suggested that environmental xenobiotics may play a role in inducing autoimmune thyroiditis and thyroid dysfunction.
3. *Eliminate exposure to xenobiotics.* One clinical approach for patients with borderline hypothyroidism would be to implement a detoxification program, focused first on eliminating the sources of toxin exposure, and then on nutritional support of phase I and phase II detoxification reactions and adequate levels of vitamin D to support balanced reactions in the immune system. The purpose of this approach would be to nutritionally support hepatic and intestinal detoxification systems, reduce body burden of stored toxins, and decrease antithyroidal antibodies produced as a consequence of "cross-talk" between the immune system with exogenous toxins.
4. *Improve the conversion of thyroxine to tri-iodothyronine (T_4 to T_3).* Nutritional agents that support proper intracellular deiodination by the Type 1 5'deiodinase enzyme include selenium as selenium methionine. Adrenal support also reduces excess production of cortisol or enhances cortisol detoxification.
5. *Improve T_3 receptor binding.* The role that T_3 appears to play is through its nuclear receptor super-family and its effects on gene transcription. T_3 also has direct effects through receptors found in the mitochondria that engage in controlling oxidative phosphorylation and energy production. These receptors interact with vitamin A and PPAR agonists like CLA, EPA, and DHA. Intake of adequate vitamin A in a preformed state, along with adequate levels of omega-3 fatty acids, plays an important role in this interaction. EPA and DHA increase thermogenesis in animals and selectively improve gene transcription related to thyroid function. Vitamin A is converted into all-*trans* retinoic acid through a series of metabolic steps. It then regulates the retinoic acid receptor that interacts with the thyroid receptors, and may help to improve thyroid hormone activity. Carnosic acid, which is one of the principal constituents in rose-

mary concentrate, was found to potentiate the effects of vitamin D and retinoic acid on monocyte differentiation.[280] Carnosic acid is a powerful antioxidant.[281] Zinc as zinc clycinate, has also been shown to be important in promoting proper thyroid function, by its role as a cofactor for the thyroid receptor.

6. *Enhance T_3 influence on mitochondrial bioenergetics.* As explained earlier, a number of important nutritional relationships improve thyroid hormone's effect on the mitochondria. Selenium supplementation in animals can improve the production of T_3 and lower autoantibodies to thyroid hormones, while improving energy production. Supplementation with selenium methionine results in improved deiodination of T_4, which may improve ATP formation by supporting improved mitochondrial activity.[282]

Supplementation and Thyroid Function

Research described in a paper in the *Journal of Endocrinology* in 1998[283] evaluated the antigoitrogenic effects of a combined supplement of vitamin E, vitamin A as beta-carotene, and vitamin C in aging animals. Results of this study suggested these vitamins, vitamin E in particular, modulate the regulatory cascades involved in the control of thyroid function.

In a placebo-controlled trial in 2001, thyroid function responded to selenium supplementation (selenium methionine), particularly in individuals with posttraumatic or stress-induced alterations of the thyroid axis. Subjects in this human clinical trial were given 500 mg of selenium daily with or without 150 mg of alpha-tocopherol and 13 mg of zinc. Supplementation resulted in modest changes in thyroid hormones with an increase in T_3 and a reduction in rT_3.[284]

This observation is consistent with the recognition that selenium, vitamin E, and vitamin C play a role in the antioxidant-sensitive T_3 effects on induced mitochondrial function.[285] Vitamin E has a protective effect against the lead-induced deterioration of 5'deiodinase activity.[286] It might, therefore, influence thyroid function positively by several mechanisms. In a clinical trial assessing the safety of high-dose, short-term supplementation of vitamin E in healthy older adults, Meydani and Blumberg reported that a daily supplement of 800 mg of vitamin E resulted in a reduction in inflammatory cytokines, but had no adverse effect on thyroid function.[287]

Another study, in chickens, also seemed to support the positive influence of antioxidants on thyroid activity at the mitochondrial level. Chickens supplemented with vitamin C and treated with the antithyroidal drug propylthiouracil, had normal thyroid function. This study suggests vitamin C improves thyroid function in animals with hypothyroidism experimentally induced through toxic exposure.[288]

Similarly, other published work suggests an interrelationship between thyroid hormones and vitamin A and zinc nutritional status. One such report suggests a causal relationship between the pathogenesis of deranged vitamin A metabolism and a low T_3 syndrome, either by interfering with T_4 entry into the tissues or by directly affecting the enzymatic conversion of T_4 to T_3.[289] Subjects in this study were stable patients with hepatic or gastrointestinal disorders that modified the absorption and metabolism of vitamin A and zinc. Animal studies indicate aging decreases the vitamin A and T_3 nuclear expression, suggesting that exogenous or supplemental vitamin A may be important for increasing retinoic acid levels in order to modulate this decreased expression.[290] A companion study, in which supplemental vitamin A was able to increase activity at the T_3 nuclear receptor in the brain of aging animals, produced the same result.[291] Other animal studies have shown nicotinamide modulates expression of thyrotropin.[292]

Natural Therapies before Pharmacology in Thyroid Dysfunction

Thyroid hormones have both gene expression and non-genomic effects on cellular metabolism. Many of these effects are clearly related to nutritional status and integrate into a larger picture that also involves psychosocial and environmental modulators that influence the HPT axis. These signaling pathways control multiple functions in the individual, translating environmental signals into physiological function. For example, cell signaling processes initiated by thyroid hormones are intertwined with the vitamin A and D signaling pathways.[293,294] Taken together, the results from limited human clinical trials, animal studies, *in vitro* work, and epidemiological evidence may strongly indicate but do not conclusively prove the hypothesis that functional modifications will serve as therapeutic interventions for improving outcome in patients with chronic thyroid dysfunctions.

Clearly, the proof of the concept is in the clinical outcome of the patient who has been evaluated and managed by a functional medicine approach. In the absence of clinical intervention studies assessing the effectiveness of this complex algorithm for the management of thyroid-related dysfunctions, the clinician must rely on an understanding of complex mechanisms, their disruptors and supporters, and on empirical clinical evidence. At worst, the effects of the nutrients listed at the levels suggested should produce no untoward effects, and there is a reasonable amount of science to indicate they should be helpful.

Fortunately, a growing evidence base provides support for this empirical approach. To summarize, we are suggesting the following steps: 1) provide adequate precursors for thyroxine formation; 2) reduce antithyroidal antibodies by lowering immune potential, improving the conversion of T_4 to T_3, and improving receptor binding of T_3; and 3) activate mitochondrial bioenergetics through balanced thyroid function. All of this may be accomplished in many patients by modification of nutriture, lifestyle, and environment.

In this review of thyroid function, we have examined the production of thyroid messenger substances, the transport of thyroid messenger substance, the issues of tissue sensitivity to the message, the intracellular response to thyroid hormones, and detoxification and excretion of messenger substances. We have delved deeply into thyroid function as an example of how functional endocrinology develops a more complex understanding of inter- and intracellular communication and cross-talk. The last essay in this chapter again addresses thyroid function, with a focus on specific clinical interventions for improving patient outcomes.

We will now attend to the adrenal hormones (focusing on DHEA HRT) and the HPA axis, growth hormone dynamics, and insulin-like growth factors, using these specific areas of investigation to further elaborate the evolving model of functional neuroendocrine-immunology.

Stress, Adrenal Function, and The HPA Axis, with a Focus on DHEA HRT

One of the environmental modulators of neuroendocrine function is physical or psychosocial stress. Interaction between the neuroendocrine system and the external environment often occurs through the senses, creating a substantial impact on the hypothalamus/pituitary/adrenal (HPA) axis.

Long-term, unremitting stress results in loss of adrenal gland reserve related to the reduced production of stress hormones like cortisol and epinephrine. Under stress, the human adrenal cortex secretes not only the essential hormones cortisol and aldosterone, but also dehydroepiandrosterone (DHEA) and large amounts of dehydroepiandrosterone sulfate (DHEA-S). The serum concentration of DHEA-S is 20 times that of serum cortisol, whereas the concentration of free DHEA is 1/20th that of cortisol. The high concentration of DHEA-S reflects its high rate of secretion by the adrenal cortex and its low rate of metabolic clearance. DHEA is produced from DHEA-S in the zona reticularis of the adrenal gland and in the liver by a sulfotransferase. Many organs that are targets of androgens and estrogens also convert DHEA-S back to DHEA; the same organs can then biotransform it into an active androgen like testosterone or estrogens.[295,296]

In normal individuals, serum concentrations of DHEA and its sulfate are highest at age 30. After age 30, concentrations of both gradually decrease. By age 70 or 80, the values are about 20% of peak values in men and 30% of peak values in women. This decrease has led to the suggestion that DHEA might be a marker compound for the effects of stress on endocrine function, and the postulate that supplementation with DHEA might help support proper endocrine function in individuals with low values of DHEA-S and DHEA.

Since the ovaries do not secrete DHEA and the testes secrete only small amounts, adults with primary or secondary adrenal insufficiencies often have very low concentrations of DHEA and its sulfate and low levels of androgens derived from DHEA.[297] In a study of men and women with severe hypopituitarism, administration of a single oral dose of 50 mg of DHEA transiently raised serum concentrations of DHEA, its sulfate, and androstenedione (known to be a precursor of both testosterone and estrogen) into the normal range for young adults.[298] It also raised the serum concentrations of estrogens and active androgens (testosterone and dihydrotestosterone), but only in the lower end of the normal range for young women (based on normals for the early follicular phase of the menstrual cycle).

Evaluating DHEA Replacement: A Model for Evaluating Pros/Cons of HRT

In 1999, Arlt et al. evaluated the psychological and biochemical effects of DHEA replacement in women with adrenal insufficiency.[299] They administered DHEA orally in a dose of 50 mg per day or placebo for four months and evaluated the effects on well-being and sexuality, as well as serum hormone values. Some of the women had primary or secondary hypogonadism, and some were postmenopausal; if they were taking estrogen-progestin replacement therapy for these concerns, they were counseled to continue the oral hormone therapy during the study. After treatment, serum DHEA, DHEA-S, and androstenedione concentrations increased from initial low values to normal, and serum testosterone and dihydrotestosterone concentrations rose to the lower limit of the normal range in the women. Serum estrogen concentrations did not change significantly, possibly because of a small increase obscured by the estrogen replacement therapy used by some of the participants. Evaluation of psychological factors by questionnaire found positive effects of DHEA on depression, anxiety, general well-being, and the physical aspects of sexuality. There was also a small but significant rise in serum insulin-like growth factor-1 concentrations (a mediator of some effects of growth hormone in the liver), and a small decrease in total and low-density lipoprotein cholesterol concentrations.

One problem with DHEA is that it serves as a precursor to androgens. Because DHEA can stimulate the synthesis of testosterone, it should be administered with caution to women who may be hyperandrogenic. Excessive use can cause acne, unwanted hair growth, or adverse influence on the menstrual cycle in women. With the passage of the U.S. Dietary Supplement Health and Education Act of 1994 (DSHEA), DHEA has become widely available, and a growing market has developed for this so-called "fountain of youth." It is often available through direct mail outlets with no recommendation for hormone or endocrine balance evaluation before administration. Promoters have claimed DHEA is a "super hormone" that can help overcome obesity; build muscle mass; prevent cancer, heart disease, and type 2 diabetes; slow aging; prevent or slow the progression of Alzheimer's and Parkinson's diseases; boost libido; strengthen the immune system; and help treat systemic lupus erythematosus.

Unfortunately, many of these claims are as yet unsubstantiated,[300] and none of them should be used to promote unmonitored use of powerful hormones without trained clinical guidance. Very few randomized clinical trials have been performed on long-term effects of DHEA in humans for these conditions. DHEA metabolism in animals is very different from that in humans. For example, primates show a higher level of adrenal steroidogenesis than do humans. Differences in metabolism of DHEA and other steroids have also been noted between humans and many animal species. Extrapolation of encouraging research results of DHEA administration studies in animals to use in humans needs careful ongoing evaluation.

The results to date suggest it may be justified to prescribe a daily dose of 5 to 20 mg of DHEA for patients with defined adrenal insufficiency, whose sexuality and well-being are subnormal, **provided** they are monitored for breast or prostatic cancer and managed by a competent clinician. It is very important to precede the administration of DHEA with salivary or serum tests for DHEA and DHEA-S, as well as testosterone and estradiol. A baseline hormone analysis is critical to establish the overall influence of DHEA on neuroendocrine balance. It is inappropriate to administer DHEA based on clinical symptoms alone. Other possible indications for replacement with DHEA include depression associated with low hormone levels and, since estrogen can be increased by DHEA, possibly postmenopausal osteoporosis.[301] In a recent placebo-controlled trial involving patients with major depression, treatment with DHEA (maximum dose of 90 mg per day) resulted in significant improvement in the Hamilton Depression Rating Score as compared to placebo.[302]

Evaluating Growth Hormone Function

Growth hormone (GH), an endogenous growth factor produced by the anterior pituitary gland, is involved primarily in skeletal and soft-tissue growth.[303] It also participates in numerous metabolic feedback loops, and has been found to be anabolic in skeletal muscle tissue,[304] lipolytic in peripheral fat stores, and induces the breakdown of glycogen in the liver.[305] Clinicians have used these effects to treat growth-deficient patients,[306] to attenuate catabolism in the aged and critically ill, and in trauma and burn patients.

As we grow older, we experience a decrease in lean body mass and bone density, and a reduction in the size of the internal organs, suggesting loss of organ reserve. These symptoms may be associated with loss of GH. The healthy young man between age 20 and 30 secretes between 0.5 and 1.0 mg of GH each day. Secretion declines by about 14% per decade. In some elderly people, GH production cannot be detected at all.[307]

GH is a peptide hormone of approximately 22 kD in molecular weight with 191 amino acids, having two disulfide bridges joining cysteines. Base sequence analysis reveals that growth hormone is homologous to both prolactin and placental lactogen. GH receptors are found in a wide variety of tissues, including muscle, bone, liver, heart, and lymphoid organs. GH induces the secretion of another hormone made by the liver called somatomedin C, or insulin-like growth factor (IGF-1). It appears that many, though not all, effects of GH are actually mediated by IGF-1.[308] Although GH concentration follows a diurnal rhythm, IGF-1 concentrations do not fluctuate in the course of a day. Consequently, IGF-1 concentration is often taken as a diagnostic indicator of GH output.

GH and IGF-1 decline with age. If GH output declines with age, it might be expected that IGF-1 concentrations would also decline. In fact, there is a close relationship between the 24-hour average output of GH and the concentration of IGF-1 in the bloodstream. In the decades between ages 40 and 80, the average IGF-1 concentration falls from 800 units per liter to 570, then to 410 units per liter and 320, respectively.[309] The reduced concentration reflects declining GH output rather than a diminished liver responsiveness to GH because injection of GH, even in elderly people, results in a rapid rise in IGF-1. Therefore, the decline of IGF-1 concentration appears to be the result of events associated with aging that can be traced back to a decline in GH secretion, which results from a decrease in the hypothalamic output of GH-releasing hormone (GHRH).

In 1990, two independent studies tested GH injections in the elderly. Both lasted six months and showed positive metabolic effects.[310] In one study involving 16 healthy men and women over age 60, IGF-1 levels rose in direct proportion to the amount of GH used. In a second study, 21 healthy men between 61 and 81 years of age also showed an increase in IGF-1 after GH injections. However, when treatment was extended in these men for a year, significant adverse side effects were noted with the GH therapy. Ten instances of carpal tunnel syndrome (24%) and two examples (9%) of gynecomastia were reported. Adverse side effects were generally limited to subjects whose IGF-1 was brought to the higher end of the normal IGF-1 range. This study suggests that for GH therapy to be effective in the elderly, great care should be taken to use a dose that brings plasma levels of IGF-1 to no higher than the 500–1000 units-per-liter range.

Growth Hormone Replacement Considerations

GH deficiency is associated with increased risk of cardiovascular mortality, and it has been suggested this is a consequence of altered lipid dynamics and arterial function related to GH deficiency.[311] GH deficiency is associated with abnormalities in plasma lipoproteins, including increased LDL and plasma triglycerides, and low HDL levels. Several studies have shown that GH replacement therapy in individuals who are GH deficient is able to lower plasma total and LDL cholesterol, as well as increase HDL.[312,313]

In 24 GH-deficient adults, GH replacement therapy was shown to elevate the activity of plasma lecithin-cholesterol acyltransferase. In this study, GH deficiency was defined as peak serum GH levels in response to insulin-induced hypoglycemia (a venous blood glucose less than or equal to 2.2 mmol per liter in the presence of hypoglycemic symptoms). Regular insulin was intravenously administered in a dose of 0.15 to 0.20 units per kilogram body weight to induce the hypoglycemia, and growth hormone levels were measured at the low blood glucose nadir. It is important to point out that these subjects were adults with demonstrated GH deficiency and, therefore, the results may not apply to older individuals with no demonstrable GH deficiency.

GH administration contributes to insulin resistance and may consequently contribute to the development of type 2 diabetes in some individuals. In a recent study, GH-deficient children who received GH therapy had no increase in type 1 diabetes, but experienced a six-fold increase in type 2 diabetes.[314] In spite of the effect of GH on insulin resistance, GH supplementation has been shown, in individuals who are GH deficient, to reduce the risk of cardiovascular disease and possibly improve well-being.[315]

These studies make a very important point about the therapeutic use of GH: it should generally be considered only for adults with established severe GH deficiency. GH administration to an individual in the normal GH range may result in adverse side effects, including type

2 diabetes and musculoskeletal problems.[316] Cardiovascular risk reduction can be achieved with nutritional and lifestyle strategies; if those efforts are unsuccessful, pharmaceutical approaches are available. The effect of GH on the structure of body fat, muscle, and bone can be addressed by other means as well, including optimum hormone replacement therapy and a structured exercise and lifestyle program.[317]

Stimulating GH Release

We know exercise induces the neuroendocrine release of GH, although the mechanism by which it does so remains unclear. A study in 2000 found the GH levels of exercising athletes were highest 30 minutes after exercise and could be elevated even with modest workloads.[318] The study data indicate that under strenuous exercise conditions, endogenous GH-releasing hormone activity causes a further increase of GH release. A GH-releasing protein-2-mediated mechanism in central neuroendocrine regulation seems to act as a booster, possibly by stimulating the effects of GH-releasing hormone, indicating a graded effect of exercise on GH activities.

Because GH secretion is controlled by both GH-releasing hormone and GH-releasing peptides as secretagogues, new therapeutic approaches focus on stimulating the secretion and balance of GH. Researchers have discovered small GH-releasing peptides that seem to work by an entirely new signaling pathway.[319] This pathway does not depend on releasing factors of hypothalamic origin. It does not involve receptors of GH-releasing hormone or a cyclic AMP-mediated signaling pathway, and its signaling potential does not diminish with age. The signaling pathway for GH-releasing peptides is activated through small 5-amino acid peptides that seem to induce GH secretion.

GH and IGF-1 Supplementation

Ongoing clinical trials are evaluating the administration of recombinant IGF-1. Although GH is diabetogenic and causes water retention, IGF-1 does not have these effects. However, there are some countervailing concerns about IGF-1. It is a potent stimulator of cell replication and thus may be associated with the induction of cancer. IGF-1 suppresses apoptosis, and most tumors express IGF-1 receptors. High IGF-1 levels in males are associated with an increased risk of prostate cancer.[320] As a whole, the clinical outcomes of supplementation with GH, IGF-1, or GH secretagogues are as yet unclear. Whatever strategy is used, levels of IGF-1 and GH should be measured prior to administration of any exogenous growth factors. Evaluating IGF-1 levels appears to be critically important in defining the hormonal milieu related to growth factors. IGF-1 levels in individuals younger than age 40 range from 800-1000 units per liter. In 60-year-olds, those levels are about 400 units per liter. It is not clear whether elevated levels of IGF-1 in older individuals are associated with significantly increased risk of prostate, breast, or other cancers. The decision to increase IGF-1 levels by administering GH should be approached with caution. The first steps in implementing a GH support strategy should be exercise, insulin balance, and DHEA support.

Melatonin and the Menopausal Female Neuroendocrine System

The onset of menopause, characterized by the cessation of menstruation, signals not only the end of fertility, but also the beginning of a multitude of alterations in the hypothalamus/pituitary/ovary relationships. The result is a shifting of the function of the neuroendocrine system, which can impact cognitive and cardiovascular function, bone density, and the risk of many age-related diseases. Figure 32.3 describes the interrelationships among various components of the neuroendocrine system in female metabolism. As Figure 32.4 shows, when a woman ages and goes through menopause, her levels of estrogens, follicle-stimulating hormone (FSH), and luteinizing hormone (LH) change dramatically.

Disturbed sleep is one feature associated with the alteration of neuroendocrine function in women moving into menopause. The sleep cycle, an important circadian rhythm that results in repair of cellular damage incurred throughout the day, is initiated by cyclical secretions of the pineal hormone melatonin. Melatonin secretion can decrease dramatically with age[321] and with disease.[322] Melatonin is known to be a very effective oxygen radical scavenger and therefore may help protect the brain against oxidative injury.[323,324]

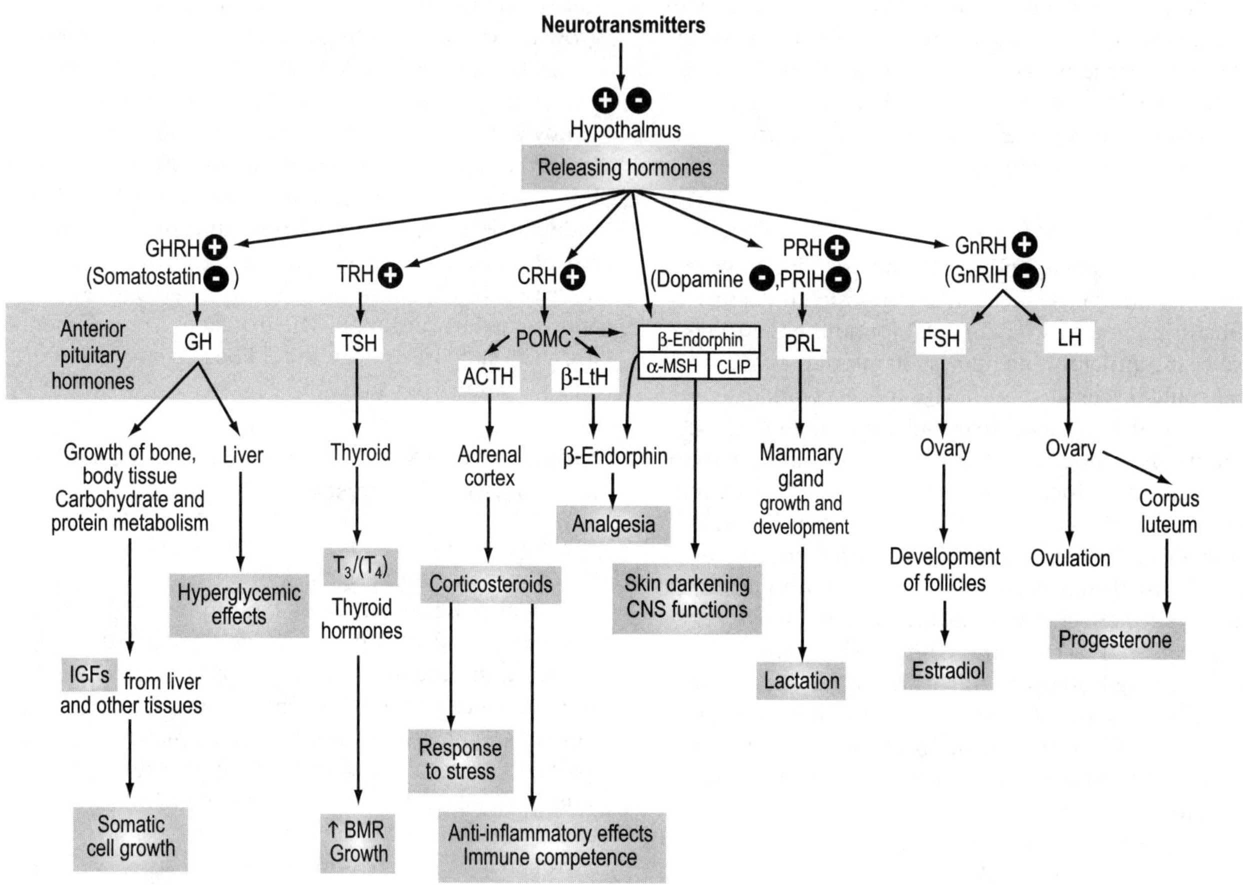

Figure 32.3 **The female neuroendocrine system**

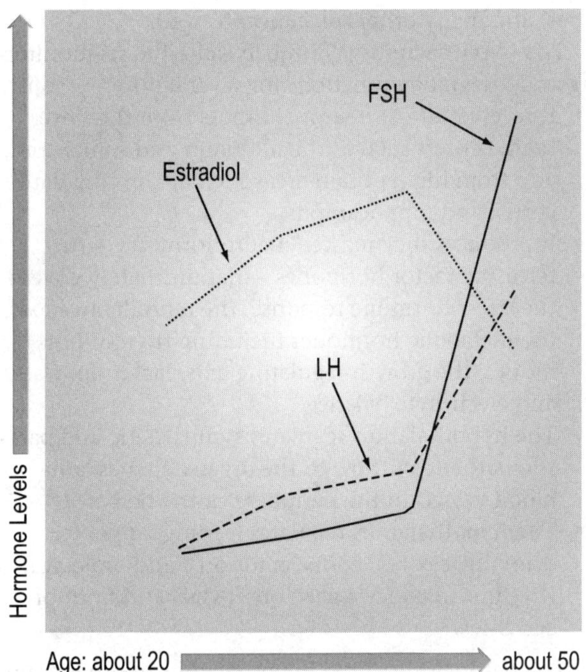

Figure 32.4 **Female homeostat**

Melatonin also has a very important effect on setting the "biological clock" of the hypothalamus. Indirectly, therefore, it influences estrogen secretion and metabolism. Normal aging is associated with both subjective and objective alterations in sleep quality in aging women and men as a consequence of changes in neuroendocrine function. The pineal release of melatonin is only a part of this story. Among the most common changes in sleep in aging individuals are decreased deep sleep (stages 3 and 4 or delta), poor slow-wave sleep, and an increase in the number of nocturnal awakenings.[325]

A report in 2000 indicated that poor slow-wave sleep results in lowered output of growth hormone and increases in evening cortisol output.[326] It appears from this research that poor sleep quality reduces growth hormone output during the important evening hours, while increasing adrenocortical output. This may argue strongly for sleep therapy and/or melatonin being of primary importance in the management of some symptoms associated with neuroendocrine aging.

The functional medicine approach to improvement of circadian rhythms and their relationship to neuroendocrine function are beautifully explained in *The Circadian Prescription* by Sidney Baker, MD.[327] In this book, he presents the concepts of rhythmic balance using food, nutrients, exercise, and breathing in setting the body's cycles such as waking, sleeping, and secretion. As an addendum to the prescription for sleep hygiene, melatonin has been used successfully as a supplement in the sleep cycle at doses from 0.1 to as much as 10 mg per day.[328]

Summary

This discussion focused on a few topics that exemplify how important an understanding of cellular messaging is in the functional medicine approach to improving endocrine function. We have emphasized the value of modifying nutrition, lifestyle, and environment in controlling hormone-related, age-dependent disorders. The modulation of neuroendocrine messenger sensitivity, immune signaling, and cellular response can have a significant impact on many age-related conditions. Even with the recent explosion of information about the functional aspects of thyroid hormone and its metabolites, the field of functional endocrinology is still in its infancy. The strength of the model is its ability to identify important interconnections among different endocrine functions and to describe how they relate to modifiable environmental, lifestyle, and nutritional factors. The weakness of the model is that these interventions have generally not been subjected to large-scale, long-term, rigorous controlled clinical trials to examine how reproducible the effects are in patients, as well as which factors may be most important to consider when evaluating hypothalamic-pituitary-thyroid-adrenal (HPTA) axis function.

One can hope that such research will be done. However, without a significant financial incentive (as is present with pharmaceutical interventions), it may be a long time before we have definitive evidence. In the meantime, we use the emerging science, the functional medicine matrix, and the logic of the "interconnected web" to highlight viable new directions in the eternal struggle to relieve suffering and improve health. There is much we can do, even with incomplete and imperfect knowledge.

The Hypothalamus-Pituitary-Adrenal Axis

Michael Lumpkin, PhD

Introduction

The bodies and minds of humans and all living creatures are constantly subjected to changing circumstances in the outside world, as well as to changes occurring inside their bodies. When these alterations—whether internal, external, or both—perturb the balance of biochemical and physiological processes that maintain the baseline activities of normal organ, tissue, and gene function, physiologists refer to such challenges to normal balance as stress. The situations or events that cause stress can be of physical, metabolic, psychological, or emotional origin. The stressors themselves can be acute and short-lived or they can be chronic, persistent, and unrelenting. When an individual experiences an acute stressor, a coordinated series of nervous, endocrine, and immune system responses are put into play to ensure the immediate survival of the individual as the internal and/or external environment changes. At the core of this critical response is the hypothalamus of the brain. The hypothalamus is the **integrative** center of the central nervous system (CNS) because it monitors neuronal, hormonal, metabolic, and immune signals arising from inside the body and compares these inputs to information being sent to it from inside and outside the body by various receptor systems for temperature, pain, pressure, electrolyte, and metabolite concentrations, and other functions. Further, the state of mind—whether one is fearful, agitated, depressed, angry, happy, amused, or contented, for instance—is also perceived by higher brain centers, and this information is projected to the hypothalamus for processing and comparison to the baseline activities of the other organ systems being monitored.

Three components of the hypothalamus lie outside the blood-brain barrier (BBB), namely, the median eminence (ME), the organum vasculosum of the lamina terminalis (OVLT), and the posterior pituitary gland (or neurohypophysis—a downgrowth of median eminence neuronal tissue). Because these portions of the hypothalamus are exposed to blood, they are therefore able to detect the concentrations of many blood-borne solutes including glucose, electrolytes (especially sodium), fatty acids, amino acids, water- and fat-soluble hormones, neurotransmitters, peptides, cytokines, chemokines, and many other substances as well.

The hypothalamus is uniquely suited to its monitoring and integrative functions for several other reasons:

- It receives direct neuronal inputs from the lower brain centers such as the midbrain and spinal cord, and from higher brain areas such as the cingulate cortex and hippocampus.
- It produces the "master" neurohormones—the releasing factor hormones—that ultimately govern the stress hormone response, the reproductive axis, the metabolic hormones including thyroid hormones, the growth regulating axis, lactation, water and electrolyte balance.
- The hypothalamus regulates sympathetic and parasympathetic outflow to the organs, tissues, and blood vessels in the periphery of the body.
- The hypothalamus regulates feeding, appetite, drinking, sex behaviors, emotions, and biological rhythms in concert with other CNS and hormonal activities.

The hard wiring of the hypothalamus to other brain structures via well-known neuronal projection pathways provides the anatomical substrates for communicating conscious thoughts, emotions, and memories to the hypothalamic integrator and governor of the so-called vegetative or visceral functions.[329] In other words, the hypothalamus, with its neuroendocrine primacy and its extensive CNS connectivity, forms a neuroanatomical basis for the mind-body (psychosomatic) connection.

The Hypothalamus and the Limbic System

The specific CNS pathways that subserve the mind-body connection are included in the limbic system,[330] in which the hypothalamus occupies a pivotal position. Information from the neocortex, where rational, factual thought takes place, flows into the cingulate cortex lying above the corpus callosum. From the cingulate gyrus, cortical nerve fibers project to the hippocampus where the learning and memory of new information are transferred to long-term memory.[331] Additional cortical projections lead to the amygdala where emotional responses are attached to the factual information and memory of past events.[332] Stated differently, the factual information arriving at the hippocampus and amygdala is placed into an interpretable and familiar context. This collective information is then projected into the hypothalamus via the fornix, the stria terminalis, and the amygdalo-fugal pathways.[333] At this point, the hypothalamus and its various intercommunicating regions (nuclei) with their respective releasing factor (hormone) neurons will elicit the specific hormonal, autonomic, metabolic, and behavioral changes that are appropriate for the physical or emotional stress being experienced. Much of the time, individuals are quite unaware of these autonomic (automatic), visceral alterations in the body's physiology. However, because of projection pathways (called the mammillo-thalamic tract) exiting from the hypothalamus, and the relay of this information to the thalamus and from the thalamus via thalamo-cortical efferents arriving back at the cerebral cortex, individuals may become aware of changes in their physiological responses to stress. This increased perception of arousal may manifest as changes in the rate of respiration, muscular tremors due to the release of sympathetic catecholamines, increased mentation and alertness, increased body temperature and perspiration, cold hands, dry mouth, changes in appetite and food preferences, increased thirst, and bowel discomfort. A person may choose to act upon or moderate these responses. The neuronal pathways of connectivity described above and their linkages to hypothalamic/autonomic signaling may provide the basis for the effectiveness of mind-body relaxation techniques such as biofeedback to address stress-related pathologies.[334]

The Hypothalamic-Pituitary-Adrenal Axis

In order to understand how so much information is coordinated by the hypothalamus, it is helpful to review the elements of the hypothalamic-pituitary-adrenal gland axis. The parvocellular neurons of the paraventricular nucleus (PVN) of the hypothalamus elaborate the "master" stress hormone, a 41-amino acid neuropeptide known as corticotropin-releasing hormone (CRH) or factor (CRF).[335] When an individual is exposed to stressful stimuli—some of which may be physical such as pain, trauma, infection, hypotension, exercise, or hypoglycemia; or others that may be psychological in nature such as bereavement, fear, personal loss, or anger—the release of hypothalamic CRH is stimulated.[336,337] The CRH in turn is released into the portal blood vessels of the ME and is carried by venous blood flow to the corticotroph cells of the anterior pituitary gland. There, the CRH binds to its receptor on the corticotrophs and stimulates the ultimate production and release of adrenocorticotropic hormone (ACTH). The ACTH enters the systemic circulation and reaches the adrenal cortex of the adrenal gland, where its stimulates the synthesis of the glucocorticoid hormone cortisol and also androgenic hormones such as androstenedione and dehydroepiandrosterone (DHEA), both of which may ultimately be converted into the more potent testosterone or dihydrotestosterone (DHT) in peripheral tissues.

Cortisol acts as an important stress hormone because it maintains blood glucose levels during a stressful "fight or flight" challenge. During stress, as more demands are placed on the body, more metabolic fuel is consumed; yet, a critical amount continues to be needed to ensure normal brain function and to supply activated organs such as the heart, lungs, and skeletal muscle with a renewable supply of substrate. In addition, the cortisol also participates with aldosterone (the mineralocorticoid hormone) in driving sodium reabsorption by the kidney tubules. This serves the important function of conserving electrolytes and water within the vasculature to help maintain blood and perfusion pressures to critical organs and tissues that are participating in the fight or flight reactions. During the stress response, the blood concentrations of cortisol will rise until the cortisol starts to exert its negative feedback effect upon both the CRH neurons and the pituitary corticotrophs that manufacture ACTH, in order to reduce their increased levels of secretion back to their normal baseline.[338] This homeostatic mechanism, when working correctly, prevents overproduction or prolonged elevations in CRH, ACTH, and cortisol.[339] Thus, metabolic substrate is only mobilized when there is a specific need during the stress response.

When an individual experiences chronic stress along with maladaptive responses or a lack of coping, cortisol levels may remain inappropriately elevated due to persistent stimulation of the CRH-ACTH-cortisol axis. Metabolically, this can take a toll on the organism. The ongoing high concentrations of cortisol may keep blood glucose levels high for prolonged periods, cause redistribution of fat from the thighs and buttocks to the abdominal and cervical regions ("buffalo hump") due to mobilization of free fatty acids; cause insulin resistance to develop; cause fluid retention and hypertension; produce proteolysis in muscle, bone, and connective tissues; and inhibit peptide and protein hormone formation (especially by the pituitary gland).[340] The persistent presence of increased cortisol will also have a profound inhibiting effect on immune system capabilities.[341] Elevated cortisol concentrations can decrease the number and functions of blood lymphocytes, eosinophils, basophils, monocytes/macrophages, and neutrophils. Further, cortisol can inhibit the production of immune cell-signaling molecules such as the proinflammatory cytokines interleukin (IL)-1, IL-2, IL-2 receptor, IL-6, tumor necrosis factor (TNF), and gamma interferon. Chronically elevated glucocorticoids can also decrease antibody and immunoglobulin production. Consequently, chronic activation of the HPA axis is associated with the development and worsening of chronic infectious diseases.

CRH as a Neurotransmitter

While CRH is best known for its neuroendocrine role in stimulating ACTH secretion from the anterior pituitary gland, CRH also acts as a neurotransmitter by stimulating sympathetic outflow from the brain and spinal cord and simultaneously inhibiting the outflow of parasympathetic activity to the periphery.[342] Part of the sympathetic response is to stimulate the adrenal medullary release of the catecholamines epinephrine and norepinephrine into the circulation. Additionally, sympathetic nerves that innervate visceral organs and tissues such as the heart, coronary arteries, peripheral blood vessels, kidney, lungs, pancreas, gastrointestinal tract, and gonads, will release their contents of norepinephrine and neuropeptide Y at these sites. The overall result is to accelerate cardiopulmonary activity by increasing heart rate, strength of cardiac contraction, arterial vasoconstriction, and blood pressure, with shunting of blood from the splanchnic vasculature to skeletal muscles, heart, and brain, and increasing the rate and depth of respiration.[343] Stimulated sympathetic catecholaminergic inputs to the liver and adipose tissue result in enhanced glycogenolysis and lipolysis, thereby supplementing the glucose and free fatty acid-elevating action of cortisol. The integrated view is that CRH is acting in its neuroendocrine capacity to supply the main metabolic substrates (via its cortisol and catecholamine stimulating action) for the CRH-directed trigger of visceral organ stimulation upon sympathetic nervous system activation after physical or psychological challenge. Other CRH-directed sympathetic targets involve the stimulation of the renal renin-angiotensin-aldosterone system and the neurosecretion of antidiuretic hormone (arginine vasopressin). These sympathetically driven hormones will act in concert with cortisol and the catecholamines to defend against volume depletion and hypotension during any homeostatically threatening situation.

Stress-related activation of CRH also alters the ratio of sympathetic to parasympathetic inputs to the gastrointestinal tract.[344] The net outcome for the stomach is an inhibition of gastric contractility and decreased emptying, leading to sensations of fullness and bloating. In the case of the colon, accelerated motility with rapid transit times for chyme and poor absorption of nutrients and water is the result. Diarrhea and inflammation of the bowel can result if the stress is of sufficient intensity and length. It has been suggested that this mechanism of stress may contribute to the development of irritable bowel syndrome and the exacerbation of Crohn's disease.[345] Such inflammatory states of the bowel may lead to the "leaky gut" syndrome with maldigested food antigens provoking inappropriate immune responses in the form of food reactions. (These issues are explored in depth in Chapters 28 and 31.)

Sympathetic noradrenergic nerve fibers also innervate immune organs such as the thymus gland, spleen, lymph nodes, bone narrow, and intestinal Peyer's patches.[346] Norepinephrine-containing nerve fibers have been seen in contact with thymocytes, B lymphocytes, and macrophages.[347] In fact, alpha and beta adrenergic receptors have been identified on these immune cells. In general, activation of the sympathetic nervous system or administration of epinephrine produces leukocytosis, lymphopenia, and suppression of natural killer (NK) cell activity. In other words, the action of catecholamines is to inhibit lymphocyte proliferation and suppress the immune response. Experimentally, it has been observed that the stress of foot shock, cold exposure, maternal deprivation, and fear may cause thymus gland involution, decreased lymphocyte proliferation and cytotoxicity, and less antibody production. Conversely, the interruption of sympathetic innervation to immune organs results in lymph node, spleen, and bone marrow cell proliferation, in addition to antigen-provoked immunoglobulin production.[348] Consequently, prolonged stress that activates CRH-driven sympathetic outflow would be expected to lead to greater susceptibility to disease, infections, and cancer in human patients with a chronically suppressed immune system.[349]

CRH and Behavior

CRH neurons are not only located in the hypothalamus but are also found in the dorsal raphe nucleus, the hippocampus, the bed nucleus of the stria terminalis, the reticular formation, periaqueductal gray, locus coeruleus, septum, and telencephalon. Due to their presence in these areas of the brain and their involvement in regulating autonomic nervous system activity and hormone secretion, CRH is well-positioned to participate in coupling these neurochemically-governed responses to corresponding stress-related behaviors. It has been observed in animal models that CRH injected into the brain produces behaviors that are typically seen when animals and humans experience stressful events:[350,351]

- Increased locomotor activity (to rapidly escape danger)
- The startle response (to orient to a threat)
- An anxiogenic-like effect
- A dose-dependent facilitation of stress-induced fighting
- A dose-dependent taste and place aversion (An interest in eating may decline and unfamiliar and threatening locations will be avoided.)

In addition, when CRH is injected into the brains of animals, they display the same signs and symptoms as humans who are suffering from major clinical depression,[352] including a lack of interest in pleasurable activities; significant changes in weight and appetite; sleep disturbances; psychomotor agitation; fatigue; and self-destructive behavior (suicidal tendencies in humans).

That CRH is indeed driving much of this symptomatology is evidenced by 1) the fact that depressed humans also have sustained 24-hour elevations of plasma cortisol, and 2) the blocking of depressive states by administration of CRH receptor antagonists in experimental animals.[353] Thus, it is no surprise that patients with chronic diseases may be depressed and that chronically depressed patients may be suffering from a multitude of disorders, all of which are likely contributed to by chronic stimulation of the HPA axis. In fact, Chrousos and Gold have developed a list of chronic disease states that are associated with increased HPA (high cortisol present) or decreased HPA (low cortisol present) activity.[354] Table 32.2 shows conditions associated with high and low HPA activity. Clearly, if the course of chronic stress and its associated disease states could be addressed at the neuroendocrine and behavioral levels of CNS CRH overstimulation, a number of downstream pathologies might be favorably impacted.

Table 32.2 **Conditions Associated with HPA Axis Dysregulation**

Associated with High HPA Activity	Associated with Low HPA Activity
Chronic stress	Adrenal insufficiency
Melancholic depression	Chronic fatigue syndrome
Anorexia nervosa	Fibromyalgia
Diabetes mellitus	Postpartum depression
Syndrome X	Post-traumatic stress syndrome
Premenstrual syndrome	Exacerbation of rheumatoid arthritis

HPA Axis and Cytokines

Immune cells produce and secrete soluble mediators known as proinflammatory and anti-inflammatory cytokines.[355] The proinflammatory cytokines not only allow immune cells to communicate with each other and mount a vigorous immune response, but they also permit the immune system to communicate with neuroendocrine systems.[356] Proinflammatory cytokines such as IL-1, IL-2, IL-4, IL-6, and TNF are, of course, variously made by macrophages, monocytes, lymphocytes, and natural killer cells. In response to foreign antigens and pathogens (infectious stress), inflammation, trauma, and psychological stress, immune cells will release their large polypeptide, proinflammatory cytokines and these will enter the systemic circulation, thereby gaining access to the hypothalamus either through specific transport mechanisms[357,358] or by passing through the circumventricular organs (i.e., the OVLT and ME) where the blood-brain barrier is absent.[359] It is also happens that microglial, astroglial, endothelial, and neuronal cells in the hypothalamus synthesize their own IL-1, IL-2, IL-6, and TNF.[360] Interestingly, systemically circulating cytokines produced in response to stress can signal the activation of hypothalamically-produced cytokines. Each of the proinflammatory cytokines discussed here has been shown to stimulate CRH activity in the hypothalamus.[361] Chronic elevations of these cytokines in the brain not only raise CRH output, but also can cause anorexia, fever, fatigue, dementia, and even neuronal death.[362,363,364] With increased CRH activity, more ACTH (and thus cortisol) is produced. An important function is served by this cortisol increase following activation of immune cell cytokine production. When homeostasis is operating correctly, the rising levels of corticosteroid will eventually dampen the very robust immune response by reducing the proliferation and secretion of cytokines from immune cells. In the short term, this is useful because it prevents the increased immune response from running amok.[365] If the immune response were to go unchecked, it could trigger autoimmune events and produce unhelpful inflammatory responses during a fight or flight situation.[366]

Sometimes, though, individuals are exposed to persistent stressors without relief. Such situations will provide more or less continuous stimulation of the CRH-ACTH-cortisol axis. The ongoing high levels of cortisol may cause damage and death to the neurons in the hippocampus that mediate cortisol negative feedback on CRH neurons. In other words, with unregulated or untreated chronic stress, excessive exposure to cortisol may disable the negative restraint on stimulated CRH secretion.[367] The consequence of this may be to produce many of the pathologies associated with CRH-driven activities. For instance, excessive CRH acting in the brain may lead to depression and other behavioral disorders. This might be accompanied by elevated cortisol that causes metabolic derangements such as hyperglycemia, insulin resistance, hypertension, and other symptomatology of the Cushingoid condition. The presence of too much glucocorticoid may impair an individual's immune status, leading to the development of infectious conditions and memory impairment due to loss of hippocampal neurons.[368]

The HPA axis is in many ways the conductor of the homeostatic symphony. It is probably apparent at this point that the CRH of the brain is intertwined in some way with virtually every physiological system of the body. Polycystic ovary disease (PCOD) is an example of chronic illness that can be used to illustrate the interconnected web of physiological systems. In fact, almost any chronic, difficult-to-treat condition might share in the cascade of events to be described. **The main principle to be learned is that any chronic perturbation to one element of the system will ripple through other components of the web.** This being the case, one must try to address the initial causes of the perturbation at the beginning of the cascade to achieve the best outcome. Of course, there may still be much utility in addressing downstream symptoms to provide some immediate relief, but the most long-lasting solutions to chronic disease probably require the most comprehensive interventions aimed at the top of the pathological cascade.

Polycystic Ovary Disease: A Possible Scenario

Many women with polycystic ovary disease (also known as polycystic ovary syndrome, or PCOS) also suffer from anxiety and depression. In many instances, these women are overweight and develop insulin resistance. The have become amenorrheic or oligomenorrheic, which results in infertility. How might all of these symptoms be related?

If depression and anxiety precede the PCOD, we could speculate that some manner of life stress, without treatment or coping skills present, stimulates the overproduction of CRH in the brain and cortisol in the body. The elevated CRH drives the development of clinical depression, elevated adrenal cortisol, and androgen production. The high cortisol levels raise blood glucose levels. The persistence of high glucose concentrations leads to excessive insulin secretion. Excessive insulin secretion may cause insulin resistance to develop. With insulin resistance comes even more pancreatic production of insulin in an attempt to compensate. The high cortisol and insulin concentrations work synergistically to cause centripetal obesity characteristic of the metabolic syndrome (syndrome X). The excessive insulin, either through insulin or insulin-like growth factor-1 (IGF-1) receptors on ovarian stromal and thecal cells, stimulates more androgen hormone production. The excess androgen is converted into estrone by the extra adipose tissue of obesity. The elevated estrone levels disrupt the normal pulsatile secretion pattern of gonadotropin-releasing hormone (GnRH). This disruption alters the proper ratio of luteinizing hormone (LH) to follicle-stimulating hormone (FSH) release from the pituitary gland. The result is that too much LH is made and not enough FSH. The elevated LH stimulates further excessive androgen production, which compounds the hyperandrogenism being driven by the increased insulin concentrations. In the face of hyperandrogenism, high estrone, and disrupted LH/FSH ratio, normal menstrual cycles cease with amenorrhea, anovulation, and infertility being the result. The patient may display virilizing characteristics due to high androgen production such as acne, hirsutism, clitoral enlargement, and male hair distribution.[369]

Figure 32.5 graphically displays this sequence of events.

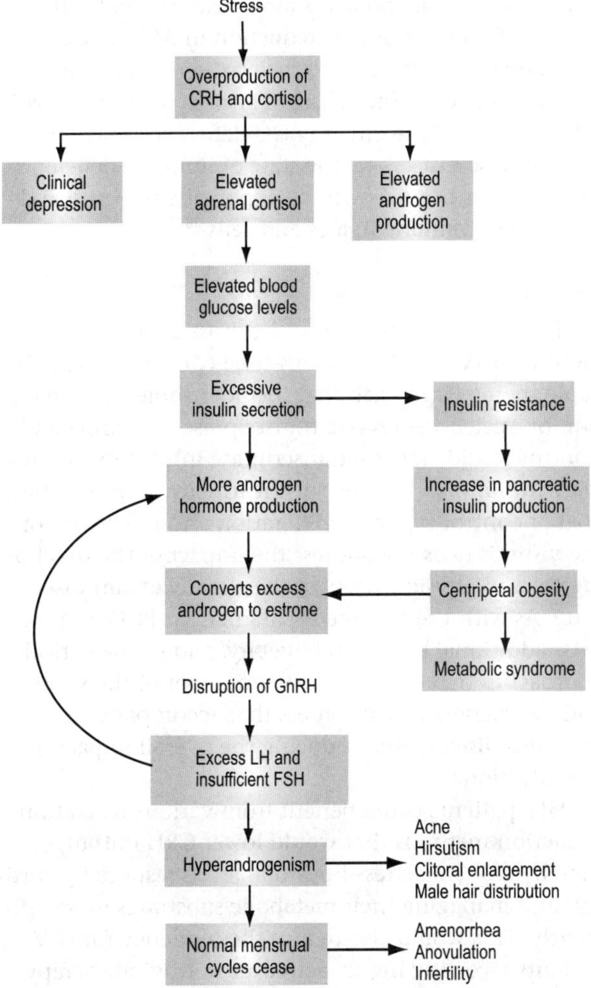

Figure 32.5 **The HPA cascade in PCOD**

Clinical Approaches to PCOD

While the classical approach to the treatment of this disease has been to use estrogen agonists and antagonists and perhaps androgen blockers, these interventions may be rather remote from important initiating factors in the cascade of decompensating events. A more comprehensive approach might involve lifestyle, dietary, and nutraceutical interventions that target more of the interconnected web of pathophysiological associations than treatment of the hyperandrogenization alone is likely to achieve.

Relaxation induction methods such as biofeedback, autogenic training, and mindfulness meditation[370,371] have been shown to reduce parameters indicative of sympathetic activation such as vasoconstriction of peripheral blood vessels, accelerated heart rate, and hypertension. Because increased sympathetic outflow is generated by CRH activation, a reduction of these parameters through relaxation methods would imply a reduction in CRH activity in the hypothalamus. From this would follow a lowering of cortisol, glucose, and insulin levels, which would reduce the overstimulation of androgen production by the adrenal cortex and the ovary. Then, less estrone would be synthesized by adipose tissue. The lowering of androgen and estrone levels could set the stage for a reestablishment of the normal pulsatile secretion of GnRH by the hypothalamus, and thus normal LH and FSH secretion patterns, followed once again by normal ovulatory cycles. All the while, the patient's psychologic and physiologic states are being improved.

Dietary and nutraceutical approaches might include increased intake of complex carbohydrates and fiber, and decreased intake of refined carbohydrates, to address the mood and metabolic disorders.[372] Chromium administration could aid both the depressive aspects of the condition as well as the insulin resistance issue.[373] Increased consumption of soy could inhibit the aromatization of excess androgen into estrone and improve the metabolic conversion of the excess estrogen into the 2-OH series rather than the more carcinogenic 16-OH series.[374] Increasing the intake of omega-3 fatty acids could combat the proinflammatory mediators brought on by the excess body fat and insulin resistance that are characteristic of PCOD. Further, omega-3 fatty acids combat depressive mood disorders.[375]

HIV/AIDS: A Probable Scenario

Patients suffering from HIV/AIDS experience not only the pathophysiological stress of the infection itself, but also the psychological stress of having a chronic, difficult-to-manage disease that carries a social stigma as well. In HIV/AIDS, inflammatory mediators are produced and lymphocyte numbers and function are impaired. The AIDS virus in peripheral and brain tissues results in significant production of the proinflammatory cytokines, especially IL-1β, TNF-α, and IL-6.[376] But the emotional stress of having this disease can also be expected to elevate proinflammatory cytokine levels. As described previously in this chapter, these cytokines will act upon the hypothalamus to stimulate the CRH-ACTH-cortisol axis,[377] and will act on the brain directly to produce sensations of fatigue, lethargy, and cachexia—symptoms that are common in AIDS patients. It also happens that CRH neurons make synaptic contact with the GnRH neurons that govern LH/FSH and thus gonadal steroid hormone synthesis. CRH axons project onto TRH neurons that govern TSH and thus thyroid hormone (T_4/T_3) synthesis by the thyroid gland. Furthermore, CRH nerve cells make synaptic contact with the GHRH cell bodies in the hypothalamus that govern growth hormone (GH) secretion and thus growth and repair of bone and soft tissues.[378]

When chronic HIV stress activates the CRH neurons, the GnRH-gonadotropin-sex steroid axis, the TRH-TSH-thyroid hormone axis, and the GHRH-GH-growth axis are all inhibited or impaired to varying degrees. In an acute stress response, this shifting of metabolic support away from reproductive and growth-promoting activities and toward the support of critical brain, heart, and skeletal muscle function enhances the likelihood of survival during a fight-or-flight situation. However, in a chronic condition such as AIDS, the persistent stimulation of the cytokine-CRH system and its negative impact on sex steroid, thyroid hormone, and GH activities can have devastating consequences that worsen the morbidity and mortality of the condition. For instance, the ongoing elevations in cortisol will further impair the protein synthesis of the pituitary hormones. This, of course, aggravates the already degraded production of hormones of the reproductive axis. In male patients with HIV/AIDS, the reduced production of testosterone by the testis may not only cause impotence, loss of libido, and infertility, but the diminution of this anabolic steroid may also contribute to the protein wasting that is often seen[379,380] and that is directly related to the imminence of death from the disease.[381]

Severely ill AIDS patients will also experience the "euthyroid sick syndrome," involving reduced production of TRH and impaired response of the thyroid gland to TSH.[382] The net result is a state of hypothyroidism that produces the well-known symptoms of lethargy, weakness, cold intolerance, dryness and pallor of skin, edema, and slowed mentation. The hormone deficiencies noted above may be accompanied by insufficient GH production due to the direct actions of the HIV virus to inhibit hypothalamic GHRH activity and because proinflammatory cytokines (such as IL-1) and CRH exert direct effects to inhibit GHRH and to stimulate somatostatin release from the hypothalamus.[383,384,385] Since GH is a protein anabolic hormone that promotes the growth of body tissues, its reduction in AIDS patients undoubtedly contributes to the wasting of lean body mass in adults and the failure of growth in children with this disorder.[386] The ongoing GH deficiency may, interestingly, also exacerbate the state of immune deficiency, since GH has been shown to support the integrity and function of immune tissues and cells.[387]

Clinical Approaches to HIV/AIDS

There is no question that the most effective treatment for HIV infection at this time continues to be the triple therapy approach that includes some combination of nucleoside reverse transcriptase inhibitors and non-nucleoside reverse transcriptase inhibitors, or protease inhibitors.[388] While this treatment addresses the goal of controlling the proliferation and infectivity of the virus, it does not address the impact of the psychological and physical stress of the already extant disease state. As with the treatment paradigm in PCOD, there exist additional behavioral, dietary, and nutraceutical approaches that could address a number of the stress and neuroendocrine disorders that accompany this insidious disease, thus reducing the overall impact of the infection.

HIV patients could benefit from various relaxation induction methods that would lower CRH output, thereby reducing stress hormone levels (especially cortisol) and managing their metabolic substrates more efficiently. This would also reduce the tendency for HIV patients receiving highly active antiretroviral therapy (HAART) to gain abdominal fat mass at the expense of lean muscle mass.

Relaxation-induced reductions in stress-elevated cytokines and CRH would also decrease the inhibitory tone exerted over LHRH, GHRH, and TRH neurons, possibly leading to increased pituitary gland output of LH, FSH, GH, and TSH that might restimulate their peripheral targets. If that goal could be achieved, it would increase the chances of elevating anabolic hormone levels of GH and testosterone (both lipolytic hormones), thereby enhancing the possibility of maintaining lean body mass and decreasing the drug-induced fat deposition. Poor wound healing would then be expected to improve due to the protein synthesis actions of these hormones. The improvement in TRH-TSH-thyroid hormone production would also be expected to increase the energy level and mental abilities of such patients. More GH production might enhance the immune status of the individual. Because the elevated proinflammatory cytokine levels in the brains of HIV patients may also cause neuronal damage and states of dementia to develop,[389] any attempts to reduce stress-activated cytokine levels could prove beneficial in this disorder.

Proinflammatory cytokines also act in the brain to cause the manufacture of reactive oxygen species (oxygen radicals) and inflammatory prostaglandins, which mediate many of the deleterious effects of the cytokines.[390] Since this is a problem in AIDS, the administration of antioxidant vitamins could be beneficial. In particular, vitamins C, E, and B complex have been shown to be effective in improving neuropsychologic disorders.[391,392,393] Most interestingly, this same combination of vitamins was recently demonstrated to delay the progression of HIV disease in women, most likely by exerting their antioxidant effects against the mediators of inflammatory processes.[394] HIV patients could also benefit from the intake of omega-3 fatty acids to help repair and protect neuronal membranes damaged by inflammatory mediators and, as in PCOD, to improve the depressive state of the patient.

Due to the protein wasting of AIDS, supplementation with amino acids in the face of improved anabolic hormone status might enhance the likelihood of restoring lean body mass. If the supplementation includes such amino acids as phenylalanine, tyrosine, and L-tryptophan, which are precursors for the synthesis of norepinephrine, thyroxine, and serotonin, respectively, then both neurological and thyroid gland functions could be better supported, as would the interactions between thyroid hormone, the CNS, and neuroendocrine systems.

With AIDS dementia, there can be compromised memory function. This could be addressed through the use of *Ginkgo biloba* to improve impaired memory in states of dementia.[395]

Obviously, in both chronic disorders mentioned above, the approaches described are not complete or exhaustive, nor is the research base for such interventions very well developed. They are offered as examples of how to view chronic disease in a more integrated and connected fashion, using our understanding of underlying mechanisms and pathways to provoke alternate considerations when designing comprehensive care for multifaceted disease states.

Summary

Chronic disease states necessarily imply chronic disruptions to homeostasis. Or, more simply, chronic disease creates chronic stress for patients. Chronic stress involves both psychological and physical reactions, setting off a cascade of events that is common to many complex, long-lasting illnesses. At the heart of stress detection is the hypothalamus, the integrative control center of actual mind-body (or brain-body) functions. With chronic stress of any kind comes the production of proinflammatory cytokines that signal increased activity of the hypothalamic-pituitary-adrenal axis. The hormones of the corticotropic axis then coordinate and manage the further activities of the brain, other neuroendocrine axes, behavior, metabolic substrates, electrolyte and water balance, and the immune system, all done in proper coordination with the demands and feedback from other organ systems.

In the acute phases of the stress response, the integrated control of the organ systems by the hypothalamic CRH system will enhance the likelihood of survival of the organism. However, if the elements of the acute stress response are not appropriately moderated or reduced in a timely fashion, the lasting stimulation of proinflammatory cytokines and CRH sets off a cascade of pathophysiological events that will negatively impact virtually every organ system to a lesser or greater degree. In the past, the approach to such massive decompensation of the patient was to treat each end-of-cascade symptom as a separate entity. However, this practice does not address the initiators of the cascade, overlooks ancillary problems, and often does not provide satisfying results to patients or their physicians. A better understanding of the factors that govern the initiation and mediation of this common cascade should help clinicians find healthier and more comprehensive avenues for managing chronic illnesses. An appreciation of the hypothalamic-pituitary-adrenal axis in stress responses and functional medicine philosophy should facilitate this goal.

Managing Insulin and Glucose Balance

Dan Lukaczer, ND

The balance between insulin and glucose is quite possibly the single most important clinical issue facing the practicing clinician today. It is clear that a substantial and growing body of evidence suggests that insulin sensitivity problems are an underlying causal factor in cardiovascular disease, stroke, type 2 diabetes, polycystic ovary syndrome (PCOS), and certain forms of cancer. Insulin resistance and hyperinsulinemia result in a cascade of biological effects; this complicated pathophysiology has been described elsewhere in this book. Here we will review a practical clinical approach to the diagnosis and treatment of this condition.

Clinical and Laboratory Diagnosis

Insulin resistance syndrome (IRS) refers to a cluster of symptoms characterized by varying degrees of glucose intolerance, abnormal HDL cholesterol and/or triglyceride levels, high blood pressure, and upper body obesity. The most obvious sign suggestive of IRS is upper body adiposity and elevated body mass index (BMI). Waist circumference >88 cm (34.5 in) in women and >102 cm (40 in) in men is an important and simple assessment.[396] However, care must be taken not to conclude that insulin resistance is exclusively seen in obese subjects, since greater than 50% of individuals with IRS are not classified as obese, and individuals may have normal insulin sensitivity with elevated BMI.[397] Recently, the Third Report of the National Cholesterol Education Program Expert Panel (2001) outlined specific criteria to diagnose metabolic syndrome.[i] These criteria are listed in Table 32.3.

[i] Metabolic syndrome does not completely encompass all aspects of insulin resistance. However, the parameters used to describe metabolic syndrome are broadly applicable. Metabolic syndrome is now widely used in research and, therefore, has become a well-recognized definition that is often used interchangeably with insulin resistance syndrome.

Table 32.3 **Criteria for the Diagnosis of Metabolic Syndrome**

A patient must have three or more of the following five criteria to be diagnosed with metabolic syndrome:

- Abdominal obesity: waist circumference >102 cm (40 in) in men and >88 cm (34.5 in) in women;
- Hypertriglyceridemia: ≥150 mg/dL (1.69 mmol/L);
- Low high-density lipoprotein (HDL) cholesterol: <40 mg/dL (1.04 mmol/L) in men, <50 mg/dL (1.29 mmol/L) in women;
- Blood pressure: ≥130/85 mm Hg;
- Fasting glucose: ≥110 mg/dL (≥6.1 mmol/L).

Published in the Third Report of the National Cholesterol Education Program Expert Panel, 2001.

Clinical observation may suggest other signs and symptoms helpful in identifying an individual with insulin resistance. Table 32.4 provides a list of commonly encountered signs and symptoms that may offer additional information in a clinical assessment.

Table 32.4 **Other Laboratory and Clinical Signs and Symptoms that May Be Suggestive of IRS**

Family history of diabetes
Gestational diabetes
Polycystic ovary syndrome (PCOS)
Infertility
Low birth weight
Sleep apnea
Sugar cravings and carbohydrate "addiction"
Sleepiness after a meal and insomnia relieved by snacking
Increased appetite following a high carbohydrate meal
Fatigue following high-carbohydrate meals
Hypoglycemia
Dietary history of high-refined carbohydrate intake
Resistant weight loss
Hirsutism, acne, and menstrual irregularities

Many individuals who develop insulin resistance maintain normal to near-normal fasting glucose control; two-hour postprandial glucose challenge test with a 75-gram glucose load may be marginally elevated, suggesting impaired glucose tolerance. Elevated fasting insulin, and/or two-hour postprandial insulin may also be important indicators of insulin resistance. However, after the onset of type 2 diabetes there may be a reduction in beta cell function and, eventually, a fall in insulin. In addition, several other laboratory signs may suggest an individual with subclinical IRS, or at high risk of developing insulin resistance. Useful additional markers that suggest IRS include elevated triglycerides and depressed HDL (triglycerides-to-HDL ratio of >3).[398] An elevated serum uric acid also appears to be associated with IRS. Recent literature also suggests a relationship between IRS and markers of inflammation, such as hsCRP.[399]

Clinical Intervention

It appears that at the core of insulin resistance is a defect in cellular sensitivity to insulin. As more light has been shed on this topic, this underlying metabolic dysregulation has become a focus for the clinician's attention.[400] Although the cellular disturbance is not completely understood at the biochemical level, modifiable factors such as obesity, exercise, and nutrition appear to play a significant role. While genetic inheritance may determine propensity to the disorder, these modifiable factors should be addressed as part of any comprehensive clinical management strategy.

Exercise, Smoking and Obesity

Exercise has profound beneficial effects on insulin resistance and should be aggressively pursued. Numerous studies support the use of exercise in the management of this condition.[401,402] Conversely, cigarette smoking plays a role in exacerbating insulin resistance in susceptible individuals.[403] Therefore, in those individuals, smoking is particularly detrimental. Increased adiposity plays a pivotal role as well, especially when concentrated around the abdomen and upper body. Adiposity/obesity induces insulin resistance in peripheral tissues; thus, weight loss (specifically fat loss) is of prime importance, and has been shown (not surprisingly) to improve insulin sensitivity.[404,405] Because of its anabolic activity, insulin and hyperinsulinemia secondary to insulin resistance may predispose to increased weight gain and difficulty with weight loss.[406] Longitudinal studies suggest that elevated insulin levels may start in childhood, with fasting hyperinsulinemia serving as a predictor of increased body weight gain and obesity.[407,408]

While adiposity is an important issue, not all insulin-resistant individuals are obese. Other factors are involved, and individuals may have normal insulin levels while still remaining overweight.[409,410] The sensitivity of insulin to stimulate glucose uptake varies widely from person to person, with the degree of obesity as only one factor.[411] Clearly, obesity, smoking, and a sedentary lifestyle increase risk for insulin resistance and should be managed aggressively; however, they are not necessarily an essential characteristic of this complex syndrome.

Nutritional Modulation

In addition to appropriate lifestyle changes, insulin and glucose balance can be promoted through dietary adjustments and the use of select nutritional supplements. The relative amounts and types of carbohydrate, protein, fat, and fiber are all important factors that influence glucose availability and insulin secretion and therefore may be important in managing IRS. Dietary recommendations for patients with insulin resistance should be individualized, with consideration given to eating habits and other lifestyle factors. Nutritional supplement recommendations are then developed to meet treatment goals and desired outcomes. Monitoring metabolic parameters, including blood glucose, lipids, blood pressure, and body weight, as well as quality of life, is crucial to ensure successful outcomes.

Food as Medicine

Macronutrients influence both glycemic and insulin response. The ratio and type of macronutrients are important considerations, yet the dietary prescription remains controversial. A high-carbohydrate, low-fat diet for type 2 diabetics has been shown in some studies to produce adverse lipid and glycemic effects. High carbohydrate diets (60–70% carbohydrate) decrease insulin receptor numbers, probably as a result of the increased insulin cellular contact and resultant receptor downregulation.[412] Some studies have shown that high-carbohydrate diets increase triglyceride and VLDL cholesterol levels, and elevate insulin and glucose concentrations in type 2 diabetics.[413,414] Fat in general has been thought to have little insulinogenic effect. However, alterations in membrane lipid composition and membrane fluidity influence important cellular functions. Studies have suggested that there is an altered membrane dynamic in type 2 diabetics as compared to normal controls, which may influence insulin action. This underscores the importance of the physiochemical properties of the cell membrane to control the activity of membrane proteins such as insulin receptors. If the decreased response to insulin is, in part, the result of a defect in characteristics or functions of the receptor caused by altered membrane fluidity, attending to membrane dynamics becomes an important therapeutic target.[415]

Fatty acids within the phospholipid bilayer help to determine the physiochemical properties of membranes that, in turn, influence cellular functions, including hormone responsiveness. Dietary fat has been shown to determine to a large extent the composition of cell membrane phospholipids. It appears that direct alterations in the fat composition of the cell membrane can induce changes in insulin responsiveness. The long-chain polyunsaturated fatty acids (PUFAs) can modulate the function of insulin receptors and glucose transporters through effects on the physical properties of the surrounding lipid environment.[416] In cultured cells, increasing cell membrane content of PUFAs increases membrane fluidity, insulin binding to receptors, and insulin action.[417] In animal models it has been shown specifically that omega-3 fatty acids (explored in depth in Chapter 27) such as eicosapentaenoic acid (EPA) and docosahexaenoic acid (DHA) have a beneficial effect on plasma insulin and lipid concentrations.[418] Conversely, saturated fats and *trans* fatty acids decrease membrane fluidity and decrease binding of insulin to its receptors.[419,420,421] When omega-3 fatty acids are substituted for other sources of fat in a high-fat diet, insulin resistance in skeletal muscle may be prevented.[422,423] In human trials, monounsaturated diets appear to mitigate against these adverse changes as well.[424] For these reasons, the high-monounsaturated fat diet (popularized as the Mediterranean Diet) has been proposed as an alternative to the high-carbohydrate diet. Studies using a lower carbohydrate, higher monounsaturated and polyunsaturated fat diet show decreased fasting glucose, insulin, and triglycerides.[425,426,427] Most, but not all,[428] studies have supported this conclusion.

Studies using dietary approaches to treat individuals with insulin resistance have been inconsistent. This may be explained in part by the wide range of physiologic effects that equal amounts of different carbohydrates may have on glucose regulation. This variation in response to carbohydrates has resulted in the study of the glycemic index (GI). The concept of GI developed as the result of intensive carbohydrate research showing that similar amounts of carbohydrate in foods did not elicit similar postprandial glycemic responses.[429,430] The GI of a food is defined as the blood glucose response to a 50-gram available carbohydrate portion of that food expressed as a percentage of the response to the same amount of carbohydrate from a standard food, which is either glucose or white bread. The GI value depends on a number of factors, such as degree of starch gelatinization, physical form of the food, acidity, food processing, and the presence, amount, and type of protein, fat, fiber, and available carbohydrate in the food. Of these, the effects of fiber and type of starch on glucose response deserve further mention.

It is well known that fiber plays an important role in affecting insulin and glucose response.[431,432] High fiber, independent of total carbohydrates, has a beneficial effect on blood glucose control and atherogenic lipoproteins.[433] It appears that soluble fibers in particular act favorably on blood insulin concentrations. Their mode of action appears to be in slowing gastric emptying and, to a lesser extent, inhibition of starch degradation in the upper small intestine.[434] The type of starch is also an important issue in GI. Because of its structure, the starch amylose, as opposed to the more common amylopectin, has a significant positive impact on insulin response in both animal and human studies.[435,436] Insulin and triglyceride levels were reduced in individuals placed on a high-amylose diet, suggesting a beneficial effect on factors involved in insulin sensitivity.[437] Studies also suggest that a low-GI dietary plan helps control blood sugar levels and leads to decreased caloric intake.[438] Overall, studies in both men and women show that diets with a low GI are associated with a lower risk of developing type 2 diabetes and heart disease.[439,440] Recently, the United Nations World Health Organization has recommended that all people base their diets on low-GI foods.

Protein may also have an impact on insulin and glucose response. Some studies have shown protein ingestion results in a blunting of the glucose rise and insulin response in normal individuals.[441] However, more recent work suggests that protein-rich foods may vary in their effect, although in general they exhibit a low to modest response.[442]

Selected Nutrients and Phytonutrients

Research has shown that many vitamins, minerals, and certain phytonutrients have the potential to improve insulin sensitivity and stabilize blood glucose levels. The mechanism of action for many of these substances has not been completely elucidated and remains under intense investigation. The following is not an all-inclusive list, but highlights some key nutrients and phytonutrients that show significant promise in their ability to modify insulin resistance.

Magnesium. Magnesium plays an important role in glucose homeostasis by altering both insulin secretion and action. Adequate intracellular magnesium concentrations may therefore allow for improvement of glucose handling.[443] Daily magnesium supplements appear to improve the behavior of hormone receptors and improve glucose transport into the cell.[444] Tissue levels of magnesium are often low in diabetics and in individuals with normal glucose disposal.[445,446,447] Low intracellular magnesium results in impairment of insulin action and a worsening of insulin resistance in hypertensives and type 2 diabetics.[448,449] A low magnesium concentration in nondiabetic subjects has been associated with relative insulin resistance, glucose intolerance, and hyperinsulinemia.[450]

Chromium. A great deal of work has been done on the relationship between chromium and glucose tolerance.[451,452] Certain lipophilic forms of chromium have been shown to increase membrane fluidity and insulin-mediated glucose uptake in cultured cells and animal models. Chromium may affect the action of insulin by influencing the rate of insulin internalization, which may regulate the synthesis or insertion of insulin receptors into the plasma membrane.[453] Chromium functions physiologically to promote the insulin responsiveness of skeletal muscle, and probably adipocytes as well. Chromium deficiency is also associated with elevated blood glucose levels, hypercholesterolemia, and the development of aortic plaques.[454] Beneficial effects of supplemental chromium on serum lipids have been reported in controlled trials.[455] Recent studies have examined the use of chromium in type 2 diabetics and suggest that fasting and postprandial blood sugar and insulin, as well as glycated hemoglobin, are significantly reduced with supplementation.[456,457]

Vanadium. Vanadyl sulfate is a salt of the mineral vanadium. Although vanadium is ubiquitous in the environment, its essentiality in humans has not been established. However, results from deficiency studies are highly suggestive of an essential role for vanadium as a nutrient in humans.[458] In both animal and human studies, vanadate and vanadyl forms of vanadium have demonstrated insulin-like effects on glucose metabolism.[459] However, its exact physiological action is not completely understood. It does not replace insulin by its action, but rather appears to activate cellular insulin receptors either by phosphotyrosine phosphorylation or via inhibition of phosphotyrosine phosphatase enzymes.[460,461] This leads to an increase in glucose transporter proteins (GLUTs) in the plasma membrane, which are essential for the transport of glucose into the cell. In human trials, vanadium has been shown to improve insulin sensitivity in type 2 diabetes at dosages of 100–125 mg/day.[462,463,464] There is currently no RDA for vanadium. The upper safe limit has been set by the U.S. Food and Nutrition Board at 1.8 mg/day; therefore, ingesting 50–100 mg long-term may be dangerous. In fact, a recent study suggested chronic exposure to high levels of vanadium reduces cognitive abilities.[465] While this was not from oral ingestion of vanadium, caution is called for in long-term supplementation with high levels of vanadium, and supplementation should be strictly monitored.

Biotin. Biotin is a vitamin that can be synthesized by microflora in the colon. Biotin deficiency has been suggested to result in an impairment of glucose tolerance. Animal studies suggest that a high biotin intake can improve the metabolism and/or utilization of glucose without the acceleration of insulin secretion from the pancreas.[466] Human studies indicate that intravenous biotin may be useful in the management of diabetes.[467] Additionally, it has been observed that high dose oral biotin (9 mg/day in divided dosages) may substantially lower fasting glucose in type 2 diabetic patients.[468] While the mechanism remains unclear, it may be due to the enhancement of the biotin-dependent enzyme, pyruvate carboxylase, and its effect on utilization of glucose in the citric acid cycle.

Conjugated linoleic acid. Conjugated linoleic acid (CLA) is a mixture of isomers of linoleic acid and is found naturally in dairy products and meats. *In vitro* models using CLA have shown effects on peroxisome proliferators (PP) similar to those seen with the class of oral insulin-sensitizing agents known as thiazolidinediones.[469,470] PPs exert their biological responses as the result of activation of a subgroup of nuclear steroid hormone receptors known as peroxisome proliferator activated receptors (PPARs). PPARs appear to modulate lipid and insulin metabolism through a variety of mechanisms, including regulation of gene expression and an increase in the mobilization and production of GLUTs. The PPAR agonist drugs, classed as thiazolidinediones, have been shown to decrease circulating glucose levels and also reverse insulin resistance.[471] CLA has been shown in animal studies to share some functional similarities to these thiazolidinediones, and has further been shown to normalize impaired glucose tolerance and improve hyperinsulinemia.[472] However, clinical human research has been inconclusive.

Alpha-lipoic acid. Animal and human studies suggest that alpha-lipoic acid (ALA) increases insulin-stimulated glucose disposal. The mechanisms of action may involve improvement of glucose transport, an increase in the number or activation of glucose transporter proteins, or an increase in non-oxidative or oxidative glucose disposal.[473,474,475,476] Recent human trials suggest that oral administration of ALA (600–1800 mg/day for four weeks) can improve insulin sensitivity in patients with type 2 diabetes.[477] Additionally, a number of trials have also been conducted using ALA in the treatment of diabetic polyneuropathy (DPN) with doses of at least 600 mg per day. Results generally demonstrate that ALA improves this condition and support the assumption that ALA might exert some of its beneficial effects unassociated with glucose disposal. One hypothesis suggests that its effects in DPN are at least partially due to improved microcirculation.[478]

Green tea. Green tea may have important effects on insulin modulation. Primary phytonutrients in green tea are the catechins and epicatechins. *In vitro* and animal studies have shown catechins to be an insulin sensitizer, pancreatic protectant, helpful in the delay of glucose absorption, and able to repress hepatic glucose production.[479,480,481,482,483] While the dosage for humans is not clear, doses of 200–400 mg/day of catechins have been used in various studies in other areas and appear to be very safe.

Cinnamon. Work on cinnamon began a few years ago with *in vitro* data that suggested this common spice had bioactive compounds that might have insulin-like effects.[484] Other *in vitro* work appeared to confirm this.[485,486] Follow-up animal experiments suggest that long-term use of cinnamon bark might provide benefit against diabetic complications.[487] Recently, the first human clinical trial was published. In this placebo-controlled study, diabetic subjects given as little as 1 g/day of cinnamon powder for six weeks showed improvements in fasting glucose, triglycerides, LDL and total cholesterol.[488]

Summary

IRS is a complex disorder that requires a multifaceted plan to manage. With estimates that over a quarter of the United States population may already have signs and symptoms suggestive of this dysfunction, relying primarily on a pharmacological approach after a frank disease such as diabetes or heart disease has been diagnosed seems far too costly and unlikely to stem the rising tide. A primary prevention and early treatment strategy should be to maintain a healthy balance between glucose and insulin throughout each person's life by focusing on diet, nutritional supplementation, exercise, and other lifestyle modifications.

Perimenopause, Menopause, and Women's Health: The Dance of the Hormones, Part II

Bethany Hays, MD

Introduction

The job of the clinician is to translate the scientific information obtained from various sources into a systematic evaluation and treatment plan for patients with specific or general complaints, or for patients who simply wish to stay healthy and enjoy a long life. Such an evaluation and treatment plan can be created in the area of female hormone therapies, despite the current fluctuations in the standard of care and the rapidly changing stream of information, by using the concepts of functional medicine.

A Clinical Approach

Although many clinicians are trained using a "protocol" approach, patient-centered care has more recently come to the forefront. Recognizing that treating individuals rather than the mean of a group (the bell-shaped curve) is a cornerstone of functional medicine.

Assessing Body Type

The first step in the assessment of the individual patient is to do a history and physical. Functional medicine—and the matrix (Chapter 34)—present a wonderfully coherent way to receive and organize the information uncovered in this process. Physical examination of patients starts when you first set eyes on them:

- Look at body size and shape (weight distribution).
- Assess skin color, temperature, and tone. Is the hand trembling or sweating when you shake it?
- Notice any visible rashes or evidence of dry skin.
- Note posture, demeanor, and movement.

Although an initial evaluation should never be done with the preconceived idea of focusing on a specific part of the functional medicine web, when the clinician finds a preponderance of clinical issues in the neuroendocrine part of the web, he/she should start the evaluation of the patient by noticing size and weight distribution. Diana Schwarzbein describes the body habitus of people with dominance of the three major hormones.[489]

1. **Adrenaline or Catecholamine**—These folks are thin, with muscle wasting in any muscles they are not specifically exercising. Fortunately, many of them are exercising; unfortunately, the purpose of their exercise and other lifestyle activities is to stay thin. Many are overexercising, with a concomitant elevation in adrenaline levels. Ironically, even in the context of increased exercise, they lose muscle mass secondary to the metabolic effects of increased adrenaline levels. The marathon runner is the prototypical adrenaline body type.
2. **Cortisol**—These folks usually move to a high cortisol neuroendocrine pattern after years of living a high-stress, high-adrenaline/catecholamine lifestyle. With elevated cortisol comes a new fat distribution around the midsection. Contrary to popular belief, the apple body shape is less likely to be an indication of high insulin and more likely to be a sign of high cortisol. After many years of high cortisol output, they may progress to a cortisol deficiency state with relative inability to respond adequately to intercurrent stresses. Allergy, as an expression of relative adrenal exhaustion, can become a major component of their symptomatology with accompanying "allergic shiners." Inflammatory symptoms also occur due to the inability to provide adequate cortisol response. If they have maintained an exercise program, they may not manifest the final step—insulin resistance.
3. **Insulin**—These folks are the insulin-resistant, and/or diabetic patients. They often put weight on everywhere. They get there one of two ways: through a high cortisol lifestyle or through dysfunctional genetics. The former will have the apple body shape of their previous high cortisol and the latter may not. In the unusual case, a client can present with insulin resistance with a thin body habitus, so be cautious!

Since there are many factors active in the production and distribution of fat and muscle mass, this approach is not 100% accurate, but it is surprising how often the body-type assessment is a useful finding in setting the course for further assessment.

Patient-centered History

After the initial assessment, the clinician should take a thorough history. (Chapter 34 provides an in-depth review of the overall patient assessment process.) Allowing patients to tell their stories, without interruption if possible, can be a valuable tool for the functional medicine practitioner. Most patients have never had an opportunity to do this without significant interruption. *Engaged listening* can create a context of safety for deeper revelations by the patient about their observations and fears related to their own bodies. (Chapter 36 explores the doctor-patient relationship in detail.)

While taking the history, the clinician should look for symptoms that suggest imbalances in major or minor hormones. A thorough **menstrual history**, including onset, frequency, length, volume, and character of flow in the past and recently, is important for the clinician assessing hormones. Other key indicators to look for include:

1. **Evidence of estrogen dominance**
   - Breast tenderness
   - Fibrocystic changes
   - Heavy periods
   - Fat distribution in the hips or thighs
   - Anxiety
   - Recent growth of fibroids
   - Presence of endometriosis or symptoms suggestive of it, such as pain or dysmenorrhea
2. **Lack of progesterone or imbalance between estrogen and progesterone**
   - Spotting before and after the period
   - Anxiety
   - Oral contraceptive use
   - Hormone replacement of estrogen only
   - Perimenopause
   - Oligo-ovulation such as in PCOS

3. **Signs of perimenopause and menopause**
   - Irregularity in menstrual cycle
   - Changes in length and flow of menstrual cycle
   - Increasing PMS symptoms
   - For postmenopausal women—when did they go through menopause; was it natural or surgical?
4. **Whether the patient has had a tubal ligation or hysterectomy with or without removal of the ovaries.** Both of these procedures can affect ovarian steroid output, either temporarily or permanently, often without the patient knowing (since the uterus is absent). Many women have been started on hormone replacement therapy before they were truly menopausal and need to be tested to confirm their true status.

A **pregnancy history** should pay attention to size of infants, complications during pregnancy, any history of infertility and how it was managed, and what kinds of problems the children are having. (A major source of stress for mothers, with accompanying neuroendocrine imbalances, is the health of their children; some functional medicine guidance about issues such as family nutrition can make huge difference in the patient's life.)

The clinician should also be looking for evidence of imbalance in other systems that affect or interact with the female hormone system:

1. **Testosterone imbalance**
   - Acne
   - Anger or aggressiveness
   - Changes in libido
   - Hair growth or loss and distribution
   - Loss of muscle mass
2. **Thyroid dysfunction**
   - Constipation
   - Low or loss of energy
   - Muscle pain or burning
   - Changes in skin or hair
   - Depression
   - Irregular bleeding
3. **Neuroactive chemical imbalance**
   - Depression
   - Anxiety
   - Hot flashes
   - ADD
   - Poor sleep
4. **Elevated adrenaline**
   - Heart palpitations
   - Anxiety
5. **Inability to secrete adrenaline** when needed (dizziness upon standing up)
6. **High cortisol**
   - Frequent colds or infections
   - Difficulty losing abdominal weight
7. **Inability to secrete cortisol** when needed
   - Allergies
   - Inflammatory diseases
   - Autoimmune diseases
   - Any problem that has been treated with corticosteroids
8. **Insulin resistance**
   - Infections or poor wound healing
   - Brain fog
   - Difficulty losing weight
   - Carbohydrate cravings
   - Excessive weight gain in pregnancy, or
   - A large-for-gestational-age baby
9. **Inflammatory conditions**
   - Dysmenorrhea
   - A history of endometriosis
   - Skin rashes
   - Arthritis and other pain symptoms

Once a picture of the patient's "functional web" has been created from the history, we proceed to the physical examination. Since most patients who come with the idea that they are there to get help with hormonal problems need a gynecologic exam, the following will be familiar to the gynecologist but incomplete from a general medical practice point of view. (A more complete approach is discussed in Chapter 34.)

Physical Examination

Important things to look for relative to endocrine function include (but are not limited to):

1. Vital signs
   - Height and weight
   - Especially palpitations or elevated pulse
   - Elevated BP
   - Orthostatic hypotension
2. Skin
   - Turgor
   - Dryness
   - Rashes
   - Hair distribution

- Flushing or mottling
- Acne

3. Thyroid
   - Enlargement
   - Loss of tissue
   - Evidence of autoimmune disease (gland consistency)
   - Tremor
   - Eye signs (e.g., exophthalmia, lid lag)
4. Breast
   - Cysts
   - Masses
   - Fibrocystic changes
   - Tenderness
   - Discharge
   - Dimpling
5. Abdominal exam
   - Abdominal obesity
   - Liver size
   - Presence of gas or constipation
   - Masses
   - Ascites
6. Vaginal exam
   - Vulvovaginal atrophy
   - Amount and type of discharge
7. Uterine exam
   - Fibroids
   - Increased size or bogginess of the corpus
   - Fixation or evidence of adhesions
8. Ovarian exam
   - Size
   - Symmetric cystic enlargement
   - Masses suggestive of endometriosis or cancer
   - Fixation or evidence of adhesions

The clinician should be looking for signs of imbalance of the major hormones (adrenaline, cortisol, and insulin), evidence of high or low estrogen effect, underproduction or overproduction (or more often overdosing) of progesterone, evidence of overproduction or effect of testosterone, hypothyroidism or less often hyperthyroidism, as well as any pathology.

Most of the other imbalances of the endocrine system will require laboratory evaluation to ferret out. However, by the end of the history and physical, the clinician should have a pretty good idea about the three major hormones, the estrogen effect, the balance between estrogen and progesterone, and the presence of excessive or inadequate testosterone.

Laboratory Evaluation

A good clinician should use both clinical evaluation and laboratory data to evaluate hormonal status. Although liberal use of laboratory evaluation can be reassuring, the idiosyncrasies of hormonal fluctuation and the limitations of laboratory testing can lead to excessive expense and unhelpful information. Therefore, the clinician must learn to use the patient's symptoms and responses to guide diagnosis and therapy.

Because of the current concerns about hormone therapy, a clinician should have a low threshold for obtaining laboratory documentation of the levels of hormone replacement once a stable regimen is established, assuring that the therapy and dosage are normalizing hormone levels and not creating non-physiologic levels.

Evaluating hormone levels is difficult at best. Which test? Which fluid(s)? When to test? Ideally, one would test the levels in the tissue of interest; however, this is not yet clinically feasible in most instances. **It is important to remember that hormone levels in various target body tissues are likely to be very different than in the body fluids tested (blood, urine, or saliva).**[490] Breast tissue for instance, especially in the area surrounding tumors, has been shown to elaborate aromatase, 17-OH-ase, and sulfatase, sometimes significantly increasing the local level of estrogens.

In addition to the absolute values of various hormones, it is important to assess the ratios of hormones that interact with each other, such as estrogen and progesterone, bound and unbound estrogen and testosterone, and 2/16-OH estrogen metabolites.

Because of the normal fluctuations of these hormones, it may be necessary to obtain multiple samples in order to average the levels over time and get an accurate picture. This is especially true premenopausally when there are dramatic fluctuations over the course of a single menstrual cycle. When evaluating multiple samples over the course of a menstrual cycle, it is most practical to obtain salivary hormone levels so that patients can do home collection of samples every few days over the course of a month. Because there is less fluctuation of testosterone over the month (except during midcycle), a single testosterone level during the month is usually adequate. This type of collection over the course of a month can be helpful to assess presence of ovulation, luteal phase deficiency (helpful in fertility patients and with certain types of menstrual abnormalities), and ratios of estrogen to progesterone that can be compared with standards.

Single salivary hormone levels can be more problematic. Although single salivary estrogen levels appear to be reliable, there is considerable debate about the interpretation of salivary progesterone levels[491,492,493,494] and testosterone levels.[495] In particular, there has been controversy about the effectiveness of transdermal progesterone in protecting the endometrium and bone, and in the appropriateness of using salivary hormone levels to monitor progesterone transdermal therapy. It is clear that salivary progesterone, while reported to reflect the levels in serum, is much higher in saliva when administered transdermally than when given by mouth. Explanation for this has been that progesterone in transdermal creams is lipophilic and is absorbed by red blood cells in capillaries, keeping serum levels low while delivering higher doses to tissues. A study by Lewis et al.[496] using 20 and 40 mg doses of progesterone transdermally showed elevated and variable salivary hormone levels and no increase in RBC membrane levels of progesterone. In addition, despite high levels of progesterone in salivary secretions, most studies show failure of secretory changes in the endometrium with transdermal progesterone regimens,[497] suggesting that levels may differ from one tissue to another. It should be noted, however, that in spite of this failure to induce secretory changes, the levels of progesterone reaching the endometrium appear to be able to prevent endometrial hyperplasia, the goal of most postmenopausal progesterone therapies.[498]

Urinary hormone levels over 24 hours allow an average level of hormone to be determined and the 2- to 16-OH estrogen ratio can be determined. Collection can be done at home, but is somewhat cumbersome for patients and must be compared to creatinine excretion to insure adequacy of collection.

Serum hormone levels correlate with perhaps the largest number of reported studies, and, in addition, serum hormone levels are more likely to be covered by insurance companies (with the right diagnostic codes, of course). They are limited by providing only a "snapshot" of the often fluctuating hormonal milieu. As stated before, serum hormone levels do not necessarily reflect the levels in target tissues and therefore reflect availability of hormone precursors perhaps more than they reflect hormone *effect*.

In summary, because of complicating variables such as the difference between blood and tissue levels of hormone, and because of the biological effect of metabolites, xenoestrogens, and nutritional estrogens, the relevance of the measured hormone levels should be assessed with some degree of circumspection. The clinician will have to determine through use which laboratory assessments to use in a given clinical picture (serum in single sample postmenopausal women whose hormones are relatively stable vs. multi-sample salivary collections in premenopausal women for the purposes of documenting ovulation or perhaps assessing hormone balance). In order to evaluate hormonal balance, hormone load, and free hormone levels, ordering serum testosterone, progesterone, 2- and 16-OH estrogens, and SHBG, all collected at the same time, will prove useful. The clinician should try several of these approaches and familiarize him/herself with an approach that seems to correlate best with the patient's symptoms and needs.

Prescribing Hormones

When prescribing hormones in my clinical practice, I am guided by the following principles:

1. Replace human hormones with bioidentical hormones.
2. Attempt to return hormone levels to "normal" physiological levels.
3. Attempt to give the hormone in the most physiological way.
4. Remember to think about other hormones that may affect the level of the hormone you wish to treat.
5. Check hormone levels by laboratory testing, if possible, to be sure you are creating normal levels.
6. Whenever possible, check downstream metabolites of administered hormones and hormones whose levels may be affected by the therapy.

Although it has been suggested that there is no evidence to prefer bioidentical hormones,[499] it is clear that laboratory evaluation of hormone therapy requires that the hormones that are given and their metabolites be measurable with the clinically available laboratory tests. This cannot be done for conjugated estrogens or the commonly used progestins. The need to be able to evaluate levels of administered hormone is particularly important given the unstable medical-legal environment relating to hormone replacement therapy in menopause.

In addition, the estrogens most used in the U.S. (conjugated equine estrogens) have a substantially different metabolism due to the large fraction of equine estrogens and the fact that because of the unsaturated B ring they are metabolized to DNA-damaging quinines.[500,501] Some metabolites of equine estrogens are stronger estrogens than their substrate.[502]

Philosophically, one would think that the path of evolution would be more reliable than the rather brief history of human intervention, so whenever possible one should try to return hormone levels to established norms for age and gender. In order to achieve the integration of these goals into practice, the following questions should be asked and (hopefully) answered prior to initiating therapy:

1. Is the gland over- or, more often, underproducing the hormone?
2. If so, is it because it is "broken" (absent or affected by autoimmune disease)?
3. If it is not "broken," is it compensating for another hormone that is abnormally low or high?

For example, it is conceivable that when adrenaline is high, thyroid will compensate to protect the heart from arrhythmias and excessive pulse rates. In this environment, administering thyroid hormone may put the heart under further stress. Without understanding this reciprocal relationship, many clinicians have had the experience of treating patients with symptoms of borderline hypothyroidism and slightly elevated TSH levels with a trial of thyroid hormone. The patient would return complaining that the cardiac and nervous symptoms were too much to handle. It is possible that these patients' low thyroid function was balancing their high adrenaline state. Attempts to "normalize" their thyroid levels failed because the intervention (thyroid replacement) inadequately assessed the total metabolic picture. Thus, basing treatment of thyroid on a clinical parameter such as low basal body temperature without consideration of the complex mix and interaction of hormones can lead to further loss of hormone flexibility. Therefore, in the appropriate clinical context, it might be advisable to address the high adrenaline (catecholamine) levels with diet, lifestyle, and supplement approaches before treating borderline hypothyroidism with thyroxine or triiodothyronine.

In menopause management, there are currently two competing philosophies: one position suggests that premenopausal women are normal and postmenopausal women are hormone deficient. The other says that premenopausal women are hormone toxic in order to have babies and postmenopausal women are normal. Depending upon which philosophy the clinician adheres to, he/she will treat postmenopausal women differently. In the first instance, the clinician will wish to return postmenopausal hormone levels to "normal" premenopausal levels; in the second, he/she will try to normalize women at a postmenopausal level of hormones. This author is an advocate of the second philosophy.

Since the WHI, there has been a growing discussion in the gynecological literature suggesting that if women are given low-dose hormone replacement they will not need progesterone therapy even if they retain their uteruses.[503] This suggests that if postmenopausal women are only replaced to a level at the lower end of the range for normal menopause (10–40 pg/mL[504]), normal progesterone levels produced by the adrenal glands could provide enough balance to prevent endometrial hyperplasia,[505] as they appear to do in unsupplemented women who maintain normal levels of hormone. If, however, adrenal progesterone (the primary source of progesterone after menopause) is being shifted instead into the production of cortisol (e.g., secondary to a stress-prone lifestyle), progesterone will need to be replaced to balance estrogen in various organ systems including breast, brain, bone, and uterus. This may also be true of women who have elevated estrogen levels due to obesity or inadequate metabolism and excretion of estrogens. These women are currently not being evaluated in any specific way and may be the true at-risk population. It is the author's suspicion that, at physiologic levels, continuous progesterone HRT will not produce insulin resistance (a potential side effect of continuous progesterone HRT), obviating the need for cycling progesterone as has been recommended by some.[506] However, since there are no randomized studies with this approach, careful monitoring of hormone levels and endometrial assessment with periodic biopsy or ultrasound should be done. Fasting insulin levels to assess the effects of progesterone on glucose metabolism would also be advisable.

Exogenously administered hormones are metabolized into "downstream" metabolites depending on

- the genetics of the CYP and phase II enzymes,
- the environmental up- and downregulators of those enzymes,

- dosage of hormone given, and
- whether the hormones are synthetic derivatives or bioidentical.

It is wise, therefore, to evaluate the downstream metabolites, as well as the hormone being administered, whenever possible. An example would be to obtain 2- and 16-OH estrogen levels before and after administering exogenous estrogen. Another would be to obtain estrogen and testosterone levels when administering pregnenolone or DHEA. Because enzyme function is often bi-directional, high doses of a hormone may flow upstream to precursors; for instance, estriol (especially when administered by mouth) has the potential to be converted to 16-OH estradiol, a much stronger estrogen.[507] The author cannot report having seen this effect with vaginally administered estriol and has inadequate experience with orally administered estriol. When evaluating the "estrogen pool," or the totality of estrogen receptor agonists, evaluation of SHBG can be useful, as it appears that levels of SHBG increase in response to many of the downstream metabolites, as well as to estrogen, estrone, and testosterone.

Balancing Hormones after Menopause

Ultimately-the role of hormone replacement is to replace or re-balance (a much more complicated prospect) missing or underproduced hormones. Since the various hormones interact with each other, it is important to try to understand whether a hormone is missing or is low because it is compensating for another hormone that is elevated or depressed.

It should also be remembered that normal levels of estrogen in postmenopausal women decline from around 30 pg/mL soon after menopause to as low as 5 pg/mL in later years. Women with undetectable levels of estrogen, however, were found to have increased risk of osteoporosis.[508] Although levels in the range of 8 pg/mL were not shown to increase the risk of endometrial cancer,[509] the higher the level of estrogen, the more likely endometrial hyperplasia is to occur unless opposing progesterone is given. Presumably, in women with low (normal) levels of estrogen, the progesterone balance is supplied by adrenal progesterone. Therefore, it might be assumed that women under stress might also be imbalanced with regard to progesterone and at higher risk for endometrial hyperplasia.

If estrogens are replaced, the level of balancing progesterone should be evaluated. If endogenous progesterone levels are low or endogenous estrogens are high, progesterone should be replaced or adrenal stress minimized to get endogenous levels back to a point of balance. When progesterone is administered vaginally, higher levels are found in the endometrium than in serum,[510] which may be important since both transdermal and transvaginal progesterone administration have been shown not to produce serum levels consistent with luteal phase. As stated previously, that does not necessarily mean that the patient is susceptible to endometrial hyperplasia or cancer. It also appears that luteal phase levels are not necessary if estrogens are replaced at low postmenopausal levels.[511] Remember, the goal is to *normalize* hormone levels. It is important to remember that after menopause estrogens come primarily from peripheral sites that may be preserved even in the absence of ovarian tissue. Testosterone comes from both the adrenals and the ovaries, about 50% from each, and may need to be replaced, especially in the case of oophorectomy. Progesterone comes primarily from the adrenals and levels can be depressed when there is a high demand for cortisol such as with stress,[512] allergy,[513] or inflammatory processes.

It is clear from the work of Hlatky, using the HERS trial data[514] and reconfirmed in the WHI,[515] that the majority (approximately 80%) of postmenopausal women do better without any hormone replacement. There are only a small number of women who will need HRT, and these are likely to be women with underfunctioning ovaries either from surgical removal, autoimmune destruction, or perhaps compensation for prolonged elevated levels of other hormones such as adrenaline; underlying imbalances of other hormones can be addressed with diet and lifestyle changes. The latter make up a significant percentage of the women who have undergone natural menopause but are complaining of hot flashes, insomnia, and anxiety/depression.

Estrogen administration. The most important symptoms that lead a woman or her practitioner to consider HRT are hot flashes,[516] insomnia,[517] and depression or anxiety.[518] Since these are all primarily brain symptoms, it is important to note that the brain is an ER-β rich organ. It would take much higher doses of estrone or estriol to engage these brain receptors and it is likely that they would have to be converted to estradiol to be effective. Nutritional phytoestrogens such as genistein and coumestrol, on the other hand, might have a beneficial effect.[519,520] This thinking has led the author to turn away from HRT containing estrone and estriol as the primary treatment for brain symptoms. The goal is to get the best, targeted effect while giving the smallest number of estrogen-like molecules, in the event that metabolism or excretion is not ideal.[521] Remember, it takes very few estradiol molecules to have a powerful effect. Although estradiol engages both the α- and β-receptors and therefore would be expected to have effects in the endometrium and breast (where growth stimulation would not be desirable after menopause), smaller doses are in the long run more physiologic and, if properly balanced with progesterone and perhaps testosterone, appear to be relatively safe.

Since the route of administration is clearly important, both in obtaining adequate blood and (brain) tissue levels and in the liver effects of these hormones, the most physiologic way to give HRT is via a route that does not produce first-pass effects in the liver. Transdermal estradiol is now readily available in commercial preparations of gels and patches. Transvaginal routes also appear effective. Although there would be a concern regarding higher levels of estrogen in the uterus when giving transvaginal estrogen, the higher uterine levels of vaginally administered progesterone, on the other hand, would be expected to be advantageous. Other routes, such as injectable and subdermal pellets, are also available, but not as acceptable to patients or as easily managed by the practitioner. Buccal estrogens via troches are available from formulating pharmacies but provide a mixture of transmembrane and gut-absorbed hormone, and thus might be expected to have increased liver first-pass effects.

Since absorption from many of these routes varies from woman to woman, dosages should be started at low levels and titrated to the normal range. Patient symptoms can be used to determine that treatment effects are in the normal range (minimal hot flashes without insomnia and **no** breast tenderness or bleeding). Following normalization of symptoms, hormone levels can be obtained.

Progesterone administration. Progesterone can be administered with commercially prepared and tested oral and transvaginal formulations, and formulating pharmacies will make transdermal, buccal, oral or transvaginal preparations. Commercially prepared transdermal creams are also available with varying amounts of USP progesterone per ounce. Levels obtained via any of these routes are highly variable due to differences in dose, absorption, and metabolism. When using progesterone primarily to protect the endometrium, rather than to support cortisol production or suppress anxiety, the vaginal route has the advantage of providing high local levels of progesterone without increasing serum levels appreciably.[522] Oral progesterone will in general have better effects on brain symptoms of anxiety because of its first pass through the liver, with subsequent production of allopregnanolone, a natural anxiolytic. While not strictly following the rule of normalizing hormones, this strategy may be temporarily helpful in women with anxiety. Women with very low cortisol output will sometimes respond to progesterone in higher doses due to progesterone's position as a cortisol precursor in the hormonal cascade. Transdermal preparations can be used and, if adequate blood levels are obtained, avoid the sedative effect of allopregnanolone in the brain. (The clinician should be aware of the potential connection between higher cortisol levels and worsening depression.)

Once symptoms suggest appropriate levels and a balance between estrogen and progesterone, levels should be obtained to determine that physiological values have actually been attained. Estradiol levels in the 15–25 pg/dl range, with adequate progesterone (greater than 0.3 ng/mL—1 ng/dL), are reasonable in the years immediately following menopause, provided there are no symptoms of hormone excess such as bleeding or breast tenderness. These levels represent early menopause to low follicular phase levels. They have been chosen somewhat arbitrarily since "normal levels" are usually obtained by measuring hormone levels in populations that have not been screened for the kinds of subtle mediating systems addressed in functional medicine such as adrenal stress, autoimmune destruction of the ovary, and testosterone and SHBG imbalances.

It is advisable to obtain informed consent with all HRT patients. On the type of regimes described above, patients should know that, while their risk of breast cancer **is** higher on any hormone replacement, their quality and length of life will be better if their hormones are balanced. If a patient is diagnosed with breast cancer while on hormone replacment, the clinician may be legally at risk if he or she cannot document such consent.

Replacing hormones after oophorectomy. In what appears to be an oversight of gargantuan proportions, women who have undergone removal of the ovaries (approximately 50–60% of all women undergoing hysterectomy, or 300,000 per year[523,524]) are often treated as simply postmenopausal. The incidence of hot flashes in these women is almost three-fold higher.[525] These premenopausal women lose estrogen, progesterone, and testosterone production compared to "normal" menopausal women. They are also likely to be much younger and have potentially higher needs for these hormones. Physicians may be unaware of the differences between the normal postmenopausal woman and the surgically-induced menopausal woman; they are often lumped together in studies. Differences between these groups were noted in the literature as early as the 1930s when a Mayo Clinic study showed that the most severe atherosclerotic disease was not found in men but in women who had been ovariectomized.[526]

It is important to note that many of the studies on animal models that contributed to the early powerful bias that hormone replacement was **healthy** after menopause were done on spayed animals, which were then replaced with estrogen and/or other combinations of hormones. It is also important to note that these animals were likely to have less genetic diversity than that seen in the American human population and therefore, at best, would represent only a subpopulation of women at risk. Finally, true to expectation, when the women in the hysterectomized arm of the WHI were analyzed, a lower incidence of breast cancer was found. This was predicted, not because there were no progestins used, but because the estradiol levels in the patients in that study would be expected to be lower, since a standardized dosage of .625 mg of conjugated equine estrogen (CEE) was given in both arms of the study. This translates to a total higher level of estrogen in the non-hysterectomized, postmenopausal women arm of WHI. Indeed, the hysterectomized ERT group had a RR of breast cancer of .77 (CI 0.59–1.01), while the risk of breast cancer in the non-hysterectomized group was 1.26 (CI 1.00–1.59).[527,528]

These findings do not prove that estrogen is safe to give without progestin; they simply indicate that normal-to-low levels of estrogen carry a lower risk of breast cancer than higher-than-physiologic levels do. And these findings do lead us to a rational approach for women who have had hysterectomy, with or without oophorectomy. The goal should be to normalize hormone levels. For women below the age of 50, normal follicular levels of 20 pg/mL to perhaps as high as 60 pg/mL should suffice. Cycling with progesterone in the luteal phase of the cycle is appropriate in the higher ranges and is less likely to lead to insulin resistance than continuous therapy.[529] These relatively lower levels of hormone may still yield higher numbers of breast cancer than had hormone not been replaced, but leaving these women in a sub-physiologic range will increase their overall morbidity and mortality. Their risk compared to normally menopausal women should be reduced.

Around age 50 and approximately every 10 years or so thereafter, hysterectomized women should be re-evaluated with serum estradiol levels, and hormone replacement should be normalized to postmenopausal levels at their newly achieved age. ERT is usually not necessary after the age of normal menopause, if estradiol levels are maintained by fat production. If this is not the case, however, ERT should be given transdermally. Progesterone will also need to be normalized in order to balance brain effects of estrogen. If brain symptoms are not a problem, estrogen alone should be given until further information is available about bio-identical progesterone in the menopause. There is inadequate support at this time to say that natural progesterone—even in high doses—supports bone growth or prevention of osteoporosis,[530,531] although physiologically this is possible. If the woman is under stress, her progesterone levels are likely to be low and she will need replacement to normalize levels. In these women, bone loss will be greater, so care should be taken to attend to normalizing hormones and using nutritional support to prevent osteoporosis.

When oophorectomy has been performed, it is important to remember that a significant drop in testosterone will occur. This is likely to cause further endocrine imbalances by increasing SHBG and binding more free estrogens and the testosterone that is available from the adrenals. Although normalizing testosterone levels has been shown to improve libido in postmenopausal women, it is not a panacea for loss of libido at midlife.

Use of estriol. Estriol has been used both orally and transvaginally with the assumption that because of its lower estrogen receptor affinity, it would be safer. Data from a case-control study in Sweden,[532] where many women have been prescribed both vaginal and oral estriol, showed an increased incidence of endometrial cancer in women taking oral estriol in doses of 1–2 mg, OR 2.0 (1.6–2.6), but no statistically significant difference in women taking the vaginal preparations of estriol or dienestrol, OR 1.2 (1.0–1.6) In this study, endometrial cancers were more likely to be lower grade and less invasive in women using estriol orally. However, there was no difference in those using vaginally delivered estriol, supporting the lack of connection to the vaginally administered hormone. Previous studies have shown that estriol in 6 mg oral doses can produce vaginal bleeding when progestins are added.[533] Studies have also shown that lower doses produce decreased symptoms and prevention of bone loss.[534]

Oral estriol is metabolized in the liver by conjugation, but is not well bound to SHBG or albumin in serum. Therefore, levels of free, biologically active estriol are significant and can lead to estrogen effects. There is also concern that orally administered estriol might be processed in a "retrograde" fashion to the much stronger 16-OH estrogens of which it is a downstream product in normal estrogen metabolism. This has not been demonstrated clinically. Vaginal estriol is much more readily absorbed; 1 mg of vaginal estriol and 10 mg of orally administered estriol appear to have similar effects. However, much lower doses of estriol are normally administered (1–2 mg orally and .5 mg twice weekly vaginally are standard doses in the Swedish study cited above). Furthermore, as the vaginal epithelium cornifies under the influence of estriol following 1–2 weeks of therapy, less of the drug is absorbed.[535] Vaginal estriol appears to be both safe and effective for urogenital symptoms.[536]

Studies suggest that vaginally administered estriol (.5 mg daily for 2–3 weeks then twice weekly) is effective in the treatment of atrophic vaginitis with minimal if any effect on the endometrium. Orally administered estriol in a daily dose of 1–2 mg is more problematic and should be considered potentially hazardous to the endometrium and possibly the breast. Occasionally, women will complain of increased hot flashes that are presumably caused by the antiestrogen SERM effect of estriol. I have also seen resolution of hot flashes, confirming the individually diverse nature of estriol metabolism.

Recently, a murine model of MS has shown potential benefit from estriol,[537] suggesting that it may be useful in autoimmune diseases. Further work will be necessary before applying this information to humans.

Replacing testosterone. Testosterone has many important functions in balancing the hormonal effects of estrogen. Testosterone has numerous effects on estrogen availability and effect. Increased testosterone decreases sex hormone binding globulin (SHBG), making both estrogen and testosterone more available to the tissues. In women who are at risk for estrogen-related tumors, or who have a tendency toward anxiety and irritability (PMS), these effects can be undesirable. It is important to note, however, that the correct level of testosterone must be maintained around .4 ng/mL.[538] When giving testosterone to women, very small doses may be adequate. Higher doses will have a negative effect on lipids, and possibly vascular compliance, as well as producing unpleasant side effects such as acne and hair loss.

There is evidence that women with higher levels of testosterone have a higher risk of breast cancer.[539] This report referred to endogenous testosterone and therefore may represent metabolic uniqueness (such as the effect of insulin on CYP 17,20 lyase in the population of women with insulin resistance—a known risk for breast and uterine cancer). Testosterone has also been shown to decrease the proliferation of mammary epithelium in oophorectomized rhesus monkeys given estrogen by increasing the ratio of ER-beta to ER-alpha and lowering MYC oncogene expression, thereby exerting an anti-estrogen effect on the mammary epithelium. Once again, it is important to first measure the levels of hormones before administering exogenous hormones to postmenopausal women and then to monitor levels during treatment, as other hormone levels (such as insulin or androstenedione) might change with treatment, creating unintended effects.

Testosterone also has central effects, increasing vasopressin, which is associated with better ability to focus (its absence has been related to ADHD and chronic fatigue) and to libido, explaining some of the positive effects of testosterone in postmenopausal women.[540]

Genomics and Hormone Balance

When family history suggests a genetic pattern of disease, such as breast or ovarian cancer, genetic testing can be both explanatory and helpful in creating therapeutic interventions. A number of SNPs have been shown to have a relationship to the production and metabolism of hormones. As we become better able to identify these genetic polymorphisms in our patients, it is important to evaluate their usefulness in formulating interventions that address manipulation of hormone levels. In a recent study in the *Journal of the National Cancer Institute*, the association between levels of sex hormones and SNPs for enzymes that regulate them was studied.[541] The results from this study suggested that only polymorphisms in the CYP19 aromatase enzyme and SHBG contributed to the variation in circulating hormone levels. (Remember that hormones in the serum do not reflect the local production of hormones.) Tumors of the breast in particular appear to be able to recruit available genes in the production of increased estrogen. This would seem more likely than that the cancer cell mutated to produce a gene that increased estrogen.

In another study,[542] multiple SNPs of interest to hormone metabolism were studied. Of these women, 66% had at least two homozygous mutant SNPs of interest. A thrombophilic pre-disposition was found in 9.9% of women, and 23% of women had at least two SNPs associated with an increased risk of breast cancer (COMT, CYP17, CYP19, CYP1A1, and CYP1B1). This would suggest that these women might be at increased risk from HRT such as was used in the WHI. The SNPs predisposing women to cardiovascular pathologies (e.g., APOE, AGT, eNOS, and PAI-1) were found in 12.3% of women. SNPs predisposing to early postmenopausal bone loss and osteoporosis (ER-alpha and VDR) were found in 26.7% of women. The authors conclude: "These data suggest that the assessment of SNPs associated with risks and benefits of estrogen/hormone therapy may be a new means to individualize counseling about and prescription of estrogen/hormone therapy in up to 66% of women." Work in this area has focused on the analysis of polymorphisms of potential functional significance in several classes of genes, including those involved in carcinogen metabolism, estrogen metabolite biosynthesis, steroid hormone receptor activation, and DNA damage response.[543]

Critical enzymes for which gene SNPs have been determined include (some of the tests are commercially available):

- **CYP1B1**—This cytochrome P450 detoxification enzyme in the liver is responsible for metabolizing a number of drugs and chemicals. When acting upon estrogen (and especially the estrogen-like horse hormones equilin and equilenin), this enzyme produces 4-OH estrogens,[544] which are rapidly converted into quinones, which are adducts of DNA. SNPs that upregulate this enzyme can increase the production of cancer-causing 4-OH estrogens.[545,546] Polycyclic aromatic hydrocarbons[547] and tobacco smoke are biotransformed through this P450 enzyme, further upregulating it. DHEA, hesperetin (a flavonoid), and resveratrol have been shown to be downregulators of this enzyme. It should be noted that studies attempting to link CYP1B1 polymorphisms and breast cancer incidence have not shown a correlation with this enzyme by itself.[548,549]
- **CYP1A1**—This enzyme is responsible for the production of 2-OH estrogens. Once methylated, these downstream metabolites are thought to be protective estrogens; the methoxylated form is currently being studied as a cancer therapy. There appear to be many variants of the CYP1A1 gene, each associated with different diseases. For instance, CYP1A1 4887A and 4889G may be precipitating factors for susceptibility to psoriatic arthritis; an additive effect was found between them.[550] CYP1A1 6235C allele carriers showed a non-significant (P=0.06) trend towards a decreased risk of ER-positive breast cancers (OR=0.65, 95% CI 0.42–1.02), but not ER-negative breast cancers.[551] In a multiple model, CYP1A1-1 MspI restriction fragment length polymorphism (RFLP) T→C (p=0.004), and CYP1A1-2 Ile462Val A→G (p=0.03), were found to be associated with significantly decreased and increased risks of breast carcinoma, respectively.[552] These subtleties add significant value to the interpretation of an assay for limited SNPs.
- **CYP3A family**—Assays for these enzyme genes are not currently available to clinicians but are responsible for 16-OH estrogens. They can be upregulated by xenoestrogens such as those found in pesticides. They appear to be upregulated in obesity.
- **MTHFR (methyltetrahydrofolate reductase)** is responsible for activating folate to 5-methyltetrahydrofolate, one of the key steps in the production of methyl groups and in conversion of homocysteine to methionine. The 677C→T variant is seen in 20% of the population. Increased folate supplementation or providing the activated folate as 5-methyl or 5-formyl-tetrahydrofolate can compensate for this abnormality. Measuring homocysteine levels after therapy confirms the effectiveness of this therapy.
- **COMT (C-O-methyl transferase)** transfers the methyl group from methionine to many substrates in the body's metabolic processes. Persons who are homozygous positive for the M-alleles of this gene

have four-fold reduction of COMT activity and are associated with slowed metabolism of dopamine, epinephrine, norepinephrine, and drugs like L-dopa.[553] They may have decreased postsynaptic catecholamine receptors and an increased risk of certain neuropsychiatric illnesses such as rapid cycling bipolar disorder, antisocial behavior, violence and suicide in schizophrenics. Activity of this enzyme has been shown to be downregulated by catechol-containing phytonutrients such as quercetin, with a subsequent increase in DNA damage.[554] However, a study by Wu et al. showed, among Asian women with lowered COMT activity, the decreased metabolism of catechins from green tea increased its antioxidant capability, thereby decreasing the incidence of breast cancer.[555] Other alleles are also associated with increased risk of breast cancer.[556] Activity of this enzyme may be improved by increasing the substrate methionine with SAMe.

- **CYP19 aromatase** is responsible for converting adrenal androgens into the estrogens estrone and estradiol. Aromatase inhibitors have recently received a great deal of attention as cancer adjunctive therapy. The inflammatory prostaglandin E2 is a potent upregulator of CYP19[557] and therefore COX-2 inhibitors such as omega-3 fatty acids or low-dose aspirin[558] may be able to decrease aromatization of adrenal steroids to estrogens.
- **CYP17 (17α-hydroxylase/17,20-lyase)** converts 17-OH progesterone and 17-OH pregnenolone to androstenedione and testosterone. This enzyme is upregulated by insulin in insulin resistance syndromes and PCOS.
- **EDH17 B2 (17β-hydroxysteroid dehydrogenase type 2)** converts androstenedione to testosterone and estrone to estradiol. It has been found in breast tissue and fat and is responsible for the conversion of adrenal steroids to estrogen in these tissues.
- **SHBG**—Two SNPs have been found that increase levels of SHBG. Since these are not available commercially, and since SHBG can be measured directly, it is important to remember that SHBG levels can be controlled genetically and not just in response to hormone levels.
- **VDR**—Recurrent references to vitamin D receptors are encountered when reviewing the literature.[559,560,561] Vitamin D appears to be important in apoptosis and therefore has an impact on epithelial cell cancers such as breast, prostate, and colon cancers. Vitamin D is also involved in immune cell apoptosis and therefore interacts with the inflammatory cells that respond to estrogen in diseases such as Th1 mediated autoimmune diseases[562,563] and osteoporosis. The vitamin D receptor in rats and mice has been shown to be estrogen sensitive.[564]
- **IL-1β**—Upregulators of the promoter sequence (31C-T) increase IL-1β, which has been shown to increase pituitary production of FSH and have an effect on LH production, which may be involved in the suppression of fertility during chronic disease.[565]
- **IL-6 (–174 G-C)** is a Th2 cytokine upregulator that has also been shown to increase FSH and LH production.
- **UGT (UDP-glucuronosyltransferase)** has been shown to have polymorphisms that can affect the levels of estrogen and testosterone in the circulation. Lowering hormone levels has been shown to increase the numbers of ER- and PR-negative cancers. Since these cancers have a worsened prognosis than the ER/PR-positive tumors, these polymorphisms might be important.
- **SULT (Sulfotransferase)** has also been shown to have polymorphisms that affect hormone availability, thus affecting the risk of ER-positive tumors.[566]

Dietary Modifications to Decrease Diseases of Estrogen Metabolism

A diet aimed at decreasing estrogen production would be expected to lower the risk of breast and uterine cancer and decrease symptoms of Th1 autoimmunity. This diet can also be helpful in PMS and may improve fertility in women with overproduction of estrogen or an estrogen-dominant imbalance of estrogen and progesterone. Metabolic functions that are diet responsive include production of estrogen by aromatase, metabolism to 2-OH vs. 16-OH estrogens, phase II methylation, sulfation, and glucuronidation, enterohepatic circulation of excreted estrogens, and the presence of xenoestrogens and phytoestrogens in the food.

A diet aimed at maintaining normal body mass index would be expected to improve hormone function and decrease the risk of estrogen-related disorders. In patients susceptible to insulin resistance, the appropriate balance of protein and carbohydrate will be important. Eating *organically grown* foods, especially hormone-free meats from animals known to concentrate xenoestrogens in the fat, would be expected to decrease exposure to xenoestrogen, as well as down-regulate CYP3A enzymes that produce 16-OH estrogens and inhibit 2 OH estrogens. Fatty acid precursors of inflammatory prostaglandins (arachidonate) concentrated in red meat, milk, and eggs, may increase PGE-2 and aromatase, so limiting these foods would be wise. Chapter 26 contains a very thorough and well-documented review of dietary influences on health, including those summarized briefly below.

Milk and Soy

Jane Plante has suggested that the epidemiology of milk drinking around the world, and the induction of high levels of IGF-1 in bGH-treated cows, make milk drinking problematic for some breast cancer patients.[567] Milk drinking has also been shown to be problematic for women at risk for ovarian cancer.[568] Substituting soy milk and adding other soy products appears to be a useful approach for many reasons and may be especially helpful for young women in preventing later cancers. Use of isoflavones not obtained from soy foods, especially in the menopause or in women who have breast cancer, is still controversial. However, accumulating data in humans appears to favor soy as a food substance in these situations, or at least to suggest they do not increase risk.

Vegetables

A diet high in cruciferous vegetables and, therefore, indole-3-carbinol would be expected to increase production of 2-OH estrogens, improving the 2-OH/16-OH ratio and lowering the estrogenic pressure in the system. Brightly colored vegetables and fruits containing antioxidants would be expected to decrease oxidative damage to DNA and to lower risks. Methylation is also important; since there are high numbers of MTHFR and COMT polymorphism carriers, a diet high in vegetables containing B vitamins would be prudent. Sulfate groups are supplied by garlic and onion and, for those able to process these foods, an advantage in sulfation of circulating estrogens could accrue.

Fiber and Fat

Rock and colleagues showed that a diet higher in fiber and lower in fat significantly decreased bioavailable estrogen.[569] The effect was primarily mediated by the fiber, which is thought to bind estrogen in the gut, preventing enterohepatic recirculation. Freshly ground organic flax seeds provide fiber, omega-6 and omega-3 precursors, and flax lignans. It is difficult to protect flax oil against oxidation and it does not reverse the common omega-3/omega-6 deficit.

Mozaffarian et al. showed that a diet high in *trans* fatty acids increased systemic inflammation in women in the Nurses Health Study.[570] Diets high in omega-3 fatty acids, as would be expected, have been shown to have the reverse effect, so it appears that a prescription of "good fats" is preferable to one of "no fat."

Sugar and Alcohol

A diet low in sugar and high in fiber would be expected to improve bacterial flora, further decreasing enterohepatic recirculation of estrogens by normalizing β-glucuronidase in the gut. D-glucarate, also found in colorful vegetables, has been shown to block glucuronidase activity and lower enterohepatic recirculation of estrogens.[571] Such a diet might also limit overgrowth of yeast with its concomitant mycoestrogens and alcohol production. Sad as it is to say, since we all seem to love sugar, a diet low in simple sugars appears to be appropriate for many reasons other than discouraging yeast growth. Sugar is the preferred substrate of cancer cells[572] and has profound effects in inducing insulin resistance. A diet low in sugar should be encouraged. Limiting alcohol to small amounts of resveratrol-containing wines (red) may help to normalize CYP enzymes affecting the ratios of 2-, 4-, and 16-OH estrogen metabolites.

Supplements

- **I3C** upregulates CYP1A1, increasing protective 2-OH estrogens,[573] and may reduce 4-OH.[574]
- Some potentially useful COX-2 inhibitors and anti-inflammatory supplements include **omega-3 fatty acids, curcumin, hops, boswellia, rosemary.**[575,576,577,578,579]
- **Curcumin** increases glutathione and induces GST.[580] **It should not be used if the patient is on cancer chemotherapy.**
- *Vitex agnus-castus* may help to balance estrogen/progesterone in premenopausal women.[581,582]
- **Silymarin** improves liver detoxification pathways.[583,584]

- **Green tea extract** and quercetin should be avoided in COMT-deficient patients, but otherwise may be helpful.[585]
- **Dong quai** is used traditionally in combination with other herbs and these combinations have not been adequately studied. In a single trial by itself it was not effective for hot flashes.[586]
- **Amino acid supplements**, especially in those patients with decreased protein intake (some vegetarians) or absorption (hypochlorhydria), improve phase II detoxification, antioxidation, and brain function.[587,588,589]
- **Activated folic acid**, B6, and B12 improve availability of methyl groups.[590,591]
- **SAMe** provides the substrate for COMT.[592]
- **Isoflavones** from soy, or other plants such as kudzu, improve 2-OH/16-OH estrogen ratios;[593] isoflavones from red clover and flax may act as SERMS. However, research is limited and results are mixed.[594]
- **Fiber and probiotics** improve gut excretion and gut flora, decreasing β-glucuronidase and its associated increased enterohepatic recirculation of estrogens and yeast overgrowth and the associated increase in mycoestrogens and ETOH production in the gut. See Chapters 28 and 31 for extensive information on gut function and flora.
- **Vitamin E** may inhibit the growth of breast cancer cells[595] and prevent oxidation of cellular fats.[596] There is limited research to suggest that vitamin E is effective against hot flashes.[597,598] A recent double-blind study suggests it is effective for dysmenorrhea.[599]
- **Vitamin D** protects bone density[600] and decreases risk of epithelial cancers such as prostate,[601] breast,[602] and colon.[603]
- **Calcium-D-glucarate** decreases β-glucuronidase and its associated increased enterohepatic recirculation of estrogens.[604,605]
- **$NaSO_4$ and Glucosamine SO_4** make sulfate groups available to bind with estrogen in biotransformation phase II excretion.
- **Antioxidant supplements** containing the full spectrum of antioxidants prevent oxidative damage to DNA. Interestingly to functional medicine clinicians, a 2004 analysis of the research suggests the following: "Clinical studies mapping the effect of preventive antioxidants have shown surprisingly little or no effect on cancer incidence. The epidemiological trials together with *in vitro* experiments suggest that the optimal approach is to reduce endogenous and exogenous sources of oxidative stress, rather than increase intake of antioxidants."[606,607] **Some antioxidants should not be used during chemotherapy or radiation therapy as they may limit the effectiveness of therapy.**

Summary

The primary purpose of the therapies discussed here is to prolong life, preserve functionality, and maintain maximum flexibility in the (human) system. The approach to achieving these important goals is to normalize as many hormones as possible using lifestyle and dietary changes, as well as bioidentical hormones in doses and routes of administration that mimic, as far as possible, natural secretion of these hormones. As our understanding of genetics and the interaction of genes and environment improves, we will be able to modify the function of hormonally important enzymes, inducing changes that may be advantageous in improving fertility and longevity, and in reducing the symptoms of women in hormonal transitions.

Fibroids and Endometriosis

Joel M. Evans, MD

A comprehensive history and physical examination, as well as a detailed understanding of hormone metabolism, set the stage for the successful management of estrogen-related disorders. Two seemingly disparate diseases, fibroids and endometriosis, are currently erroneously classified solely as disorders of hormone metabolism. Actually, they fit into the functional medicine web, which recognizes the contribution of processes such as inflammation, detoxification, and blood sugar metabolism.

Fibroids (leiomyoma), which are benign smooth muscle neoplasms, and endometriosis, which is characterized by the presence of endometrial glands and stroma outside of the lining of the uterine cavity, are both disorders of estrogen-sensitive tissues. Thus, they share common treatment strategies, such as improving estrogen metabolism both directly and indirectly.

Fibroids

Fibroids are the most common pelvic tumor in women,[608] occurring in up to 40% of women, with a higher incidence (up to 50%) in African American women.[609] They can arise in any body tissue that contains smooth muscle, but they most commonly occur in the smooth muscle (myometrium) of the uterus. Though they can be solitary, they usually are found in multiple sites within the uterus and vary in size from microscopic to the size of a melon, or even larger. Because of the large degree of variation in number, size and location of fibroids, the intensity of symptoms varies from purely asymptomatic to severely disabling with many possible manifestations,[610] including:

- Abdominal and/or pelvic pressure
- Pain
- Abnormal bleeding (if located in or causing distortion of the uterine cavity)
- Urinary frequency
- Painful intercourse
- Increase in abdominal girth
- Fatigue due to anemia
- Urinary obstruction
- Infertility
- Pregnancy complications such as preterm labor, dysfunctional labor, and abnormal fetal presentations (breech and transverse lie)

Even with this long list of possible symptoms, the majority of women with fibroids have no symptoms, and they are discovered on routine pelvic exam or ultrasound.

The cause of fibroid tumors has not yet been precisely determined. They are believed to develop from a single cell. Because of observed familial associations, genetic determinants are believed to play a role.[611] The current hypothesis is that leiomyomatous transformation is related to a mutation of a normal smooth muscle cell being influenced by estrogen, progesterone, and local growth factors. Once the smooth muscle cell undergoes leiomyomatous transformation, estrogen and progesterone receptors are found in higher concentration than in normal myometrium. Estrogen, progesterone, and growth factors are all likely involved in tumor growth, though the exact mechanisms are unclear.[612]

The long-held belief in conventional gynecology that estrogen is the primary stimulus for fibroid growth is based on clinical observations:

- Fibroids are rarely found before menarche.
- Most shrink following surgical or natural menopause.
- Most enlarge during pregnancy.
- Some enlarge with oral contraceptive use.
- Most shrink with medications that reduce estrogen levels (e.g., aromatase inhibitors).

Based on these observations, the conventional pharmacologic approach has been to decrease ovarian estrogen production by inducing a "medical menopause" with gonadotropin-releasing hormone (GNRH) agonist therapy.[613] There are two main limitations of this approach. The first is that by inducing a rapid shift into a menopausal state, symptoms of ovarian hormone deficiency can be severe. More importantly, GNRH agonist therapy is not a long-term solution, as these medications can only be prescribed for a finite amount of time (3–6 months) and, following withdrawal of the medication, the fibroids usually return to their pretreatment size.[614] Thus, the main use of GNRH agonist therapy has evolved to that of a pre-surgical intervention in cases where the surgeon feels that some reduction in fibroid size is technically advantageous (although at least one recent study indicates that there may be no significant effect in intraoperative blood loss from such treatment[615]).

The conventional gynecologic approach to fibroids that are asymptomatic (the majority of fibroids) is observation, which obviously does nothing to prevent further fibroid growth. Because observation does not address the functional imbalances that contribute to fibroid growth, many women ultimately require medical, surgical, or radiological treatments with the accompanying morbidity and even mortality associated with those approaches.

A functional approach to fibroids, therefore, first and foremost addresses asymptomatic fibroids with the objective of *preventing* future growth and *preventing* the development of symptomatology requiring medical or surgical intervention. Because of the association of estrogenic stimulation with fibroid growth, normalization of estrogen metabolism (both production and elimination) is the major point of entry into the functional medicine web for the treatment of both symptomatic and asymptomatic fibroids.

Endometriosis

Endometriosis tissue, like the endometrium from which it is derived, is estrogen sensitive and is therefore associated with painful menses. Because the endometrial tissue is located in areas other than where it is supposed to be, a local inflammatory response is created that contributes to pain and to difficulty conceiving. It is for these reasons that conventional treatment prescribes oral contraceptives (which are progesterone dominant and have the effect of creating an inactive endometrium), and anti-inflammatory medications.[616] In severe cases, GNRH agonist therapy (designed to create a medical menopause to decrease estrogenic stimulation) or surgery is indicated. Before understanding the basis for a functional approach to treatment, it is important to realize that, unlike normal endometrial tissue, which responds only to circulating estrogen, endometriosis tissue contains aromatase[617] and produces, and is stimulated by, its own estrogen. The proinflammatory prostaglandin PGE_2 is the most potent stimulator of aromatase in endometriosis tissue,[618] making normalization of PGE_2 levels and reduction of inflammation a therapeutic priority on a par with maintaining normal estrogen levels.

Since fibroids and endometriosis tissue are both estrogen sensitive and both contain aromatase, which is upregulated by PGE_2, it is easy to see how treatment goals of normalizing estrogen metabolism and inflammation are similar for both conditions.

Treatment

Before it is possible to normalize estrogen metabolism, production, and elimination (a therapeutic goal), certain physiologic parameters must be assessed. In premenopausal women, salivary testing has been shown to accurately reflect serum levels of sex steroid hormones.[619] Salivary testing offers many advantages over serum testing. Non-invasive specimen collection, which is more convenient and less expensive, allows for the multiple collections necessary to evaluate diurnal and monthly cycles. Salivary testing also reflects the bio-available fraction of hormones, which is critically important because the bioavailable form (free hormone NOT bound to sex hormone binding globulin) is the biologically active form. Since the fundamental therapeutic goal is the normalization of estrogen levels, a month-long profile will identify whether the background hormonal milieu is estrogen dominant, in which case more aggressive interventions to lower estrogen levels are required than when sex hormone levels are normal.

Since all estrogens in the body are synthesized from androgens via the enzyme aromatase, preventing stimulation of aromatase activity (which would therefore increase estrogen levels) *must* be the first step in the therapeutic strategy. Adipose tissue has aromatase activity,[620] so the elimination of excess adipose tissue through the achievement of ideal body weight plays a major role in ensuring appropriate estrogen levels. Aromatase activity is stimulated by insulin, so normalization of insulin and glucose metabolism is critical (topic discussed previously in this chapter). Additionally, insulin decreases SHBG levels, which serves to further increase circulating levels of bioavailable estrogen to stimulate fibroid growth. Fibroid cells, in contrast to normal myometrium, contain aromatase,[621] further increasing the importance of controlling insulin levels. This is true for endometriosis tissue as well.[622] Interestingly, aromatase activity in fibroids and endometriosis tissue is stimulated by the proinflammatory prostaglandin PGE_2,[623,624] making the reduction of inflammatory processes a critical goal. It is important to remember that overweight and obese women are often in an inflammatory state due to the many proinflammatory cytokines produced by adipose tissue.[625] This serves to underscore the importance of achieving ideal body weight in women with estrogen-related disorders.

Other ways to decrease aromatase activity (and decrease estrogen levels locally and systemically) include the use of pharmacologic (anastrazole and letrozole) and natural (resveratrol,[626] chrysin, soy,[627] saw palmetto, and flax lignans[628]) aromatase inhibitors.

An additional lifestyle change that can help decrease estrogen levels is eating organic foods. The goal of eating organic is to decrease exposure to estrogens that are added to foods, and to pesticides that either stimulate aromatase (atrazine) or are converted in the body to estrogen-like substances (xenoestrogens).

The next step in assessing any patient with an estrogen-sensitive syndrome (e.g., fibroids and endometriosis) is to ensure estrogen is adequately eliminated from the body. This is done by assessing the body's detoxification system (where estrogen is eliminated through the phase I and II detoxification pathways) and the health of the GI tract (where estrogen is dumped from the liver into the small intestine and dysbiosis can lead to increased beta glucuronidase levels that may increase enterohepatic recirculation of estrogen). (See Chapters 22 and 31 for in-depth discussions of detoxification.) Abnormalities of detoxification, digestion, and elimination (constipation), therefore, must be corrected if the body is to properly eliminate estrogen.

Another area of the functional medicine web that needs to be assessed and addressed is the relationship of the mind, body, and spirit. It is common knowledge, and a nearly universal experience of women and their caregivers, that stress can lead to irregular menstruation and amenorrhea through the disruption of hypothalamic and pituitary gland function, which can be associated with increased estrogen levels. Therefore, stress reduction, conflict resolution, and spiritual health are important to achieving not only hormonal regulation but also overall well-being.

It is important to note that the core functional medicine interventions to treat fibroids and endometriosis are not viewed by conventional gynecologists as treatments of choice. These interventions include:

- achieving ideal body weight (decreases aromatase and inflammation),
- eating organic (removing exogenous sources of estrogen-like compounds),
- reducing stress (optimizing pituitary function),
- optimizing insulin/glucose metabolism (decreasing stimulation of aromatase and normalizing levels of SHBG),
- decreasing inflammation (decreasing PGE_2 stimulation of aromatase), and
- normalizing detoxification, digestion, and elimination (ensuring adequate removal of estrogen from the body).

We believe that throughout this book, as well as in this particular chapter, analysis of the underlying science demonstrates that the physiology and biochemistry involved in estrogen-related disorders are of critical importance in developing treatment plans. Functional medicine practitioners, therefore, have a way to address fibroids and endometriosis while simultaneously improving their patients' overall health. Such is the wonder and beauty of functional medicine.

Neurotransmitters: A Functional Medicine Approach to Neuropsychiatry

Jay Lombard, MD

Introduction

Neurotransmitters are the chemical messages of the central nervous system. There are over 50 substances recognized as molecules that function as neurotransmitters, including peptides, nitric oxide, neurotrophic factors, and cytokines. However, we will limit the current discussion to the "classic" neurotransmitters involved in neuropsychiatry. These include the catecholamines, dopamine and serotonin; the amino acid neurotransmitters, gamma-aminobutyric acid (GABA) and glutamate; and the amine neurotransmitter, acetylcholine.

A brief overview will be provided regarding the metabolic processes involved in the synthesis and release of these neurotransmitters, their neuroanatomical locations, and the relationships of neurotransmitter imbalances to specific neuropsychiatric disorders. We will also discuss developments in the assessment of neurochemical imbalances, including indirect measures of brain activity through peripheral biomarkers and through the use of neuroimaging procedures. Unfortunately, with few exceptions, measurements of blood and urine metabolites are often an inaccurate reflection of neuronal activity. More often than not, serum and urine measurements of neurotransmitter metabolites reflect peripheral rather than central activity and should not be used to make clinical decisions concerning neurochemical imbalances in individual patients. Conversely, recent advances in PET scanning and various MRI modalities can provide useful information regarding specific structural and functional brain properties involved in the pathogenesis of neuropsychiatric disorders.

Finally, we will discuss ways in which the clinician can integrate an understanding of the relationships of specific neurotransmitter imbalances with functional brain disorders, and then modulate some of these imbalances utilizing a functional medicine approach.

Overview of the Classic Neurotransmitters

The Catecholamines

Dopamine. Dopamine is an important endogenous catecholamine that binds to specific membrane receptors and plays a key role in the control of locomotion, learning, working memory, cognition, and emotion.[629] Dopamine is synthesized in the substantia nigra and projects to cortical and subcortical limbic regions via mesocortical and mesolimbic pathways. It is synthesized by enzymatic modification of the amino acid tyrosine in a series of steps; the rate-limiting enzyme in this process is tyrosine hydroxylase. Brain tyrosine levels are usually adequate to saturate tyrosine hydroxylase and therefore precursor strategies involving exogenous tyrosine administration are not useful in enhancing dopamine synthesis or raising brain dopamine levels.[630]

There are two types of dopamine receptors, the D1 family of receptors, which are G protein coupled and stimulate adenylyl cyclase, and the D2 family, which are also coupled to G proteins but inhibit adenylyl cyclase.

From a neurobehavioral perspective, dopamine plays a critical role in motivation, reward-seeking behavior and attentional processes.[631,632] The high density of dopaminergic projections in limbic regions suggests that dopamine is also involved in orientation toward "affect-laden experience" and response to stress. Imbalances of dopamine in limbic regions have been linked to ADHD (prefrontal circuits),[633,634,635] schizophrenia (mesolimbic cortex),[636] and subcortical neuropsychiatric disorders including Tourette's syndrome[637,638] and possibly autism.[639]

Indirect measures of CNS dopamine activity, including measurements of CSF HVA (homovanillic acid) levels (the end product of dopamine metabolism), have been associated with positive symptoms of schizophrenia such as hallucinations and paranoia. More recently, SPECT and PET scan studies have provided a window into specific abnormalities of dopamine dysfunction in discrete brain regions.[640]

Nuclear brain scans can examine either perfusion or receptor occupancy and density. Perfusion studies are based on the premise that blood flow is coupled to metabolic activity and thereby inferences can be made regarding hyperfunctional or hypofunctional brain areas. Receptor studies can provide estimates of either increased or decreased receptor density in specific neuropsychiatric conditions. Examples of perfusion abnormalities include findings of reduced frontal lobe glucose utilization in adult ADHD patients.[641] In schizophrenia, receptor density measures have revealed increased D2 receptor density, supporting the notion that psychosis is related to hyperdopaminegic activity in the mesolimbic cortex.[642]

Dopamine and its receptors can be adversely affected by genetic and environmental factors. A prime example of an environmental toxin that affects dopamine is MPTP. MPTP can produce a hypodopaminergic state indistinguishable from Parkinson's disease.[643]

Serotonin. It is widely accepted that serotonin is critically important in neurobehavioral processes including mood and anxiety.[644] Serotonin is synthesized from the amino acid tryptophan via the rate-limiting step tryptophan hydroxylase. Unlike tyrosine hydroxylase (the rate-limiting step in dopamine synthesis), tryptophan hydroxylase is not saturated, and thus dietary sources of tryptophan can have a significant effect on serotonin synthesis.[645]

Serotoninergic cells are present in the brain stem and have extensive projections to limbic regions and the cortex. There are many serotonin receptor subtypes: the $5HT_{IA}$ and $5HT_3$ which predominate in limbic structures and the $5HT_2$ subtype located primarily in the neocortex. $5HT_1$ and $5HT_2$ receptors are G protein coupled where they influence cAMP levels. The $5HT_3$ receptors are ion gated and are primarily inhibitory in function.

Serotoninergic imbalances are related to mood disorders, anxiety syndromes including OCD,[646,647] PTSD and panic disorder, and autism.[648] An indirect assessment of serotonin activity can be measured through platelet serotonin binding sites. $5HT_2$ receptors are localized on platelets in the periphery, and decreased platelet serotonin binding has been observed in patients with major depression.[649]

Neuroimaging modalities, including PET and functional MRI, have revealed abnormalities in discrete anatomical regions involved in mood and anxiety disorders. For instance, in patients with major depressive disorder, reduced activity in the anterior cingulate and medial orbital frontal cortex region has been reported.[650] These limbic regions are densely innervated by serotoninergic neurons. PET scan studies utilizing a serotonin tracer molecule demonstrated significant abnormalities in serotonin synthesis in autistic children compared to controls.[651]

Like dopamine, serotonin levels are influenced by genetic and environmental factors. Functional polymorphisms of 5HT transporter genes have been associated with depression,[652] autism,[653] and (conversely) with centenarians.[654] Environmental factors such as prolonged persistent stress activate the hypothalamic-pituitary-adrenal axis (HPA) and cause hypersecretion of ACTH and cortisol (see earlier discussion in this chapter of the HPA axis). These changes may alter chaperone proteins, which are essential for maintaining serotonin receptor structural integrity, and thus lead to a hyposerotoninergic state.

Amino Acid Neurotransmitters: GABA and Glutamate

GABA is regarded as the principal inhibiting neurotransmitter in the brain. GABA is formed via a metabolic pathway called the GABA shunt. The initial step in this pathway utilizes alpha ketoglutarate, which is then transaminated to form glutamate, the immediate precursor of GABA. Glutamate is then decarboxylated by glutamic acid decarboxylase (GAD) to form GABA. Pyridoxine is the key cofactor in GAD activity, positively favoring the conversion of glutamate to GABA. Pyridoxine-deficient states are associated with low CSF GABA levels and improve with B6 administration.[655]

GABA and glutamate are ubiquitous in the CNS and have a reciprocal, ying-yang interaction of inhibition and excitation. As mentioned earlier, GABA is the principal inhibiting neurotransmitter, whereas glutamate acts as the principal excitatory neurotransmitter in the brain. Glutamate produces neuronal depolarization via binding to either NMDA, AMPA [2-amino-3-(3-hydroxy-5-methyl-4-isoxazolyl) propionic acid], or kainite receptor sites. One of the most important physiological roles of glutamate is in learning processes[656] such as synaptic remodeling and long-term potentiation (LTP), a process in which long-term memories are acquired and stored.

Glutamate is also involved in neuronal injury and apoptosis. Excessive glutamate produces a cascade of destructive molecular events, including elevated cytoplasmic and mitochondrial membrane calcium, uncoupling of the mitochondrial membrane potential, and elaboration of caspases and phospholipases. (See Chapter 30 for more on energy production and oxidative stress.) Excess glutamate has been linked to several neurodegenerative disorders including Alzheimer's disease,[657] ALS,[658] and multiple sclerosis, and neuropsychiatric disorders including epilepsy, bipolar disease,[659] migraine,[660] and schizophrenia.[661]

Measurements of GABA and glutamate in the CNS are exceedingly difficult, but inferences can be made by measurements of N-Acetyl aspartate (NAA) through magnetic resonance spectroscopy.[662,663] Decreased levels of NAA measured by MRS have been reported in the hippocampus of Alzheimer's and bipolar disorder patients, an indication of hyperglutaminergic dysfunction in these conditions.

Acetylcholine (ACH)

The neurophysiological activity of acetylcholine in the hippocampus supports its primary role in the CNS in cognitive processes. ACH is synthesized from choline and acetyl-coA via the enzyme choline acetyltransferase. Pharmacological manipulation of acetylcholinesterase, the enzyme which degrades acetylcholine, is currently employed to treat Alzheimer's disease, which is regarded as a cholinergic deficit disorder.[664]

Functional Brain Approaches in Practice

Table 32.5 provides an overview of specific strategies employed to modulate neurotransmitter imbalances in neuropsychiatric conditions.

Table 32.5 **Strategies to Modulate Neurotransmitter Imbalances in Neuropsychiatric Conditions**

Neuro-transmitter	Potential Indications	Compound
Dopamine	ADHD	Folic acid Essential fatty acids (EFAs) Vitamin A
Dopamine blockade	Schizophrenia Autism	Melatonin
GABA	Anxiety Seizures	Pyridoxine
Excess glutamate	Epilepsy Migraine Bipolar disease Neurodegenerative disease	Magnesium EFAs Melatonin
Serotonin	Depression	Folic acid EFAs 5HTP, LAC
Acetylcholine	Dementia Mild cognitive impairment	Huperzine Acetylcarnitine

Dopamine and Serotonin Imbalances: Implications for the Treatment of ADHD and Depression

Augmentation strategies used to increase dopamine for the treatment of ADHD are based on observations that dopamine levels are preferentially reduced in frontal brain regions of adult ADHD patients.[665] Furthermore, genetic abnormalities related to dopamine transporter proteins have been reported in ADHD patients,[666] supporting the concept that symptoms of ADHD may result from a relative hypodopaminergic state.

Several nutraceutical approaches have been proposed to augment the hypodopaminegic state of ADHD patients, including specific herbal supplements, amino acids, and minerals. Our discussion will focus primarily on folic acid and omega-3 fatty acids. It should be noted that neither folate nor essential fatty acids enhance dopamine levels directly. These nutraceuticals may exert their influence on postsynaptic dopamine receptor sites by enhancing the threshold of neuronal signaling.

Neurotransmitter interactions with postsynaptic receptors induce conformational changes in the receptor. Through this engagement, referred to as signal transduction, changes in the phosphorylation status of ion channels, second messenger systems such as cyclic AMP (cAMP) and gene transcription factors alter the behavior of targeted neuronal cells. An elaborate example of signal transduction is the binding of dopamine to D1 receptors. The binding of dopamine stimulates the activity of adenylyl cyclase, which in turn catalyzes the conversion of ATP into cAMP. cAMP then transfers a phosphate group to specific intracellular proteins, a process that subsequently modifies their activity.

Postsynaptic cAMP production, which occurs through agonist stimulation of the postsynaptic receptor, initiates what may be regarded as a "pro-life" signaling cascade. One of the effects of cAMP is activation of protein kinase A, an enzyme that phosphorylates many substrates including cAMP response element binding protein (CREB). Phosphorylation of CREB increases the expression of the anti-apoptotic factor BCL-2. BCL-2 inhibits apoptosis by stabilizing the mitochondrial membrane potential, inhibiting the opening of the mitochondrial permeability transition pore and preventing the release of "death-driving" cysteine proteases involved in programmed cell death.

One of the most important physiological effects of cAMP in the brain involves its regulation of heat shock proteins. Brain cells respond to adverse changes in the cellular milieu, including free radicals, insulin receptor subsensitivity, elevated temperature, and ionic imbalances, through the production of heat shock proteins. Heat shock proteins assist in the holding of newly synthesized proteins, the degradation of malformed protein, and maintenance of calcium homeostasis within the endoplasmic reticulum.[667] Neurochemical processes that augment cAMP promote the expression of heat shock proteins and enhance neuronal cell survival, whereas molecular factors that diminish cAMP reduce heat shock proteins and lead to increased risk of apoptosis.[668]

Protein phosphorylation can be regarded as a "final common pathway" involved in neurotransmitter signal transduction and may link emotional states with physical changes in the body. The relationship of catecholamine agonists with cell survival at a molecular level may help to explain the observed benefits of antidepressant therapy and decreased mortality in patients with cardiovascular disease, and perhaps why happy people seem to live longer than sad people.

In addition to receptor modification and protein conformational changes that occur through phosphorylation, methylation of phospholipids may alter activity of dopamine receptors. Richard Deth, at Northeastern University, first demonstrated that inhibiting methylation at D4 receptor sites resulted in reduced G protein activation and reduced intrinsic activity of the receptor. Conversely, increased methylation of the D4 receptor, which is enhanced by folic acid in the form of methyltetrahydrofolate, increases intrinsic dopamine activity.[669]

Clinically, folate-deficient states are associated with symptoms of depression, apathy, and impaired concentration,[670] and they have been linked to a poor response to antidepressants as well.[671] These symptoms, while nonspecific, may result from either a hypodopaminergic or hyposerotoninergic state. Folate deficiency may produce a catecholamine deficit, either through impaired methylation of postsynaptic receptors, or through folate-dependent enzymatic pathways. Folic acid is a cofactor in production of tyrosine hydroxylase, the rate-limiting factor in dopamine synthesis, and also in tryptophan hydroxylase, the rate-limiting step in serotonin synthesis. Several studies have demonstrated an inverse relationship between low folate levels and mood, as well as response rate and relapse rate to antidepressants.[672] In support of these observations, reduced blood folate levels have been correlated with reduced levels of CSF serotonin (5HIAA).[673]

Tryptophan and Brain Scrotonin

L-tryptophan is the immediate precursor to brain serotonin, a fact which has led many clinicians to employ this amino acid to treat hyposerotoninergic states, including depression, insomnia, and anxiety. The importance of tryptophan in the regulation of mood is supported by the observations that dietary depletion of tryptophan leads to increased release of hypothalamic corticotropin-releasing factor (CRF), increased plasma cortisol, and an exacerbation of depression symptoms.[674] Hypercortisolemia is a frequent finding in depressed patients and may be a consequence of a loss of normal inhibitory function of tryptophan on CRF activity.

It should be noted that dietary administration of L-tryptophan is generally an inefficient way to enhance brain serotonin production due to competitive inhibition with other large neutral amino acids to cross the blood-brain barrier. An innovative strategy to bypass this limitation involves the utilization of alpha lactalbumin (LAC). Ingestion of LAC enchances serotonin synthesis in animals and humans, lowers cortisol levels, and induces anxiolytic effects.[675]

Omega-3 Fatty Acids

Role in dopamine, serotonin, and glutamate imbalances. The omega-3 fatty acids, which are constituted in the phospholipids of all cell membranes, exert direct and indirect influences on neurotransmission through modifications at the postsynaptic receptor. They influence signal transduction by inhibiting the hydrolysis of inositol triphosphate (IP3), an effect that closely resembles the activity of lithium. Essential fatty acids also inhibit membrane phospholipase activity,[676] and reduce arachidonic acid release from neuronal cell membranes.[677] Because arachidonic acid has been demonstrated to increase glutamate release, block reuptake of glutamate, and potentiate NMDA receptors,[678] essential fatty acids may be regarded as indirect glutamate antagonists and should be considered as potential agents in excess glutamate states (bipolar disease, for example).

Omega-3 fatty-acid deficiency has been linked to diminished dopamine receptors in rats,[679] and several researchers have found a direct correlation between low plasma or membrane-bound essential fatty acids and depression.[680]

Potential neuroprotective mechanisms of omega-3 fatty acids:

- Modulation of sodium and calcium channels with reduction of electrochemically excitable tissue
- Inhibition of phospholipase activity
- Reduced synthesis and release of membrane bound arachidonic acid
- Downregulation of excitotoxic glutamate-mediated neurotransmission

Vitamin A and Hypodopaminergic States

Vitamin A has an important and often overlooked function in brain development and in the adult brain. The distribution of retinoid receptor proteins in the amygdala, hippocampus, and other paralimbic brain regions suggests that retinoid signaling plays a vital role in cognitive and affective processes. Isomers of retinoic acid induce cyclic-AMP response elemental binding protein (CREB) and stimulate the expression of brain-derived neurotrophic factor (BDNF).[681]

Brain retinoic acid acts to upregulate D1 receptors and dopamine-dependent cAMP.[682] In animals, vitamin A deficiency results in a loss of hippocampal synaptic plasticity, and deficits in spatial learning, memory, and long-term potentiation.[683]

Defects in retinoid signaling pathways have been implicated in schizophrenia.[684] Vitamin A deficiency may lead to diminished D1 receptor gene transcription. This D1 receptor hypoactivity may produce the characteristic "negative symptoms" of schizophrenia such as apathy, blunted affect, and lack of insight. D1 receptor deficits may also have a disinhibiting effect on limbic D2 receptors, leading to the "positive symptoms" of schizophrenia such as hallucinations and delusions. Vitamin A and retinoid analogs are currently being explored as novel therapeutics in schizophrenia.

Hyperdopaminergic States

There are few nutraceutical agents that can reduce or inhibit the hyperdopaminergic state associated with psychotic disorders. However, melatonin may be an exception. Melatonin is an indoleamine found in the pineal gland, where it functions to facilitate adaptive changes in circadian rhythms.[685] Melatonin has a nocturnal pattern of secretion, exerting an inhibiting influence on neurons and promoting sleep via stimulation of adenosine.

Melatonin and adenosine are potent inhibitors of dopamine and gluamate.[686] Adenosine agonists have behavioral properties similar to dopamine antagonists. Melatonin and adenosine exert neuroprotective effects on mitochondrial function and have direct effects on the mitochondrial transition pore.[687] This pore, referred to as the PTP channel, is opened in response to elevated cystolic calcium and hypoxia; it induces pro-apoptotic molecular events. The ability of melatonin to inhibit PTP channel opening within mitochondrial membranes may account for its neuroprotective properties. An additional mechanism involved in the neuroprotective effects of adenosine involves homocysteine metabolism. Elevated homocysteine has well-known adverse effects in the CNS, including upregulation of excitotoxic NMDA receptors. Homocysteine administration in animals has been demonstrated to trap adenosine as s-adenosylhomocysteine and increase cortical hyperexcitability. Thus, depressed adenosine that occurs as a consequence of elevated homocysteine may be a critical mechanism in neurodegenerative disease and stroke.[688]

Like melatonin, adenosine exhibits neuroprotective activity by signaling neurons to reduce metabolic activity and preserve mitochondrial ATP stores. Elevated adenosine, which occurs in response to ischemia and hypoxic conditions, may act to "shut cells off" and depress metabolic activity in the mitochondria as a compensatory mechanism during periods of high metabolic stress. In this conceptual model, melatonin and adenosine can be considered molecular signals associated with inhibitory processes—reduced metabolic activity, lower mitochondrial "burning of fuel," and even sleep. Support for this notion is the observation that melatonin has a hypothermic effect.[689] Melatonin deficiency has been reported in schizophrenia[690] and autism,[691,692] and administration of this hormone has been shown to improve sleep in patients with these disorders.[693,694,695]

Magnesium: An Endogenous Glutamate Antagonist

Magnesium inhibits voltage-gated NMDA receptor channels and prevents excessive neuronal depolarization.[696] Magnesium has been used successfully to treat eclampsia-related seizures,[697] migraines,[698,699] and in the setting of acute stroke as well.[700]

Acetylcholine Augmentation Approaches

There is considerable evidence that links cholinergic neurotransmission to cognitive processes and memory. In pathological states such as Alzheimer's disease, postmortem studies consistently reveal reduced choline acetyltransfense activity and a reduced number of cholinergic neurons in the basal forebrain.[701]

Current pharmacological approaches in the treatment of dementia inhibit the acetylcholine degrading enzyme, ACHe, and hence raise synaptic acetylcholine levels by preventing degradation. Huperzine A, a traditional Chinese herbal medicine, acts as a potential ACHe inhibitor with reportedly higher specificity at the active enzymatic site, longer duration of action, greater bioavailability, and fewer side effects than conventional ACHe inhibitors currently approved for the treatment of Alzheimer's disease.[702,703,704] Futhermore, Huperzine exhibits neuroprotective effects *in vitro* through noncompetitive NMDA receptor antagonism,[705] a biochemical effect that closely resembles memantine (Namenda), a drug approved for Alzheimer's patients to slow the progression of the disorder.

Carnitine, primarily in the form of acetylcarnitine, has been shown to raise brain acetylcholine levels, purportedly through stimulation of choline acetyltransferase.[706] Acetylcarnitine also inhibits mitochondrial dysfunction through its antioxidant effects and, in a recent meta analysis of 21 double-blind studies of acetylcarnitine in the treatment of cognitive impairment and mild Alzheimer's disease, showed significant efficacy vs. placebo.[707]

Additional Level of Complexity

An additional level of complexity in human neurochemistry is involved when considering how neurotransmitters exert influence on other neurotransmitters. Some examples of these interactions in both normal and diseased states include the following:

- Prefrontal dopamine inhibits limbic dopamine, an example in nature of the adage, "think before you act."
- In schizophrenia, low prefrontal dopamine "releases" limbic dopamine and leads to intense synaptic firing of emotional brain centers no longer under cortical influence.

- Serotonin can inhibit downstream effects of glutamate by enhancing calbindin, an intracellular calcium-binding agent.
- Several neurodegenerative diseases, including ALS, are associated with reduced calbindin activity in apoptotic targeted neurons.
- Nicotinic acetylcholine receptors stimulate dopamine release, enhancing attentional processes required for learning.
- A core neurobehavioral impairment in Alzheimer's disease involves reduced attention and apathy to surroundings.

Summary

Neurochemical processes exist in a dynamic equilibrium and neuropsychiatric disorders reflect an imbalance between excitatory and inhibiting influences. These imbalances are affected by genetic and environmental factors, and they produce dysfunctional states through alterations in the phosphorylation states of phospholipids and mitochondrial membranes. Inhibitory mechanisms exerted at a molecular level by GABA, serotonin, melatonin, and adenosine promote hyperpolarization; at a macromolecular level, physiological effects associated with restoration are noted. Conversely, excitatory processes, mediated primarily through glutamate, exert a depolarizing effect on neurons, which can be considered the signal of activity and stimulation. Like other examples in nature, neither state is inherently harmful or associated with pathological processes. Neuropsychiatric disease results when there is an imbalance in the dynamic homeostasis between these excitatory and inhibiting forces.

Thyroid

Lara Pizzorno, MA Div, MA Lit, LMT, and William Ferril, MD

Earlier in this chapter, a detailed discussion on the many causes and manifestations of thyroid dysfunction was provided. Here, we will focus on applying that information to the challenge of improving thyroid function in patients. Depending on the clinician's assessment of where the most significant problems lie for each patient, the eight areas of the functional medicine matrix can indicate many useful approaches for supporting and improving thyroid function.

Interpreting Laboratory Findings

Typical ranges for normal serum thyroid hormone values are:

T_4	4.8–13.2 µg/dl
Free T_4	0.9–2 ng/dl
T_3	80–200 ng/dl
TSH	0.4 to 4.0 mIU/L for those with no symptoms of an under- or overactive thyroid. If the patient is being treated for a thyroid disorder, the TSH should be between 0.3 and 3.0 mIU/L. Some people with a TSH value over 2.5 mIU/L who have no signs (that is, no other abnormal thyroid function tests) or symptoms suggestive of an underactive thyroid may develop hypothyroidism sometime in the future. Anyone with a TSH above 2.5 mIU/L, therefore, should be followed very closely by a doctor. Normal value ranges may vary slightly among different laboratories.[708] The sensitive thyrotropin assay is considered the most useful method of detecting thyroid dysfunction.[709,710,711]

When interpreting thyroid blood tests, it's important to note that results may be misleading for a variety of reasons:

- A test result within laboratory reference limits is not necessarily normal for a specific individual. A study in 2002[712] found that "each individual had a unique thyroid function" and "high individuality causes laboratory reference ranges to be insensitive to changes in test results that are significant for an individual."
- Another study of the problems associated with inter-laboratory differences used TSH and TSH with free thyroxine as examples of tests where such differences can "markedly affect the clinical interpretation of tests."[713]
- In chronic stress, high cortisol levels inhibit the pituitary's production of TSH while also causing displacement of thyroid protein off its carrier protein. Despite the fact that thyroid hormone becomes depleted, a blood test will show a normal TSH result. Patients under chronic stress should be

evaluated using their armpit temperature immediately before arising (see sidebar) and a 24-hour urine test to assess thyroid hormone levels.

- Cortisol and thyroid have a complex relationship. In normal functioning, cortisol is needed in the liver and kidneys for the conversion of T_4 to T_3. In conditions of cortisol excess (acute stress), the generalized pattern is characterized by a trend toward lowered TSH production and a blunted TSH response to TRH, a decline in T_3, and an increase in rT_3.[714] When acute stress becomes prolonged, chronic stress and adrenal exhaustion ensue, the body's ability to produce sufficient cortisol for the T_4 to T_3 conversion may become compromised, and even individuals whose thyroid gland is producing normal amounts of T_4, as determined by laboratory test, may be functionally deficient in thyroid hormone. In brief, both excess and insufficient cortisol negatively impact the conversion of T_4 to T_3, by slightly different mechanisms.
- Anxiety caused by the blood draw can temporarily increase free values of thyroid hormone. Anxiety activates the stress response, which activates lipoprotein lipase, resulting in an elevation in free fatty acid levels. Free fatty acids displace thyroid hormone from its carrier, temporarily raising free thyroid hormone levels.
- Certain medications can also inappropriately elevate levels of thyroid hormones by causing their displacement off thyroid binding globulin. These include aspirin (and other nonsteroidal anti-inflammatories),[715] phenytoin,[716] diazepam,[717] and increased blood heparin.[718]

Measuring Basal Body Temperature

Basal body temperature, which is controlled by the thyroid and can be a better indicator of how much T_3 is active inside cells than blood tests that measure T_4, is a good way of assessing basal metabolic rate. Procedure:

- Shake down a thermometer to below 95 degrees and place it by the bed before going to sleep.
- Upon waking, place the thermometer under the armpit for a full 10 minutes.
- Remain as still as possible, resting with the eyes closed.
- Record the temperature for at least three consecutive mornings, preferably at the same time of day. Menstruating women must check basal body temperature on the second, third, and fourth days of menstruation. Men and postmenopausal women can check on any three consecutive days.

Low thyroid function can have a variety of underlying causes. It's important to pin down the source of the problem and match the therapeutic approach to the patient's specific needs. Consider the following general types of dysfunction, indicated by the relationships among various laboratory findings:

1. Pituitary dysfunction is suggested by blood levels low in both T_4 and TSH.
2. If blood levels of TSH are elevated, yet T_4 levels are still low, this indicates that the pituitary has responded properly, but the thyroid gland is not responding to TSH by synthesizing T_4.
3. If TSH is elevated despite normal blood levels of T_4, this suggests an autoimmune problem resulting in subclinical hypothyroidism.
4. The presence of low basal body temperature and a high reverse-T_3-to-T_3 ratio is suggestive of Wilson's disease.
5. If both TSH and T_4 levels are normal, but clinical signs indicate low thyroid activity, this suggests inadequate conversion of T_4 to T_3 in peripheral tissues, which may be due to iodothyronine iodinase dysfunction.
6. If T_3 levels are adequate, but thyroid function is still low, this suggests an inability of T_3 to attach to receptors inside the cells and activate enzymes, due either to a malformation in T_3 (a high ratio of reverse-T_3-to-T_3 may be evidence of this situation) or the intracellular receptor sites.

Many factors can contribute to these problems. Using the information presented earlier in the chapter, we will take a "tour" of the functional medicine matrix to identify specific approaches the clinician can use to help patients improve thyroid function.

The Matrix: Environmental Inputs

Diet And Nutrients

The influence of diet upon health can scarcely be overstated (see Chapter 26), and there are many foods and nutrients that can hinder or support thyroid function.

Goitrogens may block iodine utilization. Both the isoflavones found in soybeans[719,720] and the isothiocyanates found in Brassica family vegetables[721] are goitrogens, which appear to reduce thyroid hormone output by blocking the activity of thyroid peroxidase, the enzyme responsible for adding iodine to the thyroid hormones. While soy foods and Brassica family vegetables (turnips, cabbage, broccoli, cauliflower, Brussels sprouts, mustard greens, kale, kohlrabi, rutabaga) are the primary sources of goitrogens, they are also found in small amounts in peanuts, pine nuts, millet, peaches, strawberries, spinach, and cassava root. Both isoflavones and isothiocyanates appear to be heat-sensitive, and limited research suggests cooking, specifically boiling, lowers the availability of these substances.[722,723] However, since boiling crucifers results in the loss not only of goitrogens but of important nutrients as well, patients for whom goitrogens may be problematic can be advised to briefly steam these vegetables and consume them in modest amounts.

Excess iodine. Although iodine is necessary for proper thyroid function, excessive intake of iodine can suppress TSH levels and inhibit thyroid hormone synthesis in susceptible individuals.[724] Although the RDA for iodine in adults is only 150 mcg, the average intake of iodine in the U.S. is estimated to be over 600 mcg per day (probably due to the ubiquitous use of iodized salt). Excess iodine (high urinary iodine concentration) and low TSH can be predictable factors for a recovery from hypothyroidism due to Hashimoto's thyroiditis after restricting iodine intake.[725] A case of neonatal iodine overload (from iodinated skin disinfectants) causing transient hypothyroidism was reported in 2005,[726] so care should be taken in the use of such products for infants.

Foods rich in nutrients needed for T_4 manufacture include:

- **Iodine:** sea vegetables (kelp, dulse, hijiki, nori, arame, wakame, kombu), clams, shrimp, haddock, oysters, salmon, sardines, eggs
- **Zinc:** fresh oysters, ginger root, lamb chops, pecans, split peas, Brazil nuts, whole wheat, rye, oats, almonds, walnuts, sardines
- **Vitamin E:** wheat germ oil, sunflower seeds, almonds, peanut oil, olive oil, wheat germ, peanuts
- **Vitamin A:** liver, red chili peppers, greens (collard, turnip, kale, Swiss chard, beet greens), apricots, winter squash, cantaloupe, papaya, nectarines, peaches, cod liver oil ("Free retinol is not generally found in foods. Retinyl palmitate, a precursor and storage form of retinol, is found in foods from animals. Plants contain carotenoids, some of which are precursors for vitamin A (e.g., alpha-carotene and beta-carotene). Yellow and orange vegetables contain significant quantities of carotenoids. Green vegetables also contain carotenoids, though the pigment is masked by the green pigment of chlorophyll."[727])
- **Vitamin B2** (riboflavin): Brewer's yeast, organ meats, almonds, wheat germ, wild rice, mushrooms, egg yolks
- **Vitamin B3** (niacin): Brewer's yeast, rice bran, wheat bran, peanuts with skin, liver, light meat of turkey and chicken
- **Vitamin B6** (pyridoxine): Brewer's yeast, sunflower seeds, wheat germ, tuna, liver, soybeans, walnuts, salmon, trout, lentils, lima beans, navy beans, garbanzos, pinto beans, brown rice, bananas
- **Vitamin C:** Red chili peppers, guavas, red sweet peppers, parsley, greens (collard, turnip, mustard, kale), strawberries, papaya, citrus fruits (oranges, lemons, grapefruit)

Foods rich in nutrients needed for $T_4 \rightarrow T_3$ conversion include:

- **Zinc:** fresh oysters, ginger root, lamb chops, pecans, split peas, Brazil nuts, whole wheat, rye, oats, almonds, walnuts, sardines
- **Selenium:** Brazil nuts. One Brazil nut provides approximately 139 mcg; 200 mcg/day is the recommended dosage. Excess selenium can interfere with enzyme systems related to sulfur metabolism and can be toxic in amounts greater than 900 mcg/day.[728]

Foods rich in nutrients needed for T_3 binding to intracellular receptors are those rich in Vitamin A: liver, red chili peppers, greens (collard, turnip, kale, Swiss chard, beet greens), apricots, winter squash, cantaloupe, papaya, nectarines, peaches, cod liver oil

Nutritional Supplementation Considerations For Improving Thyroid Function:

- Zinc, vitamin E, vitamin A, B2, B3, and B6 are all involved in the manufacture of thyroid hormone.
- Zinc is a cofactor in one form of the deiodinase enzyme that converts T_4 to T_3, and zinc deficiencies can prevent the proper activation of DNA programs (zinc finger malfunction).
- Low zinc levels are common in the elderly (and even more severe in the institutionalized elderly),[729] and the risk of hypothyroidism increases with age.[730,731]
- Vitamin A is also necessary for the formation of intracellular receptors for T_3.[732]

- Selenium, a cofactor in another of the deiodinase enzymes, is estimated to be markedly deficient in diets worldwide.[733,734] Selenium has been demonstrated to decrease thyroid antibody levels in autoimmune thyroid conditions[735,736] such as Hashimoto's, which is thought to constitute a significant percentage of subclinical hypothyroidism.[737]
- Antioxidant supplementation may be particularly important if environmental toxins are a potential contributing factor.[738,739,740,741] Supplementation with vitamins C, E, and *Curcuma longa* (turmeric), for example, has been shown to increase thyroid function in rats with methimazole-induced hypothyroidism.[742]

Exercise

Exercise stimulates thyroid gland secretion, increases tissue sensitivity to thyroid hormone, and is well known for its stress-relieving effects. Dieting has consistently been shown to cause a decrease in metabolic rate as the body strives to conserve fuel.[743] Exercise, unfortunately, has not consistently been shown to prevent this decline in metabolic rate in response to dieting.[744,745,746] However, the many other benefits of exercise, including both weight training (which builds muscle mass) and aerobic exercise (which improves the body's use of oxygen), have been described elsewhere (see Chapters 13 and 29), and constitute reason enough for including it in the overall program.

Xenobiotics

Exposure to toxic levels of heavy metals can interfere with thyroid function.[747] The destructive effects of heavy metals (lead, cadmium, mercury) are well documented and are discussed elsewhere in this book (see Chapters 13, 22, and 31). Lead and mercury invade the thyroid gland and disrupt the production of thyroid hormones, or induce minute alterations in their molecular structure, so they are no longer recognized by cellular receptors. Heavy metals can also impair liver and kidney function, decreasing conversion of T_4 to T_3.

In agricultural areas, the likelihood of pesticide contamination in the water is higher. Tap water may be contaminated with minute amounts of insecticides, weed killers, and artificial fertilizer. Pesticides have been shown to interfere with thyroid function and to increase cancer risk. People not only drink and cook with water, but also bathe and shower in it, thus absorbing chemicals through the digestive tract, skin, and respiration (from the vapors).

Hormone and antibiotic residues in meat and dairy products, food-borne bacteria, chemicals in cleaning products, food additives, cosmetics, and the metabolic by-products of unfriendly gut bacteria can denature thyroid hormones, producing reverse T_3, and can also impair the activity of the liver and kidneys, thus decreasing conversion of T_4 to T_3.

A significant correlation exists between smoking and Graves' disease.[748] Fluoride is a direct antagonist to, and therefore inhibits utilization of, iodine.[749]

Medications

A number of prescription drugs can affect thyroid hormone production and delivery:

- Lithium has multiple effects on thyroid hormone synthesis and secretion.[750,751]
- Certain antipsychotics can compromise thyroid function.[752]
- Amiodarone (Cordarone), which is used to treat arrhythmia, contains iodine and can induce hypothyroidism.[753,754]
- Somatostatin and dopamine inhibit TSH secretion.[755]
- Liver enzyme activity (and thus the rate of clearance of thyroid hormone) is elevated by phenytoin for seizure disorders, the antibiotic rifampin for tuberculosis, and the psychiatric medicine carbamazepine.

Trauma

- **Surgery:** Overt hypothyroidism may be caused by thyroid surgery and ablation to correct hyperthyroidism.
- **Radiation:** Ionizing radiation from medical and dental x-rays, particularly those received in childhood, can adversely affect thyroid function, as can radiation therapy for various cancers. A 2004 review indicated that "radiotherapy-induced thyroid abnormalities remain underestimated and underreported."[756]

The Matrix: Hormonal and Neurotransmitter Imbalances

Only a select few hormones directly activate or repress the genetic programs contained within the cell nucleus: steroids, vitamin A, and thyroid hormones. The relative proportion of each will determine which proteins are present or absent, and whether sufficient body protein is produced for maintenance and repair.[757] Protein provides the building blocks for the metabolically active constituents of body tissue. Examples of metabolically active protein-containing molecules dependent upon thyroid hormone activation of genes include actin, myosin, sodium/potassium ATPase, enzymes, and certain hormone receptors. Thus, low thyroid function leads to deficient regeneration information in key enzymes that perpetuate metabolism.

The formation of catecholamine receptors is dependent upon reception of thyroid hormone messages, so low thyroid function can both contribute to and mimic adrenal exhaustion. Since the thyroid message directs the activation of genes that increase the synthesis of key hormones and hormone receptors as well as metabolic enzymes, thyroid hormone deficiency sets off a chain reaction of other hormone deficiencies, accelerating the aging rate. For example, the amount of thyroid message received determines the rate of growth hormone synthesis within the pituitary.

The Matrix: Oxidation-Reduction Imbalances and Mitochondropathy

Thyroid hormones direct cellular DNA to increase the manufacture rate of cellular mineral pumps and mitochondrial combustion chamber components. ATPase is one of the enzymes dependent upon thyroid hormone activation of genes for its production. The sodium/potassium ATPase pump is responsible for trapping the energy the cell uses to charge its membrane. Body cells utilize the electrical charge within their membrane to protect themselves and to perform the cellular work of living. The more pumps, the more charge generated, and the more calories burned to maintain it. Fewer pumps lead to fewer calories burned. Fewer calories burned leads to a lower metabolic rate. [758,759]

For this reason, EKG voltage tends to be diminished, and armpit temperature before getting out of bed is less than 97.6 degrees in patients with peripheral thyroid resistance, despite normal free serum levels of T_4, T_3 and reverse T_3.[760]

No matter what the raw fuel consumed (protein, fat, or carbohydrate), the mitochondria can only burn acetate. Many thyroid problems are made worse by specific vitamin deficiencies that impede the processing of raw fuels into acetate. For this reason, common signs of thyroid deficiency, like cold intolerance and weight gain, worsen with nutritional deficiencies (see above under Environmental Inputs/Diet and Nutrients).

The higher the metabolic rate, the greater the oxidative stress. In patients with hyperthyroidism, supplementation with antioxidants such as lipoic acid and N-acetylcysteine should be considered. Interestingly, there is animal research emerging that indicates the presence of oxidative stress in hypothyroidism as well, although the data are still limited and controversial. One such study demonstrated protective effects of taurine against the oxidative stress of hypothyroidism,[761] while the other showed a similar action of vitamin E.[762]

The Matrix: Detoxification and Biotransformational Imbalances

Compounds that induce phase I activity, whether xenobiotic, drug or food, may contribute to a faster rate of clearance of thyroid hormone, increasing the need for the thyroid gland to produce more hormone to maintain normal levels. Studies suggesting that dioxin and polybrominated diphenyl ethers (PBDEs—flame retardants that are ubiquitous environmental contaminants) disrupt thyroid function have been conducted for many years on animals.[763,764,765,766,767,768] Although there are problems in assuming a direct transference of such information to humans, the consistent findings in animal research draw our attention to significant concerns with these chemicals, such as increasing thyroid hormone clearance and decreasing serum T_4 and T_3 levels.[769]

Impaired detoxification may result in recycling of estrogen, a concern particularly during pregnancy, and in perimenopause when estrogen levels may fluctuate to abnormally high levels. Higher estrogen levels increase thyroid binding globulin, making it harder for cells to access thyroid hormone.

The Matrix: Immune and Inflammatory Imbalances

Subclinical hypothyroidism may cause a slight increase in homocysteine, although the research has not been entirely consistent (the link is much better documented for overt hypothyroidism).[770,771] Other CVD risk factors, such as CRP and cholesterol, are well known to be higher in both subclinical and overt hypothyroidism.[772,773,774] Preventive measures that address the inflammatory and lipid markers should be undertaken if needed (see Chapter 27).

Adrenal function forms a determinant for the presence or absence of thyroid antibodies; thyroid autoantibodies are highly correlated with secondary adrenal insufficiency.[775]

In one study, patients with dermatitis herpetiformis were found to have significantly increased abnormalities of thyroid function tests (32% vs. 4%), with significant hypothyroidism being the most common abnormality affecting 12 of the 56 patients.[776] This is a good place to emphasize the connection between thyroid disorders and gluten intolerance, as the link has been demonstrated not only in dermatitis herpetiformis,[777] but also in many autoimmune diseases, including Hashimoto's thyroiditis.[778]

Thyroid hormone directly activates cellular DNA programs, including some responsible for the manufacture of receptors for other hormones. Without their receptors, it does little good for these hormones to arrive, as they cannot deliver their information. Diseases may arise because of receptor formation deficiency or receptor destruction. Asthma, for example, is sometimes caused by a defect in the receptors needed by epinephrine to keep the airways open.

The Matrix: Digestive, Absorptive, and Microbiological Imbalances

Digestive and absorptive functions also need to be considered. Thyroid hormone information affects GI motility; a slowing of the digestive and absorptive processes increases the opportunity for unfriendly bacteria to feed and proliferate. Dysbiotic bacteria produce beta-glucuronidase, which deconjugates estrogen, sending it back into the circulation. High levels of estrogen stimulate increased production of thyroid binding globulin, making it harder for cells to access thyroid hormone. In addition, a strong correlation exists among autoimmune diseases, intestinal permeability, and food allergy. In one study of 100 celiac patients, two also had overt autoimmune thyroid disease. After six months on a gluten-free diet, serologic autoantibody markers were undetectable in these patients.[779] In patients in whom digestive imbalances may be a contributing factor, the 4R program should be considered (see Chapter 28).

The Matrix: Structural Imbalances (Cellular Membrane)

Thyroid hormones deliver information to the cell's DNA to direct the creation of membrane pumps (sodium/potassium/ATPase pumps) that enable the cell to trap some of the energy produced in the mitochondria for useful work and charge its membrane. Thus, the formation and maintenance of a healthy cell membrane is dependent upon thyroid function.

Attention deficit-hyperactivity disorder has been linked with peripheral thyroid resistance,[780] creating inability of thyroid hormone to deliver its information at the DNA level due to defective cellular membrane receptors. Vitamin A is necessary throughout the body, including the brain, for the activation of thyroid-dependent DNA receptors.

The Matrix: Mind and Spirit

The psychoneuroimmunological connection to endocrine function is well recognized. Lack of belief in something greater than oneself, in a teleological universe, lack of support, community, love—these are the most fundamental causes of an inability to utilize stressors as spurs to the expression of a continually evolving positive vitality. Chronic stress, particularly if unmitigated by an inner spiritual harmony that assigns a positive meaning, disrupts normal thyroid function at virtually every level:

- Stress suppresses the hypothalamus' release of TRH, the pituitary's release of TSH, the thyroid gland's production of thyroid hormones.
- Chronic stress results in increased production of inflammatory cytokines that block conversion of T_4 to T_3 and—by binding to the thyroid peroxidase enzyme, thyroglobulin, and TSH receptors—can prevent the manufacture of T_4, and may also bind to the adrenal glands, pancreas, and parietal cells.

- Chronic stress promotes an overactive immune system and thus an increased likelihood that antithyroidal antibodies will be produced.
- Chronically high cortisol levels increase thyroid binding globulin levels in the bloodstream.
- Chronic stress may result in a state of adrenal exhaustion in which supplies of cortisol are depleted. Recall that cortisol is necessary for the conversion of T_4 to T_3.
- Chronic stress depletes magnesium reserves. Insufficient magnesium significantly lessens the body's ability to relax and get the deep sleep needed for repair and rejuvenation.

Sources of stress may be physical as well as emotional, including head or bodily injury, chronic allergies or infections, poor diet, or lack of sleep.

Summary

This completes our overview of potential influences on thyroid function from the perspective of mechanisms and the functional medicine matrix. From cellular messaging to the impact of diet, toxic exposures, medications, oxidative stress, GI dysfunction, and age, to the important role of stress and the life of the mind and spirit, the thyroid is vulnerable at myriad points on the matrix. The clinical benefit of a thorough understanding of underlying function and the imbalances that result from disturbed function is that those imbalances can often be redressed through the same mechanisms. In other words, diets can be changed, toxic exposures eliminated or reduced, oxidative stress improved with antioxidants, energy production increased, GI function and detoxification improved, cellular messaging supported, and stress management implemented. These are among the many potential interventions discussed throughout this book that can help practitioners improve outcomes for their patients with thyroid disease and dysfunction.

References

1. Wolff GL, Kodell RL, Moore SR, Cooney CA. Maternal epigenetics and methyl supplements affect agouti gene expression in Avy/a mice. FASEB J. 1998;12(11):949-57.
2. Selye H. Stress and the reduction of distress. JSC Med Assoc. 1979;75(11):562-66.
3. Lupien SJ, de Leon M, de Santi S, et al. Cortisol levels during human aging predict hippocampal atrophy and memory deficits. Nat Neurosci. 1998;1(1):69-73.
4. Pomara N, Greenberg WM, Branford MD, Doraiswamy PM. Therapeutic implications of HPA axis abnormalities in Alzheimer's disease: review and update. Psychopharmacol Bull. 2003;37(2):120-34.
5. Brown ES, J Woolston D, Frol A, et al. Hippocampal volume, spectroscopy, cognition, and mood in patients receiving corticosteroid therapy. Biol Psychiatry. 2004;55(5):538-45.
6. Brown ES, Varghese FP, McEwen BS. Association of depression with medical illness: does cortisol play a role? Biol Psychiatry. 2004;55(1):1-9.
7. O'Brien JT, Lloyd A, McKeith I, et al. A longitudinal study of hippocampal volume, cortisol levels, and cognition in older depressed subjects. Am J Psychiatry. 2004;161(11):2081-90.
8. MacLullich AM, Deary IJ, Starr JM, et al. Plasma cortisol levels, brain volumes and cognition in healthy elderly men. Psychoneuroendocrinology. 2005;30(5):505-15.
9. Licinio J, Gold PW, Wong ML. A molecular mechanism for stress-induced alterations in susceptibility to disease. Lancet. 1995;346:104-6.
10. Sapolsky RM, Romero LM, Munck AU. How do glucocorticoids influence the stress-responses? Integrating permissive, suppressive, stimulatory, and preparative actions. Endocr Rev. 2000;21:55-89.
11. Lee AL, Ogle WO, Sapolsky RM. Stress and depression: possible links to neuron death in the hippocampus. Bipolar Disord. 2002;4(2):117-28.
12. Sher L. Type D personality: the heart, stress, and cortisol. QJM. 2005;98(5):323-29.
13. Licinio J, Gold PW, Wong ML. A molecular mechanism for stress-induced alterations in susceptibility to disease. Lancet. 1995;346:104-6.
14. Axelrod J, Reisine TD. Stress hormones: their interaction and regulation. Science. 1984;224:452-59.
15. Heinrichs SC, Menzaghi F, Merlo Pich E, et al. The role of CRF in behavioral aspects of stress. Ann N Y Acad Sci. 1995;771:92-104.
16. Zhou D, Kusnecov AW, Shurin MR, et al. Exposure to physical and psychological stressors elevates plasma interleukin 6: relationship to the activation of hypothalamic-pituitary-adrenal axis. Endocrinol. 1993;133(6):2523-30.
17. Mastorakos G, Magiakou MA, Chrousos GP. Effects of the immune/inflammatory reaction on the hypothalamic-pituitary-adrenal axis. Ann N Y Acad Sci. 1995;771:438-48.
18. Kapcala LP, Chautard T, Eskay RL. The protective role of the hypothalamic-pituitary-adrenal axis against lethality produced by immune, infections, and inflammatory stress. Ann N Y Acad Sci. 1995;771:419-37.
19. Tache Y, Perdue MH. Role of peripheral CRF signalling pathways in stress-related alterations of gut motility and mucosal function. Neurogastroenterol Motil. 2004;16(Suppl 1):137-42.
20. Saruta M, Takahashi K, Suzuki T, et al. Urocortin 1 incolonic mucosa in patients with ulcerative colitis. J Clin Endocrinol Metab. 2004;89(11):5352-61.
21. Kempuraj D, Papadopoulou N, Stanford EJ, et al. Increased numbers of activated mast cells in endometriosis lesions positive for corticotropin-releasing hormone and urocortin. Am J Reprod Immunol. 2004;52(4):267-75.
22. Fisher JS. Are all EDC effects mediated via steroid hormone receptors? Toxicology. 2004;205(1-2):33-41.
23. Telang NT, Suto A, Wong GY, et al. Induction by estrogen metabolite 16 alpha-hydroxyestrone of genotoxic damage and aberrant proliferation in mouse mammary epithelial cells. J Natl Cancer Inst. 1992;84(8):634-38.
24. Bradlow HL, Davis DL, Lin G, et al. Effects of pesticides on the ratio of 16α/2-hydroxyestrone: a biologic marker of breast cancer risk. Environ Health Perspec. 1995;103(Suppl 7):147-50.

25. Jernstrom H, Klug TL, Sepkovic DW, et al. Predictors of the plasma ratio of 2-hydroxyestrone to 16alpha-hydroxyestrone among premenopausal, nulliparous women from four ethnic groups. Carcinogenesis. 2003;24(5):991-1005.
26. Cauley JA, Zmuda JM, Danielson ME, et al. Estrogen metabolites and the risk of breast cancer in older women. Epidemiology. 2003;14(6):740-44.
27. Wozniak AL, Bulayeva NN, Watson CS. Xenoestrogens at picomolar to nanomolar concentrations trigger membrane estrogen receptor-alpha-mediated Ca2+ fluxes and prolactin release in GH3/B6 pituitary tumor cells. Environ Health Perspect. 2005;113(4):431-39.
28. Pascussi JM, Gerbal-Chaloin S, Drocourt L, et al. Cross-talk between xenobiotic detoxication and other signalling pathways: clinical and toxicological consequences. Xenobiotica. 2004;34(7):633-64.
29. Hankinson SE, Willett WC, Manson JE, et al. Plasma sex steroid hormone levels and risk of breast cancer in postmenopausal women. J Natl Cancer Inst. 1998;90(17):1292-99.
30. Cummings SR, Lee JS, Lui LY, et al. Sex hormones, risk factors, and risk of estrogen receptor-positive breast cancer in older women: a long-term prospective study. Cancer Epidemiol Biomarkers Prev. 2005;14(5):1047-51.
31. Onland-Moret NC, van Gils CH, Roest M, et al. Cyp17, urinary sex steroid levels and breast cancer risk in postmenopausal women. Cancer Epidemiol Biomarkers Prev. 2005;14(4):815-20.
32. Pasqualini JR, Chetrite GS. Recent insight on the control of enzymes involved in estrogen formation and transformation in human breast cancer. J Steroid Biochem Mol Biol. 2005;93(2-5):221-36.
33. Hernandez L, Nunez-Villarl MJ, Martinez-Arribas F, et al. Circulating hormone levels in breast cancer patients. Correlation with serum tumor markers and the clinical and biological features of the tumors. Anticancer Res. 2005;25(1B):451-54.
34. Takada Y, Andreeff M, Aggarwal BB. Indole-3-carbinol suppresses NF-{kappa}B and I{kappa}B{alpha} kinase activation causing inhibition of expression of NF-{kappa}B-regulated antiapoptotic and metastatic gene products and enhancement of apoptosis in myeloid and leukemia cells Blood. 2005;Apr 5;[Epub ahead of print].
35. Adiloglu AK, Can R, Nazli C, et al. Ectasia and severe atherosclerosis: relationships with chlamydia pneumoniae, helicobacterpylori, and inflammatory markers. Tex Heart Inst J. 2005;32(1):21-27.
36. Markus HS, Mendall MA. Helicobacter pylori infection: a risk factor for ischaemic cerebrovascular disease and carotid atheroma. J Neurol Neurosurg Psychiatry. 1998;64:104-7.
37. Park SH, Jeon WK, Kim SH, et al. Helicobacter pylori eradication has no effect on metabolic and inflammatory parameters. J Natl Med Assoc. 2005;97(4):508-13.
38. Franceschi F, Leo D, Fini L, et al. Helicobacter pylori infection and ischaemic heart disease: an overview of the general literature. Dig Liver Dis. 2005;37(5):301-8.
39. Adiloglu AK, Can R, Nazli C, et al. Ectasia and severe atherosclerosis: relationships with chlamydia pneumoniae, Helicobacter pylori, and inflammatory markers. Tex Heart Inst J. 2005;32(1):21-27.
40. Davidson M, Kuo CC, Middaugh JP, et al. Confirmed previous infection with chlamydia pneumoniae (TWAR) and its presence in early coronary atherosclerosis. Circulation. 1998;98(7):628-33.
41. Wozniak MA, Shipley SJ, Combrinck M, et al. Productive herpes simplex virus in brain of elderly normal subjects and Alzheimer's disease patients. J Med Virol. 2005;75(2):300-6.
42. Itzhaki RF, Lin WR, Shang D, et al. Herpes simplex virus type I in brain and risk of Alzheimer's disease. Lancet. 1997;349:241-44.
43. Pepe S. Effect of dietary polyunsaturated fatty acids on age-related changes in cardiac mitochondrial membranes. Exp Gerontol. 2005;40(5):369-76.
44. Demarco VG, Scumpia PO, Bosanquet JP, et al. Alpha-lipoic acid inhibits endotoxin-stimulated expression of iNOS and nitric oxide independent of the heat shock response in RAW 264.7 cells. Free Radic Res. 2004;38(7):675-82.
45. Langmann T, Liebisch G, Moehle C, et al. Gene expression profiling identifies retinoids as potent inducers of macrophage lipid efflux. Biochim Biophys Acta. 2005;1740(2):155-61.
46. Gustafsson JA. Fatty acids in control of gene expression. Nutr Rev. 1998;56(2 Pt 2):S20-S21.
47. Luquet S, Gaudel C, Holst D, et al. Roles of PPAR delta in lipid absorption and metabolism: a new target for the treatment of type 2 diabetes. Biochim Biophys Acta. 2005;1740(2):313-17.
48. Maurin AC, Chavassieux PM, Meunier PJ. Expression of PPAR-gamma and beta/delta in human primary osteoblastic cells: influence of polyunsaturated fatty acids. Calcif Tissue Int. 2005;May 5;[Epub ahead of print].
49. Ibid.
50. Bousserouel S, Brouillet A, Bereziat G, et al. Different effects of n-6 and n-3 polyunsaturated fatty acids on the activation of rat smooth muscle cells by interleukin-1 beta. J Lipid Res. 2003;44(3):601-11.
51. Ziboh VA, Miller CC, Cho Y. Metabolism of polyunsaturated fatty acids by skin epidermal enzymes: generation of antiinflammatory and antiproliferative metabolites. Am J Clin Nutr. 2000;71(1 Suppl):361S-66S.
52. Badawi AF, El-Sohemy A, Stephen LL, et al. The effect of dietary n-3 and n-6 polyunsaturated fatty acids on the expression of cyclooxygenase 1 and 2 and levels of p2lras in rat mammary glands. Carcinogenesis. 1998;19(5):905-10.
53. Madigan C, Ryan M, Owens D, et al. Comparison of diets high in monounsaturated versus polyunsaturated fatty acid on postprandial lipoproteins in diabetes. Ir J Med Sci. 2005;174(1):8-20.
54. Miyamoto T, Kaneko A, Kakizawa T, et al. Inhibition of peroxisome proliferator signaling pathways by thyroid hormone receptor. J Biological Chem. 1997;272(12):7752-58.
55. Motojima K, Passilly P, Peters JM, et al. Expression of putative fatty acid transporter genes are regulated by peroxisome proliferator-activated receptor α and γ activators in a tissue- and inducer-specific manner. J Biological Chem. 1998;273(27):16710-14.
56. Clandinin MT, Claerhout DL, Lien EL. Docosahexaenoic acid increases thyroid-stimulating hormone concentration in male and adrenal corticotrophic hormone concentration in female weanling rats. J Nutr. 1998; 128:1257-61.
57. Singh J, Hamid R, Reddy BS. Dietary fish oil inhibits the expression of farnesyl protein transferase and colon tumor development in rodents. Carcinogenesis. 1998;19(6):985-89.
58. Davidson LA, Lupton JR, Jiang YH, et al. Carcinogen and dietary lipid regulate ras expression and localization in rat colon without affecting farnesylation kinetics. Carcinogenesis. 1999;20(5):785-91.
59. Collett ED, Davidson LA, Fan YY, et al. n-6 and n-3 polyunsaturated fatty acids differentially modulate oncogenic Ras activation in colonocytes. Am J Physiol Cell Physiol. 2001;280(5):C1066-75.
60. Ginn-Pease ME, Whisler RL. Redox signals and NF-κB activation in T cells. Free Radic Biol Med. 1998;25(3):346-61.
61. Bustamante J, Lodge JK, Marcocci L, et al. Alpha-lipoic acid in liver metabolism and disease. Free Radic Biol Med. 1998;24(6):1023-39.
62. Ibid.
63. d'Alessio P, Moutet M, Coudrier E, et al. ICAM-1 and VCAM-1 expression induced by TNF-α are inhibited by a glutathione peroxidase mimic. Free Radic Biol Med. 1998;24(6):979-87.
64. Lapenna D, de Gioia S, Ciofani G, et al. Glutathione-related antioxidant defenses in human atherosclerotic plaques. Circulation. 1998;97:1930-34.

65. Faruqi R, de la Motte C, DiCorleto PE. α-Tocopherol inhibits agonist induced monocytic cell adhesion to cultured human endothelial cells. J Clin Invest. 1994;94:592-600.
66. Plotnick GD, Corretti MC, Vogel RA. Effect of antioxidant vitamins on the transient impairment of endothelium-dependent brachial artery vasoactivity following a single high-fat meal. JAMA. 1997;278(20):1682-86.
67. Plotnick GD, Corretti MC, Vogel RA, et al. Effect of supplemental phytonutrients on impairment of the flow-mediated brachial artery vasoactivity after a single high-fat meal. J Am Coll Cardiol. 2003;41(10):1744-49.
68. Ling L, Zhao SP, Gao M. Vitamin C preserves endothelial function in patients with coronary heart disease after a high-fat meal. Clin Cardiol. 2002;25(5):219-24.
69. Gromadzinska J, Sklodowska M. Erythrocyte glutathione peroxidase and myocardial infaraction. JAMA. 1990;263(7):949-50.
70. Sarkar J, Gangopadhyay NN, Moldoveanu Z, et al. Vitamin A is required for regulation of polymeric immunoglobulin receptor (plgR) expression by interleukin-4 and interferon-γ in a human intestinal epithelial cell line. J Nutr. 1998;128:1063-69.
71. Guidoboni M, Zancai P, Cariati R, et al. Retinoic acid inhibits the proliferative response induced by CD40 activation and interleukin-4 in mantle cell lymphoma. Cancer Res. 2005;65(2):587-95.
72. Fang H, Jin H, Wang H. Effect of all-trans retinoic acid on airway inflammation in asthmatic rats and its mechanism. J Huazhong Univ Sci Technolog Med Sci. 2004;24(3):229-32.
73. Aoudjit F, Bosse M, Stratowa C, et al. Regulation of intercellular adhesion molecule-1 expression by retinoic acid: analysis of the 5′ regulatory region of the gene. Int J Cancer. 1994;58(4):543-49.
74. Choi WH, Ji KA, Jeon SB, et al. Anti-inflammatory roles of retinoic acid in rat brain astrocytes: suppression of interferon-gamma-induced JAK/STAT phosphorylation. Biochem Biophys Res Commun. 2005;329(1):125-31.
75. Strumia R. Dermatologic signs in patients with eating disorders. Am J Clin Dermatol. 2005;6(3):165-73.
76. Lee RG, Rains TM, Tovar-Palacio C, et al. Zinc deficiency increases hypothalamic neuropeptide Y and neuropeptide Y mRNA levels and does not block neuropeptide Y-induced feeding in rats. J Nutr. 1998;128:1218-23.
77. Yoshizawa K, Willett WC, Morris SJ, et al. Study of prediagnostic selenium level in toenails and the risk of advanced prostate cancer. J Natl Cancer Inst. 1998;90(16):1219-29.
78. Satia JA, King IB, Morris JS, et al. Toenail and plasma levels as biomarkers of selenium exposure. Ann Epidemiol. 2005;Jun 14;[Epub ahead of print].
79. Clark LC, Combs GF, Turnbull BW, et al. Effects of selenium supplementation for cancer prevention in patients with carcinoma of the skin. JAMA. 1996;276(24):1957-63.
80. Fujimoto N, Chang C, Nomura M, et al. Can we prevent prostate cancer? Rationale and current status of prostate cancer chemoprevention. Urol Int. 2005;74(4):289-97.
81. Zachara BA, Szewczyk-Golec K, Tyloch J, et al. Blood and tissue selenium concentrations and glutathione peroxidase activities in patients with prostate cancer and benign prostate hyperplasia. Neoplasma. 2005;52(3):248-54.
82. Lee SO, Nadiminty N, Wu XX, et al. Selenium disrupts estrogen signaling by altering estrogen receptor expression and ligand binding in human breast cancer cells. Cancer Res. 2005;65(8):3487-92.
83. Nuttall SL, Martin U, Sinclair AJ, MJ Kendall. Glutathione: in sickness and in health. Lancet. 1998;351:645-46.
84. Beckett GJ, Arthur JR. Selenium and endocrine systems. J Endocrinol. 2005;184:455-65.
85. Mancardi D, Ridnour LA, Thomas DD, et al. The chemical dynamics of NO and reactive nitrogen oxides: a practical guide. Curr Mol Med. 2004;4(7):723-40.
86. Wink DA, Vodovotz Y, Laval J, et al. The multifaceted roles of nitric oxide in cancer. Carcinogenesis. 1998;19(5):711-21.
87. Murad F. Signal transduction using nitric oxide and cyclic guanosine monophosphate. JAMA. 1996;276(14):1189-92.
88. Downey JM. The cellular mechanisms of ischeamic and pharmacological preconditioning. Cardiovasc J S Afr. 2004;15(4 Suppl 1):S3.
89. Boje KM. Nitric oxide neurotoxicity in neurodegenerative diseases. Front Biosci. 2004;9:763-76.
90. Pocernich CB, Boyd-Kimball D, Poon HF, et al. Proteomics analysis of human astrocytes expressing the HIV protein Tat. Brain Res Mol Brain Res. 2005;133(2):307-16.
91. Bulut AS, Erden E, Sak SD, et al. Significance of inducible nitric oxide synthase expression in benign and malignant breast epithelium: an immunohistochemical study of 151 cases. Virchows Arch. 2005;June 10:[Epub ahead of print].
92. Yao JK, Leonard S, Reddy RD. Increased nitric oxide radicals in postmortem brain from patients with schizophrenia. Schizophr Bull. 2004;30(4):923-34.
93. Suschek CV, Schnorr O, Kolb-Bachofen V. The role of iNOS in chronic inflammatory processes *in vivo*: is it damage-promoting, protective, or active at all? Curr Mol Med. 2004;4(7):763-75.
94. Hofseth LJ, Saito S, Hussain SP, et al. Nitric oxide-induced cellular stress and p53 activation in chronic inflammation. Proc Natl Acad Sci U S A. 2003;100(1):143-48.
95. Huang B, Zhao J, Li H, et al. Toll-like receptors on tumor cells facilitate evasion of immune surveillance. Cancer Res. 2005;65(12):5009-14.
96. Wink DA, Vodovotz Y, Laval J, et al. The multi-faceted roles of nitric oxide in cancer. Carcinogenesis. 1998;19(5):711-21.
97. Bolad I, Delafontaine P. Endothelial dysfunction: its role in hypertensive coronary disease. Curr Opin Cardiol. 2005;20(4):270-74.
98. Garhofer G, Resch H, Lung S, et al. Intravenous administration of L-arginine increases retinal and choroidal blood flow. Am J Ophthalmol. 2005;Jun 11;[Epub ahead of print].
99. Fu TL, Zhang WT, Chen QP, et al. Effects of L-arginine on serum nitric oxide, nitric oxide synthase and mucosal Na(+)-K(+)-ATPase and nitric oxide synthase activity in segmental small-bowel autotransplantation model. World J Gastroenterol. 2005;11(23):3605-09.
100. Hoshida S, Nishida M, Yamashita N, et al. Amelioration of severity of myocardial injury by a nitric oxide donor in rabbits fed a cholesterol-rich diet. J Am Coll Cardiol. 1996;27(4):902-.
101. Gauthier TW, Scalia R, Murohara T, et al. Nitric oxide protects against leukocyte-endothelium interactions in the early stages of hypercholesterolemia. Arterioscler Thromb Vasc Biol. 1995;15(10):1652-59.
102. Engelman DT, Watanabe M, Maulik N, et al. L-arginine reduces endothelial inflammation and myocardial stunning during ischemia/reperfusion. Ann Thorac Surg. 1995;60:1275-81.
103. Lerman A, Burnett JC Jr., Higano ST, et al. Long-term L-arginine supplementation improves small-vessel coronary endothelial function in humans. Circulation. 1998;97:2123-28.
104. Sakaghuchi Y, Shirahase H, Ichikawa A, et al. Effects of selective iNOS inhibition on type II collagen-induced arthritis in mice. Life Sci. 2004;75(19):2257-67.
105. Cai Y, Chen T, Xu Q. Astilbin suppresses collagen-induced arthritis via the dysfunction of lymphocytes. Inflamm Res. 2003;52(8):334-40.
106. Kawamoto EM, Munhoz CD, Glezer I, et al. Oxidative state in platelets and erythrocytes in aging and Alzheimer's disease. Neurobiol Aging. 2005;26(6):857-64.

107. Dixon LJ, Hughes SM, Rooney K, et al. Increased superoxide production in hypertensive patients with diabetes mellitus: role of nitric oxide synthase. Am J Hypertens. 2005;18(6):839-43.
108. Brown MR. Peptide biology: past, present, and future. Ann N Y Acad Sci. 1990;579:8-16.
109. Kastin AJ, Banks WA, Zadina JE. A decade of changing perceptions about neuropeptides. Ann N Y Acad Sci. 1990;579:1-7.
110. Guidi L, Tricerri A, Vangeli M, et al. Neuropeptide Y plasma levels and immunological changes during academic stress. Neuropsychobiology. 1999;40(4):188-95.
111. Ho WZ, Evans DL, Douglas SD. Substance P and human immunodeficiency virus infection: psychoneuroimmunology. CNS Spectr. 2002;7(12):867-74.
112. Scott FW, Cui J, Rowsell P. Food and the development of autoimmune disease. Trends Food Sci Technol. 1994;5:111-16.
113. Trompette A, Clauste J, Caillon F, et al. Milk bioactive peptides and beta-casomorphins induce mucus release in rat jejenum. J Nutr. 2003;133(11):3499-503.
114. Sun Z, Cade R. Findings in normal rats following administration of gliadorphin-7 (GD-7). Peptides. 2003;24(2):321-23.
115. Pert CB, Ruff MR, Weber RJ, et al. Neuropeptides and their receptors: a psychosomatic network. J Immunol. 1985;135(2 Suppl):820s-26s.
116. Pert CB, Dreher HE, Ruff MR. The psychosomatic network: foundations of mind-body medicine. Altern Ther Health Med. 1998;4(4):30-41.
117. Ember LR. Surviving stress. Chem & Eng News. 1998;76(21):12-24.
118. Joffe H, Cohen LS. Estrogen, serotonin, and mood disturance: where is the therapeutic bridge? Biol Psychiatry. 1998;44:798-811.
119. Ultra-low dose estrogen patch improves bone, appears safe for the uterus. Harv Womens Health Watch. 2005;12:6-7.
120. Gambacciani M, Vacca F. Postmenopausal osteoporosis and hormone replacement therapy. Minerva Med. 2004;95:507-20.
121. Joseph C, Kenny AM, Taxel P, et al. Role of endocrine-immune dysregulation in osteoporosis, sarcopenia, frailty and fracture risk. Mol Aspects Med. 2005;26:181-201.
122. Bai C, Schmidt A, Freedman LP. Steroid hormone receptors and drug discovery: therapeutic opportunities and assay designs. Assay Drug Dev Technol. 2003;1:843-52.
123. Edwards DP. The role of coactivators and corepressors in the biology and mechanism of action of steroid hormone receptors. J Mammary Gland Biol Neoplasia. 2000;5:307-24.
124. Norman AW, Mizwicki MT, Norman DP. Steroid-hormone rapid actions, membrane receptors and a conformational ensemble model. Nat Rev Drug Discov. 2004;3:27-41.
125. Friesema EC, Jansen J, Milici C, et al. Thyroid hormone transporters. Vitam Horm. 2005;70:137-67.
126. Berkenstam A, Gustafsson JA. Nuclear receptors and their relevance to diseases related to lipid metabolism. Curr Opin Pharmacol. 2005;5:171-76.
127. Jacobs MN, Lewis DF. Steroid hormone receptors and dietary ligands: a selected review. Proc Nutr Soc. 2002;61:105-22.
128. Blaustein JD. Minireview: Neuronal steroid hormone receptors: they're not just for hormones anymore. Endocrinology. 2004;145:1075-81.
129. Lange CA. Making sense of cross-talk between steroid hormone receptors and intracellular signaling pathways: who will have the last word? Mol Endocrinol. 2004;18:269-78.
130. Mariotti S, Sansoni P, Barbesino G, et al. Thyroid and other organ-specific autoantibodies in healthy centenarians. Lancet. 1992;339:1506-8.
131. Rose MR, Mueller LD, Long AD. Pharmacology, genomics, and the evolutionary biology of ageing. Free Radic Res. 2002;36:1293-97.
132. Rozendaal FP. [Thyreotoxicosis in the elderly: aspecific signs may cause a delay in diagnosis.] Tijdschr Gerontol Geriatr. 2005;36:77-80.
133. Rehman SU, Cope DW, Senseney AD, et al. Thyroid disorders in elderly patients. South Med J. 2005;98:543-49.
134. Rozendaal FP. [Thyreotoxicosis in the elderly: aspecific signs may cause a delay in diagnosis.] Tijdschr Gerontol Geriatr. 2005;36:77-80.
135. Kvetny J. Subclinical hyperthyroidism in patients with nodular goiter represents a hypermetabolic state. Exp Clin Endocrinol Diabetes. 2005;113:122-26.
136. van Boxtel MP, Menheere PP, Bekers O, et al. Thyroid function, depressed mood, and cognitive performance in older individuals: the Maastricht Aging Study. Psychoneuroendocrinology. 2004;29:891-98.
137. Rizzo MR, Mari D, Barbieri M, et al. Resting metabolic rate and respiratory quotient in human longevity. J Clin Endocrinol Metab. 2005;90:409-13.
138. Mariotti S, Sansoni P, Barbesino G, et al. Thyroid and other organ-specific autoantibodies in healthy centenarians. Lancet. 1992;339:1506-8.
139. Hsu HC, Scott DK. Mountz JD. Impaired apoptosis and immune senescence—cause or effect? Immunol Rev. 2005;205:130-46.
140. Chang CC, Huang CN, Chuang LM. Autoantibodies to thyroid peroxidase in patients with type 1 diabetes in Taiwan. Eur J Endocrinol. 1998;139:44-48.
141. Andersen-Ranberg K, HOier-Madsen M, Wiik A, et al. High prevalence of autoantibodies among Danish centenarians. Clin Exp Immunol. 2004;138:158-63.
142. Cooper DS. Subclinical hypothyroidism. N Engl J Med. 2001;345:260-65.
143. Surks MI, Ortiz E, Daniels GH, Sawin CT, et al. Subclinical thyroid disease: scientific review and guidelines for diagnosis and management. JAMA. 2004; 291:228-38.
144. Gharib H, Tuttle RM, Baskin HJ, et al. Subclinical thyroid dysfunction: a joint statement on management from the American Association of Clinical Endocrinologists, the American Thyroid Association, and the Endocrine Society. J Clin Endocrinol Metab. 2005;90:581-85.
145. Pollock MA, Sturrock A, Marshall K, et al. Thyroxine treatment in patients with symptoms of hypothyroidism but thyroid function tests within the reference range: randomized double blind placebo controlled crossover trial. BMJ. 2001;323:891-95.
146. Parle JV, Maisonneuve P, Sheppard MC, et al. Prediction of all-cause and cardiovascular mortality in elderly people from one low serum thyrotropin result: a 10-year cohort study. Lancet. 2001;358:861-65.
147. Krunzel TA. Thyroid function testing: dealing with interpretation difficulties. J Naturopathic Med. 2001;1:1-9.
148. Fatourechi V. Subclinical hypothyroidism: how should it be managed? Treat Endocrinol. 2002;1:211-16.
149. Diez JJ, Iglesias P, Burman KD. Spontaneous normalization of thyrotropin concentrations in patients with subclinical hypothyroidism. J Clin Endocrinol Metab. 2005 Apr 5; [Epub ahead of print].
150. Wardle CA, Fraser WD, Squire CR. Pitfalls in the use of thyrotropin concentration as a first-line thyroid-function test. Lancet. 2001;357:1013-14.
151. Basier WV, Hertoghe J, Eeckhaut W. Thyroid insufficiency. Is TSH measurement the only diagnostic tool? J Nutr Environ Med. 2000;10:105-13.
152. Zoncu S, Pigliaru F, Putzu C, et al. Cardiac function in borderline hypothyroidism: a study by pulsed wave tissue Doppler imaging. Eur J Endocrinol. 2005;152:527-33.

153. Hamano K, Inoue M. Increased risk for atherosclerosis estimated by pulse wave velocity in hypothyroidism and its reversal with appropriate thyroxine treatment. Endocr J. 2005;52:95-101.
154. Downing D. Hypothyroidism: treating the patient not the laboratory. J Nutr Environmental Med. 2000;10:101-3.
155. Gullu S, Sav H, Kamel N. Effects of levothyroxine treatment on bio chemical and hemostasis parameters in patients with hypothyroidism. Eur J Endocrinol. 2005;152:355-61.
156. Marongiu F, Cauli C, Mariotti S. Thyroid, hemostasis and thrombosis. J Endocrinol Invest. 2004;27:1065-71.
157. Soni S, Singh G, Yasir S, et al. An unusual presentation of hypothyroidism. Thyroid. 2005;15:289-91.
158. Lindsay RS, Toft AD. Hypothyroidism. Lancet 1997;349:413-17.
159. Nygaard B. Primary hypothyroidism. Clin Evid. 2003;(10):715-20.
160. Adlin V. Subclinical hypothyroidism: deciding when to treat. Am Fam Physician. 1998;57:776-80.
161. Serter R, Demirbas B, Kirukluoglu B, et al. The effect of L-thyroxine replacement therapy on lipid based cardiovascular risk in subclinical hypothyroidism. J Endocrinol Invest. 2004;27:897-903.
162. Galesanu C, Lisnic N, Teslaru R, et al. [Lipids profile in a group of hypothyroid patients vs. treated hypothyroid patients.] Rev Med Chir Soc Med Nat Iasi. 2004;108:554-60.
163. Ingenbleek Y, Bernstein L. The stressful condition as a nutritionally dependent adaptive dichotomy. Nutrition. 1999;15:305-20.
164. Riedel W, Layka H, Neeck G. Secretory pattern of GH, TSH, thyroid hormones, ACTH, cortisol, FSH, and LH in patients with fibromyalgia syndrome following systemic injection of the relevant hypothalamic-releasing hormones. Z Rheumatol. 1998;57(Suppl 2):81-87.
165. Vantyghern MC, Ghularn A, Hober C, et al. Urinary cortisol metabolites in the assessment of peripheral thyroid hormone action: overt and subclinical hypothyroidism. J Endocrinol Invest. 1998;21:219-25.
166. Riedel W, Layka H, Neeck G. Secretory pattern of GH, TSH, thyroid hormones, ACTH, cortisol, FSH, and LH in patients with fibromyalgia syndrome following systemic injection of the relevant hypothalamic-releasing hormones. Z Rheumatol. 1998;57(Suppl 2):81-87.
167. Monzani F, Caraccio N, Del Guerra P, et al. Neuromuscular symptoms and dysfunction in subclinical hypothyroid patients: beneficial effect of LT4 replacement therapy. Clin Endocrinol (Oxf). 1999;51:237-42.
168. Baumgartner A, Campos-Barros A, Meinhold H. Thyroid hormones and depressive illness: implications for clinical and basic research. Acta Med Austriaca. 1992;19(Suppl 1):98-102.
169. Chan S, Kilby MD. Thyroid hormone and central nervous system development. J Endocrinol. 2000;165:1-8.
170. Strait KA, Carlson DJ, Schwartz HL, et al. Transient stimulation of myelin basic protein gene expression in differentiating cultured oligodendrocytes: a model for 3,5,3'-triiodothyronine-induced brain development. Endocrinology. 1997;138:635-41.
171. Stoewsand GS. Bioactive organosulfur phytochemicals in Brassica oleracea vegetables—a review. Food Chem Toxicol. 1995;33:537-43.
172. Farrar GE Jr. Goiter, iodine, and cabbage. Clin Ther. 1990;12:191-92.
173. McMillan M, Spinks EA, Fenwick GR. Preliminary observations on the effect of dietary brussels sprouts on thyroid function. Hum Toxicol. 1986;5:15-19.
174. de Groot AP, Willems MI, de Vos RH. Effects of high levels of brussels sprouts in the diet of rats. Food Chem Toxicol. 1991;29:829-37.
175. Sterling K. Thyroid hormone action at the cell level. N Engl J Med. 1979;300:117-23.
176. Brent GA. The molecular basis of thyroid hormone action. N Engl J Med. 1994;331:847-53.
177. Zhang J, Lazar MA. The mechanism of action of thyroid hormones. Annu Rev Physiol. 2000;62:439-66.
178. Kelly G. Peripheral metabolism of thyroid hormones: a review. Altern Med Rev. 2000;5:306-33.
179. Kohrle J. Local activation and inactivation of thyroid hormones: the deiodinase family. Mol Cell Endocrinol. 1999;151:103-19.
180. Kohrle J. Thyroid hormone deiodinases-a selenoenzyme family acting as gate keepers to thyroid hormone action. Acta Med Austriaca. 1996;23:17-30.
181. Divi RL, Chang HC, Doerge DR. Anti-thyroid isoflavones from soybean: isolation, characterization, and mechanisms of action. Biochem Pharmacol. 1997;54:1087-96.
182. Chang HC, Doerge DR. Dietary genistein inactivates rat thyroid peroxidase *in vivo* without an apparent hypothyroid effect. Toxicol Appl Pharmacol. 2000;168(3):244-52.
183. Ishizuki Y, Hirooka Y, Murata Y, Togashi K. [The effects on the thyroid gland of soybeans administered experimentally in healthy subjects.] Nippon Naibunpi Gakkai Zasshi. 1991;67:622-29.
184. Jabbar MA, Larrea J, Shaw RA. Abnormal thyroid function tests in infants with congenital hypothyroidism: the influence of soy-based formula. J Am Coll Nutr. 1997;16(3):280-82.
185. Bell DS, Ovalle F. Use of soy protein supplement and resultant need for increased dose of levothyroxine. Endocr Pract. 2001;7:193-94.
186. Chorazy PA, Himelhoch S, Hopwood NJ, et al. Persistent hypothyroidism in an infant receiving a soy formula: case report and review of the literature. Pediatrics. 1995;96:148-50.
187. Bruce B, Messina M, Spiller GA. Isoflavone supplements do not affect thyroid function in iodine-replete postmenopausal women. J Med Food. 2003;6:309-16.
188. van der Heide D, Kastelijn J, Schroder-van der Elst JP. Flavonoids and thyroid disease. Biofactors. 2003;19:113-19.
189. Schroder-van der Elst JP, van der Heide D, Romijn JA, et al. Differential effects of natural flavonoids on growth and iodide content in a human Na*/I-symporter-transfected follicular thyroid carcinoma cell line. Eur J Endocrinol. 2004;150:557-64.
190. Kohrle J, Spanka M, Irmscher K, Hesch RD. Flavonoid effects on transport, metabolism and action of thyroid hormones. Prog Clin Biol Res. 1988;280:323-40.
191. Divi RL, Doerge DR. Inhibition of thyroid peroxidase by dietary flavonoids. Chem Res Toxicol. 1996;9:16-23.
192. Benvenga S, Ruggeri RM, Russo A, et al. Usefulness of L-carnitine, a naturally occurring peripheral antagonist of thyroid hormone action, in iatrogenic hyperthyroidism: a randomized, double-blind, placebo-controlled clinical trial. J Clin Endocrinol Metab. 2001;86:3579-94.
193. Benvenga S, Lakshmanan M, Trimarchi F. Carnitine is a naturally occurring inhibitor of thyroid hormone nuclear uptake. Thyroid. 2000;10:1043-50.
194. Friesema EC, Jansen J, Visser TJ. Thyroid hormone transporters. Biochem Soc Trans. 2005;33:228-32.
195. Safer JD, Cohen RN, Hollenberg N, et al. Defective release of corepressor by hinge mutants of the thyroid hormone receptor found in patients with resistance to thyroid hormone. J Biol Chem. 1998;273:30175-82.
196. Gurnell M, Rajanayagam O, Barbar I, et al. Reversible pituitary enlargement in the syndrome of resistance to thyroid hormone. Thyroid. 1998;8:679-82.
197. Kaneshige M, Kaneshige K, Zhu X, et al. Mice with a targeted mutation in the thyroid hormone β receptor gene exhibit impaired growth and resistance to thyroid hormone. Proc Natl Acad Sci U S A. 2000;97:13209-14.
198. Williams GR, Franklyn JA, Neuberger JM. Thyroid hormone receptor expression in the "sick euthyroid syndrome." Lancet. 1989;2(8678-8679):1477-81.

199. Lazar MA. Thyroid hormone receptors: multiple forms, multiple possibilities. Endocr Rev. 1993;14:184-93.
200. Amma LL, Campos-Barros A, Wang Z, et al. Distinct tissue-specific roles for thyroid hormone receptors β and αl in regulation of type 1 deiodinase expression. Mol Endocrinol. 2001;15:467-75.
201. Morel G, Ricard-Blum S, Ardail D. Kinetics of internalization and subcellular binding sites for T3 in mouse liver. Biol Cell. 1996;86:167-74.
202. Yang YZ, Burgos-Trinidad M, Wu Y, et al. Thyroid hormone receptor variant α2. J Biol Chem. 1996;271:28235-42.
203. Abel ED, Boers ME, Pazos-Moura C, et al. Divergent roles for thyroid hormone receptor β isoforms in the endocrine axis and auditory system. J Clin Invest. 1999;104:291-300.
204. Zhang CY, Kim S, Harney JW, et al. Further characterization of thyroid hormone response elements in the human type 1 iodothyronine deiodinase gene. Endocrinology. 1998;139:1156-63.
205. Qi JS, Desai-Yajnik V, Greene ME, et al. The ligand-binding domains of the thyroid hormone/retinoid receptor gene subfamily function *in vivo* to mediate heterodimerization, gene silencing, and transactivation. Mol Cell Biol. 1995;15:1817-25.
206. Toyoda N, Zavacki AM, Maia AL, et al. A novel retinoid X receptor-independent thyroid hormone response element is present in the human type I deiodinase gene. Mol Cell Biol. 1995;15:5100-12.
207. Wong CW, Privalsky ML. Transcriptional silencing is defined by isoform- and heterodimer-specific interactions between nuclear hormone receptors and corepressors. Mol Cell Biol. 1998;18:5724-33.
208. Kitamura S, Kato T, Iida M, et al. Anti-thyroid hormonal activity of tetrabromobisphenol A, a flame retardant, and related compounds: affinity to the mammalian thyroid hormone receptor, and effect on tadpole metamorphosis. Life Sci. 2005;76:1589-1601.
209. Tagami T, Park Y, Jameson JL. Mechanisms that mediate negative regulation of the thyroid-stimulating hormone α gene by the thyroid hormone receptor. J Biol Chem. 1999;274:22345-53.
210. Wu Y, Xu B, Koenig RJ. Thyroid hormone response element sequence and the recruitment of retinoid X receptors for thyroid hormone responsiveness. J Biol Chem. 2001;276:3929-36.
211. Lee SK. Lee B, Lee JW. Mutations in retinoid X receptor that impair heterodimerization with specific nuclear hormone receptor. J Biol Chem. 2000;275:33522-26.
212. Haluzik MM, Haluzik M. PPAR-alpha and insulin sensitivity. Physiol Res. 2005;May 24;[Epub ahead of print].
213. Hertz R, Nikodern V, Ben-Ishai A, et al. Thyromimetic mode of action of peroxisome proliferators: activation of 'malic' enzyme gene transcription. Biochem J. 1996;319:241-48.
214. Enderlin V, Alfos S, Pallet V., et al. Aging decreases the abundance of retinoic acid (RAR) and triiodothyronine (TR) nuclear receptor mRNA in rat brain: effect of the administration of retinoids. FEBS Lett. 1997;412:629-32.
215. Feart C, Pallet V, Boucheron C, et al. Aging affects the retinoic acid and the triiodothyronine nuclear receptor mRNA expression in human peripheral blood mononuclear cells. Eur J Endocrinol. 2005;152:449-58.
216. Pallet V, Azais-Braesco V, Enderlin V, et al. Aging decreases retinoic acid and triiodothyronine nuclear expression in rat liver: exogenous retinol and retinoic acid differentially modulate this decreased expression. Mech Ageing Dev. 1997;99:123-36.
217. Hayden LJ, Hawk SN, Sih TR, et al. Metabolic conversion of retinol to retinoic acid mediates the biological responsiveness of human mammary epithelial cells to retinol. J Cell Physiol. 2001;186:437-47.
218. Kurlandsky SB, Xiao JH, Duell EA, et al. Biological activity of all-trans retinol requires metabolic conversion to all-trans retinoic acid and is mediated through activation of nuclear retinoid receptors in human keratinocytes. J Biol Chem. 1994;269:32821-27.
219. Wang XD, Krinsky NI, Benotti PN, et al. Biosynthesis of 9-cis-retinoic acid from 9-cis-beta-carotene in human intestinal mucosa *in vitro*. Arch Biochem Biophys. 1994;313:150-55.
220. Limpach A, Dalton M, Miles R, Gadson P. Homocysteine inhibits retinoic acid synthesis: a mechanism for homocysteine-induced congenital defects. Exp Cell Res. 2000;260:166-74.
221. Chen H, Namkung MJ, Juchau MR. Effects of ethanol on biotransformation of all-trans- retinol and all-trans-retinal to all-trans-retinoic acid in rat conceptual cytosol. Alcohol Clin Exp Res. 1996;20:942-47.
222. Dauncey MJ, White P, Burton KA, et al. Nutrition-hormone receptor-gene interactions: implications for development and disease. Proc Nutr Soc. 2001;60:63-72.
223. Casas F, Pineau T, Rochard P, et al. New molecular aspects of regulation of mitochondrial activity by fenofibrate and fasting. FEBS Lett. 2000;482:71-74.
224. Goglia F. Biological effects of 3,5-diiodothyronine (T(2)). Biochemistry (Mosc). 2005;70:164-72.
225. Lanni A, Moreno M, Horst C, et al. Specific binding sites for 3,3'-diiodo-L-thyronine (3,3'-T2) in rat liver mitochondria. FEBS Lett. 1994;351:237-40.
226. Wrutniak-Cabello C, Casas F, Cabello G. Thyroid hormone action in mitochondria. J Mol Endocrinol. 2001;26:67-77.
227. Videla LA. Energy metabolism, thyroid calorigenesis, and oxidative stress: functional and cytotoxic consequences. Redox Rep. 2000;5(5):265-75.
228. Horrum MA, Tobin RB, Ecklund RE. Effects of 3,3',5-triiodo-L-thyronine (L-T3) and T3 analogues on mitochondrial function. Biochem Mol Biol Int. 1995;35:913-21.
229. Goglia F, Lanni A, Barth J, et al. Interaction of diiodothyronines with isolated cytochrome c oxidase. FEBS Lett. 1994;346:295-98.
230. Sterling K, Brenner MA, Sakurada T. Rapid effect of triiodothyronine on the mitochondrial pathway in rat liver *in vivo*. Science. 1980;210:340-42.
231. Mutvei A, Husman B, Andersson G, et al. Thyroid hormone and not growth hormone is the principle regulator of mammalian mitochondrial biogenesis. Acta Endocrinol (Copenh). 1989;121:223-28.
232. Pillar TM, Seitz HJ. Thyroid hormone and gene expression in the regulation of mitochondrial respiratory function. Eur J Endocrinol. 1997;136:231-39.
233. Goglia F, Moreno M, Lanni A. Action of thyroid hormones at the cellular level: the mitochondrial target. FEBS Lett. 1999;452:115-20.
234. Enríquez JA, Fernández-Silva P, Garrido-Pérez N, et al. Direct regulation of mitochondrial RNA synthesis by thyroid hormone. Mol Cell Biol. 1999;19(l):657-70.
235. Guerra C, Roncero C, Porras A, et al. Triiodothyronine induces the transcription of the uncoupling protein gene and stabilizes its mRNA in fetal rat brown adipocyte primary cultures. J Biol Chem. 1996;271:2076-81.
236. Lanni A, De Felice M, Lombardi A, et al. Induction of UCP2 mRNA by thyroid hormones in rat heart. FEBS Lett. 1997;418:171-74.
237. Lanni A, Beneduce L, Lombardi A, et al. Expression of uncoupling protein-3 and mitochondrial activity in the transition from hypothyroid to hyperthyroid state in rat skeletal muscle. FEBS Lett. 1999;444:250-54.

238. Prummel MF, Wiersinga WM. Thyroid peroxidase autoantibodies in euthyroid subjects. Best Pract Res Clin Endocrinol Metab. 2005;19:1-15.
239. Bonar BD, McColgan B, Smith DF, et al. Hypothroidism and aging: the Rosses' survey. Thyroid. 2000;10:821-27.
240. Canaris GJ, Manowitz NR, Mayor G, et. al. The Colorado thyroid disease prevalence study. Arch Intern Med. 2000;160:526-34.
241. Rooney S, Walsh E. Prevalence of abnormal thyroid function tests in a Down's syndrome population. Ir J Med Sci. 1997;166:80-82.
242. Kanavin OJ, Aaseth J, Birketvedt GS. Thyroid hypofunction in Down's syndrome: is it related to oxidative stress? Biol Trace Elem Res. 2000;78:35-42.
243. Karlsson B, Gustafsson J, Hedov G, et al. Thyroid dysfunction in Down's syndrome: relation to age and thyroid autoimmunity. Arch Dis Child. 1998;79:242-45.
244. Ivarsson SA, Ericsson UB, Gustafsson J, et al. The impact of thyroid autoimmunity in children and adolescents with Down syndrome. Acta Paediatr. 1997;86:1065-67.
245. Jaruratanasirikul S, Patarakijvanich N, Patanapisarnsak C. The association of congenital hypothyroidism and congenital gastrointestinal anomalies in Down's syndrome infants. J Pediatr Endocrinol Metab. 1998;11:241-46.
246. Sategna-Guidetti C, Bruno M, Mazza E, et al. Autoimmune thyroid diseases and coeliac disease. Eur J Gastroenterol Hepatol. 1998;10:927-31.
247. Valentino R, Savastano S, Tommaselli AP, et al. Unusual association of thyroiditis, Addison's disease, ovarian failure and celiac disease in a young woman. J Endocrinol Invest. 1999;22:390-94.
248. Cash BD, Schoenfeld P, Chey WD. The utility of diagnostic tests in irritable bowel syndrome patients: a systematic review. Am J Gastroenterol. 2002;97:2812-19.
249. Toscano V, Conti FG, Anastasi E, et al. Importance of gluten in the induction of endocrine autoantibodies and organ dysfunction in adolescent celiac patients. Am J Gastroenterol. 2000;95(7):1742-48.
250. Velluzzi F, Caradonna A, Boy MF, et al. Thyroid and celiac disease: clinical, serological, and echographic study. Am J Gastroenterol. 1998;93:976-79.
251. Ventura A, Neri E, Ughi C, et al. Gluten-dependent diabetes-related and thyroid-related autoantibodies in patients with celiac disease. J Pediatr. 2000;137:263-65.
252. Freeman HJ. T cell lymphoma of the thyroid gland in celiac disease. Can J Gastroenterol. 2000;14:635-36.
253. Licastro F, Mariani RA, Faldella G, et al. Immune-endocrine status and coeliac disease in children with Down's syndrome: relationships with zinc and cognitive efficiency. Brain Res Bull. 2001;55:313-17.
254. Sategna-Guidetti C, Volta U, Ciacci C, et al. Prevalence of thyroid disorders in untreated adult celiac disease patients and effect of gluten withdrawal: an Italian multicenter study. Am J Gastroenterol. 2001;96:751-57.
255. Morgan CA 3rd, Wang S, Mason J, et al. Hormone profiles in humans experiencing military survival training. Biol Psychiatry. 2000;47:891-901.
256. Weijl NI, Van Der Harst D, Brand A, et al. Hypothyroidism during immunotherapy with interleukin-2 is associated with antithyroid antibodies and response to treatment. J Clin Oncol. 1993;11:1376-83.
257. Komorowski J. Increased interleukin-2 level in patients with primary hypothyroidism. Clin Immunol Immunopathol. 1992;63:200-202.
258. Drugarin D, Negru S, Koreck A, et al. The pattern of a T(H)1 cytokine in autoimmune thyroiditis. Immunol Lett. 2000;71:73-77.
259. Tuzcu A, Bahceci M, Gokalp D, et al. Subclinical hypothyroidism may be associated with elevated high-sensitive c-reactive protein (low grade inflammation) and fasting hyperinsulinemia. Endocr J. 2005;52:89-94.
260. Cantorna MT. Vitamin D and autoimmunity: is vitamin D status an environmental factor affecting autoimmune disease prevalence? Proc Soc Exp Biol Med. 2000;223:230-33.
261. Lemire J. 1,25-Dihydroxyvitamin D3-a hormone with immunomodulatory properties. Z Rheumatol. 2000;59(Suppl 1):24-27.
262. Smith EA, Frankenburg EP, Goldstein SA, et al. Effects of long-term administration of vitamin D3 analogs to mice. J Endocrinol. 2000;165:163-72.
263. Sustrova M, Strbak V. Thyroid function and plasma immunoglobulins in subjects with Down's syndrome (DS) during ontogenesis and zinc therapy. J Endocrinol Invest. 1994;17:385-90.
264. Licastro F, Mocchegiani E, Zannotti M, et al. Zinc affects the metabolism of thyroid hormones in children with Down's syndrome: normalization of thyroid stimulating hormone and of reversal triiodothyronine plasmic levels of dietary zinc supplementation. Int J Neurosci. 1992;65:259-68.
265. Napolitano G, Palka G, Lio S, et al. Is zinc deficiency a cause of subclinical hypothyroidism in Down syndrome? Ann Genet. 1990;33:9-15.
266. Nishiyama S, Futagoishi-Suginohara Y, Matsukura M, et al. Zinc supplementation alters thyroid hormone metabolism in disabled patients with zinc deficiency. J Am Coll Nutr. 1994;13:62-67.
267. Olivieri O, Girelli D, Stanzial AM, et al. Selenium, zinc, and thyroid hormones in healthy subjects: low T3/T4 ratio in the elderly is related to impaired selenium status. Biol Trace Elem Res. 1996;51:31-41.
268. Porterfield SP. Vulnerability of the developing brain to thyroid abnormalities: environmental insults to the thyroid system. Environ Health Perspect. 1994;102(Suppl 2):125-30.
269. Porterfield SP. Thyroidal dysfunction and environmental chemicals-potential impact on brain development. Environ Health Perspect. 2000;108(Suppl 3):433-38.
270. Cheek AO, Kow K, Chen J, et al. Potential mechanisms of thyroid disruption in humans: interaction of organochlorine compounds with thyroid receptor, transthyretin, and thyroid-binding globulin. Environ Health Perspect. 1999;107:27378.
271. Gaitan JE, Wahner HW, Gorman CA, et al. Measurement of triiodothyronine in unextracted urine. J Lab Clin Med. 1975;86:538-46.
272. Gaitan E. Goitrogens. Baillieres Clin Endocrinol Metab. 1988;2:683-702.
273. Capen CC. Mechanisms of chemical injury of thyroid gland. Prog Clin Biol Res. 1994;387:173-91.
274. Hauser P, McMillin JM, Bhatara VS. Resistance to thyroid hormone: implications for neurodevelopmental research on the effects of thyroid hormone disruptors. Toxicol Ind Health. 1998;14:85-101.
275. McKinney JD, Pedersen LG. Do residue levels of polychlorinated biphenyls (PCBs) in human blood produce mild hypothyroidism? J Theor Biol. 1987;129:231-41.
276. Brucker-Davis F. Effects of environmental synthetic chemicals on thyroid function. Thyroid. 1998;8:827-56.
277. Klein I, Ojamaa K. Thyroid hormone and the cardiovascular system. N Engl J Med. 2001;344:501-9.
278. Hendriks H. [The presence of iodine in fucus and the thyroid gland.] Pharm Weekbl. 1972;107:565-73.
279. Phaneuf D, Cote I, Dumas P, et al. Evaluation of the contamination of marine algae (seaweed) from the St. Lawrence River and likely to be consumed by humans. Environ Res. 1999;80:S175-82.

280. Danilenko M, Wang X, Studzinski GP. Carnosic acid and promotion of monocytic differentiation of HL60-G cells initiated by other agents. J Natl Cancer Inst. 2001;93:1224-33.
281. Aruoma OI, Halliwell B, Aeschbach R, et al. Antioxidant and pro-oxidant properties of active rosemary constituents: carnosol and carnosic acid. Xenobiotica. 1992;22:257-68.
282. Zhu Z, Kumura M, Itokawa Y. Iodothyronine deiodinase activity in methionine deficient rats fed selenium-deficient or selenium- sufficient diets. Biol Trace Elem Res. 1995;48:197-213.
283. Mutaku JF, Many MC, Colin I, et al. Antigoitrogenic effect of combined supplementation with dl-alpha-tocopherol, ascorbic acid and beta-carotene and of dl-alpha-tocopherol alone in the rat. J Endocrinol. 1998;156(3):551-61.
284. Berger MM, Reymond MJ, Shenkin A, et al. Influence of selenium supplements on the post-traumatic alterations of the thyroid axis: a placebo-controlled trial. Intensive Care Med. 2001;27(l):91-100.
285. Venditti P, Daniele MC, Masullo P, et al. Antioxidant-sensitive triiodothyronine effects on characteristic of rat liver mitochondrial population. Cell Physiol Biochem. 1999;9:38-52.
286. Chaurasia SS, Kar A. Protective effects of vitamin E against lead-induced deterioration of membrane associated type-I iodothyronine 5'-monodeiodinase (5'D-I) activity in male mice. Toxicology. 1997;124:203-9.
287. Meydani SN, Meydani M, Rall LC, et al. Assessment of the safety of high-dose, short-term supplementation with vitamin E in healthy older adults. Am J Clin Nutr. 1994;60:704-9.
288. Peebles ED, Miller EH, Brake JD, et al. Effects of ascorbic acid on plasma thyroxine concentrations and eggshell quality of Leghorn chickens treated with dietary thiouracil. Poult Sci. 1992;71:553-59.
289. Morley JE, Russell RM, Reed A, et al. The interrelationship of thyroid hormones with vitamin A and zinc nutritional status in patients with chronic hepatic and gastrointestinal disorders. Am J Clin Nutr. 1981;34:1489-95.
290. Pallet V, Azais-Braesco V, Enderlin V, et al. Aging decreases retinoic acid and triiodothyronine nuclear expression in rat liver: exogenous retinol and retinoic acid differentially modulate this decreased expression. Mech Ageing Dev. 1997;99:123-36.
291. Enderlin V, Alfos S, Pallet V, et al. Aging decreases the abundance of retinoic acid (RAR) and triiodothyronine (TR) nuclear receptor mRNA in rat brain: effect of the administration of retinoids. FEBS Lett. 1997;412:629-32.
292. Ohe K, Ikuyama S, Takayanagi R, et al. Nicotinamide potentiates TSHR and MHC class 11 promoter activity in FRTL-5 cells. Mol Cell Endocrinol. 1999;149:141-51.
293. Falkenstein E, Tillmann HC, Christ M, et al. Multiple actions of steroid hormones-a focus on rapid, nongenomic effects. Pharmacol Rev. 2000;52:513-56.
294. Carlberg C. Mechanisms of nuclear signalling by vitamin D3. Interplay with retinoid and thyroid hormone signalling. Eur J Biochem. 1995;231:517-27.
295. Kroboth PD, Salek FS, Pittenger AL, et al. DHEA and DHEA-S: a review. J Clin Pharmacol. 1999;39:327-48.
296. Ibid.
297. Salek FS, Bigos KL, Kroboth PD. The influence of hormones and pharmaceutical agents on DHEA and DHEA-S concentrations: a review of clinical studies. J Clin Pharmacol. 2002;42(3):247-66.
298. Young J, Couzinet B, Nahoul K, et al. Panhypopituitarism as a model to study the metabolism of dehydroepiandrosterone (DHEA) in humans. J Clin Endocrinol Metab. 1997;82:2578-85.
299. Arlt W, Callies F, van Vlijmen JC, et al. Dehydroepiandrosterone replacement in women with adrenal insufficiency. N Engl J Med. 1999;341:1013-20.
300. Diersen-Schade DA, Cleary MP. No effect of long-term DHEA treatment on either hepatocyte and adipocyte pentose pathway activity or adipocyte glycerol release. Horm Metab Res. 1989;21:356-58.
301. Villareal DT. Effects of dehydroepiandrosterone on bone mineral density: what implications for therapy? Treat Endocrinol. 2002;1:349-57.
302. Wolkowitz OM, Reus VI, Keebler A, et al. Double-blind treatment of major depression with dehydroepiandrosterone. Am J Psychiatry. 1999;156:646-49.
303. Wajnrajch MP. Physiological and pathological growth hormone secretion. J Pediatr Endocrinol Metab. 2005;18:325-38.
304. Davidson P, Milne R, Chase D, et al. Growth hormone replacement in adults and bone mineral density: a systematic review and meta-analysis. Clin Endocrinol (Oxf). 2004;60:92-98.
305. Kann PH. Clinical effects of growth hormone on bone: a review. Aging Male. 2004;7:290-96.
306. Gola M, Bonadonna S, Doga M, et al. Clinical review: Growth hormone and cardiovascular risk factors. J Clin Endocrinol Metab. 2005;90:1864-70.
307. Kann PH. Growth hormone in anti-aging medicine: a critical review. Aging Male. 2003;6:257-63.
308. Lal S, Hart DW, Herndon DN. Challenges of growth hormone therapy: pros. Curr Opin Clin Nutr Metab Care. 2000;3:135-38.
309. Wolfe J. Growth hormone: a physiological fountain of youth? J Anti Aging Med. 1998;1:9-25.
310. Rudman D, Feller AG, Nagraj HS, et al. Effects of human growth hormone in men over 60 years old. N Engl J Med. 1990;323:1-6.
311. Beentjes JA, van Tol A, Sluiter WJ, et al. Effect of growth hormone replacement therapy on plasma lecithin: cholesterol acyltransferase and lipid transfer protein activities in growth hormone-deficient adults. J Lipid Res. 2000;41:925-32.
312. Tanriverdi F, Unluhizarci K, Kula M, et al. Effects of 18-month growth hormone (GH) replacement therapy in patients with Sheehan's syndrome. Growth Horm IGF Res. 2005;15:231-37.
313. Verhelst J, Kendall-Taylor P, Erfurth EM, et al. Baseline characteristics and response to 2 years of growth hormone replacement of hypopituitary patients with growth hormone deficiency due to adult-onset craniopharyngioma in comparison to patients with non-functioning pituitary adenoma: data from KIMS (Pfizer International Metabolic Database). J Clin Endocrinol Metab. 2005;May 31;[Epub ahead of print].
314. Cutfield WS, Wilton P, Bermmarker H, et al. Incidence of diabetes mellitus and impaired glucose tolerance in children and adolescents receiving growth-hormone treatment. Lancet. 2000;355:610-13.
315. Jeffcoate W. Growth hormone therapy and its relationship to insulin resistance, glucose intolerance and diabetes mellitus: a review of recent evidence. Drug Saf. 2002;25:199-212.
316. Bryant J, Loveman E, Chase D, et al. Clinical effectiveness and cost-effectiveness of growth hormone in adults in relation to impact on quality of life: a systematic review and economic evaluation. Health Technol Assess. 2002;6:1-106.
317. Jeffcoate W. Can growth hormone therapy cause diabetes? Lancet. 2000;355:589-90.
318. Maas HCM, de Vries WR, Maitimu I, et al. Growth hormone responses during strenuous exercise: the role of GH-releasing hormone and GH-releasing peptide-2. Med Sci Sports Exerc. 2000;32:1226-32.
319. Wu D, Clarke IJ, Chen C. The role of protein kinase C in GH secretion induced by GH-releasing factor and GH-releasing peptides in cultured ovine somatotrophs. J Endocrinol. 1997;154:219-30.
320. Platz EA, Pollak MN, Leitzmann MF, et al. Plasma insulin-like growth factor-1 and binding protein-3 and subsequent risk of prostate cancer in the PSA era. Cancer Causes Control. 2005;16:255-62.

321. Graham D, McLachlan A. Declining melatonin levels and older people. How old is old? Neuro Endocrinol Lett. 2004;25:415-18.
322. Mazzoccoli G, Carughi S, De Cata A, et al. Melatonin and cortisol serum levels in lung cancer patients at different stages of disease. Med Sci Monit. 2005;11:CR284-88.
323. Sousa SC, Castilho RF. Protective effect of melatonin on rotenone plus Ca(2+)-induced mitochondrial oxidative stress and PC12 cell death. Antioxid Redox Signal. 2005;7(9-10):1110-16.
324. Tomas-Zapico C, Coto-Montes A. A proposed mechanism to explain the stimulatory effect of melatonin on antioxidative enzymes. J Pineal Res. 2005;39(2):99-104.
325. Blackman MR. Age-related alterations in sleep quality and neuroendocrine function: interrelationships and implications. JAMA. 2000;284:879-81.
326. Van Cauter E, Leproult R, Plat L. Age-related changes in slow wave sleep and REM sleep and relationship with growth hormone and cortisol levels in healthy men. JAMA. 2000;284:861-68.
327. Baker SM. The Circadian Prescription. New York, NY; GP Putnam's Sons:2000.
328. Melatonin effective for some sleep disorders. J Fam Pract. 2005;54:493.
329. Wyss JM, vanGroen T, Canning KJ. The limbic system. In: Conn PM (ed). Neuroscience in Medicine. Philadelphia: J Lippincott, 2002; 369-387.
330. Isaacson RL. The limbic system. 2nd ed. New York: Plenum Press, 1982.
331. Wyss JM, vanGroen T, Canning KJ. The limbic system. In Conn PM (ed). Neuroscience in Medicine. Philadelphia: JB Lippincott, 2002;369-387.
332. Ibid.
333. Ibid.
334. Green E, Green A. Beyond Biofeedback. New York: Delta, 1977.
335. Taylor AL, Fishman LM. Corticotropin-releasing hormone. N Engl J Med. 1988;319:213-22.
336. Antoni FA. Hypothalamic control of adrenocorticotropin secretion: advances since the discovery of 41-residue corticotropin-releasing of actor. Endocr Rev. 1986;7:351-78.
337. Chrousos GP, moderator. Clinical applications of corticotropin-releasing factor. Ann Intern Med. 1985;102(3):344-58.
338. Grossman A. Corticotropin-releasing hormone: basic physiology and clinical applications. In: DeGroot L, ed. Endocrinology. 3rd ed. Philadelphia: WB Saunders, 1995: 341-354.
339. Dallman MF, Akana SF, Levin N. Corticosteroids and the control of function in the hypothalamus-pituitary-adrenal (HPA) axis. Ann N Y Acad Sci. 1994;746:22-31.
340. Orth DN, Kovac WJ. The adrenal cortex. In: Wilson JD, Foster DW, Kronenberg HM, Larsen PR, eds. Williams Textbook of Endocrinology. 9th ed. Philadelphia: WB Saunders, 1998: 517-664.
341. Munck A, Guyre PM, Holbrook NJ. Physiologic function of glucocorticoids in stress and their relation to pharmacologic actions. Endocr Rev. 1984;5(1):25-44.
342. Pacak K. Stressor-specific activation of the hypothalamic-pituitary-adrenocortical axis. Physiol Res. 2000;49(Suppl 1):S11-S17.
343. Freeman ME, Houpt TA. The hypothalamus. In: Conn PM, ed. Neuroscience in medicine. 2nd ed. Totowa, NJ: Humana Press, 2002: 293-345.
344. Tache Y, Martinez V, Million M, Wang L. Stress and the gastrointestinal tract III. Stress-related alterations of gut motor function: role of brain corticotropin-releasing factor receptors. Am J Physiol Gastrointest Liver Physiol. 2001;280:G6173-77.
345. Ibid.
346. Felten DL, Felten SY, Madden KS. Fundamental aspects of neural-immune signaling. Psychother Psychosom. 1993;60(1):46-56.
347. Felten SY, Felten DL. Innervation of lymphoid tissue. In: Ader R, Felten DL, Cohen N (eds). Psychoneuroimmunology. 2nd Ed. New York: Academic Press, 1991: 27-61.
348. Madden KS, Ackerman KD, Livnat S, et al. Patterns of noradrenergic innervation of lymphoid organs and immunological consequences of denervation. In: Goetz EJ, Spector N.H. (eds). Neuroimmune networks: Physiology and diseases. New York: Alan R. Liss, 1989: 1-8.
349. Turner-Cobb JM, Sephton SE, Spiegel D. Psychosocial effects on immune function and disease progression in cancer: human studies. In: Ader R, Felten DL, Cohen N (eds). Psychoneuroimmunology 3rd ed. New York: Academic Press 2001: 562-582.
350. Sutton RE, Koob GF, LeMoal M. Corticotropin releasing factor produces behavioral activation in rats. Nature. 1982;297:331-33.
351. Lenz HG. Extrapituitary effects of corticotropin-releasing factor. Horm Metab Res. 1987;16(suppl):17-23.
352. Nemeroff CB. Neuropeptides and Psychiatric disorders. Washington DC: American Psychiatric Press 1991; 29
353. Chrousos GP and Gold PW. The concepts of stress and stress system disorders. Overview of physical and behavioral homeostasis. JAMA. 1992;267(9):1244-52.
354. Ibid.
355. Dinarello CA, Mier JW. Lymphokines. N Engl J Med. 1987;317:940-45.
356. Lumpkin MD. Cytokine regulation of hypothalamic and pituitary hormone secretion. In: Foa PP (ed.). Endocrinology and Metabolism 5: Humoral factors in the regulation of tissue growth. New York: Springer-Verlag 1993: 139-159.
357. Berkenbosch F, vanRooijen N, Tilders FJH. Determining role and sources of endogenous interleukin 1 in pituitary-adrenal activation in response to stressful and inflammatory stimuli. In: DeSouza EB (ed.). Neurobiology of Cytokines-part A. San Diego: Academic Press 1993: 211-231.
358. Banks WA, Kastin AJ. Measurement of transport of cytokines across the blood-brain barrier. In: DeSouza EB (ed.). Neurobiology of Cytokines-part A. San Diego: Academic Press 1993: 67-77.
359. Ibid.
360. Olschowka JA. Immunocytochemical methods for localization of cytokines in brain. In: DeSouza EB (ed.). Neurobiology of Cytokines-part A. San Diego: Academic Press 1993: 100-111.
361. Besedovsky HO, del Rey A. Immuno-neuro-endocrine interactions: facts and hypotheses. Endocr Rev. 1996;17(1):64-102.
362. Bartfai T, Ottoson D (eds). Neuro-immunology of Fever. Oxford: Pergamon Press, 1992.
363. Hopkins SJ, Rothwell NJ. Cytokines and the nervous system I: Expression and recognition. Trends Neurosci. 1995;18(2):83-88.
364. Rothwell NJ, Hopkins SJ. Cytokines and the nervous system II: actions and mechanisms of action. Trends Neurosci. 1995;18(3):130-36.
365. Munck A, Guyre PM, Holbrook NJ. Physiologic function of glucocorticoids in stress and their relation to pharmacologic actions. Endocr Rev. 1984;5:25-44.
366. Reichlin S. Neuroendocrine-immune interactions. N Engl J Med. 1993;329(17):1246-53.
367. Sapolsky RM, Krey L, McEwen BS. The neuroendocrinology of aging: the glucocorticoid cascade hypothesis. Endocr Rev. 1986;7:284-301.
368. Sapolsky R. Stress, the Aging Brain and the Mechanisms of Neuron Death. Cambridge: MIT Press, 1992.
369. Bhasin S, Fisher CE, Swerdloff RS. Follicle stimulating hormone and luteinizing hormone. In: Melmed S (ed). The pituitary. 2nd ed. Malden, MASS: Blackwell Publishing 2002; 216-278.

370. Moser DK, Dracup K, Woo MA, Stevenson LW. Voluntary control of vascular tone by using skin-temperature biofeedback-relaxation in patients with advanced heart failure. Altern Ther Health Med. 1997;3(1):51-59.
371. Kabat-Zinn J, Massion AO, Kristeller J, et al. Effectiveness of a meditation-based stress reduction program in the treatment of anxiety disorders. Am J Psychiatry. 1992;149(7):936-43.
372. Benton D. The impact of the supply of glucose to the brain on mood and memory. Nutr Rev. 2001;59(1 Pt2):S20-21.
373. Davidson JR, Abraham K, Connor KM, McLeod MN. Effectiveness of chromium in atypical depression: a placebo-controlled trial. Biol Psychiatry. 2003;53(3):261-64.
374. Wang C, Makela T, Hase T, et al. Lignans and flavonoids inhibit aromatase enzyme in human preadipocytes. J Steroid Biochem Molec Biol. 1994;50(3-4):205-12.
375. Richardson AJ. The role omega-3 fatty acids in behavior, cognition, and mood. Scand. J Nutr. 2003;47:92-98.
376. Merill JE, Otoniel M-M. Cytokines in AIDS-associated nervous and immune system dysfunction. In: DeSouza EB (ed.) Neurobiology of Cytokines, part B. San Diego: Academic Press 1993; 243-266.
377. Lumpkin MD. Cytokine regulation of hypothalamic and pituitary hormone secretion. In: Foa PP (ed). Endocrinology and Metabolism 5: Humoral factors in the regulation of tissue growth. New York: Springer-Verlag 1993: 139-159.
378. Reichlin S. Neuroendocrinology. In: Wilson JD, Foster DW, Kronenberg HM, Larsen PR, eds. Williams Textbook of Endocrinology. 9th ed. Philadelphia: WB Saunders, 1998; 165-248.
379. Poretsky L, Can S, Zumoff B. Testicular dysfunction in human immunodeficiency virus-infected men. Metabolism. 1995;44(7):946-53.
380. Grinspoon S, Corcoran C, Lee K, et al. Loss of lean body and muscle mass correlates with androgen levels in hypogonadal men with acquired immunodeficiency syndrome and wasting. J Clin Endocrinol Metab. 1996;81(11):4051-58.
381. Kotler DP, Tierney AR, Wang J, Pierson RN. Magnitude of body-cell-mass depletion and the timing of death from wasting in AIDS. Am J Clin Nutr. 1989;50(3):444-47.
382. Reichlin S. Neuroendocrine-immune interactions. N. Engl J Med. 1993;329(17):1246-53.
383. Mulroney SE, McDonnell KJ, Pert CB, et al. HIV gp120 inhibits the somatotropic axis: A possible GH-releasing hormone receptor mechanism for the pathogenesis of AIDS wasting. Proc Natl Acad Sci U S A. 1998 95:1927-32.
384. Peisen JN, McDonnell KJ, Mulroney SE, Lumpkin MD. Endotoxin-induced suppression of the somatotropic axis is mediated by interleukin-1 and corticotrophin-releasing factor in the juvenile rat. Endocrinology. 1995;136(8):3378-90.
385. Ng TT, O'Connell IP, Wilkins EG. Growth hormone deficiency coupled with hypogonadism in AIDS. Clin Endocrinol (Oxf). 1994;41(5):689-93; discussion 693-94.
386. Kaufman FR, Gomperts ED. Growth failure in boys with hemophilia and HIV infection. Am J Pediatr Hematol Oncol. 1989;11:292-94.
387. Kelley KW. Growth hormone, lymphocytes, and macrophages. Biochem Pharmacol. 1989;38:705-13.
388. Jordon R, Gold L, Cummins C, Hyde C. Systematic review and meta-analysis of evidence for increasing numbers of drugs in antiretroviral combination therapy. BMJ. 2002;324:757-60.
389. Merill JE, Otoniel M-M. Cytokines in AIDS-associated nervous and immune system dysfunction. In: DeSouza EB (ed.) Neurobiology of Cytokines, part B. San Diego: Academic Press 1993; 243-266.
390. Reichlin S. Neuroendocrine-immune interactions. N Engl J Med. 1993;329(17):1246-53.
391. Heseker H, Kubler W, Pudel V, Westenhoffer J. Psychological disorders as early symptoms of a mild-to-moderate vitamin deficiency. Ann N Y Acad Sci. 1992;669:352-57.
392. Morris MC, Evans DA, Bienias JL, et al. Vitamin E and cognitive decline in older persons. Arch Neurol. 2002;59(7):1125-32.
393. Levitt AJ, Joffe RT. Folate, B12, and life course of depressive illness. Biol Psychiatr. 1989;25(7):867-72.
394. Fawzi WW, Msamanga GI, Spiegelman D, et al. A randomized trial of multivitamin supplements and HIV disease progression and mortality. N Engl J Med. 2004;351:23-32.
395. LeBars PL, Katz MM, Berman N, et al. A placebo-controlled, double-blind, randomized trial of an extract of Gingko biloba for dementia. North American EGb Study Group. JAMA. 1997;278(16):1327-32.
396. Ford ES, Giles WH, Dietz WH. Prevalence of the metabolic syndrome among US adults. JAMA. 2002;287:356-59.
397. Zavaroni I, Bonini L, Fantuzzi M, et al. Hyperinsulinaemia, obesity and syndrome X. J Intern Med. 1994;235:51-56.
398. McLaughlin T, et al., Use of metabolic markers to identify overweight individuals who are insulin resistant. Ann Intern Med, 2003;139(10):802-9.
399. McLaughlin T, Abbasi F, Lamendola C, et al. Differentiation between obesity and insulin resistance in the association with C-reactive protein. Circulation. 2002;106(23):2908-12.
400. Ruderman N, Chisholm D, Sunyer X, Schneider S. The metabolically obese, normal-weight individual revisited. Diabetes. 1998;47:699-713.
401. Wallace MB, Mills BD, Browning CL. Effects of cross-training on markers of insulin resistance/hyperinsulinemia. Med Sci Sports Exerc. 1997;29(9):1170-75.
402. Lampman R, Schteingart D. Effects of exercise training on glucose control, lipid metabolism, and insulin sensitivity in hypertriglyceridemia and non-insulin dependent diabetes mellitus. Med Sci Sports Exerc. 1991;23(6):703-12.
403. Ronnemaa T, Ronnemaa E, Puukka P, et al. Smoking is independently associated with high plasma insulin levels in nondiabetic men. Diabetes Care. 1996;19:1229-32.
404. Henry RR, Wallace P, Olefsky JM. Effects of weight loss on mechanisms of hyperglycemia in obese non-insulin dependent diabetes mellitus. Diabetes. 1986;35:990-98.
405. Su H-Y, Sheu W H-H, Chin H-ML, et al. Effect of weight loss on blood pressure and insulin resistance in normotensive and hypertensive obese individuals. Am J Hypertens. 1995;8(11):1067-71.
406. Odeleye OE, de Courten M, Pettitt D, Ravussin E. Fasting hyperinsulinemia is a predictor of increased body weight gain and obesity in Pima Indian children. Diabetes. 1997;46:1341-45.
407. Ibid.
408. Bao W, Srinivasan S, Berenson G. Persistence elevation of plasma insulin levels is associated with increased cardiovascular risk in children and young adults. Circulation. 1996;93:54-59.
409. Bogardus C, Lillioja D, Mott M, et al. Relationship between degree of obesity and *in vivo* insulin action in man. Am J Physiol. 1985;248 (Endorcrinol Metab II):E286-91.
410. Barnard R, Ugianskis E, Martin D, et al. Role of diet and exercise in the management of hyperinsulinemia and associated atherosclerotic risk factors. Am J Cardiol. 1992;69:440-44.
411. Zavaroni I, Bonini L, Fantuzzi M, et al. Hyperinsulinaemia, obesity and syndrome X. J Int Med. 1994;235:51-56.
412. Devynck M. Do cell membrane dynamics participate in insulin resistance? Lancet. 1995;345:336.
413. Chen YD, Coulston AM, Zhou MY, et al. Why do low-fat high-carbohydrate diets accentuate postprandial lipemia in patients with NIDDM? Diabetes Care. 1995;18(1):10-16.

414. Garg A, Bantle J, Henry R, et al. Effects of varying carbohydrate content of diet in patients with non-insulin-dependent diabetes mellitus. JAMA. 1994:271:1421-28.
415. Tong P, Thomas T, Berrish T. Cell membrane dynamics and insulin resistance in non-insulin-dependent diabetes mellitus. Lancet. 1995;345:357-58.
416. Simopoulos A. Fatty acid composition of skeletal muscle membrane phospholipids, insulin resistance and obesity. Nutr Today. 1994;1:12-16.
417. Field CJ, Ryan EA, Thomson AB, Clandinin MT. Dietary fat and the diabetic state alter insulin binding and the fatty acid composition of the adipocyte plasma membrane. J Biochem. 1988;253:417-24.
418. Luo J, Rizkalla SW, Boillot J, et al. Dietary polyunsaturated (n-3) fatty acids improve adipocyte insulin action and glucose metabolism in insulin resistant rats: relation to membrane fatty acids. J Nutr. 1996;126:1951-58.
419. Field CJ, Ryan EA, Thomson AB, Clandinin MT. Dietary fat and the diabetic state alter insulin binding and the fatty acid composition of the adipocyte plasma membrane. J Biochem. 1988;253:417-24.
420. Luo J, Rizkalla SW, Boillot J, et al. Dietary polyunsaturated (n-3) fatty acids improve adipocyte insulin action and glucose metabolism in insulin resistant rats: relation to membrane fatty acids. J Nutr. 1996;126:1951-58.
421. Medeiros LC, Liu YW, Park S, et al. Insulin, but not estrogen, correlated with indexes of desaturase function in obese women. Horm Metab Res. 1995;27:235-38.
422. Storlien LH, Ban DA, Kriketos AD, et al. Skeletal muscle membrane lipids and insulin resistance. Lipids. 1996;31(S):S261-65.
423. Storlein LH, Kraegen EW, Chisholm DJ, et al. Fish oil prevents insulin resistance induced by high fat feeding in rats. Science. 1987;237:885-88.
424. Garg A, Bantle JP. Henry RR, et al. Effects of varying carbohydrate content of diet in patients with non-insulin-dependent diabetes mellitus. JAMA. 1994;271(18):1421-28.
425. Golay A, Allaz A, Morel Y, et al. Similar weight loss with low- or high-carbohydrate diets. Am J Clin Nutr. 1996;63:174-78.
426. Garg A, Grundy S, Unger R. Comparison of effects of high- and low-carbohydrate diets on plasma lipoproteins and insulin sensitivity in patient with mild NIDDM. Diabetes. 1992;41:1278-85.
427. Cambpell, L, Marmot P, Dyer J, et al. The high-monounsaturated fat diet as a practical alternative for NIDDM. Diabetes Care. 1994;17(3):177-82.
428. Purnell J, Brunzell J. The central role of dietary fat, not carbohydrate, in the insulin resistance syndrome. Current Opin Lip. 1997;8:17-22.
429. Crapo P, Reaven G, Olefsky J. Postprandial plasma-glucose and -insulin responses to different complex carbohydrates. Diabetes. 1977;26:1178-83.
430. Jenkins DA, Wolever TM, Taylor RH, et al. Glycemic index of foods: a physiological basis for carbohydrate exchange. Am J Clin Nutr. 1981;34:362-66.
431. Philipson H. Dietary fibre in the diabetic diet. Acta Med Scand. 1983;671(suppl):91-93.
432. Landin K, Holm G, Tengborn L, Smith U. Guar gum improves insulin sensitivity, blood lipids, blood pressure, and fibrinolysis in healthy men. Am J Clin Nutr. 1992;56:1061-65.
433. Rivellese A, Giacco A, Genovese S, et al. Effect of dietary fibre on glucose control and serum lipoproteins in diabetic patients. Lancet. 1980;2:447.
434. Leclere CJ, Champ M, Boillot J, et al. Viscous guar gums lower glycemic responses after a solid meal: mode of action. Am J Clin Nutr. 1994;59(suppl):776S.
435. Kabir M, Rizkalla S, Champ M, et al. Dietary amylose-amylopectin starch content affects glucose and lipid metabolism in adipocytes of normal and diabetic rats. J Nutr. 1998;128:35-43.
436. Howe JC, Rumpler WV, Behall KM. Dietary starch composition and level of energy intake alter nutrient oxidation in "carbohydrate-sensitive" men. J Nutr. 1996;126:2120-29.
437. Behal KM, Howe JC. Effect of long-term consumption of amylose vs. amyolopectin starch on metabolic variables in human subjects. Am J Clin Nutr. 1995;61:334-40.
438. Ludwig D, Majzoub J, Al-Zabroni A, et al. High glycemic index foods, overeating and obesity. Pediatrics. 1999;103(3):e26.
439. Liu S, Manson J, Stampfer M, et al. Dietary glycemic load assessed by food-frequency questionnaire in relation to plasma high-density-lipoprotein cholesterol and fasting plasma triacylglycerols in postmenopausal women. Am J Clin Nutr. 2001;73(3):560-66.
440. Salmeron J, Ascherio A, Rimm E, et al. Dietary fiber, glycemic load, and risk of NIDDM in men. Diabetes Care. 1997;20(4):545-50.
441. Krezowski PA, Nuttall FQ, Gannon MC, Bartosh NH. The effect of protein ingestion on the metabolic response to oral glucose in normal individuals. Am J Clin Nutr. 1986;44:847-856.
442. Holt SH, Miller, JC, Petocz P. An insulin index of foods: the insulin demand generated by 1000-kJ portions of common foods. Am J Clin Nutr. 1997;66:1264-76.
443. Paolisso G, Sgambato S, Pizza G, et al. Improved insulin response and action by chronic magnesium administration in aged NIDDM subjects. Diabetes Care. 1989:12:265-69.
444. Paolisso G, Sgambato S, Gambardella A, et al. Daily magnesium supplements improve glucose handling in elderly subjects. Am J Clin Nutr. 1992;55:1161-67.
445. Elamin A, Tuvemo T. Magnesium and insulin-dependent diabetes mellitus. Diab Res Clin Pract. 1990;10:203-9.
446. Paolisso G, Sgambato S, Pizza G, et al. Improved insulin response and action by chronic magnesium administration in aged NIDDM subjects. Diabetes Care. 1989:12:265-69.
447. Schmiedl A, Schwille P. Magnesium status in idiopathic calcium urolthiasis—an orientational study in younger males. Eur J Clin Chem Clin Biochem. 1996;34:393.
448. Paolisso G, Barbagallo M. Hypertension, diabetes, and insulin resistance: the role of intracellular magnesium. Am J Hypertens. 1997;10(3):346-55.
449. Paolisso G, Sgambato S, Pizza G, et al. Improved insulin response and action by chronic magnesium administration in aged type 2 diabetes subjects. Diabetes Care. 1989:12:265-69.
450. Rosolova H, Mayer O Jr., Reaven G. Effect of variations in plasma magnesium concentration on resistance to insulin-mediated glucose disposal in nondiabetic subjects. J Clin Endorcrinol Metab. 1997;82:3783-85.
451. Linday LA. Trivalent chromium and the diabetes prevention program. Med Hypotheses. 1997;49:47-49.
452. McCarty MF. Exploiting complementary therapeutic strategies for the treatment of type II diabetes and prevention of its complications. Med Hypotheses. 1997;49:143-52.
453. Evans GW, Bowman TD. Chromium picolinate increases membrane fluidity and rate of insulin internalization. J Inorg Bio. 1992;46:243-50.
454. Anderson RA. Chromium metabolism and its role in disease processes in man. Clin Physiol Biochem. 1986;4(11):31-41.
455. Roeback JR Jr., Hla KM, Chambless L, et al. Effects of chromium supplementation on serum high-density lipoprotein cholesterol levels in men taking beta-blockers. Ann Intern Med. 1991;115:917-24.
456. Anderson R, Cheng N, Bryden, et al. Beneficial effects of chromium for people with type II diabetes. Diabetes. 1996;45:124A.

457. Anderson RA, Cheng N, Bryden NA, et al. Elevated intakes of supplemental chromium improve glucose and insulin variables in individuals with type 2 diabetes. Diabetes. 1997;46:1786-91.
458. French RJ, Jones PJ. Role of vanadium in nutrition: metabolism, essentiality and dietary considerations. Life Sci. 1992;52:339-46.
459. Ibid.
460. Shechter Y, Li J, Meyerovitch J, et al. Insulin-like actions of vanadate are mediated in an insulin-receptor-independent manner via non-receptor protein tyrosine kinases and protein phosphotyrosine phosphatases. Mol Cell Biochem. 1995;153(1-2):39-47.
461. Halberstam M, Cohen N, Shlimovich P, et al. Oral vanadyl sulfate improves insulin sensitivity in type 2 diabetes but not in obese nondiabetic subjects. Diabetes. 1996;45:659-65.
462. Goldfine AB, Simonson DC, Folli F, et al. Metabolic effects of sodium metavanadate in humans with insulin-dependent and noninsulin-dependent diabetes mellitus *in vivo* and *in vitro* studies. J Clin Endocrinol Metab. 1995;80(11);3311-19.
463. Boden G, Chen X, Ruiz J, et al. Effects of vanadyl sulfate on carbohydrate and lipid metabolism in patients with non-insulin-dependent diabetes mellitus. Metabolism. 1996;45(9):1130-35.
464. Halberstam M, Cohen N, Shlimovich P, et al. Oral vanadyl sulfate improves insulin sensitivity in NIDDM but not in obese nondiabetic subjects. Diabetes. 1996;45(5):659-66.
465. Barth A, et al. Neurobehavioral effects of vanadium. J Toxicol Environ Health A. 2002;65(9):677-83.
466. Shang H, Osada K, Maebashi M, et al. A high biotin diet improves the impaired glucose tolerance of long-term spontaneously hyperglycemic rats with non-insulin-dependent diabetes mellitus. J Nutr Sci Vitamin. 1996;42:517-26.
467. Koutsikos D, Fourtounas C, Kapetanaki A, et al. Oral glucose tolerance test after high-dose i.v. biotin administration in normoglycemic hemodialysis patients. Ren Fail. 1996;18(1):131-37.
468. Maebashi M, Makino Y, Furukawa Y, et al. Therapeutic evaluation of the effect of biotin on hyperglycemia in patients with non-insulin dependent diabetes mellitus J Clin Biochem Nutr. 1993;14:211-18.
469. Belury M, Moya-Camarena S, Liu KL, et al. Dietary conjugated linoleic acid induces peroxisome-specific enzyme accumulation and ornithine decarboxylase activity in mouse liver. J Nutr Biochem. 1997;8:579-84.
470. Moya-Camarena S, Heuvel J, Blanchard S, et al. Conjugated linoleic acid is a potent naturally occurring ligand and activator of PPARα. J Lipid Res. 1999;40:1426-33.
471. Saltiel A, Olefsky J. Thiazolidinediones in the treatment of insulin resistance and type II diabetes. Diabetes. 1996;45:1661-69.
472. Houseknecht K, Vanden Heuvel J, Moya-Camarena S, et al. Dietary conjugated linoleic acid normalizes impaired glucose tolerance in the Zucker diabetic fatty fa/fa rat. Biochem Biophys Res Commun. 1998;247(3):911.
473. Jacob S, Henriksen EJ, Schiemann AL, et al. Enhancement of glucose disposal in patients with Type 2 diabetes by alpha-lipoic acid. Arzneim-Rorsch Drug Res. 1995;45(2):872-74.
474. Jacob S, Henriksen EJ, Tritschler HJ, et al. Improvement of insulin-stimulated glucose-disposal in type 2 diabetes after repeated parenteral administration of thioctic acid. Diabetes. 1996;104:284-88.
475. Jacob S, Streeper RS, Fogt DL, et al. The antioxidant alpha-lipoic acid enhances insulin-stimulated glucose metabolism in insulin-resistant rat skeletal muscle. Diabetes. 1996;45:1024-29.
476. Streeper RS, Henriksen EJ, Jacob S, et al. Differential effects of lipoic acid stereoisomers on glucose metabolism in insulin-resistant skeletal muscle. Am J Physiol. 1997;273 (Endocrinol Metab 36):E185-91.
477. Jacob S, Ruus P, Hermann R, et al. Oral administration of RAC-alpha-lipoic acid modulates insulin sensitivity in patients with type-2 diabetes mellitus: a placebo-controlled pilot trial. Free Radic Biol Med. 1999;27(3-4):309-14.
478. Ziegler D, Reljanovic M, Mehnert H, et al. Alpha-lipoic acid in the treatment of diabetic polyneuropathy in Germany: current evidence from clinical trials. Exp Clin Endocrinol Diabetes. 1999;107(7):421-30.
479. Mori M, Hasegawa N. Superoxide dismutase activity enhanced by green tea inhibits lipid accumulation in 3T3-L1 cells. Phytother Res. 2003;17(5):566-67.
480. Kim MJ, et al. Protective effects of epicatechin against the toxic effects of streptozotocin on rat pancreatic islets: *in vivo* and *in vitro*. Pancreas. 2003;26(3):292-99.
481. Han MK. Epigallocatechin gallate, a constituent of green tea, suppresses cytokine-induced pancreatic beta-cell damage. Exp Mol Med. 2003;35(2):136-39.
482. Murase T, et al. Beneficial effects of tea catechins on diet-induced obesity: stimulation of lipid catabolism in the liver. Int J Obes Relat Metab Disord. 2002;26(11):1459-64.
483. Anderson RA, Polansky MM. Tea enhances insulin activity. J Agric Food Chem. 2002;50(24):7182-86.
484. Imparl-Radosevich J, et al. Regulation of PTP-1 and insulin receptor kinase by fractions from cinnamon: implications for cinnamon regulation of insulin signalling. Horm Res. 1998;50(3):177-82.
485. Broadhurst CL, et al. Insulin-like biological activity of culinary and medicinal plant aqueous extracts *in vitro*. J Agric Food Chem. 2000;48(3):849-52.
486. Anderson RA, et al. Isolation and characterization of polyphenol type-A polymers from cinnamon with insulin-like biological activity. J Agric Food Chem. 2004;52(1):65-70.
487. Onderoglu S, et al. The evaluation of long-term effects of cinnamon bark and olive leaf on toxicity induced by streptozotocin administration to rats. J Pharm Pharmacol. 1999;51(11):1305-12.
488. Khan A, et al. Cinnamon improves glucose and lipids of people with type 2 diabetes. Diabetes Care. 2003;26(12):3215-18.
489. Schwarzbein D. Dysinsulinemia, Accelerated Metabolic Aging and CVD. 10th International Symposium on Functional Medicine, May 2003. Institute for Functional Medicine, Gig Harbor, WA.
490. Pasqualini JR. Estrone sulfate-sulfatase and 17β-hydroxysteroid dehydrogenase activities: a hypothesis for their role in the evolution of human breast cancer from hormone-dependence to hormone-independence. J. Steroid Biochem Molec Biol 1995;53(1-6):407-12.
491. MacFarland SA. The use of Pro-Gest cream in postmenopausal women. Letter to editor. Lancet. 1998;352:905.
492. Lee JR. The use of Pro-Gest cream in postmenopausal women. Letter to editor. Lancet. 1998;352:905
493. Stevenson JC, Purdie DW. The use of Pro-Gest cream in postmenopausal women. Letter to editor. Lancet. 1998;352:90
494. Cooper AJ, Whitehead MI. Author's reply. The use of Pro-Gest cream in postmenopausal women. Letter to editor. Lancet. 1998;352:906.
495. Cefalu WT. Serum bioavailability and tissue metabolism of testosterone and estradiol in rat salivary gland. J Clin Endocrinol Metab. 1986;63(1):20-28.
496. Lewis JG. Caution on the use of saliva measurements to monitor absorption of progesterone from transdermal creams in postmenopausal women. Maturitas. 2002;31(1):1-6.
497. Wren BG, McFarland K, Edwards L, et al. Effect of sequential transdermal progesterone cream on endometrium, bleeding pattern, and plasma progesterone and salivary progesterone levels in postmenopausal women. Climacteric. 2000;3(3):155-60.

498. Leonetti HB. Topical progesterone cream has antiproliferative effect on estrogen-stimulated endometrium. Fertil Steril. 2003;79(1):221-22.
499. Boothby LA. Bioidentical hormone therapy: a review. Menopause. 2004;11(3):356-67.
500. Zhang F. The major metabolite of equilin, 4-hydroxyequilin, autoxidizes to an O-quinone which isomerizes to the potent cytotoxin 4-hydroxyequilenin-o-quinone. Chem Res Toxicol. 1999;12(2):204-13.
501. Bolton JL. Role of quinoids in estrogen carcinogenesis. Chem Res Toxicol. 1998 11:1113-27.
502. Bhavnani BR. Pharmacokinetics and pharmacodynamics of conjugated equine estrogens: chemistry and metabolism. Proc Soc Exp Biol Med. 1998;217(1):6-16.
503. Ettinger B. Effects of ultralow-dose transdermal estradiol on bone mineral density: a randomized clinical trial. Obstet Gynecol. 2004;104(3):443-51.
504. Yen S, Jaffee RB, Barbieri RL. Reproductive Endocrinology: Pathology, Pathophysiology and Clinical Management 4th Edition WB Saunders, Philadelphia 1999.
505. Ettinger B. Effects of ultralow-dose transdermal estradiol on bone mineral density: a randomized clinical trial. Obstet Gynecol. 2004;104(3):443-51.
506. Schwarzbein D. Dysinsulinemia, Accelerated Metabolic Aging and CVD. 10th International Symposium on Functional Medicine, May 2003. Institute for Functional Medicine, Gig Harbor, WA.
507. Bradlow L. Sterol biochemistry. Applied Biochemistry and Nutrition of Endocrinology; 8th International Symposium on Functional Medicine. May 2001. Institute for Functional Medicine, Gig Harbor, WA.
508. Ettinger B. Associations between low levels of serum estradiol, bone density, and fractures among elderly women: the study of osteoporotic fractures. J Clin Endocrinol Metab. 1998;130:897-904.
509. Ettinger B. Effects of ultra low-dose transdermal estradiol on bone mineral density: a randomized clinical trial. Obstet Gynecol. 2004;104:443-51.
510. Ficicioglu C. High local endometrial effect of vaginal progesterone gel. Gynecol Endocrinol. 2004 May;18(5):240-43.
511. Ettinger B. Effects of ultra low-dose transdermal estradiol on bone mineral density: a randomized clinical trial. Obstet Gynecol. 2004;104:443-51.
512. Khaksari M. Differences between male and female students in cardiovascular and endocrine responses to examination stress. J Ayub Med Coll Abbottabad. 2005;17(2):15-19.
513. Redmond AM. Premenstrual asthma: emphasis on drug therapy options. J Asthma. 2004;41(7):687-93.
514. Hlatky MA. Quality-of-life and depressive symptoms in postmenopausal women after receiving hormone therapy: results from the Heart and Estrogen/Progestin Replacement Study (HERS) trial. JAMA. 2002;287(5):591-97.
515. Hays J. Effects of estrogen plus progestin on health-related quality of life. N Engl J Med. 2003:348(19):1839-54.
516. Keenan NL. Severity of menopausal symptoms and use of both conventional and complementary alternatives Menopause. 2003;10:507-15.
517. Ibid.
518. Vliet EL. New insights on hormone and mood. Menopause Management. 1993 Jun/Jul Carrington Communications, Inc.
519. Wylie-Rosett J. Menopause, micronutrients, and hormone therapy. Am J Clin Nutr. 2005;81(suppl):1223S-31S.
520. Patisaul HB. Phytoestrogen action in the adult and developing brain. J Neuroendocrinol. 2005;17(1):57-64.
521. Friel PN. Hormone replacement with estradiol: conventional oral doses result in excessive exposure to estrone. Altern Med Rev. 2005;10(1):36-41.
522. Ficicioglu C. High local endometrial effect of vaginal progesterone gel. Gynecol Endocrinol. 2004;18(5):240-43.
523. Dicker RC, Scally MJ, Greenspan JR, et al. ACOG Practice Bulletin: Hysterectomy among women of reproductive age. JAMA. 1982;248:323-27.
524. Pokras R, Hufnagel VG. Hysterectomy in the United States, 1965-84. Am J Public Health. 1988;78:852-53.
525. Li C. Menopause-related symptoms: what are the background factors? A prospective population-based cohort study of Swedish women (The Women's Health In Lund Area Study) Am J Obstet Gynecol. 2003;189:1646-53.
526. Wuest JH Jr, Dry TJ, Edwards JE. The degree of coronary atherosclerosis in bilaterally oophorectomized women. Circulation. 1953;7(6):801-9.
527. Anderson GL. Effects of conjugated equine estrogen in postmenopausal women with hysterectomy: the Women's Health Initiative Steering Committee. JAMA. 2004;291:1701-12.
528. Writing Group for the Women's Health Initiative Investigators. Risks and benefits of estrogen plus progestin in healthy postmenopausal women. JAMA. 2002;288:321-33.
529. Schwarzbein D. Personal communication.
530. Wren BG. Transdermal progesterone and its effect on vasomotor symptoms, blood lipid levels, bone metabolic markers, moods, and quality of life for postmenopausal women. Menopause. 2003;10(1):13-18.
531. Azizi G. Effect of micronized progesterone on bone turnover in postmenopausal women on estrogen replacement therapy. Endocr Res. 2003;29(2):133-40.
532. Weiderpass E. Low-potency oestrogen and risk of endometrial cancer: a case controlled study. Lancet. 1999;353(9167):1824-28.
533. Englund DE. Endometrial effect of oral estriol treatment in postmenopausal women. Acta Obstet Gynecol Scand. 1980;59:449-51.
534. Minaguchi H. Effect of estriol on bone mass loss in postmenopausal Japanese women: a multicentric prospective open study. J Obstet Gynecol Res. 1996;22:259-65.
535. Heimer GM. Estriol absorption after long-term vaginal treatment and gastrointestinal absorption as influenced by a meal. Acta Obstet Gynecol Scand. 1984;63:563-67.
536. Dessole S. Efficacy of low-dose intravaginal estriol on urogenital aging in postmenopausal women. Menopause. 2004;11(1):49-56.
537. Palaszynski KM. Estriol treatment ameliorates disease in males with experimental autoimmune encephalomyelitis: implications for multiple sclerosis. J Neuroimmunol. 2004;149(1-2):84-89.
538. Longcope C. Editorial: Androgens, estrogens and mammary epithelial proliferation. Menopause. 2003;10(4):274-76.
539. Zeleniuch-Jacquotte A. relation of serum levels of testosterone and dehydroepiandrosterone sulfate to risk of breast cancer in postmenopausal women. Am J Epidemiol. 1997:145:1030-38.
540. Galland L. Neuroendocrine Balance in Patient Care. 8th International Symposium on Functional Medicine, 2001. Institute for Functional Medicine, Gig Harbor, WA.
541. Dunning AM. Polymorphisms associated with circulating sex hormone levels in postmenopausal women. J Natl Cancer Inst. 2004;96:936-45.
542. Tempfer CB. DNA microarray-based analysis of single nucleotide polymorphisms may be useful for assessing the risks and benefits of hormone therapy. Fertil Steril. 2004;82(1):132-37.
543. Weber BL. Low penetrance genes associated with increased risk for breast cancer. Eur J Cancer. 2000;36(10):1193-99.
544. Hayes C. 17β Estradiol hydroxylation catalyzed by human cytochrome P450 1B1. Proc Natl Acad Sci U S A. 1996;93:9776-81.
545. Li J. Estrogen carcinogenesis in Syrian hamster tissues: role of metabolism. Fed Proc. 1987;46:1858-63.

546. Liehr J. 4-hydroxylation of estrogens as a marker of human mammary tumors. Proc Natl Acad Sci U S A. 1996;93:3294-96.
547. Spink D. The effects of 2,3,7,8-tetra chlorodibenzo-p-dioxin on estrogen metabolism in MCF-7 breast cancer cells: evidence for induction of a novel 17β estradiol 4 hydroxylase. J Steroid Biochem. 1994;51:251-58.
548. DeVivo I. Association of CYP 1B1 polymorphisms and breast cancer risk. Can Epidem Biomarkers Prev. 2002;11:498-92.
549. Bailey L. Association of cytochrome P450 1B1 (CYP(1B1) polymorphism with steroid receptor status in breast cancer. Cancer Res. 1998;58:5038-41.
550. Yen JH. Cytochrome p450 1Al gene polymorphisms in patients with psoriatic arthritis. Scand J Rheumatol. 2004;33(1):19-23.
551. Miyoshi Y. Association of genetic polymorphisms in CYP19 and CYP1A1 with the oestrogen receptor-positive breast cancer risk. Eur J Cancer. 2003;39(17):2531-37.
552. Hefler LA. Estrogen-metabolizing gene polymorphisms in the assessment of breast carcinoma risk and fibroadenoma risk in Caucasian women. Cancer. 2004;101(2):264-69.
553. Lachman HM. Human catechol-o-methyltransferase pharmacogenetics: description of a functional polymorphism and its potential application to neuropsychiatric disorders. Pharmacogenetics. 1996;6:243-50.
554. Van Duursen MB. Phytochemicals inhibit catechol-o-methyltransferase activity in cytosolic fractions from healthy human mammary tissues: implications for catechol estrogen-induced DNA damage. Toxicol Sci. 2004;81(2):316-24.
555. Wu AH. Tea intake, COMT genotype, and breast cancer in Asian-American women. Cancer Res. 2003;63(21):7526-29.
556. Sazci A. Catechol-o-methyltransferase Val 108/158 met polymorphism in premenopausal breast cancer patients. Toxicology. 2004;204(2-3):197-202.
557. Brueggemeier RW. Aromatase and cyclooxygenases: enzymes in breast cancer. J Steroid Biochem Mol Biol. 2003;86(3-5):501-7.
558. Terry MB. Association of frequency and duration of aspirin use and hormone receptor status with breast cancer risk. JAMA. 2004;291(20):2433-40.
559. Peters U. Circulating vitamin D metabolites, polymorphism in Vitamin D receptor, and colorectal adenoma risk. Cancer Epidemiol Biomarkers Prev. 2004;13(4):546-52.
560. Ma J. Vitamin D receptor polymorphisms, circulating vitamin D metabolites, and risk of prostate cancer in United States physicians. Cancer Epidemiol Biomarkers Prev. 1998;7(5):385-90.
561. Hou MF. Association of vitamin D receptor gene polymorphism with sporadic breast cancer in Taiwanese patients. Breast Cancer Res Treat. 2002;74(1):1-7.
562. Liu HB. Estrogen receptor alpha mediates estrogen's immune protection in autoimmune disease. Immunol. 2003;171(12):6936-40.
563. Hayes CE. The immunological functions of the vitamin D endocrine system. Cell Mol Biol. 2003;49(2):277-300.
564. Tang S, Han H, Bajic VB. ERGDB: Estrogen Responsive Genes Database. Nucleic Acids Res. 2004;32(Database issue):D533-36.
565. Yale Department of Ob/Gyn website. Sex hormones and the immune system. http://info.med.yale.edu/obgyn/reproimmuno/projects/hormones.html
566. Pasqualini JR, Chetrite GS. Recent insight on the control of enzymes involved in estrogen formation and transformation in human breast cancer. J Steroid Biochem Mol Biol. 2005;93(2-5):221-36.
567. Plante J. Your Life In Your Hands. Thomas Dunne Books, 2000, New York, NY.
568. Cramer DW. Characteristics of women with a family history of ovarian cancer. I. Galactose consumption and metabolism. Cancer. 1994;74(4):1309-17.
569. Rock CL. Effects of a high-fiber, low-fat diet intervention on serum concentrations of reproductive steroid hormones in women with a history of breast cancer. J Clin Oncol. 2004;22(12):2379-87.
570. Mozaffarian WT. Dietary intake of *trans* fatty acids and systemic inflammation in women. Am J Clin Nutr. 2004;79(4):606-12.
571. Hanausek M. Detoxifying cancer causing agents to prevent cancer. Integr Cancer Ther. 2003;2(2):139-44.
572. Warburg O. On the origin of cancer cells. Science. 1956;123:309-14.
573. Michnovicz JJ. Changes in levels of urinary estrogen metabolites after oral indole-3-carinol treatment in humans. J Natl Cancer Inst. 1997;89(10):718-23.
574. Bradlow HL. Multifunctional aspects of the action of indeole-3-carinol as an antitumor agent. Ann N Y Acad Sci. 1999;889:204-13.
575. Wallace JM. Nutritional and botanical modulation of the inflammatory cascade—eicosanoids, cyclooxygenases, and lipoxygenases—as an adjunct in cancer therapy. Integr Cancer Ther. 2002;1(1):7-37.
576. Takada Y, Bhardwaj A, Potdar P, Aggarwal BB. Nonsteroidal anti-inflammatory agents differ in their ability to suppress NF-kappaB activation, inhibition of expression of cyclooxygenase-2 and cyclin D1, and abrogation of tumor cell proliferation. Oncogene. 2004;23(57):9247-58.
577. Lemay M, Murray MA, Davies A, et al. *In vitro* and ex vivo cyclooxygenase inhibition by a hops extract. Asia Pac j Clin Nutr. 2004;13(Suppl):S110.
578. Darshan S, Doreswamy R. Patented antiinflammatory plant drug development from traditional medicine. Phytother Res. 2004;18(5):343-57.
579. Zhu BT. Dietary administration of an extract from rosemary leaves enhances the liver microsomal metabolism of endogenous estrogens and decreases their uterotropic action in CD-1 mice. Carcinogenesis 1998;19(10):1821-27.
580. Goud VK. Effect of turmeric on xenobiotic metabolizing enzymes. Plant Foods Hum Nutr 1993;44(1):87-92.
581. Wuttke W, Jarry H, Christoffel V, et al. Chase tree (Vitex agnus-castus)—pharmacology and clinical indications. Phytomedicine. 2003;10(4):348-57.
582. Tesch BJ. Herbs commonly used by women: an evidence-based review. Am J Obstet Gynecol. 2003;188(5 Suppl):S44-55.
583. Shalan MG, Mostafa MS, Hassouna MM, et al. Amelioration of lead toxicity on rat liver with vitamin C and silymarin supplements. Toxicology. 2005;206(1):1-15.
584. Lieber CS. Silymarin retards the progression of alcohol-induced hepatic fibrosis in baboons. J Clin Gastroenterol. 2003;37(4):335-39.
585. Van Duursen MB. Phytochemicals inhibit catechol-o-methyltransferase activity in cytosolic fractions from healthy human mammary tissues: implications for catechol estrogen-induced DNA damage. Toxicol Sci. 2004;81(2):316-24.
586. Hirata JD. Does dong quai have estrogenic effects in postmenopausal women? A double-blind, placebo-controlled trial. Fertil Steril. 1997;68(6):981-86.
587. Aliciguzel Y. N-acetyl cysteine, L0cysteine, and beta-mercaptoethanol augment selenium-glutathione peroxidase activity in glucose-6-phosphate dehydrogenase-deficient human erythrocytes. Clin Exp Med. 2004;4(1):50-55.
588. Wu G. Arginine deficiency in preterm infants: biochemical and nutritional implications. J Nutr Biochem. 2004;15(8):442-51.
589. Schmedes A. Low S-Adenosylmethionine concentrations found in patients with severe inflammatory bowel disease. Clin Chem Lab Med. 2004;42(6):648-53.
590. Rampersaud GC, Bailey LB, Kauwell GP. Relationship of folate to colorectal and cervical cancer: review and recommendations for practitioners. J Am Diet Assoc. 2002;102(9):1273-82.
591. Selhub J. Folate, vitamin B12 and vitamin B6 and one carbon metabolism. J Nutr Health Aging. 2002;6(1):39-42.

592. Goodman JE, Jensen LT, He P, Yager JD. Characterization of human soluble high and low activity catechol-O-methyltransferase catalyzed catechol estrogen methylation. Pharmacogenetics. 2002;12(7):517-528.
593. Kurzer MS. Hormonal effects of soy in premenopausal women and men. J Nutr. 2002;132(3):570S-73S.
594. Kroneberg F, Fugh-Berman A. Complementary and alternative medicine for menopausal symptoms: a review of randomized controlled trials. Ann Intern Med. 2002;137:805-13.
595. Malafa MP. Vitamin E succinate promotes breast cancer tumor dormancy. J Surg Res. 2000;93(1):163-70.
596. Suarez A, Ramirez-Tortosa M, Gil A, Faus MJ. Addition of vitamin E to long-chain polyunsaturated fatty acid-enriched diets protects neonatal tissue lipids against peroxidation in rats. Eur J Nutr. 1999;38(4):169-76.
597. Wylie-Rosett J. Menopause, micronutrients, and hormone therapy. Am J Clin Nutr. 2005;81(5):1223S-31S.
598. Barton DL. Prospective evaluation of vitamin E for hot flashes in breast cancer survivors. J. Clin Oncol. 1998;16:495-500.
599. Ziaei S A randomized controlled trial of vitamin E in the treatment of primary dysmenorrhoea. BJOG. 2005;112(4):466-69.
600. Dawson-Hughes B. Racial/ethnic considerations in making recommendations for vitamin D for adult and elderly men and women. Am J Clin Nutr. 2004;80(6 Suppl):1763S-67.
601. Young MV, Schwartz GG, Wang L. et al. The prostate 25-hydroxyvitamin D-1 alpha-hydroxylase is not influenced by parathyroid hormone and calcium: implications for prostate cancer chemoprevention by vitamin D. Carcinogenesis. 2004;25(6):967-71.
602. Welsh J. Vitamin D and breast cancer: insights from animal models. Am J Clin Nutr. 2004;80(6 Suppl):1721S-24S.
603. Harris DM, Go VL. Vitamin D and colon carcinogenesis. J Nutr. 2004;124(12 Suppl):3463S-71S.
604. Walaszek Z. Metabolism, uptake, and excretion of a D-glucaric acid salt and its potential use in cancer prevention. Cancer Detect Prev. 1997;21(2):178-90.
605. Calcium-D-glucarate. Altern Med Rev. 2002;7(4):336-39.
606. Valko M, Isakovic M, Mazur M et al. Role of oxygen radicals in DNA damage and cancer incidence. Mol Cell Biochem. 2004;266(1-2):37-56.
607. Beeharry N, Lowe JE, Hernandez AR, et al. Linoleic acid and antioxidants protect against DNA damage and apoptosis induced by palmitic acid. Mutat Res. 2003;530(1-2):27-33.
608. Olufowobi O, Sharif K, Papaionnou S, et al. Are the anticipated benefits of myomectomy achieved in women of reproductive age? A 5-year review of the results at a UK tertiary hospital. J Obstet Gynaecol. 2004;24(4):434-40.
609. Akinyemi BO, Adewoye BR, Fakoya TA. Uterine fibroid: a review. Niger J Med. 2004;13(4):318-29.
610. Olufowobi O, Sharif K, Papaionnou S, et al. Are the anticipated benefits of myomectomy achieved in women of reproductive age? A 5-year review of the results at a UK tertiary hospital. J Obstet Gynaecol. 2004;24(4):434-40.
611. Vikhliaeva EM. [Molecular-genetic determinants of the neoplastic process and state-of-the-art treatment of patients with uterine leiomyoma.] Vopr Onkol. 2001;47(2):200-4.
612. Reed SD, Cushing-Haugen KL, Daling JR, et al. Postmenopausal estrogen and progestogen therapy and the risk of uterine leiomyomas. Menopause. 2004;11(2):214-22.
613. Palomba S, Orio F Jr, Russo T, et al. Long-term effectiveness and safety of GnRH agonist plus raloxifene administration in women with uterine leiomyomas. Hum Reprod. 2004;19(6):1308-14.
614. Imai A, Sugiyama M, Furui T, Tamaya T. Treatment of perimenopausal women with uterine myoma: successful use of a depot GnRH agonist leading to a natural menopause. J Obstet Gynaecol. 2003;23(5):518-20.
615. Vercellini P, Trespidi L, Zaina B, et al. Gonadotropin-releasing hormone agonist treatment before abdominal myomectomy: a controlled trial. Fertil Steril. 2003;79(6):1390-95.
616. Nasir L, Bope ET. Management of pelvic pain from dysmenorrhea or endometriosis. J Am Board Fam Pract. 2004;17:S43-47.
617. Bulun SE, Fang Z, Imir G, et al. Aromatase and endometriosis. Semin Repr Med. 2004;22(1):45-50.
618. Ibid.
619. Lawrence HP. Salivary markers of systemic disease: noninvasive diagnosis of disease and monitoring of general health. J Can Dent Assoc. 2002; 68(3):170-74.
620. Simpson ER. Sources of estrogen and their importance. J Steroid Biochem Mol Biol. 2003;86(3-5):225-30.
621. Shozu M, Murakami K, Inoue M. Aromatase and leiomyoma of the uterus. Semin Repr Med. 2004;22(1):51-60.
622. Bulun SE, Fang Z, Imir G, et al. Aromatase and endometriosis. Semin Repr Med. 2004;22(1):45-50.
623. Ibid.
624. Shozu M, Murakami K, Inoue M. Aromatase and leiomyoma of the uterus. Semin Repr Med. 2004;22(1):51-60.
625. Heber D. The linkage between obesity and prostate cancer. PCRI Insights. 2004;7(2).
626. Eng ET, Williams D, Mandava U, et al. Anti-aromatase chemicals in red wine. Ann N Y Acad Sci. 2002;963:239-46
627. Wang C, Makela T, Hase T, et al. Lignans and flavonoids inhibit aromatase enzyme in human preadipocytes. J Steroid Biochem Molec Biol. 1994;50(3-4):205-12.
628. Ibid.
629. Drozak J, Bryla J. [Dopamine: not just a neurotransmitter.] Postepy Hig Med Dosw (Online). 2005;59:405-20.
630. Pharmacology of dopamine neurons. In Psychopharmacology : the 4th Generation of Progress. Bloom FE and Kupfer DJ (Eds). Lippincott Williams & Wilkins, 4th ed. 1995.
631. Luciana M, Collins PF, Depue RA. Opposing roles for dopamine and serotonin in the modulation of human spatial working memory functions. Cereb Cortex. 1998;8(3):218-26.
632. Depue RA, Collins PF. Neurobiology of the structure of personality: dopamine, facilitation of incentive motivation, and extraversion. Behav Brain Sci. 1999;22(3):491-517.
633. Asherson P, Kuntsi J, Taylor E. Unravelling the complexity of attention-deficit hyperactivity disorder: a behavioural genomic approach. Br J Psychiatry. 2005;187:103-5.
634. Russell VA, Sagvolden T, Johansen EB. Animal models of attention-deficit hyperactivity disorder. Behav Brain Funct. 2005;1:9.
635. Krause J, la Fougere C, Krause KH, et al. Influence of striatal dopamine transporter availability on the response to methylphenidate in adult patients with ADHD. Eur Arch Psychiatry Clin Neurosci. 2005;Aug 17:[Epub ahead of print].
636. Rosin C, Colombo S, Calver AA, et al. Dopamine D2 and D3 receptor agonists limit oligodendrocyte injury caused by glutamate oxidative stress and oxygen/glucose deprivation. Glia. 2005;Aug 2:[Epub ahead of print].
637. Chou IC, Tsai CH, Lee CC, et al. Association analysis between Tourette's syndrome and dopamine D1 receptor gene in Taiwanese children. Psychiatr Genet. 2004;14(4):219-21.
638. Diaz-Anzaldua A, Joober R, Riviere JB, et al. Tourette syndrome and dopaminergic genes: a family-based association study in the French Canadian founder population. Mol Psychiatry. 2004;9(3):272-7.

639. Lam KS, Aman MG, Arnold LE. Neurochemical correlates of autistic disorder: A review of the literature. Res Dev Disabil. 2005;July 4:[Epub ahead of print].
640. Pinborg LH, Ziebell M, Frokjaer VG, et al. Quantification of 123I-PE2I binding to dopamine transporter with SPECT after bolus and bolus/infusion. J Nucl Med. 2005;46(7):1119-27.
641. Zametkin AJ, Nordahl TE, Gross M, et al. Cerebral glucose metabolism in adults with hyperactivity of childhood onset. N Engl J Med. 1990;323(20):1361-6.
642. Seeman P, Nizaik HB, Guan HC. Elevation of D2 dopamine receptors in schizophrenia is underestimated by radioactive raclopride Arch Gen Psychiatry. 1990;47(12):1170-1172.
643. Cleren C, Calingasan NY, Chen J, Beal MF. Celastrol protects against MPTP- and 3-nitropropionic acid-induced neurotoxicity. J Neurochem. 2005;94(4):995-1004.
644. Norton N, Owen MJ. HTR2A: association and expression studies in neuropsychiatric genetics. Ann Med. 2005;37(2):121-9.
645. Maes M, Jacobs MP, Suy E, et al. Suppressant effects of dexamethasone on the availability of plasma L-tryptophan and tyrosine in healthy controls and in depressed patients. Acta Psychiatr Scand. 1990;81(1);19-23.
646. Simpson HB, Fallon BA. Obsessive-compulsive disorder: an overview. J Psychiatr Pract. 2000;6(1):3-17.
647. Fallon BA, Mathew SJ. Biological therapies for obsessive-compulsive disorder. J Psychiatr Pract. 2000;6(3):113-28.
648. Lam KS, Aman MG, Arnold LE. Neurochemical correlates of autistic disorder: A review of the literature. Res Dev Disabil. 2005;July 4:[Epub ahead of print].
649. Owens MJ, Nemeroff CB. Role of serotonin in the pathophysiology of depression: focus on the serotonin transporter. Clin Chem 1994;40(2):288-95.
650. Drevets, WC, Spitznagel E, Raichle, ME. Functional anatomical differences between major depressive subtypes. In XVII International Symposium on Cerebral Blood Flow and Metabolism. Cologne, Germany, July 1995. J Cereb Blood Flow Metab. 1995;15(Suppl 1):S1-886.
651. Chugani DC. Serotonin in autism and pediatric epilepsies. Ment Retard Dev. Disabil Res Rev. 2004;10(2):112-6.
652. Sutcliffe JS, Delahanty RS, Prasad HC, et al. Allelic heterogeneity at the serotonin transporter locus (SLC6A4) confers susceptibility to autism and rigid-compulsive behaviors. Am J Hum Genet. 2005; 77(2):265-79.
653. Holden C. Neuroscience mutant gene tied to poor serotonin production and depression. Science. 2004;306(5704):2023.
654. Gondo Y, Hirose N, Arai Y, et al. Contribution of an affect-associated gene to human longevity: Prevalence of the long-allele genotype of the serotonin transporter-linked gene in Japanese centenarians. Mech Ageing Dev. 2005;Aug 8:[Epub ahead of print].
655. McCarty MF. High-dose pyridoxine as an 'anti-stress' strategy. Med Hypotheses. 2000;54(5):803-7.
656. Souder E. Neuropathology in Alzheimer's disease: target of pharmacotherapy. J Am Acad Nurse Pract. 2005;March(Suppl):3-5.
657. Poon HF, Shepherd HM, Reed TT, et al. Proteomics analysis provides insight into caloric restriction mediated oxidation and expression of brain proteins associated with age-related impaired cellular processes: Mitochondrial dysfunction, glutamate dysregulation and impaired protein synthesis. Neurobiol Aging. 2005;July 1:[Epub ahead of print].
658. Neale JH, Olszewski RT, Gehl LM, et al. The neurotransmitter N-acetylaspartylglutamate in models of pain, ALS, diabetic neuropathy, CNS injury and schizophrenia. Trends Pharmacol Sci. 2005;July 28:[Epub ahead of print].
659. Hoekstra R, Fekkes D, Loonen AJ, et al. Bipolar mania and plasma amino acids: Increased levels of glycine. Eur Neuropsychopharmacol. 2005;July 14:[Epub ahead of print].
660. D'Andrea G, Allais G, Grazzi L, Fumagalli L. Migraine with aura from pathophysiology to treatment: therapeutic strategies. Neurol Sci. 2005;26(Suppl2):s104-7.
661. Neale JH, Olszewski RT, Gehl LM, et al. The neurotransmitter N-acetylaspartylglutamate in models of pain, ALS, diabetic neuropathy, CNS injury and schizophrenia. Trends Pharmacol Sci. 2005;July 28:[Epub ahead of print].
662. Ackl N, Ising M, Schreiber YA, et al. Hippocampal metabolic abnormalities in mild cognitive impairment and Alzheimer's disease. Neurosci Lett. 2005;384(1-2):23-8.
663. Miyaoka T, Yasukawa R, Mizuno S, et al. Proton magnetic resonance spectroscopy (1H-MRS) of hippocampus, basal ganglia, and vermis of cerebellum in schizophrenia associated with idiopathic unconjugated hyperbilirubinemia (Gilbert's syndrome). J Psychiatr Es. 2005;39(1):29-34.
664. Lleo A, Greenberg SM, Growdon JH. Current pharmacotherapy for Alzheimer's disease. Annu Rev Med. 2005;Aug11:[Epub ahead of print].
665. Arnsten AF, Dudley AG. Methylphenidate improves prefrontal cortical cognitive function through α2 adrenoceptor and dopamine D1 receptor actions: Relevance to therapeutic effects in Attention Deficit Hyperactivity Disorder. Behav Brain Funct. 2005;1(1):2.
666. Roman T, Rohde LA, Hutz MH. Polymorphisms of the dopamine transporter gene: influence on response to methylphenidate in attention deficit-hyperactivity disorder. Am J Pharmacogenomics. 2004;4 (2):83-92.
667. Yu Z, Luo H, Fu W, Mattson MP. The endoplasmic reticulum stress-responsive protein GRP78 protects neurons against excitotoxicity and apoptosis: suppression of oxidative stress and stabilization of calcium homeostasis. Exp Neurol. 1999;155(2):302-14.
668. Alexandre S, Nakaki T, Vanhamme L, Lee AS. A binding site for the cyclic adenosine 3',5'-monophosphate-response element-binding protein as a regulatory element in the grp78 promoter. Mol Endocrinol. 1991;5(12):1862-72.
669. Sharma A, Waly M, Deth RC. Protein kinase C regulates dopamine D4 receptor-mediated phospholipid methylation. Eur J Pharmacol. 2001;427(2):83-90.
670. Alpert JE, Fava M., Nutrition and depression: the role of folate. Nut Rev. 1997;55(5):145-9.
671. Bolander-Gouaille C. Treatment of depression: time to consider folic acid and vitamin B12. J Psychopharmacol. 2005;19(1):59-65.
672. Alpert JE, Fava M., Nutrition and depression: the role of folate. Nut Rev. 1997;55(5):145-9.
673. Bowers MB, Reynolds EH. Cerebrospinal-fluid folate and acid monoamine metabolites. Lancet. 1972;2:1376.
674. Vielhaber K, Riemann D, Feige B, et al. Impact of experimentally induced serotonin deficiency by tryptophan depletion on saliva cortisol concentrations. Pharmacopsychiatry. 2005;38(2):87-94.
675. Markus CR, Olivier B, Panhuysen GE, et al. The bovine protein—lactalbumin increases the plasma ratio of tryptophan to the other large neutral amino acids, and in vulnerable subjects raises brain serotonin activity, reduces cortisol concentration, and improves mood under stress. Am J Clin Nutr. 2000;71(6):1536-54.
676. Stoll AL, Severus WE. Mood stabilizers: shared mechanisms of action at postsynaptic signal-transduction and kindling processes. Harv Rev Psychiatry. 1996;4(2):77-89.
677. Strokin M, Sergeeva M, Reiser G. Role of Ca2+-independent phospholipase A2 and n-3 polyunsaturated fatty acid docosahexaenoic acid in prostanoid production in brain: perspectives for protection in neuroinflammation. Int J Dev Neurosci. 2004;22(7):551-7.

678. Yu AC, Chan PH, Fishman RA; Arachidonic acid inhibits uptake of glutamate and glutamine but not of GABA in cultured cerebellar granule cells. J Neurosci Res. 1987 ;17(4):424-7.
679. Delion J, Chalon S, Guilloteau D, et al. alpha-Linolenic acid dietary deficiency alters age-related changes of dopaminergic and serotoninergic neurotransmission in the rat frontal cortex. J Neurochem. 1996;66(4):1582-91.
680. Peet M, Murphy B, Shay J, Horrobin D. Depletion of omega-3 fatty acids levels in red blood cell membranes of depressive patients. Biol Psychiatry 1998;43(5):315-9.
681. Kobayashi M, Kurihara K, Matsuoka I. Retinoic acid induces BDNF responsiveness of sympathetic neurons by alteration of Trk neurotrophin receptor expression. FEBS Lett. 1994;346(1):60-5.
682. Wang HF, Liu FC. Regulation of multiple dopamine signal transduction molecules by retinoids in the developing striatum. Neuroscience. 2005;134(1):97-105.
683. Misner DL, Jacobs S, Shimizu Y, et al. Vitamin A deprivation results in reversible loss of hippocampal long-term synaptic plasticity. Proc Nat Acad Sci. 2001;98(20):11714-9.
684. Goodman AB, Three independent lines of evidence suggest retinoids as causal to schizophrenia. Proc Natl Acad Sci. 1998;95(13):7240-4.
685. Macchi MM, Bruce JN. Human pineal physiology and functional significant of melatonin. Front Neuroendocrinol. 2004;25(3-4):177-95.
686. Zisapel N. Melatonin-dopamine interactions: from brain neurochemistry to a clinical setting. Cell Mol Neurobiol. 2001; 21(6):605-16.
687. Andrabi SA, Sayeed I, Sieman D, et al. Direct inhibition of the mitochondrial permeability transition pore: a possible mechanism responsible for anti-apoptotic effects of melatonin. FASEB J. 2004;18(7):869-71.
688. McIlwain H, Poll JD. Interaction between adenosine generated endogenously in neocortical tissue and homocysteine and its thiolactone. Neurochem Int. 1985;7:103.
689. Macchi MM, Bruce JN. Human pineal physiology and functional significant of melatonin. Front Neuroendocrinol. 2004;25(3-4):177-95.
690. Monteleone P, Natale M, La Rocca A, Maj M. Decreased nocturnal secretion of melatonin in drug-free schizophrenics: no change after subchronic treatment with antipsychotics. Neuropsychobiology 1997;36(4):159-63.
691. Tordjman S, Anderson GM, Pichard N, et al. Nocturnal excretion of 6-sulphatoxymelatonin in children and adolescents with autistic disorder. Biol Psychiatry. 2005;57(2):134-8.
692. Kulman G, Lissoni P, Rovelli F, et al. Evidence of pineal endocrine hypofunction in autistic children. Neuro Endocrinol Lett. 2000;21(1):31-34.
693. Shamir E, Laudon M, Barak Y, et al. Melatonin improves sleep quality of patients with chronic schizophrenia. J Clin Psychiatry. 2000;61(5):373-7.
694. Hayashi E. Effect of melatonin on sleep-wake rhythm: the sleep diary of an autistic male. Psychiatry Clin Neurosci. 2000;54(3):383-4.
695. Jan JE, O'Donnell ME. Use of melatonin in the treatment of paediatric sleep disorders. J Pineal Res. 1996;21(4):193-9.
696. Decollogne S, Tomas A, Lecerf C, et al. NMDA receptor complex blockade by oral administration of magnesium: comparison with MK-801. Pharmacol Biochem Behavior .1997;58(1):261-8.
697. Belfort MA. Is high cerebral perfusion pressure and cerebral flow predictive of impending seizures in preeclampsia? A case report. Hypertens Pregnancy. 2005;24(1):59-63.
698. Sandor PS, Afra J. Nonpharmacologic treatment of migraine. Curr Pain Headache Rep. 2005;9(3):202-5.
699. Mauskop A, Altura BA. Role of magnesium in the pathogenesis and treatment of migraines. Clin Neurosci. 1998;5(1):24-27.
700. Muir KW. New experimental and clinical data on the efficacy of pharmacological magnesium infusions in cerebral infarcts. Magnes Res.. 1998;11(1):43-56.
701. Gil-Bea FS, Garcia-Alloza M, Dominguez J, et al. Evaluation of cholinergic markers in Alzheimer's disease and in a model of cholinergic deficit. Neurosci Lett. 2005; 375(1): 37-41.
702. Wang R, Tang XC. Neuroprotective effects of huperzine A. A natural cholinesterase inhibitor for the treatment of Alzheimer's disease. Neurosignals. 2005;14(1-2):71-82.
703. Tang XC, Kindel GH, Kozikowski AP, Hanin I. Comparison of the effects of natural and synthetic huperzine-A on rat brain cholinergic function *in vitro* and *in vivo*. J Ethnopharmacol. 1994;44(3):147-55.
704. Hanin I, Tang XC, Kozikowski AP. Natural and synthetic Huperzine A: effect on cholinergic function *in vitro* and *in vivo*. Ann N Y Acad Sci. 1993;695:304-6.
705. Wang R, Tang XC. Neuroprotective affects of huperzine A. A natural cholinesteric inhibitor for the treatment of Alzheimer's disease. Neurosignals. 2005;14(1-2):71-82.
706. Ayala CA. Stimulation of choline acetyl transferase activity by 1- and d-carnitine in brain areas of neonate rats. J Neurosci Res. 1995;41(3):403-8.
707. Ames BN, Liu J. Delaying the mitochondrial decay of aging with acetylcarnitine Ann NY Acad Sci. 2004;1033:108-16.
708. Medline Medical Encyclopedia. Accessed at http://www.nlm.nih.gov/medlineplus/ency/article/003684.htm 7/8/05.
709. American Association of Clinical Endocrinologists. American Association of Clinical Endocrinologists medical guidelines for clinical practice for the evaluation and treatment of hyperthyroidism and hypothyroidism. Endocr Pract. 2002;8(6):457-69.
710. Bouknight AL. Thyroid physiology and thyroid function testing. Otolaryngol Clin North Am. 2003;36(1):9-15.
711. Pimentel L, Hansen KN. Thyroid disease in the emergency department: a clinical and laboratory review. J Emerg Med. 2005;28(2):201-9.
712. Andersen S, Pedersen KM, Bruun NH, Laurberg P. Narrow individual variations in serum T(4) and T(3) in normal subjects: a clued to the understanding of subclinical thyroid disease. J Clin Endocrinol Metab. 2002;87(3):1068-72.
713. Klee GG. Clinical interpretation of reference intervals and reference limits. A plea for assay harmonization. Clin Chem Lab Med. 2004;42(7):752-57.
714. Kelly G. Peripheral metabolism of thyroid hormones: A review. At Med Rev. 2000;5(4):206-333.
715. Sebe A, Satar S, Sari A. Thyroid storm induced by aspirin intoxication and the effect of hemodialysis: a case report. Adv Ther. 2004;21(3):173-77.
716. Tiihonen M, Liewendahl K, Waltimo O, et al. Thyroid status of patients receiving long-term anticonvulsant therapy assessed by peripheral parameters: a placebo-controlled thyroxine therapy trial. Epilepsia. 1995;36(11):1118-25.
717. Balon R, Pohl R, Yeragani VK, et al. The changes of thyroid hormone during pharmacological treatment of panic disorder patients. Prog Neuropsychopharmacol Biol Psychiatry. 1991;15(5):595-600.
718. Thomson JE, Baird SG, Beastall GH, et al. The effect of intravenous heparin infusions on the thyroid stimulating hormone response to thyrotrophin releasing hormone. Br J Clin Pharmacol. 1978;6(3):239-42.
719. Doerge DR, Chang HC. Inactivation of thyroid peroxidase by soy isoflavones, *in vitro* and *in vivo*. J Chromatogr B Analyt Technol Biomed Life Sci. 2002;777(1-2):269-79.

720. Doerge DR, Sheehan DM. Goitrogenic and estrogenic activity of soy isoflavones. Environ Health Perspect. 2002;110(Suppl 3):349-53.
721. Stoewsand GS. Bioactive organosulfur phytochemicals in Brassica oleracea vegetables—a review. Food Chem Toxicol. 1995;33(6):537-43.
722. Conaway CC, Getahun SM, Liebest LL, et al. Disposition of glucosinolates and sulforaphane in humans after ingestion of steamed and fresh broccoli. Nutr Cancer. 2000;38(2):168-78.
723. Rouzaud G, Young SA, Duncan AJ. Hydrolysis of glucosinolates to isothiocyanates after ingestion of raw or microwaved cabbage by human volunteers. Cancer Epidemiol Biomarkers Prev. 2004;13(1):125-31.
724. Greenspan FS. Chapter 7, Thyroid Gland, In: Greenspan FS, Gardner DG. Basic and Clinical Endocrinology, 5th ed. New York: Appleton & Lange; 1997, p. 192-262.
725. Yoon SJ, Choi SR, Kim DM, et al. The effect of iodine restriction on thyroid function in patients with hypothyroidism due to Hashimoto's thyroiditis. Yonsei Med J. 2003;44(2):227-35.
726. Khashu M, Chessex P, Chanoine JP. Iodine overload and severe hypothyroidism in a premature neonate. J Pediatr Surg. 2005;40(2):E1-4.
727. Information from the Linus Pauling Institute; accessed at http://lpi.oregonstate.edu/infocenter/vitamins/vitaminA/.
728. Institute for Functional Medicine, Clinical Nutrition, 2nd Edition. Liska D, Quinn S, eds. Gig Harbor, WA: IFM; 2004, p. 184.
729. Faure P, Ducros V, Couzy F, et al. Rapidly exchangeable pool study of zinc in free-living or institutionalized elderly women. Nutrition. 2005;21(7-8):831-37.
730. Laurberg P, Andersen S, Bulow Pedersen I, Carle A. Hypothyroidism in the elderly: pathophysiology, diagnosis and treatment. Drugs Aging. 2005;22(1):23-38.
731. Thomopoulos P.[Iodine excess and thyroid dysfunction.] Rev Prat. 2005;55(2):180-82.
732. Davis KD, Lazar MA. Selective antagonism of thyroid hormone action by retinoic acid. J Biol Chem. 1992;5:3185-89.
733. Murphy J, Cashman KD. Selenium status of Irish adults: evidence of insufficiency. Ir J Med Sci. 2002;171(2):81-84.
734. Zhang ZW, Shimbo S, Qu JB, et al. Dietary selenium intake of Chinese adult women in the 1990s. Biol Trace Elem Res. 2001;80(2):125-38.
735. Beckett GJ, Arthur JR. Selenium and endocrine systems. J Endocrinol. 2005;184(3):455-65.
736. Gartner R, Gasnier BCH, Dietrich JW, et al. Selenium supplementation in patients with autoimmune thyroiditis decreases thyroid peroxidase antibodies concentration. J Clin Endocrinol Metab. 2002;87(4):1687-91.
737. Pimentel L, Hansen KN. Thyroid disease in the emergency department: a clinical and laboratory review. J Emerg Med. 2005;28(2):201-9.
738. Prummel MF, Strieder T, Wiersinga WM. The environment and autoimmune thyroid disease. Invited review. Eur J Endocrinol. 2004;150:605-618.
739. Bacic-Vrca V, Skreb F, Cepelak I, et al. The effect of antioxidant supplementation on superoxide dismutase activity, Cu and Zn levels, and total antioxidant status in erythrocytes of patients with Graves' disease. Clin Chem Lab Med. 2005;43(4):383-88.
740. Dobrzynska MM, Baumgartner A, Anderson D. Antioxidants modulate thyroid hormone-and noradrenaline-induced DNA damage in human sperm. Mutagenesis. 2004;19(4):325-30.
741. Karbownik M, Lewinski A. The role of oxidative stress in physiological and pathological processes in the thyroid gland; possible involvement in pineal-thyroid interactions. Neuro Endocrinol Lett. 2003;24(5):293-303.
742. Deshpande UR, Joseph LJ, Patwardhan UN, Samuel AM. Effect of antioxidants (vitamin C, E and turmeric extract) on methimazole induced hypothyroidism in rats. Indian J Exp Biol. 2002;40(6):735-38.
743. Connolly J, Romano T, Patruno M. Selections from current literature: effects of dieting and exercise on resting metabolic rate and implications for weight management. Fam Pract. 1999:16(2):196-201.
744. Ibid.
745. Abdel-Hamid TK. Exercise and diet in obesity treatment: an integrative system dynamics perspective. Med Sci Sports Exerc. 2003;35(3):400-13.
746. Kaufman BA, Warren MP, Dominguez JE, et al. Bone density and amenorrhea in ballet dancers are related to a decreased resting metabolic rate and lower leptin levels. J Clin Endocrinol Metab. 2002;87(6):2777-83.
747. Greenspan FS. Chapter 7, The Thyroid Gland, In: Greenspan FS, Gardner DG. Basic and Clinical Endocrinology, 5th ed. New York: Appleton & Lange; 1997, p. 192-262.
748. Quadbeck B, Janssen OE, Mann K. [Problems and new developments in the management of Graves' disease: medical therapy.] Z Arztl Fortbild Qualitatssich. 2004;98(Suppl 5):37-44.
749. Jooste PL, Weight MJ, Kriek JA, Louw AJ. Endemic goiter in the absence of iodine deficiency in schoolchildren of the Northern Cape Province of South Africa. Eur J Clin Nutr. 1999;53(1):8-12.
750. Shulamn KI, Sykora K, Gill SS, et al. New thyroxine treatment in older adults beginning lithium therapy: implications for clinical practice. Am J Geriatr Psychiatry. 2005;13(4):299-304.
751. Vannucchi G, Chiti A, Mannavola D, et al. Radioiodine treatment of non-toxic multinodular goiter: effects of combination with lithium. Eur J Nucl Med Mol Imaging. 2005;May 4:[Epub ahead of print].
752. Feret BM, Caley CF. Possible hypothyroidism associated with quetiapine. Ann Pharmacother. 2000;34(4):483-86.
753. Saad A, Falciglia M, Steward DL, Nikiforov YE. Amiodarone-induced thyrotoxicosis and thyroid cancer: clinical, immunohistochemical, and molecular genetic studies of a case and review of the literature. Arch Pathol Lab Med. 2004;128(7):807-10.
754. Roffi M, Cattaneo F, Brandle M. Thyrotoxicosis and the cardiovascular system. Minerva Endocrinol. 2005;30(2):47-58.
755. Moura EG, Moura CC. [Regulation of thyrotropin synthesis and secretion.] Arq Bras Endocrinol Metabol. 2004;48(1):40-52.
756. Jereczek-Fossa BA, Alterio D, Jassem J, et al. Radiotherapy-induced thyroid disorders. Cancer Treat Rev. 2004;30(4):369-84.
757. Ganong, WF. Review of Medical Physiology, 19th ed. New York: Appelton-Lange, p. 303-317.
758. Ibid.
759. Pinchera, A. Endocrinology and Metabolism, McGraw Hill, 2001, p.139-216.
760. Greenspan FS. Chapter 7, The Thyroid Gland, In: Greenspan FS, Gardner DG. Basic and Clinical Endocrinology, 5th ed. New York: Appleton & Lange; 1997, p. 192-262.
761. Tas S, Dirican M, Sarandol E, Serdar Z. The effect of taurine supplementation on oxidative stress in experimental hypothyroidism. Cell Biochem Funct. 2004;Dec 22; published online. Accessed at http://www3.interscience.wiley.com/cgi-bin/abstract/109860313/ABSTRACT.
762. Sarandol E, Tas S, Dirican M, Serdar Z. Oxidative stress and serum paraoxonase activity in experimental hypothyroidism: effect of vitamin E supplementation. Cell Biochem Funct. 2005;23(1):1-8.
763. Fletcher N, Giese N, Schmidt C, et al. Altered retinoid metabolism in female Long-Evans and Han/Wistar rats following long-term 2,3,7,8-tetrachlorodibenzo-p-dioxin (TCDD)-treatment. Toxicol Sci. 2005;86(2):264-272.

764. Darnerud PO. Toxic effects of brominated flame retardants in man and in wildlife. Environ Int. 2003;29(6):841-53.
765. Hall AJ, Kalantzi OI, Thomas GO. Polybrominated diphenyl ethers (PBDEs) in grey seals during their first year of life—are they thyroid hormone endocrine disrupters? Environ Pollut. 2003;126(1):29-37.
766. Kato Y, Haraguchi K, Yamazaki T, et al. Effects of polychlorinated biphenyls, kanechlor-500, on serum thyroid hormone levels in rats and mice. Toxicol Sci. 2003;72(2):235-41.
767. Zhou T, Taylor MM, DeVito MJ, Crofton KM. Developmental exposure to brominated diphenyl ethers results in thyroid hormone disruption. Toxicol Sci. 2002;66(1):105-16.
768. Hallgren S, Darnerud PO. Polybrominated diphenyl ethers (PBDEs), polychlorinated biphenyls (PCVs) and chlorinated paraffins (CPs) in rats—testing interactions and mechanisms for thyroid hormone effects. Toxicology. 2002;177(2-3):227-43.
769. Van Birgelen AP, Van der Kolk J, Fase KM, et al. Subchronic dose-response study of 2,3,7,8-tetrachlorodibenzo-p-dioxin in female Sprague-Dawley rats. Toxicol Appl Pharmacol. 1995;132(1):1-13.
770. Sengul E, Cetinarslan B, Tarkun I, et al. Homocysteine concentrations in subclinical hypothyroidism. Endocr Res. 2004;30(3):351-59.
771. Aldasouqi S, Nkansa-Dwamena D, Bokhari S, et al. Is subclinical hypothyroidism associated with hyperhomocysteinemia? Endocr Pract. 2004;10(5):399-403.
772. Roffi M, Cattaneo F, Brandle M. Thyrotoxicosis and the cardiovascular system. Minerva Endocrinol. 2005;30(2):47-58.
773. Jublanc C, Bruckert E. Hypothyroidism and cardiovascular disease risk: role of new risk factors and coagulation parameters. Semin Vasc Med. 2004;4(2):145-51.
774. Serter R, Demirbas B, Korukluoglu B, et al. The effect of L-thyroxine replacement therapy on lipid based cardiovascular risk in subclinical hypothyroidism. J Endocrinol Invest. 2004;27(10):897-903.
775. Kasperlik-Zaluska AA, Czarnocka B, Czech W. Autoimmunity as the most frequent cause of idiopathic secondary adrenal insufficiency: report of 111 cases. Autoimmunity. 2003;36(3):155-59.
776. Gaspari AA, Huang CM, Davey RJ, et al. Prevalence of thyroid abnormalities in patients with dermatitis herpetiformis and in control subjects with HLA-B8/-DR3. Am J Med. 1990;88(2):145-50.
777. Patinen P, Hietane J, Malmstrom M, et al. Iodine and gliadin challenge on oral mucosa in dermatitis herpetiformis. Acta Derm Venereol. 2002;82(2):86-89.
778. Rousset H. [A great imitator for the allergologist: intolerance to gluten.] Allerg Immunol (Paris). 2004;36(3):96-100.
779. Mainardi E, Montanelli A, Dotti M, et al. Thyroid-related autoantibodies and celiac disease: a role for a gluten-free diet? J Clin Gastroenterol. 2002;35(3):245-8.
780. Hauser P, Zametkin AJ, Martinez P. Attention deficit-hyperactivity disorder in people with generalized resistance to thyroid hormone. N Engl J Med. 1993;328:997-1001.

Chapter 33
Stress, Spirituality, Poverty, and Community—Effects on Health

Robert J. Hedaya, MD, FAPA

Introduction

Just as one uses different levels of magnification to thoroughly examine a sample under a microscope, so must the practitioner of functional medicine become adept at assessing the patient's health using a variety of lenses and perspectives. Applying this analogy, a high-magnification lens enables one to evaluate certain aspects of the functional medicine matrix (e.g., molecular and metabolic processes involved in the restoration of health, such as hormonal regulation or detoxification pathways), while a lower-magnification but broader lens enables one to evaluate intrapsychic processes (e.g., mental constructs such as attitudes and religious beliefs), and a perspective of even lower magnification assesses the broader contextual processes involved in the restoration of health (e.g., socioeconomic status, culture, and community). In this chapter, we will explore the health impact of some intrapsychic (stress, spirituality, religion) and contextual factors (community and poverty), and then discuss some practical approaches the clinician can use to weave these essential components of health care into the clinical interaction.

Various psychosocial factors are well known to affect health.[1] A brief introduction to the topic was presented in Chapter 13. Now we will explore a few of those issues in greater depth. There is a consensus[2] based on more than 60 years of psychophysiological research that psychological and social factors are crucial determinants in a chain of events leading from psychosocial interaction to neuroendocrine-immune changes. These changes, in turn, can induce progressive disruptions of normal adaptive physiology, eventually leading to functional changes, which ultimately become involved in an interactive and reverberating feedback loop potentially affecting all levels of human function.

It is critical that the practitioner of functional medicine understand the nature of these psychosocial factors, so that he/she can treat the entire person with maximum efficacy. Clinical experience indicates that a failure to take the psychosocial aspects of the functional medicine matrix into account via adequate assessment and intervention can undermine treatment effectiveness.

Defining the Problem: What Does the Functional Medicine Practitioner Face?

Determining whether or not intervention is needed at any level of observation and identifying the types of interventions most likely to be beneficial are constant challenges for the clinician. Dysfunctional processes (discussed throughout this text) must be assessed, and promoters of and resources for change have to be selected and applied. Given the limited resources of many patients (time, money, support in the personal environment for behavioral changes, ability to self direct and maintain altered behavioral patterns), practitioners must be judicious in deciding which interventions are likely to be most effective and most likely to induce change. Unfortunately, at this time, there is a scarcity of good research (or clinical consensus) on how to decide where to "pull on the web"—that is, which intervention(s) is/are likely to produce the greatest overall benefit for the investment of time, money, and effort. It is generally true that the more points of intervention, the more likely one is to stimulate change, but maintenance of change remains a challenge. Research does indicate that involvement of the patient in decision making is beneficial to the outcome.[3]

In the following sections, we will review the concept of stress, and the impact of poverty, community, and spirituality on health, with the aim of guiding the clinician in the development of a practical and personalized approach to the integration of these considerations into clinical care.

Stress

The modern physician should know as much about emotions and thoughts as about disease symptoms and drugs. This approach would appear to hold more promise of cure than anything medicine has given us to date.
—Hans Selye[4]

Stress is the salt of life.
—Hans Selye[5]

What is Stress?

According to Selye,[6] "stress is the non-specific response of the body to any demand, and a stressor is any agent that produces stress at any time." Stressors may be loosely classified as direct physical systemic threats (e.g., starvation, heat, cold, pain, hemorrhage) or "processive" (e.g., psychosocial threats such as social defeat, separation from the maternal object, social isolation, helplessness). While direct systemic threats are not processed primarily by the cortical and limbic areas of the brain, psychosocial stressors involve higher brain functions as part of the primary processing of the sensory input.[7]

Clinically, it is important to expand the working concept of stress to include both the psychosocial factors we often think about (e.g., separation, job loss, cultural context) as well as the stress response to episodes of low blood sugar, chronic pain, or food restriction.

More recently, the concepts of stress and homeostasis have become supplanted by more specific terms and concepts. Allostasis (the ability to achieve stability through change)[8] is thought to occur via acute and chronic changes in the stress response system (neuroendocrine axes—principally the hypothalamic-pituitary-adrenal or HPA axis—and the immune, autonomic, cardiovascular, and metabolic systems). The current conceptualization is that chronic dysregulation of the HPA axis, the autonomic nervous system, and the immune system contributes to chronic alterations in metabolism and inflammation,[9] which then interact with other influences (e.g., nutrition, genetics) to cascade into specific diseases such as the metabolic syndrome, hypertension, cardiovascular disease, and even depression and cancer.[10,11]

Acute stress induces changes that are generally thought to be essential and adaptive, while chronic stress is thought to exact a higher physiological price, creating an allostatic load, defined as the long-term effect of the physiologic response to stress.[12] The acute stress response induces different biological changes in the stress response systems than those induced by chronic stress.[13]

Sensitivity to psychosocial stressors is, for many of us, an essential aspect of our biological make up, and some degree of stress is both desirable and necessary.[14] We appear to be programmed to respond to certain essential psychosocial events in a comparatively predictable manner, although significant individual variations in this reactivity, based on genetics (such as glucocorticoid receptor polymorphisms), context, and prior experience modify the manifestations of the individual response.[15]

From infancy to early adulthood, much of this response to chronic stress is not subject to modification, except by changes in the context of the individual. Infants separated from their mothers for prolonged periods display disruptions in a variety of neuroendocrine-immune functions (e.g., establishment of the normal diurnal variation in cortisol output,[16] amygdala hyperfunction,[17] alterations of markers of immune function, as well as behavioral disturbances such as excessive fear and addictive disorders).[18] Despite the broad range of disrupted neuroendocrine-immune functions, some orphans, once they are adopted, will demonstrate normalization of hypothalamic-pituitary-adrenal function.[19,20]

As we approach adulthood, however, cognitive appraisal of events and sensory input becomes possible, and we can determine, to some degree, what emotional valence (i.e., "charge" or tone) we assign to a given situation. This assignment of meaning then determines our individual definition of what is stressful, and that definition will influence our biological response. Thus, beliefs and attitudes are one focal point for stress management,[21] and studies have demonstrated beneficial effects of the cognitive-behavioral approach.[22,23,24,25]

Aside from the direct systemic stressors (e.g., hemorrhage, hypoglycemia) and obvious psychosocial stressors (e.g., trauma, separation, divorce) frequently addressed in the medical literature, other forms of stress exist. In all likelihood these have an impact on allostatic load to greater or lesser degrees in each individual. Hillman and Ventura[26] note some current cultural stressors:

> Alar on your apples; asbestos around your heating pipes; lead paint on the schoolroom ceiling; mercury in your fish; preservatives in your hot dogs; cigarette smoke in the diner; rays from the microwave; sprays, mothballs, radon, feathers, disinfectants, perfumes, exhaust gases; the glue and synthetics in your couch; antibiotics and hormones in your beef.

Hillman continues: "The greatest moral choice we can make today, if we are truly concerned with the oppressed and stressed lives of our clients' souls, is to sharpen their sense of beauty." Furthermore, if beauty is an objectification of pleasure, as George Santayana posits,[27] then with each styrofoam cup, each asphalt slab, each blank wall, each teetering telephone pole, we are, each of us, robbed of a bit of pleasure.

Beyond the "aesthetic anesthesia" described by Hillman, and beyond the fast pace of change in western society, we are often subject to other societal pressures:

- Two-income families are on the rise. Given the weakened extended family structure in many modern societies, daycare is now part of the psychosocial soil in which we grow our next generation. Our society has yet to attend to studies that demonstrate the significant effect such rearing may have on the stress response system and behavior,[28,29] as well as later psychopathology.[30]
- The quality of social relatedness predicts general health and mortality, and one's emotional adjustment to stress.[31] Unfortunately, in our mobile society, where job and residence change are the norm, the reliability of social support (scientifically defined as consisting of social networks, social relationships, and social integration[32]) as a buffer against stress has diminished.
- Additional stressors include, but are not limited to, crime, terrorism, lengthening commute times in major cities, traffic, and a bulimic diet of fear-focused media input.

Clinical Interventions—Stress

Assessment of psychosocial factors. Simply asking a patient "What are the main stresses in your life?" can be very useful. Together, the clinician and patient can generate a list of these stressors, so that they can be tracked and addressed. Such a list might read:

- marital problems
- job
- finances
- death of a close relative
- medical illness

The next step is to flesh out the complexities of each item on the list, asking questions such as:

- How long has this been going on?
- How hopeful do you feel about resolving this problem?
- What kinds of thoughts and feelings do you have when you think about this particular issue?
- What are you doing to address this problem?
- Do you think you need more help or would you like more help addressing this problem?

The clinician can use these inquiries to develop an assessment of the patient's life stresses, a sense of how the person adapts to different kinds of stress, and to build better rapport. (More on building rapport can be found in Chapter 36, which focuses on *The Healing Relationship*.) As clinicians, we can empathize with our patients' predicaments, perspectives, and feelings, via recollection of similar events in our own lives. If this understanding is checked out with the patient for validity, and if it informs the clinician's actions, the patient will feel understood and well-connected, and those feelings will pay dividends in terms of compliance.[33] While not proven, it seems intuitive that an empathic relationship between clinician and client would also aid in stress reduction and improved satisfaction for both parties.

Planning the intervention. Once the stressors have been identified and explored, the clinician and patient work together on developing an intervention plan. Asking "Which of these stresses do you think needs to be taken care of first?" will help identify the most urgent priority. Lifestyle measures useful for improving stress management include meditation, adequate nutrition and sleep, enhancement of social connectedness, and exercise. More specific interventions must be tailored to the patient's unique situation; discussion of a number of common issues and possible interventions follows.

Marital problems. The quality of a marriage is a critical variable in health maintenance.[34] Couples therapy can be useful when both partners are genuinely interested in making the partnership work. There are many varieties of couples therapy.[35] Some short-term marital therapies that have demonstrated benefit include:

- interpersonal therapy,[36] which is particularly useful when one of the partners is depressed;
- cognitive-behavioral therapy,[37] and
- emotionally focused therapy.[38]

Of utmost importance, aside from the method of therapy, is that both partners are comfortable with the choice of therapist. Therefore, when possible, the clinician should develop a referral list of several couples counselors, and strongly encourage the couple to interview several therapists before selecting one.

It is not uncommon for one partner to refuse therapy, or to have an addiction and deny any problem or need for help. In those cases, individual therapy geared to addressing a non-partnered marital relationship can still be helpful. For a client enmeshed in a relationship with an addict, 12-step groups such as Al-Anon and Codependents Anonymous can be very helpful and should be encouraged. Since it is the nature of the addict to isolate the non-addicted partner in the relationship from normal supports, these group approaches offer much needed social connection as well as education about the nature of addiction and its impact on families and couples. It is this author's experience that the nature of the particular addiction is less important than the process of addiction itself (although there certainly are differences in the effects of various addictions). In a community with a limited variety of 12-step meetings, the nature of the addiction should not preclude a referral to a 12-step group, even if it is not specific to the patient's situation.

Job stresses may be caused by a variety of factors, including threatened loss of job; interpersonal conflicts; mismatch between skills, abilities, and job requirements; shift work; and physical/environmental factors (e.g. sick building syndrome, lack of adequate breaks, inadequate light, excessive noise). It is important to assess the nature and source of the stressors so that an appropriate plan can be developed. If the client's job is threatened, does the problem reside primarily in the organization, the employee, the industry in general, or some combination thereof? Does the client have difficulty cooperating with others, manifested by a long-term history of employment problems? For that person, individual psychotherapy can be useful in addressing the problem. Sometimes vocational counseling or aptitude testing can be helpful when a change in career is being considered, as in the case of an aptitude-skill mismatch. If the situation is such that the client realistically cannot make a change, and has no behavioral options within the situation, then attitude must be addressed and coping strategies devised. This is often best done via cognitive-behavioral therapy.[39] Spiritual work on the meaning of the situation can also be beneficial, if the person is so inclined, as can increased attention to other rewarding aspects of life such as hobbies (which can make use of untapped abilities), community work, and satisfying relationships.

Shift work can be a significant stress for many people.[40] Patients may need to be educated as to the health consequences of shift work, which include increased risk of cardiovascular, gastrointestinal, and reproductive dysfunction as well as depression or exacerbation of other psychiatric conditions.[41] Support from the physician may aid in reducing shift work as much as possible; this can take the form of letters to the employer recommending limits on hours worked or case loads, and emphasizing the medical necessity of such recommendations. If the shift work is continuous, light therapy may be useful.[42]

Finances. Finances are often a very powerful stressor for clients, not only because of the realities of financial hardship, but also because in the United States the link between financial status, social status, and self esteem reflects our strongly material orientation. Patients may be as reluctant to talk about their finances as they are about their sexual habits. If the client has identified this as an area of stress, approaching the subject with some open-ended questions can be helpful. "When you think about your finances, what do you feel?" Note that the answer to this question should be one or two words, i.e., angry, scared, nervous, sad, not an analysis of the situation (which involves thoughts, rather than feelings). Responses that begin with "I feel *that* ... " mean it's important to restate and clarify the question. Explain that a feeling is usually one word: happy, anxious, tense, etc. Other useful questions on this subject include: "How often do you worry about your finances and have these feelings?" "Does your worry affect your sleep or appetite?" "Do you share these worries with anyone?" "How long have you been preoccupied with your finances?" "Has your financial situation changed and, if so, when?" "What have you tried to do about your situation?" "Have you sought any help?" "Are you doing the things you need to do?"

Many people with depression and anxiety disorders have unrealistic or exaggerated fears of financial decline. If you are concerned that this may be the case, getting collateral history from a trusted partner, parent, sibling, or caretaker, can be surprisingly useful. If it appears that the patient is unnecessarily anxious, cognitive-behavioral therapy is indicated, and the question of a depressive or anxiety disorder should be raised and explored. It is not uncommon for patients with a depressive disorder to contemplate suicide, hoping that the life insurance payment will alleviate the financial burdens of the family. This factor must be identified and given serious weight in assessment of the depressed or anxious patient who has financial concerns.

If the client is indeed under genuine financial stress, then the physician should consider making a referral to a financial counselor, or a credit repair company. People under chronic financial stress need a strategic plan of attack. They may lack the skills, prefer to avoid the overwhelming feelings of failure and loss of control, or perhaps are simply too fatigued or anxious to develop one on their own. Connecting with a qualified advisor who can guide the development of a sound financial plan can help patients regain a sense of control over the situation, which will reduce the perceived stress. In the course of the discussion, it can be useful to have the client list any possible sources of help that he or she might have overlooked (e.g., friends with financial experience).

Certain stages in life indeed are more financially taxing than others, and the experienced clinician may be comfortable in simply offering support and comfort ("Don't worry, it will pass. Every one goes through this at one time or another"). But this should not be done until the nature of the problem is clear. Incorrectly used, before a careful assessment of the realities, reassurance can be experienced as invalidating, or a minimization of the problem, with an implication that the client is "wrong" for feeling what he/she does. For patients who are very stressed, such an experience can become a significant barrier to good communications. When asked about the financial problems at the next visit, the patient may indicate that they have been handled, but this assurance may soon be followed by the patient's disappearance from the physician's practice, or by a decrease in compliance.

Death of a close relative or loved one. The death of a close relative, friend, or pet often creates stress on multiple levels. The effect of such loss depends on the degree and nature of involvement with the deceased, the nature and quality of the relationship, the manner of and preparation for the death, and the spiritual questions raised by the death. Grief counselors often assume that recovery from loss requires a period of grief work in which the ultimate goal is the dissolution of the attachment bond to the deceased. However, reviews appearing in the 1980s noted a surprising absence of empirical support for this view.[43] In fact, different cultures cope with death differently. Rather than detachment from the deceased, some cultures emphasize "transformations of attachment to the deceased."[44] Thus the clinician's role is to identify the grief state, differentiate it from depression, and help the client obtain culturally specific and appropriate support and reintegration into life, in the context of a warm and genuinely empathic concern.

Once the client has identified a loss, the clinician may ask any of the following questions to assess the extent of the impact:

- How long ago did the loss occur?
- How much, how often, and in what ways is this loss affecting you?
- Was the deceased part of your everyday life?
- What was the quality of your relationship? (Ambivalent, conflict-laden relationships are more difficult to grieve.)
- What have your previous reactions been to losses such as these?

These questions will alert the clinician to the degree of recovery from the loss, and the likelihood of a difficult recovery.

In order to differentiate grief from depression, a number of questions must be asked.

- Are you feeling primarily sad, or do you feel depressed or hopeless?
- Do these feelings come in waves, triggered by some memory of the deceased or are the feelings more constant?
- Do you find yourself focused on the deceased and missing him/her, or do you find yourself thinking more about yourself, and your future and past?
- Have you thought that you would like to join the deceased soon?
- Are you able to sleep and eat?

- Is it difficult to engage in your normal activities?
- Are you still able to experience pleasure from the activities you used to enjoy?

If the clinician is satisfied that the client is grieving and not depressed, then a referral to a grief counselor or a pastoral counselor or clergy may be appropriate. If there is an aspect of depression, then appropriate treatment of the depression should be instituted.

Illness. Illness is a stress; it can have many different manifestations in a patient's life: pain, limitations on normal functioning, impact on financial stability or self concept, changes in relationships with others, and the raising of religious, spiritual, or existential questions. Because illness has the capacity to affect one's life in such a pervasive manner, most patients will acknowledge this "burden of illness" as a stress in and of itself. When approached about these issues in a thoughtful manner (and from a functional medicine perspective), many patients immediately experience a reduction in stress because they feel that their problem is being taken seriously and underlying causes are being sought. Many patients are relieved that "pills are not being thrown at me."

The clinician, by virtue of his/her careful empathic interest, restores hope in recovery, and can assist the client in adapting to non-reversible physical changes via support groups, education, and collateral services as needed. It is also part of the practitioner's mission to remind the patient that the goal of all health care is recovery of a vibrant life, with abundant joy and happiness. Achieving this goal is both a privilege and a gift which we as healthcare providers can and must aspire to.

Even brief attention to these factors in the lives of our patients—and to the rapidly developing body of stress research—allows one to appreciate the importance of the contextual soup within which we all live, and with which our stress response systems must cope. Understanding this, it becomes important to take into account additional contextual factors that often impact health via the stress response system: community and socioeconomic status.

Community and Socioeconomic Status

While the precise definition of "neighborhood" is yet to be determined, numerous studies have found that neighborhood context, or "place," does play a role in quality of health.[45] Neighborhood context has been investigated as a factor in various aspects of health, including child development,[46] child problem behavior,[47] cardiovascular disease,[48,49,50,51] cigarette smoking,[52] mental health,[53] and overall mortality.[54] It is intuitively obvious that a community which fosters a sense of control (e.g., personal safety, good visibility, predictability), access to privacy, social support, and access to nature and other positive recreational activities would be one that fosters health. Segregating out the various factors that contribute to the effects of community and socioeconomic status (SES) on health remains a challenge,[55] yet it is clear that socioeconomic status (usually determined by education, occupation, and income) is also a major contributor to differential health outcomes in various neighborhoods.[56,57,58,59] The adverse health effects of socioeconomic position are not limited to those at the poverty level, however. In fact, the effects of social position occur at all levels of the social class hierarchy.[60] This is not surprising when we realize that our position in the social hierarchy determines the degree of control we have (or think we have) over our environment. That sense of control is related to our emotional state,[61] and our emotional state is the "crucial driving force in a chain of events leading from psychosocial interaction to neuroendocrine changes."[62] These neuroendocrine changes involve the HPA axis (see discussion in Chapter 32) and involve learned expectations of helplessness.[63]

In the attempt to determine which aspects of SES and neighborhoods most affect health, and to what degree, consideration has been given to perception of the physical environment,[64] work conditions, housing, municipal services (e.g., transportation, healthcare facilities), community norms and values, social support networks, and political empowerment as components of the impact of neighborhood context on health.[65] The mediating factors that help reduce morbidity and mortality via higher socioeconomic status are thought to vary with locale and time (e.g., higher SES is a factor in reduced exposure to infection in underdeveloped countries). Diet, nutrition, smoking, exercise, pathogen and carcinogen exposure, crime, and psychosocial factors are also significant areas of concern.[66]

The above-mentioned factors (e.g., neighborhood, perception of relative status, factors associated with poverty) are contextual, yet they operate ultimately at the level of the individual to impact health outcomes. Evidence is accumulating that there are multiple pathways by which neighborhood, poverty, and SES determine health outcomes:

- involvement of the stress response system as a result of cognitive appraisal of potential helplessness or harm (e.g., low job control),
- direct effect of health behaviors (e.g., diet, exercise, smoking),
- neighborhood effects (e.g., availability of municipal services, physical perceptions of neighborhood), and
- social support.

Given that socioeconomic status (as measured by education, occupation and income) and community (physical environment,[67] work conditions, housing, municipal services such as healthcare facilities, community norms and values, social support networks, and political empowerment) must play some role in health, the question arises: How is the practitioner of functional medicine to take these variables into consideration?

The answer to this question varies with the context within which the clinician practices. A patient population of upper income clients, for example, is likely to experience fewer issues of social hierarchy relative to the general population. Practitioners should remember, however, that high SES individuals must cope with many other major stressors, most of which are independent of position: illness, loss of a loved one, job problems, marital and family issues. Financial difficulties such as excessive debt and possible bankruptcy may also arise, and high SES patients may be less likely to admit them due to their perceived social stigma. Clients from very wealthy communities may labor under pressure to maintain their socioeconomic status and lifestyle, which is often a gauge of self esteem.

Populations with narrower income variability tend to have lower mortality rates.[68] This implies that healthcare practitioners should find out who the client compares him/herself to, and where she/he stands in the hierarchy. The impact of social status on health is determined more by perception and personal expectations than by facts. Lacking well-validated instruments, the following questions might serve as a starting point for an analysis of the **patient's perception of socioeconomic status**:

- Do you feel that the people in your life are generally more or less well off than you are?
- If you imagined a scale of 0 to 100, with 100 being the people you know who are most successful in their work and their lifestyle, where are you, currently, in your estimation? Is that a change?
- Are you satisfied with this, or do you feel bad about this sometimes?
- Where do you expect you will be on this scale in the future?

Education is easily assessed with a few straightforward questions:

- What is the highest degree you have attained?
- Are you satisfied with this, or do you feel this holds you back?
- Do you intend to get further education of any type?

Occupation may require a little more probing. Asking "What kind of work do you do?" might generate a response such as, "I work at ABC accounting corporation." The practitioner might accept this answer, but still not know whether the patient is a janitor, a clerk, an accountant, a partner, an administrator, a salesperson, or in human resources. Does he/she like what he/she does? If not, why not? Aptitude testing (to determine a more appropriate career path or job), along with skills training and work on interpersonal skills, might be important; a job change may need to be considered.

The physical environment one lives, works, and recreates in can have significant effects on all aspects of health. The biological (e.g., sanitation, water quality), psychological (crowding, privacy), social (safety, neighbors, local services), and aesthetic (trees, flowers, design, open space) aspects of community are all important. For example, a recent study of 207 elderly people living independently indicated that "a considerable number of the residents in the Silver Peer Housing facilities studied had mental health problems associated with limitations in the layout of their apartment and/or the location of the housing."[69] Practitioners who are able to make house calls (or otherwise become familiar with the cultures and communities their patients inhabit) have an advantage both in connecting with the client and in avoiding the pitfalls of making unreasonable healthcare suggestions. Asking a patient to "jog or walk around your neighborhood," without knowing whether there are concerns about crime, traffic, or air quality may be a mistake. The amount of sunlight exposure (affecting vitamin D levels and possibly seasonal affective disorder), ventilation and air quality, noise exposure affecting sleep-wake cycles (e.g., 4 am street cleaners, airplanes overhead), and access to nature are additional variables to consider. The amount of perceived control over one's environment can reinforce a sense of optimism or despair.

As practitioners, we must consider the cultural norms that drive behavior. Each community has particular characteristics with which the practitioner can become acquainted. In higher SES communities, it might be the norm to have a drink at lunch or half a bottle of wine with dinner. Immigrant or ethnic communities may connect very closely with particular foods; as we know, diet has a powerful impact on health. To elicit some of these factors, patients can be asked to identify potential obstacles to dietary or lifestyle changes they might face within their families, at work, or in their communities.

Social support networks should be assessed; questions such as the following are useful:

- Do you feel isolated or lonely?
- How well do you feel you fit in with your community?
- Where do the different members of your family live?
- Who are you closest to in your family? Where do they live? How often do you speak to or see them?
- Do you generally feel better after a visit with certain members of your family?
- When you have a problem, who do you turn to?
- What kind of friendships do you have? Are they of long or short duration?
- Have you suffered any losses of important people?
- Who do you have fun with?

Political empowerment can be defined as feeling able to influence the political events and economic decisions that affect one's community. A community with low levels of political power will suffer health consequences on a broad scale. Clinicians who empower their clients to be in charge of their health can diminish the helplessness that members of disenfranchised communities often feel. Beyond the individual level, however, there are several other factors to consider. The practitioner who works in a lower SES community might consider connecting with influential individuals within the community (e.g., the pastor of a local church) to advance educational efforts (e.g., nutrition, fitness, or general health promotion programs for adolescents) that have the potential to reach a larger number of people in a more fundamental manner than can be achieved one-on-one.

The Impact of Spirituality and/or Religion on Health

Defining Spirituality and Religion

Over the past 15 years, there has been increasing interest on the part of both patients and healthcare professionals regarding the role of religion and spirituality in the promotion of health.[70,71] While definitions of spirituality and religious practice overlap significantly, they are not interchangeable terms. Spirituality and religion are best thought of as two overlapping circles in a Venn diagram.[72] Spirituality can be defined as the search for the sacred, the sense of being connected to something greater than self, while religion may be defined as an organized, institutionalized, social mechanism for attaining the spiritual connection.

Relevance of Spirituality and Religion to Healthcare Practitioners

Human beings receive information about the world in three ways: from the food and water we ingest, from the air we breathe, and via our senses (conscious or unconscious experience, observation, and interpretation of the world and ourselves). These inputs impact the expression of our genes via complex interactive pathways. If we turn our attention to the third pathway, the senses, we recognize that the sensory input we receive is constantly evaluated by our mind and body, so that we may respond appropriately. There is an ongoing automatic and preconscious inner dialogue, so to speak: "Is this chair comfortable?" "Do I trust this person?" "Am I in danger?"

One primary filter through which we evaluate incoming sensory input is our set of beliefs and attitudes (cortical function); another is our limbic (emotional) predisposition. Support for the proposition that thinking affects emotion comes from Beck,[73] who, in formulating cognitive-behavioral theory, postulated that one's views of self, the world, and the future (the "cognitive triad") are critical determinants of one's emotional state. Numerous studies have demonstrated the effectiveness of cognitive therapy in a variety of psychiatric disorders.[74,75,76,77]

Furthermore, according to Schore,[78] "Because the right hemisphere of the brain is deeply connected into the limbic system and the autonomic nervous system, it is centrally involved in controlling vital functions supporting survival and enabling the individual to cope with stresses and challenges." Thus our automatic and rapid assessment of sensory input may be negative, neutral, or positive, but the valence of the interpretation we place on our experience is then conveyed to the deeper brain structures such as the amygdala, the hippocampus, the hypothalamic-pituitary-hormonal axes, the autonomic nervous system, the immune system,[79] and other points on the functional medicine matrix. Given a favorable assessment of sensory input, we experience pleasant feelings, such as pleasure or relief, and a corresponding physiology. A negative assessment activates a different psychophysiological response.

It is thus reasonable to conclude that the separation of mind-body that has pervaded western medicine is unfounded.[80] The mind-body is, in fact, an interactive single unit embedded in the larger sociocultural environmental context. Beliefs and attitudes can influence the entire state of the person, including physiology. Thus, religiosity and spiritual beliefs are vital issues in health promotion and are addressed within the functional medicine matrix. Body and mind are inextricably intertwined. Acknowledging these facts, researchers have sought to determine and define the effects of spirituality and religion on health.

The Evidence Concerning Health Effects of Spirituality and Religion

In a comprehensive and systematic 2001 review of the literature over the past century, Koenig assessed over 225 reports on religion and pain/disability, heart disease, blood pressure, stroke, immune/neuroendocrine function, infectious disease, cancer, and overall mortality.[81] He concluded that:

> While more research and better designed studies are needed, the vast majority of research completed to date indicates that religious beliefs and practices are associated with better mental and physical health. These associations are as consistent and robust as associations between health status and other psychosocial variables (like social support, marital status, and certain health behaviors).

In another critical review of the evidence, which differentially assessed religious/spiritual dimensions and meditation/relaxation, Seeman et al.[82] created a "levels of evidence" ranking system to evaluate the available literature. Studies were ranked according to the strength of study design (A to C). Eleven propositions relating to the hypothesized relationships between spirituality/religion and physiological markers (e.g., blood pressure, oxidative stress) were then developed. They defined four levels of evidence:

- 3 (persuasive support for the proposition, including at least three category A studies),
- 2 (reasonable evidence demonstrated by two category A studies or 3–4 category A and B studies),
- 1 (some evidence in at least one category A study, or two or more category B studies), and
- 0 (insufficient support, i.e., not even one category A or two category B studies to support the proposition).

They concluded that:

1. Meditation/relaxation is associated with better health outcomes in clinical patient populations (category 3).
2. Meditation/relaxation is associated with lower blood pressure (category 2.5).
3. Religion/spirituality is associated with lower blood pressure, less hypertension, better immune function (all category 2).
4. Meditation/relaxation is associated with lower cholesterol, lower stress hormone levels, and differential patterns of brain activity (category 2).
5. Meditation is associated with less oxidative stress, and less blood pressure and stress hormone reactivity under challenge (category 1).

In contrast to these reviews, Sloan et al,[83] in a comprehensive "though not systematic" earlier review of the empirical evidence, raised the flag of caution. While he acknowledged the great interest in the subject at hand, he pointed out that the quality of the research is marred by inadequate definition of terms, poor control of confounding variables and other covariates, a failure to control for multiple comparisons, and conflicting findings. He raised concerns about the ethical validity of intervening in a patient's life with a "non-medical agenda," and described it as an abuse of professional status. Even if religious or spiritual factors are determined to be related to health outcome, he contended that "we generally regard financial and marital matters as private and personal and not the business of medicine even if they have health implications." He therefore advocated that the religious/spiritual should remain in that private domain. Finally, he expressed concerns that "linking religious activities and better health outcomes can be harmful to patients, who already must confront the age-old folk wisdom that illness is due to their own moral failure."

In response to Sloan, Powell et al.[84] conducted another "levels of evidence" approach to the question in 2003. This review specifically excluded studies examining the link between religion or spirituality and physiological markers (e.g., blood pressure), studies examining all psychosocial outcomes (including suicide, substance abuse and depression), and studies with a variety of methodological flaws. Powell et al. concluded that while a relationship between religion or spirituality and physical health exists, it may be both more limited and more complex than some authors suggest.

Among their findings:

1. In healthy individuals (especially females) there is a dose-response correlation, where frequency of church attendance is positively correlated with approximately 25% reduction in mortality, after adjustment for demographic, socioeconomic, and health-related confounders (e.g., better diet in attenders).
2. There is inadequate support for the hypothesis that religiosity protects against disability.
3. While there is a positive correlation between weekly church attendance and reduced cardiovascular disease (myocardial infarction, angina pectoris, stroke, congestive heart failure, and congenital cardiovascular defects), a large measure of the relationship is accounted for by the healthier lifestyles adopted by churchgoers. Given the difficulty maintaining long-term lifestyle change (see section on promoting lifestyle change) by other methods, these data do support encouraging church attendance as one method of improving lifestyle factors that contribute to morbidity.
4. All five studies that qualified for review failed to support the hypothesis that religion or spirituality improves objective measures of recovery from acute illness. Three qualifying studies of intercessory prayer (prayer at a distance), although not without flaws, indicate that being prayed for improves the quality of the subjective experience during recovery from acute illness.

Integrating Spirituality in Clinical Practice

As the popular pendulum swings toward the perception of spirituality as a legitimate health-promoting factor, it is simultaneously becoming clear that facile conclusions are unwarranted and that many voids in our knowledge base remain. In the face of these cross-currents, clinicians are at the helm, obliged to navigate complex waters as clients, media, and the professional literature demonstrate increasing concern and curiosity.[85] For those practitioners who plan to integrate this important aspect of health into clinical practice, there are some key issues to consider:

When can the clinician know that a discussion of religion or spirituality is indicated? Given the trend of the data, which indicate that there is some degree and nature of interaction between religion/spirituality and health, it seems prudent to assess this factor as a point for potential intervention in the majority of patients. In the treatment of chronic diseases, the approach must be individually tailored. The clinician should determine the relative importance the patient places on the subject matter, and assess the receptivity of the patient to the issue, while asking him/herself, for example, whether the relationship between the patient and healthcare provider can "hold" the subject. The majority of the American population would welcome their physician's inquiry into their spiritual or religious practice if gravely ill.[86]

How does one explore the subject? On the front lines of medicine, statistics can only offer probabilities, and each patient must be recognized as unique. From this perspective, we might open the subject with a simple inquiry: "Mr. Jones, is spirituality or religion important to you? Is it something you would like to discuss, with me or with someone else?" In the case of a patient with chronic stress, hypertension, perhaps immune dysfunction, or an imbalance of adrenal function (such as low morning cortisol), meditation or relaxation techniques might be offered as a tool for addressing the patient's physical problems.[i] "Development of a daily meditation

[i] There are many approaches to meditation or other relaxation techniques; some clearly have a spiritual or religious connection, while others do not. It may be important to the patient to know more about those nuances. Resources are usually available in most communities, but *Full Catastrophe Living* (Jon Kabat-Zinn) outlines a structured meditation program, and is an excellent book. A less structured approach to meditation is discussed in Jon Kabat-Zinn's second book, *Wherever You Go, There You Are*. Tapes can be purchased to facilitate the learning on one's own, although live training and group practice may help patients learn the techniques more quickly and effectively.

practice, has been shown to be very helpful for many people, Ms. Jones, so that when you are stressed you will manage it better." If meditation is recommended, it should be emphasized that this is a skill that takes time to develop, but one which can have many health benefits, both mental and physical. In a patient who is depressed and/or guilt ridden, meditation (during which he/she may ruminate on negative cognitions) could be contraindicated. Similarly, I have seen religious attendance be helpful as well as harmful. In cases of trauma or guilt associated with a specific church, the clinician could support the patient's exploring other religious denominations (if the patient is so inclined).

After ascertaining whether the patient is religiously or spiritually oriented, you may want to define the difference between the two, so the patient is clear about the question. It's also important to evaluate the clinician's context—i.e., what is the nature of your relationship to the patient? Are you (the clinician) pursuing a spiritual or religious practice? Has it been helpful with your personal health issues? Do you have any negative feelings/experiences associated with religion or spirituality (e.g., being forced to go to church, abuse history within the church)? It may be appropriate to make a personal disclosure about the role of religion or spirituality in one's own life, if the relationship with the client can hold the disclosure: "A willingness to self disclosure on the analyst's part facilitates self disclosure by the patient, and therefore productive dialectical interchange between analyst and patient is maximized."[87]

What are the risks of raising the subject? Clinicians must approach the assessment of spirituality/religion with respect for the patient's autonomy, personal history, and social context. The inquiry must remain as neutral and non-judgmental as it is for any other area of inquiry. The sole goal of the inquiry must be to benefit the person's health. The clinician must be sensitive to the patient's inclinations, and conduct the discussion with respect and sensitivity. If the clinician detects resistance to the subject matter, it is very important to acknowledge the person's right not to discuss the issue, and simply let them know that, should they desire to discuss the issue in the future, the door will be open. Failure to approach the person in this manner has a high likelihood of eroding the foundation of trust in the relationship.

Where/how to set the boundary between the clinician's belief system and that of the patient can be tricky. Generally speaking, the boundary will be a function of the interaction between the clinician's belief systems and the patient's belief systems, and the clinician's function is, first, to protect the patient and, second, to guide him/her if such guidance is desired. As in all areas of clinical practice, there is a somewhat porous, interactive boundary between the physician's life, beliefs, personal history, personality style, and those same factors within the patient. Clinicians who eat properly and exercise may be more likely to focus on such issues with their patients. Consequently, a physician who manifests some mastery of these lifestyle factors can be perceived as supportive and hope-inducing by some patients; yet, for other patients, the clinician's mastery may paradoxically represent a mirror of their own imperfections. Each clinician-client interaction presents a unique interactive dynamic, a human chemical reaction. So, a clinician who considers him/herself atheist will have a different interaction with a very spiritual patient than a clinician who is him/herself very spiritually oriented. It's important to be cognizant of this interactive tension, which can be communicated by many nonverbal factors, ranging from body language to office decor.

On the other hand, a clinician-patient dyad in which both parties are members of the same religious persuasion, and perhaps of the same community, offers different potential benefits, perils, and outcomes. The clinician must therefore understand that there is no formulaic approach in this arena, and it is most important that general principles of autonomy, respect, sensitivity, and care are the clinician's guideposts.

How does the clinician establish an effective referral to a pastor or other trusted person? Once the client has indicated the desire for further discussion or exploration of the spiritual/religious realm, the clinician should help the patient determine with more precision what the needs are. If the patient is confused about allegiance to a church, referral to a pastor might be less useful and more threatening than referral to a pastoral counselor, who is trained in both the spiritual and psychological dimensions. Is the client looking for a new pastor or for training in meditation? Possibly a new religious community or a support group might be needed. As clinicians become more skilled and informed, it can be very useful to develop a resource list and a bibliography that can be offered to those who are interested. The best strategy is to address the client's needs with suggestions about resources they may have overlooked. Once these needs have been identified and a plan for action has been determined, the clinician may offer to make the initial contact (a referral) on the patient's behalf. Finally, follow up should be done on the next visit with an inquiry as to action and outcome.

What clinical outcomes can the clinician and patient expect? Because "very little apparent progress has been made within the health promotion/health education discipline [on] the development of integrated content, methods, and applications for spiritual health promotion,"[88] clinicians must extrapolate to determine the best methods of promoting health and setting reasonable expectations for outcome. Inadequate information also exists in other areas of healthcare, where clinicians must often make decisions without full information. The data seem to support the assumption that the earlier one intervenes in the multicausal chain of illness, the more beneficial the effects. Powell observed that "the effects of prayer and meditation may be more powerful in the prevention of mortality before the overwhelming force of functional impairment sets in."[89] Early life stresses as well as chronic stress result in isolation, helplessness, and consequent adoption of unhealthy lifestyles (e.g., poor diet, smoking, lowered activity levels). These lifestyle habits then interact with genetic predispositions, mediators, and triggers, resulting in disease. After a comprehensive literature survey, Hawks[90] reviewed three peer-reviewed, well-designed, reproducible, spiritually-based, comprehensive health intervention programs (the Lifestyle Heart Trial, a Stanford University School of Medicine complex psychosocial intervention in patients with metastatic breast cancer, and the stress reduction clinic of Jon Kabat-Zinn at the University of Massachusetts Medical Center). The Hawks concluded that:

> ... improved spiritual health may be associated with improved behavioral and emotional health in such areas as diet, activity levels, communication skills, treatment compliance, reduced anxiety and depression, and improved mood states. These positive behavioral and emotional improvements in turn may be associated with heart disease reversal, reduced cancer mortality, enhanced immune function, and reductions in pain and other medical symptoms.

Mind-Body Interventions in Clinical Practice

This brief review of health effects of certain mind-body factors—stress, religion and spirituality, community and poverty—indicates the complexity of the field and the multiplicity of issues that may play a role in health outcomes. It is abundantly clear that each aspect of the bio-psycho-social–spiritual web is interactive and in communication with other aspects. Much remains to be clarified before definitive guidance can be offered by the research community. What is the clinician to do?

First Things First

The practitioner's choices will be dependent, in part, on the type of clinical setting and the resources available to both clinician and client. Clinicians who practice in a private setting can "provide health education advice to individual patients, whereas clinicians in community health centers are more likely to be involved in group health promotion activities and broader community development initiatives."[91] The functional medicine practitioner needs to determine, first, how, and to what depth, he/she will be integrating this material into clinical practice. That assessment will affect the setting and style of practice, as well as the potential activities that can be integrated.

Helping Patients to Change

Next, it is good to have an awareness of the factors involved in making permanent behavior change. While it is frequently possible to assist patients in making short-term changes in lifestyle factors known to promote health (e.g., improvement of diet, addition of meditation and exercise, etc.), it is far more challenging to promote long-term lifestyle change. Recognizing this fact, in January of 2003, the National Institutes of Health, Office of Behavioral and Social Sciences Research targeted funds toward the study of factors involved in the maintenance of long-term behavioral change.[92] While clinicians wait for the results of this research initiative, certain guidelines can tentatively be suggested.

From the clinician's perspective, it is best to view change as a long-term process, involving different stages of both change and relapse. "Behavior change is rarely a discrete, single event; the patient moves gradually from being uninterested (pre-contemplation stage of change) to considering a change (contemplation stage) to deciding and preparing to make a change."[93] These stages are followed by the active change phase and then maintenance of change. Most people find themselves "cycling through" the stages of change several times (relapsing) before the change becomes truly established. A detailed discussion of the stages of change approach is provided in Chapter 36.

Emphasizing the fact that long-term change requires long-term support and follow-up, a randomized five-year outcome study of the effect of dietary change and smoking reduction in patients with angina revealed that changes were sustained at two years, but not at five years.[94] The intervention group received two years of quarterly personal health promotion from a trained nurse. This study highlights both the efficacy of short-term interventions, and the unanswered questions about induction of long-term change.

Short-term Studies of Health Promotion

Successful intervention on the nutritional level can have broad-ranging benefits on health outcomes. In a systematic and thorough review of published information on methods to change key dietary habits (fat, fiber, and fruit and vegetable intake), Bowen and Beresford[95] focused on interventions at the individual level, the family/provider, worksite interventions, and community level. Multiple studies in their review indicated that nutritional counseling, individually or in group settings, can have sustained impact on nutritional status at one year following intervention.

Another one-year follow-up reported in 2003 used biomarkers of dietary change (e.g., plasma beta carotene) to measure outcome.[96] This study supported the hypothesis that brief interventions (two 15-minute sessions, two weeks apart, supported by written materials and consisting of either behavioral or generalized nutritional counseling) can be an effective means of increasing consumption of fruits and vegetables. The behavioral intervention (which was statistically more effective in changing the biomarkers than the generalized nutritional counseling approach) was based on the "stages of change model."[97] The intervention was tailored to which stage of change the subject was considered to be in (i.e., precontemplation, contemplation, preparation for change, action, or maintenance). This individualized approach was found to be superior to the generalized nutritional approach (which pointed out the importance of healthful diet, the constituents of a nutritionally sound diet, and the effects on health). Interestingly, the effects of the interventions were similar across income groups. Based on this study, clinicians might consider assessing the client's stage of change before intervening, with the intention of offering stage-appropriate advice.

In a survey of 796 low-income people, Eikenberry and Smith[98] provided evidence that low-income individuals lack knowledge of what constitutes a healthful diet, that racial and economic differences exist in motivation for eating well (African Americans and lower-income individuals had less motivation), and that time and money were cited as the most significant barriers to healthful eating. The most common promoters of healthful eating were social factors (living alone was a frequent barrier; how one was raised was also influential) and food assistance programs. Based on this survey, and the common-sense notion that eating is generally a social activity, clinicians might consider promoting increased (or at least regular) frequency of family meals. Encouraging patients to reconnect with their cultural cuisine might be an additional incentive for some individuals to steer away from fast food, and move toward a more wholesome and meaningful diet; this might also enhance a sense of connectedness to a larger community. For adolescents, family meals can have a marked influence on a variety of behaviors. "In general, adolescents who reported more frequent family meals, high priority for family meals, a positive atmosphere at family meals, and a more structured family meal environment were less likely to engage in disordered eating."[99] Frequency of family meals has been positively correlated with reduced substance use, academic performance, self esteem, depressive symptoms, suicidal ideation, and suicide attempts.[100]

Similar results were reported from a short-term intervention for behavior change directed at reduction of cardiovascular risk factors;[101] however, due to the short duration of the intervention, the actual risk levels were not changed (with the exception of blood pressure), despite changes in behavior.

In an evidence-based review of physical activity promotion, Eakin, Glasgow and Riley[102] found that "well controlled physical activity studies have generally produced moderate short-term improvements, but these results are often less encouraging at long-term follow-up. Of significant note is the fact that all except two of the 15 studies that met the criteria for review relied on self reports of physical activity, although the two studies that used objective measures (e.g., activity monitors) corroborated the self reports. In addition there was considerable variability across studies." Physical activity-only interventions fared better in the short term, but all three of the studies with significant long-term effects were multiple risk factor interventions (e.g., diet/exercise/smoking). While conclusions are certainly premature, this could imply that long-term change is best achieved by approaching the patient's life with a broad lens. A program that utilizes multiple interventions and recognizes the whole person, including social and occupational contexts, as well as stages of change, might be most useful. Clinicians can expect significant failure rates from any approach they employ, as study attrition rates were 20–56% in the longer-term follow ups. Not surprisingly, those in poorer health, those with less education, and smokers were more likely to drop out of the studies.

Long-term Studies of Health Promotion

A more recent review of physical activity promotion studies,[103] using similar exclusion criteria (the RE-AIM model[104]), indicated that five out of nine long-term studies (six-month follow up or longer) reported positive findings for a variety of interventions (e.g., physician/nurse counseling, written materials, mailings, and telephone follow-up), varying frequency, and duration of contact. This report concludes that "the evidence about the long-term impact of single risk factor interventions and about the effect of multiple risk factor interventions" is equivocal. There is good evidence that "interventions delivered to primary care patients that address physical activity alone can achieve short-term" changes in physical activity. The author recommends that clinicians "carry out brief interventions to advise patients with health problems who could benefit from increased physical activity." (An extensive review of the health effects of increased physical activity is available in Chapter 13; Chapter 29 offers a detailed discussion of how to help patients plan and implement a physical fitness program.) In clinical practice, the clinician must follow up, at each visit, on the targeted behavioral changes, which should be prominently displayed in the patient's chart or problem list. When dealing with chronic health problems, long-term changes in health-inducing behaviors require long-term concern, monitoring, encouragement, positive reinforcement, and problem solving on the part of both clinician and client.

Summary

This review of the effects of spirituality, community, poverty, and stress on health indicates that much more research is called for to help us understand the influence of these factors on patient (and population) health. We do know, however, that there can be significant health effects, that these are complex variables, and that they are in all likelihood linked inextricably with the larger societal context within which people live. Our current system is making slow progress in quantifying factors and variables that affect quality of life and health status, but the evidence-based recommendations offer only broad guidelines. These facts make broad-based, one-size-fits-all suggestions difficult and inappropriate. Fortunately, several themes emerge from the data, to help the practitioner who wishes to expand her/his clinical practice to include direct attention to mind-body factors.

Interventions must be individualized. Individualization of care requires that we obtain more information about our patients' lives. Clinicians must find ways to acquire knowledge that, in the past, was often gained by the house call ("Hey Joe, I don't like what I am seeing in your refrigerator"). Thinking outside the box (a picture is worth a thousand words), one might ask patients for pictures of their home, their kitchen, etc. Fundamental questions must be asked: Who exactly is in the patient's intimate social network? How much contact with them are they able to have? What does their home and neighborhood look and feel like to them? What are the patient's social and personal barriers to improving specific health behaviors? What is the patient's financial situation? How does the patient feel about religion or spirituality? How does the patient experience and cope with stress (are symptoms felt in the mind, the body, or both)?

Some sort of partnership with the patient must be formed. Many patients, but certainly not all, prefer to be involved in the clinical decision-making process.[105,106] As patients age, they want more interest from their healthcare providers regarding health care.[107]

Clinicians must be realistic about what they can expect of themselves and of their clients. These expectations should be contingent on the setting and skills of the practitioner and the life setting of the client. Expectation of behavioral change must be tempered by an understanding of the long-term nature of that process, and various interventions must be tried, seeking a suitable and personalized approach for each client.

Finally, healthcare practitioners must strive to form caring, warm, empathic, genuine relationships with their clients. The clinician-patient dyad can be considered, like most relationships, a third entity that grows over time, out of the affinity that the parties develop for each other. This third entity evolves within a socioeconomic and political medium that is different for each client, and often includes a wide variety of influential third parties (e.g., clergy, therapists, insurers, courts, pastoral counselors). The nature of the partnership is influenced by all of these factors. The clinician's availability in times of urgent need can help solidify the partnership, as can genuine empathy, acceptance, warmth, appropriate humor, and a real interest in who the client is in body, mind, and spirit. It is only in the clear air of such a healing relationship that new and healthier behaviors can be nurtured.

References

1. McEwen BS. The neurobiology of stress: from serendipity to clinical relevance. Brain Research. 2000;886:172-189
2. Henry JP. The relation of social to biological processes in disease. Soc Sci Med. 1982;16(4):369-80.
3. Scheibler F, Janssen C, Pfaff H. Shared decision making: an overview of international research literature. Soz Praventivmed. 2003;48(1):11-23.
4. Selye H. Stress and holistic medicine. J of Family and Community Health 1980. Vol 3;2; 85-8.
5. Selye H. Forty years of stress research: principal remaining problems and misconceptions. Canadian Med Assoc. Journal. 115;1;1976:53-56.
6. Ibid.
7. Herman JP, Cullinan WE. Neurocircuitry of stress: central control of the hypothalamic-pituitary-adrenal axis. Trends Neurosci. 20;78-84; 1997
8. Sterling P, Eyer J. Allostasis: A new paradigm to explain arousal pathology. In: Handbook of life stress, cognition and health. S. Fisher and J Reason Eds.:New York: John Wiley & Sons. 1988. p 629-649.
9. Seematter G, Binnert C, Martin JL, Tappy L. Relationship between stress, inflammation and metabolism. Current Opinion in Clinical Nutrition and Metabolic Care 2004, 7:169-173.
10. Holden RJ, Pakula IS, Mooney PA. An immunological model connecting the pathogenesis of stress, depression, and carcinoma. Medical Hypothesis (1998);51;309-314.
11. Kune S. Stressful life events and cancer. Epidemiology 1993;4;395-397.
12. McEwen BS. Protective and damaging effects of stress mediators. NEJM, 1998;338(3):171-9.
13. Charney DS. Psychobiological mechanisms of resilience and vulnerability: implications for successful adaptation to extreme stress. Am J Psychiatry 2004;161:195-216.
14. Selye H. Forty years of stress research: principal remaining problems and misconceptions. Canadian Med Assoc. Journal. 115;1;1976:53-56.
15. Yehuda R. and McEwen BS. Protective and damaging effects of the biobehavioral stress response: cognitive systemic, and clinical aspects: ISPNE XXXIV meeting summary. Psychoneuroendocrinology (2004) 29; 1212-1222.
16. Gunnar MR, Donzella B. Social regulation of the cortisol levels in early human development. Psychoneuroendocrinology. 2002;27:199-220.
17. Teicher MH, Andersen SL, Polcari A, Anderson CM, Navalta CP. Developmental neurobiology of childhood stress and trauma. Pediatr Clin N Am 25 (2002) 397-426.
18. Charmandari EK, Kino T, Souvatzoglou E, Chrousos GP. Pediatric Stress: hormonal mediators and human development. Horm Res. 2003;59(4):161-79.
19. Yehuda R. and McEwen BS. Protective and damaging effects of the biobehavioral stress response: cognitive systemic, and clinical aspects: ISPNE XXXIV meeting summary. Psychoneuroendocrinology (2004) 29;1212-1222.
20. McEwen BS. Early life influences on life-long patterns of behavior and health. Mental Retardation and Developmental Disabilities Research Reviews. 9;149-154;2003.
21. Lazarus RS, Folkman S. Stress, appraisal, and coping. Springer Publishing Company, NY 1984.
22. Antoni MH, Cruess S, Cruess DG, et al. Cognitive-behavioral stress management reduces distress and 24 hour urinary free cortisol output among symptomatic HIV-infected gay men. Ann. Behav. Med. (2000); 22:29-37.
23. Cruess DG, Antoni MH, Kumar M, et al. Cognitive-behavioral stress management buffers decreases in dehydroepiandrosterone sulfate (DHEA-S) and increases in the cortisol/DHEA-S ratio and reduces mood disturbance and perceived stress among HIV seropositive men. Psychoneuroendocrinology (1999);24;537-549.
24. Gaab J, Blattler N, Menzi T, Pabst B, Stoyer S, Ehlert U. Randomized controlled evaluation of the effects of cognitive behavioral stress management on cortisol responses to acute stress in healthy subjects. Psychoneuroendocrinology 28 (2003) 767-779.
25. Hugdahl K. Cognitive influences on human autonomic nervous system function. Current Opinion in Neurobiology, 1996; 6; 252-258.
26. Hillman J, Ventura M. We've had a hundred years of psychotherapy, and the world's getting worse. HarperCollins Publishers, NY 1992, p 124-130.
27. Ibid, p. 130.
28. Greenspan SI. Child care research: a clinical perspective. Child Dev. 2003 Jul-Aug;74(4):1064-8.
29. Watamura SE, Donzella B, Alwin J, Gunnar MR. Morning-to-afternoon increases in cortisol concentrations for infants and toddlers at child care: age differences and behavioral correlates. Child Dev. 2003 Jul-Aug;74(4):1006-20.
30. Thadani PV. The intersection of stress, drug abuse and development. Pychoneuroendocrinology. 2002. 27; 221-230.
31. Kendler KS. Social Support: A genetic-epidemiologic analysis. Am J Psychiatry 1997;154;1398-1404.
32. Mookadam F. Arthur HM. Social support and its relationship to morbidity and mortality after acute myocardial infarction. Arch Intern Med. 2004;164;1514-1518.
33. Squier RW. A model of empathic understanding and adherence to treatment regimens in practitioner-patient relationships. Soc Sci Med. 1990;30(3):325-39.
34. Robles TF, Kiecolt-Glaser JK. The physiology of marriage: pathways to health. Physiol Behav. 2003;79(3):409-16.
35. Baucom DH, Epstein N, Gordon KC. Marital therapy: Theory, practice, and empirical status. In C. R. Snyder & R. Ingram (Eds.), Handbook of Psychological Change: Psychotherapy Processes and Practices for the 21st Century. New York: Wiley, 2000.

36. Weissman MM, Markowitz JC, Klerman GL. Comprehensive Guide to Interpersonal Psychotherapy. New York, Basic Books, 2000.
37. Baucom DH, Epstein N, LaTaillade JJ. Cognitive-behavioral couple therapy. In AS Gurman & NS Jacobson (Eds.), Clinical Handbook of Couple Therapy (3rd ed.). New York: Guilford Press, 2002.
38. Johnson S. Creating Connection: The Practice of Emotionally Focused Marital Therapy. Formerly Philadelphia: Brunner/Mazel, now New York: Taylor and Francis, 1996.
39. Beck JS. Cognitive Therapy: Basics and Beyond. New York, Guilford Press, 1995.
40. Boivin DB, James FO. Light treatment and circadian adaptation to shift work. Ind Health. 2005 Jan;43(1):34-48.
41. Scott AJ. Shift work and health. Prim Care. 2000;27(4):1057-79.
42. James FO, Walker CD, Boivin DB. Controlled exposure to light and darkness realigns the salivary cortisol rhythm in night shift workers. Chronobiol Int. 2004;21(6):961-72.
43. Bonanno GA, Kaltman S.Toward an integrative perspective on bereavement. Psychol Bull. 1999 Nov;125(6):760-76.
44. Shapiro ER. Family bereavement and cultural diversity: a social developmental perspective. Fam Process. 1996 Sep;35(3):313-32.
45. Diez Roux AV. Investigating neighborhood and area effects on health. American Journal of Public Health (2001). 91;11;1783-1789.
46. Bradley RH, Corwyn RF. Socioeconomic status and childe development. Annu Rev Psychol. 2002;53;371-99.
47. Kalff AC, Kroes M, Vles JSH, Hendriksen JGM, Feron FJM, Steyaert J, Van Zeben TMCB, Jolles J, Van Os J. Neighborhood level and individual level SES effects on child problem behavior: a multilevel analysis. J Epidemiol Community Health 2001;55:246-250.
48. Cubbin C, Hadden WC, Winkleby MA. Neighborhood context and cardiovascular disease risk factors: The contribution of material deprivation. Ethnicity and disease 2001; 11;687-700.
49. Borrell LN, Diez Roux AV, Rose K, Catellier D, Clark BL, Neighborhood characteristics and mortality in the Atherosclerosis Risk in Communities study. Int J. epidemiol. 2004;33(2):398-407.
50. Sundquist K, Malmstrom M, Johansson SE. Neighborhood deprivation and incidence of coronary heart disease: a multilevel study of 2.6.million women and men in Sweden. J Epidemiol Community Health 2004;58;71-77.
51. Diez Roux AV, Borell LN Haan M, Jackson SA, Schultz R. Neighborhood environments and mortality in an elderly cohort: results from the cardiovascular health study. J. Epidemiol. Community Health 2004;58:917-923.
52. Bergen AW, Caporaso N. Cigarette smoking. J. Natl cancer Inst. 1999;91(16);1365-75.
53. Dalgard OS, Tambs K. Urban environment and mental health: A longitudinal study. British J of Psychiatry 1997;171;530-536.
54. House JS, Lepkowski JM, Williams DR, et al. Excess mortality among urban residents: How much, for whom, and why? Am J. Public Health 2000;90(12);1898-1904.
55. Cubbin C, Hadden WC, Winkleby MA. Neighborhood context and cardiovascular disease risk factors: The contribution of material deprivation. Ethnicity and disease 2001; 11;687-700.
56. Davey Smith G, Neaton JD, Wentworth D, Stamler R, Stamler J. Mortality differences between black and white men in the USA: contribution of income and other risk factors among men screened for the MRFIT.1998.The Lancet;351;934-939.
57. Anderson RT, Sorlie P, Backlund E, et al. Mortality effects of community socioeconomic status. Epidemiology 1997;8;42-47.
58. Lin CC, Rogot E, Johnson NJ, et al. A further study of life expectancy by socioeconomic factors in the national longitudinal mortality study. Ethn Dis 2003;13;240-247.
59. Hahn RA, Eaker ED, Barker ND, Teutsch SM, Sosniak WA, Krieger N. Poverty and death in the United States. Intl. J. of Health Services 1996;26;4;673-690.
60. Adler, NE, Boyce WT, Chesney M, Folkman S, Syme L. Socioeconomic inequalities in health: No easy solution. JAMA 1993;269;3140-3145.
61. Rodin J. Aging and health: effects of the sense of control. Science 1986. 233;1271-1276.
62. Henry JP. The relation of social to biological processes in disease. Soc Sci Med. 1982;16(4):369-80. Review.
63. Kristenson M, Eriksen HR, Sluiter JK, et al. Psychobiological mechanisms of socioeconomic differences in health. Social Sciences and Medicine 2004;58;1511-1522.
64. Wilson K, Elliott S, Law M, et al. Linking perceptions of neighborhood to health in Hamilton, Canada. J Epidemiol Community Health 2004;58;192-198.
65. Cubbin C, Hadden WC, Winkleby MA. Neighborhood context and cardiovascular disease risk factors: The contribution of material deprivation. Ethnicity and disease 2001; 11;687-700.
66. Adler, NE, Boyce WT, Chesney M, et al. Socioeconomic inequalities in health: No easy solution. JAMA 1993;269;3140-3145.
67. Wilson K, Elliott S, Law M, et al. Linking perceptions of neighborhood to health in Hamilton, Canada. J Epidemiol Community Health 2004;58;192-198.
68. Wilkinson RG. Health, hierarchy, and social anxiety. Ann N Y Acad Sci. 1999;896:48-63.
69. Migita R., Yanagi H. Factors affecting the mental health of residents in a communal-housing project for seniors in Japan. Factors affecting the mental health of residents in a communal-housing project for seniors in Japan. Arch Gerontol Geriatr. 2005;41(1):1-14.
70. Koenig HG. Religion, spirituality, and medicine: how are they related and what does it mean? Mayo Clinic Proc. 2001; 76(12):1189-1191.
71. Seeman TE, Dubin LF, Seeman M. Religiosity/spirituality and health: a critical review of the evidence for biological pathways. Am Psychol. 2003;58(1):53-63.
72. Thoresen CE, Harris AHS. Spirituality and health: what's the evidence and what's needed? Ann Behav Med. 2002;24(1):3-13.
73. Beck JS. Cognitive Therapy: Basics and Beyond. New York, Guilford Press, 1995.
74. Kennedy T, Jones R, Darnley S, et al. Cognitive behaviour therapy in addition to antispasmodic treatment for irritable bowel syndrome in primary care: randomised controlled trial. BMJ. 2005;331(7514):435.
75. Wright JH, Wright AS, Albano AM, et al. Computer-assisted cognitive therapy for depression: maintaining efficacy while reducing therapist time. Am J Psychiatry. 2005;162(6):1158-64.
76. Whittal ML, Thordarson DS, McLean PD. Treatment of obsessive-compulsive disorder: Cognitive behavior therapy vs. exposure and response prevention. Behav Res Ther. 2005;May 21:[Epub ahead of print].
77. Tafet GE, Feder DJ, Abulafia DP, Roffman SS. Regulation of hypothalamic-pituitary-adrenal activity in response to cognitive therapy in patients with generalized anxiety disorder. Cogn Affect Behav Neurosci. 2005;5(1):37-40.
78. Schore AN. Affect Regulation and the Repair of the Self. NY: W.W.Norton; 2003, p. 75.
79. Rossi EL. The Psychobiology of Mind-Body Healing (revised edition). NY: W.W. Norton; 1993, p. 161.
80. Watkins A. Mind-Body Medicine: A Clinician's Guide to Psychoneuroimmunology. NY: Churchill Livingstone: 1997, p 1-25.
81. Koenig HG. Religion and medicine IV: religion, physical health, and clinical implications. Int J Psychiatry Med. 2001;31(3):321-336.

82. Seeman TE, Dubin LF, Seeman M. Religiosity/spirituality and health: a critical review of the evidence for biological pathways. Am Psychol. 2003;58(1):53-63.
83. Sloan RP, Bagiella E, Powell T. Viewpoint: religion, spirituality and medicine. Lancet. 1999;353:664-67.
84. Powell LH, Shahabi L, Thoresen CE. Religion and spirituality: linkages to physical health. Am Psychol. 2003;58 (1):36-52.
85. Daaleman TP. Special communication: religion, spirituality, and the practice of medicine. J Am Board Fam Pract. 2004;17:370-376.
86. Ehman JW, Ott BB, Short TH, et al. Do patients want physicians to inquire about their spiritual or religious beliefs if they become gravely ill? Arch Intern Med. 1999;159;1803-1806.
87. Schore AN. Affect Regulation and the Repair of the Self. NY: W.W. Norton; 2003, p. 75.
88. Hawks, SR, Hull ML, Thalman RL, Richins PM. Review of spiritual health: definition, role, and intervention strategies in health promotion. Am J. Health Promotion 1995;9(5):371-8.
89. Powell LH, Shahabi L, Thoresen CE. Religion and spirituality: linkages to physical health. Am Psychol. 2003;58 (1):36-52.
90. Hawks, SR, Hull ML, Thalman RL, Richins PM. Review of spiritual health: definition, role, and intervention strategies in health promotion. Am J. Health Promotion 1995;9(5):371-8.
91. Baum F, Kalucy E, Lawless A, Barton S, Steven I. Health promotion in different medical settings: women's health, community health and private practice. Aust N Z Public Health 1998;22;200-5
92. http://obssr.od.nih.gov/funding/Behavioral%20Change%20RFA%20Outcome.htm
93. Zimmerman GL, Olsen CG, Bosworth MF. A stages of change approach to helping patients change behavior. Am Fam Physician 2000;61:1409-1416
94. Cupples ME, McKnight A. Five year follow up of patients at high cardiovascular risk who took part in a randomized controlled trial of health promotion. Br Med J. 1999. 319;867-88
95. Bowen DJ, Beresford AA. Dietary interventions to prevent disease. Annu Rev Public Health 2002. 23; 255-286.
96. Steptoe A, Perkins-Porras L, McKay C, et al. Behavioral counseling to increase consumption of fruits and vegetables in low income adults: randomized trial. BMJ 2003;326;855-869.).
97. Prochaska JO, Velicer WF. The transtheoretical model of health behavior change. Am J Health Promot 1997;12:38-48.
98. Eikenberry N, Smith C. Healthful eating: perceptions, motivations, barriers, and promoters in low-income Minnesota communities. J am Diet Assoc. 2004;104;1158-1161.
99. Neumark-Sztainer D, Wall M, Story M, Fulkerson JA. Are family meal patterns associated with disordered eating behaviors among adolescents? J Adolesc Health. 2004 Nov;35(5):350-9.
100. Eisenberg ME, Olson RE, Neumark-Sztainer D, et al. Correlations between family meals and psychosocial well-being among adolescents. Arch Pediatr Adolesc Med 2004;158;792-796.
101. Steptoe A, Doherty S, Rink E, et al. Behavioral counseling in general practice for the promotion of healthy behavior among adults at increased risk of coronary heart disease: randomized trial. BMJ 1999;319;943-948.
102. Eakin EG, Glasgow RE, Riley KM. Review of primary care-based physical activity intervention studies: Effectiveness and implications for practice and future research. J Fam Pract 2000;49:158-168.
103. Smith BJ. Promotion of physical activity in primary health care: update of the evidence on interventions. J of Science and Medicine in Sport. 2004;7(1 suppl):67-73.
104. Glasgow RE, Vogt TM, Boles SM. Evaluating the public health impact of health promotion interventions: the RE-AIM framework. Am J Public Health 1999;89:1322-7G
105. Golin, C. DiMAtteo R, Duan N, Leake B, Gelberg L. Impoverished diabetic patients whose doctors facilitate their participation in medical decision making are more satisfied with their care. J Gen Intern Med. 2002;17:857-866.
106. Butler CC, Pill R, Stott NCH. Qualitative study of patients' perceptions of doctors' advice to quit smoking: implications for opportunistic health promotion. BMJ 1998; 316:1878-1881.
107. Richmond, R, Kehoe L, Heather N, Wodak A, Webster I. General practitioners' promotion of healthy life styles: what patients think. Aust N Z J Public Health 1996;20:195-200.

Section VII

Putting It All Together

Chapter 34
The Patient's Story; the Clinician's Thinking—A Place to Start

Michael Stone, MD and David S. Jones, MD

Introduction

Healthcare practitioners—whether modern or ancient, from Western or Eastern disciplines, physician or shaman—have always needed a system for constructing an "explanatory story" of the patient's illness. These systems can vary from a few questions and much observation (an approach characteristic of the Yupik shaman), or prolonged palpation of the pulse while listening to the breathing pattern (a Tibetan healer), to patient questionnaires accompanied by physical exam and laboratory data (the Western medical model). Whatever the tradition or training, the healer/healthcare practitioner and patient together construct a story; the most comprehensive methods integrate experiences, perceptions, observations, and objective information into a coherent, culturally-sensitive narrative. Two important outcomes are generated from a *comprehensive* patient story: (1) the patient experiences being understood within a context that is often considerably broader than the standard biomedical portrait, and (2) hope is established in the minds of both patient and practitioner that steps can be taken to change the trajectory of the present illness back toward health.

Clinical medicine really begins with the patient's story, so it is worth our time to be sure we construct that story in a way that is appropriate to the patient, to his or her complaint(s), and to the therapeutics that can be most helpful.

Most healthcare systems have a heuristic approach to this challenge—a shorthand way of directing attention that does not require continuous application of the entire, detailed decision model at every step of the process. Collecting, sorting, and focusing relevant data toward the development of a coherent story and well-founded therapeutic plan can, indeed, be cumbersome and time-consuming in the absence of an efficient model. In standard medical care, efficiency is gained by generating and sorting information through a well-established and very useful model: chief complaint, medical history of the presenting problem(s), past medical history (including important family medical history), social and work history, present medications, history of drug sensitivities, and a complete review of systems. This standard medical heuristic is organized to achieve a relatively quick and highly useful distillation of the patient's story into a "short list" of potential diagnoses; the process of selecting among those potential diagnoses (achieving the differential diagnosis) is usually facilitated by collecting further data (physical examination, laboratory measures) related to the most likely choices.

The inherent goal in this model is to narrow the inquiry down as quickly as possible to a specific diagnosis,[1] with the expectation that such a process leads fairly directly to a therapeutic plan of (usually) pharmaceutical and/or surgical intervention(s).[2] Implicit in such a model is a belief that enough of the patient's full story can be captured by a diagnosis that an appropriate and effective treatment plan can be based upon it. The organization of information into only those categories that help the clinician formulate the diagnosis and the treatment plan simplifies the process of "doctoring," and lends coherence and reproducibility to the standard medical approach.

The cost, however, of the speed and efficiency of this model is that the narrow focus precludes a comprehensive response to some of today's most common and costly conditions: chronic, complex illnesses.[3] Speed and efficiency are highly desirable in the acute care setting; however, the steady and disturbing rise in the incidence and prevalence of serious chronic diseases makes the case that those are not the best standards for non-acute circumstances.

This textbook has been devoted to the exposition of a new information-gathering-and-sorting architecture that stands on the very substantial shoulders of the standard medical paradigm, expanding it with an emphasis on principles and mechanisms that weld meaning and mechanistic explanations to the diagnosis, and deepen the clinician's understanding of the often overlapping ways things "go wrong," and what to do about it.

Any methodology for constructing a coherent story and an effective therapeutic plan in the context of complex, chronic illness must be flexible and adaptive. Like an accordion file that can compress and expand upon demand, the amount and kind of data needed will necessarily change in accordance with the patient's situation and the clinician's time and ability to piece together the underlying threads of dysfunction. In the acute setting, the clinical information requirements contract to a very slim, survival-driven set of points that provide guidance and milestones with as little extraneous information as possible in order to achieve rapid diagnosis and intervention. Relevant examples of the clinical conditions responsive to this model abound: cardiac arrest, gram-negative shock, pneumonia, herpetic corneal infection, spinal cord compression, and so forth. However, in the approach to complex chronic illness, with multiple co-morbidities, the accordion file must expand to incorporate a much larger database of relevant information. For example, the compilation of the "present illness" section of the history and physical must expand to include a thorough investigation of antecedents, triggers, and mediators (see Chapter 8), if the completed story is to develop and sustain a robust partnership between the patient and the healthcare provider. Personalized medical care without this essential investigation will fall short. There are many pathways that can lead to chronic disease; the story elements must broaden sufficiently to assess those.[4] Diagnosis is only one step in the functional medicine process; it is not, as it often is in the standard paradigm, the final step before intervention.

Traditionally, the *review of systems* assesses how the various organ systems—neurological, ENT, respiratory, cardiovascular, etc.—are functioning; it follows the questions about present illness and past medical history and often completes the initial data collection process. In the setting of complex, chronic illness, however, a new step must be inserted after the *review of systems*. In order to construct a robust response to the many issues of chronic illness, a *"review of mechanisms"* (functional medicine's *raison d'être*) must engage the clinician's attention. (As is apparent from a glance at the functional medicine matrix—discussed below—this process includes the mind-body or psychosocial mechanisms as well as the physical.) This step enables the clinician to engage in a focused review of pathways and factors that contribute to the development and perpetuation of disease. To complete the metaphor, in the *acute medical setting*, the accordion file takes on a compressed, streamlined profile, with non-essential information removed to facilitate rapid response. But in *chronic, complex disease* care, the file expands to accommodate a more comprehensive set of data elements that help the clinician understand a great deal more about the patient: environment, genetic predispositions, physiological and biochemical functionality, and body/mind/spirit influences. The end point of this expanded process is a patient story that is broader and deeper, and that contains many more indicators for both patient and practitioner in terms of developing and implementing an effective therapeutic plan.

The Functional Medicine Matrix or Web

In 1913, William Osler anticipated our ability to "study the interaction of internal secretions, their influence upon development, upon mental process and upon disorders of metabolism." He believed it would "likely prove of a benefit scarcely less remarkable than that which we have traced in the infectious diseases."[5] As we write in 2005, examples of our more sophisticated understanding of human physiology are increasingly part of our common knowledge and clinical thinking—from genetics and the genome to cytochrome P450 polymorphisms, from the symphony of cytokines involved in inflammation to emerging vitamin D research documenting its role as a humoral, immune modulator (a "hormone"). As a result, we now recognize many different opportunities for clinical intervention. Figure 34.1 depicts one way of considering the continuum of health in the functional medicine model.

Methods for helping clinicians incorporate new evidence and new ways of thinking into the pressured pace of clinical practice must be improved. Functional medicine offers an approach to the comprehensive *review of essential elements and mechanisms of disease* that incorporates "the interaction of internal secretions" and the emerging understanding of human physiology and mind-body research. Explicit in the principles of functional medicine is the concept that each patient comprises his or her own "universe" with a unique set of interconnections, potentials, diversities, and reserve capacities.[6] Also recognized is that "the body can only be understood as a whole."[7] The functional medicine principles (see Section II of this book) add a significant level of complexity to the clinical thinking process, requiring not only more data collection but also a conscious synthesizing process: Who is this patient—in detail and in whole? IFM has developed some tools to facilitate both data collection and sorting, as well as analysis/synthesis. The central organizing tool is the functional medicine *matrix* or web tool (see Figure 34.2). Further on in the chapter, we'll discuss the use of the matrix, but it's important to have the basic image in mind at this point.

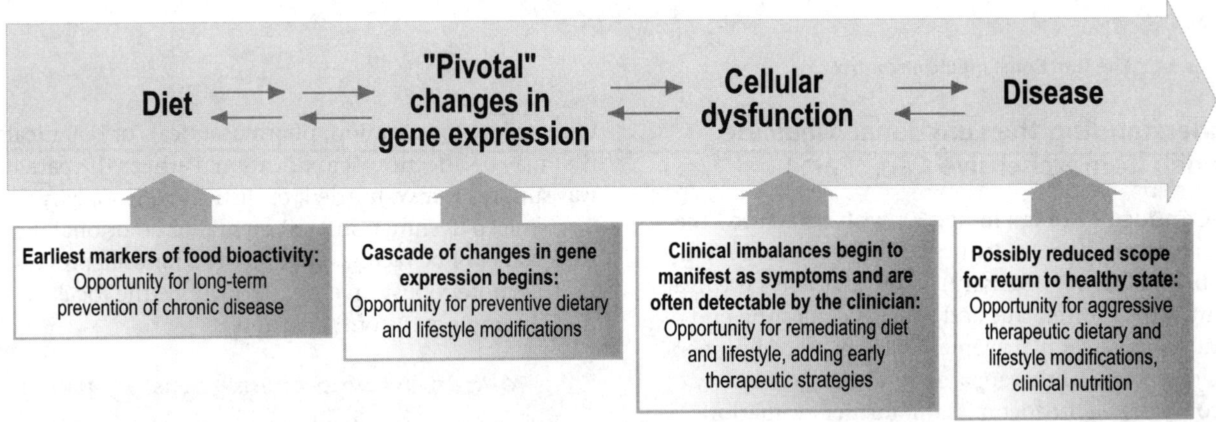

Figure 34.1 **Intervention opportunities in functional medicine**

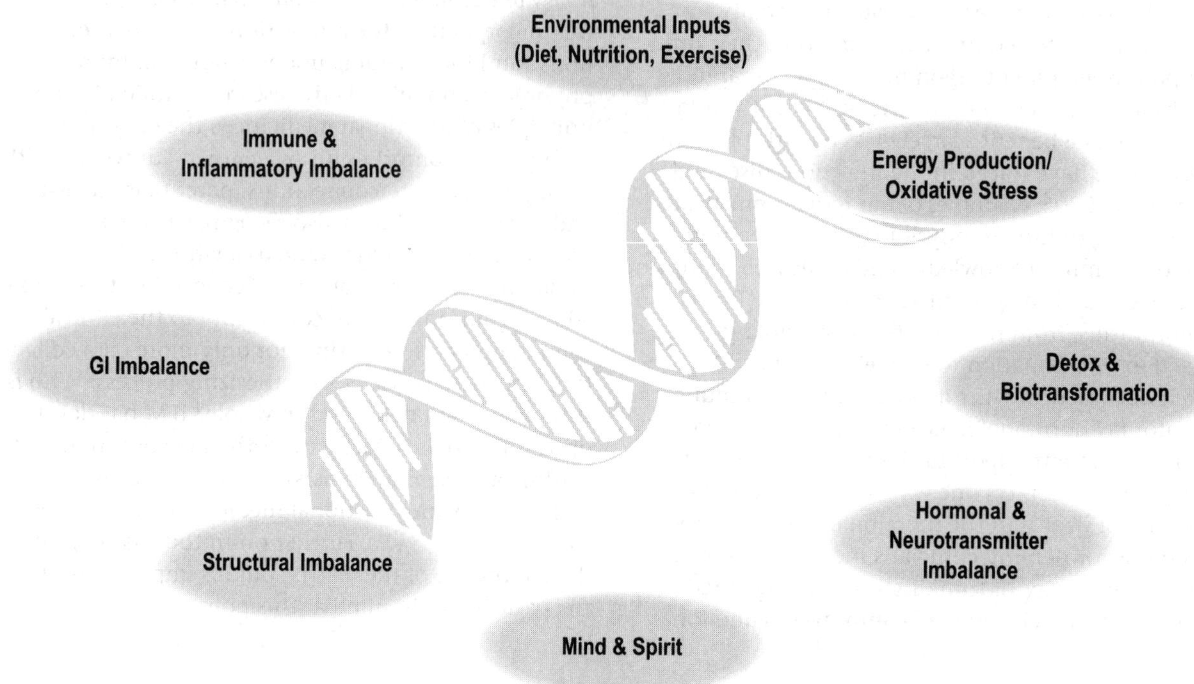

Figure 34.2 **The functional medicine matrix**

Understanding the Functional Medicine Model: Comprehensive Care, Part I

Consider a woman in her 60s with a fractured toe. The acute problem is identified, evaluated, and fixed (orthopedically, if necessary) and the patient's toe heals. Right? This is often true and usually signals the end of standard medical management. However, comprehensive care, even in this apparently simple acute case, encompasses a broader mission; further evaluation might indicate underlying contributory problems, and a preventive approach to those may prevent similar problems in the future.

Asking one basic question initiates a process that could have significant long-term health benefits for the patient: *What were the antecedents to and/or triggers of the problem?* Underlying issues may include bones weakened from vitamin D or mineral undernutrition; medication-nutrient interactions that have altered absorption or excretion of bone matrix substrate; endocrine dysfunction; chronic inflammation; lack of exercise or altered weight bearing; balance or movement problems perhaps triggered by intoxication; pharmaceuticals or botanicals that may be affecting detoxification. Perhaps the patient was simply clumsy, hurried, or distracted. If so, why? Stress, sleep dysfunction, and mental or emotional distress could all be factors. Organizing a rational process for this more robust investigation will be the focus of the remaining parts of this chapter.

Tools to Assist in Comprehensive History-taking

Before proceeding further with this case, let's imagine an entire therapeutic encounter. First of all, a critical aspect in the establishment of trust and the creation of a therapeutic alliance is cultural sensitivity to the circumstances and beliefs of the person seeking help (see Chapter 36 for an in-depth discussion on creating effective doctor-patient relationships). How a question is asked can be nearly as important as whether it was asked at all. In gathering information to illuminate the diagnosis and functional assessment, the stage is also being set for downstream issues of compliance with treatment recommendations and alliance in the therapeutic relationship. Identifying obstacles to health in the data-gathering process—whether physical, mental, emotional, or environmental—demands conscious attention, skillful interviewing, and effective listening. Table 34.1 reviews common elements of a comprehensive history; most of these points will be familiar to clinicians from many different disciplines, but it's good to have the basic context in mind, because it's what we build upon.

The history-taking can be facilitated by appropriately focused data-collection forms. Every office has these, of course, but we offer in the Appendix samples of a few forms that support a functional medicine approach:

- The *Environmental Exposure and Tolerance* questionnaire is useful if the patient has a history suggesting drug, nutrient, or environmental intolerance.
- The *Life Stress Questionnaire* will help identify issues that are known to affect emotional stress and health.
- The *3-Day Diet Record* provides a very straightforward way of assessing dietary habits, and it can be reviewed in the context of the healthy eating pyramid[8] proposed by Walter Willett. This type of record can be used to assess adequacy of diet compared to the old and new USDA food pyramids[9,10] and the vegetarian food pyramid guidelines,[11] as well as other popular diets, all of which have their own strengths and weaknesses.[12,13]
- Additional useful forms include the *Review of Organ Systems* and the *Medical Symptoms Questionnaire*, which quantifies the incidence of symptoms and their frequency (and also provides a quick measure of patient improvement, if it is re-administered at regular intervals).

Interactions and adverse reactions. Today's history-taking process is complicated by the fact that many people use multiple OTC and prescription drugs, as well as nutraceuticals of various kinds. We now know that this situation creates increased risks of intolerance and/or adverse reactions for a variety of reasons. As part of normal history taking, therefore, all herbal, pharmaceutical, and nutritional supplements should be listed in the patient's chart, updated regularly, and reviewed for possible interactions. Clinicians should be cognizant of the fact that there are now commercially available drug-drug interaction software programs, as well as drug-nutrient, nutrient-nutrient, and botanical-drug publications and programs to help in evaluating the patient's list for potential problems. An article published in 2001[14] identified 27 drugs frequently cited in adverse drug reaction studies. Among these drugs, 59%

Table 34.1 **Components of a Comprehensive History**

Chief Complaint: The current concern or problem
Present Illness: The timeline and symptoms involved with the current problem(s) and associated complaint(s); functional medicine practitioners add questions that explore any noteworthy *antecedents, triggers and mediators* of the present illness.

Past Medical and Surgical History
Review of Lifestyle and Habits
Review of Organ Systems

Considered within the context of underlying mechanisms in the areas of the functional medicine matrix:

Environmental Inputs	Structural
Oxidative Stress	Neuroendocrine
Mind/Body	Detoxification
Immune/Inflammation	GI Function

- Medical problems
- Surgeries and hospitalizations
- Traumas
- Medications
- Supplements, herbs, nutrients, homeopathics, adaptogens
- Allergies, sensitivities, or intolerance to medications, herbs, foods
- Exercise patterns
- Diet or special dietary habits:
  - What foods are regularly eaten or avoided?
  - Artificial sweeteners or fats: aspartame, sucralose, olestra
- Social, occupational, and lifestyle history:
  - Relationships (family, work, community)
  - Passions, hobbies, interests
  - Work and potential environmental exposures
  - Habits and addictions: tobacco, alcohol, caffeine, illegal drugs
  - Sexually active (if yes, practicing safe sex?)
  - Spirituality and faith
  - Preventive medicine interventions
  - Vaccinations and immunizations
- Family history
  - Genetically-linked illnesses and predispositions
  - Family behaviors or emotional tones
  - Lifestyle issues of family members

Differential Diagnosis

are metabolized by at least one enzyme with a variant allele known to cause poor metabolism. These findings are summarized in Table 34.2.

Table 34.2 Commonly Identified Drugs in Adverse Drug Reactions

Therapeutic Category and Drug Class	Specific Drug
Cardiovascular	
• Beta blockers	atenolol, metoprolol
• Angiotensin converting enzyme (ACE) inhibitors	lisinopril
• Diuretics	furosemide, hydrochlorothiazide
• Calcium channel blockers	diltiazem, verapamil
• Inotropic agents/ pressors	digoxin
Analgesics	
• NSAIDs	aspirin, piroxicam, ibuprofen, naproxen
• COX-2 inhibitors	Vioxx®, Bextra®, Celebrex®
Psychiatric	
• Tricyclic antidepressants	imipramine, nortriptyline
• SSRIs	fluoxetine
Antibiotics	
• Penicillin	amoxicillin
• Antitubercular agents	isoniazid, rifampin
• Macrolides	erythromycin
Other	
• Anticoagulants	warfarin sodium
• Corticosteroids	prednisone
• Anticonvulsants	carbamazepine, phenytoin
• Antidiabetic agents	insulin
• Bronchodilators	theophylline
• Electrolytes	potassium
• Antiemetics or antihistamines	meclizine hydrochloride

Adapted from Phillips KA, et al. Potential role of pharmacogenomics in reducing adverse drug reactions; a systemic review. JAMA. 2001;286:2270-79.

Other important factors to consider:

- Many pharmaceuticals and herbs pass through the main cytochrome P450 enzymes as substrates, and can act as inducers or inhibitors of these enzyme systems.
- In addition, the list of enzyme polymorphisms that affect the efficacy and clearance of various drugs and herbs is now extensive and is updated regularly.
- The prevalence of poor metabolizers (a function of polymorphisms in the P450 system) varies by race. A few examples will bring this point home:
  - Among Caucasians, 12% are poor metabolizers of CYP1A2 substrates, up to 6% of CYP2C9 and CYP2D19, and up to 10% of CYP2D6 substrates.
  - Among Chinese, up to 17% are poor metabolizers of CYP2C19 substrates, and <2% are poor metabolizers of CYP2D6 substrates.
  - In people with Japanese heritage, up to 23% are poor metabolizers of CYP2C19 and <2% are poor metabolizers of CYP2D6 substrates.
  - There are many genetic variants within each group of cytochrome alleles and each has its own incidence among races. For example within the CYP2D6 enzyme, there are at least 31 allele variants, with race data showing presence of allele variants in up to 50% of Chinese, 34% of African Americans, 60% of Japanese, 19% of Koreans, 50% of other Asians, and 34% of Africans. (More information on genetic variability and polymorphisms in detoxification can be found in Chapters 22 and 31.)

Genetic inheritance, diet, and combinations of drugs (and other substances) ingested are all factors in the incidence of adverse drug reactions.[15] A study published in 2003 reported that "one quarter of outpatients had adverse drug events during a three-month period … ."[16] Thirty-nine percent of the ADRs reported were classified as "ameliorable or preventable," which implies that 61% were not (given current knowledge). The most common cytochrome polymorphisms are listed in Table 34.3, and the Appendix provides an extensive listing of inhibitors and inducers of some important P450s. Clinicians do need to consider ways in which the patient's history can be evaluated for some of the most common potential problems elucidated by this complex and rapidly growing research.

Table 34.3 **Drugs Implicated in Adverse Drug Reactions Metabolized by Enzymes with Variant Alleles Associated with Poor Metabolism**

Enzyme	Drugs
CYP1A2	Carbamazepine, diltiazem, erythromycin, fluoxetine, imipramine, isoniazid, naproxen, nortriptyline, phenytoin, rifampin, theophylline, verapamil.
CYP2C9	Fluoxetine, ibuprofen, imipramine, isoniazid, naproxen, phenytoin, piroxicam, rifampin, verapamil, warfarin
CYP2C19	Fluoxetine, imipramine, isoniazid, nortriptyline, phenytoin, rifampin, warfarin
CYP2D6	Diltiazem, fluoxetine, imipramine, metoprolol, nortriptyline, theophylline.

From Phillips KA, et al. Potential role of pharmacogenomics in reducing adverse drug reactions; a systemic review. JAMA. 2001;286:2270-79.

Understanding the Functional Medicine Model: Comprehensive Care, Part II

The review of underlying mechanisms of disease (the functional medicine matrix) is where the functional medicine approach begins to significantly depart from the standard model of care, to establish a more comprehensive model. This section of the comprehensive history is best filtered through the *functional medicine matrix*, a tool that helps organize information, clarifying the level of present understanding and illuminating the need for broader investigation (an example of "knowledge-coupling" as proposed by Dr. Larry Weed[17,18]). Let's look at this methodology, as illustrated by a continuation of the "Broken Toe" case (see Figure 34.3).

The functional medicine matrix tool was developed by the Institute of Functional Medicine's Curriculum Committee through a two-year process of repeatedly asking the question: "For comprehensive evaluation of underlying elements and mechanisms of disease, what categories would need to be represented?" This question was subjected to all areas of scientific inquiry in the area of human biology including the expanding research in the importance of mind-body-spirit web-like interconnectedness with physiology. All areas of credentialed medical practice were also drawn into this web of inquiry. We have entered the 21st century with the real possibility of moving medical care from a focus on the differential diagnosis to a focus on understanding the mechanisms associated with the origins of the signs and symptoms that underlie the patient's dysfunction. In 21st century medicine, we will learn to extract the explanation from our understanding of specific antecedents, triggers, and mediators, as well as the frequency, intensity, and duration of the patient's symptoms.[19]

The Institute for Functional Medicine teaches the expanded use of the functional medicine matrix in the six-day course, *Applying Functional Medicine in Clinical Practice* (AFMCP). Information about that course can be reviewed on IFM's web page: www.functionalmedicine.org. The first step in the utilization of the matrix requires a disciplined understanding and review of each element of the matrix, connecting important signs and symptoms to their appropriate element or mechanism of action. The shorthand version of this step in the use of the matrix is illustrated in Figure 34.3 for our sample case. The web-like connections within the eight elements of the matrix will be further elaborated as we progress through this illustrative case study.

The Comprehensive Physical Exam

The physical exam is a key component of patient assessment in nearly all healthcare disciplines. Common components of the basic physical exam are listed in Table 34.4. More extensive systemic exams can be completed, depending on initial findings, specific symptoms, or specialty focus. Signs of undernutrition or altered nutrition are summarized in the Appendix and are extremely important to watch for. For example, many patients with bulimia, and between 24–76% of patients with anorexia nervosa,[20] have dermatologic and physical exam findings of multiple nutritional deficiencies; knowing what those are can help identify a serious underlying problem. Nutritional deficiencies are also common in the elderly, who have a significant risk of being deficient in at least two nutritional cofactors.[21]

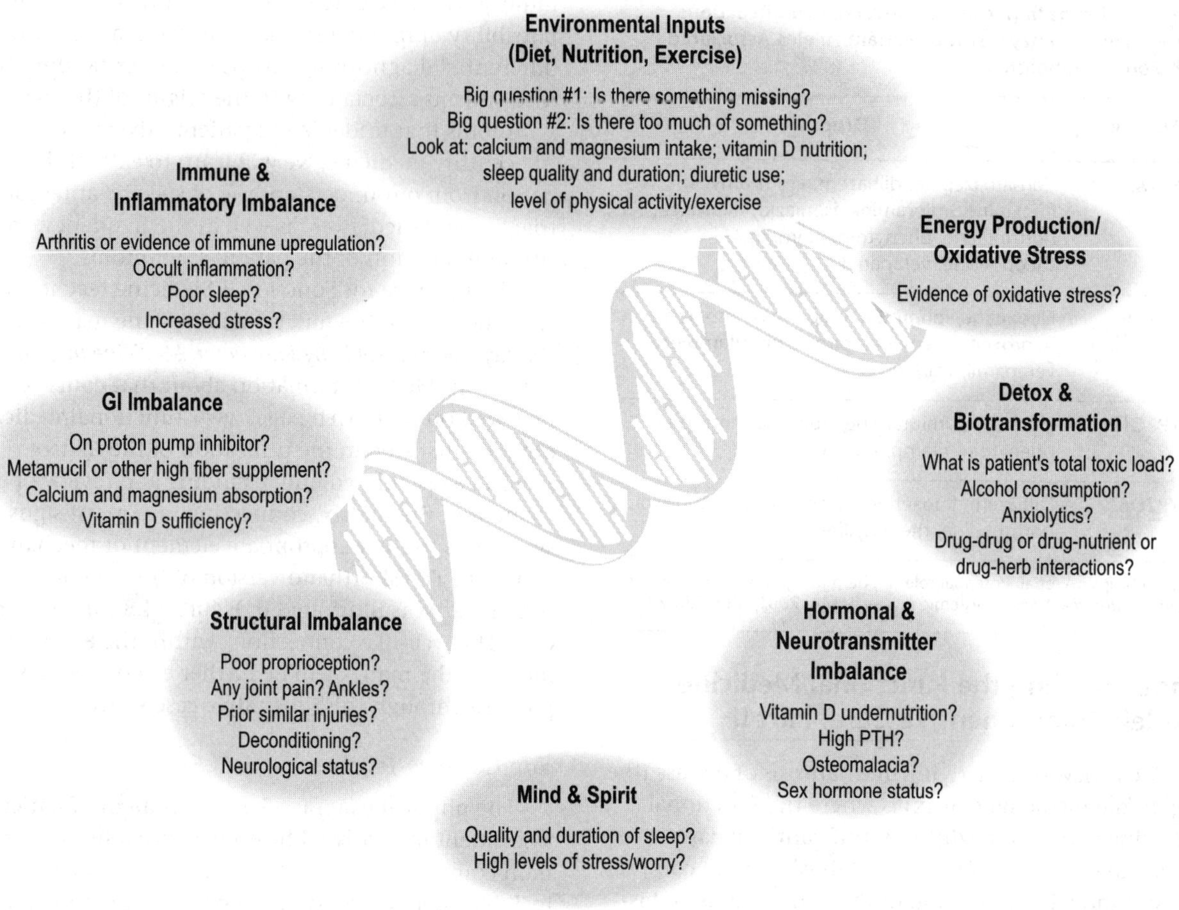

Figure 34.3 **The matrix as applied to the "Broken Toe" case**

Comprehensive history taking and physical exam from a functional medicine perspective require a different time frame and the use of additional data-gathering and sorting tools. It is impossible to investigate the patient's unique health history using a review of mechanisms, *and* perform a thorough physical, within the time constraints of a brief office visit. Recent research has documented that all primary care providers in the present healthcare environment face a significant time problem in managing patients with chronic, complex illnesses.[22] However, after the comprehensive assessment is completed, it is then possible to break further assessments and interventions into shorter segments; but a comprehensive approach to the first visit is critical.

Sidney Baker, MD tells a story about his early medical training and mentoring while serving in Kathmandu, Nepal in 1959. His senior medical tutor, before the completion of a patient workup, always asked: "Sidney, is there anything else we can do for this patient?" We suggest a similar question: "What additional information would be helpful to understand this patient?" Chapter 35 focuses on just that question, emphasizing dietary assessment and the benefits and limitations of laboratory assessment.

Table 34.4 **Common Components of the Basic Physical Exam**

General	Height, weight, blood pressure, pulse, respiratory rate, temperature, appearance, somatotype, emotional state
Head	Configuration, shape, symmetry or asymmetry, excess hair or hair loss, lesions, scars, bruits or tenderness behind the ears, tenderness on the temporal arteries, prominence of vessels
Eyes	Visual acuity, conjunctiva, sclera color, extraocular movements, visual fields by confrontation, papillary reaction to light and accommodation, iris, funduscopic examination of the lens, disks, retinal vessels, upper and lower lids
Ears	Auditory acuity, shape, external auditory canal, tympanic membranes and acoustic meatus, hearing—bone/air conduction
Nose	Air movement, nares, turbinates, polyps, septum, mucosa, drainage, rhinorrhea, smell
Mouth	Symmetry, control of lips and jaw. Oral exam: lips, mucosa, gingival plaque; normal, decayed, or missing teeth; enamel staining/color, dentures, or implants; degree of amalgams and what type, occlusion; saliva, ducts, tongue color, fissuring, tastebud lack or prominence, tonsils, pharynx, redundancy of tissue, uvula at rest and during phonation, lesions, infections
Neck	Symmetry and configuration, movement, strength; mobile and midline trachea; cervical anterior, posterior, and supraclavicular lymph nodes; thyroid, bruits, carotid pulses, muscle symmetry, masses, cysts. Suprasternal notch or supraclavicular fossa fullness. Inspect and palpate spine.
Axilla	Nodes, masses, hair presence or absence
Chest	Symmetry, excursion/movement. Palpate for tenderness of ribs, masses, maldevelopment, or crepitus.
Breasts	Symmetric, masses, cysts, tenderness, discharge, lesions on nipple
Lungs	Rate and rhythm of respiratory cycle, vital capacity, hoarseness, clarity with breathing, symmetric, rhonchi, rales, wheezes, crepitus, pleural rub, percussion symmetry
Heart	Rhythm; heart valves—sounds, murmurs, changes with position; pulses—radial, femoral, popliteal, dorsalis pedis, lateralization of the point of maximal impulse; extra sounds—rubs, clicks
Abdomen	Symmetry; liver or spleen enlargement; bowel sounds, bruits, friction rubs, tenderness, masses; percussion tenderness; rectus diastasis, hernias. Palpate the femoral and iliac arteries, abdominal aorta. Palpate lymph nodes of the inguinal canal
Back	Symmetry of station, musculature, posture. Vertebral tenderness. Range of motion of neck, thorax, lumbar spine
Musculoskeletal	Trigger-point tenderness; normal movement of the shoulders, elbows, wrists, hands, hips, knees, ankles, toes—opening/closing of hands; hips, knees, ankles, toes. Swelling, tenderness, or asymmetry of joints or tendons; signs of ligament laxity; signs of previous or current injury.
Rectal	Perianal or anal lesions, fissures, masses; sphincter tone; prostate size (males), retroflexed uterus (female)
Genitourinary	Male: scrotum, testes, epididymi, penis, glans, lesions Female: external genitalia, introitus, mucosa of the introitus, vagina, cervix; presence of rectocele/cystocele; palpation of the cervix, uterus, and adnexa; discharge or masses; ovaries present
Skin	Texture, lesions, abnormal discolorations, hair pattern; subcutaneous fat texture. Nails—dysmorphic, texture or asymmetry, marks, abnormal thickness or consistency. Nail beds—color, lesions
Neurologic	Auditory acuity, intelligence, memory, mood, speech, gait, balance, involuntary movements. Cranial nerves 1–12; cerebellar exam; frontal release signs. Deep tendon reflexes of the biceps, triceps, brachioradialis, patellar, Achilles, and plantar. Proprioception, vibratory sense; orientation, mini-mental status. Can the patient get up from sitting, walk across the room, pick up a piece of paper, walk back, and sit down?

The matrix, however, is extremely useful in identifying where the preponderance of evidence from the initial history and physical lies, and also in clarifying where further investigation (e.g., laboratory work) is needed. For example, indicators of *inflammation* on the matrix might lead the clinician to request tests for specific inflammatory markers (such as hsCRP, interleukin levels, and/or homocysteine) to help illuminate the "immune/inflammatory" processes that might be at work. Essential fatty acid levels, methylation pathway abnormalities, and organic acid metabolites help determine adequacy of *dietary and nutrient* intakes. Markers of *detoxification* (glucuronidation and sulfation, cytochrome P450 enzyme heterogeneity) can determine functional capacity for molecular biotransformation. Neurotransmitters and their metabolites (vanilmandelate, homovanillate, 5-hydroxyindoleacetate, quinolinate) and hormone cascades (gonadal and adrenal) have obvious utility in exploring "messenger molecule" balance. CT scans, MRIs, or plain x-rays extend our view of the patient's *structural* dysfunctions. The use of bone scans, dexa scans, or bone resorption markers[23,24] can be useful in further exploring the web-like interactions of the matrix. Newer, useful technologies such as functional MRIs, SPECT or PET scans open a frontier of more comprehensive assessment of metabolic function within organ systems. But it is the process of completing a comprehensive history and physical and then charting these findings on the matrix that best directs the choice of laboratory work and successful treatment.

Five Levels of Functionality: Selecting Effective Treatments

Distilling the data from the history, physical exam, and laboratory into a narrative story line that includes antecedents, triggers, and mediators can be daunting. Key to developing a thorough narrative is viewing the story through the lens of the functional medicine matrix, which facilitates organizing the story according to a set of eight common underlying mechanisms of (or influences upon) health. However, even with the matrix as an aid to synthesizing and prioritizing information, it can be very useful to consider the impact of each variable at five different levels:

1. Whole body (the "macro" level)
2. Organ system
3. Metabolic or cellular
4. Subcellular/mitochondrial
5. Subcellular/gene expression

Therapies should be chosen for their potential impact on the most central imbalances of the particular patient; evaluating interventions that are available at each of the five levels can help to identify a reasonably comprehensive set of options from which to choose. The following lists incorporate only a few examples of various types of interventions within these five different levels. The rest of this book contains many more.

1. **Whole body interventions:** Because the human organism is a complex adaptive system, with countless points of access, interventions at one level will affect points of activity in other areas as well. For example, improving the patient's sleep will beneficially influence the immune response, melatonin levels, T cell lymphocyte levels, and will help to decrease oxidative stress. Incorporating exercise markedly affects many areas of the matrix; we know that exercise reduces stress, improves insulin sensitivity, and improves detoxification, just to mention a few instances. Reducing stress (and/or improving stress management) can reduce cortisol levels, improve sleep, improve emotional well being, reduce the risk of heart disease, and so forth. Changing the diet can have myriad effects on health, from reducing inflammation to reversing coronary artery disease. (See Chapter 26 for a discussion of the many potential benefits of dietary interventions.)
2. **Organ system interventions:** These interventions are used more frequently in the acute presentation of illness. Examples include splinting; draining lesions; repairing lacerations; reducing fractures, pneumothoraxes, hernias or obstructions; or removing a stone to reestablish whole organ function. There are many interventions that improve function. For example, bronchodilators improve air exchange, thereby decreasing hypoxia, reducing oxidative stress, and improving metabolic function and oxygenation in a patient with reactive airway disease.
3. **Metabolic or cellular interventions:** Cellular health can be addressed by insuring the adequacy of macronutrients and micronutrients, the cofactors for intracellular metabolism. For example, deficiencies of folate, vitamins B6, and B12 are

widespread.[25] An individual's metabolic enzyme polymorphisms can profoundly affect his or her nutrient requirements. Providing adequate essential amino acids, vitamins, and cofactor minerals in the diet according to the patient's unique metabolic needs is essential. The frequency and impact of the greater than 50 identified enzymatic polymorphisms that are common in the population have been outlined.[26] These affect enzymatic systems in the cytosol and mitochondria. There are many more examples of appropriate nutrient interventions that should be made in the context of the patient's condition. For example, adding conjugated linoleic acid (CLA) to the diet can alter the PPAR system, affect body weight, and modulate the inflammatory response.[27,28,29] However, in a person who is diabetic or insulin resistant, adding CLA may induce hyperproinsulinemia, which is detrimental.[30,31] Altering the types and proportions of carbohydrates in the diet may increase insulin sensitivity, reduce insulin secretion, and fundamentally alter metabolism in the insulin-resistant patient. Alcohol consumption and smoking both change requirements for many of the nutrient and vitamin cofactors. Decreasing use of these substances may lower excessive demand and exert less pressure on the cellular detoxification pathways in the lungs and liver. Supporting liver detoxification pathways with supplemental glycine and N-acetylcysteine improves the endogenous production of adequate glutathione, an essential antioxidant in the central nervous system and GI tract. N-acetylcysteine also plays a role in the sulfur conjugation pathway that is important in the detoxification of acetaminophen and other substances.

4. **Subcellular/mitochondrial interventions:** There are many examples of mitochondrial nutrient-support interventions.[32,33] Inadequate iron intake causes oxidants to leak from mitochondria, damaging mitochondrial function and mitochondrial DNA. Making sure there is sufficient iron helps alleviate this problem. Inadequate zinc intake (found in >10% of the U.S. population) causes oxidation and DNA damage in human cells.[34] Insuring the adequacy of antioxidants and cofactors for the at-risk individual must be considered in each part of the matrix. Carnitine, for example, is required as a carrier for the transport of fatty acids from the cytosol into the mitochondria, improving the efficiency of beta oxidation of fatty acids and resultant ATP production. In patients who have lost significant weight, carnitine undernutrition can result in fatty acids undergoing omega oxidation, a far less efficient form of metabolism.[35] Patients with low carnitine may also respond to riboflavin supplementation.[36]
5. **Subcellular/gene expression interventions:** As will be clear to the reader of this book, many compounds interact at the gene level to alter cellular response, thereby affecting health and healing. Any intervention that alters NFκB entering the nucleus, binding to DNA, and activating genes that encode inflammatory modulators such as IL-6 (and thus CRP), cyclooxygenase 2, IL-1, lipoxygenase, inducible nitric oxide synthase, TNF-α, or a number of adhesion molecules will impact many disease conditions.[37,38] There are many ways to alter the environmental triggers for NFκB, including lowering oxidative stress, altering emotional stress, and consuming adequate phytonutrients, antioxidants, alpha-lipoic acid, EPA, DHA, and GLA.[39] Adequate vitamin A allows the appropriate interaction of vitamin A-retinoic acid with over 370 genes.[40] Vitamin D in its most active form intercalates with a retinol protein and the DNA exon and modulates many aspects of metabolism including cell division in both healthy and cancerous breast, colon, prostate, and skin tissue.[41] Vitamin D has key roles in controlling inflammation, calcium homeostasis, bone metabolism, cardiovascular and endocrine physiology, and healing.[42] Many of the finer points of the functions of vitamins A and D in health have been covered earlier in the text. Folate and B12 are key in DNA repair. Requirements vary among different patients; therefore, adequacy must be individually determined and maintained.[43]

Understanding the Functional Medicine Model: Comprehensive Care, Part III

Returning once again to the "Broken Toe" case, we must now connect the Part I data on antecedents, triggers, and mediators with the Part II assessment of underlying mechanisms to answer the key clinical question: At what levels can we intervene effectively? By this time, most of the issues mentioned below will likely have been resolved and the remaining questions will be answerable, leading to clear indications for treatment.

1. **Whole body interventions:** Depending on our findings, we may determine that the patient needs to use a balance aid, or learn some core strengthening exercises to avoid further injury. Checking for balance on a neurologic exam can be essential to configuring an appropriate secondary prevention program. If osteoporosis is a factor, dietary and exercise recommendations may be a high priority.
2. **Organ system interventions:** Splinting or immobilization by buddy taping or wearing a stiff-soled shoe reduces fracture line movement and speeds healing. Orthopedic consultation for possible pinning may be in order, depending on the fracture site and extent (i.e., great toe, middle phalanx involving the joint space). Checking for drug/nutrient interactions may uncover causes of calcium or magnesium deficiency (environmental input/diet element of the matrix). Consider determining bone density; perhaps she has significant osteoporosis. Suggest dietary changes to improve calcification and healing, timing of fiber, and calcium or magnesium supplementation. If she is on calcium, evaluate her source. Is she on a proton pump inhibitor or acid blocker that may be affecting B12 availability and absorption? Has she had prior injury and has there been a program of reconditioning? Consider gonadal function and bone strength. How is her eyesight, as well as her proprioception or vibratory sense?
3. **Cellular/metabolic interventions:** Does the patient live north of 35 degrees N, or south of 35 degrees S? What is the color of her skin? Does she get enough UV B light? Is she inside all the time? Is she always covered with clothing or sunscreen? In other words, is she at risk for vitamin D deficiency and thus secondary hyperparathyroidism, resulting in osteomalacia or osteoporosis? What is her caffeine consumption? Caffeine increases calcium and magnesium loss in the urine. Are there gut absorption problems that could affect calcium absorption? Is she taking a diuretic? Does she have indices of inflammation? TNF-α inhibitors have been associated with slowing the speed of fracture healing. Is she taking an anti-inflammatory? Anti-inflammatories can also slow the healing of fractures.[44]
4. **Subcellular/mitochondrial interventions:** Are there any obvious mitochondrial issues? Is nutrient intake adequate? Is she on a level of fixed income that is associated with poor nutrient status? Does she have adequate energy? Excessive fatigue can interfere with compliance on treatment recommendations such as exercise or physical therapy.
5. **Subcellular/gene expression interventions:** Does she have any physical exam findings or genetic history that would suggest she has an altered requirement for specific nutrients? Is she getting enough vitamin A, vitamin K, vitamin D? Does she need intervention to alter NFκB with phytonutrients, or nutritionals?[45,46]

Re-Assessment: After appraising the five levels discussed above, and assessing and initiating appropriate interventions, one last re-assessment question should be asked: What is now known with certainty, and which points on the matrix still merit further investigation? A final review of the matrix, this hologram that you have constructed, can elucidate areas that still need fleshing out, or that may not truly reflect the patient's reality. Allow yourself a frank and critical review process.

Consider referrals: No single practitioner—and no single discipline—can cover all the viable therapeutic options. Interventions will differ by training, licensure, specialty focus, and even by beliefs and ethnic heritage. However, all the specialties and disciplines can—to the degree allowed by their training and licensure—use a functional medicine approach, including integrating the matrix as a basic template for organizing and coupling knowledge and data. So, where possible, seek out other providers who have also acquired some functional medicine training. Treatment success can be affected by the cultural bias of the patient and the provider, so get to know your colleagues in other fields.

Educate yourself about what other disciplines have to offer. Should any medical specialists be involved? If you are not well trained in physical medicine, consider a chiropractor or osteopathic physician. If your experience with botanicals, supplements, and dietary interventions is limited, a naturopathic physician might be a wise choice. In-depth nutritional counseling is offered by nutritionists and registered dietitians. Acupuncture has much to offer, as does Traditional Chinese Medicine (TCM). It is beyond the mission of this book to discuss the training, scope of practice, or therapeutics of the many different healthcare approaches available today, but many publications and websites do provide such information. Regardless of what discipline you have been trained in, developing a network of capable, collaborative clinicians with whom you can co-manage challenging patients and to whom you can refer for therapies outside your own expertise will enrich the care your patients receive, and will strengthen the clinician-patient relationship. Many patients do not tell one practitioner about care they are receiving from other practitioners. Keep those lines of communication open and alive. All referral relationships should be handled with the same professionalism and courtesy.

A Concluding Short Story of Comprehensive Care

We'll let another case demonstrate the value to the patient of using a comprehensive functional medical model of care. The *Lancet* reported a case study in March 1999 in a paper titled: "A Woman Who Left Her Wheelchair."[47] A 32-year old woman had suffered for over two years with progressive muscular weakness and pain. Her standard (and very thorough) medical workup had ruled out emergency spinal crisis with appropriate imaging techniques including CT scan, MRI, and bone scan. Her neurological exam did not show sensory or motor disturbance, or muscle atrophy. Electromyography and nerve conduction studies were reported to be normal. A diagnosis eluded her physicians, except for a documented iron-deficiency anemia that was treated with iron-dextran, given intravenously. Her weakness progressed over the ensuing two years, eventually requiring use of a wheelchair.

In 1997, after two years of investigation, a new review of the present medical problem, filtered through the lens of *antecedents/triggers/mediators*, revealed a long-term history of Crohn's disease, requiring steroids by age 21, followed more recently by a small-bowel resection. She had *not* experienced the symptoms of progressive muscular weakness and pain prior to the small-bowel resection. In a *review of underlying mechanisms of illness*, the question of nutrient adequacy in the context of chronic Crohn's and small-bowel disease was raised. With small-bowel resection of one meter of ileum, bile salt loss with steatorrhea can occur; she did suffer from foul-smelling stools. A fecal sample from the patient showed 90 g of fat loss over 24 hours. A complete metabolic panel was unremarkable except for elevated values of alkaline phosphatase and markers of bone reabsorption (osteocalcin and pyridinoline cross-linked telopeptide), but with normal calcium and parathyroid hormone. Further testing demonstrated a 25-OH-Vit D level that was profoundly low (2.4 ng/mL).

Tying together the antecedent conditions, triggers, and mediators of her illness with the review of underlying mechanisms of illness, a diagnosis was made: hypovitaminosis D due to selective fat malabsorption (including fat-soluble vitamin D) after small-bowel resection for resistant Crohn's disease. A treatment plan was instigated. Her metabolic stores were repleted using parenterally administered 1,25 dihydroxyvitamin D3 with additional calcium, and a phosphate-rich diet, low in fat (meat, fish, liver and root vegetables). Within three weeks she was able to walk without assistance; her weakness and bone pain resolved and did not return.

References

1. Goldman L, Weinberg M, Weisberg M, et al. A computer-derived protocol to aid in the diagnosis of emergency room patients with acute chest pain. N Engl J Med. 1982;307(10):588-96.
2. Krumholz H, Peterson ED, Ayanian JZ, et al. Report of the National Heart, Lung, and Blood Institute working group on outcomes research in cardiovascular disease. Circulation. 2005;111(23):3158-66.
3. Holman H. Chronic disease—The need for a new clinical education. JAMA. 2004;292(9):1057-60.
4. Ibid.
5. Osler W. The rise and development of modern medicine. Chapter 4 in: The Evolution of Modern Medicine: A Series of Lectures Delivered at Yale University on the Silliman Foundation in April 1913. "The study of the interaction of internal secretions, their influence upon development, upon mental process and upon disorders of metabolism is likely to prove in the future of a benefit scarcely less remarkable than that which we have traced in the infectious diseases." p. 216.
6. Levin B, Schmidt MA, Bland JS. Functional medicine in natural medicine. Chapter 1, A Textbook of Natural Medicine, 2nd ed, Volume 1. Joseph E Pizzorno, Michael T Murray, eds. Churchill Livingston, 1999. "The functional medicine practitioners use the patient as his or her own "universe," or point of reference in which his or her unique set of interconnections, potentials, diversities, and redundancies is realized." p. 10
7. Osler W. Greek medicine. Chapter 2 in The Evolution of Modern Medicine: A series of lectures delivered at Yale University on the Silliman Foundation in April 1913. "Phaedrus replies: 'Hippocrates, the Asclepiad, says that the nature, even of the body, can only be understood as a whole' (Plato, I,311:III,270-Jowett, I,131,479)." p. 60.
8. Willet WC. Eat, Drink, and Be Healthy. The Harvard Medical School Guide to Healthy Eating. Simon & Schuster; New York, NY: 2001, p. 17. Figure 2. The Healthy Eating Pyramid.
9. Willett WC. The dietary pyramid: does the foundation need repair? Am J Clin Nutr. 1998;68:218-19.
10. Mitka M. Government unveils new food pyramid. Critics say nutrition tool is flawed. JAMA. 2005;293(21):2581-82.

11. Haddad EH, Sabate J, Whitten CG. Vegetarian food guide pyramid: a conceptual framework. Am J Clin Nutr. 1999:70(Suppl):615S-19S.
12. Freedman MR, King J, Kennedy E. Popular diets: A scientific review. Obesity Res. 2001;9(Suppl 1):1S-40S.
13. Wendland BE, Greenwood CE, Weinberg I, Young KW. Malnutrition in institutionalized seniors: the iatrogenic component. J Am Geriatr Soc. 2003;51(1):85-90.
14. Phillips KA, Veenstra DL, Oren E, et al. Potential role of pharmacogenomics in reducing adverse drug reactions; a systemic review. JAMA. 2001;286:2270-79.
15. Ibid.
16. Gandhi TK, Weingart SN, Borus J, et al. Adverse drug events in ambulatory care. N Engl J Med. 2003;348(16):1556-64.
17. Weed LL. Clinical judgment revisited. Methods Inf Med. 1999;38(4-5):279-86.
18. Weed LL. Opening the black box of clinical judgment—An overview. BMJ. 1999;319:1279-82.
19. Bland JS. Functional medicine pioneer. Altern Ther Health Med. 2004;10:74-81.
20. Hediger C, Rost B, Itin P. Cutaneous manifestations in anorexia nervosa. Schweiz Med Wochenschr. 2000;130(16):565-75. The most common dermatological findings were xerosis (71%, controls 29%), cheilitis (76%), bodily hypertrichosis (62%), alopecia (24%), dry scalp hair (48%), acral coldness (38%), acrocyanosis (33%), periungual erythema (48%), gingival changes (37%), nail changes (29%) and calluses on the dorsum of the hand due to induced vomiting (67%).
21. High KP. Nutritional strategies to boost immunity and prevent infections in elderly individuals. Clin Infect Dis. 2001;33(11):1892-900. Nutritional deficiencies in the elderly include in the community 25% undernourished., Vitamin A 2-8 %, B12 7-15%, Vitamin D2-10%, Zinc 15-25%, in the institutions 17-85% undernourished, 2-20% vitamin A deficient, 20-40% vitamin D deficient, 5-15% Vitamin E deficient.
22. Østbye T, Yarnall KS, Krause KM, et al. Is there time for management of patients with chronic diseases in primary care? Ann Fam Med. 2005;3:209-14.
23. Yu SL, Ho LM, Lim BC, Sim ML. Urinary deoxypyridinoline is a useful biochemical bone marker for the management of postmenopausal osteoporosis. Ann Acad Med Singapore. 1998;27(4):527-29.
24. Palomba S, Orio F, Colao A, et al. Effect of estrogen replacement plus low-dose alendronate treatment on bone density in surgically postmenopausal women with osteoporosis. J Clin Endocrinol Metab. 2002;87(4):1502-1508.
25. Ames BN. The metabolic tune-up: metabolic harmony and disease prevention. J Nutr. 2003;133:1544S-48S.
26. Ames BN, Elson-Schwab I, Silver A. High-dose vitamin therapy stimulates variant enzymes with decreased coenzyme binding affinity (increased Km): relevance to genetic disease and polymorphisms. Am J Clin Nutr. 2002;75(4):616-58.
27. Moya-Camarena SY, Vanden Heuvel JP, Blanchard SG, et al. Conjugated linoleic acid is a potent naturally occuring ligand and activator of PPARa. J Lipid Res. 1999;40:1426-33. These data indicate that CLA is a ligand and activator of PPAR alpha and its effects on lipid metabolism may be attributed to transcriptional events associated with this nuclear receptor.
28. Gaullier JM, Halse J, Hoye K, et al. Conjugated linoleic acid supplementation for 1 y reduces body fat mass in healthy overweight humans. Am J Clin Nutr. 2004;79:1118-25.
29. O'Shea M, Bassaganya-Riera J, Mohede IC. Immunomodulatory properties of conjugated linoleic acid. Am J Clin Nutr. 2004:79(S):1199S-206S. "Evidence suggests that the cis-9,trans-11 and trans-10,cis-12 CLA isomers exert distinct effects on immune function. Specifically, these 2 isomers have differential effects on specific T cell populations and immunoglobulin subclasses in animal and human studies."
30. Malloney F, Yeow TP, Mullen A, et al. Conjugated linoleic acid supplementation, insulin sensitivity, and lipoprotein metabolism in patients with type 2 DM. Am J Clin Nutr. 2004;80(4):887-95.
31. Riserus U, Vessby B, Arner P, Zethelius B. Supplementation with CLA induces hyperproinsulinaemia in obese men: close association with impaired insulin sensitivity. Diabetalogia. 2004;47(6):1016-19.
32. Ames, BN. The metabolic tune-up: metabolic harmony and disease prevention. J Nutr. 2003;133:1544S-48S.
33. Ames BN, et. al. High-dose vitamin therapy stimulates variant enzymes with decreased coenzyme binding affinity (increased Km): relevance to genetic disease and polymorphisms. Am J Clin Nutr. 2002;75(4):616-58.
34. Ibid.
35. Bralley JA, Lord RS: Laboratory Evaluations in Molecular Medicine. 2001. In Organic Acids, Chapter 6, p. 181. "Carnitine is required as a carrier for the transport of fatty acids from the cytosol into the mitochondria for beta oxidation. This is the dominant pathway used to derive energy from fat in most cells. When carnitine is inadequate to keep up with demand, the degradation of fatty acids takes place through an alternate, less efficient pathway known as omega oxidation."
36. Ibid.
37. Yamamoto Y, Gaynor RB. Therapeutic potential of inhibition of the NF-kB pathway in the treatment of inflammation and cancer. J Clin Invest. 2001;107(2):135-42.
38. Tak PP, Firestein GS. NF-kB: a key role in inflammatory disease. J Clin Invest. 2001;107(1):7-11.
39. Yamamoto Y, Gaynor RB. Therapeutic potential of inhibition of the NF-kB pathway in the treatment of inflammation and cancer. J Clin Invest. 2001;107(2):135-42.
40. Balmer JE, Blomhoff R. Gene expression regulation by retinoic acid. J Lipid Res. 2002;43:1773-808.
41. Holick MF. Sunlight and vitamin D for bone health and prevention of autoimmune diseases, cancers, and cardiovascular diseases. Am J Clin Nutr. 2004;80(6 Suppl):1678S-88S.
42. Ibid.
43. Ames, BN. A role for supplements in optimizing health: the metabolic tune up. Arch Biochem Biophy. 2004;423:227-34. "Three ways that health is affected: DNA damage, Km concept of poorer binding affinity, and mitochondrial oxidative decay"
44. Wheeler P, Batt ME. Do non-steroidal anti-inflammatory drugs adversely affect stress fracture healing? A short report. Br J Sports Med. 2005;39:65-69.
45. Yamamoto Y, Gaynor RB. Therapeutic potential of inhibition of the NF-kB pathway in the treatment of inflammation and cancer. J Clin Invest. 2001;107(2):135-42.
46. Vasquez A. Integrative Orthopedics. Concepts, Algorithms, and Therapeutics. 2004. In Additional Concepts and Selected Treatment, Chapter 16, p.443.
47. Mingrone G, Greco AV, Castagneto M, Gasbarrini G. A woman who left her wheelchair. Lancet. 1999;353:806.

Chapter 35
Assessment and Therapeutic Strategy—A Place to Start

- ***Elimination Diet and Laboratory Testing***
- ***Identifying Practical Interventions that Help to Normalize Multiple Symptoms***

Elimination Diet and Laboratory Testing

Dan Lukaczer, ND and Barb Schiltz, MS, RN

Introduction

"Where do I start?"
"What's the best nutritional intervention?"
"Which lab test should I order?"

These three questions are the most frequently asked by clinicians new to functional medicine. As even a quick review of the preceding chapters will attest, there is often no simple (or single) diagnosis or treatment for patients with chronic health issues. This is the bane and the boon of functional medicine. Real people, real lives, and real problems frequently don't fit neatly into simple diagnostic (or treatment) categories. There is a complexity to medicine when viewed in this way that makes it forever fascinating, challenging and new, but also frustrating because of the myriad threads that must be woven together into a coherent pattern.

When viewed through the functional medicine lens, the conventional medical model often does not approach the patient holistically, and it stops short of approaching disease from the perspective of underlying mechanisms. The functional medicine model encompasses biochemical individuality in the context of multiple mechanisms and environmental influences; the symphony (some would say cacophony) of signs and symptoms must be organized in a way that suggests a discernable pattern. The preceding chapters have provided many insights on how to approach patients from this perspective, but questions about getting down to specific actions on Monday morning may still exist. That larger vision, the bird's eye view, must be translated into pragmatic steps that any practitioner interested in this medicine can take.

Although the practice of functional medicine can be frustratingly complex when piecing together the puzzle that each new patient presents, there are, in fact, specific approaches that help make the complexity manageable. One of those—the use of the functional medicine matrix—was presented in the preceding chapter and can help to define where on the interconnected web the clinician can begin. This chapter will focus on helpful first steps and approaches that can be used to set the groundwork for more detailed evaluation and treatment to be performed subsequently. The three major topics we will cover are dietary assessment, understanding laboratory assessment, and utilizing practical interventions that work to normalize multiple systems (more "bang for the buck").

The First Step: Dietary Assessment

While the possible interventions in functional medicine are numerous, the place to start is almost invariably with food. Too often we are so enamored of the newest test or diagnostic procedure that we forget the fundamental step of assessing dietary intake. Everyone must eat. Dietary assessment can provide significant clues about the patient's problems. It has been estimated that over the course of 70–80 years of living a person consumes approximately 80–90,000 individual meals. Thousands of compounds must be inspected, recognized, broken down, packaged up, and digested or discarded. Given the enormity of this process, and the many opportunities for things to go amiss, it clearly makes sense to begin our evaluation here.

How does a clinician assess this most basic question: Is the patient eating (or not eating) in a way that has become either the cause of, or a mediating influence on, his or her presenting signs and symptoms? From a scientific perspective, the answer is often difficult to pin down. The underlying mechanisms that elicit a food reaction are complex and even controversial.[i] Food reactions can run the gamut from

- those that are immunologically mediated (immediate or delayed allergic or hypersensitivity reactions, respectively), to
- non-immunologically mediated reactions such as food intolerances or sensitivities (e.g., lactose intolerance, sulfite or salicylate sensitivity), to
- reactions secondary to the effects of certain foods on other regulatory systems (e.g., simple sugars and reactive hypoglycemia), to
- reactions associated with the effects of a specific food on bowel flora (described by Hunter as "enterometabolic" reactions[1]).

A variety of assessment techniques and tools have been used to identify these food-related reactions. Unfortunately, *none* are foolproof. Generally, the most cost-effective and accurate method of identifying reactivity to specific foods is an oligoantigenic diet followed by reintroduction or food challenge. (This is not to deny the utility of laboratory testing, which can play a very important role in patient assessment; right now, however, we are focusing on an almost universally useful and affordable approach—dietary assessment.)

Why is assessment of food reactions so important? Even a quick scan of the medical literature clarifies the connection between food and disease (see Chapter 26 for a comprehensive review of the subject). Studies have been conducted on dietary interventions in the treatment of, for example, rheumatoid arthritis,[2] irritable bowel syndrome,[3] migraine headaches,[4] attention deficit disorder,[5] infantile colic,[6] otitis media,[7] atopic dermatitis,[8] chronic urticaria,[9] and Crohn's disease.[10] All have shown a connection with food as an etiological agent, to one degree or another. While clearly not all patients in these or other conditions respond positively to a dietary approach, dietary changes can produce a sustained positive response in a subset of patients with chronic complex problems. Therefore, this is an extremely important starting point.

What is needed to carry out such a protocol? First, patients must be educated to understand that this approach can provide information essential to understanding their problems. Second, patients need to know that the approach is valid, is "do-able," and c an be accomplished within a limited time frame. Third, the clinician needs tools to easily and comprehensively test the hypothesis that diet is an influence on the patient's health.

Assessment of Food Reactions with an Elimination Diet

Diet Diary

The first step is to find out what the patient is eating regularly. This can be accomplished with the use of a three-day diet diary. A sample form is provided in the Appendix. A careful review of the diet diary will often identify foods that are eaten frequently and extensively, and therefore may be the first target for an elimination diet. However, given that food reactions often present with delayed onset of 4 to 72 hours, food diaries are not always able to clarify which particular food(s) may be the offending agent(s). The idea that one single food is culpable, while enticing, is an approach that does not generally hold up in clinical practice.

The Program

A program that eliminates certain foods or food groups from the diet for diagnostic purposes can take many forms. Simpler programs may eliminate only one or two specific foods or food groups, often focusing on specific proteins found in dairy, wheat (or all gluten-containing foods), egg, soy, pork, beef, or corn. These more narrowly focused dietary exclusion programs can be particularly useful when treating children, because they are easier to carry out than a program that eliminates many foods and food groups.

A comprehensive program that eliminates more foods may be advisable as a starting point for many

[i] There are many chapters in this book where various approaches to assessing food reactions are discussed. Please see the Index for help in locating specific content.

adult patients. A sample comprehensive elimination diet can be found in the Appendix, with a list of foods to exclude, foods to include, and a chart for recording reactions upon reintroduction. This example eliminates most foods that have been found, over time and across many patients, to produce reactions. Such a program is easily modifiable to fit individual patients and situations; it allows the practitioner to throw a broader net that is more likely to catch the right fish. The common foods eliminated in this program include gluten, dairy, beef, pork, citrus fruits, corn, eggs, soy, various food additives, and colorants. Many clinicians have used this or a similar program and have found it to be generally well tolerated.

There is really no typical or normal response. Often, a patient's primary health concerns improve significantly within the first three weeks on such a program. Additionally, patients often report other nonspecific improvements such as increased energy, mental alertness, a general sense of improved well-being, or the disappearance of symptoms they have lived with for years. It is prudent to warn patients that they may have some initial reactions to the program, especially in the first week or ten days. Such reactions are sometimes difficult to explain. They may be secondary to the so-called Herxheimer reaction,[ii] to alterations in GI function from diet-induced changes in flora, to caffeine or simple sugar withdrawal, or to other less well understood causes. Symptoms may include changes in sleep patterns, lightheadedness, headaches, joint or muscle stiffness, constipation, diarrhea, rash or pruritis. Generally, such symptoms abate in the first 7–10 days of the program and can be handled with supportive measures, including activated charcoal, Alka Seltzer Gold®, additional fiber, rest, and saunas.

While changing food habits dramatically can be a complex, difficult, and sometimes confusing process, given the proper tools, encouragement, and a circumscribed timeframe, it can be a very practical and empowering endeavor. Along with providing inspiration and clear dietary instructions, the clinician should supply patients with written information tailored to their specific program. These include an explanation of the process, general food guidelines (what to eat, what not to eat), shopping lists, and sources of hidden foods. The Appendix provides an example of some patient handouts that can be adapted for these purposes.

An elimination diet should be carried out under close supervision for an initial period of not less than three weeks. While the program is generally not calorie restricted, many patients do lose 4–6 pounds over this time. At the three-week mark, it is reasonable to proceed with a careful reintroduction of excluded foods and an evaluation of the response. However, the program can be continued uninterrupted for as long as the clinician deems necessary (and the patient is compliant). A patient who has experienced noticeable improvement in certain symptoms, and is interested in continuing without reintroducing foods that have been excluded, should be strongly encouraged. In fact, in some conditions the full extent of improvement may not be completely realized for months.[11] There are no dietary deficiencies that we are aware of that make a long-term commitment to this program contraindicated.

Reintroduction Process

When excluded foods are reintroduced, the patient should use a systematic recording method, the main features of which should be:

- A particular excluded food is chosen for reintroduction. (Often those foods that were most commonly eaten prior to the elimination diet are chosen first.)
- The food is ingested two to three times over the course of a day.
- The patient otherwise continues to eat only the foods on the current food list.
- Responses are recorded on a chart such as the one shown in the Appendix. (The patient may use different headings to correspond with whatever signs and symptoms are experienced.)
- Only one new food is introduced at a time.
- The patient waits at least two days (48 hours) before challenging a new food.
- If a reaction is noted, the patient waits until that reaction has dissipated before reintroducing another food. (If the patient is unsure whether a reaction occurred, the same food is retested in the

[ii] The Jarisch-Herxheimer reaction (often referred to as Herxheimer or Herx) is believed to be caused by gut organisms dying off at a rapid rate. Many of these organisms, or their metabolic by-products, may be absorbed into the systemic circulation as endotoxins and overwhelm the liver's ability to adequately scavenge and process. Systemic reactions can thus occur and may include joint pain, fever and malaise. These reactions were originally observed in patients with syphilis who received mercury treatment, but have also been more recently characterized in Lyme disease treatment as well. Some clinicians also refer to this phenomenon as a "detoxification" or "clearing" reaction.

same manner after the possible reaction has dissipated.)

- A reactive food is recorded and kept on the excluded list.

Many underlying mechanisms may cause reactions to a given food or food group. Genetic predisposition, impaired enzyme or acid secretion, protozoal infection, bacterial dysbiosis, medications, concurrent disease, nutritional insufficiency, and aging all can play a role. Addressing these underlying issues may eventually allow the patient to resume eating some foods to which they had previously reacted. Even fairly reactive foods may eventually be tolerated in small amounts on an occasional basis.

Evaluating the Role of Laboratory Testing in Functional Medicine

Laboratory evaluation can play a pivotal and central role in clinical practice. Among its many uses are: identification of the underlying etiology of a health condition, serving as an aid to accurate diagnosis, providing a predictive measure of future health problems, or tracking the progress a patient makes on a particular intervention. The question of what laboratory tests are useful from a functional medicine perspective seems to take on a larger and even more complicated role than in the conventional realm. In the functional medicine work-up, the clinician often looks to lab, not only for signs of pathological change, but also to assess more subtle signs of imbalance or dysfunction. Bacterial dysbiosis that may be associated with digestive or systemic complaints, functional folic acid deficiency that may be associated with a mood disorder, or estrogen/progesterone shifts that may be associated with fatigue or sleep disturbances are not completely diagnosable by laboratory measures. In fact, these laboratory evaluations, if taken outside the context of the patient's totality of signs and symptoms, may not offer significant clues.

For example, two individuals may show a modest elevation in serum homocysteine, a functional test of folic acid insufficiency. In a patient who suffers from depression, this may be a key finding in clarifying the underlying etiology of the depression. In another patient, this functional folic acid deficiency may be unassociated with any sign or symptom. While it may be useful to replete with folic acid regardless, it is a less significant finding and in fact may not be a laboratory test that one would normally request for an individual with no overt symptomatology. The research literature clearly supports the link between depression and elevated homocysteine.[12,13] However, it just as clearly shows that not all depressed individuals will have an elevated homocysteine, and not all elevated homocysteine will result in depression. It is the context within which the clinician finds the patient that is important for ordering and then interpreting that laboratory marker.

Bacterial dysbiosis is another diagnosis that should not be made out of context. Clinicians may find that patient stool cultures are often positive for unusual or non-commensal bacteria. In our experience, this finding can occur in both symptomatic and healthy individuals, and it is only within the framework of the total patient work-up that the relative importance of such results is understood. The patient may present with other relevant history such as digestive complaints following repeated courses of antibiotics, unexplained joint pain or fatigue, and dermatological symptoms. When the available information coalesces into a coherent story suggesting gut dysbiosis as an underlying cause, then the laboratory results do help in confirming the patient's problem and planning a therapeutic intervention.

While laboratory evaluation can thus be of significant importance to the functional medicine practitioner, he or she must be careful to scrutinize the utility and predictive value of each laboratory test selected. There are many laboratory tools from which to choose and there is no one lab test that will uncover the dysfunction(s) in all patients. As is always the case in good health care, functional medicine practitioners first perform a careful history and physical exam, including the review of mechanisms (described in Chapter 34), and sorting the information on the functional medicine matrix. Those findings, combined with any laboratory results selected in the initial work-up, will in large part determine where on the matrix to focus initially. For specific laboratory tests to consider in various situations, the practitioner is referred back to other sections of the book, particularly *Fundamental Clinical Imbalances* and *A Practical Clinical Approach*. The scope of this section will be to provide some general information that can be of use in selecting laboratory tests.

In functional medicine, laboratory evaluation is often on the cutting edge of clinical science. It is an area of ongoing and dynamic research that can help us assess functionality in new and exciting ways. However, a thorough understanding of variability, precision, and accuracy should be foremost in the clinician's mind when considering any new or unfamiliar laboratory assessment. Functional medicine teaches us to understand and assess fundamental physiological processes and to recognize subtle signs and symptoms in an interconnected mosaic. Basic sciences, cell physiology, animal studies, epidemiological, case-controlled, and randomized controlled trials help us arrive at reasonable conclusions and follow up with integrative interventions. When assessments and interventions do not yet have many years of valid and reproducible data behind them, the clinician (in any discipline) must use both art and science to weave together the history, physical exam, and laboratory findings and filter those conclusions through a vast array of scientific data to arrive confidently at a useful place to begin. We are always functioning in an imperfect world with incomplete data. Lab tests may be valuable even if they are not definitive; they can provide general information and clues to potential underlying problems, helping us to decipher the complex tapestry of a patient with chronic unwellness. And, we must use a reliable standard of scrutiny and evaluation in the selection of laboratory tests upon which that patient's health may depend.

Assessing the Performance of a Laboratory Test

To be used with a high degree of confidence in clinical decision making, laboratory methods must meet certain standards of statistical reliability. Simply put, a test must be reproducible over time, with variability that is limited to known parameters and is not so large that it renders interpretation of the findings problematic. That is, one must be able to assume that a change in a test result is a result of the treatment plan, not the result of wide variability in the test itself. The reliability of a test includes what are termed analytical and non-analytical factors.

Analytical factors are broken down into test accuracy, precision, sensitivity, and specificity. These basic concepts, discussed below, are the cornerstones of analytical reliability. If a given test does not have reasonable precision, accuracy, specificity, and sensitivity, it is a test with little reliability.

Measurements of *accuracy* and *precision* reveal a test's basic reliability. Accuracy and precision can be compromised by fluctuations in temperature, variability in volume sample, adequacy of reagent used, changes in environment, and/or inconsistent handling of specimens. Accuracy and precision are measured and tested through duplicate sampling and internal quality control procedures. A test is *accurate* when it measures what it was intended to measure—the true value of concentration of the substance being measured in a given sample. A test is said to be *precise* when repeated analyses on the same sample give very similar results. When a test method is precise, the amount of random variation is small. A precise test method has results that are reliably reproduced time after time. A test method can be precise (reliably reproducible) without being accurate (measuring what it is supposed to measure), or vice versa.

As a test is performed on patient specimens, its accuracy is routinely monitored with a control specimen. The control has a known test value and is analyzed alongside patient specimens, revealing whether the test measurement process is correct. Although a test that is 100% accurate and 100% precise is the ideal, in reality, tests, instruments, and personnel perform less perfectly than that. A small amount of variability does not usually detract from the test's value. The level of accuracy and precision that can be obtained is specific to each test method. For newer laboratory assessments, these measurements should be requested from the individual laboratory, and if this information is not forthcoming, or is of poor quality or high variability, one should have a healthy degree of skepticism regarding the usefulness of that test (or that laboratory).

While accuracy and precision are critical components of a lab value, a laboratory test must also be able to detect abnormalities with reasonable certainty. How likely is it that an individual has the disease or condition that the test suggests? That question is influenced by both false positives (reporting the patient has the condition when he/she does not) and false negatives (reporting the patient free of the condition when she/he is not). The clinician will want to know the chances of a test delivering either a false negative or a false positive—if those chances are too high either way, using the test may not be advisable.

To this end, labs develop and monitor statistics on each test's diagnostic *specificity* and *sensitivity*. These measurements reveal how likely a false negative or false positive result is when a particular test is performed by a specific lab. *Sensitivity* is the ability of a test to correctly identify individuals who have a given disease or disorder. For example, a certain test, such as an ova and parasite examination of stool, may have a sensitivity of 90% for diagnosing an infection with the protozoa *Blastocystis hominis*. This would mean that if 100 people known to be infected with the organism are tested by that laboratory facility, the test will correctly identify 90 of those 100 infections. The other 10 people who were tested also have the parasite, but the test will fail to detect it (the test delivers a false negative). A test's sensitivity becomes particularly important when a clinician is seeking to exclude a significant health issue that would change the intervention. In this example, believing that the organism is not present may lead to trying therapies that will not be effective for the real problem. The more sensitive a test is, the fewer false negatives it produces. In summary, a false negative fails to expose a condition that is present; a high rate of false negatives indicates the test has poor sensitivity.

Specificity is the ability of a test to correctly exclude individuals who do not have a given disease or disorder. Using a different example, testing a blood specimen for elevated IgG antibodies to egg might have a specificity of, say, 70%. If 100 individuals who are known **not** to have elevated IgG antibodies to egg are tested with that method, only 70 of those 100 people will be reported as having no antibodies. For the remaining 30%, their "abnormal" findings are a misleading false positive. That is, they do not have the condition, but were falsely reported as having it. This may result in those patients being put on a therapy for something they do not have. The more specific a test is, the fewer false positives it produces. In summary, a false positive reports the presence of a condition or disease that a patient does not have; tests with a high rate of false positives have poor specificity.

Clearly, tests that have poor specificity and/or sensitivity are of less value in correctly diagnosing a patient's condition.

Non-analytical factors are also important in predicting the usefulness of a test. They fall into two main areas: *pre-analytical variation* and *within-subject (normal) biological variation*. Pre-analytical variations are factors affecting a test's result that exclude the actual performance (precision and accuracy) of the testing protocol itself. Pre-analytical variation can be affected by sample collection, storage, transport, type of sample, and even such things as tourniquet application (in the case of blood samples). For example, whether a sample degrades at room temperature may be a significant pre-analytical variability in the test results. Laboratories should perform various tests on samples, including shipping, temperature changes, and collection variations, to determine how and whether pre-analytical variation can be limited.

Biological variation (within-subject variation or intra-individual variation) involves normal day-to-day variations in an analyte caused or affected by circadian rhythms, sleep-wake cycles, food intake, physical activity, time of year or season, stress or anxiety, and concurrent illness. For example, the assessment of high sensitivity C-reactive protein may be affected by seasonal allergies. Therefore, its evaluation as a marker for cardiovascular disease in an individual patient may be problematic unless this biological variation is accounted for.[14] Biological variation is of critical importance for the laboratory to determine; without that information, the clinician has little idea if the change in analyte being measured is significant (secondary to therapy) or random. If serum cholesterol, for example, had a known variation depending on time of year, a measurement in January might be significantly different from one in June, not because of any therapeutic intervention, but because of the natural variation from winter to summer. While this is not the case with cholesterol, there are many analytes for which biological variation has not been determined, or has been determined and has shown wide variation. Biological variation is determined, in general, by collecting a series of samples from a group of participants at regular intervals, minimizing pre-analytical and analytical variation, storing samples for batch analysis later, analyzing samples in duplicate, removing outliers, and then determining within-subject (biological) analysis of variance.

It is vital for those involved in laboratory testing to minimize analytical and pre-analytical variability and to measure and report biological variation. One must consider the influence of these factors on laboratory tests and on the interpretation of laboratory results. Clinicians considering the use of new or unfamiliar tests should request information from the laboratory on all the factors discussed above, and should examine the data before relying on the test for clinical decision making.

Identifying Practical Interventions that Help to Normalize Multiple Symptoms

Nancy Sudak, MD and Virginia Shapiro, DC

The initial functional medicine approach involves foundational recommendations that produce a positive impact on multiple systems. Many of these interventions have been extensively discussed and documented in the preceding section of this book (A Practical Clinical Approach), but still we are left with the question of how and where to begin with a particular patient. Looking for the simplest interventions that will achieve maximum impact is a reasonable starting point. Although these initial interventions may sound very basic, patients are typically quite pleased to find that implementation can produce a dramatic enhancement of well-being.

It is clear that our daily behaviors have a large impact on our health. Patients seem to understand the relationship between diet and physical activity as they relate to common diseases. We are aware of abundant evidence that dietary measures can reduce the incidence of adult onset diabetes; lifestyle changes have been shown to meaningfully outperform metformin in generating a higher rate of diabetes prevention.[15,16] Secondary prevention of myocardial infarction has also been demonstrated dramatically by dietary interventions involving omega-3 fatty acids in the GISSI Trial,[17] the DART Study, [18] and the Lyon Study.[19] The functional medicine style of practice teaches patients that their daily choices have a powerful effect on their health. Therefore, in-office patient education (a very important, albeit basic, intervention) is a critical factor in achieving success with lifestyle changes. The functional medicine model requires active patient participation, and may be challenging for those expecting passive delivery of health care.

Numerous lifestyle modifications of benefit to the patient are likely to be identified early in a functional medicine work-up. Many such changes are already familiar to most patients as recommended healthy practices, but they have not been adopted for a variety of possible reasons: unpreparedness for change; belief that low-tech interventions are unlikely to have a measurable effect; insufficient understanding of how lifestyle habits affect health; and home or work situations with little support for changing behaviors. When a practitioner or patient educator thoroughly and non-judgmentally explains the basis for lifestyle recommendations relative to the individual's specific situation, a door opens for patients to meaningfully reevaluate their daily actions.

Patients need information, instruction, and ongoing support as they integrate untried practices and abandon comfortable habits that have long undermined their health. An integral element of the art of practicing functional medicine is the ability to encourage patients without overwhelming them. An overzealous functional medicine practitioner or educator may impair the therapeutic relationship by mandating too many changes simultaneously, when a given patient may already be struggling to put new principles into operation.

No two patients are treated identically in functional medicine, but some advice is applicable to nearly every patient. The following lifestyle recommendations also meet the criterion of helping to normalize multiple systems and thus provide a better foundation for health:

- Removal of processed foods and *trans* fatty acids
- Ingestion of healthy whole-food meals at regular intervals
- Increased intake of vegetables, with moderate fruit intake
- Consumption of organically raised and locally grown foods whenever possible
- Achieving balance of macronutrients
- Removal of potential or documented food allergens
- Adequate daily intake of essential fatty acids, fiber, and pure water
- Deletion of toxic influences (including, for example, household pesticides and herbicides, toxic household and personal cleaning products, and certain cosmetics)
- Inclusion of exercise, stress management techniques, and spiritual centering in daily life.

As functional medicine practitioners, we know that poor diet, toxic overload, and overstimulation of inflammatory mediators impair proper function. Consistent application of healthier lifestyle habits optimizes broad areas of function by minimizing metabolic demand. When we restore nutrient adequacy, reduce toxic burden, and diminish excessive activation of the hypothalamic-pituitary-adrenal (HPA) axis, metabolic efficiency is more likely to normalize. Patients who have been effectively instructed on these concepts often establish early improvement of symptoms before more specific and advanced interventions are suggested.

For example, when women with a variety of menopausal or perimenopausal symptoms implement basic lifestyle modifications, they tend to report improvement in bowel function, energy, mood, and general sense of well being, as well as reduction of myofascial pain, and diminished frequency/intensity of headaches and hot flashes. When patients with extremely complex disorders and imbalances make similar changes, they often achieve substantial, sometimes astonishing improvements in their physical conditions. The power of lifestyle modification in complex illness should not be underestimated. When these measures alone are ineffective in removing barriers to proper function, further investigation and treatment are warranted.

The following case example illustrates a patient with multiple and complex areas of dysfunction and her response to some fairly simple initial interventions.

A 57-year-old woman visited our office with a chief complaint of active ulcerative colitis of 3.5 years' duration. Colonoscopy revealed extensive ulceration of her colon; multiple medications had been used unsuccessfully or were not tolerated; and her gastrointestinal specialists had stated that colon resection appeared to be her only viable long-term treatment option. Additional medical problems included osteoarthritis of her neck and right shoulder for 14 years and hypertension.

Five years previously, she had traveled overseas and returned with abdominal bloating and diarrhea, acute diffuse joint pain (reactive arthritis), iritis, and urethritis. She had been diagnosed with probable giardiasis (negative stool study) and Reiter's syndrome, experiencing symptom resolution with antibiotics. One year later, her diffuse joint pain recurred, and rofecoxib was initiated. Shortly after the addition of this medication, classic symptoms of ulcerative colitis occurred, and she was treated conventionally, without any correlation made between her colitis and the cyclooxygenase (COX)-2 inhibitor. Her medications at the time of presentation in our office included rofecoxib (4 years), atenolol (5 years), mesalamine (3 years), and mercaptopurine (1 year).

Our initial clinical assessment indicated gastrointestinal inflammation, altered intestinal permeability, and mild dysbiosis of her gastrointestinal flora. We advised a basic approach, including trial elimination of gluten grains and dairy products, avoidance of refined sugars and *trans* fatty acids, macronutrient-balanced diet, and implementation of the general bulleted recommendations itemized above. She was also started on EPA/DHA fish oil, vitamin E, zinc, carnosine, 5-methyltetrahydrofolate, a probiotic supplement, L-glutamine, and an herbal anti-inflammatory product containing extracts of hops, rosemary, and olive leaf.

After two months, her bowel function, energy level, and sense of well-being were dramatically improved. Her blood pressure had normalized and atenolol was discontinued. Rofecoxib was completely withdrawn by month four, and relief from osteoarthritis symptoms was maintained with adjunctive chiropractic care and frequency specific microcurrent therapy. She has had no recurrence of her reactive arthritis. She was eventually able to discontinue the mesalamine and mercaptopurine, and remains free of gastrointestinal symptoms over a year after initial interventions in our office.

The functional medicine approach successfully addressed her underlying inflammatory dysregulation and ultimately spared her from a total colectomy. This case is also an example of the complexity of many cases seen in functional medicine practices, in which multiple causative factors occur in layers (including iatrogenic influences). In such cases, simple initial interventions may or may not result in such complete results. When symptoms continue, patience and persistence are required as the astute clinician learns to tease apart the various components of the patient's condition to determine underlying causes.

The elimination diet (discussed earlier in this chapter) is an example of a therapeutic strategy (with a diagnostic component) that tends to produce improvement in multiple systems.[20,21,22] Patients with numerous symptoms who are employing a standard American diet often benefit from a comprehensive elimination diet, in which commonly irritating foods such as gluten grains, dairy products, corn, chocolate, peanuts, and eggs are avoided for a period of several weeks. Relief from symptoms such as migraine headaches,[23,24] fatigue, body aches, mood disturbances, irritable bowel complaints,[25,26] dermatitis, and perennial rhinitis[27] is typical during the elimination phase.

A principal mechanism underlying symptom resolution in many cases is reduction of inflammatory activation from offending foods. It is helpful to consider the central location of most of the immune system—within the gastrointestinal tract. When antigenic exposures to foods mismatched to an individual's physiology are removed, physiologic function improves. If patients find that systematic reintroduction of foods, one by one, indicates several intolerances, a functional medicine practitioner will consider the likelihood of altered intestinal permeability. Reasons underlying the passage of large molecules through the gastrointestinal mucosa will then have to be explored. (Chapters 28 and 31 provide detailed information on intestinal permeability.)

When we decipher a patient's story by constantly asking why a condition has emerged, we may eventually reach a core dysfunction that can be remediated. The process of prescribing this "simple" intervention, the elimination diet (with its diagnostic and therapeutic elements), may be represented by the scheme shown in Figure 35.1.

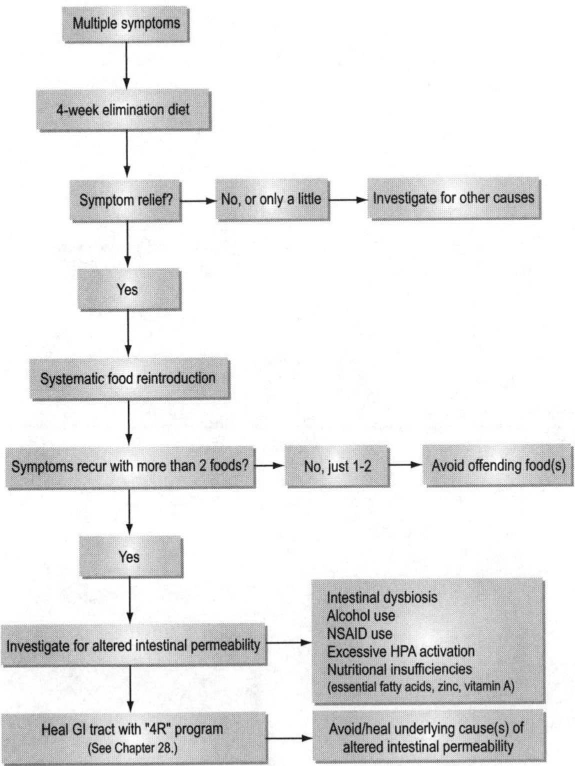

Figure 35.1 **Schema for use of elimination diet**

In summary, it behooves functional medicine practitioners and their patients to carefully consider foundational lifestyle practices when making initial assessments of patients with complex disorders or health histories. It has frequently been our experience that many medications can be reduced or eliminated through simple lifestyle modification. This should not, however, diminish the importance of thorough evaluation of the patient, appropriate to their specific condition and to the credentials and training of the practitioner. Basic changes in dietary and exercise practices can often be implemented in conjunction with more conventional treatment. In addition, many foundational lifestyle changes can be initiated without harm, while more in-depth investigations (laboratory, radiology, or others) are pending. The patient's response (or lack of response) to these basic interventions can often provide additional diagnostic information to the astute clinician, as well as provide the patient with encouraging relief of symptoms.

References

1. Hunter JO. Food allergy—or enterometabolic disorder? Lancet. 1991;24;338(8765):495-496.
2. Muller H, de Toledo FW, Resch KL. Fasting followed by vegetarian diet in patients with rheumatoid arthritis: a systematic review. Scand J Rheumatol. 2001:30(1):1-10.
3. Stefanini GF, Saggioro A, Alvisi V, et al. Oral cromolyn sodium in comparison with elimination diet in the irritable bowel syndrome, diarrheic type. Multicenter study of 428 patients. Scand J Gastroenterol 1995;30(6):535-541.
4. Mansfield LE, Vaughan TR, Waller SF, et al. Food allergy and adult migraine: double-blind and mediator confirmation of an allergic etiology. Ann Allergy. 1985;55(2):126-129.
5. Carter CM, Urbanowicz M, Hemsley R, et al. Effects of a few food diet in attention deficit disorder. Arch Dis Child. 1993(5);69:564–568.
6. Hill DJ, Hudson IL, Sheffield LJ, et al. A low allergen diet is a significant intervention in infantile colic: results of a community-based study. J Allergy Clin Immunol. 1995(6 Pt 1);96:886–892.
7. Juntti H, Tikkanen S, Kokkonen J, et al. Cow's milk allergy is associated with recurrent otitis media during childhood. Acta Otolaryngol 1999;119(8):867–873.
8. Niggemann B, Sielaff B, Beyer K, et al. Outcome of double-blind, placebo-controlled food challenge tests in 107 children with atopic dermatitis. Clin Exp Allergy 1999;29(1):91–96.
9. Henz BM, Zuberbier T. Most chronic urticaria is food-dependent, not idiopathic. Exp Dermatol 1998;7(4):139–142. Review.
10. Jones VA, Dickinson RJ, Workman E, et al. Crohn's disease: maintenance of remission by diet. Lancet 1985 Jul 27;2(8448):177-180
11. Kjeldsen-Kragh J, Haugen M, Borchgrevink CF, et al. Controlled trial of fasting and one-year vegetarian diet in rheumatoid arthritis. Lancet, 1991. 338(8772): 899-902.
12. Sachdev PS, Parslow RA, Lux O, et al. Relationship of homocysteine, folic acid and vitamin B12 with depression in a middle-aged community sample. Psychol Med. 2005;35(4):529-38.
13. Bottiglieri T. Homocysteine and folate metabolism in depression. Prog Neuropsychopharmacol Biol Psychiatry. 2005;Aug 15:[Epub ahead of print].
14. Campbell B, Badrick T, Flatman R, Kanowski D. Limited clinical utility of high-sensitivity plasma C-reactive protein assays. Ann Clin Biochem. 2002 Mar;39(Pt 2):85-88.
15. Knowler WC, Barrett-Connor E, Fowler SE, et al. Reduction in the incidence of type 2 diabetes with lifestyle intervention or metformin. N Engl J Med. 2002;346:393-403.
16. Tuomilehto J, Lindstrom J. The major diabetes prevention trials. Current Diab Rep. 2003;3(12):115-122.

17. Grundy SM. N-3 fatty acids: priority for post-myocardial infarction clinical trials. Circulation. 2003;107;1834-36.
18. Burr ML, Fehily AM, Gilbert JF, et al. Effects of changes in fat, fish, and fiber intakes on death and myocardial reinfarction: diet and reinfarction trial (DART). Lancet. 1989;2(8666):757-761.
19. de Lorgeril J, Renaud S, Mamelle N, et al. Mediterranean alpha-linolenic acid-rich diet in secondary prevention of coronary heart disease. Lancet. 1994;343(8911):1454-1459.
20. Gaby A. The role of hidden food allergy/intolerance in chronic disease. Alt Med Rev. 2001;3(2):90-100.
21. Sampson HA. Food allergy. JAMA. 1997;278(22):1888-1894.
22. Bock SA. Diagnostic evaluation. Pediatrics. 2003;111(6):1638-1644.
23. Egger J, Carter CM, Wilson J, et al. Is migraine food allergy? A double-blind controlled trial of oligoantigenic diet treatment. Lancet. 1983;2(8355):865-869.
24. Mansfield LE, Vaughan TR, Waller SF, et al. Food allergy and adult migraine: double-blind and mediator confirmation of an allergic etiology. Ann Allergy. 1985;55(2):126-129.
25. Atkinson W, Sheldon TA, Shaath N, Whorwell PJ. Food elimination based on IgG antibodies in irritable bowel syndrome: a randomised controlled trial. Gut. 2004;53(10):1459-1464.
26. Isolauri E, Rautava S, Kalliomaki M. Food allergy in irritable bowel syndrome: new facts and old fallacies. Gut. 2004;53(10):1391-1393.
27. Pastorello EA, Stocchi L, Pravettone V, et al. Role of the eliminations diet in adults with food allergy. J All Clin Immun. 1989;84(4 Pt 1):475-483.

Chapter 36
The Healing Relationship

- ▶ *Creating Effective Doctor-Patient Relationships*
- ▶ *Helping Patients Change Unhealthy Behaviors*

Creating Effective Doctor-Patient Relationships

Edward (Ted) Leyton, MD, CCFP

Introduction

In the Introduction to this book, we read the following statement:

> Functional medicine could be characterized, therefore, as "upstream medicine" or "back to basics"—back to the patient's life story, back to the processes wherein disease originates, and definitely back to the desire of healthcare practitioners to make people well, not just manage symptoms.

This begs the question of how clinicians can obtain enough of the right kind of information from patients in the relatively short period of time we are in contact with them. Patients have lived a lifetime of experiences, some good, some bad, some with significant impact, and some that are insignificant. How do we put all of this together in a frame that helps us mold a functional diagnosis and treatment plan? It has been said that 90% of all diagnoses in medicine are still made on the basis of history, symptoms, and review of systems—although we would add review of mechanisms to that list (see Chapter 34)—and that technological investigations, though frequently helpful, are most often illustrative and additive.[1]

In this chapter—indeed, in this whole section of the book—we are learning how to elicit, organize, *and use* information about the antecedents and triggers that precede the onset of symptoms, and the mediators that keep the dysfunction going. Antecedents and triggers can be amazingly diverse, ranging from motor vehicle accidents to sexual abuse, from toxic exposure and family history to limiting decisions and beliefs that patients have adopted from an early age regarding their lives. The ability to glean this information from the patient is critical to weaving the interconnected web that is so basic to the functional medicine model.

Therapy actually begins from the moment the patient enters the clinic. From the atmosphere in the waiting room to the physical posture, attitudes, beliefs, and language of the practitioner and staff, there is always a need to foster in the patient an awareness of what it means to view health as positive vitality.

Rapport

To elicit and understand the patient's story, to help people make changes that are beneficial, and to create a healing relationship, it is important to be able to develop a rapid and powerful rapport with patients, so they feel comfortable telling their stories and revealing intimate information and significant events. Rapport is the core element that enables a practitioner to glean this kind of information from patients. Without rapport, both the functional diagnosis and treatment recommendations may be flawed or ignored. We will examine the following elements of the successful doctor-patient relationship:

- What is rapport and how can it be established rapidly and respectfully?
- What questions elicit the information needed to weave the functional web or matrix, so that treatment can be successful?

- What language empowers and motivates patients in a movement toward positive vitality and wellness?
- How do we de-emphasize the pathology model to which we are accustomed?
- How do we help patients change their behaviors and lifestyles so they feel empowered, fully functional, and able to manage on their own to a large degree?

What Is Rapport?

Being in rapport is the ability to enter another person's model of the world, communicating that we truly understand that world, in a **congruent** way. Being congruent means that we express ourselves with all our senses in a unified way. You have been establishing rapport unconsciously all your life; we all learned this as we figured out how to get along with people. Now we can enhance this process by making it conscious.

In functional medicine, patients are seen as unique individuals who may not fit the pre-determined models that correspond to particular diseases or conditions. Rapport will help us elicit, in a short space of time, the patient's complete story so that we can begin formulating a treatment plan. Traditional diagnosis is usually a part of the story—at least at the outset—but it is not a primary goal, and it will not tell the full story. The initial goals are to gather information that will help to create an *individualized* picture of the patient, create a working hypothesis about the dysfunctions underlying the symptoms and complaints, and form an effective, professional bond with the patient.

Presuppositions

Presuppositions about our patients set the stage for a positive or negative relationship, and they can interfere with establishing rapport. What *you* believe will influence the course of the patient's illness or wellness, if not at the conscious level, then certainly at the unconscious level. This is demonstrated eloquently in Daniel Moerman's *Meaning, Medicine and the 'Placebo Effect,'* wherein he explores and explains the research about placebo.[2] Moerman argues that it is not so much the patient who produces the placebo effect, but rather the healthcare practitioner whose beliefs about the treatment or the patient have considerable influence on the outcome. Here are some *helpful* presuppositions (assumptions) to have about all patients:[3]

- **Patients have all the resources they need to heal.** Clearly they may not have the same *knowledge* as you do about biochemistry and metabolism, but remember that they live in their bodies, and they have had to learn many things in order to survive and function.
- **The meaning of your communication is the response you get.** If a patient gives you a signal (verbal or non-verbal) that something you have said or done has triggered a negative emotional state (see below), use that information as feedback for a different approach, because ...
- **Your personal flexibility will determine your success.** If something you are doing or saying isn't working—change it. Systems theorists have shown that the system with the most flexibility is the one that generally ends up working.[4]
- **Every behavior has a useful purpose in some context.** Patients with chronic illness sometimes develop illness behavior, which you may have learned to view as a negative trait. Remember that this behavior **serves some useful purpose** (usually unconscious) for the patient. Understanding this will help you avoid the trap of labeling anyone as a "problem patient."

Emotional States

An emotional state is *a particular way of feeling*, brought about by internal representations and physiological shifts, as a result of a person's life experience, conceptual filters, and internal map of reality, at that moment, and in that context.

Emotional states can range from depression to elation, with myriad possibilities in between: aggravation, frustration, excitement, boredom, joy, amusement, grief, and so on. Emotional states are internally generated by information that comes to us through the five senses—visual, auditory, kinesthetic, gustatory, and olfactory. The information is then processed through a variety of unconscious filters that ultimately create an internal representation of what we see, hear, taste, smell or feel. Such representations have the power to create a shift in a physiological state and can influence subsequent behavior.

A simple example will illustrate. A man is driving home on the highway from work after a stressful day. His mind is filled with thoughts about his day and anything that may have precipitated unpleasant feelings that we generally characterize as "stress." Perhaps he has a headache, neck pain, or stomach ache. As he looks out of his car window, he sees (visual representation) the sun setting in the west. He is reminded of his last vacation (past experience), when he saw a beautiful sunset, and he recalls the closeness that he felt with his wife as they watched it from their hotel balcony. As he "connects" to this past experience, he can feel his shoulders relaxing and the tension easing from his body (kinesthetic shift). This man has just changed his emotional state, fortuitously on this occasion, by changing his focus of attention and by remembering a pleasant past experience.

Most patients are in what we might call a *problem state* when they see us. They feel bad. They have to feel that way in order to communicate effectively about their problems—in other words, they have been thinking about the problem and how they are going to describe it. They have been internally rehearsing prior to the visit.

An important factor to take note of here is that we—the practitioners—are also in some kind of emotional state, and whatever it is will surely affect our interaction with the patient. So, it's good to take stock: **Consider what kind of state you are in before you see the patient.** Are you in a bad mood, or stressed out? Did the last patient trigger some bad feelings? Do you have some personal matters you are bringing to the interview? Or, on the positive side, are you relaxed, curious, and eager to discover something unique about the person you are about to see? If so, you are in an excellent state for seeing patients.

You can help yourself achieve that positive state. Remember a time when you felt **really curious** about something. Mentally imagine yourself being curious, hear what you are saying to yourself, and feel the change in your body as you do this exercise. Take a few deep breaths to relieve any tension you might have, and then greet the patient with a genuine, flexible, curiosity. This will go a long way toward building rapport and establishing a comfortable ongoing relationship with your patients.

Communication

Communication is 7% words, 38% tonality, and 55% physiology. As mentioned above, we all use our senses to take in our experience of the world. Research has shown that we use the following percentages of our senses to map our reality:[5]

- Visual—60%
- Auditory—20%
- Kinesthetic—20%
- Olfactory/gustatory— <1%

Therefore, your patients will be communicating problems to you with many of these senses, although most of us have a preferred style—most often visual, then auditory and kinesthetic.

Let's look at this a little more closely. Since we all take in the world through our senses, the type of sense we use will depend on the circumstances. For example, at a concert, the primary sense is tuned to the auditory channel. Looking at a painting requires a visual focus. Doing a workout requires a kinesthetic sense of body position and movement. When we communicate with others, we also *express ourselves* in one or more of these senses:

> Sometimes when I sit out on my deck I feel really fulfilled and content. I can **see** the vibrant colors of the blooming flowers, **and hear** the gentle trickling of the waterfall in my pond. Further off in the distance I can **hear** the fluttering of bird's wings as they play in the birdbath, while a gentle breeze **wafts** across my face bringing me the **sweet scent** of July blooms.

What's missing from this paragraph? Tonality and physiology are missing, and if you read this to yourself, you will fill them in automatically, based on your own experience. But notice that in this example the verbs or descriptive words match the nouns—that is, you see colors, hear the trickling-fluttering; feel the wafting breeze. This matching helps make the passage *congruent*. However, congruence also depends upon *tone* and *physiology* even more than the choice of words. Sarcasm is a good example of how this works—a sarcastic comment is one in which words, tonality, and expression are not balanced: "I *really* like your tie" (*sneer*). What do we tend to believe? The tone and the visual cues. If the comment is more veiled, we may just feel uneasy, or think that something "isn't quite right."

Obviously, this is important information to have, both in the context of what you hear patients saying, and how you say things to them. Some people select primarily **visual** language: "I *see* what you mean." "This *colors* my judgment." "You can *look back* on this material and notice how easily it comes to you." Others choose **auditory** images: "I *hear* what you're saying." "That *rings* a bell." "This idea is coming across *loud and clear.*" Still others use **kinesthetic** words: "I can't *grasp* that." "*Hold on* a minute!" "I'm *going to pieces.*" "I think I *have a handle* on this now."

With this information in mind, we now turn to the development of patient rapport.

Establishing Rapport

People tend to like people who are like themselves. When we meet someone new, we search for **commonality.** Rapport is created and established by pacing the individual's communication through **mirroring and matching** the key elements of a person's **physiology**—gestures, facial expressions, eye blink, breathing; **tonality**—tone, tempo, timbre, volume, pitch, pauses; and **words**—predicates (verb phrases), key words, associations.

You know you are in rapport when:

1. You are getting the outcome you want (that might be just getting along with the patient or making the patient feel comfortable), and
2. You calibrate to the person's level of comfort—that is, you keep the level of comfort relatively steady and, if discomfort arises in the patient, you change your approach so that rapport is re-established. (Sometimes when you have sufficient rapport, the relationship can tolerate a certain amount of discomfort. However, handling discomfort in the relationship is beyond the scope of this text.)

There are clearly varying degrees of rapport, as shown in Figure 36.1. In professional relationships, optimum rapport is defined in a fairly narrow band. It is important to avoid overidentification with the patient (and his or her problem) and still be able to communicate understanding and empathy. Physicians are often taught to aim for a cooler demeanor, to avoid getting "too involved." Unfortunately, this can result in a lack of rapport, generating frequent complaints from patients. In my practice, I often hear that other physicians "don't care about me, and don't listen to my concerns." I feel confident that usually the other physician does care, but because of our professional training, he or she may equate objectivity with emotional distance or coolness. I believe that maintaining understanding, openness, and empathy *without overidentification* is critical. Clinician/patient boundaries are important; clinicians must recognize that there are limits to their responsibility to and for the patient. Boundary issues regarding overidentification and sexual/romantic connections with patients are beyond the scope of this text, but have been dealt with adequately elsewhere.[6]

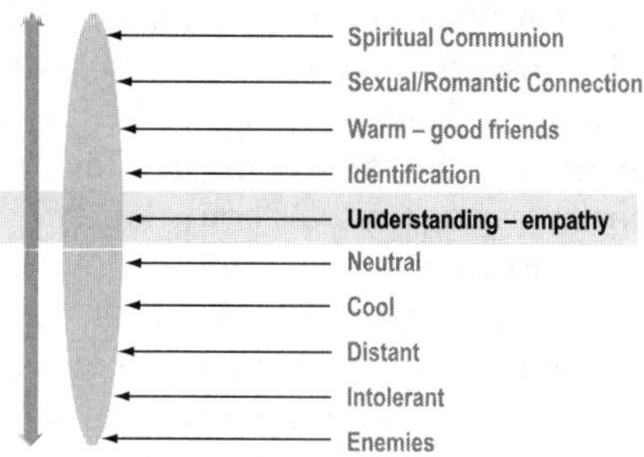

Figure 36.1 **Degrees of rapport**

Behaviors and Skills that Build Rapport

In order to build rapport, you need to develop sensory acuity. The more sensory acuity you have, the more you can calibrate to the patient's nonverbal but significant communications. We gain sensory acuity by watching, listening, and occasionally smelling and touching our patients. We use many of our senses to communicate, and also to calibrate to our patient's state. When we calibrate well, we can shift our behavior to **match and mirror** the patient, in order to gain more rapport. This is called pacing current experience.

Pacing current experience. You can learn how to match and mirror your patient's words, tone, and physiology, and thus gain sensory acuity *and* rapport at the same time. People feel more comfortable with someone who responds to them in the *same language representations* that they are using. This will lead you rapidly into a state of rapport that can—seemingly magically—produce a wealth of information in a short time. The following characteristics of certain people will help you to determine their primary representational system.

Primary Representational System	Characteristics Displayed
Visual	Thin, ectomorphic, wiry, wide-eyed, fast talkers, neat, chest breathers
Auditory	Mesomorphic, easily distracted, very verbal, even breathers
Kinesthetic	Endomorphic, lax in dress, slow talkers, diaphragmatic breathers

Pacing and then ... leading. With pacing, you begin to establish more rapport. Once rapport is established at a sufficient level, you can begin to **lead** the person. Leading is a mild challenge—have you ever paced a friend who was training to run a certain distance in a certain time? If you ran slightly ahead of him (or her), you would induce him to run faster to keep up, and then you could pace him again by running beside him. In interviewing and psychotherapy, leading may be used to help a person feel more comfortable in their surroundings, or to move them from a non-resourceful emotional state to a resourceful state. The overall process for establishing rapport through pacing is shown in Figure 36.2.

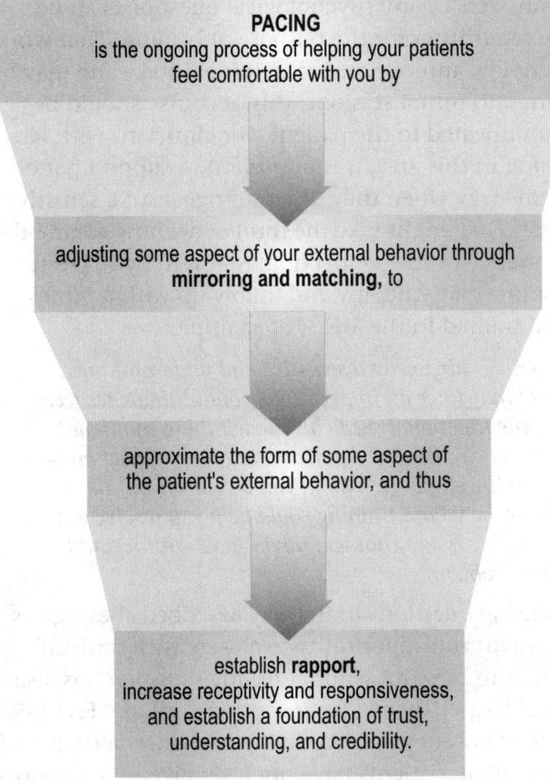

Figure 36.2 **The process of establishing rapport**

Matching is an integral part of pacing and rapport building. Table 36.1 reviews the different ways in which matching can be done.

Table 36.1 **Matching Behaviors**

Type of Matching	Behaviors
Whole Body Matching	Adjust your body to approximate the patient's postural shifts, e.g., cross legs, adjust torso angle, etc.
Partial Body Matching	Pace any stylistic use of body movements, e.g., eye blink, head shakes, head/shoulder angle, etc.
Vocal Qualities	Match shifts in tonality, tempo, volume, timbre, cadence or intonation.
Verbal Patterns	Hear and utilize sensory system language that matches and paces the representational system used by the patient (i.e., auditory, visual, or kinesthetic language).
Facial Expressions	Notice the patient's facial expressions—wrinkles, lips, eyebrows, etc.
Gestures	Respectfully match the patient's gestures.
Breathing	Adjust your breathing pattern to match the patient's.

Matching is NOT copying.
All of the above must be below the client's level of awareness.

Understanding the Story—Some Questions to Ask

Patients often provide clues about important factors in their stories in ways that can sometimes be easily overlooked when we focus too much on physical vs. emotional content. Open-ended questioning, together with listening in a non-judgmental way, will provide us with the opportunity to **really** hear what the patient is saying. Here are some open-ended questions that can elicit very useful information:

1. **When did you last feel really well?** This is an extremely important question because it takes the patient back to a time before things changed from good to bad. The answer may elicit both the temporal onset of symptoms and the **triggers or antecedents** for the functional issue. Asking the question in

this way, as opposed to focusing on when the patient began to feel sick (a more standard inquiry), requires patients to access, in memory, a time when they felt good, and that may give you important information that will help you to manage their "wellness program." If there were only one question that a clinician could ask, it might well be this one. Ensure that you do initially elicit a **wellness** description here, as it is likely that the patient will gravitate to an illness description in order to tell you what is wrong, purely out of cultural conditioning.

2. **What happened then?** This is the next question to ask because you want to elicit a sequential response that will maximize the possibility of accurately identifying antecedents and triggers. Depending upon the patient's particular way of telling stories, you will get more or less detail. Sometimes you may have to curtail too much detail, and at other times you may have to fish for more detail, remembering that you are looking for clues about triggers and antecedents.
3. **Was there anything going on in your life at that particular time that might have precipitated this [illness, pain, or other symptom]?** This question allows the patient to connect symptoms of any kind with stresses or life changes that they may have experienced. It gives them permission to make, or recall, that connection.
4. **Do you think that this [illness, pain, or other symptom] had anything to do with the fact that you [had a car accident, lost your father, became unemployed ... insert the specific event you are inquiring about]?** Again, this gives the patient permission to make connections between possible antecedents or triggers and their present symptoms. If they do make such a connection, the chances are it has some validity in their model of the world.
5. **Did anything happen to you as a child that made you feel bad?** This question is <u>very</u> open-ended, and may yield a number of results. Some patients may simply answer "no," in spite of the fact that such an answer is unlikely to be correct, since most people can recall at least one bad thing that happened to them during childhood. The "no" answer may have two possible reasons: perhaps something did happen that they don't want to talk about, or, in their map of the world, they simply don't include "bad things." Both of these have to be respected. I sometimes preface this question, particularly in patients who are presenting with gastrointestinal issues, in the following way:

> *There is research showing that some people with long-standing intestinal problems have had abuse issues as children. I don't want to suggest that that might have happened to you, but I do need to ask ...* **Did anything happen to you as a child that made you feel bad?**[7,8]

You may be thinking, "What do I do with this kind of information if I get it?" The answer will depend upon your particular clinical skills, focus of interest, and degree of comfort with exploring such issues. For those with appropriate training and interest, affirmative answers to any psychological questions can be explored further for the purpose of healing. That work may not be appropriate for an initial intake and may be deferred to future sessions; this of course should be communicated to the patient. For clinicians with less training in this area, it is important to support patients in some way when they disclose triggers of a sensitive nature. This might take the form of acknowledging the importance of the connection, followed by suggestions for appropriate therapy and follow-up with a professional trained in the area. For example:

> *This is obviously a sensitive and important area, and may have an impact upon your ultimate recovery. In the functional medicine model, these emotional factors can have a significant negative impact on our overall well-being. Would you be willing to talk to someone whose training could help you resolve any lingering issues that you might have with regard to this problem?*

Raising questions in the way described above gives the patient the opportunity to engage with difficult issues or to bow out without feeling pressure. It is also helpful to give them a future option such as, "Feel free to talk to me about this again if you change your mind." All too often, patients have not been given the opportunity to even mention such matters in a practitioner's office, let alone been given the opportunity to consider a solution.

You might wonder whether asking these kinds of questions could raise issues that are better left alone; in other words, is re-opening old wounds a good idea? I frequently find that the patient has made these connections anyway, and is relieved to know that a professional sees the importance of them. Sometimes just acknowledging this can provide such significant relief that nothing more needs to be said. This is the power of a really effective doctor/patient relationship—it becomes a healing relationship.

Motivation, Changing Behaviors, and Feedback

Language is really how we measure experience, and how we re-present our experience to others. Since our primary goal as practitioners is to help people feel better on many levels, it is important to use language that is positive and, at the same time, an honest appraisal of the situation. Transmission of hope to the patient is often essential to a good outcome.

Healing language encompasses:

- Self-empowerment
- Direction
- Motivation and feedback

Whatever the particular problems of your patients, the chances are that some aspects of their behavior will need to change in order for them to feel better. Changes may relate to diet, exercise patterns, stress management, leisure activities, or some other behavior. The functional medicine practitioner is in an advantageous position with patients because the model not only allows, but demands, that we take advantage of this "teachable moment." The functional medicine model is a generative one, in which new behaviors lead to feeling better emotionally, physically, and spiritually.

It is a good idea to assume that patients are willing to change their behavior in order to feel better. They need to begin at the appropriate "stage of change" (the subsequent discussion in this chapter addresses that topic in depth); fortunately, if that need is met and real help is offered, great progress can be made. While it is true that there are some patients with recalcitrant, addictive behaviors, it is also true that even these people usually want to change for the better. If we see a patient as an addict, rather than as someone who is capable of changing an addictive behavior, then the label "addict" tends to reinforce the belief that the condition is immutable. How can the practitioner in a general functional medicine practice help people change their unhealthy behaviors?

Motivation

People are motivated by a variety of factors. Often what brings people to practitioners is the fear of an incurable or painful condition. This at least gets them in the door, and indeed it may be a powerful motivator to do something different. However, as the person who is motivated by fear begins to get better, the impetus for the motivation decreases because the fear is no longer there. One very important factor is to ensure that the patient also has a positive **future** motivation, as well as a motivation to **move away** from the problem. You can access the desire for something positive in the future by posing some of the following questions:

- Tell me what it will be like when you are free of this problem?
- What will you be doing that is different?
- How will you be feeling that is different from the way you are feeling now?
- How will other people see you differently?
- How do you think I can help you, and what kinds of resources do you need?

Asking these questions requires that patients conceptualize future associations with wellness to sustain the changes in their lives even after fear and pain have subsided. When a patient is close to achieving initial goals, he or she can be helped to create other goals that can strengthen their motivation for the long term.

Different people motivate themselves in different ways. Here are some **un**helpful motivational styles, as outlined by Connirea Andreas in the book, *Heart of the Mind*:[9]

- **Overwhelm motivators** often select a huge goal and make it so big in their minds that they are actually unable to get started because the goal overwhelms them. If you ask what the goal "looks like" to them, they will tell you that it is very large and occupies a lot of their mental space. No wonder they feel overwhelmed. With these people it is a good idea to "chunk down" their goal into smaller, more easily obtainable portions. With weight loss, for example, aiming for small consistent losses over shorter periods of time is more effective than talking about a large weight loss over a longer period of time.
- **Dictator-style motivators** tend to talk to themselves in a negative way using language that is authoritarian and demanding. They don't get things

done because there is often a rebellious response to such demands. Generally people don't respond well to authoritarian approaches, even their own! Helping such patients create more respectful inner dialogues about their future goals can be helpful.

- **Seeing-it-done motivators.** Have you ever had trouble motivating yourself to do something you like? Probably not. We don't usually have to motivate ourselves to go to a movie, eat a meal, or go on vacation because these activities, for most of us, are enjoyable. We imagine doing them and we feel good. However, when it comes to doing the dishes, tidying our desks, or cleaning the house, the very thought can be unpleasant. The trick here is to visualize having it *done*. Seeing the house tidy, the dishes clean, the desk organized—or the exercise completed, vegetables in the refrigerator, a healthy meal actually on the table—can create a positive impetus.

Of course, these patterns are not mutually exclusive; they may vary from one context to another within a single individual. Figure 36.3 shows a general pattern for helping patients to motivate themselves.

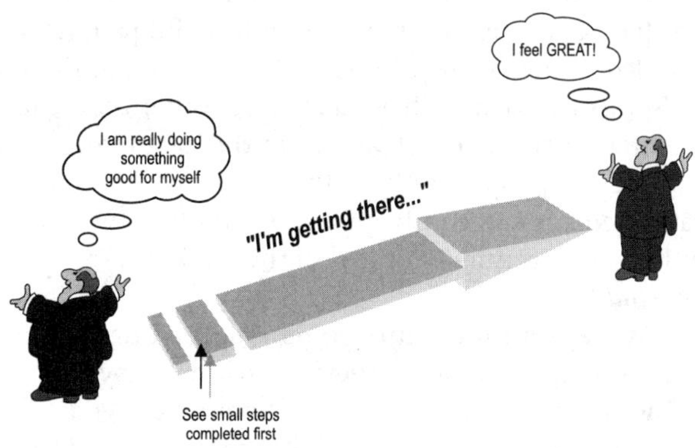

Figure 36.3 **Motivating patients**

In words, it might be phrased this way:

Pick a goal in the future that you want (e.g., weight loss). See yourself having accomplished that goal now—you are a healthy weight, wearing the clothes you like, and doing the things you like to do. Tell yourself in an encouraging internal voice how good you will feel when you get there, and how you will notice changes almost immediately that are small but pleasant. Remember to see yourself having accomplished the task. If that is too overwhelming, then see the first step clearly in your mind, and move on to each successive step as you are able.

Remember, motivating patients—and ultimately helping them to find their own effective motivation—is essential for a good outcome. People often feel overwhelmed at the thought of changing the habits of a lifetime, especially around food and exercise. However, remember that people are motivated when they enter your office. They may already be looking for a different approach and may expect you to recommend actions they can take on their own behalf, so they are primed. If you present, in an attainable way using some of the concepts outlined above, a plan for change, you enter into a partnership with them for achieving desirable goals. I find working with nutrition excellent in this regard because it often works quickly. If I have formulated the problem correctly, and the patient has carried out the instructions faithfully, by the next visit (two weeks), many patients find their symptoms have improved by as much as 50%. The Medical Symptoms Questionnaire (see Appendix) can be used as an objective measure of improvement if you ask your patients to fill it out at regular intervals. Patients can see how much better they are in black and white, so to speak. A sense of accomplishment is, in itself, a powerful motivating force.

General Language Guidelines and Giving Feedback

There is, of course, much more to be learned about how health professionals can communicate effectively with patients. Further reading from the references, or focused training, will help you move beyond this introductory information. A very useful book in this regard, particularly for health professionals, is *Irresistible Communication: Creative Skills for the Health Professional* by King, Novik, and Citrenbaum.[10] Although this book is both out of print and a little dated in its approach, it contains a wealth of useful information for communicating with patients in the healthcare setting, with excellent examples.

In thinking about the language we use with patients, it is helpful to remember that language consists not only of words strung together into sentences—we also group sentences into paragraphs or blocks of words to expand and enhance meaning. And, in oral communication, there is the final nuance, the unique way in which words and sentences are spoken (and heard), with differences in tonality, pitch, and speed, and accompanied by facial expressions and other physical manifestations. It is this complex structure that imparts such meaning to the words themselves.

In the old paradigm, we might have spoken to a patient in the following way regarding, for example, irritable bowel syndrome:

> *We have performed all the tests and they are all negative—we couldn't find anything wrong. This means you have something called irritable bowel syndrome. IBS is common; we really don't know what causes it; and there is not a lot we can do about it. You may have heard that it is caused by food allergies, but there really isn't any hard evidence for that, so I wouldn't avoid particular foods. You can eat what you want. You should increase your fiber intake and use bran or Metamucil®. Drink lots of fluids. Relaxation is sometimes helpful; take a few days off and relax. But stress doesn't cause the disease. You will likely have this for the rest of your life. I can give you some medication for the pain, and I'll see you again in a year to see how you're doing.*

All too often, this is actually a paraphrase of what is told to patients. The most common complaint I hear from patients is that they feel hopeless about this condition, and the specialist did not listen to any of their ideas about it.

Strictly speaking, what has been said in the above example is mostly true (albeit incomplete). But, we should ask ourselves, in any patient encounter, "What is my intention?" If our intention is to have the patient feeling better, then the above language needs to change.

Here is my critique of this approach:

- *We have performed all the tests and they are all negative—we couldn't find anything wrong.* Implies to the patient that there *is* something wrong, but we couldn't find it, OR there is nothing wrong and therefore,"Why are you complaining?"
- *This means you have something called irritable bowel syndrome. IBS is common; we really don't know what causes it; and there is not a lot we can do about it.* Sets the patient up to feel hopeless.
- *You may have heard that it is caused by food allergies, but there really isn't any hard evidence for that, so I wouldn't avoid particular foods. You can eat what you want.* Implies the patient can eat anything with impunity—the patient probably knows better, but may likely accede to the specialist/expert. Very few of us can truly eat exactly what we want.
- *You should increase your fiber intake and use bran or Metamucil®. Drink lots of fluids. Relaxation is sometimes helpful; take a few days off and relax.* Implies that relaxation is easily accomplished, instead of a skill to be learned. Does not address dietary approaches to increasing fiber, which can have many other benefits as well. Using approaches that help to normalize multiple systems is efficient and effective.
- *But stress doesn't cause the disease.* Implies, therefore, that stress is not really important.
- *You will likely have this for the rest of your life.* In hypnosis, this is called an embedded command—it can create a powerful negative suggestion at the unconscious level.
- *I can give you some medication for the pain, and I'll see you again in a year to see how you're doing.* Some patients interpret this as a brush-off, and it certainly doesn't create a sense of partnership in addressing the problem.

Overall, this is not an empowering communication:

1. **It provides less information than there really is about the condition.** There are approaches that can improve IBS; a number are discussed elsewhere in this book. There are dietary changes that can have multiple benefits. Training in stress management and relaxation is widely available and can be very helpful. For some patients, food sensitivities can be a problem; an elimination diet might help discover if that is the case. Exercise may help certain patients, and supplementation may help others.
2. **It leaves the patient feeling powerless.** If patients are empowered, they can be extremely effective partners in identifying triggers and mediators for this and countless other conditions. You want them working with you (and for themselves).

There are some guidelines for using language as a tool to create the outcome you and your patients want:

- **Tense.** People with chronic illness are often stuck in the past. They wish "it" hadn't happened, or it could have been different. Your language can bring them into the present and on into the future. Remember to move them forward: "What you are doing **now**, by changing your diet, will help you to feel better in the **future**. Let's imagine what that will feel like so that it becomes real for you."

- **Unconditional presuppositions.** Use **when** rather than **if.** "If" implies doubt that it might happen; "when" presupposes that it will happen—it's just a question of time and effort. For example, "**When** you start your nutrition program, you will ... ."
- **How or what, rather than why.** "Why" questions generally get us into trouble and don't lead anywhere except to more generally unhelpful information. "How" questions provide more useful information. So if a patient says, "I haven't been able to do the diet, it was just too much for me," don't ask "Why?" because that invites a list of excuses. Ask, for example:
  - "How did you actually stop yourself from starting the diet?"
  - "What would make it more likely that tomorrow you can take the first step?"

Answers to these questions should give you more information about how to help patients overcome the obstacles they have named.

- **Offer choices** that help the patient to focus on specific times and actions. For example, if a patient is beginning a lifestyle change program, say "Will you start the (nutrition, exercise) program **before or after** you go on holiday?" "What day **will** you begin?" The assumption is they will start; it's just a question of **when.**
- **Giving feedback.** The more encouraging feedback you can give, the better. Remember, your patients have been sick for a while, and they need lots of encouragement to initiate and maintain healthy changes. When you want something done differently, or you are concerned about progress, finding a respectful way to give feedback is very important. A **feedback sandwich** can work well; you sandwich any feedback that might be perceived as negative between two positive comments. For example:

I like the changes you have made to your nutrition program so far, especially the new foods you have introduced. The fact that you haven't lost weight yet is not uncommon. It would be a good idea to replace those granola bar snacks with fruit, for more energy. And keep up the good work; you are headed in the right direction!

Summary

As you review the ideas and techniques presented so far in this chapter, keep in mind that you—just as much as your patients—are now taking on the challenge of changing your behavior as a clinician. You will need to find your own motivation and reinforcement, measure your own progress, and ask for help where needed. You will need to practice; just reading about these ideas doesn't build the skills or the ability to maintain the new behaviors under stress. We have covered some important topics—**establishing and building rapport, creating good communication, and developing a healing language.** All of these can help us become more effective in our work with patients. If this work is new to you, then my hope is that you will be delightfully surprised and satisfied to learn, not immediately, perhaps, but after you have developed some skill, that your patients are responding in a different, more positive way, and accomplishing their goals with greater effectiveness. When that begins to happen, you will know that you are utilizing the tools that have been described in this chapter at both the conscious and unconscious level—they have become a part of you.

Helping Patients Change Unhealthy Behaviors

Janice M. Prochaska, MSW, PhD and
James O. Prochaska, PhD

Introduction

Healthcare providers can often become frustrated by the fact that too many of their patients have unhealthy diets, are inactive, smoke, abuse alcohol, don't manage stress effectively, and don't take their statins or antihypertensive medication as prescribed. If we don't like the way our patients are behaving, then the first thing we need to change is our own behavior. It begins by changing our mental models of behavior change. An action model has dominated medicine for more than a century. Patients are seen as changing when they quit smoking, start to exercise, or take their medications as prescribed. Action-oriented approaches are prescribed but they have little impact; for example, when healthcare systems offer action-oriented smoking cessation clinics for free, the pecentage of eligible smokers who participate annually is only 1%. We cannot impact the health of our patient populations if all we treat with the most deadly of behaviors is 1%. In this discussion, you will be introduced to a model of behavior change that can be matched to the needs of all patients and not just the minority who are ready to take action. This chapter is designed to help **you** change your mind so you can be better prepared to help your patients change their behavior.

The Transtheoretical Model of Behavior Change

The Transtheoretical Model (TTM), one of the leading approaches to health behavior change, can provide guidance in the development of interventions to increase readiness to change unhealthful behaviors. The TTM systematically integrates four theoretical constructs central to change:

1. **Stages of Change**	Readiness to practice a healthy behavior
2. **Decisional Balance**	Pros and Cons associated with a healthy behavior
3. **Self-Efficacy**	Confidence to practice and sustain the healthy behavior in difficult situations
4. **Processes of Change**	Ten cognitive, affective, and behavioral activities that facilitate the healthy behavior change

The TTM understands change as progress, over time, through a series of stages: *Precontemplation, Contemplation, Preparation, Action,* and *Maintenance.* Nearly 25 years of research on a variety of health behaviors have identified processes of change that work best in each stage to facilitate change.

The Stages of Change

Stage of change is the TTM's central organizing construct. Longitudinal studies of change have found that people move through a series of five stages when modifying behavior on their own or with the help of formal interventions.[11,12] In the first stage of change, *Precontemplation,* individuals may be unaware of the negative consequences of their behavior, believe the consequences are insignificant, have given up the thought of changing because they are demoralized, or may be defensive about the need to change. They are not intending to take action in the next six months. Individuals in the *Contemplation* stage are more likely to recognize the benefits of changing their behavior. However, they continue to overestimate the costs of changing and are ambivalent and not ready to change. Those in the *Preparation* stage are seriously considering taking action within the next 30 days, and have already begun to take small steps toward the goal. Their concern is that they will fail. Individuals in the *Action* stage are overtly engaged in modifying their problem behaviors or acquiring new, healthy behaviors. Individuals in the *Maintenance* stage have been able to sustain change for at least six months, and are faced with the challenge of sustaining the change over the long term.

Research comparing stage distributions across behaviors and populations finds that only a minority of people are in Preparation, with a majority in Precontemplation and Contemplation.[13,14] Those data suggest that if we offered all individuals action-oriented interventions that assume readiness to practice a healthy behavior, we would be mis-serving the majority who are not prepared to take action.

Stage-matched interventions can have a greater impact than action-oriented, one-size-fits-all programs, by increasing participation and increasing the likelihood that individuals will take action. Stage-matched interventions for smokers more than doubled the smoking cessation rates of the best action-oriented interventions available.[15] Stage-matched interventions have also out-performed one-size-fits-all interventions for exercise acquisition,[16] dietary behavior,[17] and mammography screening.[18]

Stage of change is generally assessed using a staging algorithm, a set of decision rules that place an individual in one of the five stage categories based on their responses to a few questions about their intentions, past behavior, and present behavior. The algorithms assess individual readiness to take action, such as to quit smoking or to exercise regularly for 30 minutes a day. The response categories place participants in one of five stages: Precontemplation (not intending to take an action such as quitting smoking in the next six months), Contemplation (intending to take action in the next six months), Preparation (intending to take action in the next 30 days), Action (already quit smoking but for less than six months), or Maintenance (quit smoking for more than six months).

Decisional Balance

Change requires the consideration of the potential gains (Pros) and losses (Cons) associated with taking action. The Decisional Balance Inventory consists of two scales, the Pros of Change and the Cons of Change. Longitudinal studies have found those measures to be among the best available predictors of future change.[19] Across more than 50 behaviors, Hall and Rossi,[20] and Prochaska, Velicer, et al.[21] found that the balance of Pros and Cons was systematically related to stage of change. The Cons of changing to a health-promoting behavior outweighed the Pros in the Precontemplation stage; the Pros surpassed the Cons in the middle stages; and the Pros outweighed the Cons in the Action stage. So the first principle of helping patients progress in Precontemplation is to increase the Pros of changing. Ask a couch potato, "What are all the benefits that you could get from regular exercise?" They can usually list four or five. Tell them there are at least 40 scientifically-documented benefits (see the Appendix). Ask them to try to double their list, and they can start changing. Let them know that there is something they can do for 30 minutes a day that can give them so many benefits.

Participants in the Contemplation stage need to lessen the Cons of changing. For quitting smoking, withdrawal is one of the big Cons. Fortunately, there are a variety of medications, such as nicotine replacement therapies, that can dramatically reduce this Con.

Self-Efficacy

Self-efficacy, or the degree to which an individual believes he or she has the capacity to attain a desired goal, can influence motivation and persistence.[22] Self-efficacy in the TTM has two components that are distinct but related: confidence to make and sustain changes, and temptation to relapse. Like decisional balance, levels of self-efficacy differ systematically across the stages of change, with subjects further along in the stages of change generally experiencing greater confidence and less temptation. Self-efficacy means having the confidence to practice the healthy behavior in a variety of difficult situations (e.g., when one is stressed, has an increased workload, or has conflicting demands).

One of the best ways to increase self-efficacy is to help the patient set realistic goals. Patients in Precontemplation will have little confidence that they can take effective action at this time. But they can have much greater confidence that they can progress to Contemplation (e.g., doubling their list of Pros). Once they start progressing, they can break out of their demoralized or defensive place, experience some success, and increase their self-efficacy. Temptations can be reduced by using strategies to cope with difficult situations, such as taking deep breaths rather than smoking as a way to reduce stress.

Processes of Change

In a comparative analysis of 24 major systems of psychotherapy, Prochaska and DiClemente[23] distilled a set of 10 fundamental processes by which people change. These 10 processes describe the basic patterns of activity that should be encouraged by clinicians to help patients change problem behaviors:

Consciousness raising	Finding and learning new facts, ideas, and tips that support the healthy behavior change
Dramatic relief	Experiencing the negative emotions (fear, anxiety, worry) that go along with unhealthy behavior risks
Self re-evaluation	Realizing that the behavior change is an important part of one's identity as a person
Environmental re-evaluation	Realizing the negative impact of the unhealthy behavior or the positive impact of the healthy behavior on one's proximal social and physical environment
Self-liberation	Making a firm commitment to change
Helping relationships	Seeking and using social support for the healthy behavior change
Counter-conditioning	Substituting healthier alternative behaviors and cognitions for the unhealthy behaviors

Reinforcement management	Increasing the rewards for the positive behavior change and decreasing the rewards of the unhealthy behavior
Stimulus control	Removing reminders or cues to engage in the unhealthy behavior and adding cues or reminders to engage in the healthy behavior
Social liberation	Realizing that the social norms are changing in the direction of supporting the healthy behavior change.

Figure 36.4 depicts our current understanding of the patterns of emphasizing particular processes as they progress through the stages.[24]

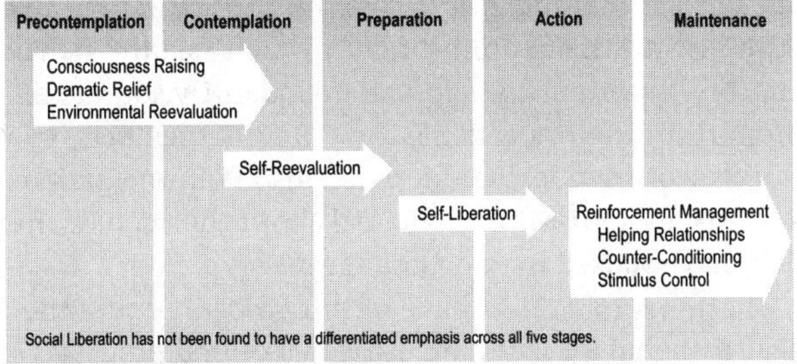

Figure 36.4 **Stages of change in which particular processes of change are emphasized**

Stage-Matched Interventions Based on the TTM

In addition to providing an assessment framework, the TTM provides a scheme for tailoring programs by matching them to the needs of patients at each stage of change for a new healthy behavior. The degree of tailoring possible depends directly on the extent of the assessment. The following are descriptions of how one could use TTM for increasing a healthy behavior through manuals, provider interventions, or internet-based programs.

Stage-Based Manuals

When only the staging algorithm is administered, tailoring can occur at the stage level. Stage-based manuals describe how self-changers progress through each stage of change, and how they recycle if they relapse. The manuals teach users about general principles of behavior change, about their particular stage of change, and the processes they can use to progress to the next stage. Appropriate sections of the manuals are matched to each stage of change and provide detail on change processes and stage-matched exercises. There are several ways to use the manuals. First, they can be read for the big picture of how people change; next, readers can turn to the section for the stage they are in and study that stage for a while. This is a good way to be sure they are heading in the right direction. Then, users can look ahead to the next stage to learn more about how to move forward. For example, if a patient in the Precontemplation stage for effective stress management is underestimating the Pros, that patient could use the section of the manual that describes dozens of documented Pros of doing effective stress management. The patient would also be encouraged to seek more information about the importance of stress management from the media and their healthcare provider.

Changing for Good[25] is a popular paperback that patients can use to help guide them through the stages of change for a broad range of health behaviors and other problem behaviors. Or a stage-based manual specific to stress management, smoking cessation, medication adherence, exercising regularly, or weight management can be viewed at www.prochange.com.

Stage-Based Provider Guidance

Healthcare providers can also tailor interventions to the patient's stage of change by administering the staging algorithm (e.g., in the waiting room). Providers can then base brief interventions on processes that are most helpful to a particular stage. For example, Precontemplators come in denying or minimizing their problems. They may be unaware of the negative consequences of their unhealthy behavior or they may be demoralized because of repeated failures in changing their behavior.

The goal for the provider is to engage Precontemplators in the change process. Lecture and confrontation won't work. Trying to pressure or persuade them to take immediate action will only make them more defensive or demoralized. As we saw earlier, just helping them to increase their awareness of the Pros of changing will help them to progress. Providers also can help Precontemplators raise consciousness by teaching them about the stages of change, and providing more information to dispel any misconceptions the patient may have. During the first appointment with Precontemplators, providers can ask if they are willing to do any of the following before the next time they meet:

- Read about the healthy behavior
- Double their list of the Pros
- Talk with someone who has successfully changed the target behavior.

Providers should reinforce the notion that their patients *have* the capacity to progress (see related discussion in the first part of this chapter). They should remind their patients that any forward movement (e.g., becoming more open to considering alternatives, becoming more aware) is progress; change does not equal action—change means progressing to the Contemplation stage.

Contemplators are thinking about changing but are not yet committed to do so. They are more likely to acknowledge that their behavior needs to be changed, but they substitute thinking about it for acting on it. They recognize the benefits of changing, but overestimate the Cons. Contemplators are ambivalent about changing and are often waiting for the magic moment. Providers can assist by acknowledging the ambivalence and working to resolve it by encouraging Contemplators to weigh the Pros against the Cons. Patients are asked to shrink Cons by comparing them to the growing list of Pros, by asking how important they are relative to the Pros, and by challenging themselves to counter the Cons. For example, time is the number one Con for regular exercise. But time becomes less of a barrier if we can get more than 40 benefits for 30 minutes. Interventions in these appointments can be more ambitious, including taking small steps toward the healthy behavior. For example, smokers in Contemplation can be given three choices to progress to Preparation:

1. Quit for 24 hours in the next month;
2. Delay the first cigarette by an extra 30 minutes; or
3. Reduce the number of cigarettes they smoke by three or four.

"Which are you most confident you can do? Great. Take it and run with it."

Providers can help by using motivational interviewing strategies like reflective listening to assist Contemplators to resolve their ambivalence by working with them to identify the negative consequences of continuing the unhealthy behavior, and by providing case examples of people who have been able to change.

Helping patients create a healthier image is important in Contemplation. Providers can encourage patients to ask themselves about their image. For example, "How do you think and feel about yourself as an inactive person? What might it be like if you became more active?"

Patients in Preparation assess the Pros as more important than the Cons, are more confident and less tempted, are developing a plan, and are more likely to participate in programs. With those in Preparation, providers need to be experienced coaches to provide encouragement. They need to coach, not lecture, and give praise, support, and recognition for taking small steps; keep interventions short, focused, and action-oriented; be available for phone support; focus on developing a plan for doing the healthy behavior; and problem solve.

Providers can enhance progress by ensuring that patients choose steps that are realistic, concrete, and measurable. Those in Preparation should be asked to put plans in writing and to role play how they will tell others about their commitment to their healthy behavior. It is important to help patients identify sources of support for their new behaviors—family members, coworkers, or friends. Providers can also help the patient to think about how they will feel about themselves after they have started making changes.

Patients in Action have recently begun doing the healthy behavior. They are using behavioral processes of change. Their confidence is building, but temptation and risk of relapse are concerns. Providers with patients in Action need to be facilitators for the behavior change. The focus is on the behavioral processes of change—counter-conditioning, stimulus control, and reinforcement management. It is also important to help patients plan ahead to prevent lapses and relapses.

Providers can help by getting patients to identify problematic beliefs and behaviors that inhibit change, and then by problem solving about positive alternatives that they believe will work for them. People, places, and things that increase the likelihood of not adhering need to be avoided or controlled (tempting cues). Reminders in both familiar and unexpected places that support the healthy behavior need to be left around—like a gym bag filled and ready to use, a picture on the desk of relaxing with friends, or pill-taking scheduled on the calendar. Those in Action also need to notice the intrinsic rewards of their healthy behavior—better health, more energy, more control of life. Patients need to reward themselves with positive statements; providers can praise achievements and help patients recognize the benefits of their efforts.

Here is a simple strategy that can help patients activate a series of important change processes. "Do you make to-do lists? OK, good. Now, for this week, write in your to-do list *walking for my heart*. Next week, *walking for my stress*. Then, *walking for my bones; walking for my brain; walking for my immune system*. Pretty soon you will be running." This technique involves self-liberation (writing down a commitment to walk); stimulus control (continue walking); and reinforcement (scratching walking off one's daily to-do list). This approach helps providers communicate to their patients that they care for them as whole people and not just as patients with a disease. Patients are being encouraged to walk not only to prevent or manage a disease like diabetes or CVD; they are encouraged to walk to enhance the health of their whole self—body, mind, and spirit.

Patients in Maintenance have high confidence, and temptations are low. They are at risk primarily in times of distress or atypical temptations. With those in Maintenance, the provider needs to be a consultant to provide advice regarding relapse prevention. Providers can do this by helping patients to cope with distress (the major cause of relapse), continuing to refine a relapse prevention plan, being available to provide support, and establishing a support system in the community. For many people, Maintenance can be a lifelong struggle—it is a dynamic not a static stage. There needs to be work to consolidate gains and increase self-efficacy through increasing coping skills.

Remember, a majority of individuals relapse to earlier stages before reaching permanent Maintenance. Your job is to make sure they don't give up on themselves and that you don't give up on them.

Intra- and Internet Expert System Program

Lengthier assessments that include each of the constructs of the TTM permit significantly more tailoring, but may be impractical in a clinic setting where competing demands limit time. We have developed computerized tailored health behavior change programs that are designed to be easy and engaging for patients to use and can be delivered over intra- or internet platforms which offer a cost-effective, easily disseminated alternative. The technical basis for these systems relies on the integration of statistical, word processing, multimedia, and database software. A system resides either on an internet server or a local network server, and can be accessed by anyone who has the appropriate address and password. Such programs are being made more available to patients through their insurers or employers. Once a patient logs onto the program, they are asked to complete a TTM assessment that evaluates stage, decisional balance, self-efficacy, and the processes of change.

During a patient's first use of the program, feedback is based on a comparison of the responses of the individual to a larger comparative sample of successful and unsuccessful individuals making the behavior change. This feedback relies only on normative comparisons, which differ by stages. The initial norms are derived from a naturalistic sample of individuals. Evaluation of the expert system provides updated norms at periodic intervals. The second and subsequent interactions compare the individual to both the normative group and to their own previous responses, and provide both ipsative (i.e., self-comparisons) and normative comparisons. The ipsative comparisons require access to the database for the results of the previous contact. The program makes individualized recommendations of change and guides the participant through the behavior change process that meets their individual needs.

The computer generated feedback also links or refers participants to sections of a stage-matched self-help interactive resource workbook. Like the stage-matched manual described above, the online integrated workbook teaches users about general principles of behavior change, as well as their particular stage of change and the processes they can use to progress to the next stage. The individualized feedback reports refer participants (via links) to appropriate sections of the workbook to provide more detail on change processes and stage-matched exercises. For example, a participant can link to the online workbook where there are testimonials about the effects of stress from people who are now effectively managing their stress, an exercise to learn about what controls one's behavior, a bulletin board listing rewards people give themselves for effectively managing stress, and substitutes for unhealthy stress management that don't involve food, smoking, or alcohol. For a sample of this program designed for stress management, please go to www.prochange.com/PDF/stress.pdf.

Summary

What is the number one reason that a majority of providers do not practice behavioral medicine? Time is number two. Reimbursement is number three. The number one reason is that two-thirds of providers have come to believe their patients cannot change or will not change. We are convinced they have become demoralized by the action paradigm.

Here is a prescription for producing a demoralized provider and a non-compliant patient. An actual case involved a 50-year-old obese male recently diagnosed with type 2 diabetes. His physician with all good intent told him, "You have to test your blood glucose twice a day, take your medication twice a day, change your diet, exercise, quit smoking, and lower your stress. Good luck!"

Two large population studies demonstrated that health behavior changes could be made simultaneously with populations of patients with diabetes by applying counseling, computers, and manuals.[26,27] But the patients were not asked to take action on these behaviors at once. Less than 10% were ready to take action on two or more of those risks. They were helped to set goals that were realistic for the stage they were in and then to use principles and processes of change to progress from one stage to the next.

As professionals, we can apply the same approach to changing our own behaviors. The goal for this chapter was to help you progress one stage toward adopting a more effective approach to functional medicine. If you have progressed just a single stage, then our time together has been worthwhile.

References

1. Adams F. Brain injury: A neuromedical overview. The Disability Reporter. 2000;Winter:19.
2. Moerman D. Medicine, Meaning and the 'Placebo Effect. Cambridge Studies in Medical Anthropology. Cambridge University Press, 2002.
3. These pre-suppositions are based on a psychological model known as Neuro-Linguistic Programming or NLP. For further reading on this topic see: O'Connor J. NLP Workbook: A Practical Guide to Achieving the Results you Want. HarperCollins UK: 2001; and O'Connor J, Seymour J. Introducing Neuro-Linguistic Programming: Psychological Skills for Understanding and Influencing People, 2nd Ed. Thorsons, London: 1993.
4. Bateson G. Steps to an Ecology of Mind: Collected Essays in Anthropology, Psychiatry, Evolution, and Epistemology. University of Chicago Press; 2000.
5. Mehrabian A, et al. Inference of attitudes from nonverbal communication in two channels. J Consult Psychol. 1967;(3):248-252.
6. Rutter P. Sex in the Forbidden Zone: When Therapists, Doctors, Clergy, Teachers and Other Men in Power Betray Women's Trust. HarperCollins: 1995.
7. Walker EA, Gelfand AN, Gelfand MD, Katon WJ. Psychiatric diagnoses, sexual and physical victimization, and disability in patients with irritable bowel syndrome or inflammatory bowel disease. Psychol Med. 1995;25(6):1259-67.
8. Ali A, Toner BB, Stuckless N, et al. Emotional abuse, self-blame, and self-silencing in women with irritable bowel syndrome. Psychosom Med. 2000;62(1):76-82.
9. Andreas C. Heart of the Mind. Real People Press: Moab, Utah: 1989.
10. King M, Novik L, Citrenbaum C. Irresistible Communication: Creative Skills for the Health Professional WB Saunders: Philadelphia, 1982.
11. DiClemente CC, Prochaska JO. Self-change and therapy change of smoking behavior: a comparison of processes of change in cessation and maintenance. Addict Behav. 1982;7:133-142.
12. Prochaska JO, DiClemente CC. Stages and processes of self-change of smoking: toward an integrative model of change. J Consult Clin Psychol. 1983;51:390-395.
13. Laforge RG, Velicer WF, Richmond RL, Owen, N. Stage distributions for five health behaviors in the United States and Australia. Prev Med. 1999;28(1):61-74.
14. Velicer WF, Fava JL, Prochaska JO, et al. Distribution of smokers by stage in three representative samples. Prev Med. 1995;24(4):401-411.
15. Prochaska JO, DiClemente CC, Velicer WF, Rossi JS. Standardized, individualized, interactive, and personalized self-help programs for smoking cessation. Health Psychol. 1993;12(5):399-405.
16. Marcus BH, Bock BC, Pinto BM, et al. Efficacy of an individualized, motivationally-tailored physical activity intervention. Ann Behav Med. 1998;20(3):174-180.
17. Campbell MK, DeVellis BM, Strecher VJ, et al. Improving dietary behavior: the effectiveness of tailored messages in primary care settings. Am J Public Health. 1994;84(5):783-787.
18. Rakowski W, Ehrich B, Goldstein MG, et al. Increasing mammography screening among women aged 40-74 by use of a stage-matched tailored intervention. Prev Med. 1998;27(5 Pt 1):748-756.
19. Velicer WF, DiClemente CC, Prochaska JO, Brandenburg N. Decisional balance measure for assessing and predicting smoking status. J Pers Soc Psych. 1985;48(5):1279-1289.
20. Hall KL, Rossi JS. Informing interventions: a meta-analysis of the magnitude of effect in decisional balance stage transitions across 43 health behaviors. Ann of Behav Med. 2003;25:S180.
21. Prochaska JO, Velicer WF, Rossi JS, et al. Stages of change and decisional balance for 12 problem behaviors. Health Psychol. 1994;13(1):39-46.
22. Bandura A. Self-efficacy: toward a unifying theory of behavior change. Psych Rev. 1977;84:191-215.
23. Prochaska JO, DiClemente CC. The Transtheoretical Approach: Crossing Traditional Boundaries of Therapy. Homewood, IL: Dorsey Press, 1984.
24. Prochaska JO, DiClemente CC, Norcross JC. In search of how people change: application to addictive behaviors. Am Psychol. 1992; 47(9):1102-14.
25. Prochaska JO, Norcross J, DiClemente C. Changing for Good. New York, NY: William Morrow and Company, Inc., 1994.
26. Jones H, Edwards L, Vallis MT, et al. Changes in diabetes self-care behaviors make a difference to glycemic control: the Diabetes Stages of Change (DiSC) study. Diabetes Care. 2003;26(3):732-37.
27. Rossi JS, Ruggiero L, Rossi S, et al. Effectiveness of stage-based multiple behavior interventions for diabetes management in two randomized clinical trials. Ann Behav Med. 2002;24:S192.

Chapter 37
Case Presentation and Extended Discussion: Metabolic Syndrome, Cardiovascular Disease, and Related Conditions

Mark C. Houston, MD, MSc, SCH, ABAAM, FACP, FAHA

Case Presentation

Fifty-five (55) year-old white male, long-distance truck driver, presents with a chief complaint of "headache, chest pain, and shortness of breath with exercise." (Table 37.1 provides a list of abbreviations used this chapter.)

Present Illness

The patient states that he began to have occipital headaches three months prior to this visit. The headaches were described as a dull ache, intermittent, but worse early in the morning and often would wake him up. The headaches were five out of ten in severity, without radiation or other associated symptoms initially, and were relieved partially by aspirin or acetaminophen. About two months prior to his visit, he had one episode of numbness and weakness in his right hand, associated with mild dizziness and posterior headache while driving his truck; it lasted for less than five minutes, resolved completely, and has not recurred since. One month ago, he noticed substernal chest pain and dyspnea while unloading his truck and also when walking up steps in his home. The chest pain was described as a "heaviness and aching" in the middle of the chest with some radiation into the left arm and hand, eight out of ten in severity and relieved by resting for three to four minutes. He also noted some shortness of breath and mild wheezing with the exertional chest pain that was so severe that he had to stop and rest. There was no cough, hemoptysis, or sputum production. He denied any other symptoms or problems.

Personal History

Social: He was born in southern Georgia where he has lived all of his life. He is married and has four children, ages 16, 20, 23, and 25. His wife recently lost her job, has been very depressed, and has started drinking alcohol heavily. They have had financial problems since then, and he has taken out a loan from the bank. He is contemplating working extra shifts for the trucking firm to pay back the loan and improve his finances. His youngest son has been arrested twice for DUI and is failing his high school classes. The patient started working as a long-distance truck driver 37 years ago, when he dropped out of high school early to support his mother after his father died of a heart attack at the age of 43. All members of his extended family moved to Texas 10 years ago and he rarely sees them or communicates with them. His wife's family lives in Mississippi, and they do not see them much either.

Habits, nutrition and exercise: The patient has smoked two packs of cigarettes per day for 40 years, drinks six beers per day, and consumes 10 to 12 cups of coffee and six soft drinks per day. He has less than one glass of tap water per day. He eats mostly in fast food restaurants with lots of "burgers, fries, fried chicken, tacos, and burritos." He hates fruits and vegetables other than potatoes, and often eats steak and mashed potatoes when he is home. His usual breakfast is a cup of coffee, a Danish, and a cigarette. He carries various types of candies and sweets in his truck to snack on during the day. He is in his truck either driving or sleeping 70% of the time. He uses the air conditioner or heater in

Table 37.1 **Abbreviations Used in Chapter 37**

A-II	Angiotensin-II	IVUS	Intravascular coronary ultrasound
ABP	Ambulatory blood pressure	LAD	Left anterior descending
ACEI	Angiotensin-converting enzyme inhibitor	LAH	Left atrial hypertrophy
ARB	Angiotensin-receptor blocker	LCX	Left circumflex
BMI	Body mass index	LDL	Low density lipoprotein
C_3	Complement 3	LP (a)	Lipoprotein (a)
CCB	Calcium channel blocker	LVH	Left ventricular hypertrophy
CHD	Coronary heart disease	MAPK	Mitogenactivated protein kinase
CSF-1	Colony stimulating factor-1	MAU	Microalbuminuria
CVD	Cardiovascular disease	MCP-I	Monocyte chemoattractant protein-I
DBP	Diastolic blood pressure	MI	Myocardial infarction
EBT	Electron beam tomography	MIP-1α	Macrophage inflammatory protein-1 alpha
eNOS	Endothelial nitric oxide synthase	MUFA	Monounsaturated fats
FBG	Fasting blood glucose	NMR	Nuclear magnetic resonance analysis
FBS	Fasting blood sugar	OGTT	Oral glucose test
FFA	Free fatty acids	PAI-1	Plasminogen activator inhibitor-1
GFR	Glomerular filtration rate	PGE	Prostaglandin E
HCT	Hematocrit	PI3-K	Phosphatidyl inositol 3 kinase
HDL	High density lipoprotein	PPAR	Peroxisome proliferator activated receptors
HS-CRP	High sensitivity C-reactive protein	PRA	Panel-reactive antibody
IBW	Ideal body weight	PUFA	Polyunsaturated fats
ICAM	Intracellular cell adhesion molecule	ROS	Reactive oxygen species
IL-6	Interleukin-6	SBP	Systolic blood pressure
ILI-B	Interleukin IB	TG	Triglyceride
IMT	Intimal medial thickness	TNF-α	Tumor necrosis factor-alpha
IR	Insulin resistance	VLDL	Very-low-density lipoprotein
IRS 1/2	Insulin receptor substrate 1 and 2	VSM	Vascular smooth muscle

the truck depending on the weather, but never has the windows open. The only exercise that he gets is when he occasionally unloads a few boxes from his truck. He states that he has been overweight since he was 21 and has gained over 30 pounds in the last 10 years. His work schedule allows little time for socializing with family and friends and he is so "stressed out" and "depressed" about his job, finances, wife, and son that he wants to be alone most of the time anyway. He has never attended any religious services or church.

Past Medical History

Hospitalizations and operations: None
Medical illnesses: Mild sinus congestion and "heartburn"
Infectious diseases: Mumps, rubella, and chickenpox as a child; otherwise, negative
Immunizations: Tetanus toxoid six years ago
Skin tests: N-isopropyl-N'-phenyl-p-phenylenediamine (IPPD) is negative
Injuries: None
Transfusions: None
Medications: Aspirin (four to five per day), acetaminophen (four per day), TUMS® (six per day) and prn over-the-counter sinus medications.
Allergies: None
Family history: Father died at 43 of a heart attack. He had hypertension and high cholesterol, smoked heavily, and was obese. Mother is alive at 83 with osteoarthritis, hypothyroidism, and hypertension. Brother is 57 and had a heart attack at age 50. He is also hypertensive and has high cholesterol. He now has severe congestive heart failure and is on disability. Sister is 49 with hypertension and high cholesterol. Grandfather died at 56 of unknown causes. Grandmother died at 71 of unknown causes.
Review of systems: Negative except for those symptoms and problems mentioned in the present illness.

Physical Exam

General: Obese, anxious, pleasant white male appearing older than his stated age.
Blood pressure: First blood pressure was 182/104 mm Hg in left arm sitting. Five minutes later the blood pressure was 176/102 mm Hg in the left arm sitting. Ten minutes later the blood pressure was 178/104 mm Hg in the right arm sitting. Twelve minutes later the blood pressure was 170/100 mm Hg in the left arm standing.
Heart rate: The initial heart rate was 92 and regular while sitting. Five minutes later the heart rate was 90 and regular while sitting. Ten minutes later the heart rate was 80 while sitting. Twelve minutes later the heart rate was 82 and regular while standing.
Temperature: 98.8° F
Respiratory rate: 16 and non-labored
Weight: 225 pounds, large frame
Height: 5 feet, 10 inches
Waist circumference: 42 inches (normal <40)
Waist-hip ratio: 1.4 (normal <1.0)
Body mass index (BMI): 32.0 kg/m2. Stage 1 obesity (normal is <25). BMI is weight in kg divided by m^2 in height.
Percent body fat: 28% (normal <16% in males)
Skin: No rash, abnormal nevi, or other lesions; normal hair and nail examination.
Head and neck: Eyes show no scleral icterus; mild erythematous scleral injection bilaterally; extraocular motion intact; and normal visual fields. Pupils are equal and reactive to light and accommodation. Vision is 20/20 bilaterally. Retina shows grade 2 Keith Wagener hypertensive changes with arteriolar narrowing and arteriolar/venous nicking. Optic discs appear normal. Ears have normal hearing with no abnormalities. Nose and mouth are erythematous without lesions. Neck shows bilateral carotid bruits, supple, no thyromegaly, neck masses, or lymphadenopathy.
Chest: Mild barrel chest; hyper-resonant to percussion; diffuse expiratory wheezes, no rales or rhonchi; no chest wall tenderness.
Cardiac: Regular rate and rhythm; increased intensity of the second heart sound, A-2 with an S4 atrial gallop sound and a II-III/VI holosystolic murmur at the lower left sternal border, but loudest at the apex with radiation to this area.
Pulses: Normal pulses in the radial, brachial, femoral, posterior tibial and dorsalis pedis bilaterally; minimal diminution of the carotid pulses bilaterally.
Abdomen: Obese, soft; normal bowel sounds; minimal tenderness in the mild epigastric area; no palpable liver, spleen or other masses; no abdominal or renal bruits.
Lymphatics: No lymph node enlargement in the cervical area, axillary, epitrochlear, inguinal or any other location.
Musculoskeletal: Normal muscle strength, tone, and flexibility.
Neurological: Mildly depressed and anxious affect; normal short- and long-term memory; normal cranial nerves; normal motor and sensory examination with normal reflexes in the upper and lower extremities bilaterally.
Genitourinary: Both testicles descended without masses or tenderness and no scrotal masses.
Rectal: Stool negative for occult blood; prostate two plus enlarged without masses or tenderness.
Extremities: No cyanosis, clubbing or edema

Nutritional Evaluation (done with diet diary and nutritionist interview)

Total daily caloric intake: 3600 KCAL
Macronutrient percentages:
- Simple and refined carbohydrates: 60%
- Crude fiber: <5 grams
- Protein: 15%
- Fats: 25%
    - Saturated fats: 82%
    - Polyunsaturated fats (PUFA): 5%
    - Monounsaturated fats (MUFA): 5%
    - *Trans* fats: 8%

Exercise

Total estimated aerobic exercise per day: 10 minutes
Resistance: No resistance exercise except for occasional lifting of boxes from his truck

Initial Lab Results

Initial visit tests for urinalysis, urea nitrogen, sodium, potassium, chloride, carbon dioxide, calcium, total protein, albumin, globulin, total bilirubin, alkaline phosphatase, AST, ALT, T_4, FT_4, FT_3, TSH, prostate specific antigen, 24-hour urine volume, and total cholesterol were within normal limits. Urine, serum, hair, and nail evaluations were performed for mercury, lead, arsenic, cadmium, etc. and were normal. The following tests were abnormal:

Sed rate by modified Westergren	42 mm/hr (normal ≤ 20)
Creatinine, 24-hour urine	2.69 g (normal range 0.63–2.50 g)
Iron binding saturation	52% (normal range 10–36%)

Cardiovascular Testing

24-hour ambulatory blood pressure monitor:
- Increased BP load and mean BP
- Systolic blood pressure (SBP): >140 mm Hg, 95% (normal load is <15%)
- Diastolic blood pressure (DBP): >90 mm Hg, 88% (normal load is <15%)
- Mean BP: 178/98 mm Hg
- No nocturnal dipping (normal decrease is SBP 10%–12% and decreased DBP 14%–17%)

Treadmill test: Positive hypertensive response to exercise, 220/112 mm Hg, with 1½ mm ST segment depression in the inferior, anterior, and lateral leads with T-wave inversion

Thallium treadmill test: Positive—anterior, inferior, and lateral perfusion defects/ischemia

Carotid artery duplex: Increased intimal medial thickness (IMT) with 60% left common carotid artery obstruction and 40% right common carotid artery obstruction

Electron beam tomography (EBT): Multi-site Ca++ – inferior, anterior, lateral. Calcium score (CAC): 485 (>99th percentile) (Figure 37.1)

Computerized arterial pulse wave analysis (age and gender adjusted):
- C-1 AC: 8, which is low (normal is >12) (large arterial compliance)
- C-2 AC: 2, which is low (normal is >7) (small arterial compliance)

Cardiac echo: Mitral regurgitation 1+ to 2+, moderate left ventricular hypertrophy (LVH), diastolic dysfunction, enlarged left atrium (LAH)

Electrocardiogram (EKG): Abnormal—sinus tachycardia, non-specific diffuse ST-T wave changes, LAH and LVH

Chest x-ray: Abnormal—hyperexpanded lung fields consistent with early emphysema; increased interstitial markings in the bases of both lungs

Renal artery duplex: Normal

Coronary arteriogram: Normal coronary arteries; no obstructive disease

Intravascular coronary ultrasound (IVUS): Severe extra-luminal atherosclerotic disease in left anterior descending (LAD), left circumflex (LCX), and right coronary arteries (Figure 37.2 shows an image that is very similar to this patient's).

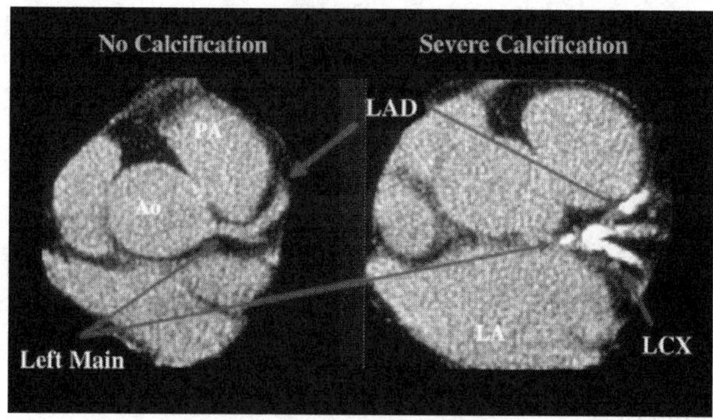

Figure 37.1 **Non-contrast EBT scan at the base of the heart**

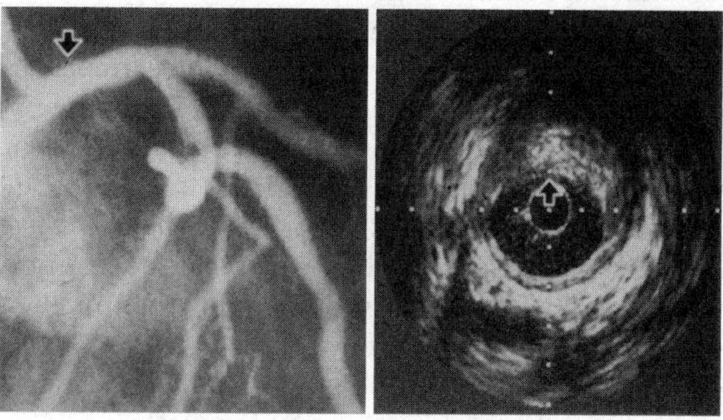

Figure 37.2 **Angiographically inapparent atheroma**

Used by permission of author. Source: Nissen, et al. In: Topol. *Interventional Cardiology Update.* 14;1995.

Standard Diagnostic Summary

Cardiovascular

Disease manifestations:

1. Hypertension: Essential/genetic/nutritional, obesity and lifestyle. High plasma renin activity (PRA), high catecholamines and cortisol. Stage 2
2. Dyslipidemia: Familial/nutritional/lifestyle. Low HDL-C, increased LDL particle number, dense/small LDL, dense/small HDL, intermediate very-low-density-lipoprotein (VLDL), elevated lipoprotein a [LP(a)] (Figure 37.3 shows an NMR lipoprotein analysis)
3. CHD: Non-obstructive, symptomatic, positive EBT, microvascular ischemia
4. Generalized endothelial dysfunction and reduced arterial compliance
5. Bilateral carotid artery disease/obstruction and increased IMT
6. Mitral regurgitation: moderate
7. LVH and left atrial hypertrophy (LAH)
8. Diastolic dysfunction
9. Resting tachycardia
10. Chest pain secondary to hypertension, LVH and microvascular angina
11. Carotid artery obstruction with history of transient ischemic attacks

Risk factors and contributing factors:

12. Homocysteinemia
13. Elevated hs-CRP (high-sensitivity C-reactive protein) and ESR (erythrocyte sedimentation rate)
14. Polycythemia
15. Elevated iron, iron stores, and percent saturation
16. Elevated fibrinogen

Renal

17. Mild renal insufficiency with MUA

Hematology

18. Leukocytosis

Endocrine

19. Obesity: Stage I—high risk
20. Insulin resistance/metabolic syndrome: Hypertension, android/central obesity (BMI, waist circumference, waist-hip ratio); increased hs-CRP; increased adipose tissue as a percentage of body weight; elevated fasting blood sugar (FBS) and 2 hour oral glucose test (OGTT), C-peptide, Hg A_1C, and insulin with impaired glucose tolerance, dyslipidemia

Gastrointestinal

21. Gastritis/Gastroesophageal reflux disease (GERD)

ENT

22. Sinusitis
23. Headaches secondary to hypertension and/or sinusitis

Pulmonary

24. Dyspnea secondary to lung disease
25. Emphysema and chronic obstructive pulmonary disease secondary to tobacco abuse

Nutritional Problems

26. Multiple micronutrient and macronutrient deficiencies
27. Reduced antioxidant defenses with increased oxidative stress
28. Caffeine abuse
29. Soft drink abuse

Genetics

30. Positive family history of premature CHD, hypertension, hyperlipidemia

Psychosocial

31. Stress, anxiety, and depression

Functional Medicine Assessment: Using the Matrix

The functional medicine matrix (presented in Chapter 34) can help to organize the multiple inter-connected elements of this patient's primary disease, the metabolic syndrome. Pathophysiology, nutrition, biochemistry, prevention, and treatment will be discussed utilizing a functional medicine approach. Following the conclusion of the Case Presentation, an extended discussion of metabolic syndrome can be found.

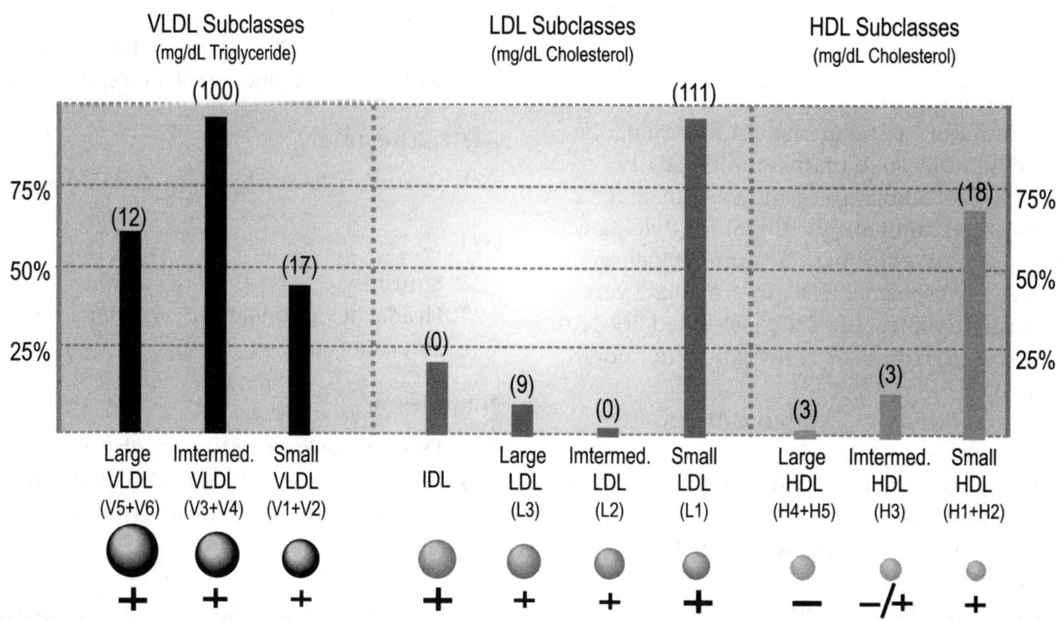

LIPOPROTEIN PANEL

Coronary Heart Disease (CHD) Risk Categories

LDL Particle Number	nmol/L	Optimal*	Near or above optimal	Borderline-High	High	Very high
	1809	under 1100	1100 - 1399	1400 - 1799	1800 - 2100	over 2100

**Goal for patients with CHD or CHD risk equivalents*

LDL Size	nm	Pattern A (large LDL)	Pattern B (small LDL)
	19.2	22.0 - 20.6	20.5 - 19.0
		Lower-Risk	Higher-Risk

Large HDL (cholesterol)	mg/dL	Negative Risk Factor	Intermediate	Positive Risk Factor
	3	greater than 30	30 -11	less than 11

Large VLDL (triglyceride)	mg/dL	Lower-Risk	Intermediate	Higher-Risk
	12	less than 7	7 - 27	greater than 27

RISK ASSESSMENT PANEL

Elevated LDL Particle Number	>1400 nmol/L	☑
Lipoprotein Traits of the Metabolic Syndrome*	≥2 traits	☑

Lipoprotein Traits of the Metabolic Syndrome*

Small LDL Pattern B (≤ 20.5nm)	Reduced Large HDL (<11 mg/dL)	Elevated Large VLDL (>27 mg/dL)
☑	☑	☐

**Elevated numbers of LDL particles and the lipoprotein traits of the metabolic syndrome affect CHD risk interactivity. Risk is highest when both are present.*

Figure 37.3 **NMR lipoprotein analysis**

Environmental Inputs: The Influence of Environment on Gene Expression

Diet: His caloric intake is excessive with incorrect proportions of macronutrients. Excessive calories and obesity contribute to vascular inflammation, endothelial dysfunction, vascular and cardiac structural abnormalities, oxidative stress, and hormonal imbalance.[1,2,3,4,5] These, in turn, contribute to his metabolic syndrome, insulin resistance, dyslipidemia, hypertension, and many other problems.[6,7,8,9,10] Adipose tissue is both the source and target of inflammatory mediators.[11,12]

Nutrition: His refined carbohydrate content is too high; crude fiber content is too low; the protein types and proportions are inappropriate; saturated and *trans* fats are disproportionately represented, with suboptimal intake of PUFA and MUFA. There is inadequate consumption of fruits and vegetables, low-fat dairy, and many micronutrients. His poor nutritional status is a major contributing factor for vascular inflammatory biology, immune dysfunction, oxidative stress with reduced oxidative defenses, mitochondrial dysfunction, hormonal imbalance, vascular structural abnormalities, and endothelial dysfunction.[13,14,15,16,17,18] These are the basic underlying pathophysiological abnormalities, for his most pressing health problems (obesity, metabolic syndrome, insulin resistance, dyslipidemia, hypertension, CHD, and vascular disease). His nutritional state creates an inflammatory, oxidatively stressed, immunologically and hormonally imbalanced environment.

Air and water: He gets little fresh air, with ventilation primarily from air conditioning and heat from his truck. He is chronically dehydrated due to excess caffeine and sodas (diuretic effects) combined with insufficient water intake. This will affect his body's ability to provide adequate hepatic metabolism, detoxification, and renal excretion of xenobiotics.

Physical exercise: He has minimal-to-no aerobic or resistance exercise and lives a very sedentary lifestyle. Exercise improves insulin resistance, vascular inflammation, vascular endothelial function and vascular structure, increases lean muscle mass, reduces adiposity, improves gastrointestinal function, hormonal balance, oxidative stress, and immune function.[19,20,21,22,23,24,25,26,27,28,29,30,31] The lack of exercise contributes to his insulin resistance, metabolic syndrome, CHD, dyslipidemia, and hypertension, as well as other health issues.

Xenobiotics: The excessive intake of aspirin and TUMS could be causing his gastric and renal problems.[32,33] The excessive TUMS (calcium carbonate) may alter blood pH, increase serum calcium, reduce phosphorous, and cause rebound gastric acidity.[34] Acetaminophen will deplete glutathione, impair hepatic metabolism, detoxification and biotransformational processes of drugs, xenobiotics and nutrients, as well as inducing hepatic and renal dysfunction.[35] The glutathione deficiency contributes to reduced oxidative defense and increases vascular inflammation and the risk for CHD and MI.[36,37]

Radiation: No obvious exposure.

Psychosocial: He has major psychosocial problems (as noted in the history) that are contributing to his health by inducing hormonal imbalances, oxidative stress, endothelial dysfunction, immune dysfunction, and inflammation, all of which contribute to his hypertension, hyperglycemia, dyslipidemia, and CHD.[38,39,40,41,42,43,44,45,46] The significant problem areas are:

- Family
- Work
- Community
- Economic status
- Stress
- Lack of support

Emotional, mind, and spirit: His life of anxiety, depression, and chronic stress creates hypercortisolism, a hypercatecholamine state, oxidative stress, and suppressed immune function, contributing to hyperglycemia, hypertension, dyslipidemia, endothelial function, and vascular disease.[47,48,49,50,51,52,53,54,55]

Hormonal and Neurotransmitter Messenger Imbalances

The patient exhibits excessive production of cortisol, catecholamines, and insulin. Each of these hormones in excess will induce inflammation, oxidative stress, and structural abnormalities, and will interfere with various biochemical and nutritional pathways that are related to his hypertension, hyperglycemia and diabetes, dyslipidemia, vascular disease, and other problems.[56,57,58,59,60,61,62,63,64,65,66,67,68]

Oxidation-Reduction Imbalances and Mitochondropathy

The mitochondria are intimately involved in insulin resistance and the metabolic syndrome.[69,70,71,72,73,74] The mitochondria are smaller, have impaired bioenergetic capacity with a defect in oxidative phosphorylation and production of adenosine triphosphate (ATP).[75,76,77] The skeletal muscle has a marked increase in the intramyocellular lipid content. The insulin resistance results in preferential metabolism of FFAs with reduced glucose utilization. The FFAs inhibit glucose uptake transporter-4 and enhance gluconeogenesis. Adipose tissue releases specific cytokines such as TNF-α and IL-6, which increase inflammation, hs-CRP, exacerbate the insulin resistance and increase FFA concentration.[78,79] TNF-α also inhibits endothelial nitric oxide (eNOS) and NO, elevating blood pressure. The FFAs increase uncoupling protein 3, which uncouples mitochondrial respiration from oxidative phosphorylation and increases oxidative stress and release of superoxide anion and subsequent ROS.[80,81,82,83,84,85,86,87,88] A genetic polymorphism, called PGC-1 (PPAR gamma coactive-1) regulates mitochondrial biogenesis and fat oxidation and is essential for the synthesis of the mitochondrial enzymes for the beta-oxidation of fatty acids.[89] PGC-1 levels are increased by weight loss, exercise, and optimal nutrition.[90,91,92]

Detoxification and Biotransformational Imbalances

The various micronutrient deficiencies noted in the antioxidant panel analysis (described at the bottom of Table 37.2, which shows the patient's lab results over 12 months) will contribute to a wide variety of abnormalities in hepatic detoxification of intrinsic toxins and xenobiotics by the cytochrome P450 system as well as other pathways.[93] In addition, many biochemical nutritional pathways will be impaired by deficiencies in B vitamins, amino acids, carnitine, vitamin D, calcium, zinc, magnesium, glutathione, CoQ10, vitamin E, and lipoic acid that will have enormous downstream effects on inflammation, immune function, hormonal and neurotransmitter function, oxidative stress, and vascular functional and structural integrity.[94] These will induce dyslipidemia, hypertension, and insulin resistance, among other problems.[95]

Table 37.2 **Patient Lab Results**

General	Initial	2 Months	6 Months	12 Months
Magnesium	1.2 mg/dL	1.8 mg/dL	2.1 mg/dL	2.4 mg/dL
WBC/HCT	12,200/55	10,400/50	8,600/46	8,200/45
Creatinine	1.6 mg%	1.4 mg%	1.2 mg%	1.1 mg%
GFR	86 cc/minute	95 cc/minute	102 cc/minute	106 cc/minute
Estimated GFR = (140 – age) x weight (Kg) / 72 x creatinine				
24 hour urine MAU	80 mgs	22 mgs	0	0
Cortisol AM	30 mcg/dL	25 mcg/dL	18 mcg/dL	16 mcg/dL
Cortisol PM	22 mcg/dL	20 mcg/dL	12 mcg/dL	10 mcg/dL
PRA	9.2 ng/ml/hr	5.1 ng/ml/hr	1.2 ng/ml/hr	0.5 ng/ml/hr
Aldosterone (serum)	30 ng/dL	25 ng/dL	20 ng/dL	18 ng/dL
24-hour urine				
Ketosteroids	12.3 mg	11 mg	10.0 mg	9 mg
Corticosteroids	5.8 mg	4.6 mg	4.1 mg	4.0 mg
Free cortisol	126 mcg	98 mcg	72 mcg	76 mcg
Norepinephrine	140 mcg	122 mcg	88 mcg	81 mcg
Epinephrine	9 mcg	8 mcg	7 mcg	6 mcg
Dopamine	498 mcg	396 mcg	324 mcg	301 mcg
Total catecholamines (*norepinephrine + epinephrine*)	149 mcg	130 mcg	95 mcg	87 mcg
Normetanephrines	580 mcg	475 mcg	392 mcg	360 mcg
Metanephrines	51 mcg	42 mcg	38 mcg	33 mcg
Total metanephrines (*normetanephrine + metanephrine*)	631 mcg	517 mcg	430 mcg	393 mcg
Vanillylmandelic acid	4.4 mg	3.9 mg	3.2 mg	3.0 mg

Table 37.2 **Patient Lab Results (Continued)**

CHD Risk Markers	**Initial**	**2 Months**	**6 Months**	**12 Months**
Homocysteine	24 micromole/L	16 micromole/L	7.7 micromole/L	6.8 micromole/L
Serum iron	220 microgm/dL	200 microgm/dL	140 microgm/dL	124 microgm/dL
Serum ferritin	460 ng/ml	390 ng/ml	180 ng/ml	150 ng/ml
Fibrinogen	580 mg/dL	500 mg/dL	340 mg/dL	302 mg/dL
HS-CRP	6	3	0.5	0.4
Glycation	**Initial**	**2 Months**	**6 Months**	**12 Months**
Fasting blood sugar	110 mg%	82 mg%	74 mg%	72 mg%
2 hour OGTT	180 mg%	140 mg%	118 mg%	110 mg%
C-peptide	4.0 ng/ml	3.0 ng/ml	1.7 ng/ml	1.3 ng/ml
Hg A_1C	6.6%	5.6%	5.1%	4/6%
Fasting insulin	44 uu/ml	32 uu/ml	20 uu/ml	5 uu/ml
NMR Lipid Profile	**Initial**	**2 Months**	**6 Months**	**12 Months**
LDL-C	94 mg/dL	58 mg%	55 mg%	52 mg%
HDL-C	24 mg/dL	34 mg%	42 mg%	44 mg%
TG	142 mg/dL	92 mg%	78 mg%	70 mg%
LP(a)	62 mg/dL	30 mg/dL	16 mg/dL	11 mg/dL
LDL particle number	1809 nmol/L	1100 nmol/L	900 nmol/L	822 nmol/L
LDL pattern	B	A	A	A
HDL pattern	Small	Large	Large	Large
VLDL pattern	Large	Small	Small	Small
Oxidative Stress	**Initial**	**2 Months**	**6 Months**	**12 Months**
CoQ10 level	1.0 ug/ml	3.4 ug/ml	3.5 ug/ml	3.5 ug/ml
Serum lipid peroxides	3.9 uM	2.8 uM	2.3 uM	2.1 uM
Urine lipid peroxides	2.4 uM	18 uM	14.9 uM	13.2 uM
Urine 8-OHdG	63 ng/ml	54 ng/ml	46 ng/ml	39 ng/ml
Total oxygen radical absorbance capacity (ORAC)	2200 uM	3000 uM	4200 uM	4400 uM
Other	**Initial**	**2 Months**	**6 Months**	**12 Months**
C-1 AC	8	14	16	17
C-2 AC	2	4	8	9

An antioxidant panel reviewing Vitamin E, B vitamins, amino acids, metabolites, fatty acids, Vitamin D, calcium, zinc, magnesium, glutathione, cysteine, selenium, and CoQ10 showed abnormal function initially (24th percentile), with steady improvements to the 50th (2 months), 70th (6 months), and 80th (12 months) percentiles for total antioxidant function.

Immune System and Inflammatory Messenger Imbalances

Adipose tissue is an active, intricate, metabolic paracrine and endocrine organ that produces a variety of "adipokines," including inflammatory mediators and hormones that result in chronic inflammation, endocrine and metabolic dysfunction manifesting as insulin resistance, glucose intolerance, diabetes mellitus, dyslipidemia, hypertension, and vascular diseases such as CHD, MI, and carotid artery obstruction.[96,97,98] The adipocytes are both a source and a target of proinflammatory signals, such as IL-6 and TNF-α.[99,100,101] IL-6 and TNF-α increase hs-CRP, which is both a CVD risk marker and mediator of the inflammatory process and is highly correlated with future cardiovascular events.[102,103] Adipose tissue— through its effective hormones, cytokines, and central nervous system mechanisms—regulates food intake, energy homeostasis, whole body insulin action and insulin sensitivity, body adiposity, carbohydrate and lipid metabolism, blood pressure, inflammation, thrombosis, and subsequent atherothrombotic disease.[104,105]

Digestive, Absorptive, and Microbiological Imbalances

The presence of gastrointestinal pathology with mucosal inflammation and leaky gut may increase absorption of allergens, bacteria such as *Helicobacter pylori*, HIV, and various periodontal microorganisms that can contribute to vascular inflammation and oxidative stress-related CVD.[106,107,108,109,110,111,112]

Structural Imbalances from Cellular Membrane Function to the Musculoskeletal System

Abnormalities in ionic membrane transport of sodium, potassium, magnesium, and calcium may result in increased intracellular content of calcium and sodium with reduced intracellular content of magnesium and potassium. These ionic concentration defects contribute to vascular and cardiac muscle dysfunction, hypertrophy and hyperplasia, reduced arterial compliance, insulin resistance, hyperglycemia, dyslipidemia, increased vascular resistance, hypertension, and subsequent CVD.[113,114,115,116]

Goals of Treatment

General:

Improve diet and nutrition.
Improve physical fitness.
Improve insulin sensitivity.
Improve cardiovascular function.
Improve antioxidant status.
Reduce oxidative stress.
Improve emotional status.

Specific:

Heart rate (resting): <70 beats per minute
Blood pressure:
- 110-120/70-75 mm Hg
- Blood pressure load <15 % of the SBP >140 mm Hg and DBP >90 mm Hg
- Re-establish normal nocturnal dipping

Dyslipidemia:
- LDL-C 60-70 mg%
- HDL >40 mg%
- TG <75 mg%
- LDL particle number <900 nmol/L
- LDL to pattern A (large)
- HDL to large pattern
- VLDL to small pattern
- LP(a) <50 mg/dl

Homocysteine: <9.0 umol/L (ideal <5.0)
hs-CRP: <0.6 mg/L
Fibrinogen: <400 mg/dL
Serum iron(Fe): <180 microgm/dL
Serum ferritin: <300 ng/ml
FBS: <90 mg% (ideal <75 mg%)
Hemoglobin A1C: <5%
2 hour OGTT: <120 mg%
C-peptide (fasting): <2 ng/ml
24 hour urine MAU: 0 (<30 mg/24 hour)
Creatinine: <1.2 mg%
Improve arterial compliance: C-1 >12.0 and C-2 >7.0
Reduce WBC: <10,000
Ideal body weight (IBW): 166 pounds
Waist circumference: <38 inches
Waist-hip ratio: <1.0
BMI: <25
Percent body fat: <16%
Hematocrit (HCT): <46%
Glomerular filtration rate (GFR): stabilize or improve
Stabilization or regression of CHD by EBT and IVUS
Reduce LVH, diastolic dysfunction, and mitral regurgitation
Improve pulmonary function
Stabilize and improve carotid artery disease

Treatment Strategies

Action steps:

Stop tobacco.
Stop caffeine, sodas, and alcohol.
Reduce or stop use of regular aspirin, acetaminophen, and TUMS.
Baby aspirin per day should be continued.
Phlebotomy for increased iron (every eight weeks until iron is normal).
Reduce to IBW: 1-to-2 pounds per week.
Aerobic exercise for 60 minutes per day and resistance exercise for 20-30 minutes per day three to four times per week.
Meditation, yoga, prayer.

Diet and nutrition:

DASH-2 diet, Paleo diet, or Mediterranean diet: 1,750–2,000 calories per day
8-10 servings of fruits and vegetables per day
30%-40% protein (fish, lean meat, fowl)
40% carbohydrates (complex, fiber) and significantly reduce refined carbohydrates

Reduce fats to 30% of calories:
Saturated fats <10%; MUFA (extra virgin olive oil), PUFA, and omega-3/6 should be ~90% of fats.
Eliminate *trans* fats entirely.
Omega-3/6 ratio—2:1 to 4:1
Fiber: >40 grams per day
Garlic: 1-2 cloves per day
Celery: 2-4 pieces per day
Sodium: 50-100 mmol per day
Potassium: 60-100 meq per day
Whey protein (hydrolyzed): 30 grams per day
Probiotic capsules: 2 bid
Nutraceuticals/vitamins/antioxidants/minerals:
Alpha lipoic acid (with biotin 2,000 micrograms): 600 mg bid
Calcium: 500 mg bid
Co-enzyme Q10: 60 mg bid
Folic acid: 1,200 micrograms per day
Fruit, vegetable and dark berry concentrate extract
L-carnitine: 1,000 mg bid
Lycopene tomato extract: 5 mg bid
Magnesium chelates: 400 mg bid
High gamma/delta mixed tocopherols: 400 IU per day
N-acetylcysteine: 1,000 mg bid
Niacin (non-flush) (IHN): 1.5 grams bid
Olive oil: 1 teaspoon bid
Omega-3 fatty acids
DHA: 1000 mg bid
EPA: 500 mg bid
Selenium: 200 micrograms per day
Taurine: 1.5 grams bid
Tocotrienols: 100 mg at bedtime
Vitamin B complex: 1 bid
Vitamin B12: 1,000 micrograms per day
Vitamin B6: 100 mg bid
Vitamin C: 250 mg bid
Vitamin D: 400 IU bid
Zinc: 25 mg per day

Case Discussion

Although this case is complex (involving many details about different assessments, re-assessments, and interventions), it exemplifies exceptionally well the impact of the interaction of genes and environment on inflammatory, immune, hormonal, oxidative stress, mitochondrial, and structural pathways in vascular pathophysiology. This patient came in with an identifiable genetic predisposition to cardiovascular disease and insulin resistance (by family history). He might never have manifested those diseases had he chosen a lifestyle that reflected an understanding of his risks and how to minimize them. Even after many years of subjecting his genes to a very poor environment, however, we were able to help him reverse his disease and regain his health.

This patient refused pharmacologic treatment. He was motivated and compliant with a nutritional and lifestyle approach, which resulted in normalization of virtually all laboratory and clinical problems over 12 months of aggressive treatment. Tables 37.2 and 37.3 present, respectively, the laboratory results and the patient visit record over the course of a year's treatment.

Utilizing the matrix helps to organize and visualize all the interconnected biochemical and physiological mechanisms that contribute to the *beginnings* of the vascular disease process. As we saw, certain mechanisms (inflammation, oxidative stress, endocrine dysfunction) were represented over and over again around the matrix, helping us to recognize where the preponderance of evidence about this patient was to be found. From there, we focused on treatments that address those common underlying pathways, thus normalizing multiple systems—in this case, without drugs.

Early diagnosis, aggressive prevention, and treatment directed at the genesis of identified functional abnormalities are more logical, efficient, and effective than directing treatment modalities at the endpoints of the clinical disease—the symptoms. Virtually none of the treatments listed above were directed toward symptoms; they were focused on restoration and normalization of function. Recognition of the downstream pleiotropic effects of nutrient imbalances, insufficiencies (for a particular patient in a particular environment), and deficiencies on the disease-development process is crucial to redirecting therapeutic emphasis. The vascular system has a finite number of ways to respond to an infinite number of insults. Identification and treatment of these initial and basic common insults will become the future of treatment in vascular medicine.

Table 37.3 **Patient Visit Record**

	Initial	2 Months	6 Months	12 Months
Weight	225 pounds	215 pounds	182 pounds	170 pounds
Blood pressure	182/104 mm Hg 176/102 mm Hg 178/104 mm Hg 170/100 mm Hg	120/76 mm Hg 118/74 mm Hg 118/72 mm Hg	112/72 mm Hg 116/74 mm Hg	110/70 mm Hg 112/72 mm Hg
BP load and dipping	Abnormal	Normal	Normal	Normal
Heart rate	92 regular 90 regular 80 regular 82 regular	74/minute	66/minute	62/minute
Waist circumference	42 inches	40 inches	36 inches	34 inches
Waist-hip ratio	1.4	0.9	0.8	0.7
BMI	32.0 kg/m^2	31 kg/m^2	26 kg/m^2	24 kg/m^2
% Body fat	28%	22%	18%	14%

Extended Discussion: Metabolic Syndrome and Cardiovascular Disease

Background

The current and expanding epidemic of obesity and the metabolic (insulin resistance) syndrome has fueled an increase in cardiovascular disease (CVD). The metabolic syndrome is an insulin-resistant state characterized by visceral obesity, hypertension, dyslipidemia, glucose intolerance, and microalbuminuria (MAU). The cardiovascular risk and complications may follow obesity by 10 or more years. Thus, escalating rates of obesity predict further substantial increases in type 2 diabetes mellitus, coronary heart disease (CHD), myocardial infarction (MI), and total CVD that are likely to rapidly eclipse rates observed throughout the 20th century in the U.S.[117,118] Environmental and lifestyle factors (inappropriate nutrition such as consumption of high-calorie foods and refined carbohydrates; reduced physical activity) as well as genetic considerations are major contributors to the metabolic syndrome and visceral obesity.[119,120]

The overall prevalence of metabolic syndrome is 24% in adults, with a higher incidence in minorities, and metabolic syndrome progressively increases with age, rising from ~7% for adults in the third decade of life to nearly 45% for those over 60 years of age.[121]

Risk Factors and Associated Conditions

Definitive associations of CVD and metabolic syndrome include a marked increased risk in CHD, MI, stroke, and total mortality that is directly proportional to the number of components of the metabolic syndrome.[122,123,124] The incident risk of CVD is greater than five-fold in subjects with four or more components, compared to those with only one component.[125] There clearly exists a continuum of risk, based on both severity of the risk factor itself and on combinations of risk factors. The metabolic syndrome and obesity are major public health and economic problems that require urgent and aggressive identification, prevention, and treatment with lifestyle modifications (nutrition, weight reduction, exercise) and pharmacologic modalities.

Definitions

The term metabolic syndrome denotes a constellation of cardiovascular risk factors related to insulin resistance and obesity with a centripetal fat pattern. Definitions have varied, but the basic elements are well validated.[126,127,128,129] National Cholesterol Education Program—Adult Treatment Panel III (NCEP-ATP-III) (2001)[130] and World Health Organization (WHO) guidelines (1999)[131,132] include hypertension, atherogenic dyslipidemia (high triglyceride, low HDL, dense LDL), obesity (elevated waist circumference, BMI, waist-hip ratio), hyperglycemia, and MAU. (See Table 37.4.) However, this definition must be expanded to recognize the underlying mechanisms: insulin resistance, inflammation, and immunologic dysfunction with increased oxidative stress, prothrombotic components, vascular endothelial dysfunction, vascular structural abnormalities, and accelerated atheroembolic disease.[133,134,135] (See Table 37.5.) Insulin resistance is the primary underlying dysfunction. The metabolic syndrome with insulin resistance and inflammation precede clinical events by decades; thus, early detection is mandatory.

Mechanisms of Action

Imbalanced vascular endothelial mediators create endothelial dysfunction and inflammation, the earliest markers of atherosclerosis. Hypertension and atherosclerosis are primarily diseases of inflammation.[136] Excess angiotensin-II (A-II) and a deficiency of nitric oxide (NO) result in vasoconstriction, growth promotion, and a prothrombotic, proinflammatory, and prooxidant state. This constellation of events is directly connected to insulin resistance, the metabolic syndrome, and the frequent clinical association of hypertension, dyslipidemia, and diabetes mellitus.[137,138,139,140,141]

Table 37.4 **Published Criteria for the Diagnosis of Metabolic Syndrome**

	National Cholesterol Education Program—Adult Treatment Panel III (NCEP-ATP-III)	World Health Organization (WHO)
Hypertension	Current antihypertensive therapy or BP >130/85 mm Hg	Current antihypertensive therapy and/or BP >140/90 mm Hg
Dyslipidemia	Plasma triglyceride level >150 mg/dL HDL-C level: Men: <40 mg/dL Women: <50 mg/dL	Plasma triglyceride level >1.7 mmol/L (150 mg/dL) and/or HDL-C level: Men: <0.9 mmol/L (35 mg/dL) Women: <1.0 mmol/L (40 mg/dL)
Obesity	Waist circumference Men: >40 inches Women: >35 inches	BMI >30 kg/m2 and/or waist/hip ratio: Men: >0.90 Women: >0.85
Glucose	Fasting blood glucose level >110 mg/dL	Type 2 diabetes or impaired glucose tolerance (IGT)
Other		Microalbuminuria (overnight urinary albumin excretion rate >20 μg/min [30 mg/g Cr])
Requirements for diagnosis	Any three of the above disorders	Confirmed type 2 diabetes or IGT and any two of the above criteria. If normal glucose tolerance, must demonstrate three of the above criteria.

Table 37.5 **Expanded Definition and Criteria: Metabolic Syndrome**

Major Criteria	
Fasting glucose	>110 mg% or hemoglobin A1C over 6.5, 2 hour PPG >140 mg%, fasting C-peptide elevated
Abdominal obesity (visceral)	Waist circumference: Men: >40 in (102 cm); Women: >35 inches (88 cm) Waist-Hip ratio: Men: >0.90; Women: >0.85 Body Fat: Men: >29% (normal is <16%); Women: >37% (normal is <22%) BMI over 30 kg/m^2
Dyslipidemia (atherogenic)	TG >130 mg% (large VLDL) (optimal is <75 mg%) HDL: Men: <40 mg%; Women: <50 mg% (small HDL) TG/HDL ratio >3.0 Small dense type B LDL with increased LDL particle number exceeding 900 (NMR) Elevated Lp(a)
Hypertension	BP >135/85 mm Hg (24 hour ABP monitoring with BP load, mean, circadian cycle and nocturnal dipping) (optimal BP 110/70 mm Hg)
Microalbuminuria	>30 mg in 24 hours or >20 ug/minute or albumin creatinine ratio >30 mg/g
Prothrombotic state	PAI-1, increased platelet activation and aggregation, fibrinogen, von Willebrand factor, Factor VII, thrombin
Insulin resistance and hyper-insulinemia	Fasting insulin, proinsulin, C-peptide
Proinflammatory state	HS-CRP, fibrinogen, IL-6, IL-1B, TNF-α, leukocytosis
Minor Criteria	
Endothelial dysfunction	
Abnormal arterial compliance	Especially small resistance arteries, low C2 compliance and increased pulse wave velocity
Left ventricular hypertrophy and diastolic dysfunction	
Hyperuricemia	
Increased vascular oxidative stress	>9 ug/L
Homocysteine	
Objective evidence of accelerated atherogenesis for age-matched gender, ethnicity and age	
Abnormalities in autonomic nervous system regulation and activation of the cardio-vascular system	

Important Points

1. This is a continuum of risk starting at BP of 110/75 mm Hg, FBS of 75 mg%, LDL of 60 mg%, TG of 75 mg%, declining HDL from 85 mg% and homocysteine of 5 μg/L. Insulin resistance and the metabolic syndrome do not start at an arbitrary cutoff level.
2. 25–30% U.S. population have metabolic syndrome.
3. Common pathogenetic factors to type 2 diabetes mellitus exist in the metabolic syndrome.

Definition for Confirmed Diagnosis

1. Three major criteria
2. Two major criteria plus two minor criteria

Insulin mediates metabolic, mitogenic and vasodilatory-vascular functions in skeletal muscle and adipose tissue, but also in the liver, brain, heart, blood vessels, pancreas, and other tissues.[142,143,144,145] Insulin resistance results in an imbalance of the mitogen-activated protein kinase (MAPK) and phosphatidyl inositol 3-kinase (PI3-K) pathways (Figure 37.4), which promotes cell proliferation and migration, thrombosis, and inflammation with increased cytokines and cell adhesion molecules. An imbalance in these pathways also reduces glucose transport in insulin-dependent tissues and decreases endothelial nitric oxide synthase/nitric oxide bioactivity.[146,147,148,149] The enhanced MAPK pathway is proatherogenic, which overrides the antiatherogenic PI3-K pathway. The roles of the insulin receptors, the mitochondria, the pancreatic beta cells, inflammatory cytokines, radical oxygen species (ROS), and free fatty acids are important in the clinical expression of insulin resistance and type 2 diabetes. Chronic insulin resistance, when followed by beta cell dysfunction and failure, eventually produces type 2 diabetes.[150,151,152,153]

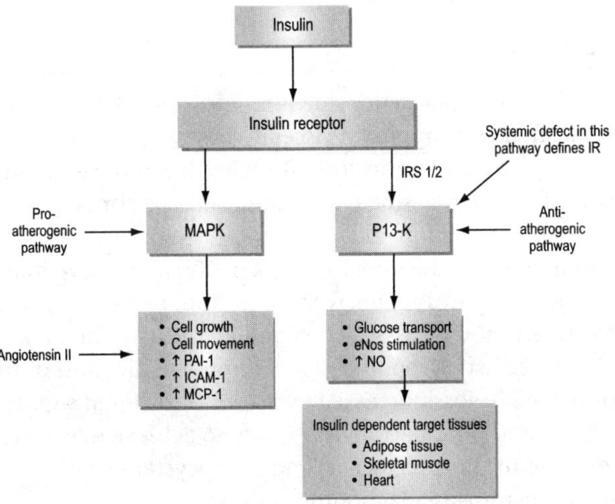

Figure 37.4 **Stimulation of the MAPK pathway in endothelial and VSM cells**

Adipose tissue is an endocrine organ that produces a variety of "adipokines," including inflammatory mediators and hormones that result in chronic inflammation, endocrine and metabolic dysfunction that manifests as insulin resistance, and the clinical diseases of hypertension, dyslipidemia, hyperglycemia, diabetes, and CVD.[154,155]

The adipocytes are both the source and the target of proinflammatory signals from various mediators such as angiotensinogen, A-II, intracellular cell adhesion molecules (ICAM), interleukin-6 (IL-6), interleukin IB (ILI-B), prostaglandin E-2 (PGE-2), monocyte chemotactant protein-I (MCP-I), colony stimulating factor-1 (CSF-1), macrophage inflammatory protein-1 alpha (MIP-1α), tumor necrosis factor-alpha (TNF-α), complement 3 (C_3), resistin, ASP (acetylation stimulating protein), leptin, FFA, lipoprotein lipase, adiponectin, chemotaxin, plasminogen activator inhibitor-1 (PAI-1) tissue factor, and other mediators.[156,157,158] The subsequent increase in high sensitivity C-reactive protein (hs-CRP is both a risk factor marker and a mediator) is highly correlated with future cardiovascular events.[159] The role of peroxisome proliferator activated receptors (PPAR) alpha and gamma are important in insulin resistance, glucose and lipid metabolism, and overall vascular function, inflammation, atherosclerosis, and hypertension.[160]

Prevention and Treatment

Prevention and treatment approaches for the metabolic syndrome and its components include early detection, aggressive nutritional intervention, nutraceuticals, supplements, vitamins, antioxidants, minerals, functional foods, weight management, aerobic and resistance exercise, moderation of alcohol ingestion, discontinuation of all tobacco products, and limited caffeine.[161,162,163]

A 6.5% weight loss reduces BP 11/6 mm Hg, glucose 17 mg/dL, triglycerides 94 mg/dL, total cholesterol 37 mg/dL at one month.[164] These changes are sustained with further decreases in BP and triglycerides at four months.[165] Exercise improves all components of the metabolic syndrome.[166,167,168,169,170,171,172,173,174,175,176,177,178]

Nutritional supplement recommendations are outlined in Table 37.6.[179] Pharmacologic therapy with antihypertensive, antidiabetic, antilipid, and anti-inflammatory medications may be required to achieve new target goals in all of the various risk factors. Although the treatment goals for risk factors continue to change, optimal goals are yet to be established. In the author's opinion, new aggressive optimal goals to achieve the best reduction in cardiovascular events are: BP <110/75 mm Hg, fasting blood glucose (FBG) ~75 mg%, LDL-C ≤60 mg%, triglyceride (TG) ≤75 mg%,

HDL >85 mg%, homocysteine <5 micromoles/L, and hs-CRP <1.0.

Table 37.6 Nutritional Supplements and Lifestyle Recommendations for Treatment of the Components of Metabolic Syndrome

1. Nutrition—establish target goals for:
   Protein, fat, carbohydrates: type, composition, percentage of calories from each source
   Glycemic index and glycemic load
   Fiber
   Calories
2. Weight loss and visceral abdominal fat reduction
3. Exercise: aerobic and resistance
4. Nutritional supplements
   Alpha-lipoic acid
   Biotin
   Carnitine
   Chromium and glucose tolerance factor (GTF)
   CoQ10
   Flavonoids
   Folate
   GLA
   Glutathione
   Green tea (contains epigallocatechin gallate, or EGCG)
   Inositol
   Magnesium
   Manganese
   MUFA (oleic acid)
   N-acetyl cysteine (NAC)
   Niacin and niacinamide
   Omega-3 FA
   Potassium
   Pycnogenol
   Selenium
   Taurine
   Vanadate
   Vitamin B12
   Vitamin B6
   Vitamin C
   Vitamin E derivatives
   Zinc

Angiotensin-converting enzyme inhibitors (ACEIs), angiotensin-receptor blockers (ARBs), and calcium channel blockers (CCBs) have the best overall profile for the pharmacologic treatment of hypertension.[180,181] The ACEIs and ARBs are preferred for patients with proteinuria or renal insufficiency. Thiazide, thiazide-like diuretics, and beta blockers may have adverse effects on glucose and lipid metabolism and should be reserved for resistant hypertension or compelling indications.[182]

Indapamide is the preferred diuretic in the metabolic syndrome due to its better antihypertensive effect and minor or no adverse effects on glucose, lipids, potassium, uric acid or renal function.[183,184,185,186] Alpha blockers and central alpha agonists may be used, but are limited due to clinical side effects.

Statins, fibrates and niacin should be used as pharmacologic monotherapy or in combination for patients with various forms of dyslipidemia.[187,188,189]

Metformin and thiazolidinediones are the preferred pharmacologic treatment of insulin resistance, glucose intolerance and type 2 diabetes, as they increase insulin sensitivity, reduce insulin levels, and improve glucose.[190,191,192]

A combination of vitamin B6 25 µg qd, B12 1,000 µg qd, and folate 800 µg qd is usually optimal treatment for elevated levels of homocysteine. Low-dose aspirin (81 mg/day), omega-3 fatty acids, mixed tocopherols, garlic (allicin), statins, ACEIs, ARBs, and possibly CCBs should be used to prevent thromboembolic problems, CVD, cardiovascular atherosclerosis, and reduce inflammation and hs-CRP.

Summary

The metabolic syndrome is an insulin-resistant state associated with lipotoxic visceral obesity, nutritional deficiencies, and unhealthy lifestyles that induce inflammation, oxidative stress, and immunologic abnormalities. It is a common condition, increasing in incidence, and is associated with a high risk of CVD. Effective management requires aggressive recognition, prevention, and treatment of CVD risk factors and identifiable vascular disease. Lifestyle modifications (improved diet and nutrition, weight loss, increased exercise), nutritional supplements, and pharmacologic therapy to achieve new goal levels of BP, lipids, glucose, and homocysteine will reduce cardiovascular complications.

References

1. Mikhail N, Tuck ML. Insulin and the vasculature. Curr Hypertens Rep. 2000;2:148-53.
2. Xu H, Barnes GT, Yang Q, et al. Chronic inflammation in fat plays a crucial role in the development of obesity-related insulin resistance. J Clin Invest. 2003;112:1821-30.
3. Szmitko PE, Wang CH, Weisel RD, et al. New markers of inflammation and endothelial cell activation. Part I and II. Circulation. 2003;108:1917-23, 2041-48.
4. Unger RH. Lipotoxic diseases. Annu Rev Med. 2002;53:319-36.

5. Wilson PWF, Grundy SM. The metabolic syndrome: practical guide to origins and treatment: part I. Circulation. 2003;108:1422-25.
6. Mikhail N, Tuck ML. Insulin and the vasculature. Curr Hypertens Rep. 2000;2:148-53.
7. Xu H, Barnes GT, Yang Q, et al. Chronic inflammation in fat plays a crucial role in the development of obesity-related insulin resistance. J Clin Invest. 2003;112:1821-30.
8. Szmitko PE, Wang CH, Weisel RD, et al. New markers of inflammation and endothelial cell activation. Part I and II. Circulation. 2003;108:1917-23, 2041-48.
9. Unger RH. Lipotoxic diseases. Annu Rev Med. 2002;53:319-36.
10. Wilson PWF, Grundy SM. The metabolic syndrome: practical guide to origins and treatment: part I. Circulation. 2003;108:1422-25.
11. Xu H, Barnes GT, Yang Q, et al. Chronic inflammation in fat plays a crucial role in the development of obesity-related insulin resistance. J Clin Invest. 2003;112:1821-30.
12. Unger RH. Lipotoxic diseases. Annu Rev Med. 2002;53:319-36.
13. Mikhail N, Tuck ML. Insulin and the vasculature. Curr Hypertens Rep. 2000;2:148-53.
14. Xu H, Barnes GT, Yang Q, et al. Chronic inflammation in fat plays a crucial role in the development of obesity-related insulin resistance. J Clin Invest. 2003;112:1821-30.
15. Szmitko PE, Wang CH, Weisel RD, et al. New markers of inflammation and endothelial cell activation. Part I and II. Circulation. 2003;108:1917-23, 2041-48.
16. Unger RH. Lipotoxic diseases. Annu Rev Med. 2002;53:319-36.
17. Wilson PWF, Grundy SM. The metabolic syndrome: practical guide to origins and treatment: part I. Circulation. 2003;108:1422-25.
18. Hsueh WA, Quinones MJ. Role of endothelial dysfunction in insulin resistance. Am J Cardiol. 2003;92:10J.
19. Gregg EW, Gerzoff RB, Caspersen CJ, et al. Relationship of walking to mortality among US adults with diabetes. Arch Intern Med. 2003;163:1440-47.
20. Brooks GA, Butte NF, Rand WM, et al. Chronicle of the Institute of Medicine physical activity recommendation: how a physical activity recommendation came to be among dietary recommendations. Am J Clin Nutr. 2004;79:921S-30S.
21. Hittel DS, Kraus WE, Tanner CJ, et al. Exercise training increases electron and substrate shuttling proteins in muscle in overweight men and women with the metabolic syndrome. J Appl Physiol. 2005;98:168-79.
22. Ziegler M, Braumann KM, Reer R. The role of jogging in the prevention and treatment of cardiovascular disease. MMW Fortschr Med. 2004;146:29-32.
23. Christ M, Iannello C, Iannello PG, Grimm W. Effects of a weight reduction program with and without aerobic exercise in the metabolic syndrome. Int J Cardiol. 2004;97:115-22.
24. Green JS, Stanforth PR, Rankinen T, et al. The effects of exercise training on abdominal visceral fat, body composition, indicators of the metabolic syndrome in postmenopausal women with and without estrogen replacement therapy: the HERITAGE family study. Metabolism. 2004;53:1192-96.
25. Jurca R, Lamonte MJ, Church TS, et al. Associations of muscle strength and fitness with metabolic syndrome in men. Med Sci Sports Exerc. 2004;36:1301-07.
26. Hawley JA, Houmard JA. Introduction-preventing insulin resistance through exercise: a cellular approach. Med Sci Sports Exerc. 2004;36:1187-90.
27. Oshida Y, Sato Y. Approach in clinical management of metabolic syndrome. Methods of exercise therapy. Nippon Naika Gakkai Zasshi. 2004;93:726-32.
28. Farrell SW, Cheng YJ, Blair SN. Prevalence of the metabolic syndrome across cardiorespiratory fitness levels in women. Obes Res. 2004;12:824-30.
29. Carroll S, Dudfield M. What is the relationship between exercise and metabolic abnormalities? A report on the metabolic syndrome. Sports Med. 2004;34:371-418.
30. Lavie CJ, Milani RV. Metabolic syndrome, inflammation, and exercise. Am J Cardiol. 2004;93:1334.
31. Franks PW, Ekelund U, Brage S, et al. Does the association of habitual physical activity with the metabolic syndrome differ by level of cardiorespiratory fitness? Diabetes Care. 2004;27:1187-93.
32. Morant SV, McMahon AD, Cleland JG, et al. Cardiovascular prophylaxis with aspirin: costs of supply and management of upper gastrointestinal and renal toxicity. Br J Clin Pharmacol. 2004;57:188-98.
33. Chaudhry MU. Milk-alkali syndrome. J Ark Med Soc. 2004;101:84-85.
34. Ibid.
35. McClain CJ, Price S, Barve S, et al. Acetaminophen hepatotoxicity: an update. Curr Gastroenterol Rep. 1999;1:42-49.
36. Winter JP, Gong Y, Grant PJ, Wild CP. Glutathione peroxidase 1 genotype is associated with an increased risk of coronary artery disease. Coron Artery Dis. 2003;14:149-53.
37. Kharb S. Low blood glutathione levels in acute myocardial infarction. Indian J Med Sci. 2003;57:335-37.
38. Gump BB, Matthews KA, Eberly LE, et al. Depressive symptoms and mortality in men: results from the Multiple Risk Factor Intervention Trial. Stroke. 2005;36:98-102.
39. Barth J, Schumacher M, Herrmann-Lingen C. Depression as a risk factor for mortality in patients with coronary heart disease meta-analysis. Psychosom Med. 2004;66:802-13.
40. Asbury EA, Creed F, Collins P. Distinct psychosocial differences between women with coronary heart disease and cardiac syndrome X. Eur Heart J. 2004;25:1695-1701.
41. Suarez EC. C-reactive protein is associated with psychological risk factors of cardiovascular disease in apparently healthy adults. Psychosom Med. 2004;66:684-691.
42. Bankier B, Januzzi JL, Littman AB. The high prevalence of multiple psychiatric disorders in stable outpatients with coronary heart disease. Psychosom Med. 2004;66:645-50.
43. Otte C, Marmar CR, Pipkin SS, et al. Depression and 24-hour urinary cortisol in medical outpatients with coronary heart disease: the heart and soul study. Biol Psychiatry. 2004;56:241-47.
44. Chrapko WE, Jurasz P, Radomski MW, et al. Decreased platelet nitric oxide synthase activity and plasma nitric oxide metabolites in major depressive disorder. Biol Psychiatry. 2004;56:129-34.
45. Suarez EC, Lewis JG, Krishnan RR, Young KH. Enhanced expression of cytokines and chemokines by blood monocytes to vitro lipopolysaccharide stimulation are associated with hostility and severity of depressive symptoms in healthy women. Psychoneuroendocrinology. 2004;29:1119-28.
46. Selley ML. Increased (E)-4-hydroxy-2-nonenal and asymmetric dimethylarginine concentrations and decreased nitric oxide concentrations in the plasma of patients with major depression. J Affect Disord. 2004;80:249-56.
47. Gump BB, Matthews KA, Eberly LE, et al. Depressive symptoms and mortality in men: results from the Multiple Risk Factor Intervention Trial. Stroke. 2005;36:98-102.
48. Barth J, Schumacher M, Herrmann-Lingen C. Depression as a risk factor for mortality in patients with coronary heart disease meta-analysis. Psychosom Med. 2004;66:802-13.
49. Asbury EA, Creed F, Collins P. Distinct psychosocial differences between women with coronary heart disease and cardiac syndrome X. Eur Heart J. 2004;25:1695-701.
50. Suarez EC. C-reactive protein is associated with psychological risk factors of cardiovascular disease in apparently healthy adults. Psychosom Med. 2004;66:684-91.

51. Bankier B, Januzzi JL, Littman AB. The high prevalence of multiple psychiatric disorders in stable outpatients with coronary heart disease. Psychosom Med. 2004;66:645-50.
52. Otte C, Marmar CR, Pipkin SS, et al. Depression and 24-hour urinary cortisol in medical outpatients with coronary heart disease: the heart and soul study. Biol Psychiatry. 2004;56:241-47.
53. Chrapko WE, Jurasz P, Radomski MW, et al. Decreased platelet nitric oxide synthase activity and plasma nitric oxide metabolites in major depressive disorder. Biol Psychiatry. 2004;56:129-34.
54. Suarez EC, Lewis JG, Krishnan RR, Young KH. Enhanced expression of cytokines and chemokines by blood monocytes to vitro lipopolysaccharide stimulation are associated with hostility and severity of depressive symptoms in healthy women. Psychoneuroendocrinology. 2004;29:1119-28.
55. Selley ML. Increased (E)-4-hydroxy-2-nonenal and asymmetric dimethylarginine concentrations and decreased nitric oxide concentrations in the plasma of patients with major depression. J Affect Disord. 2004;80:249-56.
56. Mikhail N, Tuck ML. Insulin and the vasculature. Curr Hypertens Rep. 2000;2:148-53.
57. Hsueh WA, Quinones MJ. Role of endothelial dysfunction in insulin resistance. Am J Cardiol. 2003;92:10J.
58. Otte C, Marmar CR, Pipkin SS, et al. Depression and 24-hour urinary cortisol in medical outpatients with coronary heart disease: the heart and soul study. Biol Psychiatry. 2004;56:241-47.
59. Banfi C, Cavalca V, Veglia F, et al. Neurohormonal activation is associated with increased levels of plasma matrix metalloproteinase-2 in human heart failure. Eur Heart J. 2004;Dec 17 [Epub].
60. Thomas KS, Nelesen RA, Ziegler MG, et al. Job strain, ethnicity, and sympathetic nervous system activity. Hypertension. 2004;44:891-96.
61. Maiter D. Pheochromocytoma: a paradigm for catecholamine-mediated hypertension. Acta Clin Belg. 2004;59:209-19.
62. Kendrick M. Does insulin resistance cause atherosclerosis in the post-prandial period? Med Hypotheses. 2003;60:6-11.
63. Fantidis P, Perez De Prada T, Fernandez-Ortiz A, et al. Morning cortisol production in coronary heart disease patients. Eur J Clin Invest. 2002;32:304-8.
64. Kristenson M, Kucinskiene Z, Bergdahl B, Ort-Gomer K. Risk factors for coronary heart disease in different socioeconomic groups of Lithuania and Sweden—the LiVicordia Study. Scand J Public Health. 2001;29:140-50.
65. Keltikangas-Jarvinen L, Ravaja N, Raikkonen K, et al. Relationships between the pituitary-adrenal hormones, insulin, and glucose in middle-aged men: moderating influence of psychosocial stress. Metabolism. 1998;47:1440-49.
66. Robinson LE, van Soeren MH. Insulin resistance and hyperglycemia in critical illness: role of insulin in glycemic control. AACN Clin Issues. 2004;15:45-62.
67. Aoki K, Nishina M, Yoshino A. Neuroendocrine response to critical illness and nutritional pharmacology. Nippon Geka Gakkai Zasshi. 2003;104:816-21.
68. Stentz FB, Umpierrez GE, Cuervo R, Kitabchi AE. Proinflammatory cytokines, markers of cardiovascular risks, oxidative stress, lipid peroxidation in patients with hyperglycemic crises. Diabetes. 2004;53:2079-86.
69. Mikhail N, Tuck ML. Insulin and the vasculature. Curr Hypertens Rep. 2000;2:148-53.
70. Hsueh WA, Quinones MJ. Role of endothelial dysfunction in insulin resistance. Am J Cardiol. 2003;92:10J.
71. Petersen KF, Dufour S, Befroy D, et al. Impaired mitochondrial activity in the insulin-resistant offspring of patients with type 2 diabetes. N Engl J Med. 2004;350:664-71.
72. Kelley DE, He J, Menshikova EV, Ritov VB. Dysfunction of mitochondria in human skeletal muscle in type 2 diabetes. Diabetes. 2002;51:2944-50.
73. Perseghin G, Petersen K, Shulman GI. Cellular mechanism of insulin resistance: potential links with inflammation. Int J Obes Relat Metab Disord. 2003;27:S6-S11.
74. Cleland SJ, Petrie JR, Small M, et al. Insulin action is associated with endothelial function in hypertension and type 2 diabetes. Hypertension. 2000;35:507-11.
75. Petersen KF, Dufour S, Befroy D, et al. Impaired mitochondrial activity in the insulin-resistant offspring of patients with type 2 diabetes. N Engl J Med. 2004;350:664-71.
76. Kelley DE, He J, Menshikova EV, Ritov VB. Dysfunction of mitochondria in human skeletal muscle in type 2 diabetes. Diabetes. 2002;51:2944-50.
77. Perseghin G, Petersen K, Shulman GI. Cellular mechanism of insulin resistance: potential links with inflammation. Int J Obes Relat Metab Disord. 2003;27:S6-S11.
78. Xu H, Barnes GT, Yang Q, et al. Chronic inflammation in fat plays a crucial role in the development of obesity-related insulin resistance. J Clin Invest. 2003;112:1821-30.
79. Unger RH. Lipotoxic diseases. Annu Rev Med. 2002;53:319-36.
80. Petersen KF, Dufour S, Befroy D, et al. Impaired mitochondrial activity in the insulin-resistant offspring of patients with type 2 diabetes. N Engl J Med. 2004;350:664-71.
81. Kelley DE, He J, Menshikova EV, Ritov VB. Dysfunction of mitochondria in human skeletal muscle in type 2 diabetes. Diabetes. 2002;51:2944-50.
82. Perseghin G, Petersen K, Shulman GI. Cellular mechanism of insulin resistance: potential links with inflammation. Int J Obes Relat Metab Disord. 2003;27:S6-S11.
83. Zhang CY, Baffy G, Perret P, et al. Uncoupling protein-2 negatively regulates insulin secretion and is major link between obesity, beta cell dysfunction, and type 2 diabetes. Cell. 2001;105:745-55.
84. Wang H, Chu WS, Lu T, et al. Uncoupling protein-2 polymorphisms in type 2 diabetes, obesity and insulin secretion. Am J Physiol Endocrinol Metab. 2004;286:E1-E7.
85. Chan CB, Saleh MC, Koshkin V, Wheeler MB. Uncoupling protein-2 and islet function. Diabetes. 2004;53:S136-42.
86. Hagen T, Vidal-Puig A. Mitochondrial uncoupling proteins in human physiology and disease. Minerva Med. 2002;93:41-57.
87. Schrauwen P. Skeletal muscle uncoupling protein-3 (UCP-3): mitochondrial uncoupling protein in search of a function. Curr Opin Clin Nutr Metab Care. 2002;5:265-70.
88. Schrauwen P. Oxidative capacity, lipotoxicity, and mitochondrial damage in type 2 diabetes. Diabetes. 2004;53:1412-17.
89. Petersen KF, Dufour S, Befroy D, et al. Impaired mitochondrial activity in the insulin-resistant offspring of patients with type 2 diabetes. N Engl J Med. 2004;350:664-71.
90. Ibid.
91. Kelley DE, He J, Menshikova EV, Ritov VB. Dysfunction of mitochondria in human skeletal muscle in type 2 diabetes. Diabetes. 2002;51:2944-50.
92. Perseghin G, Petersen K, Shulman GI. Cellular mechanism of insulin resistance: potential links with inflammation. Int J Obes Relat Metab Disord. 2003;27:S6-S11.
93. Groff JL, Gropper SS. Advanced nutrition and human metabolism. 3rd Ed: Wadsworth Thompson Learning;2000.
94. Ibid.
95. Wilson PWF, Grundy SM. The metabolic syndrome: practical guide to origins and treatment: part I. Circulation. 2003;108:1422-1425.
96. Xu H, Barnes GT, Yang Q, et al. Chronic inflammation in fat plays a crucial role in the development of obesity-related insulin resistance. J Clin Invest. 2003;112:1821-30.

97. Unger RH. Lipotoxic diseases. Annu Rev Med. 2002;53:319-36.
98. Grundy SM. Obesity, metabolic syndrome, and coronary atherosclerosis. Circulation. 2002;105:2696-98.
99. Xu H, Barnes GT, Yang Q, et al. Chronic inflammation in fat plays a crucial role in the development of obesity-related insulin resistance. J Clin Invest. 2003;112:1821-30.
100. Unger RH. Lipotoxic diseases. Annu Rev Med. 2002;53:319-36.
101. Grundy SM. Obesity, metabolic syndrome, and coronary atherosclerosis. Circulation. 2002;105:2696-98.
102. Xu H, Barnes GT, Yang Q, et al. Chronic inflammation in fat plays a crucial role in the development of obesity-related insulin resistance. J Clin Invest. 2003;112:1821-30.
103. Ridker PM, Buring JE, Cook NR, et al. C-reactive protein, the metabolic syndrome, and risk of incident cardiovascular events: an 8-year follow-up of 14,719 initially healthy American women. Circulation. 2003;107:391-97.
104. Xu H, Barnes GT, Yang Q, et al. Chronic inflammation in fat plays a crucial role in the development of obesity-related insulin resistance. J Clin Invest. 2003;112:1821-30.
105. Unger RH. Lipotoxic diseases. Annu Rev Med. 2002;53:319-36.
106. Pussinen PJ, Alfthan G, Tuomilehto J, et al. High serum antibody levels to Porphyromonas gingivalis predict myocardial infarction. Eur J Cardiovasc Prev Rehabil. 2004;11:408-11.
107. Gillum RF. Infection with Helicobacter pylori, coronary heart disease, cardiovascular risk factors, and systemic inflammation: the Third National Health and Nutrition Examination Survey. J Natl Med Assoc. 2004;96:1470-76.
108. Ongey M, Brenner H, Thefeld W, Rothenbacher D. Helicobacter pylori and hepatitis A virus infections and the cardiovascular risk profile in patients with diabetes mellitus: results of a population-based study. Eur J Cardiovasc Prev Rehabil. 2004;11:471-76.
109. Aceti A, Are R, Sabino G, et al. Helicobacter pylori active infection in patients with acute coronary heart disease. J Infect. 2004;49:8-12.
110. Hurwitz BE, Klimas NG, Llabre MM, et al. HIV, metabolic syndrome X, inflammation, oxidative stress, and coronary heart disease risk: role of protease inhibitor exposure. Cardiovasc Toxicol. 2004;4:303-16.
111. Manahan B. A brief evidence-based review of two gastrointestinal illnesses: irritable bowel and leaky gut syndrome. Altern Ther Health Med. 2004;10:14.
112. Kiefer D, Ali-Akbarian L. A brief evidence-based review of two gastrointestinal illnesses: irritable bowel and leaky gut syndromes. Altern Ther Health Med. 2004;10:22-30.
113. Jackson WF. Ion channels and vascular tone. Hypertension. 2000;35:173-78.
114. Barbagallo M, Gupta RK, Dominguez LJ, Resnick LM. Cellular ionic alterations with age: relation to hypertension and diabetes. J Am Geriatr Soc. 2000;48:1111-16.
115. Resnick LM, Oparil S, Chait A, et al. Factors affecting blood pressure responses to diet: the Vanguard study. Am J Hypertens. 2000;13:956-65.
116. Resnick LM, Barbagallo M, Dominguez LJ, et al. Relation of cellular potassium to other mineral ions in hypertension and diabetes. Hypertension. 2001;38:709-12.
117. Ninomiya JK, L'Italien G, Criqui MH, et al. Association of the metabolic syndrome with history of myocardial infarction and stroke in the Third National Health and Nutrition Examination Survey. Circulation 2004;109:42-46.
118. Lakka HM, Laaksonen DE, Lakka TA, et al. The metabolic syndrome and total and cardiovascular disease mortality in middle-aged men. JAMA. 2002;288:2709-16.
119. Ninomiya JK, L'Italien G, Criqui MH, et al. Association of the metabolic syndrome with history of myocardial infarction and stroke in the Third National Health and Nutrition Examination Survey. Circulation. 2004;109:42-46.
120. Lakka HM, Laaksonen DE, Lakka TA, et al. The metabolic syndrome and total and cardiovascular disease mortality in middle-aged men. JAMA. 2002;288:2709-16.
121. Ford ES, Giles WH, Dietz WH. Prevalence of the metabolic syndrome among US adults. JAMA. 2002. 16;287(3):356-59
122. Ninomiya JK, L'Italien G, Criqui MH, et al. Association of the metabolic syndrome with history of myocardial infarction and stroke in the Third National Health and Nutrition Examination Survey. Circulation. 2004;109:42-46.
123. Lakka HM, Laaksonen DE, Lakka TA, et al. The metabolic syndrome and total and cardiovascular disease mortality in middle-aged men. JAMA. 2002;288:2709-16.
124. Klein BE, Klein R, Lee KE. Components of the metabolic syndrome and risk of cardiovascular disease and diabetes in beaver dam. Diabetes Care. 2002;25:1790-94.
125. Ibid.
126. Laaksonen DE, Lakka HM, Niskanen LK, et al. Metabolic syndrome and development of diabetes mellitus: application and validation of recently suggested definitions of the metabolic syndrome in a prospective cohort study. Am J Epidemiol. 2002;156:1070-77.
127. Alberti KGMM, Zimmet PZ. Diagnosis and classification of diabetes mellitus: part 1—provisional report of a WHO consultation. Diabet Med. 1998;15:539-53.
128. The European Group for the Study of Insulin Resistance (EGIR). Frequency of the WHO metabolic syndrome in European cohorts, and an alternative definition of an insulin resistance syndrome. Diabetes Metab. 2002;28:364-76.
129. Executive Summary of the Third Report of the National Cholesterol Education Program (NCEP) Expert Panel on Detection, Evaluation, and Treatment of High Blood Cholesterol in Adults (Adult Treatment Panel III). JAMA. 2001;285:2486-97.
130. Ibid.
131. Alberti KGMM, Zimmet PZ. Diagnosis and classification of diabetes mellitus: part 1—provisional report of a WHO consultation. Diabet Med. 1998;15:539-53.
132. The European Group for the Study of Insulin Resistance (EGIR). Frequency of the WHO metabolic syndrome in European cohorts, and an alternative definition of an insulin resistance syndrome. Diabetes Metab. 2002;28:364-76.
133. Grundy SM. Obesity, metabolic syndrome, and coronary atherosclerosis. Circulation. 2002;105:2696-98.
134. Ridker PM, Buring JE, Cook NR, et al. C-reactive protein, the metabolic syndrome, and risk of incident cardiovascular events: an 8-year follow-up of 14,719 initially healthy American women. Circulation. 2003;107:391-97.
135. Creager MA, Luscher TF, Cosentino F, et al. Diabetes and vascular disease: pathophysiology, clinical consequences, and medical therapy: part I. Circulation. 2003;108:1527-32.
136. Houston MC. Vascular Biology in Clinical Practice: Hypertension, Hyperlipidemia, Atherosclerosis, Coronary Heart Disease. Hanley and Belfus, Inc.: Philadelphia; 2002.
137. Mikhail N, Tuck ML. Insulin and the vasculature. Curr Hypertens Rep. 2000;2:148-53.
138. Xu H, Barnes GT, Yang Q, et al. Chronic inflammation in fat plays a crucial role in the development of obesity-related insulin resistance. J Clin Invest. 2003;112:1821-30.
139. Szmitko PE, Wang CH, Weisel RD, et al. New markers of inflammation and endothelial cell activation. Part I and II. Circulation. 2003;108:1917-23, 2041-48.

140. Hsueh WA, Quinones MJ. Role of endothelial dysfunction in insulin resistance. Am J Cardiol. 2003;92:10J.
141. Houston MC. Vascular Biology in Clinical Practice: Hypertension, Hyperlipidemia, Atherosclerosis, Coronary Heart Disease. Hanley and Belfus, Inc.: Philadelphia; 2002.
142. Mikhail N, Tuck ML. Insulin and the vasculature. Curr Hypertens Rep. 2000;2:148-53.
143. Xu H, Barnes GT, Yang Q, et al. Chronic inflammation in fat plays a crucial role in the development of obesity-related insulin resistance. J Clin Invest. 2003;112:1821-30.
144. Szmitko PE, Wang CH, Weisel RD, et al. New markers of inflammation and endothelial cell activation. Part I and II. Circulation. 2003;108:1917-23, 2041-48.
145. Hsueh WA, Quinones MJ. Role of endothelial dysfunction in insulin resistance. Am J Cardiol. 2003;92:10J.
146. Mikhail N, Tuck ML. Insulin and the vasculature. Curr Hypertens Rep. 2000;2:148-53.
147. Xu H, Barnes GT, Yang Q, et al. Chronic inflammation in fat plays a crucial role in the development of obesity-related insulin resistance. J Clin Invest. 2003;112:1821-30.
148. Szmitko PE, Wang CH, Weisel RD, et al. New markers of inflammation and endothelial cell activation. Part I and II. Circulation. 2003;108:1917-23, 2041-48.
149. Hsueh WA, Quinones MJ. Role of endothelial dysfunction in insulin resistance. Am J Cardiol. 2003;92:10J.
150. Mikhail N, Tuck ML. Insulin and the vasculature. Curr Hypertens Rep. 2000;2:148-53.
151. Xu H, Barnes GT, Yang Q, et al. Chronic inflammation in fat plays a crucial role in the development of obesity-related insulin resistance. J Clin Invest. 2003;112:1821-30.
152. Szmitko PE, Wang CH, Weisel RD, et al. New markers of inflammation and endothelial cell activation. Part I and II. Circulation. 2003;108:1917-23, 2041-48.
153. Hsueh WA, Quinones MJ. Role of endothelial dysfunction in insulin resistance. Am J Cardiol. 2003;92:10J.
154. Xu H, Barnes GT, Yang Q, et al. Chronic inflammation in fat plays a crucial role in the development of obesity-related insulin resistance. J Clin Invest. 2003;112:1821-30.
155. Unger RH. Lipotoxic diseases. Annu Rev Med. 2002;53:319-36.
156. Ibid.
157. Grundy SM. Obesity, metabolic syndrome, and coronary atherosclerosis. Circulation. 2002;105:2696-98.
158. Ridker PM, Buring JE, Cook NR, et al. C-reactive protein, the metabolic syndrome, and risk of incident cardiovascular events: an 8-year follow-up of 14,719 initially healthy American women. Circulation. 2003;107:391-97.
159. Ibid.
160. Nestel P. Metabolic syndrome: multiple candidate genes, multiple environmental factors—multiple syndromes? Int J Clin Pract Suppl. 2003;(134):3-9.
161. Wilson PWF, Grundy SM. The metabolic syndrome: practical guide to origins and treatment: part I. Circulation. 2003;108:1422-25.
162. Tuomilehto J, Lindstrom J, Eriksson JG, et al. for the Finnish Diabetes Prevention Study Group. Prevention of type 2 diabetes mellitus by changes in lifestyle among subjects with impaired glucose intolerance. N Engl J Med. 2001;344:1343-50.
163. Diabetes Prevention Program Research Group. Reduction in the incidence of type 2 diabetes with lifestyle intervention or metformin. N Engl J Med. 2002;346:393-403.
164. Wilson PWF, Grundy SM. The metabolic syndrome: practical guide to origins and treatment: part I. Circulation. 2003;108:1422-25.
165. Ibid.
166. Gregg EW, Gerzoff RB, Caspersen CJ, et al. Relationship of walking to mortality among US adults with diabetes. Arch Intern Med. 2003;163:1440-47.
167. Brooks GA, Butte NF, Rand WM, et al. Chronicle of the Institute of Medicine physical activity recommendation: how a physical activity recommendation came to be among dietary recommendations. Am J Clin Nutr. 2004;79:921S-30S.
168. Hittel DS, Kraus WE, Tanner CJ, et al. Exercise training increases electron and substrate shuttling proteins in muscle in overweight men and women with the metabolic syndrome. J Appl Physiol. 2005;98:168-79.
169. Ziegler M, Braumann KM, Reer R. The role of jogging in the prevention and treatment of cardiovascular disease. MMW Fortschr Med. 2004;146:29-32.
170. Christ M, Iannello C, Iannello PG, Grimm W. Effects of a weight reduction program with and without aerobic exercise in the metabolic syndrome. Int J Cardiol. 2004;97:115-22.
171. Green JS, Stanforth PR, Rankinen T, et al. The effects of exercise training on abdominal visceral fat, body composition, indicators of the metabolic syndrome in postmenopausal women with and without estrogen replacement therapy: the HERITAGE family study. Metabolism. 2004;53:1192-96.
172. Jurca R, Lamonte MJ, Church TS, et al. Associations of muscle strength and fitness with metabolic syndrome in men. Med Sci Sports Exerc. 2004;36:1301-07.
173. Hawley JA, Houmard JA. Introduction-preventing insulin resistance through exercise: a cellular approach. Med Sci Sports Exerc. 2004;36:1187-90.
174. Oshida Y, Sato Y. Approach in clinical management of metabolic syndrome. Methods of exercise therapy. Nippon Naika Gakkai Zasshi. 2004;93:726-32.
175. Farrell SW, Cheng YJ, Blair SN. Prevalence of the metabolic syndrome across cardiorespiratory fitness levels in women. Obes Res. 2004;12:824-30.
176. Carroll S, Dudfield M. What is the relationship between exercise and metabolic abnormalities? A report on the metabolic syndrome. Sports Med. 2004;34:371-418.
177. Lavie CJ, Milani RV. Metabolic syndrome, inflammation, and exercise. Am J Cardiol. 2004;93:1334.
178. Franks PW, Ekelund U, Brage S, et al. Does the association of habitual physical activity with the metabolic syndrome differ by level of cardiorespiratory fitness? Diabetes Care. 2004;27:1187-93.
179. Houston MC. The role of vascular biology, nutrition and nutraceuticals in the prevention and treatment of hypertension. JANA. 2002;April (Suppl):1-71.
180. Heart Outcomes Prevention Evaluation (HOPE) Study Investigators. Effects of ramipril on cardiovascular and microvascular outcomes in people with diabetes mellitus: results of the HOPE study and MICRO-HOPE substudy. Lancet. 2000;355:253-59.
181. Dahlof B, Devereaux RB, Kjeldsen SE, et al. For the LIFE study group. Cardiovascular morbidity and mortality in the Losartan Intervention for Endpoint reduction in hypertension study (LIFE): a randomized trial against atenolol. Lancet 2002;359:995-1003.
182. Messerli FH. ALLHAT, or the Soft Science of the Secondary Endpoint. Ann Intern Med. 2003;139:777-80.
183. Ames RP. A comparison of blood lipid and blood pressure responses during the treatment of systemic hypertension with indapamide and with thiazides. Am J Cardiol. 1996;77:12b-16b.
184. Weidmann P. Metabolic profile of indapamide sustained-release in patients with hypertension: data from three randomised double-blind studies. Drug Saf. 2001;24:1155-65.
185. Teuscher AU, Weidmann PU. Requirements for antihypertensive therapy in diabetic patients: metabolic aspects. J Hypertens. 1997;15:S67-S75.

186. Weidmann PU, de Courten M, Ferrari P. Effects of diuretics on the plasma lipid profile. Eur Heart J. 1992;13 Suppl G:61-67.
187. The Scandinavian Simvastatin Survival Study Group: Randomized trial of cholesterol lowering in 4,444 patients with coronary heart disease: the Scandinavian Simvastatin Survival Study (4S). Lancet. 1994;344:1383-89.
188. Pyorala K, Pedersen TR, Kjekshus J. Cholesterol lowering with simvastatin improves prognosis of diabetic patients with coronary heart disease. Diabetes Care. 1997;20:614-20.
189. Heart Protection Study Collaborative Group. MRC/BHF Heart Protection Study of cholesterol lowering with simvastatin in 20,536 high-risk individuals: a randomized placebo-controlled trial. Lancet. 2002;360:7-22.
190. Diabetes Prevention Program Research Group. Reduction in the incidence of type 2 diabetes with lifestyle intervention or metformin. N Engl J Med. 2002;346:393-403.
191. Kirpichnikov D, McFarlane SI, Sowers JR. Metformin: an update. Ann Intern Med. 2002;137:25-33.
192. UK Prospective Diabetes Study (UKPDS) Group. Effect of intensive blood-glucose control with metformin on complications in overweight patients with type 2 diabetes (UKPDS 34). Lancet. 1998;352:854-65.

Appendix

Appendix

30 Top-Selling Drugs and 10 Top-Selling Herbal Supplements in the United States (2003)

Drugs	x 1 million scripts	Herbs
1 Lipitor	68.95	1 St. John's Wort; Hypericum perforatum
2 Synthroid	49.78	2 Echinacea
3 Hydrocodone/Acetaminophen	44.07	3 Ginkgo biloba
4 Norvasc	36.43	4 Saw palmetto
5 Zoloft	32.71	5 Feverfew
6 **Toprol XL**	29.73	6 Garlic
7 Hydrocodone/Acetaminophen*	29.65	7 Ginger
8 Zocor	29.35	8 Ginseng
9 Prevacid	28.27	9 Ephedra
10 **Amoxicillin**	27.57	10 Valerian
11 **Albuterol**		
12 Azithromycin		
13 Premarin		
14 Zyrtec		
15 **Atenolol**		
16 Levoxyl		
17 Celebrex		
18 Ambien		
19 Fosamax		
20 Allegra		
21 Nexium		
22 **Furosemide**		
23 Vioxx		
24 Singulair		
25 Ortho TriCyclen 28		
26 Neurontin		
27 Cephalexin		
28 Effexor		
29 Hydrochlorothiazide		
30 Protonix		

Bold: Common adverse drug reaction
*Different dosage than #3.

Biographical Sketches for Contributing Authors

B. Jayne Alexander, DO, is a graduate of the Kirksville College of Osteopathic Medicine located in Kirksville, Missouri. As a student she was awarded an Undergraduate Fellowship in the Department of Osteopathic Theory and Methods and following graduation served a rotating internship at the Kirksville Osteopathic Health Center. Dr. Alexander is Board Certified with Special Proficiency in Osteopathic Manipulative Medicine by the American Osteopathic Association, and is trained in traditional and biodynamic osteopathic approaches. She serves on the faculty of the Sutherland Cranial Teaching Foundation, teaches with the New England-based A. Still Sutherland Study Group, and is a clinical preceptor for osteopathic students, interns and residents. Dr. Alexander has studied functional medicine since 1983, and completed the Institute for Functional Medicine's AFMCP training in 1998 and 2001. She is currently engaged in private practice specializing in osteopathic manual medicine.

Bruce N. Ames, PhD, is a professor of the Graduate School in Biochemistry and Molecular Biology, University of California, Berkeley, and a Senior Scientist at Children's Hospital Oakland Research Institute. A member of the National Academy of Sciences, Dr. Ames served on their Commission on Life Sciences. He was a member of the board of directors of the National Cancer Institute—the National Cancer Advisory Board—from 1976 to 1982. He has received the General Motors Cancer Research Foundation Prize (1983); the Tyler Environmental Prize (1985); the Gold Medal Award, American Institute of Chemists (1991); Award for Excellence in Environmental Health Research (1995); the Honda Prize, Honda Foundation, Japan (1996); the Japan Prize (1997); the Robert A. Kehoe Award, American College of Occupational and Environmental Medicine (1997); the Medal of the City of Paris (1998); the U.S. National Medal of Science (1998); the Linus Pauling Award (2001); and the Thomas Hunt Morgan Medal from the Genetics Society of America (2004). Dr. Ames is among the few hundred most-cited scientists (in all fields), as a result of his 500+ publications.

Sidney MacDonald Baker, MD, is a 1964 graduate of Yale Medical School where he completed his specialty training in pediatrics. He is board certified in pediatrics. He has been a Peace Corps volunteer in Chad, Africa (1966-1968), an Assistant Professor of Medical Computer Science at Yale (1969-1971), a family physician in the Community Health Care Center (1971-1978) in New Haven, Conn., Director of the Gesell Institute of Human Development (1978-1985), and in private practice in Connecticut and New York. He is co-author of *Child Development* (1982), *The Years from 10 to 14* (1984), and the author of *The Circadian Prescription* (G.P. Putnam Sons, 2000) and *Detoxification and Healing* (Contemporary Books, 2003). He was co-founder in 1995 of the Defeat Autism Now! organization, with Bernard Rimland, PhD and Jon Pangborn, PhD, with whom he is co-author of *Autism: Effective Biomedical Treatments* (2005). Dr. Baker was the 1999 recipient of the Linus Pauling Award from the Institute of Functional Medicine. He is an Associate Editor of *Integrative Medicine: A Clinician's Journal*, and currently practices integrative medicine in Sag Harbor, New York.

Peter Bennett, ND, is a naturopathic physician, best-selling author, and educator. He received his doctorate in naturopathic medicine in 1987 from Bastyr University. In addition to his training as a naturopathic doctor, Dr. Bennett completed a three-year degree program in Traditional Chinese Medicine (TCM) at the Northwest Institute of Acupuncture and Oriental Medicine (NIAOM) in Seattle, WA. He is also a board certified homeopathic physician (DHANP). In 1999, Dr. Bennett co-authored the *7-Day Detox Miracle* (Prima Publishing, 2001), a safe, effective way to help people promote healing, lose weight, and increase energy. Dr. Bennett currently sees patients in Langley, BC where he focuses on providing individual biochemical assessment, and developing programs for optimum performance and recovery.

Jeffrey S. Bland, PhD, FACN, CNS. Dr. Bland's distinguished career in nutritional biochemistry has earned him international acclaim as educator, research professor, leader in the natural products industry, recognized expert in human nutrition and functional medicine, and visionary for the future of health care. Dr. Bland now serves as President and Chief Science Officer of Metagenics, Inc, and Chairman of the Board of Directors for The Institute for Functional Medicine, which he co-founded with his wife, Susan Bland, MA.

John Cline, BSc, MD, utilizes an integrative approach in his medical practice. He is medical director of the Cline Medical Centre in Nanaimo, British Columbia, Canada. He is also medical director for the Oceanside Functional Medicine Research Institute and has collaborated with Michael Lyon, MD on several research projects related to ADHD. Dr. Cline obtained a BSc in Biochemistry, followed by his MD and residency training in family medicine at the University of Calgary, Alberta, Canada. He has a particular interest in using various detoxification strategies and has taken further training through the American Board of Chelation Therapy, the American Academy of Neural Therapy, and is certified by the International Board of Clinical Metal Toxicology. In April 2005, he completed the physicians training course with the Centers for Advanced Medicine. He is writing a book for the general public about toxicity and detoxification. He has lectured extensively in the community, at medical conferences, and for The Institute for Functional Medicine.

Daniel Cosgrove, MD, earned a psychobiology degree from UCLA and received an MD degree from Washington University in St. Louis. He completed internal medicine training at the University of Utah, and became board certified in both internal medicine and emergency medicine. He holds a clinical faculty appointment at Loma Linda University School of Medicine. Dr. Cosgrove is certified by the Federal Aviation Administration as a Senior Aviation Medical Examiner. He was the Medical Director of Airstar International Air Ambulance for many years. He has published several scientific articles. He is a principal investigator in the KIMS Human Growth Hormone Study. In 1997 Dr. Cosgrove founded the WellMax Center for Preventive Medicine, which is now located at the La Quinta Resort and Club™. WellMax provides executive physicals but is best known for ongoing individualized healthcare, specializing in the early detection of disease through the creation and maintenance of a Personal Health Portfolio.

Walter J. Crinnion, ND, received his degree in naturopathic medicine from Bastyr University (Seattle, Washington) in 1982 with the first graduating class. He opened a family practice and began to specialize in allergies and in treating chronic health problems caused by environmental chemical overload. In 1985 he opened the most comprehensive cleansing facility in North America for the treatment of chemically poisoned individuals. He has published several articles in peer-reviewed journals on the topic of environmental overload. He has served on the board of directors of the American Association of Naturopathic Physicians and received their first award for in-office research in 1999, and was awarded it a second time in 2002. He is an associate professor at Bastyr University, the National College of Naturopathic Medicine in Portland, OR, and the University of Bridgeport School of Naturopathic Medicine. He is professor and director of the Environmental Medicine Center of Excellence at Southwest College of Naturopathic Medicine. In 2001, he appeared three times with Barbara Walters on ABC's "The View" and had a weekly Health Spot on Northwest Cable News from 1999 until 2003, giving viewers in Oregon, Washington, and Idaho up-to-date information on nutrition and health.

Gary Darland, PhD, received his doctorate in microbiology from the University of Washington. He is Senior Director of Clinical Biology at Metaproteomics, LLC, a division of Metagenics, Inc. Dr. Darland joined HealthComm/Metagenics after 23 years of research experience in natural products, and biochemistry and microbial genetics at Merck Research Laboratories. Research activities at Merck revolved around microbial genetics and physiology and also included work in the area of human and animal drug metabolism. Prior to joining Merck, he was a visiting Fellow at the Centers for Disease Control in the Enteric Disease Section and an assistant professor at California Polytechnic University, San Luis Obispo. These activities have led to the publication of several papers dealing with drug metabolism and the biosynthesis of natural products.

Joel M. Evans, MD, a board certified OB/GYN, is Founder and Director of The Center for Women's Health in Darien, CT, where he practices integrative obstetrics and gynecology. A frequent lecturer on complementary and alternative medicine (CAM), Dr. Evans is an Assistant Clinical Professor of Obstetrics, Gynecology and Women's Health at the Albert Einstein College of Medicine. In January 2001, he was honored as a Founding Diplomate of the American Board of Holistic Medicine. Dr. Evans' book, *The Whole Pregnancy Handbook* (Gotham Books, 2005), details his unique approach to holistic pregnancy care. Dr. Evans is on the senior faculty of The Center for Mind/Body Medicine in Washington D.C. He teaches health professionals about the medical benefits of relaxation therapies at The Center's basic and advanced training programs. He also lectures about nutrition and supplements at the Center's Cancer Guides™ and Food as Medicine conferences. Dr. Evans has a special interest in helping those affected by the tragedies of war, and participated in the Center's Mind/Body Mission to Macedonia in 1999, where he traveled to U.N. refugee camps to help Kosavar refugees. Dr. Evans also worked with the FDNY firefighters to help them handle the many stresses caused by 9/11.

William J. Evans, PhD, is director of the Nutrition, Metabolism, and Exercise Laboratory in the Donald Reynolds Department of Geriatrics at the University of Arkansas for Medical Sciences and a research scientist in the Geriatric Research, Education and Clinical Center (GRECC) at the Central Arkansas Veterans Healthcare System. He is a Professor of Geriatrics, Physiology, and Nutrition. From 1993 to 1997, he was director of the Noll Physiological Research Center at the Pennsylvania State University and, from 1982 to 1993, he served as Chief of the Human Physiology Laboratory at the USDA Human Nutrition Research Center on Aging at Tufts University. He is a Fellow of the American College of Sports Medicine, The American College of Nutrition, and an honorary member of the American Dietetic Association. Dr. Evans is the author or co-author of more than 190 publications in scientific journals. His research has examined the powerful interaction between diet and exercise in elderly people. He is the co-author of *Biomarkers: The Ten Determinants of Aging You Can Control* (Simon & Schuster, 1991) and authored *AstroFit* (Simon & Schuster, 2002). His work has been featured in numerous newspapers, including *The New York Times*, *The Boston Globe*, and *The Chicago Tribune*.

William B. Ferril, MD, received a Bachelor of Science degree in Biochemistry and his Doctorate in Medicine from The University of California at Davis. He completed his post graduate education at Sacred Heart Medical Center in Spokane, Washington. For over 19 years, Dr. Ferril has practiced medicine on the Flathead Indian Reservation and adjacent areas of Montana. It was during this posting that Dr. Ferril compiled his data for a series of books on the biochemistry of the human body. He is the author of *The Body Heals*, *Glandular Failure-Caused Obesity*, and *Why is My Doctor So Dumb? Healing 101*. Dr. Ferril resides with his wife and children in Whitefish, MT where he continues research and private practice.

Leo Galland, MD, is the recipient of the 2000 Linus Pauling Award from The Institute for Functional Medicine, for formulating key concepts underlying the discipline of functional medicine. He received his education at Harvard University and the New York University School of Medicine and trained in internal medicine at the NYU-Bellevue Medical Center. He has held faculty positions at New York University, Rockefeller University, the Albert Einstein College of Medicine, the State University of New York at Stony Brook, and the University of Connecticut. He has written over 30 scientific articles and textbook chapters and has lectured extensively on topics related to nutritional medicine, intestinal health and patient assessment. A board-certified internist, Dr. Galland is a Fellow of the American College of Physicians and the American College of Nutrition, an Honorary Professor of the International College of Nutrition, and has authored three books, *Superimmunity for Kids* (Dell, 1989), *Power Healing* (Random House, 1997), and *The Fat Resistance Diet* (Doubleday, 2006). In addition to a full-time private practice in New York City, Dr. Galland directs the Foundation for Integrated Medicine (www.mdheal.org), and Applied Nutrition, Inc., a medical software company (www.nutritionworkshop.com).

Michael D. Gershon, MD, has published over 300 scientific papers, books, and chapters. His study of the cellular basis of the neuronal control of behavior brought the enteric nervous system (ENS)—discussed in his book, *The Second Brain*—to the attention of the general public and enhanced the esteem in which neurogastroenterologists are held. He was the first to propose, and ultimately to establish, that serotonin is an enteric neurotransmitter, and he has also studied the mechanisms by which the varicella zoster virus infects cells and then is assembled into infectious particles. Dr. Gershon received his BA degree in 1958, with distinction, from Cornell University. Upon graduating from Cornell Medical School in 1963, he was awarded the Polk Prize for the best academic record and the Borden Prize for undergraduate research. He then completed postdoctoral training in pharmacology with Edith Bülbring at Oxford University (England), before returning to Cornell as Assistant Professor of Anatomy in 1967. He was promoted to Professor before leaving Cornell to accept his current position as Chair of the Department of Anatomy and Cell Biology at Columbia University's College of Physicians and Surgeons.

Patrick Hanaway, MD, is a board-certified family physician with a medical degree from Washington University (St. Louis) and residency training at the University of New Mexico. Dr. Hanaway is also a board-certified holistic physician and currently sits on the American

Board of Holistic Medicine. He received his bachelors degree from the University of Wisconsin in molecular biology and has done research and published papers in muscle biology, neurochemistry, lipid research, digestive disease, public health and prevention. Dr. Hanaway holds dual appointments as Medical Director for Family to Family: Your Home for Whole Family Health (Asheville, NC) and Medical Director for Great Smokies Diagnostic Laboratory. His current interests are in the research and clinical implementation of applied nutritional biochemistry, with an emphasis on digestion, immunology, prevention and wellness.

Bethany Hays, MD, FACOG, is an obstetrician gynecologist with a career-long passion to find the best possible forms of healing and to incorporate them into her practice. That dream has come to a new level of realization with the opening of True North, A Center for Health and Healing, in Falmouth, Maine. This unique integrative practice was created by a group of practitioners of conventional and complementary modalities after nearly four years of dreaming and planning. The addition of functional medicine to her practice has added a new dimension and new excitement for Dr. Hays as well as a passion for the biochemistry she tried so hard to forget after the first year of medical school. She is an adjunct faculty member of The Institute for Functional Medicine, where she also serves on the board of directors.

Robert J. Hedaya, MD, is a Fellow of the American Psychiatric Association and Clinical Professor of Psychiatry at Georgetown University Hospital where he teaches psychoendocrinology. He is founder of the National Center for Whole Psychiatry and is board certified by the American Board of Psychiatry and Neurology, the American Board of Adolescent Psychiatry, and certified as proficient in psychopharmacology by the American Society of Clinical Psychopharmacology. He has been a consultant to the National Institute of Mental Health. Dr. Hedaya obtained both a BA in psychology (Cum Laude, Phi Beta Kappa) and a medical degree at the State University of New York at Buffalo. Subsequently, he acquired specialized training in psychiatry at Georgetown University Hospital's Department of Psychiatry, and at the National Institute of Mental Health. Dr. Hedaya received the Physician's Recognition Award from the American Medical Association each year from 1983 through 1996. In June of 1993, 1997, and 1999, he was voted Outstanding Teacher of the Year by the Georgetown University Department of Psychiatry. He has authored *Understanding Biological Psychiatry* (Norton, 1996) and *The Antidepressant Survival Program: How to Beat the Side Effects and Enhance the Benefits of Your Medication* (Crown, 2000).

Mark C. Houston, MD, MSc, SCH, ABAAM, FACP, FAHA, is Clinical Professor of Medicine at Vanderbilt University School of Medicine, and Director of the Hypertension Institute, Vascular Biology and the Life Extension Institute, Saint Thomas Hospital in Nashville, TN. He is also Medical Director of Clinical Research, Section Chief of the Division of Nutrition, and Director of CME in the Hypertension Institute. Dr. Houston graduated from Vanderbilt Medical School, completed his medical internship and residency at the University of California, San Francisco, then returned to Vanderbilt Medical Center as chief resident in medicine. He is certified by the American Board of Internal Medicine; the American Society of Hypertension as a specialist in clinical hypertension (SCH); and the American Board of Anti-Aging Medicine (ABAAM). He completed a Master of Science degree in clinical human nutrition from the University of Bridgeport, Connecticut. He is Editor-in-Chief for the *Journal of the American Nutraceutical Association* (JANA), has published more than 120 articles and scientific abstracts, and completed over 70 clinical research studies. He co-authored the *Handbook of Antihypertensive Therapy* (Hanley and Belfus Inc., 2000), *Vascular Biology in Clinical Practice* (Hanley and Belfus Inc., 2002), and *What Your Doctor May Not Tell You about Hypertension* (Warner Books, 2003).

Mark A. Hyman, MD, is Editor-in-Chief of *Alternative Therapies in Health and Medicine*. For nearly 10 years he was Co-Medical Director at Canyon Ranch in the Berkshires, an internationally acclaimed health resort, which is an affiliated practice with Harvard University's Brigham and Women's Hospital. He graduated with a BA from Cornell University in 1982 and Magna Cum Laude from the University of Ottawa School of Medicine in 1987 and from the University of San Francisco's program in family medicine at Community Hospital of Santa Rosa. He is board certified in family medicine. He recently testified at the White House Commission on Complementary and Alternative Medicine Policy on health promotion and wellness, and met with and advised the Surgeon General on a new diabetes prevention initiative. He is on the editorial board of *Integrative Medicine: A Clinician's Journal*. Dr. Hyman combines the best of conventional and alternative medicine with a blend of science, integrity, intuition and compassion. He is co-author of *Ultraprevention, the 6-Week Plan that Will Make You Healthy for Life* (Scribner, 2003), and *The Detox Box, a Program for Greater Health and Vitality* (Sounds True, 2004). He serves on the Board of Directors for The Institute for Functional Medicine.

Mary James, ND, is a 1985 graduate of the National College of Naturopathic Medicine in Portland, Oregon. Dr. James was in private practice for several years in Portland, represented a nutraceutical company in the northeast, and has worked in medical education at Great Smokies Diagnostic Laboratory in Asheville, NC for more than 10 years. She has lectured widely within the U.S. and abroad, provided ongoing technical support to physicians, developed products, and authored an extensive array of therapeutic guides and technical articles, particularly in the areas of endocrinology and genomics. Dr. James is a member of the American Association of Naturopathic Physicians and serves on the Editorial Review Board of the *Alternative Medicine Review.*

David Jones, MD, is President of The Institute for Functional Medicine. He has practiced as a family physician with emphasis in functional and integrative medicine for over 25 years. He is a recognized expert in the areas of nutrition, lifestyle changes for optimal health, and managed care, as well as the daily professional functions consistent with the modern specialty of Family Practice. Dr. Jones is the recipient of the 1997 Linus Pauling Award in Functional Medicine. He is also the Past President of PrimeCare, the Independent Physician Association of Southern Oregon (IPASO) representing the majority of physicians in the Southern Oregon area. He is author of *Healthy Changes: Taking Charge of Your Health* (HealthComm, 1996).

Joseph J. Lamb, MD, is board certified in both internal medicine and holistic medicine. He is president of the Integrative Medicine Works in Alexandria, Virginia, and is an Assistant Clinical Professor of Medicine at George Washington University School of Medicine. Dr. Lamb works in partnership with his patients to create optimal health and well-being by using functional medical approaches including lifestyle modification, herbal and nutritional therapies, and cognitive therapy. He completed his graduate education at the Medical College of Virginia in Richmond and his residency at Presbyterian University of Pennsylvania Medical Center in Philadelphia. Dr. Lamb, a native Alexandrian, is active in his community. He is the Past President of the St. Stephen's & St. Agnes Alumni Association and the school physician at Episcopal High School in Alexandria. He is also the president of the Commonwealth Consultants Foundation, a local charity chartered to provide unique educational and social experiences for economically deserving children and young adults.

Robert H. Lerman, MD, PhD, is Medical Director of MetaProteomics, Inc., a subsidiary of Metagenics, Inc., with major emphasis on clinical research at the Functional Medicine Research Center. Previously, he was Senior Medical Advisor and Director of Medical Education for IFM, Director of Clinical Nutrition at Boston Medical Center, and Clinical Associate Professor of Medicine at Boston University School of Medicine. Dr. Lerman is board certified in internal medicine and completed fellowships in nephrology and clinical nutrition. He received his MD degree from Jefferson Medical College and a PhD in nutritional biochemistry from M.I.T. He completed a rotating internship at Letterman Army Medical Center in San Francisco and an internal medicine residency at Tripler Army Medical Center in Honolulu, and attained the rank of major in the U.S. Army Medical Corps. He was Chief of Medicine at U.S. Army Hospitals in Berlin, Germany and Vicenza, Italy and Acting Chief of Nephrology at Soroka Medical Center in Beer Sheba, Israel. He has authored and co-authored numerous papers and book chapters in addition to lecturing widely.

Edward Leyton, MD, CCFP, received his BSc (Hons.) in Biochemistry from the University of Western Ontario in 1970, and subsequently his MD degree in 1975. Since then he has trained in acupuncture with the Canadian Acupuncture Foundation (1979); gestalt therapy with the Gestalt Institute of Toronto (1976); and has followed the concepts of functional nutritional medicine as taught by Dr. Jeffrey Bland since 1982. More recently, Dr. Leyton has attained a master practitioner level in Neuro-Linguistic Programming (NLP) and is a certified hypnotherapist. He was an adjunct faculty member with The Institute of Functional Medicine, where he taught in the Applying Functional Medicine in Clinical Practice course. He is an adjunct academic staff member in the Department of Family Medicine, Queens University, Kingston, Ontario, an award recipient, and published author.

Peter Libby, MD, is the Chief of Cardiovascular Medicine at Brigham and Women's Hospital, Boston, MA, and Mallinckrodt Professor of Medicine at Harvard

Medical School. He directs the D.W. Reynolds Cardiovascular Clinical Research Center at Harvard. Dr. Libby's research currently focuses on the role of inflammation in vascular diseases such as atherosclerosis. His clinical expertise includes general and preventive cardiology, and he has published extensively in medical journals. An editor of Braunwald's *Heart Disease*, he also contributed two chapters on atherosclerosis to Harrison's *Principles of Internal Medicine*. He has held numerous visiting professorships and has delivered over 40 named or keynote lectures. Dr. Libby is a member of the Association of American Physicians and the American Society for Clinical Investigation. An active member of the American Heart Association, he has served on its Executive Committees of the Councils on Arteriosclerosis, Circulation, and Basic Science. He consults frequently to the National Heart, Lung and Blood Institute, and also served a five-year term on the Board of Scientific Councilors. Dr. Libby earned his medical degree at University of California-San Diego, and completed his training in internal medicine and cardiology at the Peter Bent Brigham Hospital.

DeAnn Liska, PhD, is Director of Technical Information and Scientific Publications at Metagenics' Functional Medicine Research Center. She received her PhD in Biochemistry from the University of Wisconsin-Madison in 1987, where she performed her graduate thesis studies on several aspects of vitamin K biochemistry. She also did postgraduate studies in the Department of Biochemistry at the University of Washington as Senior Fellow and, subsequently, Research Assistant Professor, on the subject of nutrient and growth factor effects on gene expression. Dr. Liska has authored numerous papers in peer-reviewed journals, contributed to textbooks on nutrition, is on the Biotechnology and Biomedical Device Advisory Board for the Washington Technology Center. She holds four U.S. patents. Dr. Liska has been an invited speaker at national and scientific meetings, Chair of the Nutrition Division and a member of the Scientific Advisory Panel for the American Association of Cereal Chemists (AACC). She is a member of the National Science Teachers Association and the American Medical Writers Association and serves on IFM's CME Advisory Committee.

Jay Lombard, MD, is an Assistant Clinical Professor of Neurology at Cornell Medical School and Director of the Brain Behavior Center in Pomona, NY. He specializes in Behavioral Neurology including Alzheimer's and other dementias, autism, Asperger's syndrome and ADHD. His research involves brain imaging and neuropsychopharmacology. Dr. Lombard has published several books including *The Brain Wellness Plan* (Kensington Press, 2000) and *Balance Your Brain* (Wiley, 2004), as well as numerous articles on topics related to brain health. Recently, Dr. Lombard was the medical consultant in the film, *Manchurian Candidate*, starring Denzel Washington and Meryl Streep.

Dan Lukaczer, ND, received his undergraduate degree from Duke University in 1980 and his doctorate in naturopathic medicine from Bastyr University in 1991. From 1991 to 1995, he developed and maintained a private practice. In 1996, he became Director of Clinical Research for the Functional Medicine Research Center, a division of Metagenics, Inc., and served in that capacity until 2005. He is currently working as a senior research scientist for SaluGenecists Inc., a company that is developing evidence-based expert logic health diagnostic systems using advanced computer-based technology. Dr. Lukaczer has taught, lectured and written extensively on botanical and nutritional medicine. He is a core faculty member of The Institute for Functional Medicine and serves on IFM's CME Advisory Committee.

Michael D. Lumpkin, PhD, is a tenured Professor and Chairman of the Department of Physiology and Biophysics at Georgetown University School of Medicine. He earned his doctoral degree in physiology in 1981 from the University of Texas Southwestern Medical School in Dallas. He completed NIH-sponsored postdoctoral fellowship training in neuroendocrinology at Southwestern Medical Center in 1983. Dr. Lumpkin's current research involves studying the stress-related mechanisms by which HIV/AIDS disrupts the neuroendocrine systems that regulate growth, immunity, and reproduction. From this work, he and his research group have produced a patent for treating AIDS-related wasting syndromes in adults and children. He is also a central participant in a large NIH-funded initiative to bring integrative medicine research and education to medical and graduate students at Georgetown. Dr. Lumpkin lectures extensively on the subjects of stress physiology and psychoneuroimmunology. He is an officer in two international scientific societies and serves on several boards of medical foundations. He lectures, instructs and facilitates groups in all aspects of neuroendocrinology, psychoneuroimmunology and mind-body medicine. He is a representative to the

Consortium of Academic Health Centers for Integrative Medicine. Dr. Lumpkin is the author of 180 scientific articles, book chapters, and abstracts.

Michael Lyon, BSc, MD, is Medical and Research Director for the Canadian Center for Functional Medicine located in Coquitlam, BC. He heads up a team of clinicians and researchers dedicated to biotechnology and natural health product research. He is involved in collaborative clinical research with the University of Toronto and the Imperial College of Medicine in London, England in the field of obesity, diabetes, and appetite regulation; and with the University of British Columbia in the area of childhood learning and behavioral disorders. Dr. Lyon served as an Olympics team physician (1988-1992) and was also head of a National Sport Science Committee for Sport Canada. He has a long-standing interest in toxicology and he has lectured frequently on the subject. He is the author of *Healing the Hyperactive Brain through the New Science of Functional Medicine* (Focused Publishing, 2000), and co-author of *Is Your Child's Brain Starving?* (Mind Publishing, 2002), and *How to Prevent and Treat Diabetes with Natural Medicine* (Riverhead Books, 2003).

Woody R. McGinnis, MD, was educated at Dartmouth College and the University of Colorado. After volunteer medical work in rural Peru, he practiced general medicine in Arizona for many years. In 1993, Dr. McGinnis began studying nutritional influences on behavior. Nutritional treatment of autism and other behavioral disorders became the primary focus of his practice. In 2001, Dr. McGinnis committed to full-time research in behavioral nutrition. He initiated and coordinates the Oxidative Stress in Autism Study, a first-of-its-kind university collaboration measuring a broad range of oxidative markers in the urine, blood, and central nervous system of children with autism. The urinary Mauve Factor is an area of special interest for McGinnis, who proposes that Mauve is a biomarker for oxidative stress. He resides in Ashland, Oregon, with his wife, Julia, and two sons. To balance his work, he reads, plays frisbee, does yoga, picks blueberries and generally strives to exemplify a healthful, low-oxidizing lifestyle.

Carolyn McMakin, MA, DC, is the clinical director of Integrated Pain Solutions and the Fibromyalgia and Myofascial Pain Clinic in Portland, Oregon. In addition to maintaining an active clinical practice, she teaches seminars on the use of Frequency Specific Microcurrent. She has lectured at the National Institutes of Health and at numerous conferences in the U.S., England, Canada and Australia on the subjects of fibromyalgia, and fibromyalgia associated with cervical trauma; and on the differential diagnosis and treatment of pain and pain syndromes, and sports injuries.

David Musnick, MD, is board certified in internal medicine and sports medicine with 16 years of experience. He practices in Bellevue, Washington at the Comprehensive Medical Center, an integrative medical center. His practice focuses on orthopedic and sports medicine, pain management, and functional internal medicine. An expert in exercise prescription, Dr. Musnick is the author of *Conditioning for Outdoor Fitness: Functional Exercise and Nutrition for Every Body* (The Mountaineers Books, 2004). He teaches seminars on Exercise Prescription, Orthopedic Medicine and Pain Management. Dr. Musnick is on the faculty at the University of Washington, Dept. of Sports Medicine and Orthopedics, and was the instructor of Orthopedic Medicine and Sports Medicine for five years at Bastyr University. He serves on the CME Advisory Committee for The Institute for Functional Medicine.

Joseph E. Pizzorno Jr., ND, is a leading authority on science-based natural medicine. A physician, educator, researcher, and expert spokesperson, Dr. Pizzorno was the Founding President (now Emeritus) of Bastyr University. He is also President of SaluGenecists, Inc. In 1996, he was appointed to the Seattle/King County Board of Health and the founding board of directors of the American Herbal Pharmacopoeia. In 2002, he became the founding editor of *Integrative Medicine: A Clinician's Journal*. Dr. Pizzorno was appointed by President Clinton in December 2000 to the White House Commission on Complementary and Alternative Medicine Policy and, in November 2002, was appointed by President Bush's administration to the Medicare Coverage Advisory Committee. In 2002, he was awarded "Naturopathic Physician of the Year" by the American Association of Naturopathic Physicians; in 2003, the American Holistic Medical Association recognized him as a "Pioneer in Holistic Medicine"; and in 2004, The Institute for Functional Medicine honored him with the Linus Pauling Award. Dr. Pizzorno is the author of *Total Wellness* and co-author of *A Textbook of Natural Medicine, Handbook of Natural Medicine, Encyclopedia of Natural Medicine, Natural Medicine for the Prevention and Treatment of Cancer*, and *The Encyclopedia of Healing Foods* (Atria Books, 2005).

Lara Pizzorno, MA Div, MA Lit, LMT, was among the first 10 women to graduate from Yale Divinity School with a Masters in Divinity in 1973. She earned her second Masters in Literature from the University of Washington and is also a Licensed Massage Therapist. A member of the American Medical Writers Association with more than 25 years of experience writing and editing articles, books, and website content for physicians and the public, Lara is employed as Senior Medical Editor for SaluGenecists, Inc., in Seattle. Her favorite responsibility is reviewing and summarizing the nutrition-related research each month to update The World's Healthiest Foods, a non-profit website created by SaluGenecists for the George Mateljan Foundation. Lara has attended all but one of the IFM symposia and is an AFMCP graduate. She is a contributing author to the *Textbook of Natural Medicine* (Churchill Livingstone, 3rd ed. 2005), lead author of *Natural Medicine Instructions for Patients* (Churchill Livingstone, 2002), and a co-author of *The Encyclopedia of Healing Foods* (Atria Books, 2005).

James O. Prochaska, PhD, is Director of the Cancer Prevention Research Center and Professor of Clinical and Health Psychology at the University of Rhode Island. He is the author of over 250 publications, including three books, *Changing for Good, Systems of Psychotherapy* and *The Transtheoretical Approach.* He is internationally recognized for this work as a developer of the stage model of behavior change. He is the principal investigator for over $70 million in research grants for the prevention of cancer and other chronic diseases. Dr. Prochaska has won numerous awards including the Top Five Most Cited Authors in Psychology from the American Psychology Society; an Innovator's Award from the Robert Wood Johnson Foundation and he is the first psychologist to win a Medal of Honor for Clinical Research from the American Cancer Society.

Janice M. Prochaska, MSW, PhD, is President and CEO of Pro-Change Behavior Systems, Inc. and an adjunct professor in the Department of Human Development and Family Studies at the University of Rhode Island. Her business is dedicated to the scientific development and dissemination of Transtheoretical Model-based change management programs. Through Small Business Innovation research grants from the National Institutes of Health, her company's LifeStyle management programs for depression management, regular exercise, stress management, and weight management are being disseminated through health insurance companies and employers. In addition, through an alliance with the Channing Bete Company, Pro-Change is developing effectiveness tested programs for elementary, middle, and high schools that include obesity prevention, bullying prevention, and substance abuse prevention.

Sheila Quinn, BS, has worked in health-related nonprofit organizations for more than 30 years, and in the healthcare arena itself for more than 45 years. Following twelve years as Co-founder and Vice President at Bastyr University and seven years as Executive Director of the American Association of Naturopathic Physicians, she became Senior Editor at IFM in late 2000. She has co-authored and edited many reports and publications, and was Managing Editor for IFM's *Clinical Nutrition: A Functional Approach*, 2nd edition (2004). She helped to organize the Seattle Town Hall Meeting for the White House Commission on CAM Policy in October 2000. She served on the Steering Committee for the 2001 *National Policy Dialogue to Advance Integrated Health Care: Finding Common Ground* (and co-edited the final report). She is currently Board Chair and member of both the Executive Committee and the Education Task Force for the Integrated Healthcare Policy Consortium. Through her decades of work both inside and outside the healthcare mainstream, she has become knowledgeable about health-related public policy issues and is committed to helping create a safe and effective integrated healthcare system. She attended Reed College, Stanford University, and received a BS in accounting from City University.

Robert Rountree, MD, received his medical degree from the University of North Carolina School of Medicine at Chapel Hill in 1980. He subsequently completed a residency in family and community medicine at the Milton S. Hershey Medical Center in Hershey, PA, after which he was certified by the American Board of Family Practice. He is a diplomate of the American Board of Holistic Medicine and has augmented his training with postgraduate studies in nutritional and herbal pharmacology and certification as a master practitioner of Neuro-Linguistic Programming. Dr. Rountree has provided his unique combination of traditional family medicine, nutrition, herbology, and mind-body therapy in Boulder, CO since 1983. He is co-author of three books on Integrative Medicine, *Immunotics: A Revolutionary Way to Fight Infection, Beat Chronic Illness and Stay Well* (Putnam, 2000), *Smart Medicine for a Healthier Child* (Avery Publishing, 1994) and *A Parent's Guide to Medical Emergencies* (Avery, 1997). Dr. Rountree is an adjunct faculty member at The Institute for Functional Medicine, and serves on the advisory board for the Herb Research Foundation and on the editorial boards of *The Journal of Alternative and Complementary Medicine, Alternative and Complementary Therapies*, and *Delicious! Living Magazine*.

Barb Schiltz, RN, MS, CN, has been a registered nurse for 40 years with an undergraduate degree in Foods and Nutrition and a Master's Degree in Nutrition from Bastyr University. Since 1996, she has been working as a nutrition consultant and research nurse at The Functional Medicine Research Center (FMRC) in Gig Harbor, WA, monitoring patients undergoing clinical trials for irritable bowel disease, fibromyalgia, diabetes, ADHD, and PMS. Her passion was expressed in her Master's Thesis, *The Unique Role of Carbohydrate Metabolism in Regulation of Glycemic Index*.

Virginia Shapiro, DC, DACBN, has practiced functional medicine as a chiropractor since 1985. She earned her bachelor's degree in biology at Carleton College in 1977, and her doctor of chiropractic degree at Northwestern University of Health Sciences in Minneapolis in 1985. In 1996 she completed her board certification in clinical nutrition by the American Chiropractic Board of Clinical Nutrition. A student of clinical nutrition and natural health care approaches, she has continued intensive postgraduate studies with a number of the most prominent holistic practitioners in the U.S. and the U.K. She has lectured to clinicians regarding clinical nutrition, essential fatty acid biology, nutrition in cardiovascular health, nutrition in mood and behavioral disorders, and applying functional medicine to women's hormonal health. Her successful functional medicine practice, Northland Health and Wellness in Duluth, Minnesota, provides comprehensive medical, nutritional, and chiropractic services in a joyful, compassionate, and healing environment.

Michael Stone, MD, MS, is a board certified family physician who practices in Ashland, Oregon with Leslie Stone, MD, and David Jones, MD. He has experience in rural and frontier family medicine, emergency medicine, and as a hospitalist. His undergraduate and graduate degrees are in human nutrition. He graduated from the University of Washington, and did his residency training in family practice at UCLA-Ventura, where he was chief resident, and also completed a teaching fellowship in family medicine. Dr. Stone has been an adjunct faculty at UCLA and University of Washington for primary care students in the Doctoring and RUOP programs. His career has offered him medical experiences and practice in Thailand, Alaska, eastern Sierras, Idaho, and Oregon. His interests and lectures have covered a wide range of topics, including bezoars to neonatal hypocalcemia, health issues with depleted uranium, exposure to Vitamin D and chronic disease.

Nancy Sudak, MD, completed her medical education at Case Western Reserve University in 1989, and received her residency training in family practice in Duluth, Minnesota in 1992. Board certified in both family practice and holistic medicine, she is currently in private practice in an integrated chiropractic-medical clinic in Duluth. She is a clinical instructor for the University of Minnesota School of Medicine, an active board member of the American Board of Holistic Medicine, and an editorial board member for *Integrative Medicine: A Clinician's Journal*. She attended the inaugural Applying Functional Medicine in Clinical Practice course by The Institute for Functional Medicine in 1998, which facilitated a comprehensive revitalization of her practice. She is an enthusiastic community speaker on various health-related topics.

Thomas Sult, MD, practices family and functional medicine in St. Cloud, MN. He utilizes a full range of diagnostic and therapeutic interventions ranging from ultra-fast CT and genomic testing, to lifestyle counseling and meditation. Dr. Sult is an Assistant Clinical Professor of Medicine at the Department of Family and Community Medicine, University of MN, and an instructor for the Rural Health School of Medicine, a cooperative educational outreach program of the University of MN. He is also the Medical Director of A Chance to Grow, a multidisciplinary rehabilitation clinic for brain-injured children, in Minneapolis. Dr. Sult is board certified in family medicine and holistic medicine. He is a Fellow of the American Academy of Family Medicine and a graduate of Applying Functional Medicine in Clinical Practice. While spending two years at St. Georges School of Medicine in Grenada, West Indies, he was introduced to the herbal and shamanistic customs of the Grenadian "bush doctor." Upon transfer to UCLA School of Medicine, Dr. Sult was introduced to Dr. Norman Cousins and the Division of Psychoneuroimmunology. Dr. Cousins became a close mentor to Dr. Sult and helped him form an understanding of the healing techniques he had witnessed in Grenada.

John M. Tatum, MD, is Founder and Medical Director of Optimal Health & Learning Center in Winter Park,

Florida. Dr. Tatum completed his medical degree at the Medical College of Georgia and his specialty training in psychiatry at the Shepard and Enoch Pratt Hospital in Baltimore, MD. He specializes in functional medicine, wellness, psychiatry, psychotherapy, microcurrent therapy, ADHD, learning disabilities, relationship therapy, and personal growth. He uses quantitative electroencephalograms, neurofeedback, and Tomatis Listening Therapy. He was the first to introduce and write about the synergy of combining Tomatis sound stimulation with simultaneous learning disability remediation. Although the field of psychotherapy focuses mostly on cognitive behavioral therapy, Dr. Tatum believes it is what is programmed into the deeper unconscious that causes most people their repetitive psychological problems, and this can be accessed through the body's subtle energy system. He has developed techniques for integrating bioenergetics into psychotherapy and has written and lectured on this at a national level. By using this multimodality approach and allying with the body's powerful forces for healing and growth, people can achieve levels of healing and growth not possible with a medication-only model.

Alex Vasquez, DC, ND, completed his undergraduate work in human biology by studying disorders of iron metabolism, and later published some of his findings in *Nutritional Perspectives* and *Arthritis & Rheumatism.* He graduated from Western States Chiropractic College with his Doctor of Chiropractic degree before attending Bastyr University, where he received his Doctor of Naturopathic Medicine degree. While maintaining a private practice in Seattle, Dr. Vasquez served as Adjunct Professor of Orthopedics, Rheumatology, and Radiographic Interpretation at Bastyr University, and he began work on his 486-page textbook, *Integrative Orthopedics: The Art of Creating Wellness While Effectively Managing Musculoskeletal Disorders* (Natural Health Consulting Corp., 2004). Dr. Vasquez has lectured nationally and internationally to professional audiences, and his articles and letters have been published by *Journal of the American Medical Association, British Medical Journal, The Lancet, Alternative Therapies in Health and Medicine,* and many other peer-reviewed medical journals.

David Wickes, DC, is Executive Vice President and Provost at the Western States Chiropractic College in Portland, Oregon. He graduated in 1977 from the National College of Chiropractic (NCC) and completed a two-year residency in chiropractic family practice. He chaired the Department of Diagnosis at NCC from 1980-1991, then he subsequently served as the Director of the Inpatient Facility, the Director of the Training and Assessment Center, the Dean of Clinics, the Vice President for Academic Affairs, and the Senior Vice President and Provost. He is board certified in diagnosis and internal disorders, and has been an adjunct faculty member of The Institute for Functional Medicine. He has lectured nationally and internationally on the diagnosis and management of chronic disorders.

Catherine Willner, MD, is a practicing neurologist in Durango, Colorado. She received her formal training in Neurology at the Mayo Clinic including subspecialty training in autonomic, peripheral neurology as well as pain management. She remained on staff at the Mayo Clinic until 1997, at which time she relocated to Colorado to focus her practice on functional neurology. She is board certified in neurology and in pain management. Prior to pursuing her MD degree, Dr. Willner was enrolled briefly in the National College of Naturopathic Medicine when the program was in Kansas. Her interest in biochemical individuality, nutritional biochemistry and functional medicine, though somewhat on hold during the Mayo years, is currently thriving in Durango. She is an adjunct faculty member of The Institute for Functional Medicine, and created a clinical module in Functional Neurology for IFM.

Comprehensive Elimination Diet—Sample Patient Handouts

Introduction

The Comprehensive Elimination Diet is a dietary program designed to clear the body of foods and chemicals you may be allergic or sensitive to, and, at the same time, improve your body's ability to handle and dispose of these substances.

We have called this an "Elimination Diet" because we will be asking you to remove certain foods, and food categories, from your diet. The main rationale behind the diet is that these modifications allow your body's detoxification machinery, which may be overburdened or compromised, to recover and begin to function efficiently again. The dietary changes help the body eliminate or "clear" various toxins that may have accumulated due to environmental exposure, foods, beverages, drugs, alcohol, or cigarette smoking.

In our experience, this process is generally well tolerated and extremely beneficial. We obviously hope that you will find it useful too. There is really no "typical" or "normal" response. A person's initial response to any new diet is highly variable, and this diet is no exception. This can be attributed to physiological, mental, and biochemical differences among individuals; the degree of exposure to, and type of "toxin"; and other lifestyle factors. Most often, individuals on the elimination diet report increased energy, mental alertness, decrease in muscle or joint pain, and a general sense of improved well-being. However, some people report initial reactions to the diet, especially in the first week, as their bodies adjust to a different dietary program. Symptoms you may experience in the first week or so can include changes in sleep patterns, lightheadedness, headaches, joint or muscle stiffness, and changes in gastrointestinal function. Such symptoms rarely last for more than a few days.

We realize that changing food habits can be a complex, difficult and sometimes confusing process. It doesn't have to be, and we think that we have simplified the process with information to make it a "do-able" process. Peruse this information carefully.

Bon appétit!

Guidelines

Three tables are included with these materials:

- Table 1—Foods to Include and Exclude. Eat only the foods listed under "Foods to Include," and avoid those foods shown under "Foods to Exclude." If you have a question about a particular food, check to see if it is on the food list. You should, of course, avoid any foods (listed or not) to which you know you are intolerant or allergic. Some of these guidelines may change based upon your personal health condition and history.
- Table 2—Shopping List
- Table 3—Food Reintroduction Chart

A few suggestions that may be of help:

- You may use leftovers for the next day's meal or part of a meal, e.g., leftover broiled salmon and broccoli from dinner as part of a large salad for lunch the next day.
- It may be helpful to cook extra chicken, sweet potatoes, rice, and beans, etc. that can be reheated for snacking or another meal.
- If you are consuming coffee or other caffeine-containing beverages on a regular basis, it is always wise to slowly reduce your caffeine intake rather than abruptly stop it; this will prevent caffeine-withdrawal headaches. For instance, try drinking half decaf/half regular coffee for a few days, then slowly reduce the total amount of coffee.
- Select fresh foods whenever you can. If possible, choose organically grown fruits and vegetables to eliminate pesticide and chemical residue consumption. Wash fruits and vegetables thoroughly.
- Read oil labels; use only those that are obtained by a "cold pressed" method.
- If you select animal sources of protein, look for free-range or organically raised chicken, turkey, or lamb. Trim visible fat and prepare by broiling, baking, stewing, grilling, or stir-frying. Cold-water fish (e.g., salmon, mackerel, and halibut) is another excellent source of protein and the omega-3 essential fatty acids, which are important nutrients in this diet.
- Remember to drink at least two quarts of plain, filtered water each day.

- Strenuous or prolonged exercise may be reduced during portions of this program (or even during the entire program) to allow the body to heal more effectively without the additional burden imposed by exercise. Adequate rest and stress reduction are also important to the success of this program.

Finally, anytime you change your diet significantly, you may experience such symptoms as fatigue, headache, or muscle aches for a few days. Your body needs time as it is "withdrawing" from the foods you eat on a daily basis. Your body may crave some foods it is used to consuming. **Persevere**. Those symptoms generally don't last long, and most people feel much better over the next couple of weeks.

Table 1. **Typical Foods to Include and Exclude on an Elimination Diet Program**

	Include	Exclude
Fruits	Whole fruits, unsweetened, frozen or water-packed, canned fruits and diluted juices	Oranges and orange juice
Dairy and dairy substitutes	Rice, oat, and nut milks such as almond milk and coconut milk	Dairy and eggs: milk, cheese, eggs, cottage cheese, cream, yogurt, butter, ice cream, frozen yogurt, non-dairy creamers
Grains and starch	Brown rice, oats, millet, quinoa, amaranth, teff, tapioca buckwheat, potato flour	Grains: corn and non-gluten grains: wheat, barley, spelt, kamut, rye, triticale
Animal protein	Fresh or water-packed fish, wild game, lamb, duck, organic chicken and turkey	Pork, beef/veal, sausage, cold cuts, canned meats, frankfurters, shellfish
Vegetable protein	Split peas, lentils, and all dried beans other than soybeans	Soybean products (soy sauce, soybean oil in processed foods; tempeh, tofu, soy milk, soy yogurt, textured vegetable protein)
Nuts and seeds	Sesame, pumpkin, and sunflower seeds, walnuts, hazelnuts, pecans, almonds, cashews, nut butters such as almond or tahini	Peanuts and peanut butter
Vegetables	All raw, steamed, sautéed, juiced or roasted vegetables	Corn, creamed vegetables
Oils	Cold-pressed olive, flax, walnut, safflower, grapeseed, sesame, almond, sunflower, canola, pumpkin, and coconut oils	Butter, margarine, shortening, processed oils, salad dressings, mayonnaise, and spreads
Drinks	Filtered or distilled water, non-caffeinated herbal teas, seltzer or mineral water	Alcohol, coffee and other caffeinated beverages, soda pop or soft drinks
Sweeteners	Brown rice syrup, agave nectar, stevia, fruit sweeteners, blackstrap molasses	Refined sugar, white/brown sugars, honey, maple syrup, high fructose corn syrup, evaporated cane juice, sucanat
Condiments	Vinegar, all spices, including salt, pepper, basil, carob, cinnamon, cumin, dill, garlic, ginger, mustard, oregano, parsley, rosemary, tarragon, thyme, turmeric	Chocolate, ketchup, relish, chutney, soy sauce, barbecue sauce, teriyaki, and other condiments

Read Ingredient Labels Carefully! Things to watch for:
- Corn starch in baking powder and any processed foods.
- Corn syrup in beverages and processed foods.
- Vinegar in ketchup, mayonnaise and mustard is usually from wheat or corn.
- Breads advertised as gluten-free may contain spelt, kamut, rye.
- Many amaranth and millet flake cereals have corn.
- Many canned tunas contain textured vegetable protein, which is from soy.
- Look for low-salt versions which tend to be pure tuna, with no fillers.
- Multi-grain rice cakes may not be just rice. Purchase plain rice cakes.

Table 2. **Sample Shopping List for Use with an Elimination Diet**

Fruits

Apples, applesauce
Apricots (fresh)
Bananas
Blackberries
Blueberries
Cantaloupe
Cherries
Coconut
Figs (fresh)
Grapefruit
Huckleberries
Kiwi
Kumquat
Lemon, lime
Loganberries
Mangos
Melons
Mulberries
Nectarines
Papayas
Peaches
Pears
Prunes
Raspberries
Strawberries
All the above fruits can be consumed raw or juiced.

Vegetables

Artichoke
Asparagus
Avocado
Bamboo shoots
Beets & beet tops
Bok choy
Broccoflower
Broccoli
Brussels sprouts
Cabbage
Bell peppers
Carrots
Cauliflower
Celery
Chives
Cucumber
Dandelion greens
Eggplant
Endive
Kale
Kohlrabi
Leeks
Lettuce (red or green leaf; Chinese)
Mushroom
Okra
Onions
Pak-Choi
Parsley
Potato
Red leaf chicory
Sea vegetables—seaweed, kelp
Snow peas
Spinach
Squash
Sweet potato & yams
Swiss chard
Tomato
Watercress
Zucchini
All the above vegetables can be consumed raw, juiced, steamed, sautéed, or baked.

Beans

All beans except soy
Lentils—brown, green, red
Split peas
All the above beans can be dried or canned.

Nuts & Seeds

Almonds
Cashews
Flax seeds
Hazelnuts (Filberts)
Pecans
Pistachios
Poppy seeds
Pumpkin seeds
Sesame seeds
Sunflower seeds
Walnuts
All the above seeds can be consumed as butters and spreads (e.g., tahini).

Non-Gluten Grains

Amaranth
Millet
Oat
Quinoa
Rice—brown, white, wild
Teff
Buckwheat

Vinegars

Apple cider
Balsamic
Red wine
Rice
Tarragon
Ume plum

Herbs, Spices & Extracts

Basil
Black pepper
Cinnamon
Cumin
Dandelion
Dill
Dry mustard
Garlic
Ginger
Nutmeg
Oregano
Parsley
Rosemary
Salt-free herbal blends
Sea salt
Tarragon
Thyme
Turmeric
Pure vanilla extract

Cereals & Pasta

Cream of rice
Oats
Puffed rice
Puffed millet
Quinoa flakes
Rice pasta
100% buckwheat noodles
Rice crackers and rice cakes

Breads & Baking

Arrowroot
Baking soda
Rice bran
Gluten free breads
Flours: rice, teff, quinoa, millet, tapioca, amaranth, garbanzo bean, potato, tapioca, oat, buckwheat
Rice flour pancake mix
Mochi

Flesh Foods

Free-range chicken, turkey, duck
Fresh ocean fish, e.g., Pacific salmon, halibut, haddock, cod, sole, pollock, tuna, mahi-mahi
Lamb
Water-packed canned tuna (watch for added protein from soy)
Wild game

Dairy Substitutes

Almond milk
Rice milk
Coconut milk
Oat milk

Beverages

Herbal tea (non-caffeinated)
Mineral water
Pure unsweetened fruit or vegetable juices
Spring water

Oils

Almond
Flax seed
Canola
Grapeseed
Olive
Pumpkin
Safflower
Sesame
Sunflower
Walnut

Sweeteners

Fruit sweetener (Mystic Lake Dairy, or Wax Orchards, or apple juice concentrate)
Agave nectar
Molasses, blackstrap only
Rice syrup
Stevia

Condiments

Mustard (made with apple cider vinegar)
Nutritional yeast

Table 3. **Sample Food Reintroduction Tracking Form**

Date or Day	Food		Digestion/ Bowel Function	Joint/ Muscle Aches	Headache Pressure	Nasal or Chest Congestion	Kidney- Bladder Skin Function	Energy Level
	Time	Food						

Note: Please reintroduce only one new food at a time. Ingest it 2–3 times in the same day, and then assess your response over the next 48 hours. Wait two full days to see whether you have a reaction. You may insert different headings on this chart to correspond with whatever signs or symptoms you experience. Important indicators that must be charted include: digestion, bowel function, and energy level. If you require more space, use the back of this sheet and clearly mark the day, the food, and your symptoms. If you are unsure whether you had a reaction, retest the same food in the same manner (after the two-day waiting period).

Cytochrome P450 Enzymes: Drug and Natural Product Substrates, Inhibitors, and Inducers

Cytochrome P450 1A2				
Drug Substrate		**Natural Substrate**	**Inhibitors**	**Inducers**
Acetaminophen	Riluzole	Cabbage	Amiodarone	Carbamazepine
Amitriptyline—Elavil	Ropinirole	Ginkgo leaf	Cimetidine	Charbroiled food
Caffeine	Ropivacaine	Grapefruit skin	Ciprofloxacin	Cruciferous vegetables
Chlordiazepoxide	Tacrine: Cognex	Indole-3-carbinol	Citalopram	Lansoprazole
Clomipramine—Anafranil	Theophylline—Theo-Dur	Ipriflavone	Clarithromycin	Omeprazole
Clopidogrel—Plavix	Verapamil—Calan	Nutmeg	Diltiazem	Phenobarbital
Clozapine—Clozaril	R-warfarin	Mace	Enoxacin	Phenytoin
Cyclobenzaprine— Flexeril	Zileuton—Zyflo	Ipriflavone	Erythromycin	Primidone
Desipramine—Norpramin	Zolmitriptan—Zomig	St. John's Wort	Acetaminophen	Rosemary
Diazepam—Valium			Fluvoxamine	Rifampin
Estradiol—Estrace			Hops	Ritonavir
Flutamide			Isoniazid	Smoking
Fluvoxamine—Luvox			Ketoconazole	St. John's Wort
Haloperidol—Haldol			Methoxsalen	
Imipramine—Tofranil			Mexiletine	
Levobupivacaine			Nalidixic acid	
Mexiletine—Mexitil			Norethindrone	
Mirtazapine—Remeron			Norfloxacin	
Naproxen			Omeprazole	
Nortriptyline			Oral contraceptives	
Olanzapine—Zyprexa			Paroxetine	
Ondansetron—Zofran			Tacrine	
Pentazocine—Talwin			Ticlopidine	
Propafenone			Troleandomycin	
Propranolol—Inderal			Zileuton	

Cytochrome P450 2C9				
Drug Substrate		**Natural Substrate**	**Inhibitors**	**Inducers**
Amitriptyline—Elavil	Omeprazole	Ipriflavone	Amiodarone	Aprepitant
Carvedilol	Ondansetron—Zofran	St. John's Wort	Chloramphenicol	Carbamazepine
Celecoxib	Phenytoin		Cimetidine	Phenobarbital
Clomipramine—Anafranil	Piroxicam		Clopidogrel	Primidone
Clopidogrel—Plavix	Rosiglitazone		Cotrimoxazole	Rifampin
Clozapine—Clozaril	Sildenafil		Delavirdine	Rifapentine
Desogestrel	Sulfamethoxazole		Disulfiram	
Diazepam—Valium	Tacrine—Cognex		Efavirenz	
Diclofenac	Tolbutamide		Fenofibrate	
Dronabinol	Torsemide		Fluconazole	
Estradiol (Estrace)	Valdecoxib		Fluorouracil	
Fluoxetine—Prozac	Valsartan		Fluoxetine	
Flurbiprofen	Verapamil— Calan		Fluvastatin	
Fluvastatin—Lescol	Voriconazole		Fluvoxamine	
Formoterol	S—Warfarin—Coumadin		Gemfibrozil	
Glimepiride	Zafirlukast		Imatinib	
Glipizide	Zileuton-Zyflo		Isoniazid	
Glyburide			Itraconazole	
Grepafloxacin—Raxar			Ketoconazole	
Ibuprofen			Leflunomide	
Imipramine—Tofranil			Lovastatin	
Indomethacin			Metronidazole	
Irbesartan			Milk Thistle	
Losartan—Cozaar			Modafinil	
Mefenamic acid			Omeprazole	
Meloxicam			Paroxetine	
Mirtazapine—Remeron			Sertraline	
Montelukast			Sulfonamides	
Naproxen			Ticlopidine	
Nateglinide			Voriconazole	
			Zafirlukast	

Cytochrome P450 2C19				
Drug Substrate		Natural Substrate	Inhibitors	Inducers
Amitriptyline—Elavil	Phenytoin		Citalopram	Carbamazepine
Carisoprodol	Progesterone		Delavirdine	Norethindrone
Cilostazol	Proguanil		Efavirenz	Phenobarbital
Citalopram	Propranolol—Inderal		Felbamate	Phenytoin
Clomipramine—Anafranil	Rabeprazole		Fluconazole	Prednisone
Cyclophosphamide	Teniposide		Fluoxetine	Rifampin
Desipramine—Norpramin	Thioridazine		Fluvastatin	
Diazepam—Valium	Tolbutamide		Fluvoxamine	
Esomeprazole	Voriconazole		Indomethacin	
Formoterol	R-warfarin		Isoniazid	
Hexobarbital			Ketoconazole	
Imipramine—Tofranil			Letrozole	
Indomethacin			Modafinil	
Lansoprazole—Prevacid			Omeprazole	
Mephobarbital			Oxcarbazepine	
Moclobemide			Paroxetine	
Nelfinavir			Sertraline	
Nilutamide			Telmisartan	
Omeprazole			Ticlopidine	
Pantoprazole			Topiramate	
Pentamidine			Voriconazole	

Cytochrome P450 2D6				
Drug Substrate		**Natural Substrate**	**Inhibitors**	**Inducers**
Amitriptyline—Elavil	Meperidine	Ginkgo leaf	Amiodarone	Carbamazepine
Amphetamine	Methadone	Ginseng, Panax	Bupropion	Ethanol
Atomoxetine	Methamphetamine	St. John's Wort	Celecoxib	Phenobarbital
Bisoprolol	Methoxyamphetamine		Chloroquine	Phenytoin
Carvedilol	Metoprolol		Chlorpheniramine	Primidone
Cevimeline	Mexiletine—Mexitil		Cimetidine	Rifampin
Chlorpromazine	Mirtazapine—Remeron		Citalopram	Ritonavir
Chlorpropamide	Morphine		Clomipramine	St. John's Wort
Clomipramine—Anafranil	Nortriptyline		Cocaine	
Clozapine—Clozaril	Olanzapine		Desipramine	
Codeine	Ondansetron— Zofran		Diphenhydramine	
Cyclobenzaprine—Flexeril	Oxycodone		Fluoxetine	
Desipramine—Norpramin	Paroxetine		Fluphenazine	
Dexfenfluramine	Perphenazine		Halofantrine	
Dextromethorphan	Pindolol		Haloperidol	
Dolasetron	Propafenone		Hydroxychloroquine	
Donepezil—Aricept	Propoxyphene		Imatinib	
Doxepin	Propranolol—Inderal		Levomepromazine	
Encainide	Quetiapine		Methadone	
Fenfluramine	Risperidone		Moclobemide	
Fentanyl—Duragesic	Thioridazine		Norfluoxetine	
Flecainide	Tramadol		Paroxetine	
Fluoxetine—Prozac	Trazodone		Perphenazine	
Fluphenazine	Venlafaxine		Propafenone	
Fluvoxamine—Luvox			Propoxyphene	
Formoterol			Quinacrine	
Galantamine			Quinidine	
Haloperidol—Haldol			Ranitidine	
Hydrocodone			Ritonavir	
Imipramine—Tofranil			Sertraline	
Lidocaine			Terbinafine	
Maprotiline			Thioridazine	

Cytochrome P450 3A4				
Drug Substrate		**Natural Substrate**	**Inhibitors**	**Inducers**
Alfentanil	Dronabinol	American elder	Acitretin	Aminoglutethimide
Almotriptan	Dutasteride	Bishop's weed	Amiodarone	Acetaminophen
Alprazolam	Efavirenz	Bitter orange	Amprenavir	Carbamazepine
Amitriptyline—Elavil	Ergotamine	Cat's claw	Aprepitant	Dexamethasone
Amiodarone	Erythromycin	Chamomile	Cimetidine	Efavirenz
Amlodipine	Esomeprazole	DHEA	Ciprofloxacin	Ethosuximide
Amprenavir	Estrogens, contraceptives	Echinacea	Clarithromycin	Garlic
Aprepitant	Ethinyl estradiol	Elder root	Cyclosporine	Glucocorticoids
Atorvastatin	Ethosuximide	Garlic	Danazol	Glutethimide
Bepridil	Etonogestrel	Ginkgo leaf extract	Delavirdine	Griseofulvin
Bexarotene	Etoposide	Goldenseal	Diltiazem	Modafinil
Bromocriptine	Exemestane	Licorice	Diethyl-dithiocarbamate	Nafcillin
Budesonide	Felodipine	Milk thistle	Efavirenz	Nevirapine
Buprenorphine	Fentanyl—Duragesic	Red clover	Eleuthera	Oxcarbazepine
Buspirone	Fexofenadine	Red yeast	Erythromycin	Phenobarbital
Busulfan	Finasteride	Saw palmetto	Acetaminophen	Phenytoin
Cannabinoids	Flutamide	St. John's wort	Fluconazole	Primidone
Caffeine	Fluticasone	Valerian	Fluoxetine	Rifabutin
Carbamazepine	Fulvestrant	Wild cherry bark	Fluvoxamine	Rifampin
Cevimeline	Galantamine		Gestodene	Rifapentine
Chlorpheniramine	Haloperidol—Haldol		Grapefruit	St. John's Wort
Cilostazol	Hydrocodone		Indinavir	
Cisapride	Hydrocortisone		Imatinib	
Citalopram	Ifosfamide		Isoniazid	
Clarithromycin	Imatinib		Itraconazole	
Clindamycin	Imipramine—Tofranil		Ketoconazole	
Clomipramine—Anafranil	Indinavir		Metronidazole	
Clonazepam	Isradipine		Methylprednisone	
Clopidogrel—Plavix	Itraconazole		Miconazole	
Cocaine	Ketoconazole		Mifepristone	
Cyclobenzaprine—Flexeril	Lansoprazole—Prevacid		Milk Thistle	
Cyclophosphamide	Letrozole		Nefazodone	
Cyclosporine	Levobupivacaine		Nelfinavir	
Dapsone	Lidocaine		Nicardipine	
Delavirdine	Lopinavir Loratadine		Nifedipine	
Desogestrel	Losartan—Cozaar		Norethindrone	
Dexamethasone	Lovastatin		Norfloxacin	
Dextromethorphan	Methadone		Norfluoxetine	
Diazepam—Valium	Methylprednisolone		Oxiconazole	
Dihydroergotamine	Miconazole		Prednisone	
Diltiazem	Midazolam		Quinine	
Disopyramide	Mifepristone		Ritonavir	
Docetaxel	Mirtazapine—Remeron		Roxithromycin	
Dofetilide	Modafinil		Saquinavir	
Dolasetron	Mometasone		Sertraline	
Donepezil—Aricept	Montelukast		Synercid	
Doxorubicin				

Cytochrome P450 3A4 (Continued)				
Drug Substrate		Natural Substrate	Inhibitors	Inducers
Nateglinide	Salmeterol		Troleandomycin	
Nefazodone	Saquinavir		Verapamil	
Nelfinavir	Sertraline		Voriconazole	
Nevirapine	Sibutramine		Zafirlukast	
Nicardipine	Sildenafil		Zileuton	
Nifedipine	Simvastatin			
Nimodipine	Sirolimus			
Nisoldipine	Tacrolimus			
Nitrendipine	Tamoxifen			
Nortriptyline	Temazepam			
Norethindrone	Testosterone			
Omeprazole	Tiagabine			
Ondansetron—Zofran	Tolterodine			
Oral contraceptives	Toremifene			
Oxybutynin	Tramadol			
Paclitaxel	Trazodone			
Pantoprazole	Triazolam			
Pimozide	Trimetrexate			
Pioglitazone	Valdecoxib			
Prednisolone	Verapamil- Calan			
Prednisone	Vinblastine			
Progesterone/Progestins	Vincristine			
Quetiapine	Vinorelbine			
Quinidine	Voriconazole			
Quinine	R-warfarin			
Rabeprazole	Zaleplon			
Repaglinide	Zileuton-Zyflo			
Rifabutin	Ziprasidone			
Rifampin	Zolpidem			
Ritonavir	Zonisamide			

Detailed Review of Systems

General	Fever, weight loss, weight gain. Are you at the weight you want? How much time do you exercise per day _____, per week _____? Hours of sleep per night? Any problems with sleep?
Head	Headaches, migraine, trauma, vertigo, syncope, convulsive seizures.
Eyes	Visual loss or color blindness, diplopia, hemianopsia, trauma, inflammation, glasses (date of refraction). Cataracts, decreased vision or blindness at night.
Ears	Deafness, tinnitus, vertigo, discharge from the ears, pain, mastoiditis, operations. Sounds you have trouble hearing.
Nose	Coryza, rhinitis, sinusitis, discharge, obstruction, epistaxis, polyps, deviation of septum, operations.
Mouth	Soreness of the mouth or tongue, gingivitis, change in taste, tooth pain, aphthous ulcers.
Throat	Sore throats, tonsillitis, voice changes, hoarseness, polyps, difficulty swallowing.
Neck	Swelling, suppurative lesions, enlargement of the lymph nodes, goiter, stiffness, limitation of motion.
Breasts	Development, lactation, trauma, lumps, pains, discharge from nipples, gynecomastia, changes in nipples, soreness, previous biopsies.
Respiratory	Pain, shortness of breath, wheezing dyspnea, nocturnal dyspnea, orthopnea, cough, sputum, hemoptysis, night sweats, pleurisy, bronchitis, tuberculosis (history of contacts), pneumonia, asthma, other respiratory infections—coccidioidomycosis, histoplasmosis exposures.
Cardiovascular	Palpitation, tachycardia, irregularities of rhythm, pain in the chest, exertional dyspnea, paroxysmal nocturnal dyspnea, orthopnea, cough, cyanosis, ascites, edema. Intermittent claudication, cold extremities, phlebitis, postural or permanent skin color changes. Hypertension rheumatic fever, chorea, syphilis, diphtheria. When you exercise how fast do you get your heart rate? _____% Maximal predicted heart rate (220 - age = _____). Wheezing with exercise. Problems walking up a hill. Do you get short of breath or have chest pain when vacuuming, raking, or shoveling snow or dirt?
Gastrointestinal	Appetite, anorexia, dysphagia, nausea, eructations, flatulence, abdominal pain or colic, vomiting, hematemesis, jaundice (pain, fever, intensity, duration, color of urine and stools), stools (color, frequency, consistency, odor, gas, cathartics), hemorrhoids—internal/external. Change in bowel habits.
Genitourinary	Color of urine, polyuria, oliguria, nocturia, dysuria, hematuria, pyuria, urinary retention, urinary frequency, incontinence, pain or colic, passage of stones or gravel. Menstrual history: Age of onset, frequency of periods, regularity, duration, amount of flow, leukorrhea, dysmenorrhea, date of last normal and preceding periods, date and character of menopause, postmenopausal bleeding. Pregnancies: Number, abortions, miscarriages, stillbirths, chronologic sequence, complications of pregnancy. Venereal history: Chancre, bubo, penile or vaginal discharge. Treatment of venereal diseases. Sexual history: Age of onset of sexual relations, single partner or number of partners, libido, ability to orgasm, erectile dysfunction, sexual preference, satisfaction. Fertility issues?

Nervous system	Disturbances of smell (1), visual disturbances (2,3,4,6); orofacial paresthesias and difficulty in chewing (5); facial weakness and taste disturbances (7); disturbances in hearing and equilibrium (8); difficulties in speech, swallowing and taste (9,10,12); limitation in motion of neck (11). Motor system: Paralysis, atrophy, involuntary movements, convulsions, gait, incoordination Sensory system: Pain, lightning pain, girdle pain, paresthesia, hypesthesia, anesthesia. Autonomic system: Control of urination and defecation, sweating, erythema, cyanosis, pallor, reaction to heat and cold.
Mental status	Describe reactions to and influence of parents, siblings, spouse, children, friends and associates, sexual adjustments, successes and failures, illnesses. Lability of mood, hallucinations, grandiose ideas, sleep disturbances. How is your memory—short term, long term? Any memory frustrations?
Skin	Color, pigmentation, temperature, moisture, eruptions, pruritus, scaling, bruising, bleeding. Hair: Color, texture, abnormal loss or growth, distribution. Nails: Color changes, brittleness, ridging, pitting, curvature or white spots.
Lymph nodes	Enlargement, pain, suppuration, draining sinuses, location.
Bones, joints, muscles	Fractures, dislocations, sprains, arthritis, myositis, pain, swelling, stiffness, migratory distribution, degree of disability, muscular weakness, wasting, or atrophy. Night cramps.
Hematopoietic	Anemia (type, therapy, and response), lymphadenopathy, bleeding (spontaneous, traumatic, familial).
Endocrine	History of growth, body configuration and weight. Size of hands, feet, and head, especially changes during adulthood. Hair distribution, skin pigmentation, weakness, goiter, exophthalmos, dryness of skin and hair, intolerance to heat or cold, tremor. Polyphagia, polydipsia, polyuria, glycosuria. Secondary sex characteristics, impotence, sterility, treatment. Sun exposure/week.
Immunologic and allergy	Dermatitis, urticaria, angioneurotic edema, eczema, hay fever, vasomotor rhinitis, asthma, migraine, vernal conjunctivitis. Seasonal incidence of previous conditions. Known sensitivity to pollens, foods, danders, or drugs. Previous skin tests and their results. Results of tuberculin tests and others. Desensitization, vaccinations and immunizations. Lyme disease. Mold sensitivities. HIV exposures or concerns. Hepatitis exposures or concerns.

Adapted from Degowin EL and Degowin RL. Bedside Diagnostic Examination. 3rd Edition. Macmillan Publishing Co.,1975, p. 24-26.

Environmental Sensitivity Questionnaire

Are you bothered by:

	YES	NO		YES	NO		YES	NO
Gasoline fumes	❑	❑	Hair spray	❑	❑	Tobacco smoke	❑	❑
Diesel exhaust	❑	❑	Cosmetics	❑	❑	Cats	❑	❑
Smell of rubber	❑	❑	Perfume	❑	❑	Dogs	❑	❑
Soaps	❑	❑	Dust	❑	❑	Mold-indoor	❑	❑
Detergents	❑	❑	Fabric stores	❑	❑	Mold-outdoor	❑	❑
Chlorinated water	❑	❑	New car smell	❑	❑	Tree pollen	❑	❑
Moth balls	❑	❑	Air conditioners	❑	❑	Grass pollen	❑	❑
Asphalt/tar	❑	❑	Newsprint	❑	❑	Ragweed pollen	❑	❑

Do you have or use any of the following at/near home or work?

	Home	Work		Home	Work		Home	Work
Spring water	❑	❑	Kerosene space heater	❑	❑	Animals	❑	❑
Well water	❑	❑	Forced hot air heat	❑	❑	Exterminator	❑	❑
Water purifier	❑	❑	Electric blanket	❑	❑	Moth balls	❑	❑
Damp cellar	❑	❑	Feather pillow	❑	❑	Mold on:	❑	❑
Wooded area	❑	❑	Foam rubber pillow	❑	❑	Shower curtain	❑	❑
Swamp	❑	❑	Feather/down	❑	❑	Basement walls	❑	❑
Power lines	❑	❑	Comforter	❑	❑	First story walls	❑	❑
Microwave transmitter	❑	❑	Coat/Jacket	❑	❑	Second story walls	❑	❑
Smoke stacks	❑	❑	Stuffed upholstery	❑	❑	Garage under living space	❑	❑
Dump	❑	❑	Polyester blend in:	❑	❑	Urea formaldehyde	❑	❑
Gas stove	❑	❑	Sheets	❑	❑	Insulation	❑	❑
Gas furnace	❑	❑	Pillow cases	❑	❑	Other: ____________		
Gas hot water heater	❑	❑	Pajamas	❑	❑			
Gas dryer	❑	❑	Shirts	❑	❑	____________		
Wood stove	❑	❑	Skirts	❑	❑			
Coal stove	❑	❑	Pants	❑	❑	____________		

Please check appropriate selections about carpeting in your home:

	Bedroom		Family Room		Living Room		Bathroom	
	YES	NO	YES	NO	YES	NO	YES	NO
None	❑	❑	❑	❑	❑	❑	❑	❑
Area rugs	❑	❑	❑	❑	❑	❑	❑	❑
Wall-to-wall	❑	❑	❑	❑	❑	❑	❑	❑
Wool	❑	❑	❑	❑	❑	❑	❑	❑
Synthetic pad	❑	❑	❑	❑	❑	❑	❑	❑
Glued down	❑	❑	❑	❑	❑	❑	❑	❑
How old is carpeting?	❑	❑	❑	❑	❑	❑	❑	❑
On slab?	❑	❑	❑	❑	❑	❑	❑	❑
Ever damp or wet?	❑	❑	❑	❑	❑	❑	❑	❑
Moldy?	❑	❑	❑	❑	❑	❑	❑	❑
Linoleum?	❑	❑	❑	❑	❑	❑	❑	❑

Health Benefits of Exercise

System	Increases	Decreases
Cardiovascular	HDL cholesterol Cardiac output Fibrinolytic activity in Response to venous occlusion Increases arteriolar diameter	Serum triglycerides Heart rate CRP Incidence of cardiac arrest Coronary mortality Coronary artery occlusion Peripheral arteriolar resistance Blood pressure
Endocrine		
Diabetes	Improves glucose tolerance Concentration of insulin receptors	Insulin requirements
Hyperlipidemias	HDL cholesterol	Serum triglycerides
Metabolic rate	Increases Caloric expenditure Proportion of lean body mass	Proportion of fat Body weight
Mood	Endorphins	Depression scores
Respiratory disease	Exercise endurance Cognition Work tolerance VO2 max	Breathlessness
Skeletal	Bone retention Muscle mass Sleep Balance Muscle strength Coordination	Number of falls
Overall health	Mobility, strength, endurance Overall longevity	Chronic disease risk Desire for alcohol, smoking

Recommended Reading:

Boule NG, Kenny GP, Haddad E, et al. Meta-analysis of the effect of structured exercise training on cardiorespiratory fitness in Type 2 diabetes mellitus. Diabetologia. 2003 Aug;46(8):1071-1081.

Castaneda C, Gordon PL, Parker RC, et al. Resistance training to reduce the malnutrition-inflammation complex syndrome of chronic kidney disease. Am J Kidney Dis. 2004 Apr;43(4):607-616.

Craft LL, Perna FM. The benefits of exercise for the clinically depressed. Prim Care Companion J Clin Psychiatry. 2004;6(3):104-111.

Karlsson M. Does exercise reduce the burden of fractures? Acta Orthop Scand. 2002 Dec;73(6):691-705.

Nestle M. Exercise and Work Performance, Chapter 50, p. 271 in Nutrition in Clinical Practice. Jones Medical Publication. 1985.

Okura T, Nakata Y, Tanaka K. Effects of exercise intensity on physical fitness and risk factors for coronary heart disease. Obes Res. 2003 Sep;11(9):1131-1139.

Rochester CL. Exercise training in chronic obstructive pulmonary disease. J Rehabil Res Dev. 2003 Sep-Oct;40(5 Suppl 2):59-80.

Sato Y, Nagasaki M, Nakai N, et al. Physical exercise improves glucose metabolism in lifestyle-related diseases. Exp Biol Med (Maywood). 2003 Nov;228(10):1208-1212.

Seguin R, Nelson ME. The benefits of strength training for older adults. Am J Prev Med. 2003 Oct;25(3 Suppl 2):141-149.

Internet-based Resources for the Healthcare Practitioner

http://medicine.iupui.edu/flockhart/
This site provides a table that is designed as a hypothesis testing, teaching and reference tool for physicians and researchers interested in drug interactions that are the result of competition for, or effects on, the human cytochrome P450 system.

PDR net for physicians
http://www.pdr.net/pdrnet/librarian/
Database containing 15 full text journals, PDR drug book, PDR drug interactions book. Medical news is also posted, and Medline can be accessed. Free to some health professionals.

MD consult
http://www.mdconsult.com
A library of 48 full text journals, 36 books, medical news, and Medline access. Subscription. Free 10-day trial for physicians.

Medscape
http://www.medscape.com/px/splash
Access to 62 full text journals, many non-journal periodicals and professional publications, Medline, online medical textbooks, and journal scanning to extract highlights from recent literature within chosen fields. Conference listings; direct CME offerings; news items.

WebMD
http://www.webmd.com
Consumer-focused content. Medscape is their physician content site. This site provides access to a wide array of physician-focused and medical office Internet-based services.

Databases, Research, and Scientific Resources

Organizing Medical Networked Information (OMNI)
http://omni.ac.uk/
OMNI offers free access to a searchable catalogue of Internet sites covering health and medicine.

Merck Manual
http://www.merck.com/mrkshared/mmanual/home.jsp
This website provides access to the 17th edition of the Merck Manual.

Harvard Department of Molecular and Cellular Biology
http://mcb.harvard.edu/Biolinks.html

Rosenthal Directory of Databases
www.rosenthal.hs.columbia.edu/Databases.html
This website provides a compilation of established sources in the U.S., Europe and Asia, designed to facilitate research by both professionals and the public in clinical, biomedical, review, meta-analytical or survey research. Many of the databases listed do charge a fee.

MedWeb Plus
http://medwebplus.com/about.html
From the site: Our goal at MedWebPlus is to give users tools to quickly locate and assimilate good and reliable information covering the entire spectrum of healthcare.

Cancer Detection and Prevention Online
http://www.cancerprev.org/
This is an International Society for Preventive Oncology (ISPO) website that offers access to current and past issues of Cancer Detection and Prevention journals. $225 annual subscription fee. Some free browsing.

Pesticides, Metals, & Chemical
http://vm.cfsan.fda.gov/~lrd/pestadd.html
This is U.S. FDA/Center for Food Safety and Applied Nutrition (CFSAN) website provides information regarding pesticides, metals, and chemical contaminants in food(s).

BioMedNet
http://www.biomednet.com/
This website provides information for biological and medical researchers. It offers access to a full-text library (over 170 biological and medical journals), and BioMedLink (evaluated and annotated database of internet resources for biological and medical researchers). Access to Medline reviews of 3500 websites. Free registration.

Medical Biochemistry Subject List
http://web.indstate.edu/thcme/mwking/subjects.html
This website offers details on specific biochemistry and medical subjects.

Elsevier Science
http://www.elsevier.nl/
This website provides access to purchasing of research publications and journals in the physical, life and social sciences.

The Lancet
http://www.thelancet.com/

British Medical Journal
http://bmj.com/
All articles of BMJ are available for free online.

NLM Clinical Trials Database
http://clinicaltrials.gov
Location, design, purpose, criteria and other information on NIH clinical trials.

PubMed
http://www.ncbi.nlm.nih.gov/PubMed/
National Library of Medicine; free access to Medline.

USDA Nutrient Database
http://www.nal.usda.gov/fnic/cgi-bin/nut_search.pl
This interface allows simple searches on the USDA Nutrient Database

General Resources

National Center for Complementary and Alternative Medicine (NCCAM)
http://nccam.nih.gov
This is a NIH website offering fairly comprehensive information regarding alternative therapies. Includes Consensus Reports, research, clinical trials, database links.

NIH Office of Dietary Supplements
http://odp.od.nih.gov/
The International Bibliographic Information on Dietary Supplements (IBIDS) is a NIH website produced by the Office of Dietary Supplements (ODS). It offers a database of published, international, scientific literature on dietary supplements, including vitamins, minerals, and botanicals. Search can be limited to peer-reviewed publications.

Herb Research Foundation (HRF)
http://www.herbs.org/
A nonprofit research and educational organization focusing on herbs and medicinal plants.

American Botanical Council's Herbal Information
http://www.herbalgram.org/
This website provides information about herbs that have been compiled from a number of reputable scientific sources including the German Commission E Monographs, Botanical Safety Handbook, and numerous clinical trials that have been referenced in HerbalGram, their quarterly publication.

Healthfinder
http://www.healthfinder.gov
This website provides consumer health and human services information developed by the U.S. Department of Health and Human Services. It provides access to selected online publications, clearinghouses, databases, websites, and support and self-help groups.

NIH Consumer Health Information
http://health.nih.gov/
This website provides access to consumer publication titles specific to certain conditions/diseases.

HealthGate
http://www.healthgate.com/
This website provides patient and consumer information regarding drugs and vitamins, symptoms and medical tests, and general health. It also provides access to Medline. Provider of web-enabled technology and services for healthcare organizations, including hospitals.

Medherb
http://medherb.com/
This website of Medical Herbalism, a quarterly journal of clinical herbalism. It provides links to medical information and to any resource relevant to medicinal herbs or herbalism practiced in clinical settings, plus sample articles on hundreds of herbs.

The World Lecture Hall
http://www.utexas.edu/world/lecture/
This website provides links to pages created by faculty worldwide who are using the web to deliver university-level academic courses in any language.

Food Allergy and Anaphylaxis Network (FAAN)
http://www.foodallergy.org/
This website provides access to FAAN, a nonprofit organization established to increase public awareness about food allergy and anaphylaxis. It offers, among other things, a bimonthly newsletter, product alerts, and updates on food allergy.

Dr. Duke's Phytochemical and Ethnobotanical Databases
http://www.ars-grin.gov/duke/
Database of phytochemical ingredients for herbs and spices.

http://www.essentialfats.com
This website presents information about the role of essential fatty acids in health and disease. It includes discussions on fatty acid analysis, research results, new diagnostic and treatment approaches of fatty acids in such areas as lipid abnormalities and inflammatory bowel disease.

Other Useful Sites

- http://commons.ucalgary.ca/mercury (Video on the toxic neurologic effects of mercury)
- http://ods.od.nih.gov (Office of Dietary Supplements Database)
- http://vm.cfsan.fda.gov/~frf/sea-mehg.html (EPA Report of Mercury Levels in Seafood)
- www.ajcn.org (American Journal of Clinical Nutrition)
- www.alternative-therapies.com (Alternative Therapies in Health and Medicine)
- www.bmj.com (British Medical Journals)
- www.bruceames.org (researcher in aging and nutrition)
- www.cdc.gov/exposurereport (Second National Report on Human Exposure to Environmental Chemicals)
- www.celiac.com (resource for celiac disease and gluten-free diet)
- www.cfsan.fda.gov/~dms/admehg3.html (EPA Mercury Fish Advisory)
- www.cmbm.org (The Center for Mind Body Medicine)
- www.consumerlab.com (Consumer Lab: Independent Assays of Supplements)
- www.ehponline.org (Environmental Health Perspectives)
- www.ewg.org (Environmental Working Group)
- www.ewg.org/reports/bodyburden (Study of Body Burden of Toxins)
- www.functionalmedicine.org (The Institute for Functional Medicine)
- www.healthjourneys.com (resource for audio recordings to support mind body healing)
- www.imconsortium.org (The Consortium of Academic Health Centers for Integrative Medicine or CAHCIM)
- www.jama.com (Journal of the American Medical Association)
- www.nap.edu/books/0309071402/html (Toxicological Effects of Methyl Mercury, 2000; National Academy of Sciences Press)
- www.ncbi.nlm.nih.gov/entrez (National Library of Medicine—Pub Med)
- www.nccam.nih.gov (National Center for Complementary and Alternative Medicine)
- www.nejm.org (New England Journal of Medicine)
- www.padmamedia.com (practical products to support an authentic life and the healing arts)
- www.whccamp.hhs.gov (White House Commission on Complementary and Alternative Medicine Policy. Final Report, March 2002)
- www.yourcancerrisk.harvard.edu (a risk assessment questionnaire)

Food Resources

- www.vitalchoice.com (Vital Choice Seafood—wild salmon and other food products)
- www.whfoods.org (World's Healthiest Foods)
- www.diamondorganics.com (source for home delivery of organic and healthful foods)

Supplement Companies and Distributors

(There are many to choose from; here are a few to get started with.)

- www.biotics research.com
- www.collegepharmacy.com
- www.designsforhealth.com
- www.douglaslabs.com
- www.emersonecologics.com
- www.integrativeinc.com
- www.metabolicmaintenance.com
- www.metagenics.com
- www.nordicnaturals.com
- www.protherainc.com
- www.thorne.com
- www.tidhealth.com
- www.vitalnutrients.net
- www.xymogen.com

Laboratory Testing and Diagnostic Resources

- www.doctorsdata.com (testing for heavy metal toxicity and other nutritional and metabolic disorders)
- www.enterolab.com (home stool gluten sensitivity testing)
- www.geimatron.com (electron beam tomography scanning for evaluation of calcium scores of the heart to assess cardiovascular risk)
- www.genovations.com (genetic testing for SNPs)
- www.gsdl.com (testing for digestive, immune, nutritional, endocrine, and metabolic function)
- www.igenex.com (specialized testing for detecting chronic infections such as Lyme Disease with PCR technology)
- www.immunolabs.com (IgG food sensitivity testing)
- www.immunoscienceslab.com (immunological and infectious diseases assessments)
- www.liposcience.com (nuclear medicine spectroscopy for the assessment of lipid particle size; assessing cardiovascular risk factors)
- www.melisa.org (immunotoxicology of heavy metals)
- www.metametrix.com (nutritional and metabolic testing)
- www.prometheus-labs.com (testing for gluten-related disease)
- www.questdiagnostics.com (common conventional laboratory testing)
- www.questest.com (self-testing)
- www.spectracell.com (functional analysis of essential micronutrients)
- www.yorkallergyusa.com (IgG food sensitivity testing)

Life Stress Questionnaire

Name ______________________________ Date ______________

During the past two years, have you had any of the following things happen to you? If so, simply circle one of the numbers following those items (and only those items that apply to you). Circle only one number after each event which has occurred in your life recently.

	LIFE EVENT	POINT VALUE		
		Slight	Moderate	Great
Example:	Change in social activities	10	15	20
	Change in sleeping habits	10	15	20
	Change in residence	10	15	20
1	Change in social activities	10	15	20
2	Change in sleeping habits	10	15	20
3	Change in residence	10	20	30
4	Change in work hours	15	20	25
5	Change in church activities	15	20	25
6	Tension at work	20	25	30
7	Small children in the home	20	25	30
8	Change in living conditions	20	25	30
9	Outstanding personal achievement	25	30	35
10	Problem teenager(s) in the home	25	30	35
11	Trouble with in-laws	25	30	35
12	Difficulties with peer group	25	30	35
13	Son or daughter leaving home	25	30	35
14	Change in responsibilities at work	25	30	35
15	Taking over a major financial responsibility	25	30	35
16	Foreclosure of mortgage or loan	25	30	40
17	Change in relationship with spouse	30	35	40
18	Change to different line of work	30	35	40
19	Loss of a close friend	30	35	45
20	Gain of a new family member	35	40	45
21	Sex difficulties	35	40	45
22	Pregnancy	35	40	50
23	Change in health of family member	40	45	50
24	Retirement	40	45	55
25	Loss of job	45	50	55
26	Change in quality of religious faith	45	50	55
27	Marriage	45	50	55
28	Personal injury or illness	45	50	65
29	Loss of self-confidence	55	60	70
30	Death of a close family member	50	60	70
31	Injury to reputation	50	60	75
32	Trouble with the law	55	65	75
33	Marital separation	55	65	85
34	Divorce	65	76	120
35	Death of spouse	80	100	
36	Other (invalid in family; drug or alcohol problem, etc.)	______	______	______
37	Other: ______________________	______	______	______
	Total of three columns	______	______	______

Scoring System
(1) Greater than 300, highly significant life stress
(2) 200–300, significant life stress
(3) 150–200, moderate life stress
(4) Less than 150, low life stress

Medical Symptoms Questionnaire

Name: ______________________________________ Date: ___________________

Rate each of the following symptoms based upon your typical health profile for:

❑ Past 30 days ❑ Past 48 hours

Point Scale
0 - Never or almost never have the symptom
1 - Occasionally have it, effect is not severe
2 - Occasionally have it, effect is severe
3 - Frequently have it, effect is not severe
4 - Frequently have it, effect is severe

HEAD	_______ Headaches _______ Faintness _______ Dizziness _______ Insomnia	Total _______
EYES	_______ Watery or itchy eyes _______ Swollen, reddened or sticky eyelids _______ Bags or dark circles under eyes _______ Blurred or tunnel vision (does not include near- or far-sightedness)	Total _______
EARS	_______ Itchy ears _______ Earaches, ear infections _______ Drainage from ear _______ Ringing in ears, hearing loss	Total _______
NOSE	_______ Stuffy nose _______ Sinus problems _______ Hay fever _______ Sneezing attacks _______ Excessive mucus formation	Total _______
MOUTH/THROAT	_______ Chronic coughing _______ Gagging, frequent need to clear throat _______ Sore throat, hoarseness, loss of voice _______ Swollen or discolored tongue, gums, lips _______ Canker sores	Total _______
SKIN	_______ Acne _______ Hives, rashes, dry skin _______ Hair loss _______ Flushing, hot flashes _______ Excessive sweating	Total _______
HEART	_______ Irregular or skipped heartbeat _______ Rapid or pounding heartbeat _______ Chest pain	Total _______

LUNGS	________	Chest congestion	Total ________
	________	Asthma, bronchitis	
	________	Shortness of breath	
	________	Difficulty breathing	
DIGESTIVE TRACT	________	Nausea, vomiting	Total ________
	________	Diarrhea	
	________	Constipation	
	________	Bloated feeling	
	________	Belching, passing gas	
	________	Heartburn	
	________	Intestinal/stomach pain	
JOINTS/MUSCLE	________	Pain or aches in joints	Total ________
	________	Arthritis	
	________	Stiffness or limitation of movement	
	________	Pain or aches in muscles	
	________	Feeling of weakness or tiredness	
WEIGHT	________	Binge eating/drinking	Total ________
	________	Craving certain foods	
	________	Excessive weight	
	________	Compulsive eating	
	________	Water retention	
	________	Underweight	
ENERGY/ACTIVITY	________	Fatigue, sluggishness	Total ________
	________	Apathy, lethargy	
	________	Hyperactivity	
	________	Restlessness	
MIND	________	Poor memory	Total ________
	________	Confusion, poor comprehension	
	________	Poor concentration	
	________	Poor physical coordination	
	________	Difficulty in making decisions	
	________	Stuttering or stammering	
	________	Slurred speech	
	________	Learning disabilities	
EMOTIONS	________	Mood swings	Total ________
	________	Anxiety, fear, nervousness	
	________	Anger, irritability, aggressiveness	
	________	Depression	
OTHER	________	Frequent illness	Total ________
	________	Frequent or urgent urination	
	________	Genital itch or discharge	

GRAND TOTAL ____________

Physical Signs Indicative or Suggestive of Undernutrition

Normal Appearance	Signs Associated with Undernutrition	Symptoms and Conditions	Corrective Nutrients
General: Well nourished, not obese	Wasted, skinny, or obese	Sarcopenia	Calorie, protein
Hair: shiny, firm, not easily plucked	Lack of shine, dull, dry, thin, sparse, fine flag sign, easily plucked, alopecia, corkscrew hairs	Easily plucked hair, alopecia Dry, brittle hair Corkscrew hairs Menke's Steely Hair Alopecia Changes in hair color, slow hair growth	Protein Protein biotin Vitamin C Copper Biotin Manganese
Face: skin color uniform, smooth, not swollen	Skin color loss, depigmentation, skin dark over cheeks and malar and supraorbital pigmentation. Flakiness of the skin of the nose and mouth, swollen face, enlarged parotid glands, nasolabial seborrhea, greasy, scaling dermatitis, butterfly distribution.	Dry and scaly, flaky, pain Nasolabial seborrhea Psoriasiform rash Pallor Follicular hyperkeratosis Perifollicular hemorrhage Easy bruising Hyperpigmentation Petechiae Seborrheic dermatitis	Vitamin A, zinc Essential fatty acids Vitamin A, zinc Iron B12 folate Vitamin A, EFA Vitamin C Vitamin K or C Niacin Vitamin C and K Riboflavin, vitamin B6 and zinc
Eyes: bright, clear, no sores in corners of eyelids, membranes pink, moist. No prominent blood vessels or mounds of tissue on sclera	Pale conjunctiva, or conjunctival redness, Bitot's spots, angular palpebritis, conjunctival xerosis, corneal xerosis, kerato malacia, corneal scarring, circumcorneal injection, xerophthalmia	Night blindness Photophobia, xerosis Conjunctival Inflammation Retinal field defect Xerophthalmia, keratomalacia, Bitot's	Vitamin A, zinc Vitamin A, zinc Riboflavin and Vitamin A Vitamin E Vitamin A
Lips: smooth, not chapped or swollen	Cheilosis, angular fissures or scars	Cheilosis, angular fissures, scars	Riboflavin, pyridoxine, niacin
Tongue: Deep red in appearance; not swollen or smooth	Swelling, scarlet or raw tongue, magenta, smooth, swollen sores, hyperemic, hypertrophic papillae, atrophic papillae, no glossitis, no filiform papillary atrophy	Glossitis (smooth) red tongue Decreased taste or smell, hypogeusia Tongue fissuring Tongue atrophy	Riboflavin, pyridoxine, niacin, folic acid, B12, iron Zinc Niacin Riboflavin, niacin, iron
Teeth: No cavities; no pain, bright	Missing or erupting abnormality, grey or black spots (fluorosis), cavities	Missing enamel Dental caries	Calcium Fluoride

Normal Appearance	Signs Associated with Undernutrition	Symptoms and Conditions	Corrective Nutrients
Gums: healthy, red, do not bleed, not swollen	Spongy and bleed easily, recession of gums Swollen, red, friable gums, periodontal disease	Bleeding gums	Vitamin C, riboflavin Vitamin D
Face/neck: Face not swollen	Thyroid enlargement, goiter: parotid enlargement Neck dermatosis—broad band or dark collar	Goiter Parotid enlargement Casel's Necklace	Iodine Thiamin Pellagra-Niacin
Skin: No rashes, swellings, dark or light spots, no bruising	Xerosis, follicular hyperkeratosis, flaking skin, edematous dermis, dark discolorations; red swollen pigmentation of exposed areas—pellagrous dermatosis, dyspigmentation, petechiae, fat atrophy, or vasculitis, bilateral symmetric dermatitis, acrodermatitis enteropathica	Dry and scaly, flaky, pain Nasolabial seborrhea Psoriasiform rash Pallor Follicular hyperkeratosis Perifollicular hemorrhage Easy bruising Hyperpigmentation Dryness and xerosis Pellagrous dermatosis Impaired wound healing	Vitamin A, zinc Essential fatty acids Vitamin A, zinc Iron, B12, folate Vitamin A, EFA Vitamin C Vitamin K or C Niacin Biotin, linoleic acid, zinc Niacin Vitamin C, A, zinc, protein, omega-6 FA
Nails: Firm, pink	Koilonychia, brittle, ridged, splinter hemorrhages, Beau's lines, leukonychia, pale nail beds, onycholysis, chronic paronychia	Koilonychia Transverse depigmentation White pitting—leukonychia Psoriatic nails Beau's lines Pale nail beds Meuhreke's lines Splinter hemorrhages Onycholysis Chronic paronychia	Iron, copper, zinc, protein Protein Zinc Vitamin D Zinc Iron Protein Vitamin C Iron, niacin Zinc
Musculoskeletal system: good muscle tone; some fat under the skin; can walk and run without pain	Muscles have wasted appearance, baby's skull bones are thin and soft (craniotabes); round swelling of the front and side of the head (frontal bossing); epiphyseal enlargement. Small bumps on both sides of the chest wall on the ribs. Beading of ribs, delayed closing of the anterior fontanelle, knock-kneed or bow legs, bleeding into the muscle. Enlarged wrists. No pretibial edema, Rachitic rosary, subperiosteal hemorrhages, myopathy, pigeon breast deformity.	Edema Bone tenderness Bone/Joint pain Muscle pain Joint swelling Cramping Myofascial back pain Atrophic muscles Decreased grip strength Osteomalacia, osteoporosis Rickets, rachitic rosary Calf muscle tenderness	Protein, thiamin Vitamin D Vitamin A, D, C Thiamin Vitamin C Calcium, potassium, magnesium Vitamin D Protein Protein, vitamin D Vitamin D, calcium Vitamin D Thiamin

Normal Appearance	Signs Associated with Undernutrition	Symptoms and Conditions	Corrective Nutrients
Cardiovascular system: Normal heart rate and rhythm; no murmurs or abnormal rhythms, normal blood pressure for age	Tachycardia, cardiomegaly, arrhythmia, frequent premature atrial or ventricular contractions, hypertension	High output failure Congestive heart failure Hypertension Palpitations, arrhythmia Cardiomegaly	Thiamin Coenzyme Q10 Calcium, potassium, magnesium, vitamin D Thiamin, magnesium, CoQ10, K, calcium Selenium, thiamin
Respiratory	Tachypnea, wheezing	Reactive airways	Magnesium
Circulation: No pallor, vascular spasm, claudication	Pallor, pale conjunctiva, stocking glove cyanosis	Anemia, hemolytic Anemia, microcytic hypochromic Anemia, megaloblastic Prolonged clotting time Intermittent claudication Stocking glove cyanosis without edema	Vitamin E Copper, iron Folate, vitamin B12 Vitamin K Thiamin
Gastrointestinal tract: No palpable organs or masses	Liver enlargement; enlargement of the spleen, dysphagia, and achlorhydria.	Ascites Hepatomegaly Diarrhea Ileus Plummer Vinson syndrome	Protein Protein, fat Zinc, niacin, dysbiosis Potassium Iron
Nervous system: psychological stability, normal reflexes, normal position and vibratory sense. Cranial nerves intact, normal smell, taste, and night vision	Mental irritability and confusion, burning and tingling of the hands and feet- paresthesias, hyperesthesias, impaired position and vibratory sense; weakness and tenderness of muscles with altered gait or inability to walk; decrease and loss of normal ankle, knee reflexes. Dementia.	Dementia Acute disorientation Nystagmus Ophthalmoplegia Wide-based gait Peripheral neuropathy Loss of vibratory sense Loss of position sense Tetany Paresthesias Wrist or foot drop Diminished reflexes Convulsions Ataxia, with loss of ankle knee reflexes Weakness, inability to walk Paresthesias about the lips, tongue, fingers Carpopedal spasm Circumoral and extremity paresthesias	Thiamin, B12, folate, niacin Phosphorus, niacin Thiamin Thiamin Thiamin, B12 Thiamin, pyridoxine, vitamin E, B12 B12 B12 Calcium, magnesium Thiamin, B12, omega-3 Thiamin Iodine Magnesium, vitamin B6 Thiamin, B12, vitamin E Omega-3 Calcium Calcium, magnesium Phosphorus

Three-Day Diet Diary

Please complete this Three-Day Diet Diary for three consecutive days within a week before your scheduled visit. Please include one weekend day.

- Record information as soon as possible after the food has been consumed.
- Describe the food or beverage consumed e.g., milk—whole, 2%, or nonfat; toast—whole wheat, white, buttered; chicken—fried, baked, breaded, etc. Record the amount of each food consumed using standard measurements as much as possible, such as 8 ounces, 1/2 cup, 1 teaspoon, etc.
- Include any added items. For example: tea with 1 teaspoon sugar, potato with 2 teaspoons butter, etc.
- Please record all beverages, including water. List them in the "Beverage" category.

Diet Diary

Name: ______________________________ **Date:** ______________

Time	Food	Amount	Time	Beverage	Amount

Index

NOTE: An *f* after a page number denotes a figure; a *t* denotes a table.

B

C

D

G

H

O

S

W

X

Y

Z